Kidney and Pancreas Transplantation

Kidney and Pancreas Transplantation

Ernesto Pompeo Molmenti MD PhD MBA
Vice Chairman, Department of Surgery
Director, Transplant Program
North Shore-LIJ Health System
Long Island, New York, USA

Professor, Departments of Surgery and Medicine
Hofstra North Shore–LIJ School of Medicine
Long Island, New York, USA

Forewords

Michael J Dowling

Lawrence G Smith

Ron Shapiro

JAYPEE The Health Sciences Publishers
New Delhi | London | Philadelphia | Panama

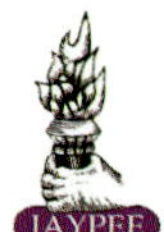

Jaypee Brothers Medical Publishers (P) Ltd

Headquarters

Jaypee Brothers Medical Publishers (P) Ltd
4838/24, Ansari Road, Daryaganj
New Delhi 110 002, India
Phone: +91-11-43574357
Fax: +91-11-43574314
Email: jaypee@jaypeebrothers.com

Overseas Offices

J.P. Medical Ltd
83, Victoria Street, London
SW1H 0HW (UK)
Phone: +44-2031708910
Fax: +02-03-0086180
Email: info@jpmedpub.com

Jaypee-Highlights.
Medical Publishers Inc
City of Knowledge, Bld. 237
Clayton, Panama City, Panama
Phone: +1 507-301-0496
Fax: +1 507-301-0499
Email: cservice@jphmedical.com

Jaypee Medical Inc.
The Bourse
111 South Independence Mall East
Suite 835, Philadelphia, PA 19106, USA
Phone: +1 267-519-9789
Email: jpmed.us@gmail.com

Jaypee Brothers
Medical Publishers (P) Ltd
17/1-B Babar Road, Block-B
Shaymali, Mohammadpur
Dhaka-1207, Bangladesh
Mobile: +08801912003485
Email: jaypeedhaka@gmail.com

Jaypee Brothers
Medical Publishers (P) Ltd
Shorakhute, Kathmandu
Nepal
Phone: +00977-9841528578
Email: jaypee.nepal@gmail.com

Website: www.jaypeebrothers.com
Website: www.jaypeedigital.com

Inquiries for bulk sales may be solicited at: jaypee@jaypeebrothers.com

Kidney and Pancreas Transplantation

First Edition: **2015**
ISBN: 978-93-5152-339-0
Printed at Ajanta Offset & Packagings Ltd., New Delhi.

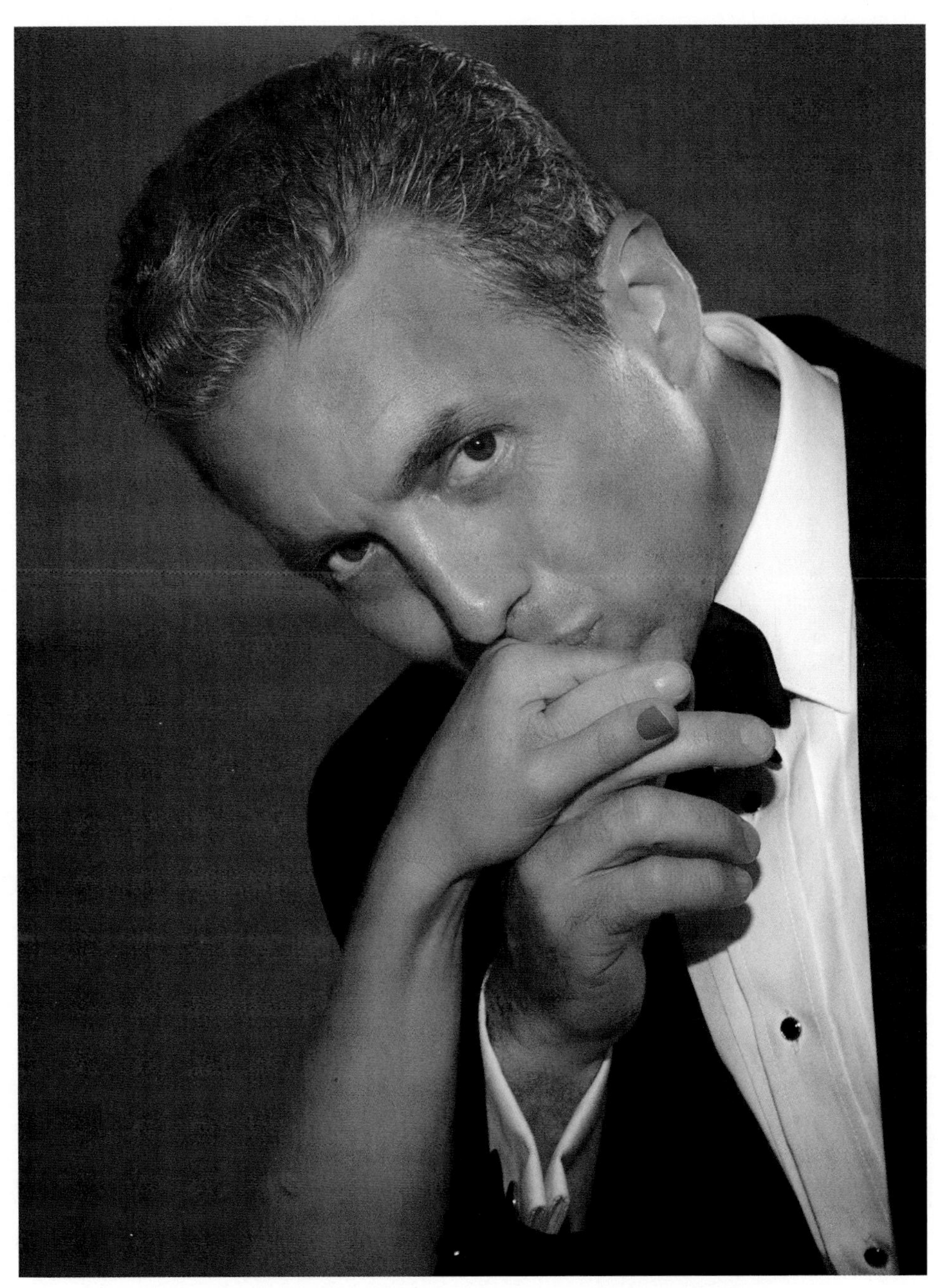

To my bright and beautiful wife Christine Louise.

We become victims of what we underestimate, ignore, and disregard.

Molmenti

Contributors

Stergiani Agorastos BS
Research Assistant
Laboratory for Behavioral and
Molecular Neuroimaging
Feinstein Institute for Medical Research
North Shore-LIJ Health System
Hempstead, New York, USA

Rajesh K Ahlawat MBBS MS MCh MNAMS
Chairman
Division of Urology and Renal Transplantation
Medanta Kidney and Urology Institute
Medanta the Medicity
Gurgaon, Haryana, India

Khalid Al Meshari MD FACP
Consultant
Renal Transplant Nephrologist
Director, International Affairs Office Corporate Level
King Faisal Specialist Hospital
Kingdom of Saudi Arabia

Asha Alex MD
Division of Transplant Surgery
Department of Surgery
North Shore-LIJ Health System
Hempstead, New York, USA

Mohini Alexander MD
Consulting Nephrologist
Valley Nephrology Associates
Manteca, California, USA

Nicole M Ali MD
Attending, Division of Nephrology
Department of Medicine
North Shore-LIJ Health System
Hempstead, New York, USA

Viren Amin MD
Attending, Department of Medicine
North Shore-LIJ Health System
Hempstead, New York, USA

Leo I Amodu MD MPH
Resident, Department of Surgery
North Shore-LIJ Health System
Hofstra North Shore-LIJ School of Medicine
Hempstead, New York, USA

Mashael Anizi MD
Foundation Doctor
Bart's and the Royal London
North East Thames Foundation School
London, England

Richard Barnett MD
Attending Physician in Nephrology
North Shore-LIJ Health System
Associate Professor of Medicine
Hofstra North Shore-LIJ School of Medicine
Hempstead, New York, USA

Pablo César Bassan MD
General and Thoracic Surgeon
Military Central Hospital
Medical Chief, Health Department
National Military School
Assistant Professor of Surgery
University of Buenos Aires and University of Salvador
Buenos Aires, Argentina

Amit Basu MD
Attending
Division of Transplant Surgery
Department of Surgery
North Shore-LIJ Health System
Hempstead, New York, USA

David Bernstein MD
Chief, Division of Hepatology and
Center for Liver Diseases
North Shore-LIJ Health System
Professor of Medicine
Hofstra North Shore-LIJ School of Medicine
Hempstead, New York, USA

Mahendra Bhandari MS MCh FAMS FNASc DSc MBA
Director, Robotic Surgery Education and Research
Vattikuti Urology Institute, Henry Ford Hospital
Detroit, Michigan, USA
CEO, Vattikuti Foundation
Honorary Professor
Centre Biomedical Research
Sanjay Gandhi Postgraduate Institute Campus, India

Madhu Bhaskaran MD
Medical Director, Transplant Program
North Shore-LIJ Health System
Associate Professor of Medicine and Surgery
Hofstra North Shore-LIJ School of Medicine
Hempstead, New York, USA

Louise Bongiorno MS RD CSR CDE
Dietician, Division of Transplant Surgery
North Shore-LIJ Health System
Hempstead, New York, USA

Joaquin A Cagliani MD
Department of Surgery
North Shore-LIJ Health System
Hofstra North Shore-LIJ School of Medicine
Hempstead, New York, USA

Kellie Calderon MD
Transplant Nephrologist
Department of Medicine
North Shore-LIJ Health System
Assistant Professor of Medicine
Hofstra North Shore-LIJ School of Medicine
Hempstead, New York, USA

Renee Cercone

Nirupama Chandel PhD
Department of Medicine
Feinstein Institute for Medical Research
North Shore-LIJ Health System
Hempstead, New York, USA

Nataliya Chorny MD
Attending, Division of Pediatric Kidney Center
Department of Pediatrics
North Shore-LIJ Health System
Assistant Professor of Pediatrics
Hofstra North Shore-LIJ School of Medicine
Hempstead, New York, USA

Gene F Coppa MD
Chairman, Department of Surgery
North Shore University Hospital and
Long Island Jewish Medical Center
Senior Vice President, Surgical Services
North Shore-Long Island Jewish Health System
Executive Director
Surgical Service Line
John D Mountain MD
Professor of Surgery
North Shore-LIJ Health System
Hempstead, New York, USA

Catherine D'Agostino MD
Attending
Department of Radiology
North Shore-LIJ Health System
Associate Director
Body Imaging Fellowship Program
Assistant Professor of Radiology
Hofstra North Shore-LIJ Health System
Hempstead, New York, USA

Maximiliano de Rodrigo MD
Instructor in Surgery
Hospital Interzonal General de Agudos
"Dr. Oscar Alende" (HIGA)
Esophageal and Gastric Surgery
Mar del Plata, Argentina

Craig Devoe MD
Associate Attending
Division of Hematology and Oncology
Monter Cancer Center
Department of Medicine
North Shore-LIJ Health System
Assistant Professor of Medicine
Hofstra North Shore-LIJ School of Medicine
Hempstead, New York, USA

Yosef D Dlugacz PhD
Senior Vice President/Chief
Clinical Quality
Education and Research
North Shorc-LIJ Health System
Assistant Professor of Science Education
Hofstra North Shore-LIJ School of Medicine
Hempstead, New York, USA

Cinthia B Drachenberg MD
Director, Electron Microscopy Laboratory
Department of Pathology
Professor of Pathology
University of Maryland School of Medicine
Baltimore, Maryland, USA

Regina S Druz MD FACC FASNC
Clinical Associate Professor of Cardiology
Hofstra North Shore-LIJ School of Medicine
Hempstead, New York, USA

Alicia Eubanks
Masters Program
University of Southern Florida
Tampa, Florida, USA

Antonette S Flecha PharmD
Clinical Pharmacist, Division of Transplant Surgery
North Shore-LIJ Health System
Assistant Professor of Surgery
Hofstra North Shore-LIJ School of Medicine
Adjunct Professor of Clinical Pharmacy
St. John's University-College of Pharmacy
Hempstead, New York, USA

Timothee Freisen MD
Attending, Finney Trimble
Surgical Associates
Greater Baltimore Medical Center
Baltimore, Maryland, USA

Dominick Gadaleta MD
Associate Chairman
Department of Surgery
Chief, General Surgery
Director, Bariatric Surgery
Department of Surgery
North Shore-LIJ Health System
Assistant Professor of Surgery
Hofstra North Shore-LIJ School of Medicine
Hempstead, New York, USA

Larry Gellman MD
General, Laparoscopic and Bariatric Surgery
Chief, Division of Minimally Invasive Surgery
Co-Director, Bariatric Surgery
North Shore-LIJ Health System
Hempstead, New York, USA

Charmaine Gentles NP
Bariatric Clinical Liaison
Department of Surgery
North Shore-LIJ Health System
Hempstead, New York, USA

George Georgiev BS
Clinical Research Associate, Sr.
Institute for Cellular Transplantation
Department of Surgery
University of Arizona
Tucson, Arizona, USA

Matthew Giangola MD
Resident, Surgical Residency Program
Department of Surgery
Postdoctoral Research Fellow
Feinstein Institute for Medical Research
North Shore-LIJ Health System
Hempstead, New York, USA

Veronica Claudia Gigena MD
General Surgeon, Military Central Hospital
Medical Associate Professor
Buenos Aires University
2nd Chief of General Ultrasound and Doppler
Military Central Hospital
Buenos Aires, Argentina

Michael J Goldstein MD FACS
Chief, Kidney Transplantation
Miami Transplant Institute
Jackson Memorial Hospital
Executive Director
Life Alliance Organ Recovery Agency
University of Miami
Associate Clinical Professor of Surgery
University of Miami Miller School of Medicine
Miami, Florida, USA

Evelina Grayver MD FACC
Attending, Department of Cardiology
North Shore-LIJ Health System
Assistant Professor of Medicine
Hofstra North Shore-LIJ School of Medicine
Hempstead, New York, USA

Stuart Greenstein MD
Attending, Division of Transplant Surgery
Department of Surgery, Montefiore Medical Center
Director, Outreach and Program Development
Professor of Surgery, Albert Einstein College of
Medicine of Yeshiva University
New York, New York, USA

Blaine Greenwald MD
Vice Chairman, Combined Department of Psychiatry
Long Island Jewish Medical Center and
North Shore University Hospital
Medical Director, The Zucker Hillside Hospital (ZHH)
Director, Geriatric Psychiatry Division, ZHH
North Shore-LIJ Health System
Associate Professor of Psychiatry
Hofstra North Shore-LIJ School of Medicine
Hempstead, New York, USA

Richard J Grieco MD
Clinical Vice Chairman
Department of Anesthesia
North Shore-LIJ Health System
Assistant Professor of Radiology
Hofstra North Shore-LIJ School of Medicine
Hempstead, New York, USA

Angelika Gruessner MS PhD
Professor of Public Health
Division of Epidemiology and Biostatistics
Mel and Enid Zuckerman College of Public Health
University of Arizona
Tucson, Arizona, USA

Christine E Gruessner BA
Medical Student
University of Arizona
Tucson, Arizona, USA

Rainer Gruessner MD PhD
Professor and Chairman
Department of Surgery
University of Arizona
Tucson, Arizona, USA

Stefan A Gruessner BA BS
Medical Student
University of Arizona
Tucson, Arizona, USA

W Mark Hamilton MD
Attending Staff Radiologist
Baylor University Medical Center
Dallas, Texas, USA

David A Hirschwerk MD
Attending
Division of Infectious Disease
Department of Medicine
North Shore-LIJ Health System
Assistant Professor of Medicine
Hofstra North Shore-LIJ School of Medicine
Hempstead, New York, USA

Ezra Israel MD
CEO, American Medical Diagnostics
Mount Sinai Health System
New York, New York, USA

Wooju Jeong MD
Senior Urologist, Vattikuti Urology Institute
Henry Ford Health System
Detroit, Michigan, USA

Kenar D Jhaveri MD
Attending, Division of Nephrology
Department of Medicine
North Shore-LIJ Health System
Associate Professor of Medicine
Hofstra North Shore-LIJ School of Medicine
Hempstead, New York, USA

Louis R Kavoussi MD
Chairman, Department of Urology
North Shore-LIJ Health System
Medical School Chairman
Department of Urology
Waldbaum Gardiner Professor of Urology
Hofstra North Shore-LIJ School of Medicine
Hempstead, New York, USA

Liise Kayler MD MS
Attending, Division of Transplant Surgery
Department of Surgery
Montefiore Medical Center
Associate Professor of Clinical Surgery
Albert Einstein College of
Medicine of Yeshiva University
New York, New York, USA

Adam Khader MD
Resident
Surgical Residency Program
Department of Surgery
Postdoctoral Research Fellow
Feinstein Institute for Medical Research
North Shore-LIJ Health System
Hempstead, New York, USA

Edward Kraus MD
Attending
Division of Nephrology/Transplant
Department of Medicine
Johns Hopkins Medicine
Associate Professor of Medicine
Johns Hopkins School of Medicine
Baltimore, Maryland, USA

Prathik Krishnan MD
Division of Transplant Surgery
Department of Surgery
North Shore-LIJ Health System
Hempstead, New York, USA

Ramesh Kumar MD
Clinical Fellow
Vattikuti Urology Institute
Henry Ford Health System
Detroit, Michigan, USA

Michael Kuncewitch MD
Resident
Surgical Residency Program
Department of Surgery
Postdoctoral Research Fellow
Feinstein Institute for Medical Research
North Shore-LIJ Health System
Hempstead, New York, USA

Alexander Lee MD
Program Director
Interventional Cardiology Fellowship
Department of Cardiology
North Shore-LIJ Health System
Assistant Professor of Medicine
Hofstra North Shore-LIJ School of Medicine
Hempstead, New York, USA

Jessica Lee MD
Resident
Department of Obstetrics-Gynecology
North Shore-LIJ Health System
Hempstead, New York, USA

Ashwani Malhotra PhD
Senior Research Scientist, Division of Nephrology
Department of Medicine
Associate Investigator
Feinstein Institute for Medical Research
North Shore-LIJ Health System
Hempstead, New York, USA

Prashant Malhotra MD
Attending, Division of Infectious Disease
Department of Medicine, North Shore-LIJ Health System
Hempstead, New York, USA

Carlos E Marroquin MD FACS
Chief, Division of Transplant Surgery and Immunology
Department of Surgery, Fletcher Allen Health Care
Associate Professor of Surgery
University of Vermont College of Medicine
Burlington, Vermont, USA

Sabeen F Mekan MD
Attending, Division of Hematology-Oncology
Department of Medicine, North Shore-LIJ Health System
Assistant Professor of Medicine
Hofstra North Shore-LIJ School of Medicine
Hempstead, New York, USA

Marcelo Mendez Jr MD
Resident, Department of Internal Medicine
Mount Sinai Beth Israel Hospital
New York, New York, USA

Mani Menon MD
Professor of Urology
The Raj and Padma Vattikuti Distinguished Chair
Director, Vattikuti Urology Institute
Detroit, Michigan, USA

Andrew W Menzin MD
Vice Chairman for Academic Affairs
Department of Obstetrics and Gynecology
North Shore University Hospital and
Long Island Jewish Medical Center
North Shore-LIJ Health System
Professor of Obstetrics and Gynecology
Hofstra North Shore-LIJ School of Medicine
Hempstead, New York, USA

Pranjal Modi MS MCh
Professor of Urology
Head of Transplantation Surgery
H.L. Trivedi Institute of Transplantation Sciences
Ahmedabad, Gujarat, India

Christine Sardo Molmenti MPH PhD
Postdoctoral Research Fellow and
Postdoctoral Research Scientist
Department of Epidemiology
Mailman School of Public Health
Herbert Irving Comprehensive Cancer Center
New York-Presbyterian
Columbia University Medical Center
New York, New York, USA

Divya Monga MD
Assistant Professor
Division of Nephrology, Department of Medicine
University of Mississippi Medical Center
Jackson, Mississippi, USA

Robert A Montgomery MD DPhil
Chief, Division of Transplantation
Director
Johns Hopkins Comprehensive Transplant Center
Johns Hopkins Medicine
Professor of Surgery
Johns Hopkins School of Medicine
Baltimore, Maryland, USA

Raghava B Munivenkatappa MBBS
Attending Surgeon
Division of Transplantation
Department of Surgery
Johns Hopkins Medicine
Baltimore, Maryland, USA

Thangamani Muthukumar MD
Division of Nephrology and Hypertension
Department of Medicine
Department of Translational Medicine
New York Presbyterian Hospital
Assistant Professor of Medicine
Weill Medical College of Cornell University
New York, New York, USA

David Nagata MD
Internal Medicine
St. Luke's Fruitland Clinic
Fruitland, Indiana, USA

Jeffrey M Nicastro MD
Vice President
Clinical Services, Surgery Service Line
Vice Chairman, Department of Surgery
Chief
Division of Acute Care Surgery
Program Director, General Surgery
Residency, Department of Surgery
North Shore-LIJ Health System
Assistant Professor of Surgery
Hofstra North Shore-LIJ School of Medicine
Hempstead, New York, USA

Julia Nunley MD FAAD FACP
Professor and Program Director
Department of Dermatology
Medical College of Virginia Hospital
Virginia Commonwealth University
Richmond, Virginia, USA

Christopher Palestro MD
Chief
Division of Nuclear Medicine and
Molecular Imaging
Department of Radiology
North Shore-LIJ Health System
Professor of Radiology
Hofstra North Shore-LIJ School of Medicine
Hempstead, New York, USA

Abeed Pall MD FRCP
Consultant, Renal Transplant Physician
Section Head, Adult Transplant Nephrology
Department of Kidney and Pancreas Transplantation
King Faisal Specialist Hospital & Research Centre
Ridayh, Saudi Arabia

Gabriel Pantol MD
Chairman, Neurology Section
Cape Fear Valley Health System
Fayetteville, North Carolina, USA

John C Papadimitriou MD PhD
Director, Anatomic Pathology
Department of Pathology
University of Maryland Medical Center
Professor of Pathology
University of Maryland School of Medicine
Baltimore, Maryland, USA

RoseMarie Pasmantier MD
Attending Endocrinologist
Department of Medicine
Veterans Affairs New Jersey Healthcare System
East Orange, New Jersey, USA

Pallavi Patri MD
Instructor
Division of Hypertension and Nephrology
Department of Medicine
NewYork-Presbyterian/Weill Cornell Medical Center
New York, New York, USA

Andreas Paul MD
Chairman
Department of General, Visceral and
Transplantation Surgery
University of Duisburg-Essen
Essen, Germany

John Pellerito MD
Vice Chairman, Clinical Affairs
Director
Peripheral Vascular Laboratory
Department of Radiology
North Shore-LIJ Health System
Associate Professor of Radiology
Hofstra North Shore-LIJ School of Medicine
Hempstead, New York, USA

Benjamin Philosophe MD PhD
Clinical Chief
Division of Transplantation
Department of Surgery
Johns Hopkins Medicine
Professor of Surgery
Johns Hopkins School of Medicine
Baltimore, Maryland, USA

Barbara Ponieman MD
Attending
Department of Psychiatry
North Shore-LIJ Health System
Assistant Professor of Psychiatry
Hofstra North Shore-LIJ School of Medicine
Hempstead, New York, USA

Jose Prince MD
Attending, Division of Pediatric Surgery
Department of Surgery
Director, Minimally Invasive Surgery
Cohen Children's Medical Center of New York
Institute Researcher, Feinstein
Institute for Medical Research
North Shore-LIJ Health System
Assistant Professor of Surgery
Hofstra North Shore-LIJ School of Medicine
Hempstead, New York, USA

Arnold Radtke MD
Associate Professor
Department of General and Transplant Surgery
University of Muenster
Muenster, Germany

Salil R Rajayer MBBS
Resident
Department of Internal Medicine
Woodhull Medical and Mental Health Center
New York University School of Medicine
New York, New York, USA

Prejith P Rajendran MBBS
Division of Transplant Surgery
Department of Surgery
North Shore-LIJ Health System
Hempstead, New York, USA

Poornima Ramadas MD
Division of Transplant Surgery
Department of Surgery
North Shore-LIJ Health System
Hempstead, New York, USA

Andrea Restifo RN MPA
Associate Executive Director, Administration
North Shore University Hospital
North Shore-LIJ Health System
Hempstead, New York, USA

Lee Richstone MD
System Vice Chairman, Department of Urology
Chief of Urology
North Shore-LIJ Health System
Associate Professor of Urology
Hofstra North Shore-LIJ School of Medicine
Hempstead, New York, USA

Horacio L Rodriguez Rilo MD PhD
Professor of Surgery, Immunology, Cell Biology, Physiology, Mechanical and Aerospace Engineering
Director, Islet Cell Transplant Program
Director, Cell Transplant Institute
Associate Director
Arizona Diabetes Center
University of Arizona School of Medicine
Tucson, Arizona, USA

Ezequiel Rodríguez Reimundes MD
Attending
Department of Internal Medicine and Intensive Care
Nyon Hospital
Nyon, Switzerland

Mala Sachdeva MD
Attending, Division of Kidney Diseases and Hypertension
Department of Medicine
North Shore-LIJ Health System
Assistant Professor of Medicine
Hofstra North Shore-LIJ School of Medicine
Hempstead, New York, USA

Ankita Sagar MD
Chief Resident
Department of Internal Medicine
North Shore-LIJ Health System
Hempstead, New York, USA

Sonu Sahni MD
Research Assistant
Division of Pulmonary, Sleep and Critical Care Medicine
North Shore-LIJ Health System
Hempstead, New York, USA

Simpa S Salami MD
Resident
Department of Urology
The Arthur Smith Institute for Urology
North Shore-LIJ Health System
Hempstead, New York, USA

Michael J Schwartz MD
Associate Residency Program Director
Director
Robotics and Minimally Invasive Surgery
Smith Institute for Urology
North Shore-LIJ Health System
Assistant Professor of Urology
Hofstra North Shore-LIJ School of Medicine
Hempstead, New York, USA

Dorry Segev MD PhD
Attending Surgeon
Division of Transplantation
Associate Vice Chair of Research Department of Surgery
Johns Hopkins Hospital
Associate Professor of Surgery
Johns Hopkins University School of Medicine
Associate Professor of Epidemiology
Johns Hopkins Bloomberg School of Public Health
Baltimore, Maryland, USA

David Serur MD
Medical Director
The Rogosin Institute Transplantation Program
Associate Attending Physician
New York-Presbyterian Hospital/Weill Cornell
Associate Professor of Clinical Medicine
Weill Medical College of Cornell University
New York, New York, USA

Surya V Seshan MD
Attending, Department of Pathology
New York Presbyterian Hospital
Professor of Clinical Pathology and Laboratory Medicine
Weill Cornell Medical College
New York, New York, USA

Christine Sethna MD
Division Chief, Pediatric Nephrology
Cohen Children's Medical Center of New York
North Shore-LIJ Health System
Assistant Professor of Pediatrics
Hofstra North Shore-LIJ School of Medicine
Hempstead, New York, USA

George Sgourakis MD PhD FACS
Staff Specialist General Surgeon
Korgialenion-Benakion, Red Cross Hospital
Athens, Greece

Hitesh H Shah MD
Director
Nephrology Fellowship Program, Department of Medicine
North Shore-LIJ Health System
Associate Professor of Medicine
Hofstra North Shore-LIJ School of Medicine
Hempstead, New York, USA

Iuliana Shapira MD
Attending, Division of Oncology
Department of Medicine, North Shore-LIJ Health System
Associate Professor of Medicine
Hofstra North Shore-LIJ School of Medicine
Hempstead, New York, USA

Ron Shapiro MD
The Robert J Corry Chair in Transplantation Surgery
Thomas E Starzl Transplantation Institute
Professor of Surgery, University of Pittsburgh School of Medicine
Pittsburgh, Pennsylvania, USA

Pravin C Singhal MD
Chief
Emeritus Nephrology
Kidney Diseases and Hypertension
North Shore-LIJ Health System
Professor of Medicine
Hofstra North Shore-LIJ School of Medicine
Hempstead, New York, USA

Narendra Singh MD
Intensivist
Division of Critical Care Surgery
Department of Surgery
North Shore-LIJ Health System
Hempstead, New York, USA

Eric J Siskind MD
Chief Resident
Surgical Residency Program, Department of Surgery
North Shore-LIJ Health System
Hempstead, New York, USA

Patrick R Smith BA EMT-P
Center for Learning and Innovation
North Shore-LIJ Health System
Hofstra North Shore-LIJ School of Medicine
Hempstead, New York, USA

Akshay Sood MD
PGY-I Urology Resident
Vattikuti Urology Institute, Henry Ford Health System
Detroit, Michigan, USA

Georgios C Sotiropoulos PhD FACS FEBS
Professor of Surgery and Transplantation
Department of General, Visceral and
Transplantation Surgery, University Hospital Essen
Essen, Germany

William Stewart DDS
Chief
Division of Dental Medicine
North Shore-LIJ Health System
Assistant Professor of Dental Medicine
Hofstra North Shore-LIJ School of Medicine
Hempstead, New York, USA

Keith Sultan MD
Attending, Division of Gastroenterology
Hepatology and Nutrition, Department of Medicine
North Shore-LIJ School of Medicine
Assistant Professor of Medicine
Hofstra North Shore-LIJ School of Medicine
Hempstead, New York, USA

Arunabh Talwar MD FCCP
Attending Physician, Division of Pulmonary
Sleep and Critical Care Medicine
North Shore-LIJ Health System
Professor of Medicine
Hofstra North Shore-LIJ School of Medicine
Hempstead, New York, USA

Donato F Tramontozzi RPh
Auburndale Pharmacy, Inc.
Flushing, New York, USA

Megan L Troxell MD PhD
Associate Professor of Pathology
Oregon Health & Science School of Medicine
Portland, Oregon, USA

Roberto M Verzaro MD PhD FACS
Program Director, General Surgery
Vannini Hospital in Rome, Instructor, General Surgery
Residency Program, University of Rome La Sapienza
Rome, Italy

Mariano Volpacchio MD
Head, Computed Tomography
Hospital de Clinicas Jose de San Martin
Universidad de Buenos Aires
Head, Body Imaging, Centro de Diagnostico
Dr. Enrique Rossi
Buenos Aires, Argentina

Ping Wang MD
Vice Chairman for Research, Department of Surgery
North Shore-LIJ Health System
Head, Center for Translational Research
The Feinstein Institute for Medical Research
Professor of Surgery and Molecular Medicine
Hofstra North Shore-LIJ School of Medicine
Hempstead, New York, USA

Joseph S Weiner MD PhD

Attending Physician
Department of Psychiatry
North Shore-LIJ Health System
Associate Professor of Clinical Psychiatry and Medicine
Hofstra North Shore-LIJ School of Medicine
Hempstead, New York, USA

Jay Weinstein MD

Attending
Division of Internal Medicine
Department of Medicine
North Shore-LIJ Health System
Assistant Professor of Medicine
Hofstra North Shore-LIJ Health System
Hempstead, New York, USA

Robin J Warshawsky MD

Associate Chairman
Department of Radiology
North Shore-LIJ Health System
Assistant Professor of Radiology
Hofstra North Shore-LIJ School of Medicine
Hempstead, New York, USA

Collaborators

Radiology Chapters

Eran Ben-Levi MD

Karen S Black MD

Alexander J Blood BA

Grazyna Bober RDMS

Dennis Burgos RDMS

Brian J Burke MD

Drew M Caplin MD

Jesse Chusid MD MBA

Regina S Druz MD FACC

Adam L Evans MD

Bilha Chesner Fish MD

Barak Friedman MD

Eric J Gandras MD

Veronica Claudia Gigena MD

Evelina Grayver MD FACC

Craig R Greben MD FSIR

Gregory M Grimaldi MD

Brett Helfner MD

John J Hines MD

Asaph CJ Levy BS

Pamela Lombardi MD

Saiedeh Maghool RDMS

Jessica Moon RDMS

James B Naidich MD

Jason J Naidich MD

Diana Navi RDMS

Radha Persaud RDMS

Amalia Pose BS RDMS

Daniel Putterman MD

David R Rosman MD

Kathrin Sakni RDMS

Lindsay Schwartz RDMS

Priya K Shah MD

Rakesh D Shah MD

Eric J Siskind MD

Branson Sparks

Karen Torres BS RDMS

Gene G Tronco MD

Biana Trost MD

Robert Villani MD

Rona F Woldenberg MD

Pey-Jen Yu MD

Input and Strategic Design

Adam Aponte MD MSc FAAP
Matthew A Bank MD
Eileen Bishop MD
Sabina Figari Bizzotto
Sylvester M Black MD PhD
Fouad N Boctor MD PhD
John Chang MD
John D Chelico MD MA FACP
Charles Choy MD
Christian Coppa
James M Crawford MD PhD
Salvatore Cumella MD
Suzanne El-Sayegh MD FACP
Lara Fishbane

Patrick J Gannon PhD
Maria D Georgiades MD
Gary Giangola MD FACS
Lawrence R Glassman MD
Azzour D Hazzan MD
Jerrold Hirsch PhD
Susana Hong MD
E Ilamathi MD FACP FNKF
Mitchel C Jacobs MD FACP
Sam H James MD
Jasmeet Kaur MD
Nancy Kheck PhD
Y H Kieso-Chelico MSCR
Mark Kissin MD

Michael W Kleeman DO FACS
Jeffrey A Kraut BA MBA
K V Krishnasastry MD
Dana Lustbader MD FCCM
Jerzy Macura MD
Anna Mathew MD
Joseph Mattana MD
James C Maurer MD
Alexia Molmenti
Hebe Molmenti MD PhD
Luis A Molmenti MD PhD
Octavio Molmenti
Luis F Morales MD
Cameron Moser

Samuel Packer MD
Frank and Linda Perlman
Rajasekhar Perumalla MD
John Platz MD
Lauren E Procaccino
James Sardo MD
Todd L Slesinger MD FACEP
Laurence N Spier MD
Joel Stern NH PhD
James Sullivan MD
Hugo Villar MD
Robert S Waldbaum MD
Rimda Wanchoo MD

Manuscript Evaluation

A Abdurakhmanov BA
Haris S Ahmed MD
Khalid K Al-Talib MD FACP
Eden Amdemichael MD
Maxine Ames
S Sandeep Anantha MD
Evan R Ashley AOS NREMT-P
Krassimir Atanassov MD
Coney Bae MD
Meade P Barlow MD
Cerdi Beltrė BA
Dron Bhandari MBBS
Omar D Bholat MD FACS
Vinoth Birabaharan BS
Daina A Blitz
Alexander J Blood BA
Mark S Blum MD
Dana E Bregman BA
Joaquin A Cagliani MD
Shayna Carp
Alexandra M Cerutti MD

Ashley Chandler
Jennifer S Chang MD
Sebastian Choi
Pablo Ciaravino MD
Chris Cipolla
Romain Cosandre MD
Catherine M De Stio BS
Gary Deutsch MD
Jordan A Dienstag BS
Charles M Ekstein MD
Annalise R Ellis MHA
Melissa D Fana MD
Diego Lucas Fernández MD
Hannah C Gannon
Julian Gannon
Victoria M Gilbert BS
Katherine M Giovinazzo
Andrew J Godwin MD
Ayush Goel
Alex D Gold
Jamie Golden MD

Michael J Golia MD
Ilana Golovaty MS RD
Edwin Goncharuk
Ekjot S Grewal BA
Benjamin Guzik BA
Lindsay Hahn
Jeffrey Hallock
Majid Hamidi BS
Justin P Henneman MS
Mallory J Highstein BA
Jacob Hirsch
Hannah B Hoffman BA
Lauren Hoffman
Jared M Hutson MD
Mitchell Jacobs MD
Sapna Jairath MD MHA
Nicholas Jandovitz PharmD
Vivek Jayaschandran MBBS
Trevor R Jones
Rohan Jotwani
Aditya Kadiyala MD MPH

Ameneh D Kalani MD
Sanjay D Kalra
Bilge D Kalyon MD
Irena Karanetz MD
Matthew Katz
Naixin Kang MD
Mamata Khanal MD
Armen Kasabian MD
Shachar Kenan MD
Brian Koch
P Praveen Kolumam MBBS
Amie J Kraus MD
Adam M Kressel MD
Marc D Krokowski MPA
Minh Le Nguyen MD
David Leon BS
Rachelle Y Leong MD
Sam Leung MD
Asaph CJ Levy
Leandro A Lumermann MD
Frances L Mabrey BA

Sulynn Machado BA

Reshmi Madankumar BS

Jonathan R Mallen BS

B T Manekshana MD MSc

Osvaldo Marcenaro BS RT(R)

Laura W Marinelli MD

Christine Mathew

Lauren E Mathew

Jessica E McSharp BS

Barbara Mellace

Marcelo Mendez Jr MD

Jenna S Meriggi

Robert T Metzler BS

Marni A Mishler MD

Munazza Mohammad MD

Víctor A Moon MD

Nikhil Mulchandani MD

Clancy Mullan BS

M Y Mutawakkil BSc

Lakshmi Nambiar MD

Kusuma Nio MD

Jolanta Barbara Norelli BA

Homaira Omar ANP MBA

Alisha R Oropallo MD

Adam I Ovadia BA

Thomas Panetta MD

Madhavan Parvathy MBBS

Lauren Michele Paster MD

Jennifer N Peacock MD MPH

Shabana Perveen MD

Soniya N Pinto MBBS

Darci Pitchon MD

Lauren M Plumley MD MPH

Sahil Rawal

Deepa Ramadurai BA

Abhita T Reddy BA

Sameer Rehman MBBS

John P Ricci MD

Melissa K Robinson MD

Jesus Rosado

Joshua E Ross MD

Benjamin Russo

Emil Sameyah MD

Syed M Sayeed MD

Christopher Scavelli

Christina Scelfo BS

Tony Shao MD

Ilya Shnaydman MD

Adam W Shen MD

Lauren Shikowitz-Behr MD

Louis R Spiegel MD

Sharon S Stanley MD

Shawn Swift MPA

Neil Tanna MD MBA

Santo P Terranova DO

N P J Theckumparampil MD

Patrick Touhy BA

Mary Bridget Tracey

Maureen Tracey

Richard O Tyrell MD

Mario Vega MD

Ricardo Vega MD

H Franco Veglia MD

John Wagner MD

Heath A Walden MD

Steven Weintraub MD

Georgia T Xenophontos

Harry Zemon MD FACS

Foreword

In 2007, the North Shore-LIJ Health System opened a kidney transplant center at North Shore University Hospital in Manhasset, the first transplant program serving residents of New York State's Nassau and Queens counties. Transplant surgery was available in Manhattan and on eastern Long Island, but it put an undue burden on patients and family members from Nassau and Queens, who had to travel for surgeries and pre- and postoperative care.

Our goal with the program was twofold: ensure broader access to state-of-the-art, patient-centered kidney transplant surgery and provide the very best surgical and postoperative care available anywhere.

To lay the groundwork for the new program, we assembled the region's foremost kidney transplantation team led by renowned surgeon and organ transplantation expert Ernesto P Molmenti, MD PhD MBA. The results speak for themselves.

In less than a decade, under Molmenti's direction, the interdisciplinary transplantation team has developed a reputation for delivering the highest quality of kidney transplant care in both inpatient and outpatient settings. It has been an important evolution in organ transplant care for the entire tri-state region.

Molmenti is a distinguished surgeon, internationally recognized author and educator, who mentors surgical and nephrology residents and medical students as a Professor of Surgery and Medicine at the Hofstra North Shore-LIJ School of Medicine in New York.

He shares his clinical expertise in the comprehensive textbook *Kidney and Pancreas Transplantation*. I trust you will find it to be an invaluable resource and reference.

Michael J Dowling
President and Chief Executive Officer
North Shore-LIJ Health System
New York, USA

Foreword

Molmenti and his coauthors have produced *Kidney and Pancreas Transplantation*, which deals with the medical, surgical, and short- and long-term care of these patients. The chapters cover an extraordinary breadth of subjects ranging from patient selection, medical care, and surgical techniques to health policy and quality of care. It is noteworthy that the field of transplantation, which used to be the business only of select tertiary care facilities, now is a medical intervention that has returned so many patients to their community caregivers that it is an essential area of learning for virtually all physicians. *Kidney and Pancreas Transplantation* utilizes some novel ways to transmit the essential "need to know" information in a readily accessible format. The book is filled with outstanding tables, bullet points, illustrations, photos, histopathology, and radiology. The text is concise and the key elements of each section are easily focused on by the reader.

Thus, I would compliment the authors not only on producing the textbook in a cutting-edge area of medical practice but also in exploring an innovative and highly effective way to transmit that information. Anyone interested in understanding the basis of these highly complex areas of medical and surgical practice will find this book extraordinarily useful.

Lawrence G Smith MD MACP
Dean, Hofstra North Shore-LIJ School of Medicine
Physician-in-Chief, North Shore-LIJ Health System
Long Island, New York, USA

Foreword

Molmenti and his colleagues have written a detailed and comprehensive textbook on *Kidney and Pancreas Transplantation*. Classic textbooks have historically gone over the details of recipient selection, donor selection, technical aspects, medical management issues, discussions of immunosuppression, outcomes, and complications after transplantation, and this book describes these topics in meticulous detail, using a format that combines both outline and text as needed, with a number of detailed photographs and figures. However, as the field of transplantation has matured, it has acquired bureaucratic structures related to outcomes assessment and quality improvement, and a modern textbook needs to include a discussion of all of these associated topics. One of the virtues of this book is its inclusion of all of these areas so as to provide a truly comprehensive overview of all aspects of *Kidney and Pancreas Transplantation*. This book is written for all professionals actively engaged in the field, including fellows, attendings, nurses, and administrators, and provides a broadly based reference for anyone with a serious interest in *Kidney and Pancreas Transplantation*.

Molmenti was one of my fellows during his training in transplantation, and one of the most satisfying aspects of teaching is the success of one's students. I am proud of Molmenti's accomplishments and delighted that he has put together such a well constructed textbook.

Ron Shapiro MD
Professor of Surgery
Robert J Corry Chair in Transplantation Surgery
Associate Clinical Director
Thomas E Starzl Transplantation Institute
University of Pittsburgh,
Pittsburgh, Pennsylvania, USA

Preface

This new text is intended to be the most comprehensive, up-to-date book published on the topic of *Kidney and Pancreas Transplantation*. It examines the entire gamut of considerations for transplantation, including candidate evaluation, surgical techniques, and complications. We present practical and focused information in a concise, easy-to-read format for busy practitioners.

We have written the text for a multidisciplinary audience and feature contributions from imaging specialists, surgeons, pathologists, anesthesiologists, and dermatologists. Unique topics include epigenetics, imaging, complications, pathology, dermatologic manifestations, obesity and metabolic syndromes, and cutting-edge material on robotic surgical techniques. We also offer extensive coverage of living and deceased donor kidney considerations. This text will be a definitive resource for all members of the transplant team and is intended to encourage a spirit of teamwork among all.

Conveniently divided into 22 sections including 72 chapters, the text is richly illustrated with full-color figures and photos that clearly illustrate step-by-step surgical procedures and key concepts.

We are delighted that you have taken the time to consider our book and hope that you find it very useful.

Molmenti

Acknowledgments

We are grateful for the ongoing support of:

Mr and Mrs John and Janet Raggio/Janet and John Raggio Nephrology Institute
Mr John Raggio and Donna R Kesselman MD
Mr and Mrs John and Lindsay Raggio
Ms Lauren Raggio and Mr Kyle Hall
Mr and Mrs Michael and Donna Mazzei/NuBest Salon and Spa
Mr and Mrs Jamie and Violet Mazzei/NuBest Salon and Spa
Mr and Mrs Leland and Lise Hirsch

We would like to acknowledge for their professional development and support:

Alice Fornari EdD RD
Director of Faculty Development
North Shore-LIJ Health System
Associate Dean of Educational Skills Development
Hofstra North Shore-LIJ School of Medicine
Associate Professor of Science Education, Population Health and Family Medicine

Victor Fornari MD
Director, Division of Child and Adolescent Psychiatry
North Shore University Hospital and Long Island Jewish Medical Center
(including Zucker Hillside Hospital and Cohen Children's Medical Center)
Professor of Psychiatry & Pediatrics
Hofstra North Shore-LIJ School of Medicine

We would also like to acknowledge for their interest and enthusiasm:

Mr and Mrs Rocco F Andriola Esq
Mr and Mrs Chris and Angela Paradysz

We would like to thank and acknowledge the following for their continuous support:

Alessandro Bellucci MD
Steven Fishbane MD
Richard Schwarz MD

We would like to thank the following collaborators for their invaluable contribution ensuring the accuracy of this work:

Hannah Millward Fisher MLS
Robert E Fisher MLS

We would like to thank the following for the tireless effort preparing this work:

Claudia Cassidy

Transplant Team:

Barry Kristen NP; Bongiorno Louise MS RD CSR CDE; Brown Hoshane; Cappello Joan LMSW; Cascone Barbara BS; Cassidy Claudia AAS; De Barros Irene P; DeFlorio Patricia NP; Flecha Antonetta PharmD; Goldstein Marlene LCSW; Green Kathleen RN; Hernandez Freddy BA; John Tess MSN; Kiernan Lisa RN; Mayvaldov Evgenia NP; Martocci Maude RN; Minogue Elizabeth LCSW; Moore Tracy LCSW; Morgan Ruth M DC; Reyes Julissa; Reynoso Celenia BS; Russo Linda RN; Sendach Jon MPA FACHE; Siegel-Joffe Rachel B LCSW; Somerville Susan RN; Williams Amanda R; Wilson Petrian; Wrynn Barbara RN; Zoll Kristin LMSW

Contents

SECTION 16 Cutaneous Manifestations

***Editor**: Julia R Nunley*

PART 2 PANCREAS TRANSPLANTATION

SECTION 17 Overview

SECTION 18 Operative Technique: Pancreas Recipient

SECTION 19 Complications

SECTION 20 Pathology

***Editor**: Cinthia B Drachenberg*

SECTION 21 Radiology

***Editors**: Mariano Volpacchio, Catherine D'Agostino, Christopher Palestro, W Mark Hamilton, Robin J Warshawsky, David Nagata, Maximiliano de Rodrigo, John Pellerito, Ernesto P Molmenti*

PART 3 ISLET CELL TRANSPLANTATION

SECTION 22 Islet Cell Transplantation

Editor: *Horacio Rilo*

PART 1 KIDNEY TRANSPLANTATION

Section 12 Basic Science

- Epigenetics in Transplantation
- Ischemia Reperfusion

Section 13 Pediatric Kidney Transplantation

- Pediatric Kidney Transplantation

Section 14 Pathology

- Renal Transplant Pathology

Section 15 Radiology

Pre-Transplant

- Candidate Imaging
- Donor Evaluation

Post-Transplant

- Collections
- Parenchymal Imaging
- Urologic Imaging
- Vascular Imaging
- Infections and Malignancies
- Various Findings

Section 16 Cutaneous Manifestations

- Dermatologic Manifestations of Kidney Disease

CHAPTER 1

Overview of Kidney Transplantation

Christine Sardo Molmenti, Ernesto P Molmenti, Madhu Bhaskaran, Nicole Ali, Amit Basu, Eric Siskind, Viren Amin, and Collaborators

OVERVIEW

Benefits of Kidney Transplantation

The main benefits of transplantation (for those who qualify for the procedure) are:

- Improved survival
- Improved quality of life
- From a public health financial perspective, kidney transplantation is cost-effective when compared to chronic dialysis

Other Observations

- Pre-emptive (prior to starting dialysis) transplantation provides the best outcomes
- Risk of death is directly proportional to time on dialysis
- As in all medical and surgical procedures, no guarantees can be provided with respect to outcomes and/or results
- Transplant candidate: Before transplantation
- Transplant recipient: After transplantation

Transplantation: A Multidisciplinary Team Approach

Transplantation entails a multidisciplinary team approach that includes but is not limited to:

- Transplant Center Director
- Transplant Administrator
- Transplant Coordinator
- Transplant Financial Coordinator
- Transplant Independent Living Donor Advocate/Team (at institutions performing live donor transplants)
- Transplant Nephrologist
- Transplant Pharmacist
- Transplant Social Worker
- Transplant Surgeon
- Transplant Unit Staff Nurses
- Consulting Specialists (cardiology, infectious diseases, psychiatry, endocrinology, others)
- Referring Physicians

Evaluation

Medical, surgical, psychiatric, social and financial conditions are considered when determining candidacy.

Waiting List

- Once approved for transplantation, candidates are placed on a waiting list
  - Regular re-evaluations are required, especially when approaching the top
- Being in the waiting list for a deceased donor does not guarantee transplantation
  - Events such as strokes and myocardial infarctions may disqualify candidates

Donors

- Kidneys can be obtained from live or deceased donors
- Live donor kidneys are generally associated with better outcomes than those of deceased donors

Facts About Live Donation

- Donor safety and well-being constitute the main priority when considering live donor transplantation
- Communications between potential donors and the transplant center should always be kept confidential (unless otherwise authorized by the donor)

Positive Aspects of Living Donation

- Short waiting time
- Elective procedure
- Improved graft and recipient outcomes
- Potentially improved genetic compatibility
- Psychological benefit for donors (and recipients)

Risks Involved in Living Donation

- Donor surgical, medical, psychiatric, social and financial risks
- Complications may be short and/or long lasting

Blood Typing

- Donor and recipient must be ABO identical or compatible (unless otherwise addressed prior to transplantation) (Table 1)
- Transplantation across incompatible blood types is possible but requires intensive preparation both before and after transplantation

Outcomes After Transplantation

- Graft and patient survival rates vary from center to center
- National and transplant center-specific outcomes are publically reported

Complications

The benefits of kidney transplantation may be diminished or totally obliterated by potential complications associated with the transplant surgery and/or with the transplant process.

Table 1: Blood type compatibility

Recipient ABO	Compatible donor ABO
O	O
A	A, O
B	B, O
AB	AB, A, B, O

Transfusion of Blood Products and Transplantation of an Organ

- Exposure to biological products (such as an organ transplant and blood products) is associated with the potential for transmission of infections (such as hepatitis B, hepatitis C, human immunodeficiency virus (HIV)/acquired immunodeficiency syndrome (AIDS), West Nile virus, swine flu, Chagas' disease, rabies, malaria), malignancies (such as cancers and lymphomas), and/or other pathologies
- Receiving blood products may lead to sensitization, adversely affect receiving future transplants

Biopsies

- Routinely obtained percutaneously under local anesthesia
- Complications include but are not limited to bleeding, injury to blood vessels, injury to abdominal organs or other structures (such as bowel or nerves), hematuria, pain, infections, urinary leaks, arterio-venous fistulas, hematomas, loss of the kidney, death, etc.

Delayed Kidney (graft) Function (DGF)

- Has been reported to be associated with:
  - Increased incidence of rejection
  - Diminished graft and patient survival
  - Increased costs
  - Prolonged hospitalization
  - Increased complexity of care (including but not limited to biopsies and dialysis)
- Occasionally, the kidney may not function at all, requiring re-transplantation

Immunosuppression

- Life-long immunosuppression (unless organ failure occurs prior to death) is required
- Immunosuppression medications can have interactions with other medications (both prescription and over-the-counter medications) as well as with herbal medications, supplements, foods and beverages
- Prior to starting or discontinuing any medications recipients should check with their transplant centers

Potential Side Effects of Immunosuppression

The potential side effects of immunosuppression include but are not limited to:

- Acne
- Adverse reactions to prolonged sunlight

- Agitation
- Anemia
- Anxiety
- Arthritis
- Cardiovascular events
- Cataracts
- Cough
- Cushingoid features ("moon-face" and "buffalo hump" among others)
- Decreased ability of the blood to clot
- Diabetes/hyperglycemia
- Gastrointestinal complaints
- Gout
- Gingival hyperplasia
- Hair loss/thinning
- Headaches
- Hirsutism
- Hypertension
- Hypercholesterolemia
- Hyperglycemia
- Increased appetite
- Infections
- Interactions with prescription, over-the-counter, and herbal medications as well as with foods and beverages
- Joint and bone pain
- Malignancies
- Mood swings
- Muscle weakness
- Nephrotoxicity
- Neurological events
- Noncompliance
- Osteoporosis
- Pancreatitis
- Paresthesias
- Progressive multifocal leukoencephalopathy
- Skin peeling on palms and feet
- Swelling of feet, hands, abdomen or face
- Tremors
- Trouble sleeping
- Unusual and/or unwanted fat deposits
- Vascular disease
- Weight gain
- White cell count and platelet abnormalities
- Other side effects

Long- and Short-Term Success

- Long- and short-term success is dependent but not limited on:
  - Organ quality
  - Recipient medical condition
  - Patient compliance
  - Surgical and medical complications
  - Episodes of rejection
  - Age and health of the recipient
  - Quality of the allograft
- Over half of recipients die with a functioning graft
  - Recipient mortality is frequently associated with:
    - Cardiovascular disease
    - Infections

Vaccines

- Prior to receiving any vaccines (or being in close contact with children or adults who have recently received vaccines) recipients should consult with their transplant center
- Attenuated pathogens that lead to immunity in immunocompetent individuals can be associated with full-blown disease in immunosuppressed ones

FURTHER READING

1. Hariharan S, Johnson CP, Bresnahan BA, et al. Improved graft survival after renal transplantation in the United States, 1988 to 1996. N Engl J Med. 2000;342(9):605-12. PMID: 10699159.
2. National Kidney Foundation.
   Available from: http://www.kidney.org/index.cfm
3. Organ Transplant Interpretive Guidelines Update. Center for Medicaid and State Operations/Survey & Certification Group.
   Available from: http://www.cms.gov/Medicare/Provider-Enrollment-and-Certification/SurveyCertification-GenInfo/downloads/SCLetter08-25.pdf

CHAPTER 2

Diagnoses and Diagnostic Categories for Kidney Transplantation

Nicole Ali, Eric Siskind, Ernesto P Molmenti

DIAGNOSES AND DIAGNOSTIC CATEGORIES FOR KIDNEY TRANSPLANTATION[1,2]

Congenital, Rare Familial and Metabolic Disorders

- Congenital obstructive uropathy
- Cystinosis
- Fabry's disease
- Hypoplasia/Dysplasia/Dysgenesis/Agenesis
- Medullary cystic disease
- Nephrophthisis
- Prune belly syndrome

Diabetes

- Diabetes Type I: Insulin dependent/juvenile onset
- Diabetes Type II: Insulin dependent/adult onset
- Diabetes Type I : Non-insulin dependent/juvenile onset
- Diabetes Type II: Non-insulin dependent/adult onset

Glomerular Diseases

- Anti-glomerular basement membrane (GBM)
- Thin basement membrane disease
- Chronic glomerulonephritis: Unspecified
- Chronic glomerulosclerosis: Unspecified
- Focal glomerular sclerosis (Focal Segmental–FSG)
- Idiopathic/Post-infectious crescentic glomerulonephritis
- Rapid progressive glomerulonephritis (RPGN)
- HIV nephropathy
- Immunoglobulin A (IgA) nephropathy
- Hemolytic uremic syndrome
- Membranous glomerulonephritis
- Mesangiocapillary 1 glomerulonephritis
- Mesangiocapillary 2 glomerulonephritis
- Systemic lupus erythematosus
- Alport's syndrome
- Amyloidosis
- Membranous nephropathy
- Goodpasture's syndrome
- Henoch-Schonlein purpura
- Wegener's granulomatosis

Hypertensive Nephrosclerosis

Hypertensive nephrosclerosis

Neoplasms

- Incidental carcinoma
- Lymphoma
- Myeloma
- Renal cell carcinoma
- Wilms' tumor

Polycystic Kidneys

Polycystic kidneys

Renovascular and Other Vascular Diseases

- Hepatorenal syndrome
- Cholesterol embolization

- Chronic nephrosclerosis: Unspecified
- Malignant hypertension
- Polyarteritis
- Progressive systemic sclerosis
- Renal artery thrombosis
- Scleroderma

Retransplant/Graft Failure

Retransplant/Graft failure

Tubular and Interstitial Diseases

- Pre BM transplantation total body irradiation
- Drug related interstitial nephritis
- Lithium toxicity
- Acquired obstructive nephropathy
- Analgesic nephropathy
- Antibiotic-induced nephritis
- Cancer chemotherapy-induced nephritis
- Chronic pyelonephritis/Reflux nephropathy
- Gout
- Nephritis
- Nephrolithiasis
- Oxalate nephropathy
- Radiation nephritis
- Acute tubular necrosis
- Cortical necrosis
- Calcineurin inhibitor nephrotoxicity
- Heroin nephrotoxicity
- Sickle cell anemia
- Sarcoidosis
- Urolithiasis

Other

- Rheumatoid arthritis
- Familial nephropathy

REFERENCES

1. OPTN-HRSAhttp://optn.transplant.hrsa.gov/organ Datasource/about.asp?display=Kidney
2. Adult Kidney Transplant Candidate Registration Worksheet. Form Approved: O.M.B No 0915-0157 Expiration Date 3/31/2015

CHAPTER 3

Kidney Transplant Recipient Evaluation: Outcome Based Approach

Madhu Bhaskaran, Ankita Sagar, Eric Siskind, Nicole Ali, Amit Basu, et al.

INTRODUCTION

Kidney transplantation offers improved survival and better quality of life for patients with end-stage renal disease (ESRD). However this is dependent on successful transplantation outcomes. A thorough transplant recipient evaluation should address modifiable risk factors (for resolution) and nonmodifiable risk factors (for informed consent or exclusion of candidates). Factors affecting perioperative outcome as well as long-term post-transplant outcome are to be addressed to ensure a smooth perioperative and optimal post-transplant course for the recipient. Factors affecting mortality and perioperative morbidity as well as short-term survival of recipient or allograft will have a major negative impact on the benefit of kidney transplantation as a treatment option.

FACTORS AFFECTING PERIOPERATIVE MORTALITY

- Life-threatening cardiovascular event
  - Infarction
  - Arrhythmias
  - Congestive heart failure
- Coagulopathy causing bleeding
- Hypercoagulable states causing blood clots and fatal pulmonary embolism
- Severe pre-existing lung disease
- Fatal gastrointestinal bleeding
- Fatal cerebrovascular event
- Pre-existing infection leading to postoperative sepsis
- Postoperative infection causing sepsis

FACTORS AFFECTING PERIOPERATIVE MORBIDITY AND PROLONGED HOSPITAL STAY

- Nonfatal acute coronary event
- Deep vein thrombosis
- Postoperative bleeding-operative site or gastrointestinal requiring transfusion
- Lung disease leading to prolonged intubation and intensive care unit (ICU) stay and complications related to it
- Postoperative pneumonia causing respiratory failure
- Postoperative urinary infection causing sepsis
- Mechanical complications related to surgery
  - Arterial or venous obstruction
  - Ureteral obstruction or leak
  - Bladder injury
  - Visceral (bowel) injury
  - Vascular compromise of the lower extremity
- Poor preoperative functional status
- Obesity predisposing to perioperative complications

FACTORS AFFECTING MORBIDITY AND MORTALITY IN THE DELAYED POST-TRANSPLANT PERIOD

- Cardiovascular
- Compliance with medications
- Progression of co-morbid conditions
  - Chronic hepatitis

- New opportunistic infections
  - Pneumocystis jiroveci pneumonia
  - Cytomegalovirus (CMV)
  - BK polyomavirus (BKV)
  - Parvovirus B19
  - Opportunistic fungal infections
  - Mycobacterium tuberculosis
- Recurrent kidney disease
  - Focal segmental glomerulosclerosis (FSGS)
  - Membranoproliferative glomerulonephritis (MPGN)
  - Lupus nephritis
  - Thrombotic microangiopathy
- Post-transplant malignancies
  - Lymphoma
  - Skin malignancies
  - Native kidney neoplasm

OUTCOME BASED APPROACH TO RECIPIENT EVALUATION (TABLE 1)

Apart from a detailed history stressing medical, surgical and immunological risk factors affecting the outcome of transplantation and a full physical examination by the nephrology/transplant surgery team, the following categories comprehensively address the above mentioned factors affecting short- and long-term outcome of transplant recipients:

- Cardiovascular risk evaluation
  - Echo, nuclear stress test and electrophysiology studies
    - Severe valvular disease, active coronary artery disease, severe pulmonary hypertension and high risk of arrhythmias are major causes for perioperative mortality and impact short- and long-term outcome. Low ejection fraction (< 40%), reversible ischemia on nuclear perfusion scan and arrhythmogenicity may place a candidate into high risk group with unfavorable outcome unless these are addressed
  - Cardiac catheterization in selected cases: Long duration of being on dialysis (5 or more years), diabetes mellitus, nuclear scan suggestive of ischemia are indicators that may suggest need for coronary angiogram to improve risk assessment and risk mitigation strategies
    - Pre-ESRD patients pose a special risk of contrast nephropathy pushing them into dialysis and risk versus benefit consideration often requires a detailed discussion with the primary nephrologist, cardiologist and the informed patient
- Cancer screening
  - Age appropriate cancer screening is noncontroversial
    - Mammogram, PAP smear (Papanicolaou test), prostate-specific antigen (PSA), prostate exam, colonoscopy
  - Chest computed tomography (CT) scan in smokers is an example of special circumstances in the setting of transplant evaluation. Most transplant programs prefer to get chest CT than to ignore the risk
  - Screening for native kidney neoplasia by imaging is again often practiced in the pretransplant setting and appears to be reasonable
- Compliance screening
  - Compliance with medications and follow-up are closely linked to optimal outcome
  - Prior history of noncompliance, substance use, young age, psychiatric illnesses, lack of social and financial support are factors which impact compliance
  - Communication with dialysis unit team and nephrologist may clarify state of compliance over a period of time that can help determine possibility of noncompliance post-transplant
- Infectious diseases
  - Positive purified protein derivative (PPD): Test quantiferon, ID evaluation and Isoniazid (INH) therapy
  - Hepatitis B, hepatitis C positive: viral load, abdominal sonogram, Alfa fetoprotein level and hepatology evaluation for liver biopsy. Chronic active hepatitis, cirrhosis and high suspicion for hepatocellular cancer will be high risk for renal transplant
  - HIV positive: Transplantation offered by centers specializing in such patients with controlled disease. Needs close monitoring of tacrolimus, cyclosporine and sirolimus levels and adjustment of doses due to high interaction with protease inhibitors
- Imaging
  - Chest X-ray, abdomen and pelvis sonogram, magnetic resonance angiography (MRA) for screening for aneurysm (patients with polycystic kidneys)
  - Incidental findings on imaging are investigated to exclude active or dormant infection or neoplasia
- Nutritional evaluation
  - To ensure optimal pre- and post-operative nutritional outcome and dietary advice post-transplant
- Social work evaluation
  - Important variable determining the outcome of transplantation
- Financial evaluation
  - Ensures ability to continue medications and follow-up medical care to achieve optimal outcome
- Specialist consultations and special circumstances
  - *See* Table 1

Table 1: Recipient evaluation

Risk factor	Investigations	Radiology	Consults	Actions
Cardiovascular/ Cerebrovascular risk	EKG, Echocardiogram, Nuclear stress test with perfusion imaging	Coronary angiography (if indicated) Carotid Doppler (If indicated) MRA for aneurysms (Recipients with polycystic kidney disease)	Cardiology, electrophysiology if risk of arrhythmias	Predictors of poor transplant outcome: Low ejection fraction (< 40%), severe untreated coronary artery disease, severe pulmonary hypertension, AICD, Severe valvular heart disease, Low blood pressure pre dialysis (<100 mm Hg systolic), Recent coronary intervention with deployment of stent (within 6 months); Significant carotid stenosis Give aspirin perioperatively, continue plavix in patients on it
Cancer screening	PSA, PAP smear, Colonoscopy, Serum immunofixation (recent ESRD of unclear etiology)	Chest X-ray Chest CT (smokers) Abdominal Sonogram Mammogram	Dermatology Gyn Pap smear GI (colonoscopy) Oncology (previous history of cancer)	High risk: Prior cancers High incidence of cancers in the family Prior h/o immunosuppression for other reasons (lupus, nephritic syndrome)
Compliance screening	Age, Prior h/o noncompliance, Substance use, Psychiatric illness history	Tox screen	Social work; Dialysis unit Social work; Psychiatry	High risk of noncompliance pretransplant may lead to poor outcome post-transplant
Hepatitis C or Hepatitis B	Panel A, B Viral load PCR, Alfa fetoprotein	Abdominal sonogram	GI/hepatology consult	Cirrhosis, Chronic active hepatitis, High alfa fetoprotein: High risk of poor outcome after transplant Antiviral treatment pretransplant
Positive PPD	Quantiferon gold	CXR	ID	
Smoker, Sleep apnea	PFT, Sleep study	Chest CT	Pulmonary	Uncontrolled sleep apnea and continued smoking—poor outcome
Coumadin therapy	PT/INR		Hematology	Informed consent regarding possible risk of bleeding and need for transfusion

Contd...

Contd...

Risk factor	Investigations	Radiology	Consults	Actions
Hypercoagulable state	Hematology work up: Protein C, Protein S, Antithrombin III, Prothrombin gene mutation, Factor V leiden, Antiphospholipid antibody		Hematology	Hypercoagulable state may lead to primary nonfunction from allograft thrombosis
Incidental finding of lung nodule	Chest CT/ biopsy if indicated		Pulmonary, oncology	
Incidental adrenal nodule	Functional studies-catecholamines, metanephrines		Endocrinology	
Incidental native kidney nodule		CT/MRI	Urology, oncology	
Peripheral vascular disease		Lower extremity Doppler/ Angiogram if indicated	Vascular consult	Informed consent regarding possible lower extremity ischemia
Lower urinary tract abnormalities, prostate disease	PSA	CT abdomen/pelvis, urodynamic study	Urology	
Prior history of Cancer		Imaging as appropriate	Oncology, breast surgery (if breast ca), GU (prostate ca/ renal cancer)	Informed consent regarding risk of recurrent disease with immunosuppression
Prior history of vasculitis/Lupus	ANA, Anti-DS DNA titer, C3, C4 level, ANCA, Anti-GBM		Rheumatology	Increased risk if active disease
Risk of recurrent kidney disease	Review of prior kidney biopsy		Nephrology	Increased risk of recurrence with FSGS, MPGN
History of CVA, Seizures	Review of medications	Carotid Doppler, Brain imaging-CT/MRI	Neurology	Major interaction of tacrolimus with anticonvulsants
Inflammatory bowel disease/malabsorption, short bowel			Gastroenterology	Increased risk of allograft rejection due to malabsorption of immunosuppressive medications

(AICD: Automatic implantable cardioverter defibrillator; ANA: Antinuclear antibody; Anti-GBM: Anti-glomerular basement membrane antibody; ANCA: Anti-neutrophil cytoplasmic antibody; Anti-dsDNA: Anti-double stranded DNA; CT: Computed tomography; CXR: Chest X-ray; EKG: Electrocardiogram; ESRD: End-stage renal disease; FSGS: Focal segmental glomerular sclerosis; GI: Gastrointestinal, GU: Genitourinary; Gyn: Gynecologic; MRA: Magnetic resonance angiography; MRI: Magnetic resonance imaging; PFT: Pancreatic function test; PPD: Purified protein derivative; PSA: Prostate-specific antigen).

IMMUNOLOGICAL RISK EVALUATION

- Conventional immunological risk
  - Tissue typing to determine degree of human leukocyte antigen (HLA) mismatch
  - Lymphocyte cross match

    Detects preformed cytotoxic antibodies
  - Donor-specific antibodies

    Detects preformed donor-specific anti HLA antibodies
- Special circumstances that require individualized discussion of immunological risk
  - Desensitized recipients
  - ABO incompatible transplantation

- Re-transplantation after failed allograft
- Zero mismatched transplant
- Experimental immunological protocols

DONOR-DERIVED RISK

- Risk of allograft dysfunction
  - Older donor
  - Long cold ischemia time
  - Anatomic abnormalities in donor kidney or ureter
  - Extended criteria donor
  - Donor after cardiac death
- Risk of transmission of disease
  - Neoplasia
  - Infection

Informed consent for kidney transplantation involves discussion of donor-derived risk and answering questions based on available data on the donor.

CHAPTER 4

Sample Recipient Evaluation Form

Ernesto P Molmenti, Nicole Ali, Amit Basu, Madhu Bhaskaran

Below is a sample recipient evaluation form. It constitutes only a possible way to address the intake information. It should be modified according to the specific needs of each program.

PATIENT NAME

I personally saw and examined this patient. My history and physical is based on my own examination and interaction with the patient and those present with him/her, on available medical records, as well as on the reports and observations of other members of the team.

Date of birth: ___ year old
Gender:
Race/Ethnicity:
Date of service: **Time:**
Chief complaint: End-stage renal disease. Presents to be evaluated for kidney transplantation.

PHYSICIAN REQUESTING CONSULTATION

Nephrologist:
- Name: ....
- Address: ....
- Telephone number: ....

Primary care physician:
- Name: ....
- Address: ....
- Telephone number: ....

Other physicians:
....

Location of encounter:
☐ Outpatient office (Address) ....
☐ Hospital (Address) ....
☐ Other ....

Others Present:
....
....

Cause of kidney failure:
- Date of diagnosis of kidney failure:
- Date of start of dialysis (hemo/peritoneal):
- Date of diagnosis of hypertension (if any):
- Date of diagnosis of diabetes (if any):
- Previous kidney transplant:

Cardiac history:
Previous transfusion of blood products:
History of deep vein thrombosis (DVT)/arteriovenous dialysis access thrombosis/ miscarriages:
Course complicated by/past medical-surgical history:
....
....
....
....

Name:
DOB:

Allergies:

Pain scale (0–10, with 10 being worst pain):

Current medications:

....

....

....

....

Family history:

Father: age ☐ alive ☐ deceased Cause of death/illnesses:

Mother: age ☐ alive ☐ deceased Cause of death /illnesses:

Family history of kidney disease: ☐ Yes ☐ No

Siblings, other:

Social history:

Occupation:
☐ Single ☐ Married ☐ Divorced ☐ Separated
☐ Widowed ☐ Other

Children? ☐ No ☐ Yes (how many):

Potential live donors?

Habits:
Smoking: ☐ No ☐ Yes (Amount):
Drinking: ☐ No ☐ Yes (Amount):
Drug use: ☐ No ☐ Yes (Amount):

Studies reviewed:

. . . .

. . . .

. . . .

. . . .

Review of systems:

General: ( ) Weight changes ( ) Fevers or chills (+) As per HPI
Head, ears, nose and throat: ( ) trauma ( ) As per HPI

Eyes: ( ) Wears glasses ( ) As per HPI

Skin: ( ) Rashes ( ) Tattoos ( ) Scars ( ) As per HPI

Neck: ( ) Pain/Stiffness ( ) As per HPI

Pulmonary: ( ) Cough ( ) Wheezing ( ) As per HPI

Cardiac: ( ) Shortness of breath ( ) Chest pain ( ) As per HPI

Gastrointestinal (GI): ( ) Nausea ( ) Vomiting ( ) Diarrhea ( ) Constipation ( ) As per HPI

Genitourinary (GU): ( ) Urine output: cups/day ( ) Pre-dialysis ( ) Hematuria ( ) UTI (+) As per HPI

Gynecological: ( ) N/A ( ) Regular menstrual periods ( ) Postmenopause ( ) As per HPI

Neurological: ( ) Headache ( ) Seizures ( ) Fainting spells ( ) As per HPI

Psychological: ( ) Hallucinations ( ) As per HPI

Endocrine: ( ) Diabetes ( ) Hypothyroidism ( ) As per HPI

Hematological: ( ) Adenopathy ( ) As per HPI

Physical examination:
T: **BP:** **P:** **Resp:** ☒ As per nursing notes
Height: **Weight:** **BMI:**
☐ Well-developed
☐ Well-nourished
☐ No acute distress

Head, ears, nose and throat:

( ) Normocephalic ( ) Atraumatic.

Eyes: ( ) Sclerae anicteric

Neck: ( ) Supple ( ) No carotid bruits.

Chest: ( ) Clear to auscultation

Heart: ( ) Regular rate and rhythm ( ) Murmur ( ) Systolic ( ) Diastolic

Abdomen/GI: ( ) No guarding ( ) Soft ( ) Non-tender ( ) No hepatomegaly

Extremities: ( ) Intact femoral pulses ( ) Lower extremity edema ( ) Wounds

( ) Fistula ( ) Graft: ( ) Right arm ( ) Left arm ( ) Right forearm ( ) Left forearm ( ) Thigh

Neurological: ( ) Alert and oriented, responds to questions appropriately ( ) Able to ambulate without assistance.

Psychological: ( ) No evidence of aberrant behavior.

Hematological: ( ) No cervical/inguinal lymph adenopathy.

ASSESSMENT/IMPRESSION

Based on the above findings, I believe kidney transplantation should be considered as a treatment option for this patient's end-stage renal disease.

We should proceed with our protocol evaluation for kidney transplantation.

PLAN

I have discussed with the patient at length the risks and benefits of transplantation. Patient is aware that transplantation is a process that requires a life-long commitment, and that it is a personal choice to proceed with it rather than to remain with alternative treatments such as dialysis. Patient understands that the two major benefits of

Name:
DOB:

transplantation include prolonged survival and improved quality of life. I have mentioned to the patient that organs from live donors in general do better than those of deceased donors. We will attempt to place the kidney on the right side, but if that is not possible may need to go to the contralateral side.

Patient is aware that he/she will need to take immunosuppression medications in order to preserve the kidney for as long as the organ is functioning in order to prevent rejection. Patient is aware that immunosuppression is required in addition to his/her baseline medications and in addition to other medications such as antimicrobials. The immunosuppression levels will probably be decreased with time. Patient is aware that immunosuppression levels are usually at their highest during the first 6 months, which is coincident with the period of the greatest incidence of rejection and complications. Patient is aware as well that immunosuppression side-effects include but are not limited to the onset or worsening of diabetes, allograft damage, increased incidence of all types of infections, increased incidence of all types of malignancies but most prominently of the skin and hematological, neurological illness and pathologies.

Patient is aware that the incidence of malignancies in non-functioning kidneys is higher than in those with normal function. Patient is also aware that immunosuppression will make this incidence even higher. Patient instructed to have screening imaging exams on a regular basis in order to detect such tumors at an early stage.

Patient is aware that it is possible to have children after transplantation (for those in childbearing age). We have instructed patient to wait until there is stable kidney function, and to notify us in advance so we can discontinue teratogenic medications, including but not limited to mycophenolic compounds.

Patient is aware that the average survival of transplanted kidneys is approximately 13 years, and that a second kidney transplant will probably be required especially in younger patients.

Patient is aware that the benefits of transplantation may be diminished or totally cancelled by potential complications associated with the surgery itself and/or with the transplant process. Patient is aware that the treatment of complications may require among other interventions, the need for reoperations, the need for placement of internal and/or external catheters and/or drains, the need for radiological interventional procedures, the need for transfusion of blood products, or observation. Patient is aware that such potential complications include, but are not limited to:

- Bleeding
- Infections with bacteria, viruses, fungi and parasites
- Leaks of urine
- Ureteral and vascular strictures
- Thrombosis of the organ associated with twisting of the blood vessels, rejection, occlusion from events such as intimal flaps and unintentional malpositioning of sutures during the surgery, low blood pressure, or other events, both known and/or unknown
- Cardiac events
- Injury to blood vessels associated with the transplant surgery that may lead to attempts to revascularize an extremity
- Injury to nerves, either temporary or long-lasting
- Fluid collections requiring external and/or internal drainage
- Delayed function of the kidney, requiring dialysis for a period ranging from days to months, or in some cases non-function of the kidney

Patient is aware that he/she may require transfusion of blood products. Patient is aware that such transfusion of blood products as well as the transplant organ itself may be associated with transmission of infections (such as hepatitis B, hepatitis C, HIV, West Nile virus), malignancies, and/or other pathologies.

FURTHERMORE, PATIENT AND THOSE PRESENT IS/ARE AWARE OF THE FOLLOWING FACTS REGARDING HIS/HER SPECIFIC CASE

- The underlying factors that led to failure of the native kidneys will also affect the transplanted kidney (except in rare instances such as polycystic kidney disease)
- The wound will be closed with widely spaced stitches after the surgery to decrease the incidence of infections. Dressing changes will be required. If the skin edges heal unevenly, a plastic procedure may be necessary
- Patient instructed to ambulate frequently, not to lay immobile for prolonged periods of time, and not to cross legs for prolonged periods of time in order to prevent the formation of deep venous thromboses (a life-threatening condition)
- Patient has met with other members of the transplant team as stated in their corresponding notes
- Other:

Name:
DOB:

SPECIFIC ISSUES

As previously stated, we should proceed with our routine protocol transplant evaluation. In addition, based upon my evaluation, I believe the following should be addressed prior to transplantation:

- Cardiac evaluation—all candidates
- Hypercoagulable evaluation—if history of DVT/thrombosis/miscarriages/SLE
- Other:

I have answered all of the patient's questions as well as all questions of those present with the patient. The patient understands we can offer no guarantees and agrees to proceed. Once all of this is completed, the patient should be presented to the multidisciplinary transplant selection committee for a decision whether to proceed with listing and transplantation.

Name:
DOB:

CHAPTER 5

Fluids and Electrolytes

Richard Barnett, Ezequiel Rodríguez Reimundes, RoseMarie Pasmantier, Asha Alex

INTRODUCTION

There are 17,000 new renal transplant recipients and more than 170,000 end-stage renal disease (ESRD) patients with a functional kidney graft per year in the US. The challenges of optimizing therapy for these patients are formidable. Most of them, at some point in their course, manifest a variety of fluid and electrolyte disorders that require attention. The skilled practitioner is required to be knowledgeable in the management of renal transplant recipients in the preoperative, postoperative and maintenance periods. The immediate postoperative period is particularly complex as acute renal failure (ARF), abrupt changes in glomerular filtration rate (GFR), and specific problems resulting from the unique characteristics of the immunosuppressive agents need to be considered.

This chapter will focus principally on adult patients undergoing solitary kidney transplantation.

- Less than 10% all US recipients are younger than 18 years of age
- Less than 10% are dual renal/other organ transplants

While 80% of new recipients are already on maintenance dialysis, an increasing number represent "pre-emptive" transplants; their disparate requirements will be reviewed.

The major topics to be considered include:

- Disorders of salt and water metabolism
- Potassium homeostasis
- Acidosis
- Hypomagnesemia
- Hyperuricemia
- Abnormalities of calcium, phosphorus and bone homeostasis

PREOPERATIVE CONSIDERATIONS

Pre-Emptive Transplant Recipients

Increasing numbers of recipients who undergo pre-emptive transplantation have GFRs less than 20 mL/min. Most of these patients never receive preoperative optimization with dialysis. It is likely that we will be encountering more of these individuals with recent evidence demonstrating improved graft and patient survival compared to recipients maintained on dialysis.[1] It is beyond the scope of this topic to review in detail the medical management of patients with chronic kidney disease (CKD) IV and V.

The judicious use of diuretics and in the case of patients with chronic congestive heart failure (CHF) angiotensin-converting-enzyme (ACE) inhibitors/angiotensin receptor blocker (ARB) therapy to improve left ventricular (LV) function has become standard treatment.

- Goal: to avoid volume overload before surgery
- Acute dialysis is seldom indicated because of the effectiveness of loop diuretics even in the face of GFRs less than 10 mL/min
- Combined with metolazone, the vast majority of pre-emptive patients are able to maintain acceptable volume status
  - Metolazone may exacerbate hyponatremic tendencies in patients with advanced CKD by effects on urinary dilution
- Overall free water clearance is reduced in advanced renal failure, but most individuals present preoperatively with sodium levels in excess of 130 mEq/L
  - Sodium concentrations substantially less than this require therapy usually involving water restriction and loop diuretics

- Hemodialysis can effectively raise plasma sodium levels but the rapid rate of correction may have adverse consequences

With reduced GFR, hypokalemia and hypomagnesemia are rarely encountered but occasionally require acute supplementation.

- More frequently, hyperkalemia is noted with goal of maintaining levels less than 5 mEq/L
- The K^+ excreting properties of loop diuretics and/or metolazone may be aided by concurrent sodium bicarbonate therapy which exerts its effect primarily by trapping K^+ in the distal nephron
- Hyperkalemia is the most frequent electrolyte disorder in these patients requiring preoperative hemodialysis

Mitigation of progressive acidosis with bicarbonate therapy to maintain levels in the 20–25 mEq/L range has become more common, with mounting evidence of its benefit in slowing the progression of chronic renal failure (CRF).[2]

- Preoperative evaluation of HCO_3^-, less than 20 or more than 30 should include a blood gas [arterial blood gas (ABG) or venous blood gas (VBG)] to ascertain a major respiratory component
  - Elevated HCO_3^- levels may be encountered with overzealous diuretic and HCO_3^- therapy, but is also observed in patients with CO_2 retention resulting from chronic obstructive pulmonary disease (COPD) or obstructive sleep apnea. These latter disorders are important preoperative conditions, which should be recognized prior to major surgery
  - Decreased HCO_3^- usually results from the increased anion gap acidosis of advanced CRF, but acute respiratory alkalosis could indicate worsening heart failure, pneumonia, sepsis or pulmonary embolus

Phosphate levels are typically well-controlled with binder therapy.

- Hyperphosphatemia is rarely a contraindication for surgery
- Hypophosphatemia is frequently consequent to overzealous binder therapy and should be addressed
  - Levels less than 2 mmol/L may predispose to intraoperative rhabdomyolysis, particularly in association with pre-existing renal failure, statins and hypothyroidism

Calcium levels are managed well with vitamin D and/or calcium supplementation.

- Normal ionized calcium levels may optimize intraoperative cardiac function and vasoreactivity
- Hypercalcemia is rarely a consideration in pre-emptive patients
  - Management: Discontinue vitamin D and/or Ca^{2+} containing PO_4^{3-} binders

End-Stage Renal Disease Patients

In many respects, the preoperative fluid and electrolyte management of prospective renal transplant recipients with ESRD is less complex.

Volume overload, hyperkalemia and acidosis are readily mitigated with standard dialytic therapy.

- Most practitioners avoid hemodialysis on the day of transplant surgery to decrease complications relating to volume depletion and hypokalemia
- There may be delay in graft function for patients undergoing hemodialysis within the 24 hours before surgery[3]

In patients with longstanding ESRD, hyperparathyroidism and hypercalcemia may be important considerations.

- Hypercalcemia associated with hyperparathyroidism is controlled increasingly with calcimetic therapy[4]
- The value of parathyroidectomy prior to transplant surgery in ESRD is controversial and should probably be reserved for the most severe cases, which cannot be medically managed

POSTOPERATIVE CONSIDERATIONS

The challenges of managing the fluid and electrolyte disorders in new renal transplant recipients are significant. Substantial disparities in pre-existing medical conditions, initial graft function and immunosuppression regimen require a very individualized approach.

Areas that must be carefully considered include:

- Volume regulation
- Sodium disorders-hyponatremia
- Potassium disorders
- Acid-base balance
- Calcium and phosphate metabolism

Volume Regulation

Most patients are volume optimized prior to surgery. Consequently the third spacing, altered vasoreactivity and perioperative blood loss results in many recipients sustaining central volume depletion immediately following surgery.

Volume Depletion

- Management: In absence of volume overload, urine output less than 20 cc/hour, and relative hypotension, volume supplementation with crystalloids should be seriously considered
- "Volume challenges" are recommended:
  - Consists of several 500 cc intravenous saline boluses each administered over 30 minutes while carefully assessing vital signs, O_2 saturation, development of gallop or rales, and urine output
  - Failure to respond with a brisk increase in urine volume should prompt a vigorous search for other entities including heart failure, postoperative hemorrhage, and urinary obstruction
- Urinary chemistries (Na^+, K^+, Cl^-, Cr, osm) should be obtained, but high urinary sodium may reflect diuretic therapy as well as acute tubular necrosis (ATN). In prerenal, high aldosterone states the low urinary Na^+ usually parallels $C1^-$, while K^+ is significantly higher. Uosm more than 300 may reflect a high antidiuretic hormone (ADH) state reflecting significant volume depletion
- The use of low-dose dopamine and diuretics to augment urine volume is common and controversial as they may delay renal function improvement[5]
- Delayed graft function is still the diagnosis of exclusion and is more commonly observed in kidneys harvested from deceased donors

Volume Overload

- Management in the early postoperative period is done conservatively with volume restriction, preload reduction and supplemental oxygen
- Standard preload reduction measures:
  - Nitrates
  - Loop diuretics
  - Control of hyperglycemia
  - Noninvasive positive pressure ventilation.
- In the context of volume overload and anuria, hemodialysis for volume optimization should not be delayed. Withholding dialysis in this setting may lead to respiratory failure requiring ventilator support
  - The relationship of dialysis membrane "sensitization" in exacerbating delayed graft function is tenuous at best. Patients requiring dialysis after transplant however have significantly worse outcomes[6]
  - The well-defined risks of invasive ventilation also include respiratory infections, which may be particularly resistant to therapy in these immunosuppressed patients

Sodium Disorders

- Distal function is substantially altered in new grafts

  Hypernatremia:
  - Seldom observed; may be associated with polyuria when loop diuretics are employed and/or reflect recovery of delayed graft function
  - Hypercalcemia and hypokalemia may limit ADH effect in the distal tubule
  - Responds to water supplementation and treatment of underlying causes

  Hyponatremia:
  - Far more commonly hyponatremia is observed
  - Volume overload is the most common cause in the postoperative setting
  - Free water clearances may be reduced, particularly in the setting of delayed graft function. Further stimulation of ADH and the renin-angiotensin-aldosterone axis will favor hyponatremia and edema formation
  - Management:
    - Intravenous and oral water restriction indicated in mild hyponatremia
    - In volume overload, loop diuretics may enhance water excretion in contrast to the thiazides and metolazone
  - Dialysis is an option in patients with delayed graft function
    - It may be necessary to adjust the dialysate sodium concentration to avoid wide osmolar swings in patients with Na^+ less than 125 mEq/L
  - Because of the insulin resistant state in the perioperative period in part related to high dose corticosteroids, hyperglycemic shift of intracellular water dilutes the extracellular compartment, with resultant hyponatremia
    - Glycemic control may be important for surgical outcomes in individuals undergoing renal transplantation[7]
  - Hyponatremia in association with hyperkalemia and a rising creatinine in the immediate postoperative period may be a sign of an obstructive uropathy and/or urinary leak and should be investigated with an imaging study[8]

Potassium Disorders

Hyperkalemia

- Frequently encountered in the initial postoperative period

- Causes of limited K^+ excretion:
  - Decreased glomerular or tubular function
  - Cellular release of potassium from tissue breakdown
  - Stress/steroid induced hypercatabolism
  - Acidosis
  - Insulin deficiency
- Medications used routinely following transplant surgery that cause hyperkalemia:
  - Calcineurin inhibitors[9]
  - Beta blockers
  - Trimethoprim sulfamethoxazole
  - Heparin
- Obstructive uropathy with consequent aldosterone resistance should be assiduously evaluated in resistant hyperkalemia, and is not always accompanied by oliguria
  - Management:
    - Mitigate the underlying cause(s)
    - Remove offending medications
- Nonobstructed patients with improving graft function
  - Management: insulin, HCO_3^-, and K^+ restriction
  - Kayexalate is a poor remedy in the immediate postoperative period
- Hyperkalemia in association with hyponatremia and a rising creatinine in the immediate postoperative period may be a sign of a urinary leak and or urinary obstruction and should be investigated with an imaging study[8]
- Treatment of severe and life-threatening hyperkalemia:
  - Aggressively intravenous (IV) calcium
  - Insulin
  - Sodium HCO_3^-
  - Aerosolized beta agonists
  - Hemodialysis, if necessary

Hypokalemia

- Regularly encountered as consequence of diuretic therapy. Associated with metabolic alkalosis, insulin treatment, polyuria, and beta agonist treatment
- Management:
  - Calcineurin inhibitors mitigate urinary potassium losses
    - The diarrhea associated with mycophenolate may facilitate gastrointestinal K^+ losses although it is unclear whether the calcineurin inhibitors offset this effect in the colon
  - Removal of dietary K^+ restrictions and oral K^+ supplements is generally sufficient

Hypomagnesemia

- Usually associated with hypokalemia and diuretic therapy
- Limits tubular K^+ reabsorption, may contribute to cyclosporine nephrotoxicity[10]
- In the immediate postoperative period, we aim to maintain magnesium levels in blood at around 2 mg/dL

Acid Base Abnormalities

Respiratory Acidosis

- Common in the immediate postoperative period while patients are under the influence of residual anesthetic, sedatives and narcotic analgesics
- Transplant recipients with obesity, COPD and obstructive sleep apnea may be at increased risk; require prolonged intensive observation

Respiratory Alkalosis

- Should provoke a prompt evaluation of underlying causes
- Pain and anxiety = diagnoses of EXCLUSION
  - Prompt recognition and treatment is essential
- Causes:
  - Volume overload is the major significant cause following surgery
    - Exuberant fluid administration and resolving capillary leak can elevate central filling pressures
  - Congestive heart failure (CHF) with or without associated acute myocardial infarction (MI) needs to be considered
  - Other etiologies encountered several days later include:
    - Bacterial infection/sepsis
    - Severe anemia
    - Pulmonary embolus
- Diagnosis:
  - The increased sensitivity of ultrasound techniques, brain natriuretic peptide measurements and troponin assays has vastly simplified the workup
- Management:
  - Preload reduction with nitrates, morphine, positive pressure ventilation (preferably noninvasive), diuretics and dialysis are variably employed depending upon condition severity

Metabolic Acidosis

- Generally mitigated by successful engraftment
- The ability of the distal tubule to acidify urine usually improves over time
- Management:
  - Mild postoperative acidosis seldom requires aggressive supplementation or dialysis to repair the "HCO_3^- deficit"
  - Calcineurin inhibitors may specifically limit acid excretion
- Mild acidosis is well-tolerated and by virtue of the Bohr Effect improves oxygen delivery
- Lactic acidosis with increased anion gap should be excluded when indicated, as impairments in tissue perfusion and oxygenation require prompt intervention
- Diabetic ketoacidosis (DKA) may initially be observed in Type II as well as Type I individuals in the setting of stress, high dose glucocorticoids and calcineurin inhibitors
  - The development of DKA several days after renal transplant, particularly associated with respiratory alkalosis and lactic acidosis should be treated presumptively for severe infection and evaluated for acute MI

Metabolic Alkalosis

- Seldom problematic
- Not as common, as the forces favoring acidosis usually limit severity
- Alkalosis associated with vomiting or nasogastric suctioning is uncommon with the widespread use of H_2 blockers or proton-pump inhibitors
- Management:
  - Diuretic associated volume depletion and hypokalemia in patients with good graft function responds to saline and potassium replacement

Phosphate Metabolism

- The rapid restoration of endogenous renal function may have profound effects on plasma PO_4^{3-} levels
- Secondary or even tertiary hyperparathyroidism can promote considerable PO_4^{3-} excretion, which may be exacerbated by tubular effects of the calcineurin inhibitors. FGF-23 may be particularly important in the PO_4^{3-} wasting seen in the early postoperative period[11]
- Management:
  - Withholding phosphate binders until the magnitude of this process becomes evident, is a reasonable strategy as mild hyperphosphatemia is well-tolerated
  - Many individuals require supplementation when PO_4^{3-} is at or less than 2 mmol/L
  - Consideration should be given to increasing the oral intake of dark colas (with high content of phosphorus) and phosphate-rich foods

Calcium Metabolism

- Alterations in Ca^{2+} are difficult to predict in advance
- Contributing factors:
  - Skeletal resistance
  - Parathyroid hormone (PTH)-mediated proximal tubular reabsorption
  - Calcineurin inhibitor induced renal calcium wasting[12]
- Management of hypocalcemia:
  - In the early postoperative period: calcium supplementation with or without vitamin D is usually sufficient
  - In hypophosphatemic patients: calcium carbonate is preferred as it is less effective in binding intestinal PO_4^{3-} than calcium acetate
  - In patients with concomitant hyperparathyroidism: severe hypercalcemia may be observed shortly after transplantation following normalization of 1,25 vitamin D levels
    - Use of cinacalcet may be invaluable in this setting and mitigate the requirement for urgent parathyroidectomy

LONG-TERM STRATEGIES

Many of the fluid and electrolyte disorders experienced by renal transplant recipients in the months and years following engraftment reflect the common challenges faced by individuals with moderate to severe CKD. It is beyond the scope of this section to deal with the general management of renal insufficiency. Nonetheless, there are problems specific for kidney transplant patients that are worth reviewing.

Volume Regulation

Sodium retention and varying degrees of volume overload are regularly encountered in the renal transplant population.

- Significant contributors:
  - Chronic graft dysfunction, obstructive uropathy, medications and CHF
- Diagnosis:
  - The routine office-based use of sonographic techniques has substantially improved the recognition of obstructive uropathy

- The high cardiovascular risks in established transplant patients related to CKD and calcium phosphate disorders requires vigilance for coronary artery disease and valvulopathies
- Management:
  - Treat underlying urinary obstruction in these individuals largely dependent on a solitary kidney
  - Therapy of CHF frequently involves use of loop diuretics. However, renal hypoperfusion related to LV dysfunction may cause the cardiorenal syndrome associated with significant decreases in GFR. The concurrent use of diuretics with ACE inhibitors or ARBs in this setting may be especially deleterious. Renal transplant recipients are particularly susceptible to acute kidney injury (AKI) in the context of *volume depletion*
  - Immunosuppressive agents (i.e. mycophenolate), and opportunistic (i.e. cytomegalovirus) and nosocomial (i.e. Clostridium) infections favor gastrointestinal (GI) losses predisposing to volume depletion
  - Calcineurin inhibitors as well as ACE inhibitors/ARB alter glomerular hemodynamics predisposing to loss of autoregulation of renal blood flow
  - The role of ACE inhibitors/ARB in long-term preservation of graft function remains to be fully defined. They provoke efferent arteriolar vasodilatation, which decreases intraglomerular pressure reducing proteinuria and limiting the progression of interstitial fibrosis and tubular fibrosis/atrophy. However, in the setting of volume depletion these medications predispose to further GFR reduction and AKI
  - Calcineurin inhibitors provoke afferent arteriolar vasoconstriction reducing GFR and predisposing to AKI in the setting of volume depletion
  - Moreover, diarrhea increases the enterohepatic circulation of tacrolimus leading to toxic concentrations. The combination of diarrhea and volume depletion in association with ACE inhibitors/ARB therapy leads to a high risk of AKI[13] and metabolic acidosis. Calcineurin inhibitors further contribute to AKI in this setting
  - Prompt discontinuation of, as well as prudent volume restitution should be considered
- Management:
  - Volume and electrolyte repletion
  - Treatment of underlying infection and/or diarrhea
  - Prompt discontinuation of ACE inhibitors/ARB
  - Calcineurin-inhibitor dose reduction and strict monitoring of serum concentrations

Hyperkalemia and Acidosis

The association of hyperkalemia and normal anion gap acidosis (renal tubular acidosis) reflects distal tubular dysfunction and/or hypoaldosteronism.

Causes

- Calcineurin inhibitors diminish urinary K^+ and acid secretion largely by affecting cortical collecting Na^+-K^+ ATPase although impairment of aldosterone secretion may contribute[9]
- ACE inhibitors/ARB, beta-blockers, spironolactone, other potassium sparing diuretics and Bactrim® may contribute to hyperkalemia
- Obstructive uropathy is typically associated with distal tubular dysfunction. Hyponatremia is frequently present
- Chronic rejection (formerly chronic allograft nephropathy) is frequently associated with distal tubular dysfunction
- Adrenal insufficiency is rare in patients under glucocorticoids maintenance treatment. However, in the context of sepsis and other stress situations (i.e. surgery) relative adrenal insufficiency may be observed. Rapid tapering of corticosteroids may also predispose

Management: methods to enhance K^+ excretion include:

- Dose reduction or withdrawal of the above mentioned medication
- Addition of a loop diuretic
- Prudent extracellular volume repletion
- Evaluation of adrenal axis if adrenal failure is suspected
- Addition of a "stress dose" of glucocorticoids in septic shock or major surgery
  - Sodium HCO_3^- supplementation
  - Has added benefits of improving distal luminal electronegativity and thus enhancing K^+ trapping
  - Systemic acidosis may also be mitigated
  - It is unclear if HCO_3^- supplementation may decrease the progressive loss of nephrons observed in nontransplanted patients with CRF
  - At this point it seems prudent to maintain HCO_3^- levels in the normal ranges in transplanted CKD patients with supplementation when required

Electrolyte Disorders Associated with Calcineurin Inhibitors

The calcineurin inhibitors (tacrolimus and cyclosporine) have numerous shared effects on electrolyte homeostasis largely secondary to actions on the renal tubule.

- Distal K^+ and H^+ secretion can be impaired and contribute to hyperkalemia and acidosis
- Calcium excretion may be augmented by these agents,[12] although frequently mitigated by coexisting hyperparathyroidism
- Interestingly, cyclosporine may aggravate the PO_4^{3-} wasting associated with elevated PTH states
- Magnesium reabsorption may be impaired and low plasma levels may be implicated in some of the nephrotoxicity observed with these agents[10]
  - Management:
    - Mg^{2+} supplementation in such circumstances is warranted
    - Use of amiloride is not advisable as its limitation of distal Mg^{2+} losses is counterbalanced with enhanced susceptibility to hyperkalemia
- Cyclosporine can raise serum uric acid levels and provoke gout attacks in susceptible individuals[14]
  - Management:
    - Concurrent treatment with diuretics may augment any tendencies for developing symptomatic gout

Phosphate and Calcium

Successful renal transplantation reverses many of the abnormalities associated with hyperparathyroidism.

- Furthermore the functioning graft with plentiful alpha-1 hydroxylase restores vitamin D metabolism toward normal
- Chronic dialysis patients, who may be considered for parathyroidectomy, often improve sufficiently after transplantation to avoid a surgical approach
- The duration of dialysis therapy may relate to persistent abnormalities in Ca^{2+} and PO_4^{3-} levels following transplantation

Despite improvements in management of ESRD dialysis patients, significant hypercalcemia associated with hyperparathyroidism is observed and may be associated with adverse graft outcomes.

- Management:
  - The large experience of most nephrologists with the calcimimetic agent cinacalcet has promoted its use in transplant patients[4]
    - It is probably premature to firmly recommend this approach versus parathyroidectomy. Most clinicians will initially opt for medical therapy
  - Severe, refractory hypercalcemia, typically noted either in the early post-transplant period or in more established patients however strongly warrants surgical considerations
  - Parathyroidectomy, of course, has its own challenges including hypocalcemia and adynamic bone disease. It is beyond the scope of this section to outline the lack of consensus in the management of post-transplant bone disease

Hypophosphatemia following successful transplantation tends to improve over time.

- Some of this may relate to progressively decreased FGF-23 levels[11]
- Management:
  - Persistent hypophosphatemia is generally managed with oral phosphate supplementation and PO_4^{3-} rich foods and beverages
  - Although elevated PTH levels are associated with this PO_4^{3-} wasting, use of cinacalcet to limit PTH-mediated PO_4^{3-} losses in this setting has not been well established

FURTHER READING

1. Danovitch GM. Handbook of Kidney Transplantation. Philadelphia: Lippincott Williams and Wilkins; 2007.
2. Rose BD, Post TW. Clinical Physiology of Acid-Base and Electrolyte Disorders. 5th edition. New York: McGraw Hill; 2001.
3. Schrier RW. Renal and Electrolyte Disorders. 7th edition. Philadelphia: Lippincott Williams and Wilkins. 2010.
4. Taal MW, Chertow GM, Marsden PA, et al. Brenner and Rector's The Kidney. 9th edition. Mosby, US: Saunders; 2010.

REFERENCES

1. Liem YS, Weimar W. Early living donor kidney transplantation: a review of the associated survival benefit. Transplantation. 2009;87(3):317-8.
2. Mahajan A, Simoni J, Sheather SJ, et al. Daily oral sodium bicarbonate preserves glomerular filtration rate by slowing its decline in hypertensive nephropathy. Kid Int. 2010;78:303-9.
3. Van Loo AA, Vanholder RC, Bernaert PR, et al. Pretransplantation hemodialysis strategy influences early renal graft function. J Am Soc Nephrol. 1998; 9(3):473-81.
4. Kruse AE, Eisenberger U, Frey FJ, et al. The calcimetic cinacalcet normalizes serum calcium in renal transplant patients with persistent hyperparathyroidism. Nephrol Dial Transplant. 2005;20(7):1311-4.
5. Lassnigg A, Donner E, Grubhofer G, et al. Lack of renoprotective effects of dopamine and furosemide during cardiac surgery. J Am Soc Nephrol. 2000;11(1):97-104.
6. Shoskes DA, Cecka JM. Deleterious effects of delayed graft function in cadaveric renal transplant recipients independent of rejection. Transplantation. 1998;66:1697-701.
7. Van den Berghe G, Wouters P, Weekers F, et al. Intensive insulin therapy in critically ill patients. N Engl J Med. 2001;345(19):1359-67.

8. Molmenti, Ernesto. Personal communication.
9. Kamel KS, Ethier JH, Quaggin S, et al. Studies to determine the basis for hyperkalemia in recipients of a renal transplant who are treated with cyclosporine. J Am Soc Neph. 1992;2(8):1279-84.
10. Miura K, Nakatani T, Asai T, et al. Role of hypomagnesemia in chronic cyclosporine nephropathy. Transplantation. 2002;73(3): 340-7.
11. Sirilaks S, Chatsrisak K, Ingsathit A, et al. Renal phosphate loss in long term kidney transplantation. Clin J Am Soc Nephol. 2012;7(2):323-31.
12. Niijenhuis T, Hoenderop JG, Bindels RJ. Downregulation of Ca(2+) and Mg(2+) transport proteins in the kidney explains tacrolimus (FK506) induced hyperclciuria and hypomagnesemia. J Am Soc Nephrol. 2004;15(3): 549-57.
13. Stirling C, Houston J, Robertson S, et al. Diarrhoea, vomiting and ACE inhibitors:—an important cause of acute renal failure. J Hum Hypertens. 2003;17(6):419-23.
14. Abbot KC, Kimmel PL, Dharnidharka V, et al. New onset gout after renal transplantation: incidence, risk factors and implications. Transplantation. 2005;80(10):1383-91.

CHAPTER 6

Cardiac Evaluation

Alexander Lee, Mashael Al Anizi, Evelina Grayver, Regina Druz, Nicole Ali

INTRODUCTION

The failing kidney affects multiple organ systems in the body as it becomes ineffectual in clearing toxins, producing hormones, and metabolizing substrates. Frequently, the cardiovascular system is affected in patients with chronic kidney disease (CKD), leading to significant morbidity and mortality. Cardiovascular disease (CVD) remains the leading cause of mortality (over 35%) in end-stage renal disease (ESRD) patients on dialysis.[1] In a review of the Medicare population, the incidence of acute myocardial infarction (AMI) increases with time for both patients on the waiting list and those after transplant.[2] Although the overall risk of AMI is lower after both deceased donor and living donor transplantation, the relative risk of myocardial infarction (MI) is highest in the early postoperative period.[2] In consideration of patients who are renal transplant candidates, the risk of cardiovascular events is not only prevalent during the perioperative period but also spans the pre- and post-transplant continuum. Thus, cardiovascular risk assessment in this special population must take into consideration not only perioperative risk but their annual risk as well.

CORONARY ARTERY DISEASE PREVALENCE AND CARDIOVASCULAR MORTALITY

There is an increased prevalence of coronary artery disease (CAD) and higher annual cardiovascular mortality in patients with ESRD on dialysis. Although cardiovascular mortality is lower post-transplant compared to patients with ESRD or mild to moderate CKD, it remains two-fold greater than that of the general population.[3] The prevalence of angiographically significant CAD may range from 25% to 85% varying with age and the presence or absence of longstanding diabetes.[4] In addition, those with ESRD tend to have more numerous and severe coronary artery lesions compared to patients without CKD.[4]

Chronic kidney disease has been strongly associated with MI. The combination of disease of both these vital organs becomes particularly problematic in this patient group, enhancing their mortality risk in the event of a MI. Evidence suggests that a decline in renal function reduces survival rates in the period following a MI compared to a population with normal renal function.[3]

The evidence concludes that not only is CAD more prevalent amongst patients with CKD, it is also more likely to cause death in the interval following a cardiovascular event.

CARDIOVASCULAR RISK FACTOR MODIFICATION IN PATIENTS WITH CHRONIC KIDNEY DISEASE

In 1948, the Framingham Heart Study under the direction of what is now the National Heart, Lung and Blood Institute (NHLBI) took on the task of identifying common factors that contribute to CVD. Since its inception, the study identified several major risk factors associated with CVD: high blood pressure, high cholesterol, diabetes, smoking, obesity, and physical inactivity.[5] This study did not consider renal disease as a risk factor but many studies since then have concluded that CKD is an independent risk factor for the development of CVD, and is in fact a coronary heart disease (CHD) equivalent.[6] The Framingham risk factors for CHD are useful when considering optimal medical therapeutics in patients with renal disease, as its modification impacts positively on survival and health in this population. In an article by McCullough, he reviewed therapeutic opportunities to improve cardiovascular care in patients with renal disease and its potential clinical impact.[4] The following are recommendations for modifiable risk factors and aspirin use in patients with renal disease:

- Hypertension: Blood pressure should be well-controlled (systolic blood pressure <130 mm Hg) for prevention of cardiovascular events and death. Renin-angiotensin-aldosterone system blocking agents in particular angiotensin-converting enzyme inhibitor (ACEI) and angiotensin receptor blocker (ARB) if tolerated should be used for its cardiovascular effects and possible preservation of kidney function. Beta-blockers may help as an anti-ischemic agent in patients with CAD or as part of optimal medical therapy in congestive heart failure (CHF) patients
- Cholesterol: Ensure optimal lipid control for primary prevention of cardiovascular events and death through diet, statins, and or fibrates and aim for levels: low-density lipoprotein cholesterol (LDL-C) <100 mg/dL, triglycerides <150 mg/dL and high-density lipoprotein cholesterol (HDL-C) >40 mg/dL (male) and >50 mg/dL (female)
- Diabetes: Optimize blood sugar control (glycohemoglobin < 7.0 mg/dL) for reducing rates of microvascular disease such as retinopathy and potentially clinically relevant atherosclerotic disease (AMI, stroke, CVD death)
- Smoking cessation: Smokers have a two to four times risk for development of CHD compared to nonsmokers. Smoking is an independent risk factor for sudden cardiac death in patients with CHD
- Weight: Maintenance of a healthy weight [body mass index (BMI) ≤25 kg/m^2]
- Exercise: Encourage exercise as a sedentary lifestyle is a risk factor for heart disease
- Homocysteine: Reduction in homocysteine levels may aid to reduce the risk of CVD and death, and may be achieved by supplements of folic acid, vitamin B6 and B12
- Antiplatelets: Aspirin 81 mg daily or clopidogrel 75 mg daily if intolerant to aspirin should be used without reservation if indicated, even in those awaiting cadaveric renal transplants

Patients with renal disease need to be treated more aggressively and in a proactive manner according to the rationale that they have an increased vulnerability to CVD, which may be undiagnosed.

CORONARY ARTERY DISEASE EVALUATION IN RENAL TRANSPLANT CANDIDATES

In light of the prevalence and associated mortality of CAD in the CKD population, it stands for good reason to ensure this risk is assessed in all patients with kidney failure who are candidates for transplant, allowing for appropriate and timely management to ensue when applicable. Asymptomatic patients should be seen on an annual basis after initial evaluation to monitor for CVD whilst on the waiting list. Cardiac evaluation should be revisited sooner if a patient develops symptoms suggestive of ischemic heart disease or heart failure. Some key points of consideration in evaluating the pretransplant patient include:

- Optimize medical regimen for risk factor modification
- Patients may be divided into those with pre-existing CAD and those without
- Whether the patient has active symptoms of CAD or heart failure may guide testing strategy
- All patients should have an electrocardiogram (ECG) and assessment of their cardiac function (echocardiogram) as part of their initial assessment
- Stress testing should be considered in patients with moderate or potentially high-risk CAD risk factors or in those with pre-existing CAD (asymptomatic)
- Patients who are potentially high risk for CAD (by symptoms or risk factors) or have symptomatic CAD should be considered for cardiac catheterization with coronary angiography
- Special considerations may be necessary for patients who are deemed high risk and who are not on dialysis
- Right and left heart catheterization should be offered in patients with significant systolic dysfunction [left ventricular ejection fraction (LVEF) ≤40%] to better understand the hemodynamics of their failing heart as patients with similar ejection fractions may have very different hemodynamic profiles
- Patients with structural heart disease need proper assessment, evaluation, and follow-up
- Finally, cardiac testing and risk stratification strategies should take into consideration the individual patient's clinical condition and their comorbidities

Purpose of CAD screening in renal transplant candidates include not only assessment of perioperative surgical risk but also assessment of risk for major adverse cardiovascular events during the pre- and post-transplantation periods. Coronary revascularization [coronary artery bypass graft (CABG) or percutaneous coronary intervention (PCI)] when indicated should be performed prior to renal transplant.

Noninvasive Testing

Myocardial perfusion studies (MPS) and stress echocardiography are commonly used for risk stratification. Although well-studied in the general population, the sensitivity and specificity of these tests in ESRD patients may be more variable and thus less precise. In a study by Patel et al. on patients who had pretransplant stress single-photon emission computed tomography (SPECT) myocardial perfusion imaging, those with normal images had significantly higher cardiac event-free survival rate (97%) than those with abnormal images (87%) at 42 months ($p = 0.006$).[7] In a meta-analysis of MPS and dobutamine stress echocardiography (DSE) for stratifying cardiac risk among candidates for kidney or kidney-pancreas transplantation, the presence of reversible defects was associated with an increased risk of MI (diabetics) and cardiac death (diabetics and nondiabetics), whereas fixed defects were associated with an increased risk of cardiac death but not MI.[8] Thus, proper screening and stress testing in transplant candidates serve an important role in risk stratification and subsequent management. Risk of findings on noninvasive testing using criteria defined for traditional exercise stress tests:[9]

- Low-risk stress test: Cardiac mortality of less than 1% per year
- Intermediate-risk stress test: 1–3% per year cardiac mortality
- High-risk stress test: Greater than 3% per year cardiac mortality

The use of dobutamine echocardiography has been an accepted standard for stress imaging in this patient population but it has its own limitations. The specific noninvasive screening method for CAD detection and risk stratification is largely dependent on the institution and their level of expertise. Clinical judgment with institutional considerations must be exercised in all cases in selecting the most appropriate noninvasive testing strategy.

Invasive Testing

The use of coronary angiography as part of the pretransplant cardiac assessment, especially in patients at high risk for CAD allows for the diagnosis and understanding of the extent and severity of coronary disease, which has been correlated with subsequent mortality in patients with ESRD evaluated for renal transplant. Jones et al. conducted a study to explore the relationship between CAD, transplantation status and subsequent mortality in ESRD patients undergoing evaluation for renal transplantation.[10] The study included 253 patients at high risk for CAD who underwent coronary angiography and can be summarized as follows:

- Cohorts divided in three groups:
  - Group 1 ($n = 127$): No vessel with ≥50% stenosis
  - Group 2 ($n = 56$): One vessel with ≥50% stenosis
  - Group 3 ($n = 70$): Two or more vessels with ≥50% stenosis
- Long-term survival was determined with median follow-up of 3.3 years
- Group 2 and 3 had older age and higher diabetes mellitus (DM), peripheral vascular disease (PVD), and dyslipidemia
- Survival was worse in Group 3 compared to Group 1 ($p < 0.0001$)
- Each of the subgroups had better survival with renal transplant ($p < 0.001$)
- Although the degree of CAD is related to subsequent mortality, transplantation is associated with better survival regardless of the extent and severity of CAD
- Thus, the presence of CAD should not exclude ESRD patients from consideration for this therapy

Under current appropriate use criteria for diagnostic catheterization, preoperative coronary evaluation in stable patients prior to solid organ transplantation received a median appropriate use score of 5, where a median score of 4–6 is assigned an appropriateness rating of "uncertain for specific indication" (test *may* be generally acceptable and *may* be a reasonable approach for the indication).[9] Given the lack of clinical evidence in supporting the routine use of coronary angiography in all patients prior to renal transplant, diagnostic catheterization with coronary angiography used as an initial strategy in cardiac risk assessment should be reserved only for patients who are deemed *high risk*. In a single center retrospective study of adult renal transplant patients, significant risk factors for perioperative MI were age more than 50, pre-existing CAD, and DM.[11] Diabetic patients with CAD were at especially high risk for perioperative cardiac events, thus a more aggressive approach, which may include coronary angiography prior to transplant, is warranted. However, every transplant candidate must be reviewed on an individual basis.

STRATEGIES IN CARDIOVASCULAR ASSESSMENT IN THE TRANSPLANT CANDIDATE

Several algorithms have been proposed in assessing patients who are awaiting transplant. However, there is a general lack of consensus as to the most optimal strategy in cardiac risk assessment and thus subsequent cardiovascular outcomes. Many follow the guidelines

Flowchart 1: Risk stratification strategy for potential kidney transplant candidates with known coronary artery disease

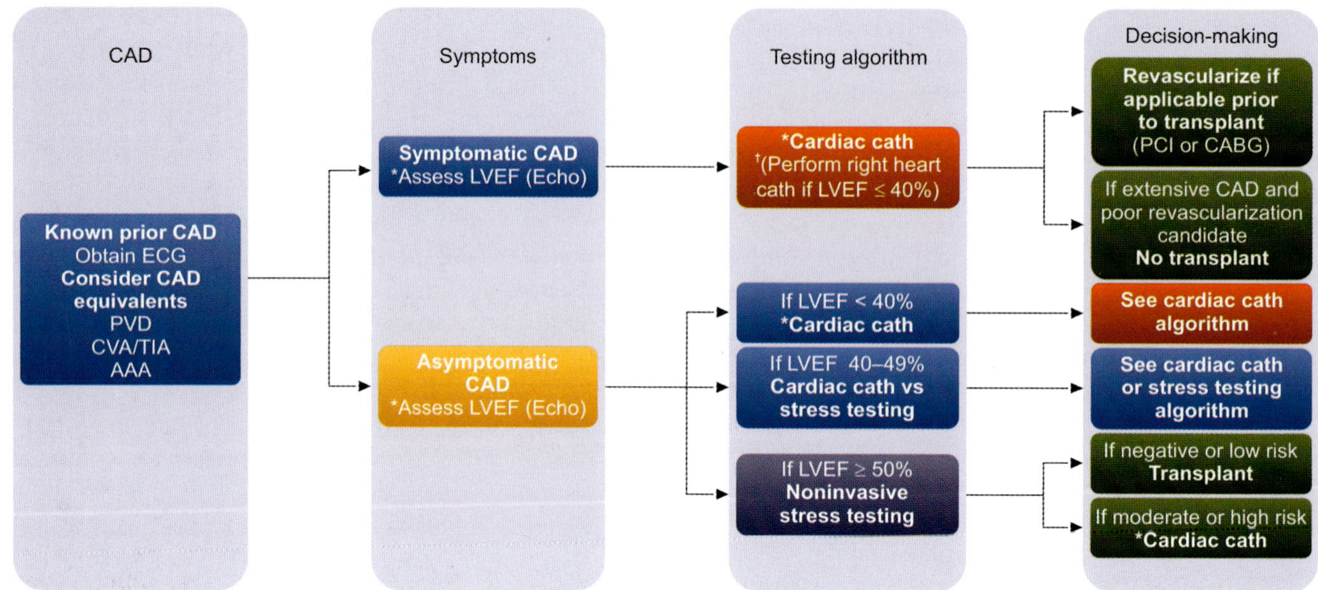

(CAD: Coronary artery disease; PVD: Peripheral vascular disease; TIA: Transient ischemic attack; AAA: Abdominal aortic aneurysm; LVEF: Left ventricular ejection fraction; CABG: Coronary artery bypass graft; PCI: Percutaneous coronary intervention).

†Assessment of hemodynamics including cardiac index should be recommended when considering transplantation in patients with LVEF ≤40%.

*Careful consideration of which patients are able to undergo cardiac catheterization and coronary angiography when indicated must be individualized. Consider cardiac catheterization with coronary angiography in patients with newly diagnosed LV systolic dysfunction if patient potentially able to tolerate contrast use (previously on dialysis). Consider initial noninvasive stress testing in patients who currently are not on dialysis.

set forth by the American College of Cardiology Foundation (ACCF)/American Heart Association (AHA) for noncardiac surgery.[12] But careful review and consideration of the ACCF/AHA Guideline for Assessment of Cardiovascular Risk in Asymptomatic Adults would also provide additional practicality in assessment of the pretransplant patient with special attention given to global coronary and cardiovascular risk scoring systems and thus risk factors considered.[13] In 2012, a scientific statement from the AHA and the ACCF on cardiac disease evaluation and management among kidney and liver transplantation candidates was published.[14] In its review of previously published recommendations, there is a general consensus that symptomatic patients require further testing. Less consistency exists when considering the asymptomatic patient. The scientific statement provided recommendations and highlighted several key elements from each of the available published consensus-based recommendations for cardiac risk assessment before kidney transplantation in asymptomatic patients.[12,15-18] Some of the key aspects may be summarized as follows:

- The specific number of risk factors needed to prompt testing remains to be determined. However, patients with at least three clinical or *relevant risk* factors are considered reasonable for testing
- Relevant risk factors include: Age more than 60 years, diabetes, prior CVD, more than 1 year on dialysis, LV hypertrophy, smoking, hypertension and dyslipidemia
- Patients with diabetes or prior ischemic heart disease should undergo testing
- Other notable clinical risk factors or *high-risk* features include: PVD, cerebrovascular disease, LVEF less than or equal to 40%, and history of MI
- Coronary angiography should be performed for positive stress test results. However, current evidence does not support prophylactic coronary revascularization in asymptomatic patients unless there is high-risk surgical anatomy

The following algorithm for testing incorporates several key aspects of prior recommendations,[12,13,15-18] including the latest statement from AHA/ACCF[14] but with an additional emphasis on defining anatomy and hemodynamics in those that may be in high-risk subsets. The proposed strategy places particular importance on the presence (Flowchart 1) or absence (Flowchart 2) of pre-existing coronary disease, symptomatology, and potential

Flowchart 2: Risk stratification strategy for potential kidney transplant candidates without pre-existing coronary artery disease

No CAD

No prior CAD
Obtain ECG
Assess risk factors
Age
DM
Dialysis >1 year
Smoking
FH
HTN
Chol
LVH

CAD risk assessment

Low risk
Normal ECG
Age < 45 Male
Age < 55 Female
No DM
No CAD or CHF symptoms

Intermediate risk
Normal ECG
Age ≥45 M and DM
Age ≥55 F and DM
or ≥3 Risk factors
No CAD or CHF symptoms

High risk
CAD or CHF symptoms
Evidence of prior MI (abnormal ECG)
DM ≥ 20 years

Testing algorithm

*Assess LVEF (Echo)
If LVEF ≥50%
Consider other risk factors

*Assess LVEF (Echo)
If LVEF <50%
Consider further testing

See asymptomatic CAD algorithm

See cardiac cath algorithm

Decision-making

Transplant

Consider stress testing algorithm if other risk factors present

See stress testing algorithm

May consider initial stress testing if patient not on dialysis

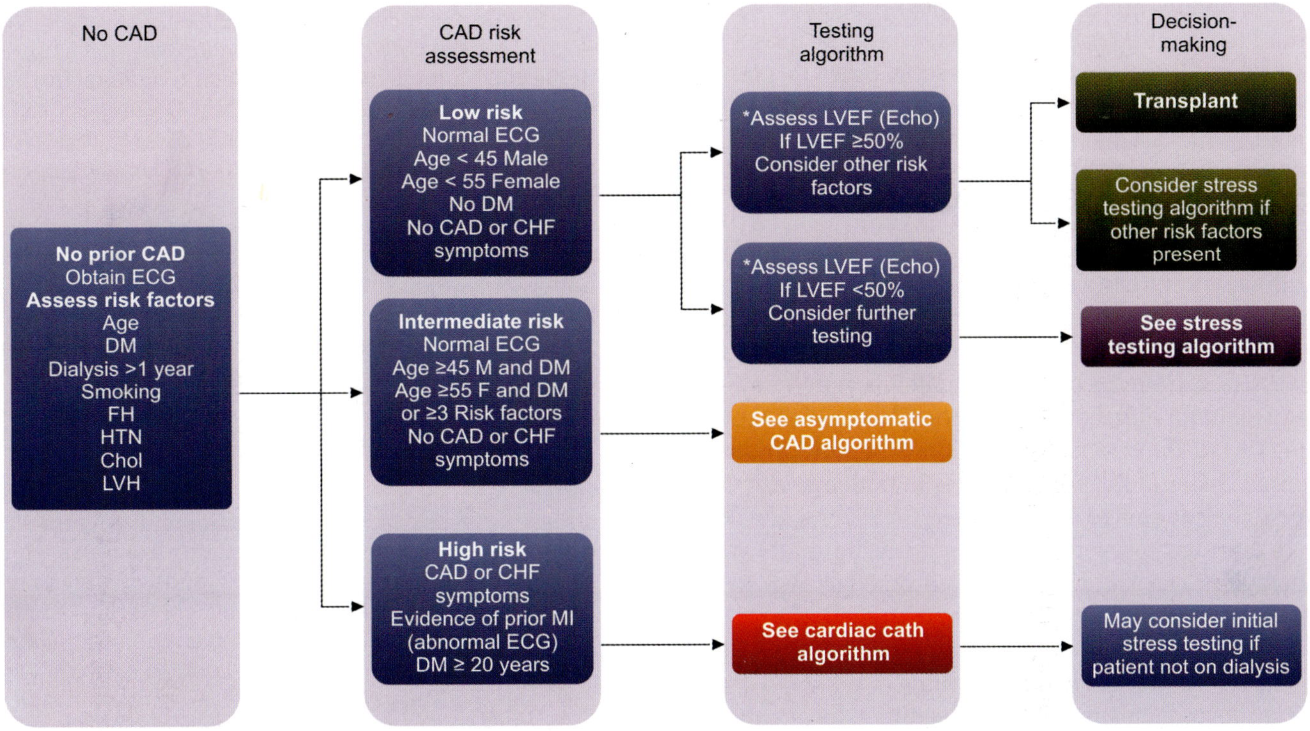

(CAD: Coronary artery disease; DM: Diabetes mellitus; FH: Family history; HTN: Hypertension; LVH: Left ventricular hypertrophy; CHF: Congestive heart failure; MI: Myocardial infarction; LVEF: Left ventricular ejection fraction).

risk category derived from risk factors and test results with special attention to left ventricular systolic function. Despite the lack of evidence in this population, patients with *high-risk* coronary anatomy, which may be defined as significant myocardium at risk, should be considered for revascularization prior to kidney transplantation. In a retrospective analysis, patients with moderate to severe ischemia on preoperative thallium scanning who underwent selective coronary revascularization prior to major vascular surgery had significantly improved long-term survival.[19] All patients should receive cardiovascular risk factor modification and medical optimization.

SPECIAL CONSIDERATIONS

Patients with structural heart disease including valvular disorders need to be evaluated appropriately and based on severity treated accordingly. Surgery when indicated should be performed prior to renal transplant. Evaluation of such patients may need to include transesophageal echocardiography and/or right and left heart catheterization studies.

Patients with at least moderate pulmonary hypertension may need further assessment with right and left heart catheterization to rule out an underlying cardiac etiology. An echocardiogram may be repeated after additional dialysis sessions with goal of reaching a more euvolemic state to reassess pulmonary hypertension prior to invasive testing. Patient should undergo pulmonary evaluation if there is no evidence of an underlying cardiac etiology.

POST-TRANSPLANT CARE AND FOLLOW-UP

Renal transplant improves but does not diminish the risk of CVD or cardiovascular events. Cardiovascular disease (about 30%) remains the leading known cause of death with graft function in adult patients after kidney transplant with highest rates in the early post-transplant period.[20,21] Cardiovascular risk reduction strategies should include regular screening for new onset diabetes and optimal glycemic control, lipid monitoring and management, and blood pressure control.[22] Immunosuppressive agents used for antirejection may lead to the development of diabetes, hypertension, dyslipidemia and obesity.

Patients with pre-existing cardiac conditions especially those with an underlying cardiomyopathy need very close monitoring of their volume status both intraoperatively and in the immediate post-transplant period to avoid volume overload and heart failure decompensation. Routine follow-up in the early post-transplant period should be required for all patients, especially those with pre-existing ischemic heart disease in order to monitor their cardiovascular status with hopes of optimizing their overall cardiovascular risk and outcomes.

CONCLUSION

There is a general lack of consensus on the approach to cardiovascular risk assessment in patients with CKD, especially in asymptomatic patients. Despite prior support for CKD as a risk factor for development of CVD,[6] the 2013 ACC/AHA Cardiovascular Risk Guideline noted that risk assessment for a first atherosclerotic CVD (ASCVD) event using CKD is *uncertain* at present time.[23] Future studies in optimal risk stratification strategies in patients with CKD need to be conducted and validated.

In summary, several key points can be made when considering cardiac evaluation and management in the transplant candidate:

- Patients with ESRD are at an increased risk for developing CAD and cardiovascular events
- Cardiovascular disease is the leading known cause of death in transplant recipients with functioning grafts with the highest rates in the early post-transplant period
- An aggressive approach to medical management of CAD and/or its risk factors is necessary to optimize outcomes for patients both in the pre- and post-transplant periods
- Cardiac evaluation and subsequent management or intervention in transplant candidates must take into consideration both potential short- and long-term risks and benefits
- Diagnostic testing should be driven by symptoms and by clinical risk factors, with an increase need for testing in patients with the highest risk or in those with an increased number of risk factors
- Regular testing should be performed annually in asymptomatic patients who are deemed *high risk* for ongoing screening and risk stratification while on the waiting list and post-transplantation
- End-stage renal disease patients with significant CAD appear to gain more benefit from revascularization than conservative management with stronger evidence supporting symptomatic patients and those with high-risk anatomy
- Finally, patients with ESRD, especially with concomitant CAD should be followed closely and managed aggressively to reduce future cardiovascular events

REFERENCES

1. U.S. Renal Data System: USRDS. 2013 Annual Data Report. Atlas of ESRD, Cardiovascular Disease, Figure 4.1. Bethesda: National Institutes of Health, National Institute of Diabetes and Digestive and Kidney Diseases; 2013.
2. Kasiske BL, Maclean JR, Snyder JJ. Acute myocardial infarction and kidney transplantation. J Am Soc Nephrol. 2005;17:900-7.
3. Gupta R, Birnbaum Y, Uretsky BF. The renal patient with coronary artery disease: current concept and dilemmas. J Am Coll Cardiol. 2004;44:1343-53.
4. McCullough PA. Evaluation and treatment of coronary artery disease in patients with end-stage renal disease. Kidney Int. 2005;67 Suppl 95:S51-8.
5. Dawber TR, Meadors GF, Moore FE Jr. Epidemiologic approaches to heart disease: the Framingham Study. Am J Public Health Nations Health. 1951;41(3):279-81.
6. Sarnak MJ, Levey AS, Schoolwerth AC, et al. Kidney disease as a risk factor for development of cardiovascular disease. A statement from the American Heart Association Council on Kidney and Cardiovascular Disease, High Blood Pressure Research, Clinical Cardiology, and Epidemiology and Prevention. Circulation. 2003;108:2154-69.
7. Patel AD, Abo-Auda WS, Davis JM, et al. Prognostic value of myocardial perfusion imaging in predicting outcome after renal transplantation. Am J Cardiol. 2003;92(2):146-51.
8. Rabbat CG, Treleaven DJ, Russell JD, et al. Prognostic value of myocardial perfusion studies in patients with end-stage renal disease assessed for kidney or kidney-pancreas transplantation: a meta-analysis. J Am Soc Nephrol. 2003; 14(2):431-9.
9. Patel MR, Bailey SR, Bonow RO, et al. ACCF/SCAI/AATS/AHA/ASE/ASNC/HFSA/HRS/SCCM/SCCT/SCMR/STS 2012 Appropriate use criteria for diagnostic catheterization. A report of the American College of Cardiology Foundation Appropriate Use Criteria Task Force, Society for Cardiovascular Angiography and Interventions, American Association for Thoracic Surgery, American Heart Association, American Society of Echocardiography, American Society of Nuclear Cardiology, Heart Failure Society of America, Heart Rhythm Society, Society of Critical Care Medicine, Society of Cardiovascular Computed Tomography, Society for Cardiovascular Magnetic Resonance, and Society of Thoracic Surgeons. J Am Coll Cardiol. 2012; 59:1995-2027.
10. Jones DG, Taylor AM, Enkiri SA, et al. Extent and severity of coronary disease and mortality in patients with end-stage renal failure evaluated for renal transplantation. Am J Transplant. 2009;9:1846-52.
11. Humar A, Kerr SR, Ramcharan T, et al. Peri-operative cardiac morbidity in kidney transplant recipients: incidence and risk factors. Clin Transplant. 2001;15:154-8.
12. Fleisher LA, Beckman JA, Brown KA, et al. ACC/AHA 2007 guidelines on perioperative cardiovascular evaluation and care for noncardiac surgery: a report of the American

College of Cardiology/American Heart Association Task Force on Practice Guidelines (Writing Committee to Revise the 2002 Guidelines on Perioperative Cardiovascular Evaluation for Noncardiac Surgery). J Am Coll Cardiol. 2007;50:e159-241.

13. Greenland P, Alpert JS, Beller GA, et al. 2010 ACCF/AHA guideline for assessment of cardiovascular risk in asymptomatic adults: a report of the American College of Cardiology Foundation/American Heart Association Task Force on Practice Guidelines. J Am Coll Cardiol. 2010;56:e50-103.
14. Lentine KL, Costa SP, Weir MR, et al. Cardiac disease evaluation and management among kidney and liver transplantation candidates. A scientific statement from the American Heart Association and the American College of Cardiology Foundation. J Am Coll Cardiol. 2012;60(5):434-80.
15. Abbud-Filho M, Adams PL, Alberu J, et al. A report of the Lisbon Conference on the care of the kidney transplant recipient. Transplantation. 2007;83 Suppl:S1-22.
16. K/DOQI Workgroup. K/DOQI clinical practice guidelines for cardiovascular disease in dialysis patients. Am J Kidney Dis. 2005;45 Suppl:S1-153.
17. Kasiske BL, Cangro CB, Hariharan S, et al. The evaluation of renal transplantation candidates: clinical practice guidelines. Am J Transplant. 2001;1 Suppl 2:3-95.
18. EBPG Expert Group on Renal Transplantation. European best practice guidelines for renal transplantation. Section I: evaluation, selection and preparation of the potential transplant recipient. I.5. Risk factors/relative contra-indications. Nephrol Dial Transplant. 2000;15 Suppl:3-38.
19. Landesberg G, Mosseri M, Wolf YG, et al. Preoperative thallium scanning, selective coronary revascularization, and long-term survival after major vascular surgery. Circulation. 2003;108:177-83.
20. U.S. Renal Data System: USRDS. 2013 Annual Data Report. Atlas of ESRD, Transplantation, Figure 7.26. Bethesda: National Institutes of Health, National Institute of Diabetes and Digestive and Kidney Diseases; 2013.
21. Lentine KL, Hurst FP, Jindal RM, et al. Cardiovascular risk assessment among potential kidney transplant candidates: approaches and controversies. Am J Kidney Dis. 2010;55(1):152-67.
22. Kidney Disease: Improving Global Outcomes (KDIGO) Transplant Work Group. KDIGO clinical practice guideline for the care of kidney transplant recipients. Am J Transplant. 2009;9 Suppl 3:S1-157.
23. Goff DC Jr, Lloyd-Jones DM, Bennett G, et al. 2013 ACC/AHA guideline on the assessment of cardiovascular risk: a report of the American College of Cardiology/American Heart Association Task Force on Practice Guidelines. Circulation. Nov 2013.

CHAPTER 7

Pulmonary Evaluation

Arunabh Talwar, Sonu Sahni

INTRODUCTION

Patients with chronic renal failure due to various mechanisms are prone to significant pulmonary comorbidities. Patients that are selected to undergo renal transplant must have thorough preoperative pulmonary evaluation to assess pulmonary status and to determine risk of postoperative pulmonary complications (Flowchart 1). It is important to identify these patients and make sure that they are treated more aggressively. Postoperative pulmonary complications in nonthoracic surgery patients have been seen in 2–19% of patients.[1] This chapter attempts to outline the preoperative pulmonary assessment of renal transplant patients.

Preoperative Risk Factors

- Chronic obstructive pulmonary disease (COPD)
- Age
- Obesity
- Smoking
- New York Heart Association (NYHA) greater than class II pulmonary hypertension
- Obstructive sleep apnea (OSA)
- Nutrition status

Obesity

Obesity has been recognized by the American Medical Association (AMA) as a diseased state that is a risk factor

Flowchart 1: Management protocol pulmonary evaluation in renal transplant patients

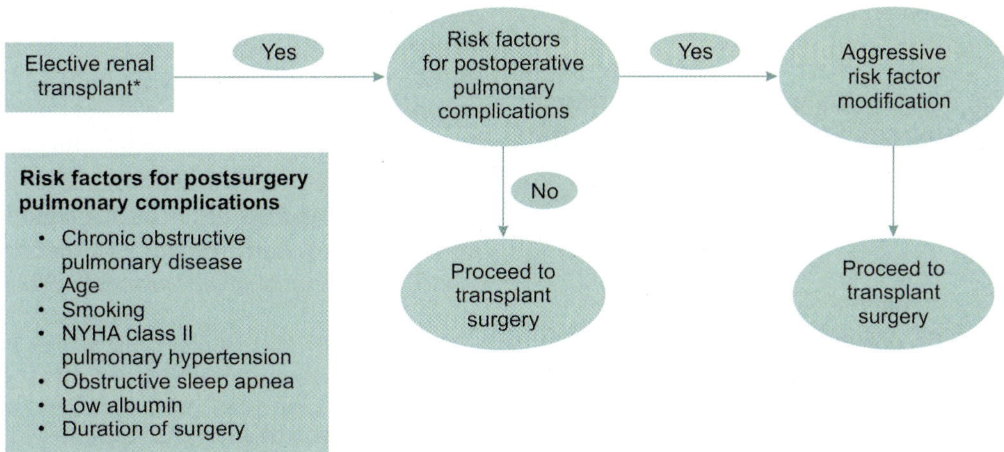

*Smoking cessation for > 6 weeks if current smoker; short acting Beta 2 agonist and systemic corticosteroid treatment for bronchial reactivity, if needed.

for all surgical patients. Obesity is defined as a body mass index (BMI) greater than or equal to 30 kg/m^2. Obesity has been shown to cause post-transplant surgical complications, and delayed graft function[2] and it demonstrated a negative effect including graft failure within the first year post-transplant.[3]

Excess abdominal fat (central or visceral obesity), which is found above the waist, is related to increased risk of diabetes and heart disease. In men, a waist greater than 40 inches and in women, more than 36 inches is of concern. Obesity leads to:

- Decreased lung volumes after surgery is a principal cause of postoperative pulmonary complications
- Obesity predisposes to OSA, diabetes mellitus and hypertension
- Also a risk factor for delayed graft function
- Obese renal transplant recipients suffer more surgical complications, including wound infections, delayed wound healing, lymphoceles and perinephric hematomas
- Management includes diet, exercise and nutritional counseling

PULMONARY COMPLICATIONS IN CHRONIC RENAL FAILURE PATIENTS

- Pneumonia
  - Patients who are living with chronic kidney disease (CKD) are prone to pneumococcal pneumonia. Infectious complications are the second leading cause of hospitalization in the end-stage renal disease (ESRD) population. Preventive health care measures have centered on routine influenza and pneumococcal pneumonia vaccinations as the best way to reduce potential morbidity and mortality from these infectious events[4]
- Pulmonary edema
  - Patients with CKD have a low urinary output and therefore may be prone to developing severe pulmonary edema due to fluid volume overload
- Pleural effusions
  - Pleural effusions are common in hospitalized patients, especially those receiving chronic hemodialysis while waiting for renal transplants. Heart failure is the most common cause. Other conditions such as parapneumonic effusions may require prompt thoracentesis as these effusions often cannot be reliably differentiated clinically. In addition, since these patients have a reduced humoral and cellular immunity, there is delay in diagnosis because of an attenuated clinical response[5]
- Pulmonary function testing (PFT) abnormalities (restrictive or obstructive defects)
  - Pulmonary function may be abnormal in chronic renal failure patients due to various mechanisms such as fluid overload, infections, pleural effusions, pulmonary hypertension, etc.[6] Concomitant restrictive or obstructive disease processes may cause intraoperative complications
  - Up to 88% of chronic renal failure patients showed pulmonary function abnormalities which improved significantly after transplantation. Improvement was seen in mean vital capacity and small airways, as shown by low maximal mid-expiratory flow rates, which tended to improve after renal transplantation.[7] Decreased diffusion capacity of carbon monoxide (DLCO) may be due to anemia, pulmonary hypertension or concomitant restrictive ventilatory defect
- Pulmonary calcifications
  - Pulmonary calcifications subsequent to secondary hyperparathyroidism occur primarily in the alveolar septa and to a lesser extent in the arterial and bronchial walls. Up to 60% of patients with ESRD on dialysis may develop this condition. The majority of them are asymptomatic with no apparent chest X-ray changes. In the few who become symptomatic, a high resolution computed tomography (CT) scan of the lungs followed by a radionuclide scan will confirm the presence of lung deposits

PULMONARY HYPERTENSION IN CHRONIC RENAL FAILURE

Preoperative assessment must include evaluation for pulmonary hypertension. Pulmonary hypertension is defined as mean pulmonary artery (PA) pressure greater than or equal to 25 mm Hg or systolic PA pressure and pulmonary arterial hypertension holding the extra criteria of a pulmonary capillary wedge pressure less than or equal to 15 mm Hg. It is a chronic, progressive condition of pulmonary vascular remodeling, leading to right heart failure and ultimately death, if left untreated.[8] Pulmonary hypertension in CKD patients is typically associated with left heart disease. Patients with CKD often also have a variety of risk factors predisposing them toward pulmonary venous congestion, including systemic hypertension, left ventricular hypertrophy (LVH), ischemic heart disease, and left ventricular (LV) diastolic dysfunction.[9] Effort should be maintained to stabilize underlying cardiac condition prior to surgery. In patients with pulmonary hypertension; elevated mean right atrial pressure, decreased cardiac index and elevated mean pulmonary artery pressure are associated with a poor prognosis.[10]

In patients that have pulmonary arterial hypertension (WHO Group 1 Pulmonary Hypertension) treatment needs to be optimized and monitored. This population tends to be on phosphodiesterase-5 inhibitors (sildenafil, tadalafil) or in a combination of endothelin receptor blockers (ambrisentan, bosentan, macitentan) or prostacyclin derivatives (treprostinil, iloprost and epoprostenol derivatives). Patients that have undergone renal transplantation are on immunosuppressives like cyclosporine. Cyclosporine has been found to have a drug-drug interaction with bosentan as well and ambrisentan leading to dangerously increased plasma concentrations of the drug.[11,12]

SMOKING

Tobacco use is an issue in patients with chronic renal disease. Smoking has pleotropic detrimental effects on almost every organ in our body an association with increased risk of cardiovascular disease (CVD). Smoking is also associated with post-transplant cancer which should intensify efforts to help patients quit smoking. Studies have estimated that between 15% and 17% of individuals with CKD who are initiated on dialysis report current tobacco use, and between 24% and 46% report previous tobacco uses.[13] Individuals with CKD already have rates of cardiovascular mortality 20–40 times greater than the general population.[14] Smoking adds to this cardiac risk, as it has been found to be an independent risk factor for cardiovascular morbidity and mortality, and overall mortality among individuals with CKD and those receiving dialysis.[15] The benefits of smoking cessation can also include preservation of renal function in individuals with CKD, but not receiving dialysis.[16]

Smoking Cessation

Due to the detrimental effects that smoking has on general health as well and the chronic renal disease patients, it is important to make an effort to promote smoking cessation. Both nonpharmacologic and pharmacologic interventions exist and should be utilized in the proper setting. Evidence suggests that a combination of psychosocial counseling and pharmacotherapy be utilized including therapies such as bupropion, varenicline and nicotine replacement. The use of these medications can increase an individual's chance of abstinence. A combination of counseling and pharmacotherapy may achieve the highest abstinence rates.[17]

Nonpharmacologic Therapies

Several counseling methods, including counseling by health professionals, telephone quit lines, individual counseling, group counseling, and computer program or internet counseling have demonstrated efficacy.[17] It is recommended that advice to quit and brief counseling be performed by a health professional at any and all contact with a smoker.[17] Intensive interventions, with person-to-person communication for four or more sessions may be more effective to achieve smoking abstinence than other nonpharmacologic methods.[17] In the setting of CKD, personal contact by dialysis health care professionals makes the dialysis unit an ideal setting for smoking cessation interventions.

Pharmacologic Intervention

The first step in pharmacologic management is over-the-counter pharmacotherapy which is composed of nicotine replacement therapy (NRT). Nicotine replacement therapy aids with physiologic nicotine withdrawal by simulating nicotine levels inhaled from smoking. NRT is available in a variety of products, including gum, lozenges, patches and inhalers. Dosing of NRT is based on the average number of cigarettes smoked per day. Dosing parameters differ for each NRT product. Smokers with CKD may use the usual doses of NRT, and experience similar adverse effects to nicotine as individuals with normal renal function.[18]

Prescription medications for smoking cessation include bupropion and varenicline. Bupropion is a dopamine and norepinephrine reuptake inhibitor that increases dopamine activity. Patients who have not quit after seven weeks of therapy are considered to be nonresponsive.[17] Contraindications to bupropion use include alcohol abuse, previous seizures and history of head trauma, stroke, or brain injury because of bupropion's ability to decrease the seizure threshold (Product Information: Zyban®, bupropion, 2008).

Varenicline is another option for smoking cessation and is a partial agonist/antagonist at the alpha-4 beta-2 nicotine receptor. Safety in patients with serious psychiatric illness such as schizophrenia, bipolar, and major depression have not been established. Individuals taking varenicline are 1.7 times more likely to quit than those taking NRT.[19] Close follow-up with smokers initiating therapy with bupropion or varenicline is necessary to determine if patients are experiencing any psychiatric side effects. Both these drugs possess renal excretion and dosing should be carefully monitored in the kidney transplant population. The doses of both varenicline and bupropion must be reduced as kidney function decreases.[18] In addition, it is important to realize that many of these patients may be on immunosuppressive therapy such as cyclosporine which may lead to increased concentration and increased risk of seizures with bupropion use.

OBSTRUCTIVE SLEEP APNEA

Obstructive sleep apnea is defined as the occurrence of at least five apneas/hypopneas (temporary cessation of breathing) in one hour. Symptoms typically associated with OSA include snoring, excessive daytime somnolence and restless sleep. Male gender, smoking and alcohol consumption, obesity and aging are known factors associated with a higher propensity for OSA.[20] Obstructive sleep apnea is associated with a number of medical comorbidities including hypertension, heart failure, myocardial infarction, diabetes mellitus, gastroesophageal reflux disease, stroke and CKD.[21,22]

There is a strong association between CKD and OSA, and sleep studies in ESRD patients have identified increased prevalence of sleep apnea both obstructive and central in origin.[23] Consequences of sleep apnea such as increased renal sympathetic activity, intermittent hypoxia, hypertension, accelerated atherosclerosis, production of postinflammatory cytokines, endothelial dysfunction and proteinuria may contribute to the progression of CKD. End-stage renal disease patients with sleep apnea on peritoneal dialysis (PD) have lower nocturnal arterial oxygen saturation during nights on PD than on other nights; hence PD may also adversely affect cardiovascular risk.[24]

All patients with OSA should undergo a continuous positive airway pressure (CPAP) titration. The regular use of CPAP may prevent the progression of nephropathy by ameliorating glomerular hyperfiltration. Long-term CPAP reduces blood pressure and plasma renin and angiotensin II levels.[25,26] Lifestyle changes, alteration of sleep hygiene parameters and reduction of obesity have a significant role in reducing overall OSA severity and associated vascular risks, these strategies are often difficult to offer and monitor in patients with chronic renal failure.[27]

Both anesthesia and postoperative analgesic measures can negatively affect OSA outcomes. The effects of anesthesia, sedation and analgesics may work similarly, increasing the risk of detrimental effects to patients with OSA. The potential perioperative risks to OSA patients include increased morbidity and mortality, as well as difficult intubation and postoperative respiratory distress/obstruction.[28] Patients may have to be initiated postoperatively on CPAP after the intubation process.

RISK REDUCTION STRATEGIES FOR POSTOPERATIVE COMPLICATIONS

Preoperative Measures

- Cessation of smoking for at least 8 weeks before surgery
- Treat airflow obstruction
- Treat respiratory infections (if any) and optimize vaccinations
- Educate patients for lung-expansion maneuvers
- Evaluate for pulmonary hypertension and optimize medication prior to surgery

Intraoperative Measures

- Limit duration of surgery to less than 3 hours
- Use laparoscopic procedures (if possible)

Postoperative Measures

- Adequate postoperative pain control
- Early mobilization
- Chest physical therapy (deep breathing and incentive spirometry)
- Continuous positive airway pressure (CPAP) in patients with known OSA during and after surgery
- Manage pulmonary hypertension

REFERENCES

1. Fisher BW, Majumdar SR, McAlister FA. Predicting pulmonary complications after nonthoracic surgery: a systematic review of blinded studies. Am J Med. 2002;112(3):219-25.
2. Johnson DW, Isbel NM, Brown AM, et al. The effect of obesity on renal transplant outcomes. Transplantation. 2002;74(5):675-81.
3. Schwarznau A, Matevossian E, Novotny A, et al. Outcome of living donor renal transplantation in obese recipients. Transplant Proc. 2008;40(4):921-2.
4. U.S. Renal Data System: USRDS 2008 Annual Data Report: Atlas of Chronic Kidney Disease & End-Stage Renal Disease in the United States, Vol. 2, Bethesda, MD, National Institutes of Health, National Institute of Diabetes and Digestive and Kidney Diseases, 2008.
5. Jarratt MJ, Sahn SA. Pleural effusions in hospitalized patients receiving long-term hemodialysis. Chest. 1995; 108(2):470-4.
6. Prezant DJ. Effect of uremia and its treatment on pulmonary function. Lung. 1990;168(1):1-14.
7. Sidhu J, Ahuja G, Aulakh B, et al. Changes in pulmonary function in patients with chronic renal failure after successful renal transplantation. Scand J Urol Nephrol. 2007;41(2):155-60.

8. Galie N, Hoeper MM, Humbert M, et al. Guidelines for the diagnosis and treatment of pulmonary hypertension: the Task Force for the Diagnosis and Treatment of Pulmonary Hypertension of the European Society of Cardiology (ESC) and the European Respiratory Society (ERS), endorsed by the International Society of Heart and Lung Transplantation (ISHLT). Eur Heart J. 2009;30(20):2493-537.
9. Hayashi SY, Rohani M, Lindholm B, et al. Left ventricular function in patients with chronic kidney disease evaluated by colour tissue Doppler velocity imaging. Nephrol Dial Transplant. 2006;21(1):125-32.
10. Batal O, Khatib OF, Dweik RA, et al. Comparison of baseline predictors of prognosis in pulmonary hypertension in patients surviving ≤2 years and those surviving ≥5 years after baseline right-sided cardiac catheterization. Am J Cardiol. 2012;109(10):1514-20.
11. Shitara Y. Clinical importance of OATP1B1 and OATP1B3 in drug-drug interactions. Drug Metab Pharmacokinet. 2011;26(3):220-7.
12. Spence R, Mandagere A, Richards DB, et al. Potential for pharmacokinetic interactions between ambrisentan and cyclosporine. Clin Pharmacol Ther. 2010;88(4):513-20.
13. Longenecker JC, Coresh J, Powe NR, et al. Traditional cardiovascular disease risk factors in dialysis patients compared with the general population: the CHOICE Study. J Am Soc Nephrol. 2002;13(7):1918-27.
14. Culleton BF, Larson MG, Wilson PW, et al. Cardiovascular disease and mortality in a community-based cohort with mild renal insufficiency. Kidney Int. 1999 ;56(6):2214-9.
15. Foley RN, Herzog CA, Collins AJ. Smoking and cardiovascular outcomes in dialysis patients: the United States Renal Data System Wave 2 study. Kidney Int. 2003;63(4):1462-7.
16. Chuahirun T, Simoni J, Hudson C, et al. Cigarette smoking exacerbates and its cessation ameliorates renal injury in type 2 diabetes. Am J Med Sci. 2004;327(2):57-67.
17. Fiore MC, Jaén CR. A clinical blueprint to accelerate the elimination of tobacco use. JAMA. 2008;299(17):2083-5.
18. Manley HJ, Stack NM. Smoking cessation therapy considerations for patients with chronic kidney disease. Nephrol Nurs J. 2008;35(4):357-63, 394.
19. Stapleton JA, Watson L, Spirling LI, et al. Varenicline in the routine treatment of tobacco dependence: a pre-post comparison with nicotine replacement therapy and an evaluation in those with mental illness. Addiction. 2008; 103(1):146-54.
20. Epstein LJ, Kristo D, Strollo PJ, et al; Adult Obstructive Sleep Apnea Task Force of the American Academy of Sleep Medicine. Clinical guideline for the evaluation, management and long-term care of obstructive sleep apnea in adults. J Clin Sleep Med. 2009;5(3):263-76.
21. Nieto FJ, Young TB, Lind BK, et al. Association of sleep-disordered breathing, sleep apnea, and hypertension in a large community-based study. Sleep Heart Health Study. JAMA. 2000;283(14):1829-36.
22. Shahar E, Whitney CW, Redline S, et al. Sleep-disordered breathing and cardiovascular disease: cross-sectional results of the Sleep Heart Health Study. Am J Respir Crit Care Med. 2001;163(1):19-25.
23. Chakravorty I, Shastry M, Farrington K. Sleep apnoea in end-stage renal disease: a short review of mechanisms and potential benefit from its treatment. Nephrol Dial Transplant. 2007;22(1):28-31.
24. Shneerson J, Wright J. Lifestyle modification for obstructive sleep apnoea. (Cochrane Review). Cochrane Database Syst Rev. 2001;(1):CD002875.
25. Kinebuchi S, Kazama JJ, Satoh M, et al. Short-term use of continuous positive airway pressure ameliorates glomerular hyperfiltration in patients with obstructive sleep apnoea syndrome. Clin Sci (Lond). 2004;107(3):317-22.
26. Gupta RM, Parvizi J, Hanssen AD, et al. Postoperative complications in patients with obstructive sleep apnea syndrome undergoing hip or knee replacement: a case-control study. Mayo Clin Proc. 2001;76(9):897-905.
27. Saarelainen S, Hasan J, Siitonen S, et al. Effect of nasal CPAP treatment on plasma volume, aldosterone and 24-h blood pressure in obstructive sleep apnoea. J Sleep Res. 1996;5(3):181-5.
28. Gupta RM, Parvizi J, Hanssen AD, et al. Postoperative complications in patients with obstructive sleep apnea syndrome undergoing hip or knee replacement: a case-control study. Mayo Clin Proc. 2001;76:897-905.

CHAPTER 8

Hematologic Evaluation

Mashael Al Anizi, Sabeen F Mekan, Craig Devoe

PREOPERATIVE IDENTIFICATION AND PROPHYLAXIS OF THE HYPERCOAGULABLE PATIENT

Major Thrombophilic Risk Factors

- History of more than or equal to two arterial-venous access thromboses
- Prior allograft thrombosis
- Multiple miscarriages
- Prior deep vein thrombosis (DVT) or pulmonary embolism (PE)
- Positive family history

Additional Clinical Risk Factors

- Estrogen replacement
- Collagen vascular diseases
- Diabetes mellitus
- Malignancy
- Age over 40 years
- Obesity
- Nephrotic syndrome
- Chronic tobacco use
- Hepatitis C virus

Mechanical Risk Factors[1]

- Arterial diameter size (differs with body size)
- Multiple renal arteries
- Stenosis of the donor renal artery
- Atherosclerosis in donor or recipient
- Surgical trauma
- Acute rejection
- Prolonged cold ischemia time with reperfusion damage

Pharmacologic Risk Factors

- Erythropoietin can increase thrombosis risk
- Calcineurin inhibitors (CSA > FK 506) increase thrombophilia
- Cyclosporin A (CSA) can increase Factor VIII and tissue factor (TF), in addition to reducing Protein C
- Orthoclone 3 (OKT3) has been associated with intrarenal thrombosis

Types of Hereditary and Acquired Thrombophilia

- Activated protein C (APC) resistance (Factor V Leiden 'FVL')
- Prothrombin gene mutation
- Proteins C and S and Antithrombin III deficiency
- Factor VIII, IX, XI elevation
- Homocysteine elevation (*MTHFR* gene)
- Lipoprotein (a)
- Antiphospholipid syndrome (APLS): Beta 2 Glycoprotein 1 (B2GP1), Anticardiolipin (ACL) and Lupus anticoagulant
- Prothrombin and fibrinogen gene mutations
- Heparin-induced thrombocytopenia (HIT)

Reported Effects of Hereditary and Acquired Thrombophilia

- Factor V Leiden (FVL): Increases risk of DVT three-fold, with a graft loss 3.3 times more prevalent than patients without FVL
- Prothrombin gene mutation
  - 3.1 × increased risk of DVT
  - 7.4 × increased risk of graft loss
- Protein S deficiency is associated with renal graft loss, arterial and venous thromboses
- Hyperhomocysteinemia increases occurrence of coronary artery disease three-fold if levels of homocysteine surpass 30 µmol/L. It may increase occurrence of DVT, but increase in graft loss has not been reported
- Antiphospholipid syndrome (APLS): Up to 19% serology positive prevalence in chronic renal failure (CRF)
- Antiphospholipid syndrome in combination with Hepatitis C virus (HCV) infection with high titers exceeding 40 GPL has been found to increase incidence of graft loss and DVT
  - Risk is enhanced in patients with a prior history of thrombosis

Incidence of Post-Transplant Thrombosis[2]

- Renal transplant is associated with an 8% risk of DVT/PE within the first month postrenal transplant
  - The incidence peaks at 4 months
- Primary graft thrombosis risk is between 1% and 7%
- Factor V Leiden
  - Thirty-nine percent of patients with heterozygous mutation have had a venous thromboembolism (VTE) compared to 6–15% of patients without the mutation
  - Three to four times increased risk of allograft thrombosis or DVT over the first 6 months
  - Three times increased risk of graft rejection
- Factor V Leiden increases risk of chronic graft dysfunction
- Prothrombin gene mutation decreases graft survival (66 compared to 149 months)
- Hyperhomocysteinemia increases risk for thromboembolism
  - Risk increase up to 22 × when combined with other hypercoagulable factors
- Many renal transplant patients have elevated homocysteine levels and are generally resistant to lowering with vitamin supplement (which has no known benefit at the moment)
- Patients with APLS and a history of thrombosis have an increased risk of graft failure and thrombosis, as well as an increased risk of arterial and venous thrombosis
- Patients with APLS without history of thrombosis did not have graft failure

Rejection and Thrombosis[3]

- Factor V Leiden, Protein C (< 60%), Protein S (< 60%), ATIII (< 70%) are all risk factors for renal allograft acute rejection
  - 70% compared to 41% within 6 months of renal transplantation
- Peripheral arterial and venous events are also increased
  - 67% compared to 28%
- Prophylactic use of heparin and warfarin was shown to decrease allograft thrombosis from 4% down to 1.6%

PRETRANSPLANT SCREENING FOR HEREDITARY THROMBOPHILIA[4]

Hypercoagulability in the recipient may cause renal graft thrombosis, a potentially preventable outcome if risk factors are identified preoperatively.

- Only 1.4% of patients with no prior history of thrombosis were subsequently found to have a hypercoagulable state whose first manifestation was a renal allograft thrombosis
- Due to the low risk and the substantial cost to perform comprehensive hypercoagulable panel testing, it is not cost-effective to obtain a complete panel on a patient with no prior history of thrombosis

Hereditary Thrombophilia

- Protein C, S and ATIII deficiency are unlikely in patients over 45 years with no personal or familial history of thrombosis
- In renal failure patients:
  - Factor V Leiden has a prevalence of approximately 6%
  - Antiphospholipid syndrome of 19%5
  - Activated protein C resistance (APCR) of 6%

Proposed Screening Guidelines

- If major thrombophilia risk factors are *absent*:
  - Screen for APL (since APL serology prevalence is up to 19%)
  - If candidate under 45 years, screening for Protein C & S and ATIII is too low of a yield

- If major thrombophilia risk factors are *present*:
  - Evaluate for APLS and FVL (Age < 45 only) first because these are the most common
  - If above negative, then consider ATIII, protein C & S activities
  - If above negative, consider prothrombin gene and homocysteine

General VTE Prophylaxis Recommendations[1,5]

- For *laparoscopic* urologic procedures, the risk of VTE appears to be low, anticoagulant thromboprophylaxis may increase the bleeding risk
- *Routine thromboprophylaxis* is recommended for more extensive, open procedures including nephrectomy

Venous Thromboembolism Prophylaxis

- Thromboprophylaxis options to consider for higher risk patients include the following:
  - Low dose unfractionated heparin (LDUH)
  - Low molecular weight heparin (LMWH)
  - Fondaparinux
  - Graduated compression stockings (GCS)
  - Intermittent pneumatic compression (IPC)
- Commencing GCS with or without IPC just prior to surgery and then adding LMWH or LDUH (for renal transplant) postoperatively is used even though this approach has not been formally evaluated in this patient population
- For patients at high risk for *bleeding*, a similar approach is suggested: starting GCS with or without IPC just before the procedure and then adding LMWH or LDUH when the bleeding risk decreases
- With the current brief lengths of hospitalization for major urologic procedures, the risk of post-hospital discharge, symptomatic VTE is likely increased
- However, continuation of thromboprophylaxis after hospital discharge has not been evaluated in these patients

Renal Impairment and Anticoagulant Dosing

- Renal function should be considered when making decisions about the use and/or dose of LMWH, fondaparinux, and other antithrombotic drugs that are cleared by the kidneys, particularly in elderly patients, patients with diabetes mellitus and those at high risk for bleeding (Grade 1A)
- Depending on the circumstances, we recommend one of the following options in this situation: avoiding the use of an anticoagulant that bioaccumulates in the presence of renal impairment, using a lower dose of the agent, or monitoring the drug level or its anticoagulant effect (Grade 1B)

Dosing of Heparin

- While these reviews concluded that the administration of heparin, 5,000 U three times a day was more efficacious than 5,000 U twice a day *without* increasing the rate of bleeding, this was based on indirect comparisons
- There are no reported studies that directly compared these two LDUH regimens

Proposed Guidelines for Anticoagulation

There are scarce published data available for anticoagulation in renal transplant patients. However, following considerations would be recommended:

- Adjust the anticoagulation to the severity of the HCS
- Borrow concepts from other know HCS
- Identify the level of risk in the patient:
  - Very High Risk: Patients with a history of arterial thrombosis; APLS with thrombosis; ATIII with prior thrombosis. Give full dose of unfractionated heparin [partial thromboplastin time (PTT) 2–3 times the normal] and warfarin lifelong
  - High Risk: Patients with a history of venous thrombosis with identified hypercoagulable state (*PT* gene, FVL, Protein C/S; ATIII without prior thrombosis). Give low dose unfractionated heparin (PTT 1.5–2 × normal) and warfarin lifelong with target INR = 2.0–2.5
  - Intermediate Risk: History of venous thrombosis with no identified disorder; history of SLE; ACL or LA positive but no prior thrombosis; hypercoagulable states with no prior venous thrombosis; multiple disorders. Give low dose unfractionated Heparin (PTT 1.5-2) + ASA 325 mg daily on discharge lifelong (Warfarin to be considered for multiple risk factors)
  - Low Risk: History of less than two dialysis-access thromboses; all others. Give subcutaneous heparin and ASA 325 mg daily on discharge for at least 30 days

Bleeding

- Partial thromboplastin time (PTT) may not be routine in the preoperative setting at some institutions

- A good bleeding history is more important than a PTT test for screening. Caveats include:
  - Unreliable patients
  - Inadequate history taking
  - Recently acquired abnormalities
  - Patients who have never been "provoked" to bleed (no prior surgeries)
- Since renal transplant/donation is thought to be a fairly high bleeding risk procedure, a proper bleeding history needs to be well-documented and well-considered before preoperative PTT is abandoned

ADDITIONAL COMMENTS

- Our routine approach (in the absence of hypercoagulability, pre-existing anticoagulation, or contraindications) is to administer low-dose unfractionated heparin immediately prior to the transplant and continued until discharge from the hospital
- We routinely apply inflatable pneumatic compression devices to both lower extremities during the entire surgery and continue their use during the entire length of hospital stay at all times except when ambulating
- In cases of recipients on anticoagulation (for valid indications), we perform the transplant surgery while fully anticoagulated. We believe that the risk of discontinuing/reversing anticoagulation exceeds its potential benefits. The use of postoperative intravenous heparin is difficult to regulate, and can result in over-anticoagulation and hemorrhage
- In cases of recipients taking clopidogrel, aspirin or similar agents (for valid indications), we proceed with the transplant surgery without discontinuing them (unless contraindicated by the manufacturer). We believe that the risk of discontinuing reversing anticoagulation exceeds its potential benefits
- We routinely administer aspirin prior to the transplant (except in instances where it may be contraindicated) and continue it postoperatively
- We perform a hypercoagulable workup in all patients with a diagnosis of lupus (irrespective of their history of thrombosis), two or more vascular access thrombosis, DVT, and two or more miscarriages

REFERENCES

1. Andrassy J, Zeier M, Andrassy K. 'Do we need screening for thrombophilia prior to kidney transplantation?' Nephrol Dial Transplant. 2004;19(Suppl 4):64-8.
2. Bockenstedt American Society of Hematology Annual Conference Education Book. 2006.
3. Heidenreich S, Dercken C, August C, et al. High rate of acute rejections in renal allograft recipients with thrombophilic risk factors. J Am Soc Nephrol.1998;9:1309-13.
4. Friedman GS, Meier-Kriesche HU, Kaplan B, et al. 'Hypercoagulable states in renal transplant candidates: impact of anticoagulation upon incidence of renal allograft thrombosis.' Transplantation. 2001;72:1073-8.
5. Guyatt et al. Antithrombotic therapy and prevention of thrombosis, 9th ed: American College of Chest Physicians evidence-based clinical guidelines. Chest 2012:141(2) suppl:7S-47S.

CHAPTER 9

Gastroenterology and Hepatology Evaluation

Keith Sultan, Iuliana Shapira, David Bernstein

INTRODUCTION

The gastroenterology (GI) and hepatology evaluation prior to renal transplantation focuses on three key areas:

1. Age appropriate screening of asymptomatic individuals for colon and rectal cancer.
2. Evaluation and management of benign conditions which may cause complications post-transplantation.
3. Diagnosis and management of apparently asymptomatic liver disease; particularly hepatitis B, hepatitis C, cirrhosis.

COLON CANCER SCREENING

The lifetime risk of colon cancer is approximately 5% in the general, Western population.[1] Most of these cancers are believed to arise from precancerous polyps which can be found in up to 20% of average risk individuals by the age of 50 years.[2] Current guidelines stress the importance of identification of these premalignant lesions, the removal of which markedly decreases the subsequent risk of colon cancer.[3-5] This is the preferred cancer *prevention* strategy, in contrast to cancer *detection* alternatives such as fecal hemoccult testing.[6]

- Colon cancer screening in the general population is associated with decreased cancer rates and improved survival
- Colon cancer screening is generally recommended to begin at age 50 years, with 45 years appropriate in the African American population
- Screening modalities in the average risk population range from fecal hemoccult testing to colonoscopy

Post-transplant immunosuppression is associated with an overall increased risk of malignancies. This increased risk extends to colon cancer. The largest study to date from Engels et al. published in 2011 examined the risk of malignancy associated with solid organ transplantation.[7] The authors reviewed the US scientific registry of 175,732 transplant recipients between the years of 1987 and 2008, of which 58.4% were kidney transplants. Among GI malignancies, gallbladder, small intestine, esophageal and gastric cancer showed increased rates and significantly elevated standardized incidence ratios (SIR's). This was true as well for colon cancer, with an SIR of 1.24. Colon cancer was by far the most common GI malignancy seen in the post-transplant population, with the number of cases exceeding the combined total of all other GI malignancies.

There also appears to be an earlier age of onset and poorer survival due to colon and rectal cancer in the post-transplant population.[8] A recent 30-year review of over 5,603 transplant cases (62% kidney transplant recipients) from the University of Wisconsin database showed an increased 10-year incidence of colon and rectal cancer in the transplant cohort, (incidence ratio = 2.6.) The data also revealed a marked decrease in the 5-year postcancer diagnosis survival rate. Compared to a 5-year survival rate of 63.5% observed in the general population from the National Cancer Institute Survival, Epidemiology, and End Results (SEER) database, the transplant cohort had an observed 5-year survival rate of 30.7%. Cancer diagnosis in the transplant group occurred at a median age of 58.7 years (32.4–78.2), with 11 patients diagnosed before the age of 50 years. By comparison, the SEER median age at diagnosis was 72.0 years.[9]

- Post-transplant immunosuppression significantly increases the risk of colon cancer
- Colon cancer post-transplantation occurs at a younger age than in the general population
- Colon cancer occurring post-transplantation is associated with worse outcomes

Currently available transplant guidelines recommend age-appropriate colon and rectal cancer screening prior to transplantation. The Canadian Society guidelines recommend "screening" without specifying a preferred screening modality.[10] The European Association of Urology guidelines,[11] updated in 2009, recommend colonoscopy every 5 years, or annual fecal blood testing. Though not explicitly stated, this recommendation applies to post-transplant surveillance, not to pretransplantation screening.

Given the clear increased risk of cancer post-transplant, we recommend age-appropriate colonoscopy rather than other modalities prior to transplantation. Although not currently validated by any prospective data, we also agree with the recommendation for continued colonoscopy surveillance every 5 years post-transplantation.

- Current guidelines recommend age appropriate cancer screening prior to transplantation
- Colon cancer screening pretransplantation should be performed with colonoscopy, with a goal of cancer prevention

SCREENING FOR NONCOLON/RECTAL INTESTINAL CANCERS

- There are no guidelines currently for screening in the US population
- There is an increased risk of GI cancers post-transplantation
- There is no recommendation for screening for noncolon/rectal cancer in the pre- or post-transplant population

SYMPTOM-BASED EVALUATION

"Screening" by definition involves an investigation of an asymptomatic person or population. GI symptoms are common in the general population, with most due to functional rather than structural disease. These complaints are even more common in patients prior to kidney transplantation.[12] While as many as 15% of the population fulfill criteria for irritable bowel syndrome, very few have colitis, diverticulitis or other small bowel/colonic structural diseases. Though as many as 20% may report complaints such as reflux or dyspepsia, less than 1% per year will actually develop peptic ulcer disease.[13,14]

As in the general population, evaluation by colonoscopy, endoscopy, imaging or other studies should not be a knee jerk response to each individual complaint (i.e. not every patient with diarrhea needs a colonoscopy). When in doubt however, we do recommend investigating complaints rather than continued observation.

MANAGEMENT FOLLOWING DIAGNOSIS

There is very little data on the appropriate management of benign GI conditions prior to transplantation. Inactive, nonmalignant disease is rarely an immediate contraindication to proceeding with renal transplantation. For example, asymptomatic cholelithiasis is not felt to pose a significant risk for patients post-transplant.[15] Diverticulitis however, should it recur postoperatively, may result in worse outcomes, likely due to the effects of immune suppression.[16] Cases of new onset inflammatory bowel disease (IBD) have been noted post-transplant, but this is not felt to be the result of immunosuppressant treatment.[17] On the contrary, IBD is the result of an overactive immune response to native gut flora, and would theoretically benefit from the post-transplant medications.[18]

Recent Canadian Society of Transplantation consensus guidelines address several nonmalignant GI conditions. The guidelines assign the "strength of evidence" Grade A through Grade E for each of their recommendations.

- Upper endoscopy in patients with complaints suspicious for peptic ulcer disease (PUD). (Grade C—The existing evidence is conflicting, but other factors may influence decision making)
- Treatment and confirmation of healing for known PUD. (Grade C)
- Gallstones are not a contraindication to transplant (Grade A-There is good evidence to support)
- Consideration for cholecystectomy for patients with suggestive symptoms of cholecystitis, and for patients with a past history of cholecystitis (Grade C)
- Consideration for elective surgery for patients with past diverticulitis (Grade C)
- Avoiding transplantation within 6 months of acute pancreatitis, and within 1 year of a bout of chronic pancreatitis. (Grade C)
- Avoiding transplantation in cases of active IBD (Grade C)

Asymptomatic Liver Disease

Liver disease is a major source of co-morbidity in the renal transplant population. All dialysis patients routinely undergo hepatitis B and C screening, with hepatitis B vaccination provided to those without active disease or confirmed immunity. If this information is not available, it should be obtained, along with a recent complete blood count including platelet count and a complete chemistry panel including aspartate aminotransferase (AST), alanine transaminase (ALT), alkaline phosphatase, total bilirubin levels and an abdominal sonogram.

Cirrhosis

The single most important aspect of the liver workup involves determining the patient's risk for cirrhosis. In cases of known cirrhosis, it is recommended that the patient not undergo kidney transplantation alone but rather be referred for dual kidney/liver transplant evaluation.

Most patients will not present with a known prior history of cirrhosis. If the evaluation raises suspicion of cirrhosis, a liver biopsy should be recommended. While a liver biopsy may be subject to sampling error, it is considered the gold standard and superior to commercially available serum noninvasive markers of fibrosis.

- Thorough history for liver disease or risk factors for liver disease
- Hepatitis B and C serologies, complete blood count, complete liver chemistries, liver imaging
- Liver biopsy if cirrhosis is suggested by evaluation
- Evaluation for liver/kidney dual transplantation if cirrhosis is present

Chronic Hepatitis B

Through an aggressive vaccination program, the United States has seen a steady decline in the rate of hepatitis B in the dialysis population. Recent data has shown that the rate of hepatitis B surface antigenemia in the dialysis population may now be less than 1%.[19] In those living or born in hepatitis B endemic regions of the world, rates may be higher.[20]

Detection of chronic hepatitis B is important in assessing the risk of cirrhosis, with some advocating liver biopsy of all chronically infected transplant candidates.[21] Patients with detectable hepatitis B virus should be started on anti-viral therapy to prevent fulminant hepatitis once immunosuppression begins.[22] Chronic hepatitis B when appropriately managed is not considered a contraindication to renal transplant.[23-25]

Those at highest risk for reactivation include those who are hepatitis B surface antigen (HBsAg) positive, with or without detectable levels of hepatitis B virus DNA (HBV-DNA) or HBeAg in the blood. While some patients may do well with a "pre-emptive" strategy that involves close serologic follow-up (i.e. monitoring of DNA and liver enzyme levels post-transplantation), most authors and current guidelines favor a more aggressive "prophylactic" approach of treatment prior to transplant and then lifelong after surgery. Studies have shown the benefit of Lamivudine prophylaxis used in this setting.[26,27] However, given the common progression to drug resistance over time with lamivudine, we recommend tenofovir for prophylaxis, for which resistance rarely develops.[28] For a patient on dialysis the dose would be 300 mg postoperative every 7 days following dialysis, with dosing adjusted to creatinine post-transplant. Entecavir may be used as well.

A much lower risk of reactivation is seen in those patients who are HBsAg negative and anti-HBc positive. Anti-viral therapy is not recommended in patients who are HBsAg negative, anti-HBc positive unless there is detectable HBV-DNA.

- Chronic hepatitis B is not a contraindication to transplantation
- Prophylactic therapy with tenofovir or entecavir is recommended for all HBsAg positive patients
- Prophylactic therapy is not indicated for HBsAg negative, anti-HBc positive patients

Chronic Hepatitis C

Like hepatitis B, there is a high incidence of chronic hepatitis C in the prerenal transplant and dialysis population.[29] As with hepatitis B, current guidelines either suggest or recommend liver biopsy for all chronic hepatitis C patients prior to renal transplantation to determine the extent of disease. In our own practice we do not send patients automatically for biopsy, but only do so in cases where there is clinical suspicion.

While renal transplant patients with chronic hepatitis C have been noted to have a poorer prognosis than those without hepatitis C, their long-term morbidity and mortality may still be superior to those with hepatitis C who remain on dialysis.[30-32] As such, chronic hepatitis C is not a contraindication to renal transplantation.

Finally, it is controversial whether there is a benefit to anti-viral treatment of hepatitis C prior to renal transplantation. Currently, renal failure is a contraindication to the use of ribavirin which is part of the standard triple therapy regimen of pegylated interferon, ribavirin and a protease inhibitor. There have been some data to suggest that interferon therapy pretransplantation, with or without viral clearance, may be of long-term benefit in this population, but treatment in this setting is not standard. The use of interferon post-transplantation is contraindicated as it has been associated with an increased risk of graft rejection.

- Chronic hepatitis C is not a contraindication to transplantation
- Current standard of care treatment including ribavirin is contraindicated in the setting of renal failure
- Interferon-based treatment is generally contraindicated post-transplant

REFERENCES

1. Jemal A, Siegel R, Xu J, et al. Cancer statistics. CA Cancer J Clin. 2010;60:277-300.
2. Ferlitsch M, Reinhart K, Pramhas S, et al. Sex-specific prevalence of adenomas, advanced adenomas, and colorectal cancer in individuals undergoing screening colonoscopy. JAMA. 2011;306:1352-8.
3. Thiis-Evensen E, Hoff GS, Sauar J, et al. Population-based surveillance by colonoscopy: effect on the incidence of colorectal cancer. Telemark Polyp Study I. Scand J Gastroenterol. 1999;34:414-20.
4. Muller AD, Sonnenberg A. Prevention of colorectal cancer by flexible endoscopy and polypectomy. A case-control study of 32,702 veterans. Ann Intern Med. 1995;123:904-10.
5. Zauber AG, Winawer SJ, O'Brien MJ, et al. Colonoscopic polypectomy and long-term prevention of colorectal-cancer deaths. N Engl J Med. 2012;366:687-96.
6. Rex DK, Johnson DA, Anderson JC, et al. American College of Gastroenterology guidelines for colorectal cancer screening 2009 (corrected). Am J Gastroenterol. 2009;104:739-50.
7. Engels EA, Pfeiffer RM, Fraumeni JF, et al. Spectrum of cancer risk among US solid organ transplant recipients. JAMA. 2011;306:1891-901.
8. Papaconstantinou HT, Sklow B, Hanaway MJ, et al. Characteristics and survival patterns of solid organ transplant patients developing de novo colon and rectal cancer. Dis Colon Rectum. 2004;47:1898-903.
9. Johnson EE, Leverson GE, Pirsch JD, et al. A 30-year analysis of colorectal adenocarcinoma in transplant recipients and proposal for altered screening. J Gastrointest Surg. 2007;11:272-9.
10. Knoll G, Cockfield S, Blydt-Hansen T, et al. Canadian Society of Transplantation: consensus guidelines on eligibility for kidney transplantation. CMAJ. 2005;173:S1-25.
11. Kalble T, Lucan M, Nicita G, et al. EAU guidelines on renal transplantation. Eur Urol. 2005;47:156-66.
12. Hammer J, Oesterreicher C, Hammer K, et al. Chronic gastrointestinal symptoms in hemodialysis patients. Wien Klin Wochenschr. 1998;110:287-91.
13. Sung JJ, Kuipers EJ, El-Serag HB. Systematic review: the global incidence and prevalence of peptic ulcer disease. Aliment Pharmacol Ther. 2009;29:938-46.
14. Sipponen P, Varis K, Fraki O, et al. Cumulative 10-year risk of symptomatic duodenal and gastric ulcer in patients with or without chronic gastritis. A clinical follow-up study of 454 outpatients. Scand J Gastroenterol. 1990;25:966-73.
15. Melvin WS, Meier DJ, Elkhammas EA, et al. Prophylactic cholecystectomy is not indicated following renal transplantation. Am J Surg. 1998;175:317-9.
16. Reshef A, Stocchi L, Kiran R, et al. Case-matched comparison of perioperative outcomes after surgical treatment of sigmoid diverticulitis in solid organ transplant recipients vs. immunocompetent patients. Colorectal Dis. HPB (Oxford). 2006;8(Suppl 2):3-256.
17. Parameswaran S, Singh K, Nada R, et al. Ulcerative colitis after renal transplantation: A case report and review of literature. Indian J Nephrol. 2011;21:120-2.
18. Brown SJ, Mayer L. The immune response in inflammatory bowel disease. Am J Gastroenterol 2007;102:2058-69.
19. Finelli L, Miller JT, Tokars JI, et al. National surveillance of dialysis-associated diseases in the United States, 2002. Semin Dial. 2005;18:52-61.
20. Wang C, Sun J, Zhu B, et al. Hepatitis B virus infection and related factors in hemodialysis patients in China—systematic review and meta-analysis. Ren Fail. 2010;32:1255-64.
21. Kalia H, Fabrizi F, Martin P. Hepatitis B virus and renal transplantation. Transplant Rev (Orlando). 2011;25:102-9.
22. Grotz W, Rasenack J, Benzing T, et al. Occurrence and management of hepatitis B virus reactivation following kidney transplantation. Clin Nephrol. 1998;49:385-8.
23. Ohishi W, Chayama K. Prevention of hepatitis B virus reactivation in immunosuppressive therapy or chemotherapy. Clin Exp Nephrol. 2011;15:634-40.
24. Vallet-Pichard A, Fontaine H, Mallet V, et al. Viral hepatitis in solid organ transplantation other than liver. J Hepatol. 2011;55:474-82.
25. Hoofnagle JH. Reactivation of hepatitis B. Hepatology. 2009;49:S156-65.
26. Loomba R, Rowley A, Wesley R, et al. Systematic review: the effect of preventive lamivudine on hepatitis B reactivation during chemotherapy. Ann Intern Med. 2008;148:519-28.
27. Katz LH, Fraser A, Gafter-Gvili A, et al. Lamivudine prevents reactivation of hepatitis B and reduces mortality in immunosuppressed patients: systematic review and meta-analysis. J Viral Hepat. 2008;15:89-102.
28. Snow-Lampart A, Chappell B, Curtis M, et al. No resistance to tenofovir disoproxil fumarate detected after up to 144 weeks of therapy in patients monoinfected with chronic hepatitis B virus. Hepatology. 2010;53:763-73.
29. Pereira BJ, Levey AS. Hepatitis C virus infection in dialysis and renal transplantation. Kidney Int. 1997;51:981-99.
30. Periera BJ, Wright TL, Schmid CH, et al. The impact of pretransplantation hepatitis C infection on the outcome of renal transplantation. Transplantation. 1995;60:799-805.
31. Fabrizi F, Martin P, Dixit V, et al. Hepatitis C virus antibody status and survival after renal transplantation: meta-analysis of observational studies. Am J Transplant. 2005;5:1452-61.
32. Pereira BJ, Natov SN, Bouthot BA, et al. Effects of hepatitis C infection and renal transplantation on survival in end-stage renal disease. The New England Organ Bank Hepatitis C Study Group. Kidney Int. 1998;53:1374-81.

CHAPTER 10

Nutritional Care

Louise Bongiorno

INITIAL NUTRITION ASSESSMENT[1]

- Anthropometrics: Height, weight, muscle and fat stores, body mass index (BMI), % standard, usual, and desired or ideal body weight (%SBW; %UBW, %DBW, %IBW), waist circumference and weight change %/trends
- Patient history: Medical, surgical, social
- Biochemical data and all relevant values [e.g. electrolytes, A1c and self-monitoring of blood glucose levels (SMBGs), blood pressure (BP), glomerular filtration rate (GFR), serum albumin and inflammation markers, anemia and fluid markers, lipid panel, markers for bone metabolism and renal bone disease
- Food allergies or Intolerances
- Intake: Diet history for analysis of macronutrients and micronutrients, e.g. energy, protein, carbohydrates (CHOs), amount and types of fat, sodium (Na) and fluid intake, potassium (K), calcium (Ca), and phosphorus (P) intake
- Medications: Check patient's reported intake against current Rx list and any OTC items used (including vitamins, minerals, and self-Rx'd dietary supplements, e.g. herbals/botanicals)
- Nutritional supplements: Protein modulars, high calorie enteral formulas
- Knowledge, beliefs or attitudes: Previous diet education, Perceptions re: current illness and associated diet recommendations, Readiness to change lifestyle behaviors
- Lifestyle patterns: Eating patterns, food preferences, frequency and type of restaurant fare, cultural and religious impact on diet/cuisine, and physical activity
- Factors affecting access to food (food security): Food-related resources, support of family/friends, patient's ability to shop/cook (ADLs)

PRETRANSPLANT OBJECTIVES[2]

- Optimize nutritional status prior to surgery
- Avoid or correct malnutrition
- Achieve target BMI:
- Most transplant departments have BMI cut-offs for eligibility such as BMI ≥ 18.5 and < 40 for recipients, and ≥ 18.5 and < 35 for donors
- Achieve acceptable lab values
- Fluid and blood pressure control
- Manage co-morbidities
- Education:
  - One-on-one education with patient re: any current, necessary interventions; often involves educating a patient's family member(s) or a caregiver
  - A brief introduction to the Post-Transplant Diet Plan, i.e. changes to expect if/when the patient does have surgery including: the potential side effects of immunosuppression Rx's, the pertinent food/drug interactions, and the need to focus on food safety skills, all of which will be reviewed before surgery and reinforced after surgery
  - Make patient aware that adherence to the immune suppression Rx regimen is critical; that non-adherence could result in the early and unnecessary loss of an otherwise functioning allograft
  - Make patient aware that while the post-transplant diet will likely be more liberal than their current CKD or dialysis diet, any underlying conditions (e.g. diabetes, hypertension, etc.) will still need to be managed
- The Nutrition Assessment helps to determine the patient's initial eligibility for transplant surgery
  - Re-assessments factor in to continuity of care all the way through post-transplant follow-up

Protein Energy Malnutrition (PEM)

- Frequent in chronic kidney disease (CKD) patients
- Caused/exacerbated by:
  - Disordered metabolism, diet restrictions, uremia induced anorexia, poly-pharmacy and treatment-related gastrointestinal (GI) distress, losses of nutrients/vitamins during dialysis, and fatigue from the rigors of dialysis treatment
- Chronic kidney disease—not on dialysis
  - Usually on controlled protein diet pre-dialysis (i.e. adequate, but not excessive protein intake) to preserve renal function
  - While energy needs remain typical for age—liberalize as needed
- Chronic kidney disease—on dialysis
  - Energy and protein needs are increased in dialysis diet plans due to losses during dialysis treatments, liberalize further as needed
  - Avoid any unnecessary dietary restrictions

Weight Management

- If candidate's BMI is above the acceptable range, weight loss support options should be offered; a weight reduction plan must be closely supervised and include adjustments appropriate to the patient's CKD or dialysis diet priorities
- Potential donors are usually very healthy individuals who may require weight reduction to meet eligibility standards
- When weight reduction for potential recipients or donors may take many months (or years) to achieve via traditional methods — because of sheer volume or failed attempts — bariatric options are deemed appropriate and should be offered
- If underweight and/or protein-energy malnourished, repletion needs can be achieved via:
  - Diet plan adjustments — i.e. liberalizing the diet as much as is medically feasible
  - Nutritional supplements (oral)
  - Nutrition support, i.e. tube feeds via GI tract (enteral) or parenteral nutrition
  - Nutrition support is rarely necessary in the acute-post-transplantation period because the progression to solid foods usually occurs within 1-3 post-operative days and the length of hospitalization may be < 5 days
  - When nutrition support is needed, the decision to begin parenteral nutrition (PN) should be made only after failed attempts at adequate intake via the oral and enteral routes or when using the oral or enteral route is contraindicated, and only when the need for PN is expected to be for more than one week[2]
- Early nutrition support is indicated for a nutritionally high risk recipient unable to achieve adequate intake via diet and oral supplements prior to transplantation
  - Aggressive nutrition support in these cases reduces mortality rates[3]
- Any patient (pre- or postoperative), who is unable to sustain adequate intake to meet calorie and protein needs after 5 days is considered a candidate for some type of nutritional intervention, depending on the patient's nutritional status, degree of catabolism, and amount of intake deficit
- Dialysis patients are recommended to take a renal vitamin, daily (after treatment) to replace losses of water soluble vitamins during dialysis
- A vitamin can be beneficial, also, for any patient on a low-calorie diet plan for weight reduction
  - Renal vitamin for a potential recipient
  - Standard one-a-day type multi-vitamin for a potential donor

POST-TRANSPLANT OBJECTIVES (ACUTE PHASE)[2,3]

- Acute phase is the period during the first 8 weeks following transplantation
- Meet increased energy and protein requirements associated with metabolic stress of surgery, wound healing and high doses of immune-suppression Rx(s)
- Provide high fluid intake for adequate hydration with high urine output encountered with good allograft function
- Correct electrolyte imbalances:
  - Hypophosphatemia and/or hypomagnesemia (often seen after surgery with good allograft function)
  - Hyperkalemia (often seen with delayed allograft function)
- Correct for glucose intolerance
  - Consider the addition of NPH to address poor glycemic control due to the addition of prednisone, as NPH matches the timed activity of prednisone very closely and it may be the best choice for the patient who has otherwise had good glycemic control on their current DM Rx regimen, without disturbing the balance of that underlying regimen[4]
  - The consistent CHO diet component will need to be added to the diet order for patients with pre-existing DM or new onset diabetes after transplant (NODAT)

  - Of note, more and more transplant programs are opting to use a prednisone free or an extremely short-lived Rx for prednisone (induction only) in their immunosuppression regimens; thus, limiting the incidence of hyperglycemia and other side effects
- Address GI side effects of immune-supression Rx(s)
- Pre-discharge education reviewing post-transplant diet plan self-management skills — including food safety review
- Maintain protein stores
- Prevent infections
- Promote wound healing

Potential Nutritional Effects of Immune-Suppression Drugs

- Hyperglycemia
- Hyperlipidemia
- Glucose intolerance
- Hypertension
- Hyperkalemia
- Interference with vitamin D metabolism/Osteoporosis
- Sodium retention
- Increased appetite/weight gain
- Gastrointestinal side-effects
- Immune-suppression Rx(s)
  - Food safety issues
  - Interactions:
    - Avoid pomegranate and grapefruit products, and be aware that grapefruit juice is added to some commercial citrus-flavored soda products
    - Caution patients about chronic use of products that boost the immune function, e.g. green tea

POST-TRANSPLANT OBJECTIVES (CHRONIC PHASE)

- Chronic phase (aka: maintenance phase) follows the acute phase for the life of the functioning allograft
- Maintain an overall satisfactory nutritional status
  - Adequate macro- and micro-nutrients
- Management of chronic disease risk factors and pre-existing or residual CKD conditions—including: bone health and control of blood glucose (BG), lipids, and blood pressure (BP)
- Prevent/minimize side-effects of immune-suppression Rx therapy:
  - Increased appetite combined with less restrictive diet that can lead to unplanned, undesirable weight gain
  - Increased serum lipid and glucose levels
  - Increased blood pressure and fluid retention
  - Potential for stomach ulcers and bone disease
- Address post-transplant concerns including:
  - Osteoporosis (OP)
  - Hyperlipidemia
  - Obesity
  - New onset diabetes after transplant (NODAT)
  - Challenges to pre-existing diabetes
  - Hypertension

THERAPEUTIC DIET PLANS

All patients with CKD (including post-transplant patients) are at high risk for cardiovascular disease (CVD). Mortality is often associated with a cardiac event.

- The "therapeutic lifestyle change" or "TLC diet" can improve a patient's lipid profile and may be instrumental in limiting CVD risk, and associated morbidity and mortality
- For patients who need diabetes prevention or management, diabetic self-management behaviors including controlled CHOs, a consistent CHO load, emphasis on complex CHO choices, weight management, and increased physical activity can be incorporated
- A sodium restriction to control BP and/or fluid volume is already a part of the diet plans used for patients with CKD including those on hemodialysis (HD)
- A sodium controlled diet can be helpful also for post-transplant patients with hypertension, and these patients may benefit further by following the "dietary approaches to stop hypertension diet" (DASH Diet)
  - The DASH Diet is low in Na, but rich in other minerals. Therefore, it should not be used by patients with CKD stages 3–4, patients on dialysis, or post-transplant patients with a failing allograft
- All of the therapeutic Diet Plans mentioned can be utilized and are often melded together to improve a patient's outcomes, as appropriate
  - This multi-layered approach should not seem overwhelming to a patient and should be presented in continuity as a single "diet plan" tailored to their needs
  - Patients with CKD stages 3-4, patients on dialysis, and post-transplant patients with a failing allograft may still benefit from a diet plan that incorporates recommendations from many of the therapeutic diets mentioned even though they will need to be adjusted to some degree to allow for the patient's renal diet plan priorities

THERAPEUTIC LIFESTYLE CHANGE (TLC) DIET GUIDELINES

- Increase:
  - Whole plant foods: for fiber, vitamins and minerals, choosing mostly plant protein, whole grains and phytochemically-rich produce (utilizing fresh vegetables more than whole fruit may be best for weight and glycemic control)
  - Healthy fats: emphasis on Mono-unsaturated and Omega 3
- Decrease:
  - Animal foods: Limit saturated fats and dietary cholesterol
  - Processed foods: Trans fats and sodium
  - Moderate portion sizes

Note: The preceding sections addressed data collection (for assessment) and broad goals for pre- and post-transplant patients. Table 1[1,2,5,6] addresses specific goals used by the RD in the medical nutrition therapy (MNT) process. These target-goals represent a safe and appropriate starting point from which the RD can make adjustments, as necessary, individualizing the nutrition care plan for each patient.

Table 1: Medical nutrition therapy (MNT) summary guidelines table

	Protein (g/kg[a]/day)	Energy (kcals[b]/kg/day)	Calcium (g/day)	Sodium (g/day)	Potassium (g or mg/day)	Phosphorus (mg/day)	Fluid (liters/day)
CKD Stages 3–4	0.6–0.8; 50% HBV	23–35 adjust to avoid loss of LBM	1–1.5; if binder Rx used, < 2 including all Calcium sources	< 2.4	No limit unless serum level is above normal range	800–1000 or 10–12 mg/g of needed protein	Maintain fluid balance UO plus 1 L, if needed
(with DM-N)[f]	0.8–0.9; 50% HBV[1,6]	Adjust to achieve or maintain a DBW					
HD	1.2*; 50% HBV	30–35; Typically: 35 for patients < 60 yo and 30 for patients 60 yo or older	Daily limit including binder load < 2	2–3 generally; 2–4 if ≤ 1 L UO; ≤ 2 if anuric/ oliguric	Individualize limit, using 40 mg/kg/day	800–1000 or 10–12 mg/g of needed protein; or < 17 mg/kg/ day	UO plus 1 L; Limit IDWGs
(with DM-N)		Adjust to achieve/ maintain a DBW		2–2.4	2–3; adjust to serum levels (goal: renal range)		
PD	1.2–1.3*; 50% HBV	30–35; including kcals from dialysate[d] Typically: 35 for patients < 60 yo and 30 for pts > or = 60 yo	Daily limit including binder load < 2	Generally, 2-3 maintain fluid balance; minimize hypertonic exchanges	Unrestricted if serum level is in renal range; a K supplement may be needed; most patients tolerate typical intake, i.e. 2–4	800–1000 or 10–15 mg/g of needed protein	Maintain balance PD patients usually tolerate a typical intake of 1–3 L/day depending on UO/UF/BP
(with DM-N)		Adjust to achieve/ maintain a DBW		DM-N with no HTN: 2–4 DM-N with HTN: < 2.4		with DM-N: 10–12 mg/g of needed protein	
Post-transplant (Acute phase)[c]	1.3–2.0	30–35; may increase with postoperative complications	1.2–1.5; If DM-N: 0.8–1.5; individualize per metabolic needs	No restriction unless BP or fluid dictates; DM-N & no HTN: ≤ 3; DM-N & HTN: ≤ 2.4	Unrestricted unless hyperkalemic 2–4 g if hyperkalemic	DRI[e]; may need supplementation to normalize serum levels	Limited only by graft function; generally unrestricted
Post-transplant (Chronic phase)	0.8–1.0 Use CKD 3–4 guidelines for limit on protein if chronic graft failure occurs after transplant	Adjust kcals to achieve or maintain DBW	1.2–1.5; If DM-N: 0.8–1.5; individualize per metabolic needs	Usually not restricted; If HTN + edema: 2-4; DM-N & no HTN: ≤ 3; DM-N & HTN: ≤ 2.4	Unrestricted unless hyperkalemic	DRI	Limited only by graft function; generally unrestricted

(g: Grams; kg: Kilograms; kcals: Kilocalories (calories); mg: Milligrams; CKD: Chronic kidney disease; HBV: High biological value (some protein foods); LBM: Lean body mass; Pt or pt: Patient; DM-N: Diabetes Mellitus-Nephropathy; UO: Urine output; HD: Hemodialysis; PD: Peritoneal dialysis; yo: Years old; K: Potassium; pts: Patients; DBW: Desired or desirable body weight; HTN: Hypertension; DRI: Dietary reference intake (recommended dietary allowance or adequate intake))

* 1.2–1.5 g protein/kg/day during catabolic stress.

Note: Renal range refers to targets for lab values for pts on dialysis that vary from standard ranges, clinical practice guidelines for renal lab targets are based on the best evidence available (see references 5, 6)
Source: Table Data are from references 1, 2, 5 and 6

TABLE NOTES:

a. The RD will pick the reference weight to be used in calculations for the pt's estimated needs that is most appropriate. The RD can use current body weight (CBW) as measured, adjusted body weight (ABW), i.e. CBW adjusted for amputation or obesity, ideal body weight (IBW) based on the Metropolitan Life Insurance – mortality data (weight tables) or use the HAMWI Method (a specific calculation yielding an IBW based on gender and height with the result ("n") as calculated and the range: n(+ or –) 10%. An RD may also use a standard body weight (SBW) based on the National Health and Nutrition Examination Survey (NHANES II) tables that describe the median body weight of average Americans from 1976 to 1980 for height, age, sex and frame size. However, there are "cautions" associated with these choices, e.g. using a CBW for a patient on HD will likely reflect fluid weight accumulated between HD treatments, and although NHANES II data is validated and standardized and uses a large database of ethnically-diverse groups, data is provided only on what individuals weigh, not what they should weigh in order to reduce morbidity and mortality. Using the "Caution" examples mentioned, you can see that any one of these "body weight" choices might be the best one to use for a given patient (or not), and RD discretion comes into play.

b. Similarly, RDs use discretion re: ranges for calories and protein grams based on a patient's metabolic stressors, age, gender and level of physical activity. The following considerations come into play: Actual measured weight, History of weight changes (both long-term and recent), Serial weight measurements, monitored longitudinally, with adjustments for suspected impact of edema, ascites and polycystic organs. The RD will then educate patients using terms they can understand re: goals or limits. The RD will analyze the patient's current intake, monitor labs, and then help the patient to cut or add the number of servings of specific foods to a level that is tolerated or optimal. For example, the RD will use a number of ounces of meat, fish, or poultry/day and describe what a 1, 2 or 3 ounce serving looks like, or display a food model that represents a ½ cup size serving, e.g. for fruits and vegetables and the number of servings recommended/day from a designated (e.g. low potassium) list.

c. Aside from CHO control in a diet order, as needed, the RD should not be too quick to recommend dietary restrictions during the first week post-transplant surgery because fluid status and lab values will quickly change as allograft function "kicks in".

d. PD calories absorbed from dialysate are calculated and subtracted from the patient's total kcal needs to guide the pt for appropriate energy intake from diet, and since the PD calories absorbed are from dextrose (refined CHO) simple sugars should also be limited in the diet.

e. Guidelines for micronutrients (vitamins and trace minerals) are not addressed in this chapter, but may be seen in references 2,3, and 4. Of note, because of the chronic anemia and Mineral Bone Diseases associated with CKD, pre-transplant patients often have shifts in their Rx regimen following protocols for anemia and bone therapy, e.g. Rx changes in Iron and Vitamin D {both 25 (OH)D and 1,25 $(OH)_2D$ or vitamin D analogs}, and these protocol details can also be seen in references 2, 4 and 5.

f. Generally for patients with DM, 50–60% of daily kcals from CHOs, 20–30 g/day of dietary fiber, 25–35% of daily kcals as fat, but < 7% of kcals from saturated fat and emphasis on sources with monounsaturated fatty acids (MUFAs) like those in olive or canola oils, < 200 mg/day dietary cholesterol, and protein needs will vary based on medical status.

REFERENCES

1. American Academy of Nutrition and Dietetics Evidence Analysis Library. Evidence-based Nutrition Practice Guideline on Chronic Kidney Disease Executive Summary of Recommendations-July 2010 at http://www.adaevidencelibrary.com/topic.cfm?cat=3927&library=EBG and copywrited by the Academy. accessed 09-2013
2. Byham-Gray L, Stover J, Wiesen, K. A Clinical Guide to Nutrition Care in Kidney Disease. 2nd ed. Chicago, IL: American Dietetic Association; 2013. ISBN: 9780880914703
3. Danovitch, GM, (Ed.) Handbook of Kidney Transplantation, 5th edition. "Nutrition in the Kidney Transplant Recipient" by Susan Weil, RD, CSR Kidney Transplant Program - David Geffen School of Medicine at UCLA, Los Angeles, California. Philadelphia: Lippincott, Williams & Wilkins, a Wolters Kluwer business; 2010.
4. Knutsen, PG, ACNS, BC, CDE, presenter, "Transplant Diabetes & Glucose Management: How Sweet It Is" NATCO Seminar: Donation and Transplantation Academy A Multi-Disciplinary Approach. Tempe, Az October 10/2013
5. KDIGO clinical practice guideline for the care of kidney transplant recipients. Am J Transplant. 2009 Nov;9 (Suppl 3): S1-155. at http://www.kdigo.org/clinical_practice_guidelines/pdf/TxpGL_publVersion.pdf. accessed 08/2013
6. National Kidney Foundation. KDOQI Clinical Practice Guideline for Diabetes and CKD. at http://www.kidney.org/professionals/KDOQI/guidelines_diabetesUp/diabetes-ckd-update-2012.pdf. accessed 08/2013

CHAPTER 11

Obesity, Metabolic Surgery and Transplantation

Timothee Friesen, Charmaine Gentles, Larry Gellman, Dominick Gadaleta

THE OBESITY EPIDEMIC

Obesity leads to a reduced life expectancy and often to an increase in multiple health problems.[1] It is caused by excess body fat accumulation, and is generally defined as a body mass index (BMI in kg/m^2) greater than 30. Morbid obesity is defined as a BMI greater than 40, or a BMI greater than 35 with co-morbidities.

Obesity is a growing problem both in the United States and around the world. According to the World Health Organization, there were 1.6 billion overweight and 400 million obese adults worldwide in 2005.[2] In the United States, the prevalence of obesity (men/women) increased from 11/16% in the 1960s, to 21/26% in 1994, and 32/34% in 2004.[3] The acceleration of the problem has affected the super obese (BMI > 50) even more severely: between 1986 and 2000, their prevalence has grown by over 500%.[4]

The trends among renal transplant recipients are similar to the national trend: between 1987 and 2001, the proportion of renal transplant recipients categorized as obese increased by 116%.[5]

MORBID OBESITY LEADS TO SOLID ORGAN FAILURE

Morbid obesity is a well-known risk factor for multiple medical problems such as diabetes and hypertension, which in turn can cause proteinuria, nephrotic syndrome and chronic kidney disease (CKD).[6] Stressed kidneys are further damaged by co-morbidities such as untreated diabetes, hypertension and dyslipidemias.[7]

In addition to this indirect relationship, there is likely also a direct relationship between obesity and kidney disease. Based on a 15–35 year cohort of over 300,000 members of Kaiser Permanente of Northern California aged 18 or older, the increase in the rate of end-stage renal disease (ESRD) was proportional to the increase in BMI, independently of hypertension or diabetes.[8]

Obesity is a major risk factor for liver disease as well. The prevalence of nonalcoholic steatohepatitis (NASH) and nonalcoholic fatty liver disease (NAFLD) in obese diabetics is 50% and 85%, respectively, compared to 3% and 25% in the rest of the population.[9] NAFLD caused by obesity-related insulin resistance is the third most common cause of liver disease in the United States.[10]

OBESITY RISKS TO TRANSPLANT DONORS AND RECIPIENTS

Obesity impacts short- and long-term renal transplant recipient outcomes negatively. In a review of over 27,000 kidney transplant recipients on the United Network for Organ Sharing (UNOS) database, Gore found that recipient obesity was associated with an increased risk of wound dehiscence, treatment for acute graft rejection (AGR) and delayed graft failure (DGF).[11] Extremes of body habitus were also associated with worse graft survival. Yoo also showed that donor obesity negatively affected liver transplant postoperative graft outcomes, although it did not impact overall graft survival.[12]

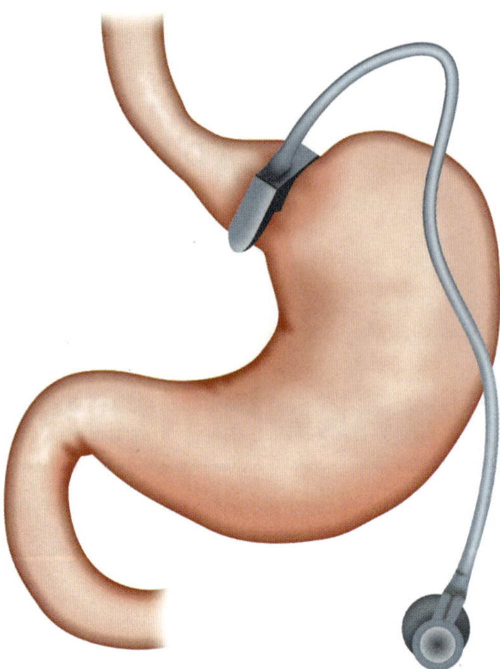

Fig. 1: Adjustable gastric band.
Source: Timothee Friesen

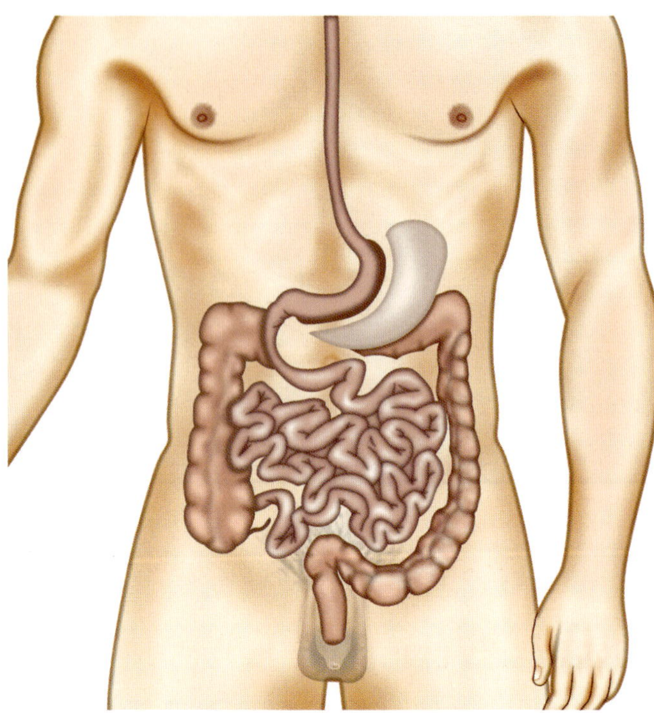

Fig. 2: Vertical sleeve gastrectomy.
Source:Timothee Friesen

In a US study evaluating over 23,000 liver transplant recipients also using the UNOS database, Nair found that obesity significantly affected long-term post-transplant survival.[13] Short-term mortality and primary graft non-function were significantly higher both in the severely and morbidly obese patients.

Although it acknowledges that there is limited data for exclusion from kidney transplantation based on obesity (since even obese patients benefit from transplantation), the existing practice guidelines issued by the American Society of Transplantation recommend a BMI of less than 30 prior to transplantation.[14] A recent survey of 67 US kidney transplant centers showed that virtually all used BMI as a selection criterion, with a range of 35–45 as the upper limit to initiate an evaluation.[15]

SURGICAL OPTIONS FOR WEIGHT LOSS

The three laparoscopic bariatric procedures that are most commonly performed in the United States are the adjustable gastric band, the vertical sleeve gastrectomy, and the Roux-en-Y gastric bypass.

The adjustable gastric band (Fig. 1) is placed around the proximal portion of the stomach laparoscopically. It is connected to a subcutaneous port, which is accessed percutaneously to adjust the tightness of the band. The typical excess weight loss is 55%, but patients need to be committed to regular band adjustments. The procedure has a low postoperative mortality rate (0.1%), but complications such as band slippage, erosion, noncompliance, and tubing malfunction require reoperation in 25–50% of patients.

The laparoscopic vertical sleeve gastrectomy (Fig. 2) is a restrictive procedure that involves the removal of approximately 60% of the stomach, leaving behind a sleeve-shaped portion of stomach. It is considerably easier to perform than a gastric bypass, since there is only one staple line and no intestinal anastomosis, and there are no implants. The typical excess weight loss is 60%, the complication rate is less than 10%, and the postoperative mortality is 0.19%.

The laparoscopic Roux-en-Y gastric bypass (Fig. 3) is a restrictive and malabsorptive procedure that involves the creation of a small proximal gastric pouch and of two anastomoses. The first one is between the pouch and the jejunum, and the second one is between the jejunum and the jejunum. The duodenum and proximal small bowel are bypassed. Typical excess weight loss is 65%, and complications include marginal ulcers, internal hernias, and nutritional deficiencies.

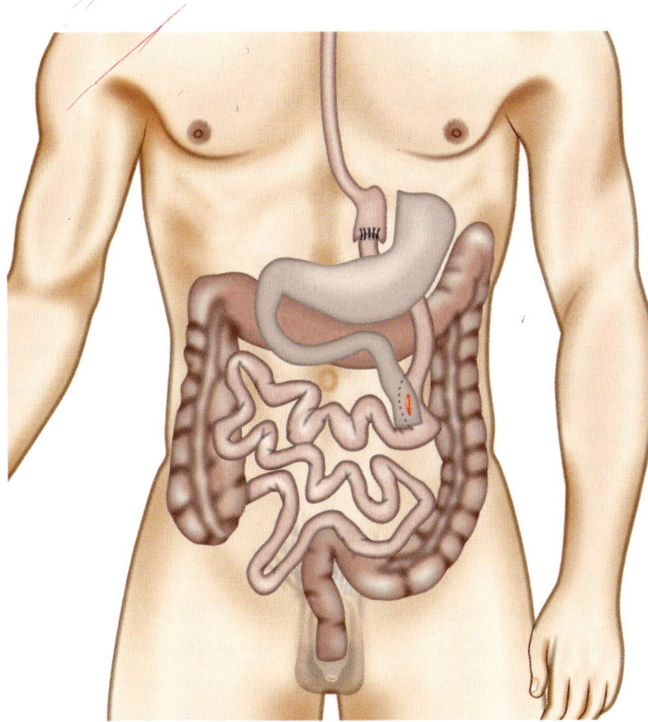

Fig. 3: Roux-en-Y gastric bypass.
Source: Timothee Friesen

WEIGHT LOSS SURGERY IN TRANSPLANT CANDIDATES AND RECIPIENTS

Several meta-analyses support a superior efficacy of bariatric surgery compared to nonsurgical therapy in achieving sustained weight loss in morbidly obese patients.[16] The 1991 NIH Consensus Conference concluded that surgical interventions, including Roux-en-Y gastric bypass, are the most appropriate treatment for obesity as defined by a BMI greater than 40 or a BMI greater than 35 with co-morbidities. Surgery must be performed in the setting of a multidisciplinary clinic with psychiatric and nutritional evaluation and education, and all patients must have long-term follow-up.

Bariatric surgery has been shown to help obese patients with solid organ failure become transplant candidates. A retrospective review[17] studied 15 patients with ESRD or endstage liver disease (ESLD)/cirrhosis who were not transplant candidates because of their BMI. They underwent laparoscopic Roux-en-Y gastric bypass or laparoscopic sleeve gastrectomy respectively. After a mean follow-up of 9 months, the excess weight loss was 61% for ESRD and 33/61% for ESLD/cirrhosis patients. There was no change in the albumin level of the liver failure patients and there were no mortalities. Fourteen of the fifteen patients became transplant candidates.

Bariatric surgery has been shown to be safe in kidney and liver transplant recipients as well.[18] A study[19] of 188 kidney transplant candidates and recipients registered with the United States Renal Data System (USRDS) who underwent open Roux-en-Y gastric bypass surgery between 1991 and 2004, had outcomes similar to patients without kidney disease in terms of excess weight loss and perioperative mortality. A Columbian study[20] of five postrenal transplant patients who underwent laparoscopic gastric bypass between 2002 and 2008, showed adequate renal allograft survival with dramatic improvements in co-morbidities, such as hyperlipidemia, insulin requirements, and hypertension. The decreased absorption of immunosuppressive medications did not result in higher doses requirements.

REFERENCES

1. Haslam DW, James WP. Obesity. Lancet. 2005;366(9492): 1197- 209.
2. World Health Organization. Obesity and overweight. Geneva: WHO, September 2007.
3. Ogden CL, Yanovski SZ, Carroll MD, et al. The epidemiology of obesity. Gastroenterology. 2007;132:2087-102.
4. Sturm R. Increases in clinically severe obesity in the United States, 1986-2000. Arch Intern Med. 2003;163(18):2146-8.
5. Friedman AN, Miskulin DC, Rosenberg IH, et al. Demographics and trends in overweight and obesity in patients at time of kidney transplantation. Am J Kidney Dis. 2003;41:480-7.
6. Wang Y, Chen X, Song Y, et al. Association between obesity and kidney disease: A systematic review and meta-analysis. Kidney Int. 2008;73(1):19-33.
7. Killackey M, Zhang R, Sparks K, et al. Challenges of abdominal organ transplant in obesity. South Med J. 2010;103(6):532-8.
8. Hsu CY, McCulloch CE, et al. Body mass index and risk for end-stage renal disease. Ann Intern Med. 2006;144:21-28.
9. Wolf AM, Busch B, et al. Histologic changes in the liver of morbidly obese patients: Correlation with metabolic parameters. Obesity Surgery. 2005;15:228-37.
10. Schreuder T, Verwer BJ, Van Nieuwkerk CM, et al. Nonalcoholic fatty liver disease: An overview of current insights in pathogenesis, diagnosis and treatment. World J Gastroenterology. 2008;14:2474-86.
11. Gore JL, Pham PT, Danovitch GM, et al. Obesity and outcome following renal transplantation. Am J Transplant. 2006;6:357-63.
12. Yoo HY, Molmenti E, Thuluvath PJ. The effect of donor body mass index on primary graft nonfunction, retransplantation rate, early graft and patient survival after liver transplantation. Liver Transpl. 2003;9(1):72-8.
13. Nair S, Verma S, Thluuvath PJ. Obesity and its effect on survival in patients undergoing orthotopic liver transplantation in the United States. Hepatology. 2002;35(1):105-9.

14. Kasiske BL, Cangro CB, Hariharan S, et al. The evaluation of renal transplantation candidates: clinical practice guidelines. Am J Transplant. 2001;1(suppl 2):3-95.
15. Pondrom S. The AJT report: News and issues that affect organ and tissue transplantation. Am J Transplant. 2012; 12:1663-4.
16. Buchwald H, Avidor Y, Braunwald E, et al. Bariatric surgery: A systematic review and meta-analysis. JAMA. 2004;292:1724-37.
17. Takata M, Campos G, Ciovica R, et al. Laparoscopic bariatric surgery improves candidacy in morbidly obese patients awaiting transplantation. Surg Obes Relat Dis. 2008;4: 159-65.
18. Tichansky DS, Madan AK. Laparoscopic roux-en-y gastric bypass is safe and feasible after orthotopic liver transplant. Obesity Surgery. 2005;15:1481-6.
19. Modanlou KA, Muthyala U, Xiao H, et al. Bariatric Surgery among kidney transplant candidates and recipients: Analysis of the United States renal data system and literature review. Transplantation. 2009;87(8): 1167-73.
20. Arias RH, Mesa L, Posada JG, et al. Kidney transplantation and gastric bypass: A better control of comorbidities. Obes Surg. 2010;20:851-4.Apiducit ilicia ipsunt as quam volendi digent, num aritia voluptat.

CHAPTER 12

Infections

David A Hirschwerk, Prashant Malhotra

INTRODUCTION – KEY POINTS

- Infections are an important cause of morbidity and mortality in kidney transplant recipients

Prior to Transplantation

- Identify potential infectious issues in both donors *and* recipients
- Identify and evaluate both donors and recipients for past, present and potential infections
- Confirm that recipients are properly vaccinated

Post-Transplantation

- Some early recipient infections may be donor-derived
- Recognizing the time course of infections provides useful information, and should be carefully considered
- Prophylaxis and treatment of acute rejection may alter/frame shift the timeline of infections
- The severity of immunocompromise should always be evaluated—based on:
  - Time from transplant
  - Type/dose of immunosuppression
  - Presence of recent rejection
  - Use of T-cell inhibiting agents

DIAGNOSTIC POINTS

- Transplant recipients may present with altered inflammatory responses to infection
- Common infections may present in uncommon ways
- Clinicians must approach transplant patients with a high degree of suspicion for infection, and consider that infection may be present until proven otherwise
- Concurrent infections (more than one single pathogen) are more likely in transplant patients than in the general population
- The differential diagnosis of potential pathogens is more extensive in transplant patients than in nonimmunocompromised individuals
- Have a low threshold for both enhanced imaging studies and biopsies. Imaging studies and biopsies should be obtained *early* in order to make a prompt definitive diagnosis and establish an adequate therapeutic approach—if in doubt, image and biopsy
- It may be difficult to distinguish between colonization and active infection

IMMUNOLOGIC DEFICIT—T-CELL INHIBITION LEADS TO INCREASED RISK OF OPPORTUNISTIC INFECTIONS

- Immunosuppression, although necessary to protect the transplanted kidney from rejection, increases the risk of infections
- Most immunosuppressive agents are associated with T-cell depletion, reduced T-cell activation, or inhibition of T-cell proliferation
- The net result of immunosuppression is reduced cell-mediated immunity
- Immunosuppression levels are the greatest from month one to six post-transplant, as well as during any subsequent episodes of rejection that require intensified immunosuppression
- Measurement of CD4+ T-helper cells is not as predictive of opportunistic infections in transplant recipients as it is in patients with HIV/AIDS

CLINICAL PREDICTORS OF POST-TRANSPLANT INFECTIONS

- Structural abnormalities
  - Ureteral strictures
  - Fluid collections
  - Foreign bodies
- Environmental exposures
  - Heavy burden of exposure to opportunistic pathogens
  - Live vaccines
- Degree of immunosuppression

DONOR/RECIPIENT SCREENING

- Human immunodeficiency virus
- Hepatitis B
- Hepatitis C
  - Testing for blood-borne viruses (HIV, Hepatitis B, Hepatitis C) should be performed on the recipient and the donor no more than 2 weeks prior to transplant (and by nucleic acid testing (PCR)) to avoid potential transfer of infection from a donor recently exposed and in the "window period"
- Cytomegalovirus (CMV)
- Toxoplasma
- Epstein-Barr Virus (EBV)
- Human T-lymphotropic virus (HTLV-1) (controversial)
- *Strongyloides*-serology or stool assay (in recipients from endemic regions)
- Latent tuberculosis infection (tuberculin skin test or QuantiFERON Gold assay)
- *Coccidiomycosis* (in recipients from endemic regions)

VACCINATIONS

- All *LIVE* vaccines should be administered *at least 4 weeks prior to transplantation*
- Transplant recipients are less likely to mount immunologic responses to vaccines after transplantation
- Hepatitis B, Pneumococcal, Varicella (live vaccine), Influenza vaccines should be provided to all recipients *prior to* transplantation

ANTIMICROBIAL PROPHYLAXIS POST-TRANSPLANT

Trimethoprim-Sulfamethoxazole (TMP-SMX)

- Single strength tablet daily
- Reduced likelihood of
  - *Pneumocystis jiroveci*
  - *Toxoplasmosis*
- Provides some protection versus standard bacterial pathogens that cause urinary tract infections post-transplant
- May provide some protection versus *Nocardia, Listeria, Legionella*

Acyclovir

Prophylaxis against Herpes simplex virus (HSV) 1 & 2—the most common viral pathogen to cause infections postrenal transplant (in the absence of prophylaxis).

Valganciclovir

- Prophylaxis against Cytomegalovirus (CMV)
- Also active against HSV
- If used for CMV, acyclovir is not given

GENERAL TIMETABLE OF POST-TRANSPLANT INFECTIONS

First Month

- Non opportunistic infections
- Same as commonly encountered postoperative infections in nontransplant surgical patients
  - Urinary tract infections
  - Wound infections
  - Abscesses
  - Intravenous (IV) catheter/line infections
  - Bacterial Pneumonia(including ventilator associated or aspiration)
  - *C. difficile* infection
  - Infections related to anastomotic leaks or ischemia
- Herpes simplex virus infections (very rare if patient taking antiviral prophylaxis)

Months 1–6

- Early post-transplant period
- Opportunistic infections
- Cytomegalovirus
- *Pneumocystis*
- *Aspergillus*
- Endemic mycosis (*Histoplasmosis, Blastomyces*, etc.)
- *Cryptococcus*
- *Listeria*
- *Endemic fungi*
- Post-transplantation lymphoproliferative disorder (PTLD), associated with EBV, seen most commonly in most immunocompromised patients

Beyond Month 6

- Late post-transplant period
- Immunosuppression levels typically are reduced
- Most infections caused by community acquired pathogens
- Similar incidence of infections but with a higher incidence than in the non-immunosuppressed population
- Less common to see opportunistic infections (though still possible and more likely than in immunocompetent individuals)

PATHOGENS OF IMPORTANCE IN KIDNEY TRANSPLANT RECIPIENTS

- Cytomegalovirus
- BK Virus
- Cryptococcus
- Pneumocystis jiroveci pneumonia (PCP)
- Toxoplasmosis
- Listeria
- West Nile Virus
- Aspergillosis
- Tuberculosis
- *Nocardia* sp

URINARY TRACT INFECTIONS/ PYELONEPHRITIS OF THE TRANSPLANTED KIDNEY

- Most common bacterial infection in kidney transplant recipients
- Low threshold for imaging of the graft to exclude ureteral abnormalities, fluid collections, and hydronephrosis (may require percutaneous nephrostomy tube placement or ureteral stenting)
- Recognition of role of resistant pathogens causing infections in this population (higher incidence of extended spectrum beta-lactamase (ESBL) organisms)
- Pathogens are often resistant to quinolones
- Quinolones should not be relied upon for empiric therapy in acutely ill patients with sepsis presumed to be derived from the urinary tract)

PNEUMONIAS/RESPIRATORY VIRAL INFECTIONS

- Community acquired respiratory viral infections (influenza, rhinovirus, metapneumovirus, parainfluenzae) may present with atypical and sometimes severe manifestations and have longer courses than in nonimmunocompromised individuals
- Transplant recipients will "shed" viruses for longer periods of time, which has implications for hospital infection control restrictions
- Adenoviral infections may present with upper/lower respiratory infections, hepatitis, hemorrhagic cystitis
- Most respiratory viral infections can be diagnosed by nasopharyngeal swabs and respiratory virus testing assays (DFA or PCR techniques are the most common ones)
- Bacterial pneumonias (e.g. pneumococcal, *H. influeanzae*) may be seen more commonly

CYTOMEGALOVIRUS PRESENTATIONS POST-TRANSPLANT

- Recipients should either:
  - Receive valganciclovir for 100 days (prophylactic strategy) post transplant, undergo periodic check for CMV viremia — Valganciclovir should be started if viremia is detected (pre-emptive strategy)
- Recipients in CMV donor negative/recipient negative cases can receive prophylaxis against HSV alone (acyclovir) as CMV in these cases is rare in this setting (unless new person to person infection post-transplant)
- Cytomegalovirus disease is most common in CMV donor positive/recipient negative cases
- Valganciclovir can lead to granulocytopenia

Cytomegalovirus Presentation

- Cytomegalovirus viremia without any symptoms
- Cytomegalovirus viremia with fever, lethargy, hepatitis, bone marrow suppression
- End organ damage—gastrointestional (GI) (colitis), pneumonitis (rare-except in donor +/recipient negative cases and recipients with high CMV viral load)
- Cytomegalovirus encephalitis—rare
- Characterized by a low white blood cell count, and liver function test (LFT) abnormalities

Cytomegalovirus Diagnosis

- Viral PCR testing in of serum sample
- Pathology of biopsied tissue with characteristic "owl eyes-viral inclusions"
- A diagnosis of CMV infection should be pursued in patients with gastrointestinal disease-colonoscopy/ upper endoscopy with biopsy should be considered even in those patients with non-detectable CMV viral load

Cytomegalovirus Treatment

- Intravenous (IV) ganciclovir, PO valganciclovir
- Intravenous foscarnet and cidofovir utilized in patients intolerant of ganciclovir or in cases of resistance to these agents has developed—more common to be seen in CMV donor positive/recipient negative cases that have high levels of CMV in the serum
- Treat with antivirals until disease controlled clinically and virus suppressed to nondetectable levels

BK VIRUS

- Reactivation may be caused by intensified immunosuppression
- Can be associated with nephropathy, but often incidental viral shedding
- Diagnosis may require biopsy with immunohistochemistry, though correlation of positive urine or serum PCRs with clinical presentation may be helpful
- Treatment involves reduction of immunosuppression
- Cidofovir has antiviral activity and may be used in convincing cases of BK nephropathy when lowering immunosuppression is unsuccessful

TUBERCULOSIS PRE KIDNEY TRANSPLANT

- Potential recipients should be screened for latent tuberculosis (TB) infection prior to transplant
- Latent TB should ideally be treated prior to transplant
- Consideration should be given to delaying transplantation until at least some treatment for latent TB infection is administered (often not necessary to complete full course of treatment prior to proceeding with transplant)

TUBERCULOSIS POST KIDNEY TRANSPLANT

- Active tuberculosis usually occurs from reactivation of latent TB
- Reactivation is as much as 75 times more likely than in the general population
- The diagnosis of TB is most common in the first year post-transplant
- High incidence of extrapulmonary and disseminated disease

PNEUMOCYSTIS JIROVECI PNEUMONIA

- Most common in first 6 months to 1 year post-transplant in patients not taking prophylaxis
- Can also be seen in patients recently treated for an acute episode of rejection
- Typically presents as interstitial pneumonitis progressing to alveolar infiltrates in the absence of pleural effusions
- Elevated lactate dehydrogenase (LDH) (non-specific), days/weeks of fevers/cough/chest pain are clues to the diagnosis
- Diagnosis made by bronchoscopy—although lung biopsy often needed to increase yield—sensitivity of bronchoalveolar lavage (BAL) lower than in AIDS patients presenting with PCP
- Treatment with high doses of IV trimethoprim/sulfamethoxazole (usually with corticosteroids)
- Patients allergic to sulfas can be treated with IV pentamadine, atovaquone
- Pneumocystis jiroveci pneumonia is extremely rare in patients receiving prophylaxis with TMP/SMX, dapsone, atovaquone
- Recent reports of late cases of PCP are emerging, occurring after 1 year of transplantation in patients not taking prophylaxis
- We advocate lifelong prophylaxis with TMP-SMX

VARICELLA ZOSTER VIRUS (VZV)

- Increased risk in transplant patients
- Localized cutaneous disease is most common, usually respects midline of the body
- Vesicular/papular lesions on an erythematous base
- Cutaneous disseminated disease and visceral disease are more common in transplant recipients
- Treatment with acyclovir or its derivatives

CRYPTOCOCCUS

- Encapsulated yeast
- Ubiquitous in the environment
- Pigeon (and other birds) droppings and soil commonly harbor the organism
- Organism is inhaled and subsequently disseminates
- Lungs and central nervous system often affected
- Central nervous system (CNS) infection should always be ruled out (spinal tap), even in patients with no CNS manifestations

- Usually causes meningoencephalitis, less frequently pneumonitis and skin-soft tissue disease
- Treatment with amphotericin B (monitor in renal transplant recipients) together with 5-FC—triazoles can also be considered (fluconazole, voriconazole)—all interact with immunosuppressants—raising levels of calcineurin inhibitors

LISTERIA

- Foodborne pathogen
- Pathogen that takes advantage of reduced cell mediated immunity
- Meningitis, mid-brain abscesses-rhomboencephalitis
- Diagnosis by blood cultures, cerebrospinal fluid (CSF) analysis, brain biopsy
- Treatment: With Ampicillin, TMP-SMX if penicillin allergic

WEST NILE VIRUS

- Single-stranded RNA flavivirus
- Mosquito transmitted
- Most severe disease occurs in the elderly and the immunocompromised
- Encephalitis with high morbidity/mortality
- Diagnosis by lumbar puncture—cerebrospinal fluid (CSF) with lymphocytic predominance, elevated protein, normal glucose, Immunoglobulin M (IgM) West Nile antibodies
- PCR of West Nile virus in CSF
- West Nile IgM in blood
- No definitive treatment so counseling, prevention is critical

PARVOVIRUS

- Deoxyribonucleic acid (DNA) virus with bone marrow tropism
- Infects pronormoblast cells leading to aplastic crisis and profound anemia
- Diagnosis by parvovirus PCR (more reliable than Parvovirus IgM serology)
- Treatment with IV immunoglobulin

TOXOPLASMOSIS

- Rare protozoal infection
- Can develop as reactivation in patients exposed/infected pretransplant (Toxo IgG +)
- Can develop in recipients who are Toxo IgG- who receive grafts from Toxo IgG+ donors—although much less common in kidney recipients than in heart transplant recipients
- More frequent in highly immunocompromised recipients (such as those given induction treatment or being treated for acute rejection)

NOCARDIA

- Soil pathogen
- Ubiquitous in the environment
- Can cause pneumonia, brain abscess, skin-soft tissue infection
- Diagnosis by biopsy suspicious lesions
- Treatment with TMP-SMX—high doses with prolonged treatment

EPSTEIN-BARR VIRUS

- Herpes virus—as such becomes latent after initial infection
- Most adults will have evidence of prior exposure/infection by the time they undergo transplantation
- Uncommon cause of acute infection in transplant patients
- Reactivation often associated with PTLD

STRONGYLOIDES

- Immune suppression may cause reactivation
- Presents as a multisystem illness complicated by severe hyperinfections—including bacteremia, meningitis, urinary tract infections and pneumonias from enteric organisms
- Diagnosis by visualization of larvae by direct microscopy of stool, urine, bronchoalveolar fluid, upper intestinal fluid or biopsy specimens
- Treatment with thiabendazole
- Pretransplant screening for patients from endemic regions highly recommended

IMMUNE RECONSTITUTION

- As immunosuppressant doses are lowered and the immune system reconstitutes in the setting of infections, a paradoxical worsening of the clinical manifestations can sometimes be observed
- Treatment with corticosteroids may be necessary to manage this phenomenon

FURTHER READING

1. Cannon RM, Ouseph R, Jones CM, et al. BK viral disease in renal transplantation. Curr Opin Organ Transplant. 2011;16(6):576-9.
2. De Keyzer K, Van Laecke S, Peeters P, et al. Human cytomegalovirus and kidney transplantation: a clinician's update. Am J Kidney Dis. 2011;58(1):118-26.
3. DeVault GA, King JW, Rohr MS, et al. Opportunistic infections with Strongyloides stercoralis in renal transplantation. Rev Infect Dis. 1990;12(4):653-71.
4. Danziger-Isakov L, Kumar D, T Infectious Diseases Community of Practice. Vaccination in Solid Srgan transplantation. Am J Transplant. 2013;13(Suppl 4):311-7.
5. Dubberke ER, Burdette SD. Clostridium difficile Infections in Solid Organ Transplantation. Am J Transplant. 2013;13(Suppl 4):42-9.
6. Fishman JA. Infection in solid-organ transplant recipients. N Engl J Med. 2007;357:2601-14.
7. Fishman JA, Emery V, Freeman R, et al. Cytomegalovirus in transplantation—challenging the status quo. Clin Transplant. 2007;21(2):149-58.
8. Goto N, Oka S. Pneumocystis jirovecii pneumonia in kidney transplantation. Transpl Infect Dis. 2011;13(6): 551-8.
9. Gallon LG, Leventhal JR, Kaufman DB. Pretransplant evaluation of renal transplant candidates. Semin Nephrol. 2002;22(6):515-25.
10. Hibberd PL, Rubin RH. Renal transplantation and related infections. Semin Respir Infect. 1993;8(3):216-24.
11. Issa NC, Fishman JA. Infectious complications of antilymphocyte therapies in solid organ transplantation. Clin Infect Dis. 2009;48:772-86.
12. Marchand S, Tchernia G, Hiesse C, et al. Human parvovirus B19 infection in organ transplant recipients. Clin Transplant. 1999;13(1 Pt 1):17-24.
13. Malhotra P, Rai SD, Hirschwerk D. Duration of prophylaxis with trimethoprim-sulfamethoxazole in patients undergoing solid organ transplantation. Infection. 2012; 40(4):473-5.
14. Minari A, Husni R, Avery RK, et al. The incidence of invasive aspergillosis among solid organ transplant recipients and implications for prophylaxis in lung transplants. Transpl Infect Dis. 2002;4(4):195-200.
15. Nelson CA, Zunt JR. Tuberculosis of the central nervous system in immunocompromised patients: HIV infection and solid organ transplant recipients. Clin Infect Dis. 2011;53(9):915-26.
16. Patel R, Paya CV. Infections in solid-organ transplant recipients. Clin Microbiol Rev. 1997;10(1):86-124.
17. Randhawa P, Brennan DC. BK virus infection in transplant recipients: an overview and update. Am J Transplant. 2006;6(9):2000-5.
18. Subramanian AK. Antimicrobial prophylaxis regimens following transplantation. Curr Opin Infect Dis. 2011; 24(4):344-9.
19. Smith SR, Butterly DW, Alexander BD, et al. Viral infections after renal transplantation. Am J Kidney Dis. 2001 Apr;37(4):659-76.
20. Singh N, Huprikar S, Burdette SD, et al. Donor-derived fungal infections in organ transplant recipients: guidelines of the American Society of Transplantation, infectious diseases community of practice. Am J Transplant. 2012;12(9):2414-28.
21. Schaffner A. Pretransplant evaluation for infections in donors and recipients of solid organs. Clin Infect Dis. 2001;33(Suppl 1):S9-14.
22. Vilchez RA, Fung J, Kusne S. Cryptococcosis in organ transplant recipients: an overview. Am J Transplant. 2002;2(7):575-80.
23. Weigt SS, Gregson AL, Deng JC, et al. Respiratory viral infections in hematopoietic stem cell and solid organ transplant recipients. Semin Respir Crit Care Med. 2011;32(4):471-93.
24. Yu X, Han F, Wu J, et al. Nocardia infection in kidney transplant recipients: case report and analysis of 66 published cases. Transpl Infect Dis. 2011;13(4):385-91.
25. Yacoub R, Nader Kassis Ak. Urinary Tract Infections and Asymptomatic Bacteriuria in Renal Transplant Recipients. J Glob Infect Dis. 2011; 3(4):383-9.

CHAPTER 13

Oral Health Evaluation Prior to Transplant Surgery

William Stewart

"It is often stated that oral disease is the most common disease of mankind and quite possibly the one disease that all humans have in common..."

—*Oral Health in America 2000*[1]

Dental caries and periodontal disease are the most common infectious diseases in the United States.[2] All transplant patients should be considered to have these diseases to some extent. Both dental caries and periodontal disease are chronic in nature but they can have acute episodes that can be serious. In the acute phase, the infectious process follows the facial planes and can be life-threatening if the swelling restricts the airway.

In addition to dental caries and periodontal disease, there are lesions of the oral mucosa that should be evaluated prior to surgery. Close to 40,000 Americans will be diagnosed with oral or pharyngeal cancer this year. Oral cancer has a 5-year survival rate of 52%, a higher death rate than ovarian, brain, testicular, kidney, cervical, skin and liver cancer.[3]

For the transplant surgeon seeking to optimize the patients overall health prior to surgery, there are several potential problems from the oral cavity that must be considered. First, an acute episode of an odontogenic infection prior to surgery may result in a delay in the surgery and further compromise the patient's health. The more severe and extensive the dental caries and periodontal disease the more likely this event may occur. Second, severe periodontal disease over time decreases the support of tooth and the tooth becomes mobile and an aspiration risk especially during intubation for general anesthesia. Finally, chronic dental infections can cause transient bacteremia, especially during dental treatment. If the surgeon feels that the bacteremia is a potential a risk to the transplanted organ, then this infection should be resolved prior to the transplant.

An oral evaluation consisting of a complete oral examination and dental radiographs should be performed prior to surgery. The oral evaluation should be focused on potential problems that dental infections may cause in the period prior to the surgery and the immediate post-operative recovery period. Not only should the presence of dental disease should be noted but severity and the extent of the disease should be assessed.

Dental caries in the initial stages is not always visible clinically and can only be detected through dental radiographs (Fig. 1). If not treated early the dental caries advances and dark spots can be seen on the teeth as the infection penetrates the tooth structure (Fig. 2). Within the tooth is the blood supply and innervation, if the infection reaches this level there is pain and the infection has pathway to the deeper structure of the face. The dark spots that are accompanied with the destruction of tooth structure when visible on clinical examination means that the dental caries is advanced there is a greater potential for an acute episode of an odontogenic infection (Fig. 3).

DENTAL CARIES (FIGS. 1 TO 5)

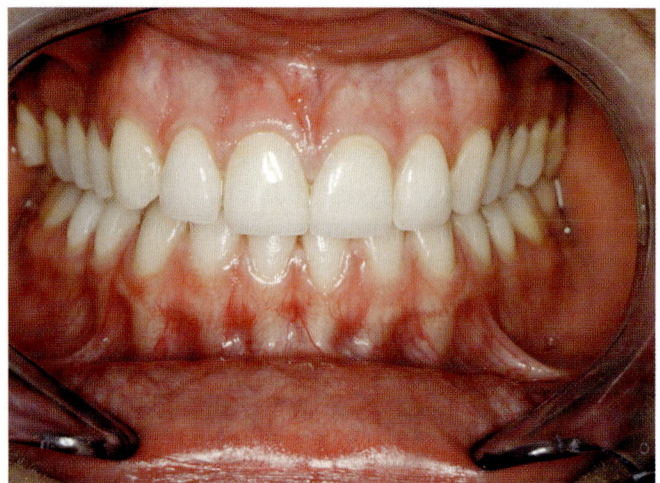

Fig. 1: Healthy dentition.

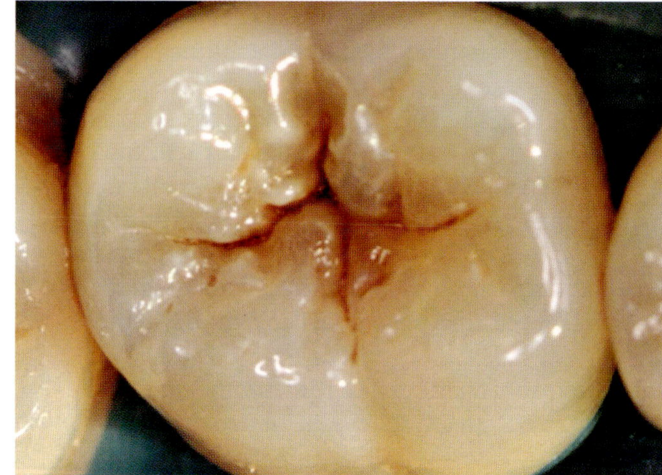

Fig. 2: Early disease—dark spots.

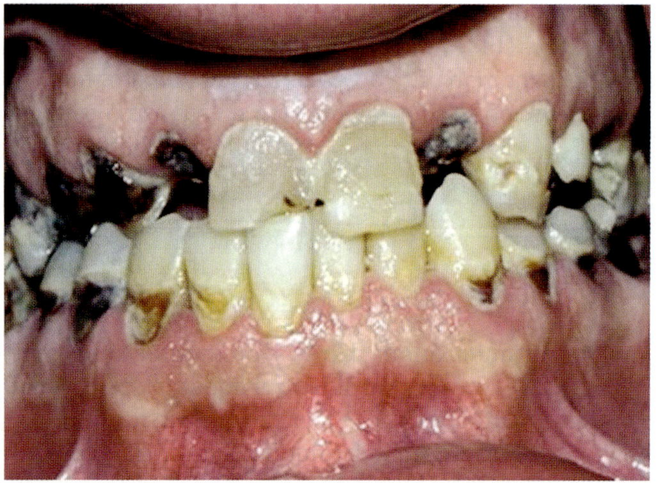

Fig. 3: Severe and extensive disease—dark spots with tooth destruction.

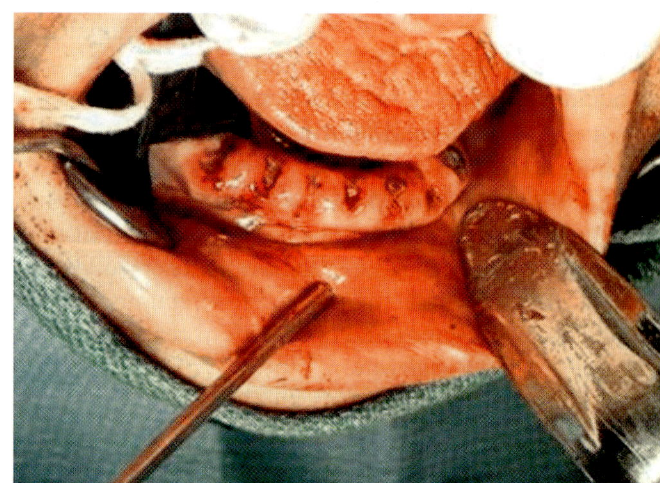

Fig. 4: Advanced disease—only root tips remaining very likely to cause acute infection.

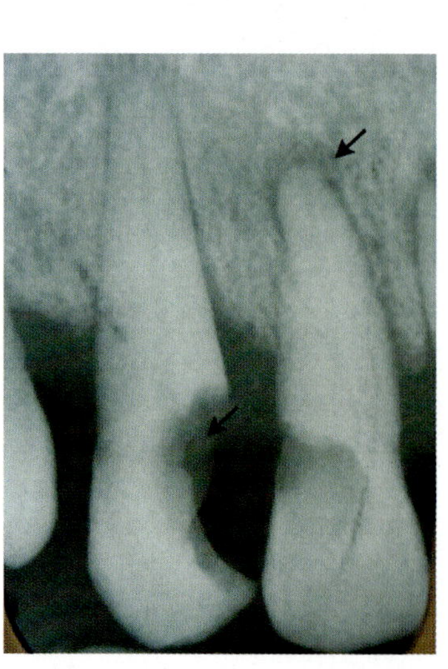

Fig. 5: Radiographic—radiolucent lesions in teeth and bone from dental infection.

PERIODONTAL DISEASE (FIGS. 6 TO 9)

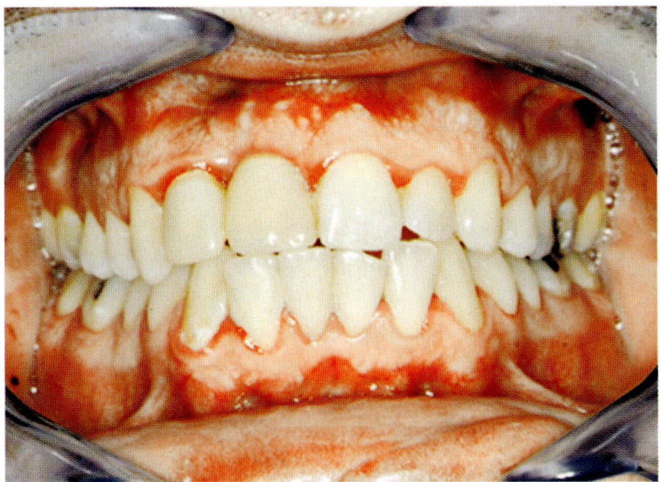

Fig. 6: Early periodontal disease—redness and bleeding of gingival tissue.

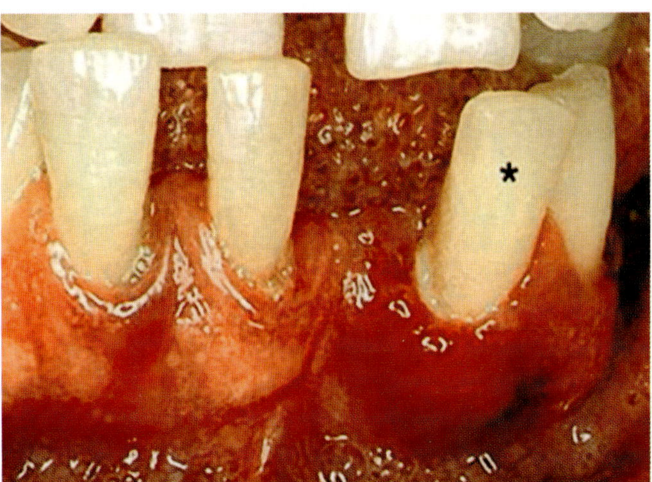

Fig. 7: Moderate periodontal disease—loss of tissue around tooth.

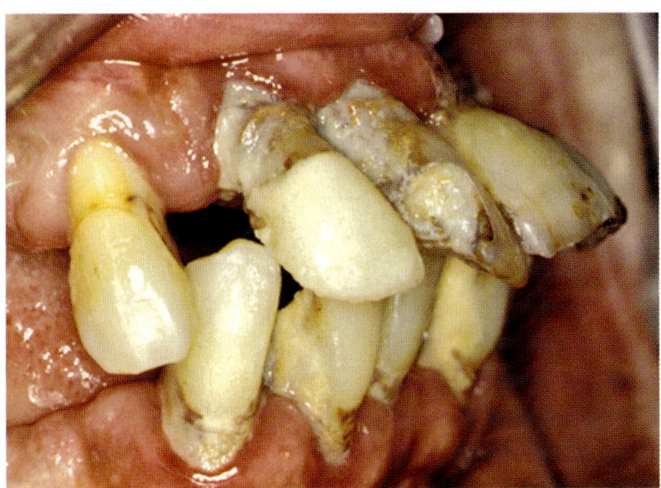

Fig. 8: Advanced periodontal disease—mobility (aspiration risk).

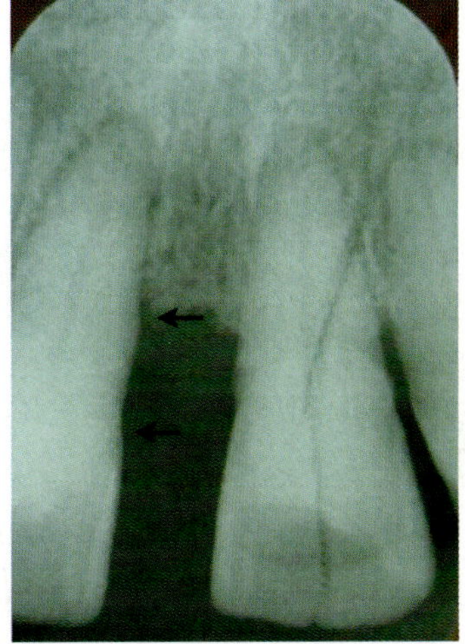

Fig. 9: Radiographic—loss of bone that supports tooth.

Periodontal disease is widely prevalent and can first be seen as redness around the teeth (Fig. 6). As the disease progresses there is a loss of tissue around the tooth and the teeth appear longer (Fig. 7). Severe periodontal disease is marked the mobility of teeth (Fig. 8). Periodontal disease is less likely to cause odontogenic facial infection but does have the same potential. The dental treatment of periodontal disease can cause transient bacteremia and this must be considered prior to surgery.

Finally, intraoral lesions must be evaluated prior to surgery. There are a great variety of lesions in the oral cavity; most will not be a problem before surgery. However, special attention must be made of ulcerative lesions in the oral cavity that do not have obvious cause. For example, a dental prosthesis may cause an irritation of the oral mucosa that is easily resolved and is not suspicious. On the other hand, an irritation without the prosthesis can be highly suspicious and should be considered for a biopsy (Fig. 13).

FACIAL SWELLING DUE TO ODONTOGENIC INFECTION (FIGS. 10 AND 11)

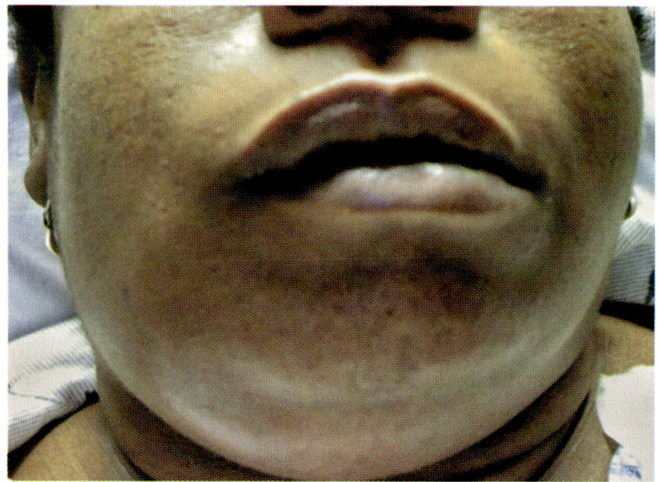

Fig. 10: Extraoral swelling—buccal space infection.

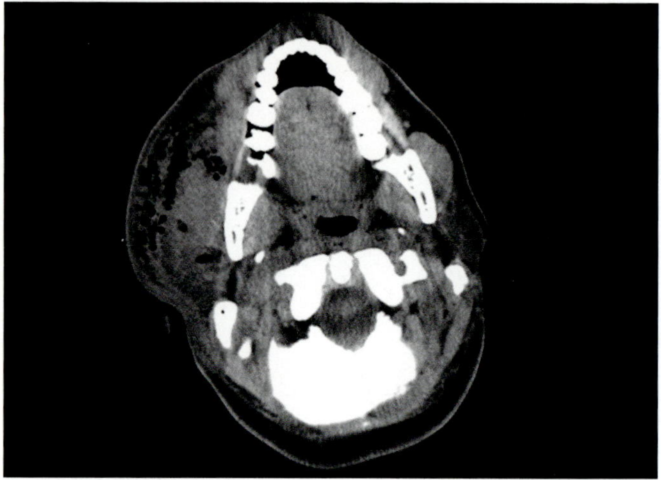

Fig. 11: Corresponding computed tomography (CT) scan.

ORAL PATHOLOGY (FIGS. 12 AND 13)

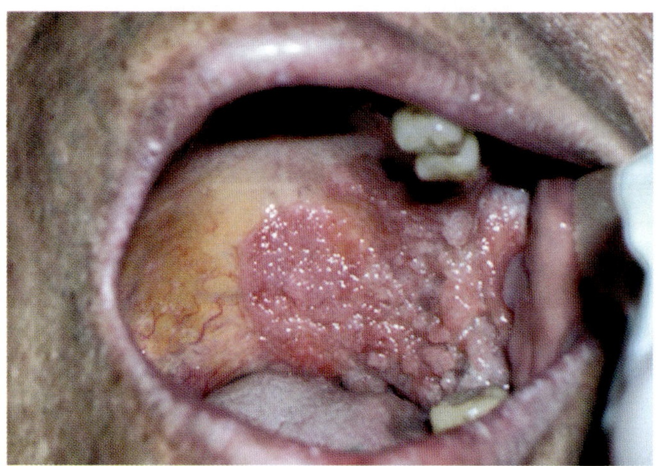

Fig. 12: Red lesions.

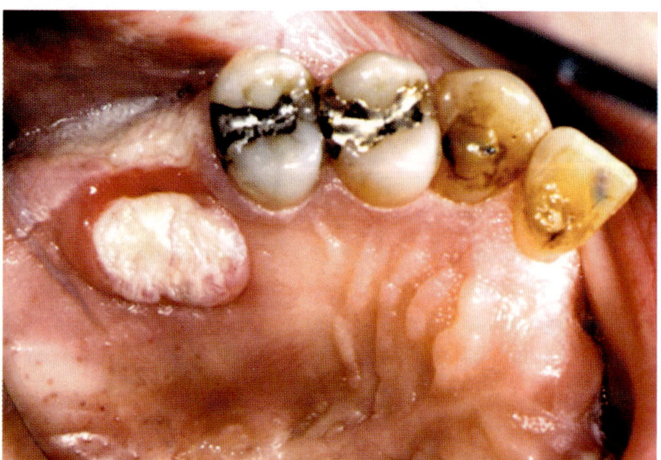

Fig. 13: White lesions.

The patient's level of oral health care is also important in determining if treatment will be required. Patients who can identify a dentist that they see on a regular basis and participate in the own oral health care are more likely to have their oral disease well controlled and are less likely to need treatment prior to surgery.

Identifying patients more likely to require dental treatment prior to surgery will allow a more expeditious referral, allow the treatment to be rendered prior to surgery and prevent the dental conditions from interfering with a good surgical outcome.

For the most part a presurgical dental evaluation is all that will be necessary. However, a clinical oral examination may help to identify patients more likely to need dental treatment. The need for dental treatment will be based on the severity, the extent of the disease and the previous level of care. The following areas need to be evaluated.

Severity of Disease

- Dental caries—visible signs of decay dark areas on teeth with evidence destruction of tooth structure
- Periodontal disease—redness, loss of support or mobility of teeth
- Oral lesions—any lesion should be followed, but there must be special attention to ulcerative lesions without apparent cause

Extent of Disease

Number of teeth exhibiting evidence of disease.

Level of Care

Lack of an identifiable dental provider that is seen on a regular basis.

There are several dental treatment options to remove sources of infection from the oral cavity. Patients, who have advanced dental disease, would require at least some of the teeth to be extracted. The treating dentist has two main concerns in rendering this treatment, the coagulation status of the patient and susceptibility of the patient to infections during treatment. In terms of homeostasis, multiple extractions require coordination between the providers especially if transfusions of blood products are needed to control postoperative bleeding. The healing period after extractions is generally 2–3 weeks. Recommendations as to antibiotic prophylaxis may be required depending on the patient's immune status and the ability to resist infections.

Disease of the oral cavity rarely prevents transplant surgery. However, if the disease is severe and extensive, intervention may be required. The following photographs demonstrate several examples of dental disease that can be seen during a clinical oral examination that require immediate attention and need for early referral for treatment.

REFERENCES

1. U.S. Department of Health and Human Services. Oral health in America: a report of the surgeon general—executive summary. Rockville, MD: U.S. Department of Health and Human Services, National Institute of Dental and Craniofacial Research, National Institutes of Health, 2000.
2. Beltrán-Aguilar ED, Barker LK, Canto MT, et al. Surveillance for dental caries, dental sealants, tooth retention, edentulism, and enamel fluorosis—United States, 1988-1994 and 1999-2002. MMWR Surveill Summ. 2005; 54:1.
3. Oral Cancer Foundation. [online] Available at http://www.oralcancerfoundation.org/facts/[Accessed July, 2013].

CHAPTER 14

Deceased Donor Management

Michael J Goldstein

THE CREATION OF THE ORGAN DONATION SYSTEM

Organ donation began well before the system created to support it. Dr Joseph Murray, a plastic surgeon from The Peter Bent Brigham Hospital in Boston, performed the first organ transplant in 1954.[1] The successful transplant placed a living identical twin's kidney into his brother well before the science of immunosuppression and the United Network for Organ Sharing (UNOS) system for organ donation and transplantation. Deceased organ donation and transplantation followed this milestone in 1962 at the same hospital with the first successful deceased donor kidney transplant. In 1969, physicians and scientists formed the Southeast Organ Procurement Foundation (SEOPF) as a membership and scientific organization for transplant professionals in Richmond, Virginia.[2] This organization became the foundation for a formal organ donation system in the United States. Many years later in 1977, SEOPF implemented the first computer-based organ matching system, dubbed the "UNOS". SEOPF established the Kidney Center in 1982, the predecessor of the UNOS organ center, for round-the-clock assistance in placing donated organs. UNOS, the agency for overseeing the national practice of donation and transplantation today, was created in 1984 after the National Organ Transplant Act (NOTA) was enacted.[3]

DONATION AND THE LAW

The foundation of our national organ donation system is based on the fundamental concept of "the gift". The uniform anatomical gift act was adopted in 1968, and amended through the years. This important legislation defined the donated organ as a gift and contains guidance on who may give, to whom gift may be given, how the gift is given and documented, how the gift may be revoked and immunity from liability in the process.[4] Furthermore, the President's council on determination of death enacted the Uniform Determination of Death Act in 1980. This Federal mandate was critical in defining death from either circulatory arrest or cessation of all neurologic function or brain death.[5] The adoption of NOTA in 1984 was the basis for the creation of the modern US system for organ donation. This legislation mandated formation of non-for-profit organ procurement organizations (OPO). It established the UNOS to oversee the organ procurement transplant network (OPTN), created the scientific registry for transplant recipients (SRTR), and defined requirements for transplant centers. Most importantly, NOTA defined the term "Organ" for donation purposes and prohibited organs for purchase.[3]

THE RIGHTS OF THE DONOR

The Uniform Anatomical Gift Act (UAGA) legally protects the right of the individual to become an organ donor. This act, revised many times and upheld by the states, legally protects the written authorization of the individual to become an organ donor. This concept of "first person authorization" (FPA) has been challenged numerous times by distraught family members and has been upheld by the justice system to protect the individual's right to become an organ donor after death if formally declared. Each state in the US has a donation "opt-in" registry for people to legally declare their wishes to become an organ donor. Without FPA on a state registry or the knowledge of an individual's known wish about organ donation, OPOs must approach the authorized party or next-of-kin to give authorization on behalf of the deceased individual to become an organ donor. The state UAGA defines the authorized party most responsible for acting on behalf of the deceased.[4]

UNDERSTANDING AND DEFINING BRAIN DEATH

The concept of brain death has been a double-edged sword for the donation process. The definition of brain death allows for the recovery of organs with the least amount of ischemic injury, thus promoting the best immediate organ function in the recipient. Prior to this definition, organs were only recovered for donation after the cessation of cardiac or circulatory function, now referred to as donation after circulatory determination of death (DCD). This process of DCD still occurs today in the US, but represents only 11% of the organ donor pool.[6] The disadvantages of the brain death definition are the limits in the number of medically suitable brain dead donors in the US for organ donation, the deleterious medical consequences of brain death on organ function in the donor, and the variability in the declaration process leading to missed opportunities and confusion around the "mystique" with public scrutiny.

Death by cessation of neurologic function or brain death was not defined legally until 1981. The Harvard ad hoc committee on irreversible coma first described the concept of brain death in 1967.[7] The concept of brain death for the purposes of organ donation has been one of the most challenging concepts for both medical professionals and the public. Brain death is defined as the irreversible cessation of all brain and brain stem functions. The challenge for medical professionals has been to establish a uniform practice for the declaration of brain death. Recently revised guidelines by the American Academy of Neurology have provided clarity on this subject.[8] Public misunderstanding of brain death remains an important challenge leading to many missed opportunities for organ donation. Some of the reasons for public discontent are related to cultural and religious beliefs. In addition, the declaration process for brain death is less tangible for family members to understand and confirm than the more obvious appearance of circulatory death.

THE TRANSITION FROM PATIENT TO DONOR

There is a critical period during which the strategy for medical professionals must shift from attempting to save the patient to salvaging and protecting organ function in a potential organ donor. The clinical presentation of advanced neurologic injury from head trauma, stroke, or anoxia begins with catastrophic brain injury management from the critical care team. The transition to consider potential organ donation begins with identified clinical triggers for which to notify the local OPO. The center for medicare and medicaid services (CMS) had mandated in 1998 conditions for participation for all hospitals to report all deaths and impending deaths to the local OPO for the purposes of improving organ donation.[9] It is an obligation for all medical professionals in CMS participatory hospitals to identify early clinical triggers for potential donation and refer these patients to the OPO. These clinical triggers differ among donation service areas, but may include patients with Glasgow coma scale (GCS) less than or equal to 5, those that appear to be without neurologic reflexes and will undergo brain death testing, planned ventilator withdrawals, and circulatory deaths.[10]

Once the patient is identified to have advanced neurologic injury and the referral for donation is made, the medical team at the donor hospital will begin the determination of brain death according to hospital policy. During this period, medical teams may frequently de-escalate the intensity of critical care support for medical futility reasons. It is during this period that significant metabolic and hemodynamic derangement may ensue due to the loss of neurologic function. At this time and even prior, it is necessary for the critical care team to consider the somatic survival of the organs for potential donation and anticipate and prevent deterioration of function after brain death. This brain death period is the most critical for the medical management of the potential organ donor.

The real potential for organ donation is never actually realized due to failures at many points in the transition from patient to donor. Some potential is lost in the identification and recognition phase for those that are never referred or are referred for donation too late. Other potential is lost in the authorization for donation phase, during which OPO professionals must interact with the authorized party to ask for donation authorization. Furthermore, the consequences of brain death lead to loss of potential donors from medical failures. Ultimately only 25–40% of potential donors are actually realized.

MEDICAL CONSEQUENCES OF BRAIN DEATH

The process of brain death has many complicating features. First, there is variability in the definition and declaration process among donor hospitals and by state law. Second, the rate of progression of brain death can dramatically alter the normal physiologic homeostatic milieu.[11] Pathophysiologic changes preceding brain death include cardiovascular instability in up to 80% of patients, as well as pulmonary and renal compromise.[12] Eighty-four percent of failed donors developed severe hypotension, leading to shock and organ loss. In addition, brain death leads to diabetes insipidus, disseminated intravascular coagulation, arrhythmias, hypothermia, hypoxia and acidosis.[13] These changes are directly related to endocrine failure at the level of the hypothalamic-pituitary axis.[14] The prevalence of anterior pituitary dysfunction approaches 30% of patients after traumatic brain injury.[15] The estimated circulating hormone reduction ranges from 15% to 80% in adrenal, thyroid, vasopressin and gonadal hormones.

Brain death involves not only hormonal and hemodynamic changes for the donor organs, but immunologic and inflammatory changes as well. Organs from deceased donors demonstrate inferior function and portend worse graft survival than organs from living donors. Studies have shown that the process of brain death creates a systemic proinflammatory response creating an end-organ inflammatory state. Kidney allografts after brain death release proinflammatory mediators granulocyte colony-stimulating factor, interleukin (IL)-6, IL-9, IL-16, and monocyte chemotactic protein-1 after reperfusion, suggesting a process that started in the donor.[16] Clinical studies of inflammation after brain death show evidence of tissue inflammation in kidney, liver, heart and lung transplantation.[17] Kuecuek et al. verified this proinflammatory process after brain death by studying the transcription of proinflammatory cytokines in living donors and in brain dead donors (DBD). The DBD had a significantly higher levels of tissue proinflammatory cytokines compared with living donor controls. Furthermore, deceased donors treated with corticosteroids expressed significantly reduced tissue and serum proinflammatory cytokines.[18] This link between brain death and a proinflammatory storm offers potential therapeutic advantage with predonation modulation of the immune system of the DBD.

HORMONAL AND ENDOCRINE SUPPORT

An important component to advanced medical management of the deceased donor is anticipation and prevention of the known complications mentioned previously. Restoring the circulating endocrine factors lost after hypothalamic/pituitary injury plays a key role in this prevention. This evidence dates back to 1987 by work from Novitzky describing profound benefits in donors treated with a hormonal cocktail of thyroid hormone, corticosteroids and insulin. Donors with hormonal treatment realized much improved cardiac output, reducedlactic acidosis, reduced hypotension, reduced hypothermia and increased opportunity for donation.[19] Research studies and clinical evidence have led to hormone replacement becoming part of standardized donor management upon declaration of brain death. Vasopressin is added to the endocrine support of the brain dead donor for the prevention and treatment of diabetes insipidus and refractory hypotension.

MAINTAINING SOMATIC SURVIVAL

The physiology of maintaining hemodynamic stability during donor management involves the interaction among the systemic capacitance, the pump and the systemic resistance. Systemic capacitance is the effective circulating volume or central venous pressure. This is usually the component most likely leading to hypotension when ineffectively managed. Critical care teams frequently treat initial hypotension with vasopressors inappropriately when volume resuscitation has not been satisfactory completed. In approaching donors with hypotension, we must consider hypovolemia secondary to the following:

- Blood loss
- Third spacing
- Diuretic treatment for reduction in intracranial pressure
- Diabetes insipidus
- Hyperglycemia

The pump represents our cardiac function. The reduction in cardiac contractility and cardiac output should be considered along with the restoration of circulating volume. Direct compression of the hypothalamic/pituitary access may cause an initial rush of circulating catecholamines or catecholamine "storm" followed by systemic depletion. Direct myocardial injury develops from high levels of circulating catecholamines, followed by a decline in inotropic support for cardiac contractility. Furthermore, other concomitant cardiac injuries should be considered related to cause of death, such as, contusion, tamponade or ischemic injury. Restoration of cardiac output is critical for adequate oxygen delivery for good end-organ function. Treatment is aimed at restoring right heart filling pressures, providing inotropic support with epinephrine, dobutamine, milrinone and/or calcium infusion.

Systemic resistance refers to the impedance of our arterial vascular resistance. The systemic resistance is necessary to generate an adequate blood pressure for perfusion. Refractory hypotension despite volume resuscitation should generate consideration for spinal shock, catecholamine depletion, adrenal failure and sepsis. Typically vasopressor support is necessary to increase vascular resistance.[20]

DONOR MANAGEMENT GOALS (TABLE 1)

The ongoing management of the brain-injured patient should not be unique for organ donation, but for all patients, and should reflect optimum ICU care.[21] There have been a number of standardized donor management strategies that have been published over the years.[20,22-25] There has been great variability in the OPO management strategies among the 58 OPOs, leading a team of donation leaders from California to call for a national sharing of donor-management goals (DMG).[26] Malinoski and colleagues developed 10 DMGs to provide guidance for OPO staff to improve the somatic health of deceased donor organs (Table 1). In the first retrospective study of DMGs and organ outcomes, this team of researchers established a relation between the number of goals met and OTPD. Of the DMGs introduced, there is evidence that oxygenation and cardiac ejection fraction are important factors leading to more organs transplanted when goals are met.[26] Other parts of the country had similar findings when employing the same set of DMGs to the local donor pool.[27] These innovative strategies have been shown to enhance the predonation organ quality, thereby providing in-situ organ resuscitation before the period of ischemia develops at the time of organ procurement.

Table 1: Donor management goals for NYODN

Critical care end point/donor management goals
MAP 60–110 mm Hg
CVP 4–10 mm Hg
EF > 50%
Vasopressor use ≤ 1
Arterial blood gas 7.3–7.5 pH
$PaO_2:FiO_2$ > 300 on PEEP = 5
Serum Na < 155 mEq/L
Blood glucose < 150 mg/dL
Urine output (averaged > 4 hours) 0.5 mL/kg/h or greater

(CVP: Central venous pressure; EF: Ejection fraction; MAP: Mean arterial pressure; NYODN: New York Organ Donor Network; PEEP: Positive end-expiratory pressure).

MINIMIZING RISK IN ORGAN DONATION

Inherent in the donation process is a risk of donor-transmitted disease to organ recipients. First, and foremost, in the process before we even consider organ quality is the assessment and minimization of risk of disease transmission. This risk evaluation is done through medical chart review, interviewing the patient's family and obtaining a medical/social history, physical exam of the donor, and vital radiologic and laboratory assessments for infections, malignancies and prior exposures through serologic testing.

Over the years, OPOs have become more aggressive at pursuing donors that were excluded in the past. The number of absolute contraindications have essential been reduced to only two, HIV and active extracranial malignancy.[28] There are numerous, rare and dangerous infections that should be considered high risk for transmission of disease, such as rabies, acute demyelinating viral encephalitis, amebic encephalitis, and lymphocytic choriomeningitis virus (LCMV). The NYODN infectious disease consultants have created a "Red flag" list (Table 2) to assist in identification of donor signs or symptoms that may increase donor risk.

Table 2: NYODN Red-flag indicators for organ donors

Encephalitis	Atypical diffuse rash +/– edema
Viral meningitis	Recent travel and clinical picture c/w Dengue fever
Cerebral edema of unknown etiology	Febrile illness with hemolytic anemia, +/– GI symptoms (possible Babesiosis)
Sepsis of unknown etiology	Infection/colonization with resistant bacteria
Flu-like illness or viral syndrome	Positive Chagas serology
Clinical picture c/w Guillain-Barré	Positive Strongyloides serology
Lymphopenia	Positive PPD/Quantiferon
Rare/unusual infectious disease	Cysticercosis
Recent unexplained weight loss	Ehrlichiosis

(GI: Gastrointestinal; PPD: Purified protein derivative).

Donation after Circulatory Determination of Death

Patients with advanced neurologic injury that do not deteriorate to brain death or those with terminal neuromuscular disease may be candidates for DCD. The general trigger for DCD is the consideration for removal of mechanical ventilatory support by either the next-of-kin or the patient him/herself. Once the end-of-life decisions have been made and either the patient or the AP has given authorization for organ donation, an assessment is made by the OPO for DCD candidacy. Each OPO and donor hospital has different standards for eligibility. In general there is a reasonable age restriction for those under 60 years due to transplant center selection bias. Furthermore, the patient must be evaluated for the potential for circulatory arrest within a specified time period after ventilator withdrawal, usually 60 minutes. This clinical assessment includes respiratory drive, hemodynamic stability, stability of airway, and comorbid conditions.

The success of DCD requires strict separation of the donation process from the end-of-life care given to the patient. Donor management, contrary to brain-dead donors, is not performed by the OPO since the patient is still alive. Medical support and comfort care is given to the patient by the donor hospital critical care team until the time of circulatory arrest. Do not resuscitate (DNR) orders must be observed to ensure that the end-of-life care is isolated from the donation process. The ventilator withdrawal process is usually performed in the operating room or in a perioperative suite to minimize the period of warm ischemia between circulatory arrest and organ recovery. A member of the critical care team is responsible for the extubation of the patient and providing comfort treatment to the patient. Systemic heparin is given for prevention of thrombus formation during circulatory failure. The members of the procurement team, excluding the donor management coordinator are far removed from the process of extubation to ensure that death is not hastened for the purpose of donation. The responsible physician declares death, after identification of circulatory arrest either by pulseless electrical activity (PEA) or asystole. A mandatory pause is required to ensure irreversibility prior to organ recovery, usually 5 minutes, but this varies by hospital. The DCD process may be ethically and emotionally challenging for members of the medical and OPO team. Excellent communication and collaboration among all team members is necessary for success.

Role of the Critical Care Team

The optimal management of the organ donor requires a proactive, multidisciplinary team. The team must be composed of collaborative members of the donor hospital and the OPO. Donor hospital team members should include intensivists, emergency medicine physicians, critical care nurses, respiratory therapists, pulmonologists, cardiologists, social workers, pastoral care workers. OPO team members should include transplant coordinators, family support providers, hospital development workers, clinical managers, and medical director. The primary focus for the donor hospital team is for early recognition for donor potential and timely referral to the OPO. It is the responsibility of the donor hospital team to provide declaration of brain death when appropriate, followed by collaboration with the OPO staff to provide optimal family and donor support.

REFERENCES

1. Watts G. Joseph Murray: innovative surgeon and pioneer of transplantation The Lancet 2011;377(9770) 987.
2. http://www.seopf.org/intro.htm.
3. PUBLIC LAW 98-507-OCT. 19, 1984 98 STAT. 2339.
4. National Conference of Commissioners on Uniform State Laws. 2009. Revised Uniform Anatomical Gift Act.
5. Uniform Determination Of Death Act National Conference Of Commissioners On Uniform State Laws 645 North Michigan Avenue, Suite 510 Chicago, Illinois 60611.
6. www.hrsa.gov/communitiesofpractice/AtaGlance/organdonation.pdf.
7. Landmark article Aug 5, 1968: A definition of irreversible coma. Report of the Ad Hoc Committee of the Harvard Medical School to examine the definition of brain death. JAMA. 1984;252(5): 677-9.
8. Evidence-based guideline update: determining brain death in adults: report of the Quality Standards Subcommittee of the American Academy of Neurology. Neurology. 2010;74(23): 1911-8.
9. http://www.gao.gov/products/OGC-98-58.
10. Organ/Tissue Donor Referral Triggers. New York Organ Donor Network. 2012.
11. Power BM, Van Heerden PV. The physiological changes associated with brain death-current concepts and implications for treatment of the brain dead organ donor. Anaesth Intensive Care. 1995;23(1):26-36.
12. Nygaard CE, Townsend RN, Diamond DL. Organ donor management and organ outcome: a 6-year review from a Level I trauma center. J Trauma. 1990;30(6):728-32.
13. Grossman MD, Reilly PM, McMahon D, et al. Who pays for failed organ procurement and what is the cost of altruism? Transplantation. 1996;27;62(12):1828-31.

14. Powner DJ, Boccalandro C, Alp MS, et al. Endocrine failure after traumatic brain injury in adults. Neurocrit Care. 2006;5(1):61-70.
15. Schneider M, Schneider HJ, Stalla GK. Anterior pituitary hormone abnormalities following traumatic brain injury. J Neurotrauma. 2005;22(9):937-46.
16. de Vries DK, Lindeman JH, Ringers J, et al. Donor brain death predisposes human kidney grafts to a proinflammatory reaction after transplantation. Am J Transplant. 2011;11(5):1064-70.
17. Barklin A. Systemic inflammation in the brain-dead organ donor. Acta Anaesthesiol Scand. 2009;53(4): 425-35.
18. Kuecuek O, Mantouvalou L, Klemz R, et al. Significant reduction of proinflammatory cytokines by treatment of the brain-dead donor. Transplant Proc. 2005;37(1):387-8.
19. Novitzky. Transplantation.1987;43:852-4.
20. Wood KE, Becker BN, McCartney JG, et al. Care of the potential organ donor. N Engl J Med. 2004;351(26): 2730-9.
21. Mascia L, Mastromauro I, Viberti S, et al. Management to optimize organ procurement in brain dead donors. Minerva Anestesiol. 2009;75(3):125-33. Epub 2008 Jan 24.
22. United Network for Organ Sharing: Donor Management Critical Pathway. [online] Available from http://www.unos.org [Accessed July 2013].
23. Zaroff JG, Rosengard BR, Armstrong WF, et al. Consensus conference report: maximizing use of organs recovered from the cadaver donor: cardiac recommendations, March 28-29, 2001, Crystal City, Va. Circulation. 2002;106(7):836-41.
24. Mascia L, Pasero D, Slutsky AS, et al. Effect of a lung protective strategy for organ donors on eligibility and availability of lungs for transplantation: a randomized controlled trial. JAMA. 2010;304(23):2620-7.
25. Hadjizacharia P, Salim A, Brown C, et al. Does the use of pulmonary artery catheters increase the number of organs available for transplantation? Clin Transplant. 2010;24(1):62-6.
26. Malinoski DJ, Daly MC, Patel MS, et al. Achieving donor management goals before deceased donor procurement is associated with more organs transplanted per donor. J Trauma. 2011;71(4):990-6.
27. Franklin GA, Santos AP, Smith JW, et al. Optimization of donor management goals yields increased organ use. Am Surg. 2010;76(6):587-94.
28. http://optn.transplant.hrsa.gov/PoliciesandBylaws2/policies/pdfs/policy_2.pdf.

CHAPTER 15

Donor Kidney Scoring Systems

Raghava B Munivenkatappa, Benjamin Philosophe

The benefits of renal transplantation for patients with end-stage renal disease on hemodialysis are well established, but currently there is a significant shortage of organs available for transplantation. In an effort to increase the size of the donor pool, donors that may have been excluded from donating previously are currently accepted. However, uses of these marginal kidneys have increased incidence of delayed graft function (DGF), acute rejection and have resulted in lower graft survival. Several strategies have been proposed to identify the donor risk factors that can impact allograft outcomes. Several donor clinical[1-3] and histopathological[4,5] scoring systems have been used to predict graft function. This has implications for organ utilization and potential to improve graft survival with proactive modification of immunosuppression.

Biopsy evaluation of donor kidney is particularly important for marginal organs to determine organ suitability. Although significant progress has been made in the field, controversy still remains regarding the value of individual pathologic parameters to predict graft outcome. Currently, donor selection is primarily based on degree of glomerular sclerosis, interstitial fibrosis, and vascular pathology.

MARYLAND AGGREGATE PATHOLOGY INDEX

Maryland aggregate pathology index (MAPI)[5] is an aggregate pathology score that is based on the evaluation of donor pathological features that are predominantly related to ischemic and hypertensive injury affecting glomeruli and vessels. The model comprises of five pathologic elements and was developed using a large cohort of deceased donor kidneys and validated using a different cohort. The histologic elements that were shown to statistically impact graft outcome included 15% or higher glomerulosclerosis, any degree of arteriolar hyalinosis, arterial sclerosis with a wall to lumen ratio in interlobular arteries of more than 0.5 (equivalent to BANFF > cv2 lesion), cortical scar, and presence of periglomerular fibrosis of arterial sclerosis (Figs. 1A to E). Points were assigned to each of these histopathologic variables based on the hazard ratio for graft loss obtained from Cox proportional hazard univariate analysis (Table 1). Interstitial fibrosis was not included in the MAPI score because it did not correlate with graft outcome. Assessment of interstitial fibrosis has poor reproducibility in interobserver and intraobserver variability studies.[6]

The MAPI score ranges from 0 to 15 points. A receiver operating curve analysis indicated that scores of 7 and 11 were sensitive threshold cutoffs for grouping MAPI scores into low, intermediate and high risk for graft failure. The 5-year graft survival for kidneys with MAPI scores from 0–7 (low risk) was 90%; for those with scores of 8–11 (intermediate risk), 63%; and for those with scores from 12 to 15 (high risk), 53%. Further validation of the MAPI scoring system was done by its prospective use in independent cohorts of deceased donors from two separate transplant centers. Overall, the MAPI score performs better as a predictor of graft survival than the Kidney Donor Risk Index, a clinical scoring system.[7]

NYBERG DECEASED DONOR SCORING SYSTEM AND IMPROVED SCORING SYSTEM (ISS)

Nyberg et al.[1] reviewed clinical parameters of 90 non-machine perfused deceased donors (DD) and recipients from center 1 to develop an donor scoring system with 30 day iothalamate creatinine clearance (30DCL) as

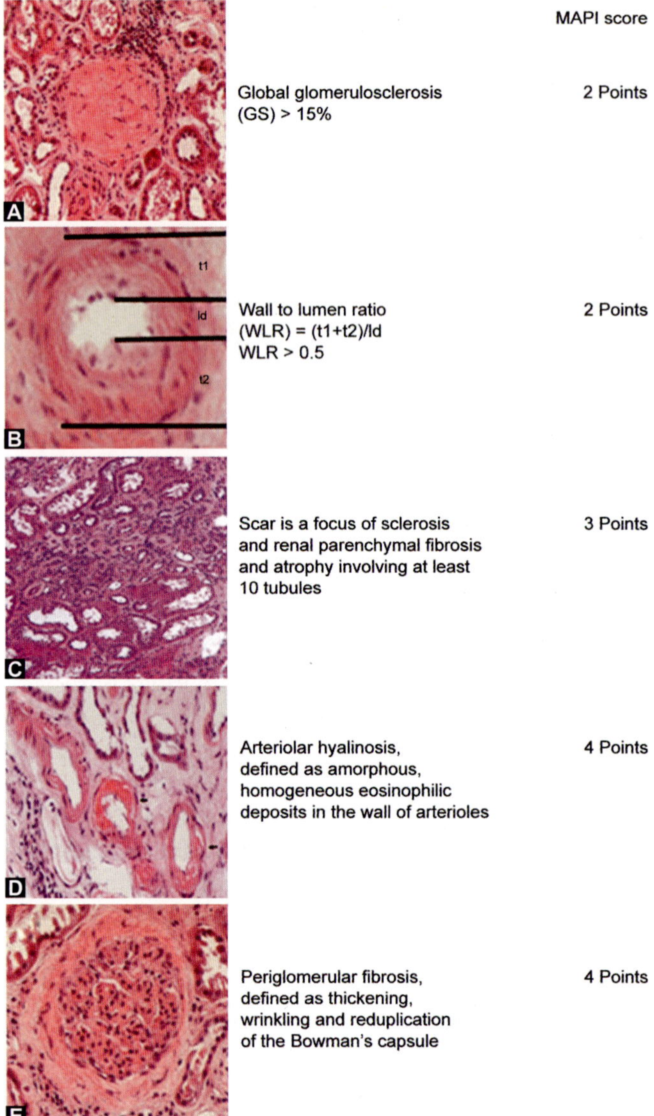

Figs. 1A to E: MAPI pathological features as observed on pre-implantation frozen sections. (A) Global glomerulosclerosis; (B) Measurements for arterial wall-to-lumen ratio (WLR) calculation, including the thickness of two walls (t1 and t2) and the luminal diameter (ld); WLR = (t1 + t2)/ld; (C) Scar with features of interstitial fibrosis, tubular atrophy and glomerulosclerosis; (D) Arteriolar hyalinosis); (E) Periglomerular fibrosis.

endpoint. The Nyberg Deceased Donor Scoring System (DDS) was validated with 141 DD donor and recipient pairs from a second independent center and prospectively applied to a new set of 26 donor and recipient pair from center 1.

- Clinical donor parameters for DDS that significantly correlated with 30DCL
- Cerebral vascular accident (CVA) as cause of death (6 points); others (0 point)
- History of hypertension in years (0 years = 0 point; 1–9 years = 3 points; ≥ 10 years = 6 points)
- Cockcroft-Gault estimated creatinine clearance (mL/min)(≥ 90 = 0 points; 80–89 = 1 point; 70–79 = 2 points; 60–69 = 3 points; 50–59 = 4 points; < 50 = 6 points)
- Donor age (< 50 = 0 points; 50–54 = 1 point; 55–59 = 2 points; 60–64 = 3 points; 65–69 = 4 points; >70 = 6 points)
- History of diabetes mellitus (DM) 3 points versus 0 for no DM
- Cold ischemia time in hours (< 12 = 0 points; 12–24 = 1 point; 25–36 = 2 points; > 36 = 3 points)
- Severity of renal artery plaque (None = 0 points; mild = 1 point; moderate = 2 points; severe = 3 points)
- The DDS which ranged between 0–32 was stratified into four grades A (0–5 points), B (6–10 points), C (11–15) and D (≥ 16)

In 2003 the DDS was modified into the improved scoring system (ISS)[3] by analysis of clinical information from 34,324 patients from UNOS scientific renal transplant registry. The donor parameters that correlated with 6 months creatinine clearance were used to develop the ISS. These include:

- Donor age (< 30 = 0 points; 30–39 = 5 point; 40–49 = 10 points; 50–59 = 15 points; 60–69 = 20 points; >70 = 25 points)
- History of hypertension in years (None = 0 point; yes; duration unknown= 2 points; ≤ 5 years = 2 points; 6–10 years = 3 points; >10 years = 4 points)
- Cerebral vascular accident as cause of death (3 points); others (0 point)
- human leukocyte antigen (HLA) mismatch (0 = 0 point; 1–2 = 1 points; 3–4=2 points; 5–6 = 3 points)

The ISS which ranges from 0–39 was stratified into four grades A (0–9 points), B (10–19 points), C (20–29) and D (30–39). The scores > 20 had poor graft function and graft survival at 6-year. The score of 20 and greater was suggested as a cutoff for marginal donor kidneys.

KIDNEY DONOR RISK INDEX

Kidney donor risk index (KDRI)[2] is a continuous donor scoring system which was developed by analyzing 69,440 donor recipient pair data from scientific renal transplant registry in order to measure the risk of the various factors known to influence graft failure. KDRI consists of fourteen donor and transplant parameters, each found to be independently associated with graft failure or death.

Table 1: Individual histopathologic parameters and MAPI scores

Pathology variable	Univariate hazard ratio	P	Index score Present	Index score Absent
Hyalinosis of glomerular arterioles	3.93	0	4	0
Glomerulosclerosis ≥ 15%	1.87	0.009	2	0
Interlobular artery wall to lumen ratio ≥ 0.5	2.05	0.008	2	0
Periglomerular fibrosis	4.09	0.002	4	0
Scar	2.58	0.011	3	0

Based on the hazard ratio an index score value was attributed to each parameter and were added resulting in the Maryland aggregate pathology index (MAPI). Score ranges from 0–15.

The 10 donor parameters include age, race, history of hypertension, history of diabetes, serum creatinine, CVA as cause of death, height, weight, donation after cardiac death, and positive hepatitis C virus status. The four transplant parameters include HLA-B and HLA-DR mismatch, cold ischemia time, double or en bloc transplants.

Formula to Calculate KDRI

KDRI = Exp(−0.0194XI [age < 18 year]X[age−18 year] +0.0128X[age-40 year] + 0.0107XI[age > 50 year]X[age-50 year]+0.179XI [race=African American]+0.126XI [hypertensive]+0.130XI [diabetic]+0.220X[serum creatinine >1 mg/dL]−0.209XI [serum creatinine >1.5 mg/dL] X[serum creatinine-1.5 mg/dL]+0.0881XI [cause of death =cerebrovascular accident]−0.0464X[{height-170 cm}/10] −0.0199XI[weight < 80 kg]X[{weight_80kg}/5]+0.133XI [donation after cardiac death] +0.240XI [hepatitis C positive]-0.0766XI [HLA-B mismatch=0]-0.0610X I [HLA-B mismatch=1]−0.130XI [HLA-DR mismatch = 0]+0.0765XI [HLA-DR mismatch=2]+0.00548X[cold ischemia time-20 hour]−0.364XI[en bloc transplant]−0.148XI [double kidney transplant]), where I (A) is set to 1 if condition A applies to the donor kidney of interest (i.e. if the donor kidney of interest possesses condition A), and otherwise it is set to 0.

- Reference donor with KDRI of 1 = Age = 40, non-African American, serum creatinine 1.0 mg/dL, non-hypertensive, nondiabetic, cause of death other than cerebrovascular accident, height 170 cm, weight more than or equal to 80 kg, brain dead donor (not donation after cardiac death), and HCV negative
- Reference transplant = two mismatches at the HLA-B locus and one mismatch at the HLA-DR locus, with > 20 hour of cold ischemia time
- The KDRI score reflected the rate of graft failure relative to that of a reference donor
- The graft survival for the highest KDRI quintile (>1.45) had an adjusted 5-year graft of 63%, compared with 82% and 79% in the two lowest KDRI quintiles (< 0.79 and 0.79- < 0.96, respectively)

REMUZZI SCORE

The subjective semi-quantitative scoring system was created as a result of a consensus by an international panel of pathologists.[4]

- For evaluation of donor kidneys > 60 years of age
- To estimate number of nephrons and the suitability of the organ as single or dual transplant
- Score ranged between a minimum of 0 to a maximum of 12 with 0 being normal pathology and 12 indicating severe renal pathology
- Four renal parenchyma parameters were considered namely:
  - Glomerular global sclerosis (GS) (0 = absent, 1≤ 20% GS, 2 = 20–50% GS and 3 ≥ 50% GS)
  - Degree of tubular atrophy (TA) (0 = absent, 1 ≤ 20% TA, 2 = 20–50% TA and 3 ≥ 50% TA)
  - Degree of interstitial fibrosis (IF) (0 = absent, 1 ≤ 20% IF, 2 = 20–50% IF and 3 ≥ 50% IF)
  - Degree of arterial and arteriolar narrowing (0 = absent, 1 = increased wall thickness but to a degree that is less than the diameter of the lumen, 2 = wall thickness that is equal or slightly greater to the diameter of the lumen, 3 = wall thickness that far exceeds the diameter of the lumen with extreme luminal narrowing or occlusion)
- Donor kidney organs with scores of ≤ 3 were used as single transplants, 4–6 scores were used as dual transplants and > 7 were discarded

REFERENCES

1. Nyberg SL, Matas AJ, Rogers M, et al. Donor scoring system for cadaveric renal transplantation. Am J Transplant. 2001;1(2): 162-70.
2. Rao PS, Schaubel DE, Guidinger MK, et al. A comprehensive risk quantification score for deceased donor kidneys: the kidney donor risk index. Transplantation. 2009;88(2):231-6.
3. Nyberg SL, Matas AJ, Kremers WK, et al. Improved scoring system to assess adult donors for cadaver renal transplantation. Am J Transplant. 2003;3(6):715-21.
4. Remuzzi G, Grinyo J, Ruggenenti P, et al. Early experience with dual kidney transplantation in adults using expanded donor criteria. Double Kidney Transplant Group (DKG). J Am Soc Nephrol. 1999;10(12):2591-8.
5. Munivenkatappa RB, Schweitzer EJ, Papadimitriou JC, et al. The Maryland aggregate pathology index: a deceased donor kidney biopsy scoring system for predicting graft failure. Am J Transplant. 2008;8(11):2316-24.
6. Mazzucco G, Magnani C, Fortunato M, et al. The reliability of pre-transplant donor renal biopsies (PTDB) in predicting the kidney state. A comparative single-centre study on 154 untransplanted kidneys. Nephrol Dial Transplant. 2010 Oct;25(10):3401-8.
7. Raghava Munivenkatappa SS, Malat G, Ranganna K, et al. Validation of the Maryland Aggregate Pathology Index (MAPI) on preimplantation biopsies (PIB) as a predictor of graft outcome at two independent transplant centers. A J Transplant.10(4):156.

CHAPTER 16

Deceased Donor Considerations

Georgios C Sotiropoulos, Andreas Paul

PROLONGED COLD ISCHEMIA TIME

- Prolonged cold ischemia time has been reported to be associated with impaired graft survival
- In our experience, satisfactory outcomes have been observed in the setting of cold ischemia time more than or equal to 20 hours with:
  - Grafts from donors under 60 years of age
  - In first-time recipients
- Induction therapy with an interleukin-2 antagonist is preferred

ELDERLY DONORS

- Transplantation of kidneys from donors more than or equal to 75 years of age is controversial
- In our experience, satisfactory outcomes can be potentially achieved with such kidneys in elderly recipients when:
  - Dual kidney grafting is used
  - In the absence of:
    - Re-transplantation
    - Surgical complications

HYPOTHERMIC MACHINE PERFUSION

Continuous pulsatile hypothermic machine perfusion has been found to be associated with:

- Reduced risk of delayed graft function and improved graft survival in the first year after transplantation
- Reduced rate of never-functioning kidneys and improve the 1-year graft survival rate of kidneys with delayed graft function (DGF) for kidneys from donors aged more than or equal to 65 years
- Improved quality-adjusted life-years while reducing costs
- Reduced risk of DGF and improved 1-year graft survival and function of expanded criteria donors (ECD) kidneys
- Reduced risk of DGF and better early graft function up to 1 month after transplantation of donor after cardiac death (DCD) kidneys

CENTERS FOR DISEASE CONTROL AND PREVENTION (CDC) HIGH RISK DONORS

Extended Criteria Donors

- The acceptance of high risk centers for disease control and prevention (CDC) donors extended criteria donors (ECD) is based on each individual transplant center guidelines
- Recipients should always be made aware of this fact and provided with the necessary information
- Counseling specific to each circumstance should always be provided if requested by the candidate
- Thorough documentation is required as per UNOS guidelines

DONORS UNDER 5 YEARS OF AGE

- Donors in this category can be transplanted en bloc or independently
- Outcomes of single grafts seem to be satisfactory in pediatric recipients

TRANSPLANTATION SIMULTANEOUS WITH IMPLANTATION OF VASCULAR GRAFTS

- Atherosclerotic disease is almost universally encountered in kidney transplant recipients
- Occasionally, simultaneous reconstruction with vascular prosthetic grafts (such as aortofemoral bypass grafting) may be required to achieve improved arterial flow to both graft and lower extremity of the recipient
- These procedures were found to be safe and to optimize outcomes
- It is recommended that an experienced vascular surgeon be involved in the procedure

FURTHER READING

1. Gallinat A, Feldkamp T, Schaffer R, et al. Single-center experience with kidney transplantation using deceased donors older than 75 years. Transplantation. 2011;92(1):76-81.
2. Gallinat A, Moers C, Treckmann J, et al. Machine perfusion versus cold storage for the preservation of kidneys from donors ≥ 65 years allocated in the Eurotransplant Senior Programme. Nephrol Dial Transplant. 2012;27(12):4458-63.
3. Gallinat A, Paul A, Minor T, et al. Optimized outcomes for renal allografts with cold ischemic times of 20 h or greater. Int Urol Nephrol. 2012;44(5):1417-23.
4. Gallinat A, Sotiropoulos GC, Witzke O, et al. Kidney grafts from donors ≤5 years of age: Single kidney transplantation for pediatric recipients or en-bloc transplantation for adults? Pediatr Transplant. 2013;17(2):179-84.
5. Groen H, Moers C, Smits JM, et al. Cost-effectiveness of hypothermic machine preservation versus static cold storage in renal transplantation. Am J Transplant. 2012; 12(7):1824-30.
6. Jochmans I, Moers C, Smits JM, et al. Machine perfusion versus cold storage for the preservation of kidneys donated after cardiac death: a multicenter, randomized, controlled trial. Ann Surg. 2010;252(5):756-64.
7. Moers C, Smits JM, Maathuis MH, et al. Machine perfusion or cold storage in deceased-donor kidney transplantation. N Engl J Med. 2009;360(1):7-19.
8. Ozçelik A, Treckmann J, Paul A, et al. Results of kidney transplantation with simultaneous implantation of vascular graft. Transplant Proc. 2007;39(2):509-10.
9. Treckmann J, Moers C, Smits JM, et al. Machine perfusion versus cold storage for preservation of kidneys from expanded criteria donors after brain death. Transpl Int. 2011;24(6):548-54.

CHAPTER 17

Infectious Risks Associated with Donors

Dorry Segev

HISTORY

- Based on 1994 guidelines published by the Centers for Disease Control and the Public Health Service (from Morbidity and Mortality Weekly Report titled "Guidelines for preventing transmission of HIV through transplantation of human organs")
- Patients who fall into seven behavioral categories are categorized as high risk for infectious transmission of HIV or hepatitis C virus (HCV) (colloquially referred to as "CDC high risk")
- The "CDC high risk donor" designation is collected by the organ procurement and transplantation network (OPTN) and reported to the organ procurement organizations (OPOs), physicians, and patients considering the organ
- The OPTN requires that the OPO give the physicians the information, and that the physicians provide the patients the information (with appropriate informed consent specific to the high infectious risk designation)

BEHAVIORAL CATEGORIES

- Men who have had sex with another man (MSM) in the preceding 5 years
- Persons who report nonmedical intravenous, intramuscular or subcutaneous injection of drugs (IDU) in the preceding 5 years
- Persons with hemophilia or related clotting disorders who have received human-derived clotting factor concentrates
- Men and women who have engaged in sex in exchange for money or drugs (commercial sex workers, CSW) in the preceding 5 years
- Persons who have had sex in the preceding 12 months with any person described above or with a person known or suspected to have HIV infection
- Persons who have been exposed in the preceding 12 months to known or suspected HIV-infected blood through percutaneous inoculation or through contact with an open wound, nonintact skin, or mucous membrane
- Inmates of correctional systems

IN PRACTICE

- These donors make up around 10% of the current donor pool
- Discard rates are higher for these donors, despite the fact that they are high-quality donors (other than the risk of unintended transmission of HIV or HCV, which turns out to be quite low, *see* below)

TESTING

- Two major testing methods are available: antibody testing (ELISA) and nucleic acid testing (NAT)
- Nucleic acid testing is not required by the OPTN, and is not even available in some OPOs
- A national survey suggested that use of NAT increases physician willingness to accept organs from CDC infectious risk donors

- A consensus conference concluded that there is insufficient evidence to require NAT, particularly because of high false-positive rates (which put organs at high risk for discard)
- The window period is the time between acquisition of the infection and serologic detectability; for example, if the window period is 7 days, and the donor is tested on the 20th of the month, any infection the donor acquired between the 14th and the 20th would not be detected
- The window period becomes relevant for donors with ongoing risky behavior
- The window period depends on the disease (HIV versus HCV) and the testing method (ELISA versus NAT); for HIV, it is around 3 weeks for ELISA and 1 week for NAT; for HCV, it is around 9 weeks for ELISA and 1 week for NAT
- The risk if undiagnosed HIV and HCV (and as a result, unintended transmission) exists for all donors, but is supposedly higher for those classified as "CDC high risk"

RISK OF INFECTION

- In general, the risk of infection is very low, particularly in the context of the risk of other complications of transplantation as well as the risk of not undergoing the transplant
- Based on a meta-analysis, the estimated risk of undetected HIV infection in a donor tested with NAT is 4.2 per 10,000 donors for MSMs, 4.9 for IDUs, 2.7 for CSWs, and less than 1 per 10,000 for other categories
- Based on a meta-analysis, the estimated risk of undetected HCV infection in a donor tested with NAT is 3.5 per 10,000 donors for MSMs, 32.4 for IDUs, 12.3 for CSWs, 12.3 for individuals having sex with categories #1–4, and less than 1 per 10,000 for other categories

TRANSMISSIONS

- At the time of writing, there was only one reported transmission of HIV through deceased donor solid organ transplantation since 1986
- This transmission of both HIV and HCV occurred in 2007 from one donor into 4 recipients
- This isolated transmission resulted in physician response out of proportion to the transmission risk

PATIENT COUNSELING

- Using a Markov decision process model (available at www.transplantmodels.com/IRD), it is possible to assist patients in making the choice of "accept the infectious risk organ currently being offered" or "wait on the waiting list for the next non-infectious risk offer"
- For most patient phenotypes, there is a significant survival advantage from accepting an infectious risk organ

CHAPTER 18

Live Donor Evaluation

Mala Sachdeva

The following evaluations should be performed for a potential living kidney donor:

- Medical, including individualized cardiac assessment
- Psychosocial
- Ethical/Legal

Donor evaluation can be divided into:

ASSESSMENTS TO PROTECT THE HEALTH AND SAFETY OF THE DONOR

Medical Assessment

Age

- Advanced age (defined as age above 65), may be associated with decreased recipient graft and patient survival; both recipient and donors should be fully informed in regard to potential long-term disadvantages
- Younger than 18 years are generally excluded due to uncertain future long-term consequences of donation, and possible maturity level of the potential donor

Diabetes Mellitus

- Initiate screening with hemoglobin A1c (A1c), and/or fasting blood glucose (FBG)
- A two hour oral glucose tolerance test [2h-oral glucose tolerance test (OGTT)] should be performed in donors with:
  - Abnormal hemoglobin A1c or FBG
  - History of gestational diabetes
  - Family history of diabetes mellitus
- Diabetic donors should be excluded (A1c ≥ 6.5%, fasting glucose ≥ 126 mg/dL (7.0 mmol/L), 2h-OGTT ≥ 200 mg/dL (11.1 mmol/L), or a person with classic symptoms of hyperglycemia or a random plasma glucose ≥ 200 mg/dL (11.1 mmol/L)
- Prediabetic donors (A1C of 5.7–6.4%, fasting glucose of 100 mg/dL [5.6 mmol/L] to 125 mg/dL [6.9 mmol/L]) or a 2h-OGTT value of 140 mg/dL [7.8 mmol/L] to 199 mg/dL [11.0 mmol/L]) should discouraged from donating and must be counseled on lifetime risk of developing diabetes and end stage kidney disease, and lifestyle modifications

Hypertension

- Obtain two blood pressure readings on separate occasions
- Twenty-four hour ambulatory blood pressure monitoring can confirm any abnormal blood pressure reading or concern
- Prehypertensives (blood pressure ranging from 120 mm Hg to 139 mm Hg systolic and/or 80–89 mm Hg diastolic) should be identified and counseled; uncertainty on whether to exclude them as potential donors still exists as they are at increased risk of developing hypertension, kidney disease from hypertension, and cardiovascular disease
- Hypertensive donors who are on one medication or whose blood pressure is well-controlled with dietary means can be accepted with great caution
- A donor on one medication can be accepted as long as blood pressure had been well controlled for at least 6 months prior to evaluation and there is no evidence of target organ damage including:
  - Microalbuminuria
  - Left ventricular hypertrophy or other cardiac disease
  - Ophthalmologic changes

- A donor with a history of hypertension on two or more medications, should generally be excluded
- Due to a genetic predisposition to developing hypertension, individuals with a family history of hypertension must be counseled
- Caution with accepting donors with prehypertension or hypertension who are African American or Hispanic

Prehypertensives or Hypertensives must be Counseled on Possible Long-term Consequences of Donating

Pregnancy

- Pregnant patients are excluded
- All female potential donors of childbearing age who are contemplating future pregnancy should be counseled on the potential risks of donating including:
  - Gestational diabetes
  - Gestational hypertension
  - Preeclampsia
  - Prematurity
  - Fetal loss
- A high level of surveillance and monitoring is suggested for all pregnant women postdonation

Renal Assessment

Glomerular Filtration Rate

- Obtain a 24-hour urine for creatinine clearance on all donors; ensure accurate collection
- Further evaluation with radionuclide methods can be performed
- Majority transplant centers cutoff for glomerular filtration rate (GFR) is less than 80 mL/min/1.73 m^3

Proteinuria

- Assess proteinuria with a 24-hour urine collection; ensure accurate collection
- Cutoff for exclusion varies from greater than 150 mg/day to 300 mg/day, depending on transplant center policy

Hematuria

- Assess with a urinalysis
- If significant microscopic hematuria then determine the etiology:
  - Dysuria, urinary frequency and the presence of pyuria can suggest a urinary tract infection; confirm with urine culture
  - In men, prostate issues should be ruled out
  - In women, make sure the urine specimen was not taken at the time of menstruation
  - African American patients should be screened for sickle cell disease or trait
  - Family history of renal disease including polycystic kidney disease, thin basement membrane disease, or Alport's syndrome or the presence of concomitant proteinuria can suggest an underlying glomerular cause of hematuria in the donor
- Renal ultrasound should be able to reveal most structural causes
- Consider renal biopsy
- If there is a family history of renal cell carcinoma or strong smoking history evaluate for malignancy with a urologic evaluation, urine cytology and cystoscopy

Nephrolithiasis

- Determine the number of stones the potential donor has formed in the past
- If the disease has been quiescent and there are no abnormalities in metabolic or radiologic testing, then donating can be acceptable with information of the lifetime risk for developing another stone
- If there is a history of recurrent episodes of nephrolithiasis, the donor should be discouraged from donating
- Donors with a strong family history of nephrolithiasis but asymptomatic can likely be accepted but must be cautioned about their lifetime increased risk of developing a kidney stone
- A 24 hr urine for stone analysis can be performed if the donor has a history of kidney stones or is found to have asymptomatic stone on imaging

Lifestyle Assessment

Obesity

- All donors should have their height and weight and a body mass index (BMI) calculated
- Majority of transplant centers exclude potential donors with a BMI over 35 kg/m^2
- If BMI is over 30 kg/m^2 but less than 35 kg/m^2:
  - Counsel on lifestyle modifications especially weight loss, diet, and exercise
  - Intense counseling on long-term associations of obesity with the development of hypertension, diabetes mellitus, metabolic syndrome and kidney disease, including end stage renal disease

Smoking

- Currently not a contraindication to donate
- Donors should be counseled on smoking cessation due to long-term health risks

High Risk Behavior

- Behavioral screening consists of:
  - Sexual history
  - Substance abuse/drug history
- Mandatory infectious disease testing—namely hepatitis B virus (HBV), hepatitis C virus (HCV) and HIV
- Issues of concern:
  - Promiscuity
  - Incarceration
  - Men or women who have had sex in exchange for money or drugs
  - Donors with history of blood transfusions or any human-derived clotting factor concentrates
  - Homosexual men
  - Anyone exposed to or who has had sexual relations with someone at risk for, or with HIV, HCV or HBV
  - Donors with a history of hemophilia
  - Intravenous, intramuscular or subcutaneous drug use

Psychosocial Assessment

Psychosocial History

- Examined on multiple levels by the independent living donor advocate, social worker, physician and psychiatrist
- Evaluates the psychological, social and emotional stability of the donor
- Establishes the relationship between the donor and the recipient
- Ensures that the donor is not threatened in any way and that there is no gain, either financial or personal
- Other donor and family relationships should be addressed, with evaluation of the donor's social support system
- Potential economic losses are addressed
- Education level, socioeconomic status and religious beliefs should be evaluated

Psychiatric History

- An in depth evaluation of the donor's current mental condition
- Evaluate for any history of any psychiatric disorder, childhood or adolescent problems, suicidality, homocidality, inpatient psychiatric hospitalizations or outpatient psychiatric evaluations
- A thorough assessment of any medications that they were taking or currently taking

Ability to Give Informed Consent

- Donors must demonstrate competence and understanding regarding the donation process
- The donor should demonstrate understanding of the recipient's illness and should understand the other options for the recipient, including deceased donor transplantation or dialysis
- The donor should be able to demonstrate understanding of the nephrectomy including the risks and benefits to the recipient, the risks and benefits to the donor, the postoperative course, the short and long-term outcomes associated with nephrectomy
- The donor should demonstrate that he is free of coercion or any outside influence and that his decision to donate is voluntary
- The donor must also be made aware of his right to reconsider donation at any point during the evaluation, of his right to opt out with a medical excuse, and of the confidentiality of the donation process

ASSESSMENTS TO PROTECT THE HEALTH AND SAFETY OF THE RECIPIENT

Medical

Infection

- Donors must be screened for active and past communicable infections:
  - Human immunodeficiency virus 1 and 2 (HIV-1 and HIV-2)
  - Human T lymphotropic virus type-1 (HTLV-I) and type-2 (HTLV-II)
  - Hepatitis A, hepatitis B, hepatitis C
  - Syphilis
  - Toxoplasmosis
  - Cytomegalovirus (CMV), epstein-barr virus (EBV), herpes simplex virus (HSV), varicella zoster virus (VZV)
- Any of the above active infections would be a contraindication to donate

- A positive testing for HIV, HCV, hepatitis B surface antigen (HBsAg), or anti-HBc, IgM positivity would be a contraindication to donate
- Hepatitis B core antibody IgG positivity in a HbsAg negative donor carries a small risk of transmission and such donors should be excluded
- Being anti-Hbs positive is not a contraindication as this could signify vaccination or long-term immunity; history can elicit the etiology
- Having past infection with toxoplasmosis, CMV, VZV, HSV or EBV is not a contraindication to donate
- Screen for *Strongyloides*, *Trypanosoma Cruzi*, West Nile Virus, tuberculosis if the donor is from an endemic area or history suggests an infectious disease

Malignancy

- Donation entails a potential risk of transmission of malignancy to the immunosuppressed recipient
- Age appropriate health maintenance should be performed:
  - All women who are sexually active or those above 18 years of age should have pap smears and pelvic examinations
  - Women over age 50 should have a mammogram
  - Prostate-specific antigen (PSA) screening is now controversial for the general population, however in a male donor over age 50, prostate screening testing should likely be performed with digital rectal examination and PSA
  - Adults over age 50 should have screening for colorectal cancer using fecal occult blood testing, sigmoidoscopy or colonoscopy
  - If there is a family history of malignancy, screening should be done at an earlier age after discussion with the donor

Renal

- The risk of the recipient receiving a suboptimal kidney exists if the donor kidney function is compromised or if there is any underlying glomerular pathology in the donor kidney (*see* donor section)

Lifestyle

- Assessment of donor high risk behavior is important to decrease the transmission of communicable diseases (*see* donor section)

FURTHER READING

1. Mandelbrot DA, Pavlakis M, Danovitch GM, et al. The Medical Evaluation of Living Kidney Donors: A Survey of US Transplant Centers. Am J Transplant. 2007;7:2333-43.
2. Sachdeva M, Bhaskaran M, Molmenti EP, et al. Approach to the pretransplant evaluation of the living kidney donor. J Transplantation. 2011;2011: 245738.

CHAPTER 19

Psychiatric Evaluation of Live Donors

Joseph S Weiner, Blaine Greenwald

GOALS

Goals of the psychiatric evaluation of prospective live kidney donors:

- To determine the decisional capacity of the donor to consent to the donation process
- To explore factors that may influence the exercise of free will in donating, even in the presence of decisional capacity
- To determine whether there is sufficient psychiatric and psychological strength along with financial and social stability to prevent harm from the burdens of donation

STAFFING

- Evaluation is preferably performed by a psychiatrist, board-certified in psychosomatic medicine
- The psychiatrist is part of the renal donor evaluation team, which is distinct and independent from the clinical team that evaluates the potential recipient
- The psychiatric evaluation is done after the initial medical evaluation, in case the potential donor is excluded based on medical factors
- All potential donors must be evaluated in their native language. The donor is evaluated either by a psychiatrist fluent in the relevant language or by the use of a telephone-based translation service and a two-headset telephone, which enables simultaneous communication between the potential donor and psychiatrist on one phone and the translator at the other end of the phone call

WHO IS EVALUATED?

- All potential living renal donors must undergo a psychiatric evaluation
- We have evaluated several types of living donors: genetically related (e.g. sibling), legally related (e.g. spouse), emotionally but not legally related (e.g. friend), not related (i.e. "altruistic" or "Good Samaritan"), and organ exchangers[1]
- Potential donors must be over 18 years of age

ETHICAL CONSIDERATIONS[1-3]

- Autonomy (the right to donate, decisional capacity, informed consent, freedom from coercion)
- Beneficence (the recipient can benefit from the donation medically; the donor can benefit emotionally)
- Nonmaleficence (the recipient has sufficient biopsychosocial support and psychological strength to not be unduly harmed by the burdens of donation)

PROCESS OF THE EVALUATION

- While some programs administer formal psychometric testing,[5] our program conducts a clinical interview based on: (1) DSM-5 diagnostic criteria, (2) well-accepted criteria for the determination of decisional capacity, (3) clinical exploration to determine that the well-accepted principles of bioethics are met prior to donation

Content of the Evaluation and the Assessment Protocol

- The psychiatric evaluation of the potential donor is a standardized process, based on an assessment protocol[1,4,6]
  - Education and socioeconomic status
  - Religious history
  - Donor's understanding of the recipient's illness
  - Knowledge of the transplant surgery
  - How the decision to donate was made
  - Relationship between the donor and recipient
  - Dynamics of the donor-recipient relationship after transplant
  - Reaction of others to the decision to donate
  - Awareness of the right to reconsider donating
  - Economic effect of donation
  - Completed medical procedures to determine donor suitability
  - Medical history
  - Surgical history
  - Medications
  - Allergies
  - Past psychiatric history
  - Family medical and psychiatric history
  - Social history, including the use of alcohol and illicit drugs
  - Review of systems
  - Coping style and personality style
  - Complete mental status exam
  - Diagnostic impression
  - Specific comments on the following:
    - Any evidence of suicidality or homicidality?
    - Is the patient psychosocially suitable to be a live renal donor and why?
    - Does the patient have decisional capacity to give informed consent to donate?
    - Is there evidence of coercion?
    - Is there evidence of a financial motive for the donor's participation?
    - Is there evidence of an imbalanced and/or subservient relationship between the potential donor and recipient?
    - What are the opinions of the donor's mental health providers, if he or she is undergoing mental health treatment?
    - If the patient has a history of psychiatric illness, is the risk of recurrence of this illness or associated adverse outcomes minimal, should there be complications from the donation?
    - If the donor has a history of alcohol or other substance abuse or dependence, is there evidence of long-term stable abstinence with a low risk of exacerbation?
  - Conclusions and clearly stated recommendations

PSYCHIATRIC EVALUATION OF LATINO LIVE DONORS

Barbara Ponieman

The psychiatric assessment of a Latino live donor must be performed by a culturally trained psychiatrist. Latinos are the largest ethnic group in the United States with 14.5% of the total population and the fastest growing minority.

The Latino population in the US is identified as a high-risk group for the development of mental health illness, including depression, anxiety and substance abuse. Latinos endure difficulties due to:

- Stressors related to immigration
- Separation from family of origin
- Acculturation including adaptation to the new culture
- Isolation
- Language barriers
- Low socioeconomic status
- Lack of access to culturally sensitive mental health treatment centers
- Lack of medical insurance
- Higher prevalence for the development of chronic illnesses (diabetes)

US born Latinos and long-term residents (13 years or more) have higher rates of mental illness than recent Latino immigrants.

The decision to become a transplant live donor can accentuate the stressors this minority has to endure. The evaluation of the Latino live donor is a unique opportunity to:

- Identify psychiatric symptoms
- Identify family members in need of services
- Educate on mental health issues
- Discuss mental health services available and options for treatment

Latino patients do not use mental health services. Less than 10% of Latinos with mental health disorders contact health providers. The difficulties to access mental health services are identified as:

- Few Spanish speaking professionals
- Lack of culturally sensitive mental health services
- Stigma and consumer fears of experiencing discrimination
- Discomfort about disclosing sexual orientation or gender identity concerns
- Latinos first report symptoms to clergy
- Latinos have a high tolerance for mental health symptoms in their family members
- Lower health literacy among Latinos

Knowledge of the Latino Culture can be a helpful tool. Once mental health issues or the risk to develop mental health issues have been identified, appropriate referrals should be made. This culture has had very little erosion as Latinos group themselves in geographic areas in the US. The main characteristics of this culture help the Live Donor with support as:

- Family has a central role
- Latinos support the improvement of the whole group (familia, la raza) above all
- Latinos are a diverse group that shares more similarities than differences
- Cultural themes unify Latinos (immigration, family, music, language)
- Language plays a central role in communication

FURTHER READING

Psychiatric Evaluation of Latino Live Donor

1. Buki LP. The Latino Patient by Nilda Chong Creating Infrastructures for Latino Mental Health Department of Health and Human Services. CDCP. NIMH-Office for research on disparities and Global Mental Health.

REFERENCES

Psychiatric Evaluation of Live Donors

1. Olbrisch ME, Benedict SM, Haller DL, et al. Psychosocial assessment of living organ donors: clinical and ethical considerations. Prog Transplant. 2001;11(1):40-9.
2. Walton-Moss BJ, Taylor L, Nolan MT. Ethical analysis of living organ donation. Prog Transplant. 2005;15(3):303-9.
3. Abecassis M, Adams M, Live Organ Donor Consensus Group, et al. Consensus statement on the live organ donor. JAMA. 2000;284:2919-26.
4. Leo RJ, Smith BA, Mori DL. Guidelines for conducting a psychiatric evaluation of the unrelated kidney donor. Psychosomatics. 2003;44:452-60.
5. Jendrisak MD, Hong B, Shenoy S, et al. Altruistic living donors: evaluation for nondirected kidney or liver donation. Am J Transplant. 2006;6(1):115-20.
6. New York State Transplant. Council. NY State Committee on Quality Improvement in Living Kidney Donation. NYS DOH, December 2007. (Section IV C. Psychosocial Evaluation).

CHAPTER 20

Transplant Immunology

Pallavi Patri, Thangamani Muthukumar

INTRODUCTION

Kidney transplantation, as a therapeutic option in patients with end-stage kidney disease, offers superior quality of life and reduction in long-term morbidity and mortality as compared with maintenance dialysis.[1] The major barrier to successful transplantation is the recipient's immune response directed against the donor kidney. Knowledge of the biologic processes involved in recipient's recognition of the allograft and advances in cross-match techniques and immunosuppression have contributed to significant improvement in allograft survival over the years from 10% in the 1960s to over 90%.[2,3]

The focus of this chapter is to outline the major immune processes of allograft recognition and the methods used to define patient's immune profile. Cross-match techniques, determination of sensitization against the donor and methods to identify rejection are also described.

RECOGNITION OF ALLOGRAFTS

Human Leukocyte Antigen System

- The major histocompatibility complex (MHC) is a gene cluster located on chromosome 6 which encodes highly polymorphic proteins known as human leukocyte antigens (HLAs)
- The HLA system allows for the differentiation between self and nonself and therefore is the major mechanism by which the recipient immune system recognizes the allografts
- The HLA gene products are membrane-bound glycoproteins that are divided into two major classes: HLA Class I and HLA Class II

Human Leukocyte Antigens Class I

- The HLA Class I gene products are expressed on the surface of all nucleated cells
- The HLA Class I molecules present peptides from intracellular proteins to cytotoxic CD8+ T-lymphocytes, i.e. donor leukocytes during transplantation present internally processed peptides of the donor HLA Class I molecule to circulating recipient CD8 T cells
- A Class I molecule consists of two noncovalently associated chains:
  - A polymorphic α-heavy chain composed of a cytoplasmic, transmembrane and an extracellular component that is made up of 3 separate regions: $\alpha1$, $\alpha2$ and $\alpha3$; between $\alpha1$ and $\alpha2$ is a groove within which peptides of up to 8–10 amino acids are bound
  - A nonpolymorphic $\beta2$ microglobulin chain
- There are three major HLA Class I genes: HLA-A, HLA-B and HLA-C

Human Leukocyte Antigens Class II

- The HLA Class II gene products are expressed on antigen-presenting cells (APCs) such as dendritic cells, macrophages and B lymphocytes
- The HLA Class II gene expression can also be induced in other cell lines including vascular endothelial cells, epithelial and mesenchymal cells

- A Class II molecule consists of two covalently bound chains of similar weight; a polymorphic α chain and a polymorphic β chain
  - The resulting dimer contains a cytoplasmic, transmembrane and an extracellular component
  - The peptide-binding groove is formed between the extracellular components of the two chains
- The HLA Class II molecules present peptides from extracellular proteins to CD4 T cells, i.e. recipient APCs endocytose donor cell components including HLA Class I and II molecules which are then processed into peptides and are presented to circulating recipient CD4 T cells
- There are three major HLA Class II alleles: HLA-DP, HLA-DQ, HLA-DR

Antigen presentation pathways (Fig. 1)

- There are two major pathways by which the immune system recognizes the allograft as foreign: direct allorecognition and indirect allorecognition
  - Direct allorecognition: The pathway by which donor APCs present donor HLA molecules to recipient T cells
  - Indirect allogrecognition: The pathway by which recipient APCs present donor HLA molecules to recipient T cells
- Direct allorecognition is thought to be the major pathway involved in acute rejection whereas the indirect allorecognition pathway may be more important in chronic rejection

Human leukocyte antigens typing and matching

- A patient's HLA profile consists of two sets of alleles which are codominantly expressed; each set, referred to as a haplotype, is inherited from each parent (Fig. 2)
- HLA typing for kidney transplant is usually performed for three different alleles: HLA-A, HLA-B and HLA-DR and therefore six different antigens (3 from each parent) are identified for each patient

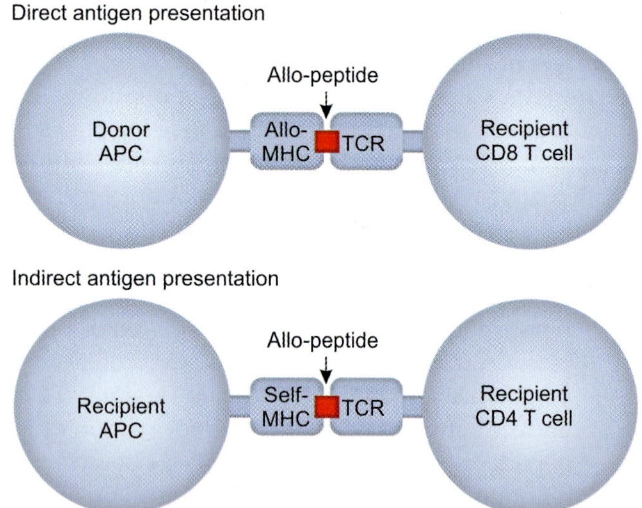

Fig. 1: Antigen presentation pathways. There are two major pathways by which the immune system recognizes the allograft as foreign: direct allorecognition and indirect allorecognition. In direct allorecognition the donor antigen presenting cells present donor HLA molecules to recipient T cells. Direct allorecognition is thought to be the major pathway involved in acute rejection. In indirect allorecognition the recipient antigen presenting cells present donor HLA molecules to recipient T cells. This pathway may be more important in chronic rejection.

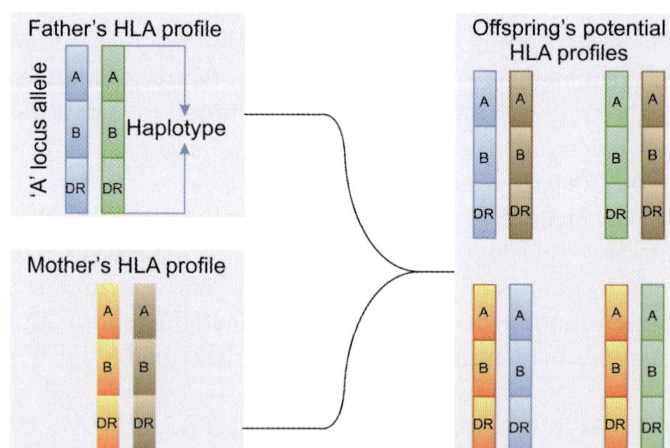

Fig. 2: Segregation of human leukocyte antigens (HLA) in a family. A patient's HLA profile consists of two sets of alleles which are codominantly expressed; each set, referred to as a haplotype, is inherited from each parent. HLA typing for kidney transplant is usually performed for three different alleles: HLA-A, HLA-B and HLA-DR and therefore six different antigens (3 from each parent) are identified for each patient. Among related donors HLA matching is considered in terms of haplotypes. Among unrelated donors or deceased donors HLA matching is considered in terms of antigens at the three different alleles (6 antigens). Immunologically, a 6-antigen matched deceased donation is not the same as a 2-haploidentical living-related donation. Similarly, due to differences in minor histocompatibility antigens, donation between 2-haploidentical siblings is not the same as donation between identical twins.

- The degree of HLA compatibility has an impact on long-term graft survival[4]
- There are two major methods by which HLA typing can be performed:
  - Serology-based typing
    - Recipient lymphocytes are mixed with serum containing antibodies to a wide range of HLA antigens
    - Limitations of this method include the inability to comprehensively screen individuals as anti-sera has been developed mostly in Caucasian populations and the need for viable recipient lymphocytes
  - Deoxyribonucleic acid (DNA) typing
    - There are several deoxyribonucleic acid typing techniques in use today: sequence-specific primers (SSP), sequence-specific oligonucleotides (SSOPs) and sequencing-based typing (SBT)
    - SSP uses primers that are specifically designed to detect different HLA alleles which then undergo amplification via polymerase chain reaction (PCR) when binding occurs
    - SSOP uses labeled nucleotide probes that bind DNA sequences specific to HLA alleles
    - The major limitations of both SSP and SSOP methods are that they can only identify known HLA alleles
    - SBT does not require knowledge of the sequence of the HLA allele and can be used to identify new HLA alleles; while this is the most comprehensive method available in HLA typing it is time-consuming and expensive

Minor Histocompatibility Antigens

- The HLA system is the major barrier for transplantation; however 2-haplotype matched siblings, unlike identical twins can still experience rejection of the allograft
- This is thought to be mediated by minor antigens such as those encoded by the MICA gene (MHC Class I-related Chain A) also located on chromosome 6
- The MICA gene products are structurally similar to HLA Class I molecules but do not associate with β-2 microglobulin
- MICA antigens are highly polymorphic and can be expressed on a variety of cells including monocytes, epithelial cells and endothelial cells
- Transplant recipients who receive well MHC matched kidneys and have MICA-antibodies have been found to have worse graft survival than those without these antibodies[5]

Blood Type Matching

- ABO blood group evaluation must be performed prior to transplantation as the ABO blood group antigens are strong immunologic antigens
- The same principles with respect to ABO groups apply for allograft transplantation as with blood transfusions, i.e group O is considered the universal donor and AB the universal recipient
- Due to the disproportionate number of recipients from certain blood groups on the waiting list, blood group compatibility as opposed to complete matching determines organ distribution
- Rh matching is not required as these proteins are mostly expressed only on red blood cells
- ABO incompatible transplants have been successfully performed with use of pretransplantation desensitization protocols that involve drugs such as rituximab, splenectomy or plasmapheresis with the aim of reducing circulating antibodies
- Blood group A2 has been found to have a lower immunologic risk as compared to blood groups A1 or B due to lower expression of the A2 antigen on graft endothelium; A2 kidneys therefore can be transplanted into O or B recipients successfully without desensitization protocols

Cross-Match Testing

Complement-Dependent Cytotoxicity Assay

- Screens for preformed antibodies in the recipient that can immediately react against the donor kidney
- Complement-dependent cytotoxicity (CDC) assay involves the following steps:
  - Recipient serum is mixed with T lymphocytes and with B lymphocytes separately isolated from the donor
  - Complement is added to the mixture in microplates
  - In the presence of preformed antibodies that bind to the donor lymphocytes, complement is activated resulting in cell death
  - The degree of cell death can be quantified and is given a numerical value; 0 (no significant cell death), 2 (20% cell death), 4 (40% cell death), 6 (60% cell death) or 8 (> 80% cell death)
  - A value of 2 or greater is considered a positive result
- Anti-human globulin (AHG) can be added to the reaction to enhance concentration of antibody binding and therefore increase sensitivity of the assay

Table 1: Interpretation of complement-dependent cytotoxicity (CDC) cross-match results

T cell CDC	B cell CDC	Interpretation	Implication
Negative	Negative	Absence of Class I and Class II antibodies at loads high enough for complement fixation and cytotoxicity	Can proceed to transplant
Negative	Positive	Probable presence of Class II antibodies or low level Class I antibodies	Can proceed to transplant
Positive	Positive	Presence of Class I antibodies and may have Class II antibodies as well	Contraindication to transplant
Positive	Negative	Likely technical error	Test should be repeated

- The CDC assay does not discriminate between immunoglobulin (Ig) G- and IgM-mediated reactions (latter thought to be mostly auto-antibodies)
- The assay can be modified to inactivate IgM antibodies so as to distinguish between IgG and IgM reactions
  - Immunoglobulin M antibodies occur as pentamers held together by disulfide bonds; these can be broken by heating (at 63°C for 10 minutes) or by use of reducing agents such as 2-mercaptoethanol or dithiothreitol
  - These modifications however, can also inactivate low levels of IgG antibodies
- Results of CDC assays can be interpreted as follows (Table 1):
  - T lymphocyte CDC assay tests for presence of HLA Class I antibodies
  - B lymphocyte CDC assay tests for presence of both HLA Class I and HLA Class II antibodies
  - B lymphocyte positive CDC assay that becomes negative following treatment with heat or with a reducing agent suggests the presence of IgM antibodies or presence of low-level IgG antibodies
  - T lymphocyte CDC assay is generally considered a prerequisite for all renal transplantations—a positive result is usually an absolute contraindication for transplantation
  - Positive B lymphocyte CDC assay with a negative T lymphocyte CDC assay likely indicates presence of Class II antibodies and/or low-level Class I antibodies; this is not considered an absolute contraindication for transplantation but is associated with lower long-term graft survival
  - Positive T lymphocyte CDC assay with a negative B lymphocyte CDC assay is likely a technical error associated with poor B cell viability and should be repeated

Flow Cytometry

- Does not depend on complement fixation or high-titer antibodies and is more sensitive antibody assay than CDC
- Flow cytometry involves the following steps:
  - Recipient serum is mixed with both T and B lymphocytes from the donor
  - The cells are incubated with fluorescent labeled anti-CD3 and anti-CD19 antibodies to distinguish T and B lymphocytes
  - A reporter fluorescent anti-human IgG antibodies is then added that will detect binding of alloantibodies
  - The flow cytometer distinguishes the combined fluorescence of the anti-CD3 or anti-CD19 with the anti-human IgG
  - A greater median channel shift based on the combined fluorescence indicates a positive result; the number of channel shifts required to label a test as positive has not been standardized
- Standard flow cytometry does not detect presence of IgM antibodies and does not distinguish between complement fixing and noncomplement fixing antibodies
- In a sensitized patient, a negative CDC with positive flow cytometry has been associated with poorer allograft survival as compared to negative flow cytometry
- There is conflicting data about the impact of a positive B lymphocyte flow cytometry in setting of a negative T lymphocyte flow cytometry on graft outcome

Solid Phase Assays for Donor Specific Antibodies

- Allow for the identification of antibodies in the recipient to specific HLA antigens
- Two methods available: Enzyme-linked immuno sorbent assay (ELISA) based and fluorescent microsphere based (Luminex®)
- The ELISA assay involves the following steps:
  - Specific purified HLA antigens are immobilized in individual wells of a microplate
  - Recipient serum is incubated in each well
  - A second anti-human IgG antibody linked to an enzyme is added

  - The addition of a substrate for this enzyme will result in a colored product if the second anti-human IgG antibody binds to the anti-HLA antibody
  - This colored product can then be quantified and reported as a positive result
- The fluorescent microsphere-based assay involves the following steps:
  - Specific synthetic HLA antigens are immobilized on fluorescent microspheres
  - Recipient serum is incubated with the microspheres
  - A second fluorescently labeled anti-human IgG antibody is added
  - The combined fluorescence of the bound anti-human IgG to the HLA-antigen-alloantibody complex can be quantified as the mean fluorescence intensity (MFI)
  - The level of MFI above which a test result is considered positive has not been standardized
- Solid phase assays are commonly used to identify IgG antibodies and do not distinguish complement fixing from noncomplement fixing antibodies
- Multiple studies have found an association between donor-specific antibodies (DSA) and increased risk of antibody-mediated rejection
- Both preformed and post-transplant de-novo DSA are associated with decreased graft survival[6,7]

Panel-Reactive Antibody Testing

- The panel-reactive antibody (PRA) test uses lymphocytes from 100 blood donors that represent the population of potential donors
- Similar to the CDC assay as described above, recipient serum is incubated with the panel of donor lymphocytes and cell lysis against each donor is tabulated such that if cell lysis occurs in half of the samples then the PRA result is 50%
- The standard PRA assay does not provide representation of all HLA Class I and II antigens and does not provide specificity on the HLA antigen that the reaction is directed against
- The PRA can be combined with solid phase assay methods to identify the specific HLA-antigen that the antibody is directed against which is then labeled an "unacceptable antigen"
- The frequency of unacceptable antigens in the national donor pool is used to compute a CPRA (calculated PRA)for a recipient who allows an approximation of the likelihood of compatibility between the recipient and donor

Allograft Rejection

- The gold standard for diagnosis of rejection is an allograft biopsy with 10 or more glomeruli and one artery available for evaluation
- The incidence of hyperacute rejection has significantly decreased with the advent of pretransplant CDC cross-match testing
- Acute allograft rejection broadly falls into two categories as defined by the Banff classification system (Table 2): Acute T cell-mediated rejection (ACR) and acute antibody-mediated rejection (AMR)
- ACR and AMR can occur concomitantly and the presence of both portends poorer graft survival
- The Banff criteria do not include all forms of rejection. An example of one such type of rejection is plasma cell-rich acute rejection, where the interstitial and tubular inflammation is composed primarily of plasma cells along with lymphocytes which portend a poor prognosis

Acute T Cell-Mediated Rejection

- This is the most common form of early rejection
- ACR is identified by the presence of tubulitis (> 4 mononuclear cells/tubular cross section) and graded based on the severity of interstitial inflammation and intimal arteritis (infiltration of lymphocytes in arterial wall)
- When there is interstitial inflammation and only mild tubulitis with less than 4 mononuclear cells/tubular cross section with no intimal arteritis, the biopsy findings do not meet criteria for ACR and are categorized as "borderline changes" suspicious for ACR

Acute Antibody-Mediated Rejection

- Detection of classical pathway complement split product C4d binding to the peritubular capillary endothelium has been found to be a marker of AMR
- AMR is identified by the presence of all three of the following features:
  - The presence of morphological changes in the allograft (acute tubular necrosis or peritubular capillaritis or intimal arteritis)
  - Immunopathological evidence of antibody action (peritubular capillary C4d deposition or immunoglobulin and complement in arterial necrosis)
  - Circulating DSA
- If only two of the above three features are present then the biopsy findings are suspicious for AMR

Table 2: Banff classification of acute rejection

Banff 4: Acute T cell mediated rejection	Banff 2: Acute antibody mediated rejection
Grade 1A	1. *Morphological evidence of kidney injury*
>25% interstitial inflammation (i2, i3) AND foci of moderate tubilitis (t2)	A. Acute tubular necrosis or
Grade IB	B. Neutrophils and/or mononuclear cells in peritubular capillaries and/or glomeruli, and/or capillary thrombosis or
>25% interstitial inflammation (i2, i3) AND foci of severe tubilitis (t3)	C. Intimal arteritis/fibrinoid necrosis/intramural or transmural inflammation in arteries
Grade IIA	2. *Immunopathological evidence of antibody action*
Mild to moderate intimal arteritis (v1)	A. Presence of C4d in peritubular capillaries or
	B. Immunoglobulin and complement in arterial necrosis
Grade IIB	3. *Serological evidence of circulating antibodies*
Severe intimal arteritis involving >25% (v2) of luminal area	A. Antibodies to donor HLA or
	B. Antibodies to donor endothelial antigens
Grade III	All 3 criteria are necessary to make a diagnosis of antibody mediated rejection; 2 out of 3 criteria makes a diagnosis of suspicious for antibody mediated rejection
Transmural arteritis and/or arterial fibrinoid changes with accompanying lymphocyte infiltration (v3)	
Definitions	
i score: i0 (<10% parenchymal inflammation), i1 (10 to 25% parenchymal inflammation), i2 (25 to 50% parenchymal inflammation), i3 (>50% parenchymal inflammation)	
t score: t0 (no mononuclear cells in tubules), t1(foci of 1–4 mononuclear cells/tubular across section), t2 (foci of 5–10 mononuclear cells/tubular across section), t3 (foci of >10 mononuclear cells/tubular across section)	
v score: v0(no arteritis), v1 (mild to moderate intimal arteritis in one arterial cross section), v2 (severe intimal arteritis with at least 25% luminal area lost), v3 (transmural arteritis and/or arterial fibrinoid change with lymphocytic infiltrate)	

Chronic Rejection

- The all-encompassing term "chronic allograft nephropathy" is no longer included in the Banff categorization
- There are three forms of chronic rejection now identified by Banff:
  - Chronic active T cell-mediated rejection defined by presence of arterial intimal fibrosis and formation of neo-intima
  - Chronic active antibody-mediated rejection defined by presence of peritubular capillary C4d staining, circulating DSA and morphologic evidence of chronic tissue injury (glomerular basement membrane double contours and/or peritubular capillary basement membrane multilayering and/or fibrous intimal thickening in arteries and/or interstitial fibrosis/tubular atrophy)
  - Interstitial fibrosis/tubular atrophy without the additional findings as above

Noninvasive Assays to Detect Allograft Rejection

- Gene expression based biomarkers in urine have been developed that allows for noninvasive assessment of allograft status
  - The measurement of urinary cell granzyme B and perforin mRNA levels, which are indicative of cytotoxic T cell activity, have been found to be sensitive and specific markers for acute T cell-mediated rejection
  - The measurement at the biopsy of urinary cell FoxP3 RNA levels, which are indicative of regulatory T cell activity, have been found to predict reversal of acute rejection with high sensitivity and specificity and identified patients at risk for graft failure within 6 months of an episode of acute rejection
- The Cylex™ Immuknow® assay identifies cell-mediated immune responses in patients on immunosuppression by quantifying the amount of adenosine triphosphate (ATP), produced by activated recipient T cells *in vitro*

- A low level of ATP (< 225 ng/mL) indicates lower global T cell function and therefore a low cell-mediated immune response; a high level of ATP (≥ 525 ng/mL) conversely indicates higher global T cell function and therefore a robust cell-mediated immune response; values in between these indicate a moderate response
- Some studies have found a correlation between the Cylex assay results and acute rejection;[8] however, a recent study has not found an association between a single time point assay result and future development of acute rejection or opportunistic infections[9]

FURTHER READING

1. Danovitch G. Handbook of Kidney Transpalntation. 5th edition. Lippincott Wiliams & Wilkins. 2010.
2. Dunn PP. Human leucocyte antigen typing: techniques and technology, a critical appraisal. Int J Immunogenetics. 2011;38(6):463-73.
3. Hartono C, et al. Noninvasive diagnosis of acute rejection of renal allografts. Curr Opin Organ Transplant. 2010;15(1):35-41.
4. Mulley WR, Kanellis J. Understanding crossmatch testing in organ transplantation: A case-based guide for the general nephrologist. Nephrology (Carlton). 2011;16(2):125-33.
5. Picascia A, et al. Luminex and antibody detection in kidney transplantation. Clin Exp Nephrol. 2012; 16(3):373-81.
6. Sis B, et al. Banff '09 meeting report: antibody mediated graft deterioration and implementation of Banff working groups. Am J Transplant. 2010;10(3):464-71.
7. Suthanthiran M et al. Urinary-cell mRNA profile and acute cellular rejection in kidney allografts. NEJM 2013; 369(1):20-31.

REFERENCES

1. Wolfe RA, et al. Comparison of mortality in all patients on dialysis, patients on dialysis awaiting transplantation, and recipients of a first cadaveric transplant. NEJM. 1999;341(23):1725-30.
2. Murrey JE. Conference on human kidney transplant: proceedings. Transplantation. 1964;2:147-65.
3. Organ Procurement and Transplantation Network (OPTN) and Scientific Registry of Transplant Recipients (SRTR). OPTN/SRTR 2010 Annual Data Report. Rockwille, MD: Department of Health and Human Services, Health Resources and Services Administration, Healthcare Systems Bureau, Division of Transplantation. 2011.
4. Opelz G and Döhler B. Effect of human leukocyte antigen compatibility on kidney graft survival: comparative analysis of two decades. Transplantation. 2007;64(2): 137-43.
5. Zou, et al. Antibodies against MICA antigens and kidney-transplant rejection. NEJM 2007; 357(13):1293-300.
6. Lefaucheur, et al. Preexisting donor-specific HLA antibodies predict outcome in kidney transplantation. JASN 2010; 21(8):1398-406.
7. Loupy A et al. Complement-binding anti-HLA antibodies and kidney-allograft survival. NEJM. 2013;369(13):1215-26.
8. Kowalski, et al. Immunodiagnostics: evaluation of functional T-cell immunocompetence in whole blood independent of circulating cell numbers. J. Immunotoxicol 2007; 4(3):225-32.
9. Huskey, et al. Single time point immune function assay (immuknow) testing does not aid in the prediction of future opportunistic infections or acute rejection. CJASN 2011; 6(2):423-9.

CHAPTER 21

Immune Risk Profiling

Khalid Al Meshari, Abeed Pall

Uncontrolled donor-specific alloimmune response mediates renal allograft injury that leads to graft loss. Immune risk profiling of kidney transplant recipients seeks to identify immunologically appropriate donor-recipient pair that will result in immunologically successful transplantation.

PURPOSE

- Prevention of hyperacute rejection
- Minimization of acute cellular rejection (ACR) and acute antibody-mediated rejection (AMR)
- Provision of a guide to immunosuppressive strategies
- Provision of a tool for prognostication of long-term patient and graft outcomes

APPROACH

A standardized four-step approach:

- Establish donor-recipient ABO blood group compatibility
- Establish donor-recipient human leukocyte antigens (HLA) compatibility
- Decide on ABO and HLA-compatible (conventional) or ABO and/or HLA-incompatible (unconventional) transplantation
- Stratify immunological risks

DONOR-RECIPIENT ABO BLOOD GROUP COMPATIBILITY

The goal of establishing donor-recipient ABO compatibility is to prevent hyperacute rejection.

- ABO blood group antigen system is the first established histocompatibility barrier to kidney transplantation
- ABO antigens are expressed on vascular endothelium
- "Natural" antibodies of immunoglobulin M (IgM) and G (IgG) classes (isohemagglutinins) are developed early in life (usually beyond 6 months of age) against A, B, and AB antigens that are not expressed on own erythrocytes (e.g., O blood group recipient forms isohemagglutinins against A and B blood group antigens)
- In case of ABO-incompatible kidney transplantation, the isohemagglutinins bind to their targeted antigens on vascular endothelium and they trigger complement dependent antibody mediated injury (hyperacute rejection)
- Both donor and recipient are typed for ABO blood group antigens
- In conventional kidney transplantation, the following kidney allocation rules are applied:
  - Donor-recipient ABO identity or compatibility is applied in living donor (LD) transplantation
  - Donor-recipient ABO identity is applied in deceased donor (DD) transplantation. Identity and not compatibility is applied in DD transplantation to account for the disproportionate distribution of certain blood group recipients on DD list

DONOR-RECIPIENT HLA COMPATIBILITY

Similar to ABO compatibility, the goal of establishing donor-recipient HLA compatibility is to prevent hyperacute rejection.

- HLA system is the second established histocompatibility barrier (positive donor-specific HLA cross-match) to kidney transplantation
- HLA antigens class I (A, B, C) and class II (DR, DQ, DP) are expressed on vascular endothelium

- "Acquired" antibodies of IgG class are developed against disparate HLA antigens through blood transfusions, multiple pregnancies, and previous organ transplantation
- In case of HLA-incompatible kidney transplantation, the preformed HLA antibodies bind to their targeted antigens (class I and/or II HLA antigens) on vascular endothelium and they trigger complement-dependent antibody-mediated injury (hyperacute rejection)
- The laboratory methodology required for establishing donor-recipient HLA compatibility are:
  - Donor and recipient molecular (DNA-based) HLA typing
  - Donor T cell complement-dependent cytotoxicity (CDC)/antihuman globulin-augmented (AHG CDC) cross-match
  - Donor B cell CDC cross-match or pronase-digested (PD) three-color B cell flow cross-match
  - Recipient HLA single antigen (SA) antibody detection by solid phase immunoassay (SPI)

Compatibility is established by the demonstration of negative cross-match and the absence of donor-specific HLA antibody by SA testing.

IMMUNOLOGICAL RISK STRATIFICATION FOR ABO AND HLA-COMPATIBLE (CONVENTIONAL) TRANSPLANTATION

The goal of immunological risk stratification in conventional transplantation is double fold:

- Minimize the incidence of ACR and AMR by providing a guide to immunosuppressive strategies
- Prognosticate long-term patient and graft survival
- The laboratory methodology required for risk stratification are:
  - Recipient panel reactive antibody (PRA) screening (preferably by flow PRA or equivalent)
  - Donor and recipient molecular (DNA-based) HLA typing of A, B, DR, and DQ loci
- High-risk candidates (require intense immunosuppression, usually with T cell depleting induction agent):
  - Sensitized (positive flow PRA)
  - Retransplant
  - DD transplant
  - Historically positive, currently negative cross-match
  - Significant HLA mismatch
- Intermediate-risk candidates (less intense immunosuppression, usually with non-T lymphocyte depleting induction agent):
  - Nonsensitized
  - First LD transplant
  - Minimum HLA mismatch
- Low-risk candidates (no need for induction therapy):
  - Nonsensitized
  - First LD transplant
  - Zero HLA mismatch
- Donor and recipient HLA class II (DR and DQ) matching has been shown to improve long-term patient and graft survival:
  - For recipient with multiple LDs, the donor with the better DR and/or DQ match with the recipient is selected
  - For recipients on the DD list, assign more points for those with better DR and/or DQ matching with the DD

ABO-INCOMPATIBLE TRANSPLANTATION

- Diagnostic prerequisites:
  - Subtyping for blood group A antigens (A1 or A2). The density of expression of A1 on tissues including vascular endothelium is higher than A2
  - Quantification of isohemagglutinin titer
  - C4d staining of renal allograft biopsy

IMMUNOLOGICAL RISK STRATIFICATION FOR ABO-INCOMPATIBLE TRANSPLANT

- The goal is double fold:
  - Prevention of hyperacute rejection
  - Minimization of ACR and acute AMR
- Major risk factors:
  - Donor blood type: Difficulty: A1 > B> A2
  - Recipient blood type: Difficulty: O > A or B
  - Recipient isohemagglutinin titer: Difficulty: High baseline isohemagglutinin titer
- High-risk candidates:
  - A1 or A1B donor
  - O recipient
  - Young recipient
  - High baseline isohemagglutinin titer
- Low-risk candidates:
  - A2 or A2B donor
  - A or B recipient
  - Old recipient
  - Low baseline isohemagglutinin titer
- In general, all recipients of ABO-incompatible kidney transplantation require preconditioning (desensitization) regimen prior to transplantation. The goal of

desensitization is to lower the donor specific isohemagglutinin titer to an acceptable level. Desensitization consists of apheresis (plasma exchange or immunoadsorption), intravenous immunoglobulin (IVIg), and anti-CD20 antibody
- Recipients of A2 or A2B donor kidneys might not require desensitization, especially if the baseline isohemagglutinin titer is low

HLA-INCOMPATIBLE TRANSPLANTATION

- Diagnostic prerequisites:
  - Donor T cell CDC/AHG CDC cross-match
  - Donor B cell CDC cross-match or PD three-color B cell flow cross-match
  - Recipient HLA SA antibody detection by SPI
  - Donor and recipient molecular (DNA-based) HLA typing for all class I and II loci (A, B, C, DR, DQ, and DP)
  - C4d staining for renal allograft biopsies

IMMUNOLOGICAL RISK STRATIFICATION FOR HLA-INCOMPATIBLE TRANSPLANT

- The goal is double fold:
  - Prevention of hyperacute rejection
  - Minimization of ACR and acute AMR
- Risk stratification: The clinical and immunological history of the recipient combined with the HLA antibody testing determines the immunological risk for HLA-incompatible transplantation
  - Clinical and immunological history
    - Transplants: Antigen exposure/immunological response
    - Pregnancies: Determine paternal HLA
    - Recent or large number of blood transfusions
    - Number of HLA mismatches with the current donor
    - Child→mother, husband→wife (with prior conception)
    - Nature of HLA mismatch: Repeat, highly immunogenic (e.g., A2)
  - HLA immunological profile
    - High risk: Positive T cell AHG CDC or B cell CDC cross-match with positive T and/or B flow cross-match and positive donor-specific antibody (DSA) by SPI
    - Intermediate risk: Negative T cell AHG CDC and negative B cell CDC cross-match with positive T and/or B flow cross-match and positive DSA by SPI
    - Low risk: Negative T cell AHG CDC and negative B cell CDC cross-match with negative T and/or B flow cross-match and positive DSA by SPI
- In general, all recipients of HLA-incompatible kidney transplantation require preconditioning (desensitization) regimen prior to transplantation. The goal of desensitization is to lower the donor-specific HLA antibody to an acceptable level. Desensitization consists of different combinations of apheresis (plasma exchange or immunoadsorption), IVIg, and anti-CD20 antibody

FURTHER READING

1. Meshari KA, Alshaibani K, Hamawi K, et al. The kidney transplant program at King Faisal Specialist Hospital and Research Centre. Clinical Transplants 2005;10:119-29.
2. Meshari KA, Pall A, Chaballout A, et al. Outcome of Desensitization in HLA and ABO incompatible living donor kidney transplantation: A single centre experience in more than 100 patients. Transplantation Proceedings 2013;45:1423-26.
3. Montgomery RA, Locke JE, King KE, et al. ABO incompatible renal transplantation: A paradigm ready for broad implementation. Transplantation 2009;87(8):1246-55.
4. Montgomery RA, Phil D, Lonze B, et al. Desensitisation in HLA incompatible kidney recipients and survival. N Engl J Med 2011;365:318-26.
5. Opelz G, Dohler B. Association of HLA mismatch with death with a functioning graft after kidney transplantation: A collaborative transplant study report. AJT 2012;12:3031-38.
6. Saw CL, Heaney DL, Gebel HM, et al. Relevance of antibody screening and crossmatching in solid organs, hematopoietic stem cell transplant and blood transfusion. Handbook of Human Immunology, Second Edition, CRC Press, pages 565-88.
7. Zachary AA, Houp JA, Vega R, et al. Evaluation of the humoral response in transplantation. Manual of Molecular and Clinical Laboratory Immunology, Seventh Edition, American Society of Microbiology Press, pages 1215-27.

CHAPTER 22

HLA and ABO Desensitization

Robert A Montgomery

DESENSITIZATION

Goal

- Lower donor-specific antibody (DSA) levels at a range safe for transplantation
  - Human leukocyte antigen (HLA) antibodies below a positive CDC AHG cytotoxic cross-match
  - Isohemagglutination immunoglobulin G (IgG) titers ≤ 16

Two Major Protocols

- High-dose intravenous immunoglobulin (IVIg)
  - Protocols for both live and deceased donor transplant recipients
  - 2 g IVIg/kg infused monthly until
    - Favorable cross-match results
    - 4 doses (main effect seen after the first dose)
  - Has a durable effect on HLA antibody that lasts for months and increases transplant rates
  - It may be more effective when combined with anti-CD20
  - Allows for transplantation of sensitized patients with no live donors
- Plasmapheresis with low-dose IVIg
  - Hopkins protocol includes every other day plasmapheresis and low-dose IVIg (100 mg IVIg/kg)
  - Plasmapheresis depletes HLA antibody and IVIg prevents new endogenous synthesis
  - At least 2 post-transplant sessions
    - More sessions may be required based on DSA levels
    - Aim to achieve DSA strength below positive flow cross-match
  - DSA levels rebound within days of discontinuing plasmapheresis if the transplant is not performed so this is usually only an option for patients with live donors
  - DSA is often eliminated after post-transplant plasmapheresis, especially DSA to class I antigens
  - 25% of patients will have a antibody-mediated rejection (AMR) after desensitization and most of these AMR episodes respond to additional plasmapheresis and IVIg

Anti-CD20

- Used selectively in high-risk donor–recipient combinations
  - Depletes memory B cells in secondary lymphoid tissues and peripheral blood
  - May prevent recall responses for which memory exists
  - Does not affect long-lived plasma cells that are residents in the bone marrow and do not express CD20
  - Splenectomy remains a rescue option in severe AMR (approximately 8% of cases)
  - Other compounds such as eculizumab and bortezomib are also considered

ABO-Incompatible Outcomes

- Outcomes are usually comparable to ABO-compatible transplants with a slight increase in early graft losses due to severe AMR
- ABO-incompatible pairs with ABO:O recipient
  - Isohemagglutinin titer ≤ 128:
    - Desensitization achieved without excessive plasmapheresis or immunoadsorption

- Isohemagglutinin titer > 128:
  - Kidney paired donation may be a better option
  - If a match in a kidney paired donation pool is not found in a reasonable length of time, proceed with desensitization

Positive Cross-Match Outcomes

- Transplantation of HLA-sensitized patients with live donors after desensitization provides a survival advantage when compared with waiting for a compatible kidney
- Usually inferior to negative cross-match transplants
- 25–40% incidence of AMR
- Class I > class II DSA elimination after engraftment
- 1-year post-transplant glomerulopathy after engraftment
  - 22% in the absence of AMR
  - 44% in instances of early AMR

Paired Donation

- Allows for the exchange of kidneys among incompatible pairs
- Blood-type skewing is present in incompatible donor pools:
  - High incidence of O recipients
  - Low incidence of O donors

List Donation

- The live donor of an incompatible pair donates to the individual at the top of the corresponding compatible UNOS list in return for the intended recipient being awarded priority for a compatible deceased organ
- Given the high incidence of incompatible pairs with A donors and O recipients, a net egress of O deceased donor kidneys could potentially occur

Compatible Pairs

- Including compatible pairs in paired donation pools allows for a greater number of matches due to the increase entry of O donors into the pool
- Benefits to compatible pairs for participation includes:
  - Altruistic reasons
  - Potential for a better organ (such as a younger donor)

Non-Directed Donors

- Inclusion of donors with nondesignated recipients into paired donation pools allows for:
  - A greater number of transplants
  - A greater number of transplants per donor than in instances of directed donations
  - No requirement for a reciprocal match
  - The amelioration of blood-type skewing

Domino Paired Donation

- A non-directed donor allows for a series of transplants ending in donation to the deceased donor pool
- Transplants are performed simultaneously to
  - Prevent donors from changing their mind
  - Prevent recipients from becoming ineligible due to medical reasons

Nonsimultaneous, Extended, and Altruistic Donor Chains

- A transplant chain is started with a non-directed donor
- The last donor in the chain acts as a "bridge" to start a new chain
- Transplants are not performed simultaneously

DESENSITIZATION AND/OR PAIRED DONATION

- Kidney paired donation and desensitization should be considered as complementary approaches
- The choice of one or the other is based on two factors:
  - Difficulty finding a suitable donor in a paired donation
  - Difficulty achieving desensitization
- ABO:O donors are associated with improved chances in paired donation
- Highly sensitized patients who have a high strength of HLA reactivity benefit from a hybrid technique using paired donation followed by desensitization in which the best donor (against whom the recipient has the lowest strength of DSA) is chosen from the paired donation pool and the patient is desensitized against that donor with better outcomes and less plasmapheresis

ABO: O Recipient/ABO: A Donor

- Most frequent incompatible association
- Associated with prolonged waiting times
- Desensitization probably the best option

ABO: A/ABO: B Combinations

Paired donation probably the best option

Highly Sensitized and ABO Incompatible

- Desensitization and/or paired donation based on donor/recipient characteristics
  - Paired donation
    - ABO: O donor and low recipient PRA and/or
    - High recipient DSA and repeat mismatches
  - Paired donation and desensitization
    - ABO: AB donor and high recipient PRA and
    - High recipient DSA and repeat mismatches
  - Desensitization
    - ABO: AB donor and high recipient PRA and/or
    - Low recipient DSA and no repeat mismatch

FURTHER READING

1. Montgomery RA. Renal transplantation across HLA and ABO antibody barriers: integrating paired donation into desensitization protocols. Am J Transplant 2010;10: 449–57.
2. Montgomery RA, Lonze BE, King KE, et al. Desensitization in HLA-incompatible kidney recipients and survival. N Engl J Med 2011;365:318–26.

CHAPTER 23

Kidney Paired Donation

David Serur

GOALS OF KIDNEY PAIRED DONATION (KPD)

- Patients with an ABO-incompatible potential living donor or a cross-match-positive living donor have traditionally been relegated to waiting on the deceased donor list
- While desensitization is available for some ABO-incompatible patients and some cross-match-positive patients, it comes at the price of an increase in immunosuppression and the risks of infection and malignancies
- KPD obviates the need for this excess immunosuppression by providing the recipient with an ABO-compatible donor or a donor to which they are not cross-match positive
- Even with a KPD it is at times difficult to find matches for the extremely highly sensitized patients, those with 98-100% calculated panel reactive antibodies (cPRA). These patients may benefit from the combined approach of desensitization and KPD
- Currently KPD transplants account for 500 transplants per year, about 10% of all living transplants in the United States
- It is estimated that with a fully functional national KPD program 3000 extra transplants would be facilitated per year

HISTORY OF KPD

- The idea of KPD was first introduced in 1986 by Dr Felix Rapaport of New York when he suggested an international exchange of kidneys
- The first KPD program was initiated in South Korea in 1991. It was a single center program, computer matching was not used, and 129 transplants were facilitated over 11 years
- The first exchanges in the United States were performed in 2000 in New England and at Johns Hopkins University
- The Dutch KPD program was initiated in 2004 utilizing seven centers throughout the country. Computer matching was initiated and match runs were performed every 3 months. The Dutch center performed 128 transplants over 5 years. The transplants occurred simultaneously and the donor traveled to the recipient center
- In the United States, the New England Program for Kidney Exchange (NEPKE) was founded in 2004 followed by the paired donation network (PDN) and the alliance for paired donation (APD). The first nonsimultaneous extended altruistic donor (NEAD) chain was performed by Dr Michael Rees of APD in 2007. The chain was 10 transplants long and occurred over several months. APD has performed 155 transplants to date
- The national kidney registry (NKR) was formed in 2008 and facilitated over 500 transplants in 4 years utilizing nondirected altruistic donors (NDDs) to start chains of various lengths. Next, the UNOS KPD pilot program was initiated in 2010 incorporating many features of the other exchanges

HOW KPD WORKS

- Incompatible pairs of patients are enrolled in a KPD registry. Chains can be simple two-way or three-way exchanges or longer. A nondirected donor often starts a KPD chain, which ends with a bridge donor at the end who can start another chain (Fig. 1). This NEAD chain may continue for several months but eventually ends with a bridge donor donating to the deceased donor list thus closing the chain

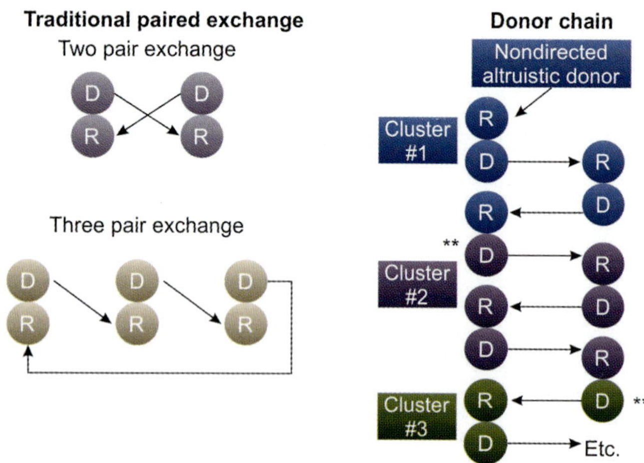

Fig. 1: Traditional paired exchange and donor chains.
**Bridge donors. With permission from the National Kidney Registry

- The donor and recipient ABO and human leukocyte antigen (HLA) are recorded and the recipient's HLA antibodies are entered. Each center decides which antigens are "unacceptable" to their recipient so that donors in KPD with those antigens will not be offered to that recipient. Having an accurate record of the donor antigens and the recipient antibodies allows for a virtual cross-match to occur that is predictive of what the real cross-match would show
- The recipients may express certain preferences such as age of donor and level of match that they are willing to accept
- Once several pairs are enrolled a computer match run takes place and a match offer is made to the centers that have matching pairs. A match run may occur as frequently as everyday to every 3 months depending on the program. Once the centers decide to accept the match offer donor blood is sent to the receiving centers in order to perform a real cross-match
- Once cross-matches are negative a logistics call is scheduled with all centers involved to plan for transportation of the organs as well as coordination with the organ procurement organizations (OPOs) and couriers involved in the exchange
- Because of the complexity of the multicenter exchange, the surgeries are usually nonsimultaneous using the honor system to ensure that donors do not back out. A donor is expected to donate but can never be forced to donate even after his intended recipient receives a kidney. There have been instances of donors backing out in the last minute but they are infrequent

CONSENT

- It is important to speak about KPD early in the donor evaluation process. This may decrease feelings of pressure that might occur if KPD is first presented after incompatibility is determined
- The donor should be made aware that he will likely never meet or even hear about the actual recipient of his kidney (unless mutually agreed upon by all parties)
- Consent includes the risks of shipping a kidney, the potential for last minute cancellations, and unexpected redirection of the kidney to a different recipient
- The donor must know about the frequent need for reblood draws for cross-matching and the changes in OR dates as so many donors and recipients in different centers are involved in chains

COMPUTER MATCHING

- Computer software based on "optimization"
- Optimization is a branch of mathematics that helps decide how to obtain the most results from a limited resource such as kidney transplants. It is also used in airline scheduling and in medical residency matching
- Computer match runs can be generated daily, weekly, or monthly. It is reasonable to perform a computer match run every time a new pair of patients are entered into the system
- After a match run, a match offer to the centers may or may not be offered based on the number of transplants it would provide. It may be prudent to await an offer that will include not only a high number of transplants but also hard to match patients with high cPRA

TRANSPORTING THE KIDNEY

- Just as in deceased donor transplants the kidney needs to be transported to the recipient hospital
- Transported by local OPO or via a courier company who hand it off to the airline. After arrival at its destination, the kidney is again picked up by the local OPO or the courier and brought to the awaiting hospital OR
- A GPS device is attached to the kidney box and it is tracked until it arrives at destination
- Extra donor blood is included in the kidney box for cross-matching with a new recipient were the intended recipient to suffer an unexpected medical event rendering them unable to receive the transplant
- Living donor kidneys can tolerate cold ischemic times 14 hours and more. The delayed graft function (DGF) rate for kidneys in KPD is 4%, same as traditional living donor DGF rate of 4%

- It is preferred for the kidney to travel and not the donor. Disadvantages of donor travel are that it is costly to the donor, the donor is exposed to a new hospital with a surgical/medical team that they are not familiar with, and the donor does not have his family around to help him recover. Following transplant, complications would be a challenge to address if the donor lived far from the hospital in which he donated

ETHICAL CONSIDERATIONS

- Some have argued that the hesitant donor has fewer opportunities to back out as he cannot invoke ABO incompatibility as reason to withdraw from the exchange
- The donor in KPD perhaps has more pressure to donate as backing out of the exchange will result in many people not getting transplanted as opposed to just one person not getting transplanted
- The deceased donor list is potentially disadvantaged as the NDD is donating to the living donor pool and not to the deceased donor transplant (DDT) list. However, a KPD chain initiated by an NDD eventually closes with a bridge donor donating to the DDT list. In this way, the DDT list is in fact benefited by KPD

THE O RECIPIENT PROBLEM

- The blood type O patient is disadvantaged in KPD. The blood type O recipient requires a blood type O donor but blood type O donors can usually donate to their own recipients so very few O donors are available in KPD. The exception to this is when there is a blood type O donor that is cross-match positive with his recipient
- The best solution to this problem is to incorporate compatible pairs into KPD namely pairs that have an O donor
- Very highly sensitized patients, even if they are non-blood type O, can wait long in KPD just as they do on the DDT list. A strategy utilizing desensitization in addition to enrollment in KPD can benefit these patients

COMPATIBLE PAIRS

- Including compatible pairs in KPD, especially those with O donors, can be a great benefit to others in KPD, especially the stranded O recipients. More matches will be available and more O recipients will get transplanted
- The recipient of the compatible pair might benefit as well by receiving a better matched kidney, or perhaps a younger kidney than his own donor

FINANCIAL ASPECTS

- As of now there is no uniform way of paying for KPD. A typical model will have the following features:
- The donor center allocates all costs for the donor evaluation to their Medicare cost report
- The donor center bills the recipient center for the nephrectomy
- Transportation of the donor organ is billed to the recipient center
- Donor complications are the responsibility of the donor center. The donor center bills the recipient's insurance or the recipient center according to agreements made pretransplant
- Medicaid patients are disadvantaged as Medicaid will not pay for out-of-state physician fees if the KPD donor is out-of-state
- Some have proposed that, as in deceased donor transplant, there should be a standard acquisition charge (SAC) for transplantation within KPD. This upfront cost will be financed by Centers for Medicare & Medicaid Services (CMS) for identifying and procuring the living donor kidney

THE IDEAL NATIONAL KPD PROGRAM

- One program for the country with a large pool of donor/recipient pairs. All other programs retired
- State-of-the-art software and frequent computer matching
- Compatible and incompatible pairs are entered into the system allowing for greater match offers and alleviating disadvantages to O recipients
- CMS would finance the system, allowing more transplants to occur and save on dialysis costs

FURTHER READING

1. de Klerk M, Witvliet MD, Haase-Kromwijk BJ, et al. Hurdles, barriers and successes of a national living donor kidney exchange program. Transplantation 2008;86:1749–53.
2. Dew MA, Jacobs CL, Jowsey SG, et al. Guidelines for the psychosocial evaluation of living unrelated kidney donors in the United States. Am J Transplant 2007;7: 1047–54.
3. Gentry SE, Segev DL, Simmerling M, et al. Expanding kidney paired donation through participation by compatible pairs. Am J Transplant 2007;7:2361–70.

4. Huh KH, Kim MS, Ju MK, et al. Exchange living-donor kidney transplantation: merits and limitations. Transplantation 2008; 86:430–5.
5. NKR website: www.kidneyregistry.org/index.php. Accessed Nov 15, 2012.
6. Optimization. http://optimizedmatch.com./learn_opt.php. Accessed Nov 15, 2012.
7. Rapaport FT. The case for a living emotionally related international kidney donor exchange registry. Transplant Proc 1986; 18:5–9.
8. Rees MA, Kopke JE, Pelletier RP, et al. A nonsimultaneous, extended, altruistic-donor chain. N Eng J Med 2009;360: 1096–101.
9. Rees MA, Schnitzler MA, Zavala EY, et al. Call to develop a standard acquisition charge model for kidney paired donation. Am J Transplant 2012;12:1392–7.
10. Ross LF, Rubin DT, Siegler M, et al. Ethics of a paired kidney-exchange-program. N Engl J Med 1997;336:1752–5.
11. Segev DL, Veale JL, Berger JC, et al. Transporting live donor kidneys for kidney paired donation: initial national results. Am J Transplant 2011;11:356–60.
12. Serur D, Charlton M. Kidney Paired Donation 2011. Progress in Transplantation 2011;21:215–8.
13. Woodle ES, Daller JA, Aeder M, et al. Ethical considerations for participation of nondirected living donors in kidney exchange programs. Am J Transplant 2010;10: 1460–67.

CHAPTER 24

Pharmacology

Antonette S Flecha, Donato F Tramontozzi

IMMUNOSUPPRESSION

- The primary goal of immunosuppression is the establishment of an environment in which the immune system (although weakened) continues to function while not rejecting the transplant allograft
- Prophylaxis of opportunistic infections is necessary given the weakened immune response

INDUCTION IMMUNOSUPPRESSION

- Intense immunosuppressive therapy utilized at the time of transplantation
- Induction agents include:
  - Corticosteroids
  - Simulect (basiliximab)
  - Campath (alemtuzumab)
  - Thymoglobulin (antithymocyte rabbit)
  - ATGAM (thymocyte equine)
  - Nulojix (belatacept)
  - Discontinued drugs: Orthoclone OKT3 (muromonab-CD3) and Zenapax (daclizumab)

Corticosteroids: Solu Medrol (Methylprednisolone) and Deltasone (Prednisone)

- Suppresses cell-mediated and antibody-mediated immunity
- High doses cause adrenal suppression
- Side effects include but are not limited to leukocytosis, hyperglycemia, osteoporosis, edema, hypertension, increased appetite, and insomnia. In rare instances may cause psychosis
- Solu Medrol is the intravenous (IV) formulation—utilized at induction
- Prednisone is the oral formulation—initiated once patient tolerates oral medications
- Prednisone is converted in the liver to active prednisolone (important if patient has hepatic insufficiency and/or failure)

Simulect (Basiliximab)

- Chimeric monoclonal antibody (MAB)
- Binds to the α-chain of the interleukin 2 receptor of activated T cells
- Dose: 20 mg given IV at time of surgery and a second dose given on postoperative day 4

Campath (Alemtuzumab)

- MAB
- Binds to CD52—antigen on the surface of B and T lymphocytes, monocytes, macrophages, natural killer cells, and some granulocytes
- Causes antibody dependent cell-mediated lysis
- Dose is 30 mg IV once at the time of surgery

Antithymocyte Globulin Rabbit (Thymoglobulin)

- Polyclonal antibody
- Targets T cells
- Active T-cell clearance from the circulation and suppression of T-cell activation
- Not as selective as a MAB
- Dose: 1.5 mg/kg IV daily typically for 3–7 days (institution specific)
- Usual maximum daily dose is 150 mg
- Rabbit origin
- Associated with fewer side effects than equine antibodies

Antithymocyte Globulin Equine (ATGAM)

- Polyclonal antibody
- Lymphocyte-selective immunosuppressant
- Alters the effectiveness of T lymphocytes involved in humoral immunity

Belatacept (Nulojix)

- Selective T-cell blocker that binds to CD80 and CD86 on antigen presenting cells
- Inhibits T lymphocyte proliferation and the production of cytokines
- Used both as induction and maintenance immunosuppression
- Infusion as maintenance once every 28 days
- All patients must be screened for Epstein-Barr Virus (EBV) serology
- Should not be administered to recipients not previously exposed to EBV—increased risk of post-transplant lymphoproliferative disease (PTLD) in EBV-negative recipients

MAINTENANCE IMMUNOSUPPRESSION

- Transplant recipients usually receive a combination therapy to allow for smaller doses of each agent
- Such combination has the potential to decrease the incidence of side effects
- Immunosuppression levels are adjusted based on timing and function
  - In the absence of rejection, levels are lowered
- Immunosuppression should be continued for life or until failure of the allograft
  - Discontinuation of immunosuppression is associated with loss of the graft
  - Only in exceptional instances and under strict medical supervision can an attempt be made to discontinue immunosuppression in a recipient with a functioning graft
- In its simplest form, maintenance immunosuppression consists of:
  - Calcineurin inhibitor (CNI)
  - Corticosteroids
  - Usually a third drug is added (such as a mycophenolic compound)
- Given that there are multiple possible maintenance combination regimens, the choice is up to each transplant center based on its experience and preference

Prograf (Tacrolimus)

- CNI
- Also known as FK 506 (based on its testing phase denomination)
- Trough levels are routinely monitored
  - Range: 5–20 ng/mL
- Binds intracellular protein FKBP-12
- Forms a complex that prevents phosphatase activity of calcineurin
- Prevents dephosphorylation and translocation of activated T cells (T cells initiate gene transcription and lymphokines)
- Inhibits T-lymphocyte activation
- Side effects include but are not limited to headache, tremors, and nephrotoxicity over time
- Available both as IV and oral formulations
  - Dose conversion is roughly 1/4 total daily oral dose given IV
  - IV formulation has a high risk of CNS side effects, including seizures

Neoral/Gengraf (Cyclosporine Modified) Sandimmune (Cyclosporine Nonmodified)

- Also a CNI
- Similar mechanism of action to Prograf
- Inhibits T lymphocyte activation by blocking of interleukin 2 and other cytokines
- Non-modified Cyclosporine (CSA) is poorly absorbed
- Modified CSA is slightly better absorbed
  - (25% nonmodified to 30% modified)
- Modified CSA is the preferred agent
- Trough levels are routinely monitored
  - Range: 150–400 ng/mL
- Side effects include but are not limited to gingival hyperplasia, hirsutism, hypertension, tremors, and nephrotoxicity over time
- Available as both IV and (liquid or capsule) oral formulations
  - Dose conversion is roughly 1/3 total daily oral dose given IV

Myfortic [Mycophenolic Acid (MPA)] and Cellcept [Mycophenolate Mofetil (MMF)]

- Antimetabolites
- Inhibit B- and T-cell proliferation and antibody production by inhibiting their de novo pathway of purine synthesis

- Adjunct therapy to CNI
- MPA: Typical dose is 360–720 mg orally twice daily
  - Enteric coated
  - May have decreased GI side effects
- MMF: Typical dose is 500–1000 mg orally twice daily
- Side effects for both compounds include but are not limited to:
  - Leucopenia
  - GI side effects (such as diarrhea, nausea, vomiting, and cramping)
  - Often dose dependent
- MPA is available in tablet form only
- MMF is available as tablet, liquid, and IV formulations

Rapamune (Sirolimus)

- Inhibits T-cell activation and proliferation as well as antibody production
- Trough levels are routinely monitored
  - Range: 10–20 ng/mL
- Side effects include but are not limited to elevations in cholesterol and triglycerides levels as well as opportunistic infection, hypersensitivity reaction, and potential for rhabdomyolysis
- If used in combination with cyclosporine, maintain at least a 4-hour separation in dosages

ADDITIONAL AGENTS

Rituxan (Rituximab)

- Administered in instances of antibody-mediated rejection and/or desensitization prior to transplantation
- Binds to CD20 antigen of B cells, destroying them
- Can activate latent hepatitis B
- Common side effects include but are not limited to infusion reactions, diarrhea, infection, and lymphopenia

Velcade (Bortezomib)

- Administered in instances of antibody-mediated rejection and/or desensitization prior to transplantation
- Inhibits the 26S proteasome in cells, leading to inhibition of plasma cells
- Common side effects include but are not limited to thrombocytopenia, leucopenia, and hypotension

Intravenous Immunoglobulin (IVIg)

- Administered in instances of antibody-mediated rejection and/or desensitization prior to transplantation
- Exact mechanism of action is unknown
- Common side effects include but are not limited to hypersensitivity reaction, and infusion reactions

Soliris (Eculizumab)

- Administered in instances of antibody-mediated rejection
- Binds to complement protein C5, and inhibits the terminal complement complex
- Common side effects include but are not limited to headache, diarrhea, and both viral and bacterial infections
- Serious cases of meningitis postadministration have been reported, so patient should be vaccinated for meningitis at least 14 days prior to use
- Paroxysmal nocturnal hemoglobinuria has also been reported

PROPHYLAXIS OF OPPORTUNISTIC INFECTIONS

Valcyte (Valganciclovir)

- Prophylaxis against cytomegalovirus (CMV) infection
- Administered immediately post-transplant for at least 3 months
- Risk of CMV infection increases depending on a recipient and donor CMV status
- Common side effects include but are not limited to headache and leucopenia

Bactrim (Sulfamethoxazole/Trimethoprim)

- Administered to prevent *Pneumocystis jiroveci* (PCP), aka, *Pneumocystis carinii* pneumonia
- Common side effects include but are not limited to rash and sensitivity to sunlight

Mepron (Atovaquone)

- Alternative to Bactrim for PCP prophylaxis
- Available in an oral liquid formulation
- Common side effects include but are not limited to rash, nausea, and insomnia

NebuPent (Pentamidine)

- Alternative to Bactrim and Mepron for PCP prophylaxis. Not a drug of choice
- Available as inhalation only
- Must be administered with Respirgard II Nebulizer
- Dose is 300 mg inhaled every 28 days
- Common side effects include cough, shortness of breath, anorexia, dizziness, and fatigue

Diflucan (Fluconazole)

- Prophylaxis for systemic fungal infections
- Hepatically metabolized
- Inhibits the CYP-450 system, leading to an increased level of certain drugs, including both tacrolimus and cyclosporine
- Common side effects include but are not limited to vomiting, abdominal pain, and headaches

Mycelex Troche (Clotrimazole)

- Used to prophylaxis against oral candidiasis
- Same drug class as fluconazole but with minimal systemic absorption and minimal inhibition of the CYP 450 system
- Common side effects include but are not limited to nausea, vomiting, abdominal pain, and diarrhea

Mycostatin Suspension (Nystatin)

- Alternative to Mycelex for oral candidiasis prophylaxis
- Must be orally rinsed and ingested for effective prophylaxis
- Suspension must be shaken well before each use

FURTHER READING

1. http://www.micromedexsolutions.com/micromedex2/librarian/keywords: Nystatin, Tacrolimus, Cyclosporine, Clotrimazole, Fluconazole, Pentamidine, Atovaquone, Bactrim, Valganciclovir, Eculizumab, Intravenous Immunoglobulin, Velcade, Rituxan, Rapamune, Cellcept, Myfortic, Belatacept, antithymocyte. Accessed October 10-15th, 2012.

CHAPTER 25

Anesthesia

Richard J Grieco

INTRODUCTION

Candidates for renal transplantation are selected from patients with end-stage renal disease (ESRD) caused by glomerular disease, diabetes mellitus, hypertensive kidney disease, polycystic kidney disease, other familial or congenital diseases, and tubulointerstitial disease. Despite concerns about the recurrence of disease in the donor kidney, it has generally been only slowly progressive. Kidney transplantation confers a 40–60% decrease in death rate compared with patients remaining on dialysis, thus proving to be one of the most important, cost-effective ways of treating ESRD. The graft survival rate is > 88% at 3 years among cadaver kidney transplant recipients, and approximately 93% in living donor recipients.

PATHOPHYSIOLOGY

The kidneys receive about 25% of cardiac output. They are essential for acid-base balance, adjusting body fluid volumes, electrolyte composition, and hemoglobin concentration. Patients who demonstrate glomerular filtration rates < 30 mL/min/1.72 m^2 (normal 120 mL/min/1.72 m^2) begin to retain fluid and electrolytes and show an increase in nitrogenous wastes in the blood, mainly urea. When measured urine production declines to < 400 cc/day, the patient is unable to excrete dietary fluid and electrolyte loads and abnormalities in Na^+, K^+, Ca^{++}, Mg^{++}, and phosphate can develop. The most dangerous being hyperkalemia.

There are multiple pathophysiologic and metabolic changes that occur in patients with ESRD. Deranged renal handling of Na^+ and fluids leads to volume expansion and hypertension. Altered levels of vasoactive substances lead to local and systemic changes in arterial tone. Increased systemic vascular resistance may be caused by hyperreninemia. Quite often, hypertensive damages to the kidney create the vicious cycle for escalating hypertension. ESRD can also promote worsening atherosclerosis as uremia can lead to changes in lipid metabolism resulting in reduced levels of protective high-density lipoproteins and increased serum triglycerides. With respect to diabetes mellitus, this disease process is the cause of ESRD in nearly 30–40% of cases and nephropathy can develop in nearly 60% of diabetics that are insulin dependent.

Other salient pathophysiologic issues in patients with ESRD are delayed gastric emptying secondary to chronic uremia. As such, all patients presenting for kidney transplantation should be considered to have full stomachs despite adequate preoperative fasting. Further, a qualitative defect in platelet aggregation exists in the uremic patient, and a bleeding tendency has long been recognized.

INDICATIONS/CONTRAINDICATIONS

Prolonged time on dialysis in the patient with ESRD can have adverse consequences on organ systems. Ideally, those patients identified with progressive renal failure should receive a kidney transplant before beginning dialysis. Unfortunately, with an average wait time in the United States longer than 3 years for a renal allograft, most patients receiving renal transplants have ESRD that has progressed to the point where dialysis is required. Comorbidities previously thought to be contraindications to transplantation now are considered acceptable. Patients with HIV infection and those infected by hepatitis C virus, both previously considered contraindications, now enjoy success rates comparable to noninfected patients.

Further, patients older than age 65 now receive renal transplants with outcomes similar to younger patients, and patients with advanced congestive heart failure do better with renal transplantation compared with those treated medically with dialysis. Patients considered poor candidates for transplantation are those with disseminated malignancies, active drug abuse, active infection, and complete thrombosis of the vena cava and iliac veins. Patients with a history of mental retardation who are unlikely to take their medications postoperatively and those patients who have a history of noncompliance constitute relative contraindications to transplantation.

ORGAN MATCHING AND ALLOCATION

There are several tests that are performed prior to transplantation to evaluate graft versus host compatibility. The first assay performed will determine major blood group (ABO) compatibility. The ABO blood group antigens behave as very strong histocompatibility antigens. As such, ABO-incompatible allografts have long been considered an impossibility as ABO-incompatible kidneys will fail rapidly if nothing is done to reduce the amount of antibody directed against the incompatible antigen in the recipient's serum. However, by using a combination of anti-B cell therapy and plasmapheresis, success is now reported. A second test determines the human leukocyte antigens (HLAs) profile of the recipient. At one time, HLA compatibility was considered to be the most crucial because transplants between individuals who shared many HLA antigens were more likely to avoid graft refection than those who did not share HLA antigens. Because of modern immunosuppression regimens, this has all changed allowing for excellent immunologic outcome even in the setting of complete HLA mismatch. As a result, HLA testing is now of much lesser value. It is now used to primarily determine which of several donors has the best histologic match to the intended recipient. Finally, a cross-match is done by mixing the recipient blood with donor blood cells to determine the presence or absence of preformed reactive antibodies against donor antigens. In prospective recipients who have antibodies directed against multiple HLA antigens, it is difficult to find an appropriate donor with a negative cross-match. Many patients, however, can be treated with desensitization strategies to reduce the burden of circulating antibodies including plasmapheresis, infusion of random donor immune globulin, and anti-B cell monoclonal antibodies. Experience is now accumulating with these protocols to allow for successful outcomes.

PREOPERATIVE PREPARATION

If possible, recipients should be dialyzed prior to surgery to correct volume status and electrolyte imbalances. Patients who are not maintained on dialysis usually produce sufficient urine volume to prevent fluid overload. To estimate volume status, the practitioner can compare a patient's current weight with their "dry weight," which hemodialysis patients usually know. Patients undergoing hemodialysis just prior to surgery may be at risk of significant hypotension on induction of anesthesia as their volume status may be suboptimal. Potassium levels should also be reviewed prior to surgery. Levels > 5.5 mEq/L may necessitate a delay in surgery and correction of potassium levels.

Cardiac evaluation should include a preoperative ECG and stress test in those patients with newly diagnosed ESRD unrelated to diabetes. A stress echocardiogram or a cardiac catheterization may be indicated in those patients with long-standing ESRD associated with diabetes and those patients with symptoms suggestive of coronary artery disease (CAD).

In patients with noninsulin-dependent diabetes, it should be determined when antiglycemic agents were last taken. Oral agents should not be taken the day of surgery because of the potential for unrecognized hypoglycemia under anesthesia. Brittle insulin-dependent diabetics are at risk of the development of ketosis and intraoperative acidemia. An indwelling arterial catheter will allow for frequent blood glucose and acid–base measurements in these patients. Insulin infusions can be utilized to maintain blood sugar levels between 90 and 110 g/dL if necessary.

SURGICAL PROCEDURE

The transplanted kidney is usually placed in the external iliac fossa after the common and external iliac arteries and veins are exposed in the retroperitoneum. The renal vein is anastamosed first in an end to side anastamosis. The renal artery is then anastamosed to the internal or external iliac artery. The final stage of the procedure is anastamosing the donor ureter to the patient's bladder.

ANESTHETIC MANAGEMENT

Although regional anesthesia has been successfully used, general anesthesia is most often selected for renal transplantation to provide stable hemodynamics, predictable depth of anesthesia, and excellent muscle relaxation. General anesthesia also provides the advantage of mechanically maintaining the patient's ventilation that may become compromised by surgical retraction limiting diaphragmatic excursion. Further, uremic platelet dysfunction and residual heparin from preoperative dialysis have limited use of regional anesthesia for kidney transplantation.

Standard American Society of Anesthesiologists monitors may be all that is needed for these procedures. Patients with more significant comorbidities may require more extensive monitoring with central venous pressure (CVP) or continuous arterial pressure monitoring, or both. Patients with symptomatic CAD or a history of congestive heart failure may benefit from pulmonary artery catheter or transesophageal echocardiography (TEE) monitoring. A common general anesthetic approach is to combine volatile anesthetics with nitrous oxide and short-acting opioids. The choice of induction agent depends on the relative health of the patient, volume status, presence of cardiovascular disease, and/or autonomic neuropathy. Relatively healthy patients will tolerate propofol at 2–3 mg/kg, whereas etomidate at 0.2 mg/kg might be a better alternative in patients who are hemodynamically compromised. The volatile anesthetic administered does not predictably influence renal function after kidney transplantation. However, the metabolism of sevoflurane has been implicated in renal toxicity by the generation of "compound A" from the breakdown of this agent by barium or sodium hydroxide. Studies have shown that fresh gas flow rates of > 4 L/minute will essentially eliminate any deleterious effects of sevoflurane toxicity.

Rapid sequence induction may be indicated in diabetic patients with gastroparesis. The use of succinylcholine is not absolutely contraindicated in patients with ESRD. After an intubating dose of succinylcholine, serum potassium elevation is the same in patients with and without ESRD, approximately 0.6 mEq/L. With an initial serum K^+ concentration < 5.0 mEq/L, this increase can be tolerated without significant cardiac risk.

Cisatracurium and atracurium are metabolized by plasma cholinesterase and spontaneous Hofmann degradation. These relaxants are attractive selections as their clearance from the plasma is independent of renal function. Patients with ESRD have an increased sensitivity to rocuronium and vecuronium. Although, these drugs are primarily metabolized by the liver, the duration of these agents may be prolonged if large doses are used. Pancuronium depends on the kidney for elimination and will have a prolonged duration of action in patients with ESRD.

Narcotics must be used cautiously in renal transplant recipients. Specifically, meperidine (Demerol) metabolism leads to the production of normeperidine that can significantly accumulate and lead to seizures. Further, a metabolite of morphine, morphine-6-B-glucoronide, which is normally excreted by the kidney has opioid agonist activity. This agent can therefore cause respiratory depression with long-term use in patients with renal failure. Fentanyl, sufentanil, alfentanil, remifentanil, and hydromorphone are safe alternatives.

CVP monitoring can be utilized to guide the volume and rate of crystalloid infusions. Optimizing hydration status during the intraoperative period will maximize renal blood flow and improve early function of the transplanted kidney.

To enhance urine formation by the newly transplanted kidney, diuretics are frequently administered. Mannitol, an agent that is freely filtered but not reabsorbed by the nephron, causes an osmotic expansion of urine volume. It also protects the cells lining the renal tubule. This medication is frequently administered to donors before harvesting as well as to recipients intraoperatively at doses of 0.25–1.0 g/kg. Loop diuretics, such as furosemide, cause an excretion of large volumes of urine with high electrolyte content by blocking the action of Na^+/K^+ pumps in the ascending loop of Henle. "Renal dose" dopamine (2–3 mg/kg/min) can be used to increase urine output, but its use is controversial in the denervated, newly transplanted kidney.

Upon release of the vascular clamp from the newly transplanted kidney, venous drainage from the legs as well as renal preservative fluid from the transplanted organ containing acid metabolites, potassium, and vasodilating chemicals from previously ischemic tissues is released into the circulation. This may cause hypotension, arrhythmias, and cardiac arrest due to sudden hyperkalemia. Communication between the surgeon and anesthesia provider is essential during this portion of the procedure, as well as heightened vigilance.

It is recommended to increase the systolic blood pressure to > 120 mm Hg prior to reperfusion of the transplanted kidney. Vasopressors such as ephedrine or neosynephrine can be infused as well as boluses of intravenous fluid to accomplish this goal. Plasmalyte is superior to either Ringer lactate or normal saline in maintaining acid-base balance in patients with ESRD, and its use is recommended.

IMMUNOSUPPRESSION

There are different phases of immunosuppression after transplantation. In the immediate post-transplant phase, potent induction immunosuppression is required to prevent rejection. By using multiple immunosuppressive agents targeting multiple sites in the immune response cascade, lower doses of each class of medications may be used. Agents typically employed include corticosteroids, an antimetabolite, a calcineurin inhibitor, and monoclonal or polyclonal antibodies.

Corticosteroids exert their immunosuppressive effects through multiple pathways resulting in inhibition of the activation of T cells. They function as both induction and maintenance immunosuppressive agents. Antimetabolites, such as mycophenolate, inhibit T- and B-cell proliferation. In general, these drugs are used to prevent rejection, not to treat active acute rejection. Calcineurin inhibitors, such as cyclosporine, are potent immunosuppressants that also inhibit T-cell activation as well as proliferation of B lymphocytes. They are considered to be a vital component of immunosuppressive regimens following transplantation. Monoclonal antibody therapy with an agent such as basiliximab has the unique ability to selectively inhibit T-cell populations that are activated at the time of transplantation, without affecting existing T-cell immunity to other antigens. As such, existing cellular immunity to other viruses is left intact. Polyclonal antibodies are potent immunosuppressive agents used for induction of immunosuppressive therapy and in the treatment of established rejection. They act by depleting circulating lymphocytes. Because they are polyclonal, they affect T cells, B cells, and natural killer cells. A common agent used in this regard is Thymoglobulin, a rabbit polyclonal antithymocyte globulin. Administration of this class of agent can lead to side effects including fever, chills, skin rashes, hypotension, acute respiratory distress, and anaphylaxis as well as neutropenia and thrombocytopenia. These side effects should be closely monitored for, and may be minimized by pretreatment with acetaminophen and diphenhydramine.

POST-TRANSPLANT MANAGEMENT

Urine output should be carefully measured postoperatively. Allografts from living donors typically have excellent immediate function with marked diuresis. Serum creatinine is closely monitored and typically decreases over 7–10 days. Those from deceased donors with longer cold ischemia may not have immediate function due to ATN. Ultrasound can be useful to evaluate for vessel thrombosis, perinephric fluid collection, or hydronephrosis if suspected. Knowledge of pretransplant blood pressures are helpful in targeting post-transplant blood pressure requirements to maintain adequate perfusion. The post-transplant patient typically requires a blood pressure > 120/80 mm Hg. Blood glucose measurements should be performed on a regular basis as hyperglycemia may be exacerbated by the administration of corticosteroids. Optimal blood glucose control in the postoperative period has been shown to decrease morbidity and mortality. Further, post-procedure monitoring of serum sodium, potassium, bicarbonate, calcium, magnesium, and phosphorus is routine. Prophylaxis against deep vein thrombosis with subcutaneous heparin as well as the administration of proton pump inhibitors or H2 receptor blockers to prevent gastric ulcers should also be considered.

CHAPTER 26

Live Donor Nephrectomy

Michael J Schwartz, Simpa S Salami, Lee Richstone, Louis R Kavoussi

PATIENT SELECTION

There are primary basic criteria that must be met for a patient to be considered as a potential renal donor:

- Absence of kidney disease
- Absence of transmissible malignancy
- No active infection

Secondary criteria for consideration include:

- Absence of significant medical comorbidities that could affect long-term renal function
- Good mental health
- Absence of communicable diseases (HIV, hepatitis, etc.)

LIVING DONOR EVALUATION (TABLES 1 AND 2)

Volunteers for renal donation require a thorough screening evaluation to ensure both physical and mental health. Discussion of perioperative risks and potential long-term morbidity of renal donation is a critical step before initiating medical evaluation.

- In long-term studies assessing the outcome of patients undergoing donor nephrectomy, creatinine clearance has been demonstrated to be 70–80% of the preoperative levels[1]
- In general, the risk of developing hypertension and chronic kidney disease is comparable to the general population.[2] However, certain patient populations have clear increased risk of developing chronic renal insufficiency including obese patients, those with preexisting hypertension and diabetics.[3-5] Most transplant programs will exclude these patients from renal donation
- Risk for developing CKD and hypertension is a spectrum, and exceptions are made in certain instances for the medically complex (extended criteria) renal donor with relatively low estimated long-term risk[6,7]
- In general, the risks to the potential donor patient are considered relatively low. With appropriate patient selection and recipient preparation, the probability of successful allograft is high enough such that the risks of donation are felt to be acceptable. The mortality risk of renal donation is estimated at 0.02–0.03%[8,9]

Preoperative evaluation involves a multidisciplinary approach, the primary goal of which is to determine if there is significant risk to normal renal function following donor nephrectomy (Tables 1 and 2). Internal

Table 1: Initial donor screening

Medical history and physical examination
Blood Pressure
ABO blood group
Serum chemistry, complete blood count, urinalysis

Table 2: Secondary donor screening (if initial screen satisfactory)

Estimated glomerular filtration rate
Infectious serology
Cardiac evaluation if appropriate (EKG, echo, stress testing, etc.)
Routine cancer screenings if not recently performed (prostate, breast, colon, cervical)
Pregnancy testing
Diabetic screening
Radiologic studies (abdominal sonogram, chest X-ray, CT angiography)
Psychiatric evaluation

medicine/nephrology, radiology, and donor surgeons are part of the standard donor evaluation. Additional medical subspecialists may also be required to evaluate specific conditions in the patient's medical history, particularly with prior history of malignancy to confirm no evidence of disease. Cardiologists are also becoming a more common part of preoperative evaluation, particularly as older patients (over the age of 50) are considered as potential donors with increasing frequency. If the screening is satisfactory and the patient meets criteria for donation, CT angiogram is typically employed to evaluate the renal vascular anatomy and to screen for any relevant renal pathology (stones, cystic lesions, etc.).

Preexisting microscopic hematuria is not a contraindication to renal donation with appropriate urologic evaluation to rule out malignancy preoperatively. This should include urine cytology, cystoscopy, and upper tract imaging such as renal sonography, CT, or MRI. Renal biopsy may also be considered by the evaluating nephrologist if the urologic evaluation is unrevealing.

ABO incompatibility and positive cross-match are also no longer strictly prohibitive for renal donation. Paired donor-swap programs and altruistic donor chains have made more renal donations possible in circumstances where direct donation could not otherwise occur.[10,11] In addition, improved immunosuppressive protocols have broadened the field of acceptable candidates for directed renal donation.[12]

KIDNEY SELECTION

- Kidney size
- Functional discrepancy
- Renal vascular anatomy

If there is a size or functional discrepancy between the kidneys, the donor is always left with the better functioning kidney. However, in most cases, the kidneys are of approximately equivalent size and function, and the renal vascular anatomy plays the most significant role in determining side of surgery for donor nephrectomy. In instances with single renal arteries bilaterally, the left side is typically preferred due to the longer associated renal vein. If one renal unit has multiple renal arteries, the kidney with the single renal artery is favored to simplify the arterial anastomosis for the recipient. For women who may become pregnant in the future, the right kidney should be considered strongly for donation due to the more frequent occurrence of hydronephrosis and pyelonephritis during pregnancy on the right side.

TECHNIQUE FOR DONOR NEPHRECTOMY

Laparoscopic donor nephrectomy (LDN) is considered standard of care for renal donor patients and preferred to open donor nephrectomy because of:

- Decreased analgesic requirement
- Decreased length of hospital stay
- Earlier return to work
- Superior cosmetic outcome

The disadvantages reported are:

- Increased operating time
- Increased need for special equipment
- Longer warm ischemia time
- Delayed graft function (Jacobs et al., 2004; Barry, 2005)[20,21]

These disadvantages are mainly reported in early experience with laparoscopic donor surgery as compared with open. With experience, the operative time and warm ischemia time improve and can often be equivalent or superior to open surgery.

PRIMARY OBJECTIVES OF RENAL DONOR SURGERY

1. Safety of the donor patient
2. Maintain the function of the allograft

The generous use of intravenous fluids helps to keep the donor kidney well perfused during the procedure. The use of osmotic diuretics (mannitol) also carries theoretical advantages of:

- Preventing cellular reperfusion injury
- Scavenging free radicals that are associated with reperfusion

PATIENT PREPARATION

The authors' preference for patient preparation is a clear liquid diet on the day prior to surgery along with one bottle of magnesium citrate in the afternoon prior to the procedure.

Equipment and Surgical Team

For a left LDN, the laparoscopic tower and monitor are placed on the left side of the patient with the surgical team on the right side. Placement of additional cautery, irrigation, and insufflation equipment is otherwise at surgeon discretion. The surgical technician is positioned on the side of surgery with the instrument table at the foot of the patient.

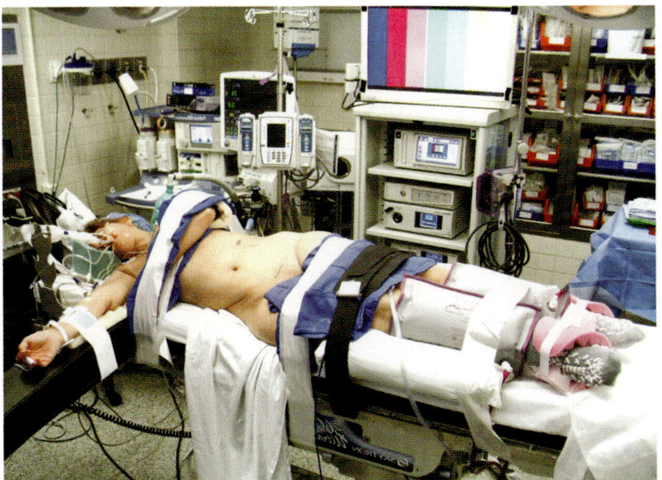

Fig. 1: Positioning for left laparoscopic donor nephrectomy. Gel rolls support the patient's scapula, flank and buttocks (not visible). A pillow supports the knees and foam padding supports the ankles, the flexed elbow and the outstretched arm. The patient is secured to the operating table using 3" silk tape and the safety strap. Sequential compression stockings are used for DVT prophylaxis.

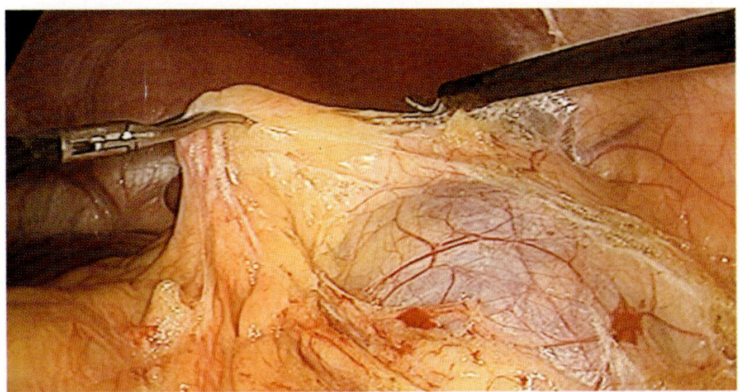

Fig. 3: The white line of Toldt is incised to allow for medial reflection of the colon. The kidney is seen within Gerota fascia that is initially left intact.

Patient Positioning (Fig. 1)

Sequential compression stockings are placed and engaged prior to the induction of anesthesia. Following induction of general anesthesia with endotracheal intubation, a Foley catheter is placed. The anterior abdomen is shaved from the xiphisternum to the pubic symphysis. A mini-Pfannenstiel incision is marked with the patient supine. The patient is positioned in a modified lateral decubitus position with the donor kidney side elevated approximately 30° with a large gel roll. The patient is secured to the table with silk tape across at points just above the xiphisternum, just below the anterior superior iliac spines, and the lower legs. The contralateral arm is placed on a padded armrest secured to the operative table, and the ipsilateral arm is positioned and secured in a neutral position, folded over the chest. Additional gel and foam padding is used to protect all pressure points. Patient's skin is prepared and draped in normal sterile fashion. It is not necessary to flex the table or use an axillary roll in this position. If the donor surgeon prefers more of a true flank position, an axillary roll is necessary.

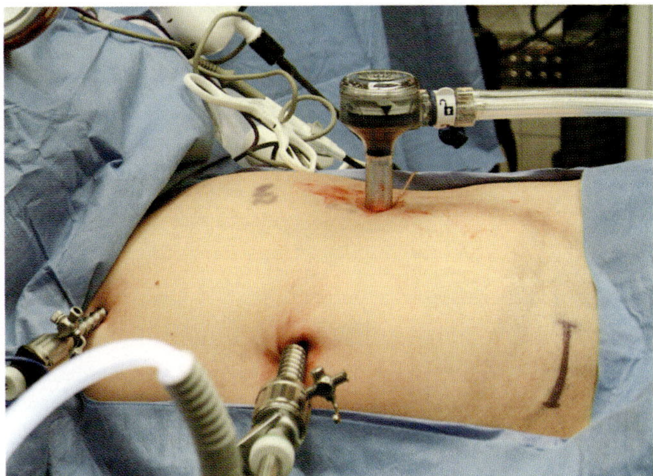

Fig. 2: Port placement for laparoscopic left donor nephrectomy. An 11-mm trocar is placed in the umbilicus to accommodate the camera. A 6-mm subxiphoid trocar and a 12-mm trocar are used for instrumentation. A previously marked 4.5 cm extraction site is shown that was marked with the patient supine prior to positioning.

Operative Procedure: Left Laparoscopic Donor Nephrectomy Port Placement (Fig. 2)

Pneumoperitoneum is induced with a Veress needle placed through the umbilicus and the abdomen is insufflated to 15 mm Hg. Three laparoscopic ports are placed: 11-mm umbilical port (camera), a 12-mm left lateral port roughly 2 fingerbreadths medial and superior to the ipsilateral anterior superior iliac spine, and a 5-mm subxiphoid port. The ports are placed in a triangular configuration for a left donor nephrectomy.

Colon Reflection and Mobilization (Fig. 3)

The peritoneum is divided with monopolar cautery shears along the line of Toldt. A combination of sharp, blunt and cautery dissection is used to reflect the colon and expose the kidney within Gerota fascia. Traction and countertraction is provided by the nonworking hand. Care is taken not to enter Gerota fascia yet at this point to facilitate dissection. It is also important to avoid initiating

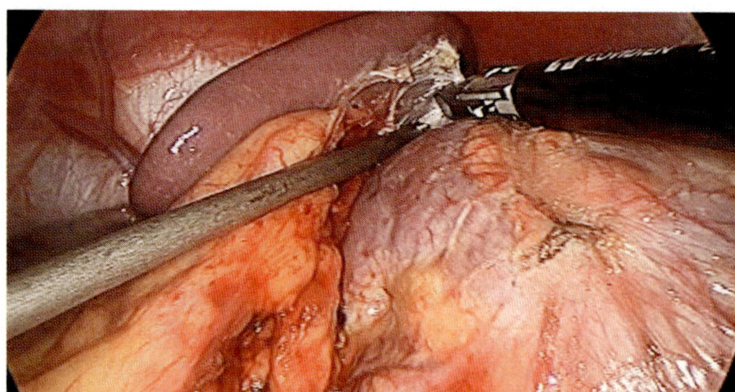

Fig. 4: Splenic attachments are freed using a combination of blunt dissection and bipolar cautery, here using the Ligasure device.

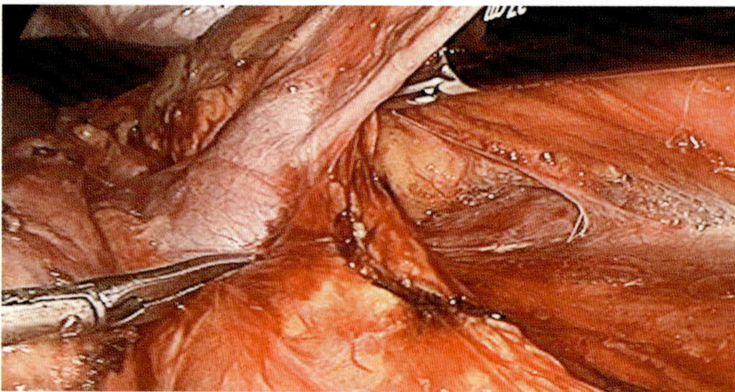

Fig. 5: Anterior traction on the kidney away from the psoas muscle shows the main left renal vein with the gonadal vein coming together with the main vein inferiorly.

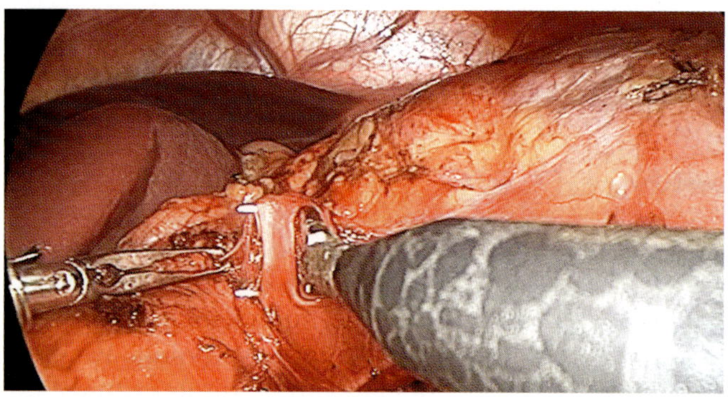

Fig. 6: Now superior to the main left renal vein, the adrenal vein has been dissected using the 10-mm right angle to free it from surrounding connective tissue, allowing it to be clipped and divided.

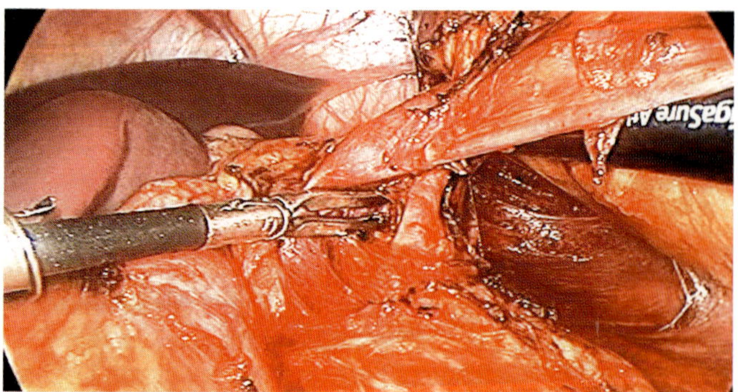

Fig. 7: Dissection behind the left renal vein reveals the main left renal artery, just lateral to is origin at the aorta.

a plane of dissection behind the kidney in order to preserve the lateral attachments. This will be helpful in preventing the kidney from dropping over the hilar vessels when performing later dissection.

Splenic Mobilization (Fig. 4)

Splenocolic and splenorenal ligaments almost always require division to allow for medial reflection of the spleen and pancreatic tail. This step dramatically improves exposure of the renal hilar vessels.

Dissection of Gonadal and Renal Veins (Figs. 5 and 6)

The left gonadal vein should now be visible below the lower pole of the kidney, overlying the left psoas muscle. It is dissected out superiorly to its insertion into the renal vein. The renal vein is then dissected, a process often expedited with employment of the suction-irrigator for blunt dissection. Anterior traction on the kidney is critical to place gentle traction on the hilum itself, both accelerating the dissection and allowing for safe visualization of the major vessels. The major tributaries (gonadal, lumbar, and adrenal veins) of the renal vein are exposed and ligated using titanium clips. Care must be taken to leave ample room medially along the vein for application of the vascular stapler later during the procedure away from any clips.

Dissection of the Renal Artery (Figs. 7 and 8)

Clipping the venous branches of the left renal vein often allows the left renal artery to become visible in the field if it had not yet been seen. The renal artery should be visible posterior to the renal vein. Preoperative CT angiogram often helps in localization of accessory renal arteries if present. The renal arterial dissection is carried out, with tissue surrounding it divided with bipolar electrocautery. Attempts should be made to expose the renal artery as close to its origin as possible.

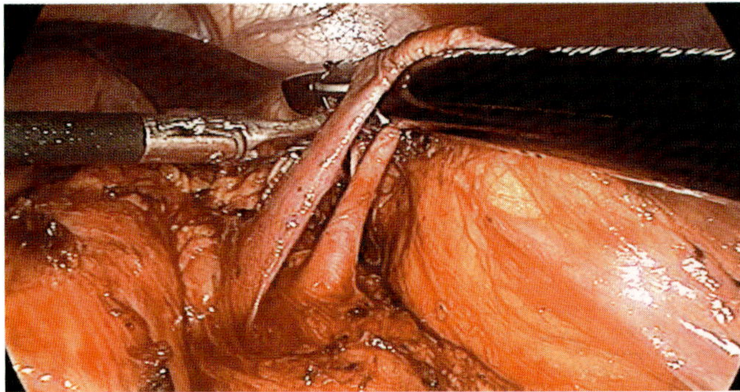

Fig. 8: The renal hilum, now fully dissected and ready for division and ligation later in the surgery.

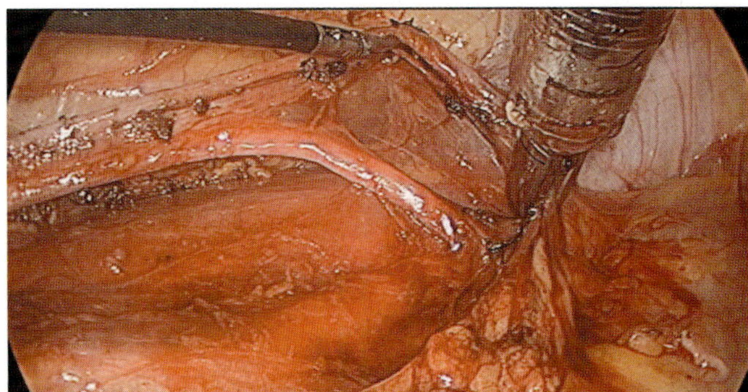

Fig. 9: The ureter is dissected to the level of the iliac bifurcation. Attention is given to not skeletonize the ureter extensively, which may impact on the blood supply and transplant anastomosis with the recipient bladder.

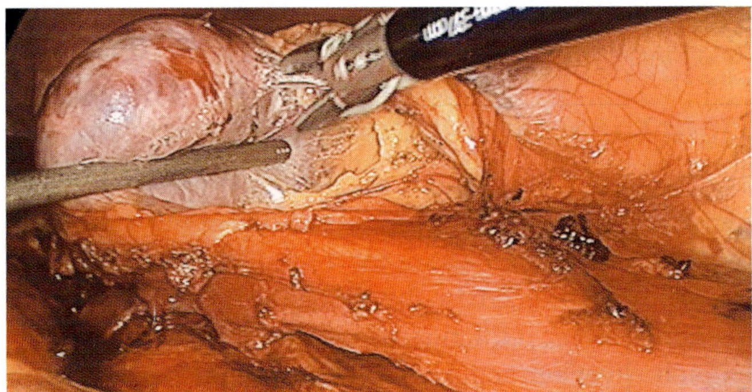

Fig. 10: Gerota fascia is entered and the kidney is freed from any surrounding fat intracorporeally.

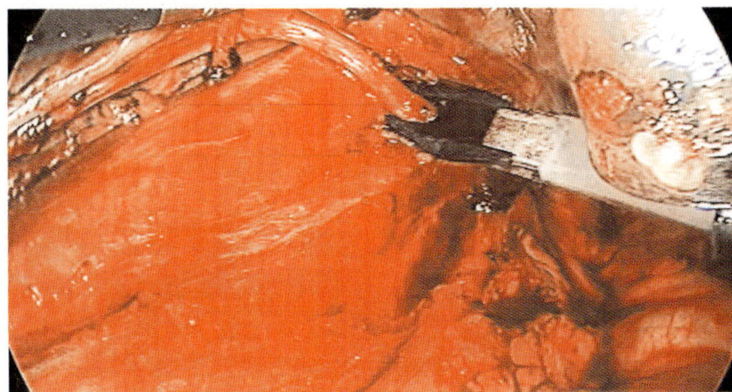

Fig. 11: Ligation of the ureter at the level of the iliac vessels using a 10-mm clip applier.

Dissection of the Ureter (Fig. 9)

The ureter is typically first visualized just behind the gonadal vein below the lower pole. It is critical to preserve adequate periureteral tissue to protect the ureteral blood supply. The dissection of the ureter is carried out distally to the level of the iliac bifurcation, with the division of the ureter at this site to be performed later in the procedure.

Dissection of the Kidney (Fig. 10)

The authors prefer entry into Gerota fascia at this point to free the kidney of the perirenal fat intracorporeally. Bipolar cautery is used to free the kidney's inferior, lateral, superior, medial and posterior attachments. The only remaining attachments at this point are the renal hilar vessels and ureter, and the kidney is now ready to be removed.

Creation of an Extraction Site

A mini-Pfannenstiel incision is made at the previously marked site. The length of the required extraction site is usually between 4 and 6 cm, depending on the size of the kidney and the patient body habitus. The rectus fascia is opened in the midline, but the peritoneum is left intact. A 15-mm port is inserted to accommodate the specimen retrieval bag. At this point, the back table for renal preservation and transplant surgical team are confirmed to be ready to receive the kidney prior to performing ureteral or hilar vessel ligation.

Ligation of the Ureter (Fig. 11)

The ureter is now clipped and divided. Diuresis is confirmed.

Ligation of the Renal Artery (Fig. 12)

The artery is ligated using 3–4 10-mm titanium clips or endoscopic vascular stapler. Use of Hem-o-lok clips for ligation of the renal artery has been reported as associated with bleeding complications and death, is contraindicated, and should NOT be used.

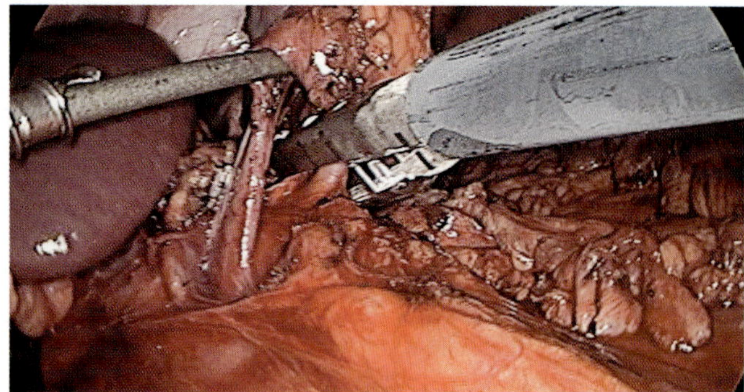

Fig. 12: An endovascular GIA multifire stapling device is used to ligate and divide the left renal artery. This can also be accomplished using 3–4 10-mm titanium clips.

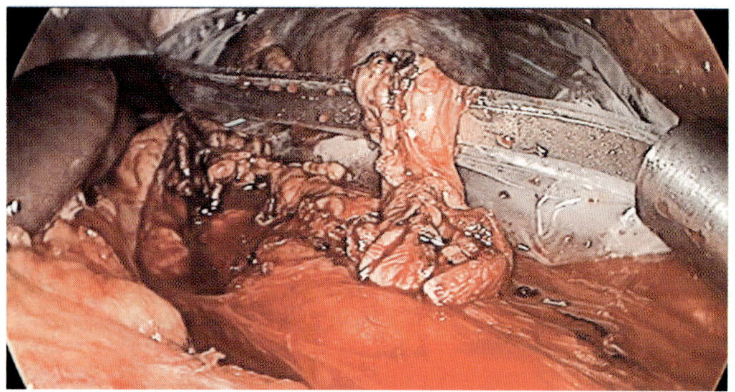

Fig. 14: The kidney and ureter are placed into an Endo Catch specimen retrieval bag that has been brought through the mini-Pfannenstiel extraction site.

Ligation of the Renal Vein with Stapling Device (Fig. 13)

The vein is then ligated using an endoscopic vascular stapler.

Specimen Extraction and Delivery (Fig. 14)

The donor kidney is placed in an Endo Catch bag and immediately extracted through the mini-Pfannenstiel incision. It is placed in ice slush where the transplant surgeon team will initiate the cold preservation process prior to immediate or delayed transplantation into the recipient.

Closure

The fascia at the extraction site is closed and the abdomen is reinsufflated. The renal hilum and fossa, staple lines, and clips on vessels are inspected for bleeding; the spleen and adrenal gland should also be inspected for injury/bleeding. The colon is returned to its normal position;

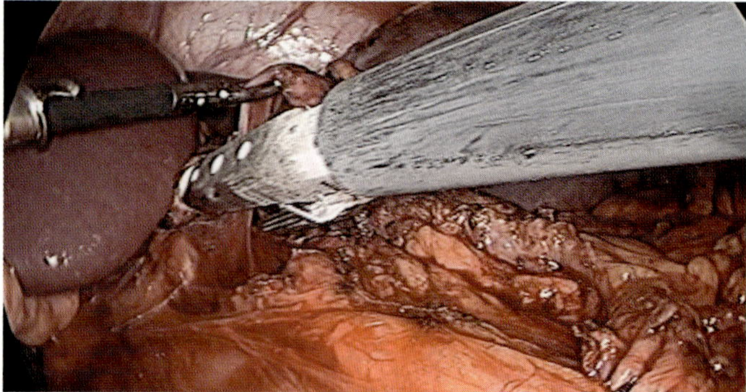

Fig. 13: Ligation of the left renal vein using a reloaded endovascular GIA multifire stapler.

and the incisions are closed. Fascial closure is performed for any cutting trocar sites >10 mm. No surgical drains are necessary unless injury to the pancreas is suspected.

Right Laparoscopic Donor Nephrectomy

The location of the monitor, the patient, the surgical team, incisions, and trocar placements are exact mirror images of what is described above for a left LDN. An additional 3-mm trocar placed in the subxiphoid region may be needed for liver retraction using a locking grasper. Alternatively, liver retraction may be accomplished using an additional 5-mm trocar in the anterior axillary line. Following nephrectomy, the liver should be closely inspected for any traction related injury and hemostasis.

Postoperative Care

Early mobilization on the day of surgery is encouraged. Patient is started on clear liquid diet and advanced as tolerated once return of bowel function is confirmed with passage of flatus or bowel movement. Pain is controlled with a combination of analgesics (oral/parenteral). The Foley catheter is removed on postoperative day 1 for a trial of void. Patients are usually discharged from the hospital on postoperative day 1 or 2.

Open Donor Nephrectomy

Open renal surgery for kidney donation is rarely performed, but donor surgeons should be familiar with open renal surgery in the case that open conversion is required. The most common reason for conversion to open renal surgery is vascular injury, and frequency of conversion is related to surgical volume and operative experience.[13]

If open conversion is required, a standard flank incision or a subcostal incision may be used to gain exposure. The operative table may also be flexed to open the space

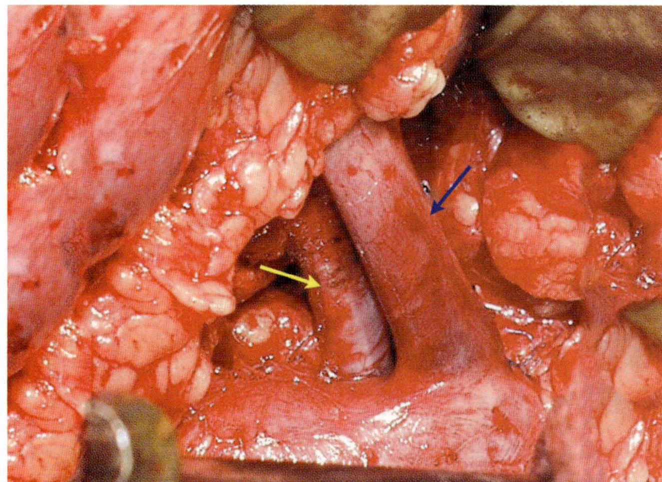

Fig. 15: Open live donor nephrectomies are infrequent since the development of the laparoscopic approach. The photograph (left) shows an open right nephrectomy, where the renal artery (yellow arrow) and renal vein (blue arrow) are ready to be clamped and transected.

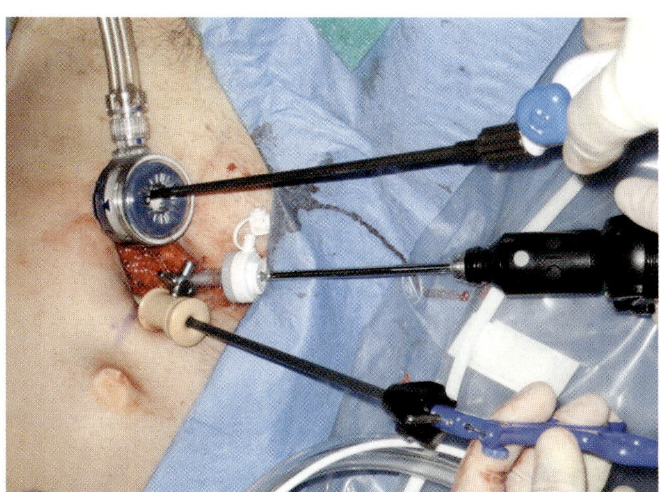

Fig. 17: Photograph of LESS donor nephrectomy with ports in place through the single mini-Pfannenstiel incision.

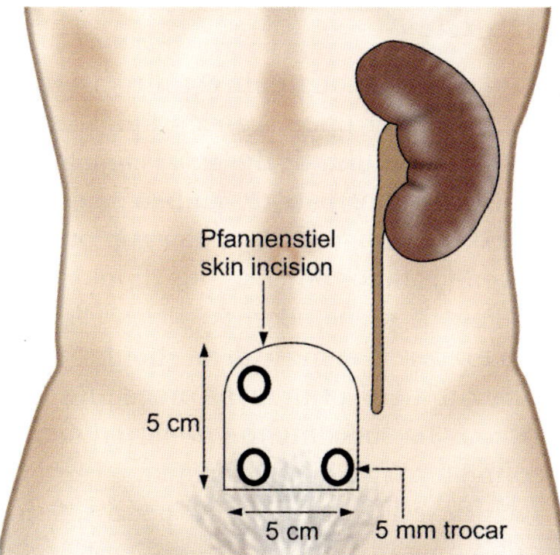

Fig. 16: Port site placement for LESS donor nephrectomy using a mini-Pfannenstiel incision. Once the incision is created, the plane between the rectus fascia and subcutaneous fat is developed to allow for port placement, maintaining triangulation albeit in much closer proximity than with the standard laparoscopic approach.

between the anterior superior iliac spine and the costal margin. In the case that significant bleeding is encountered during LDN, pressure may be applied to the affected area with a blunt laparoscopic instrument, while the open exposure is obtained. A self-retaining retractor is used to retract the abdominal wall and additional retractor blades may be applied to optimize exposure. Once hemostasis is achieved, the donor surgery may be continued, following the same principles described above for the standard laparoscopic operation. The kidney is freed from its surrounding connective tissue attachments and the ureter is dissected to the level of the iliac bifurcation prior to its ligation, again making sure to preserve the periureteral tissue to maintain blood supply. The renal hilar vessels are skeletonized (Fig. 15), and once the transplant team is ready to receive the kidney, the hilar vessels are ligated. Vessel ligation may be accomplished using multiple 0 silk ties or with the vascular stapler that may already be on the surgical field if the case was converted from a laparoscopic approach.

Laparoendoscopic Single Site (LESS) Donor Nephrectomy

Single site surgery has been employed for donor nephrectomy using a periumbilical or Pfannenstiel incision. It has been shown to be associated with reduced postoperative pain and has a potential advantage of improved cosmetic outcome. We have employed the Pfannenstiel approach because it has the potential to offer both advantages of decreased postoperative pain and can leave the patient without any easily visible scars thus improving patient satisfaction.[19] In addition, the port placement (Figs. 16 and 17) allows the surgeon to avoid the additional cost of purpose-built single site surgical devices and maintains the ability to triangulate, albeit with much closer port placement than conventional LDN. However, early series have also shown disadvantages of increased operative and warm ischemia time.

The sequence of surgical steps for the procedure is essentially identical to conventional LDN, but extensive experience with donor nephrectomy is critical prior to attempting a single site procedure. There should be a low threshold for conversion to conventional laparoscopic surgery as any potential compromise to the allograft is unacceptable.

CONCLUSION

The principles of donor nephrectomy are consistent, regardless of whether open, conventional laparoscopic, or LESS approach is utilized. The goal is first and foremost the safety of the donor patient, and second to maintain the function of the allograft. The latter is promoted by the use of intravenous fluids and osmotic diuretics during the procedure. Patient preparation is a clear liquid diet on the day prior to surgery along with one bottle of magnesium citrate on the afternoon prior to the procedure.

Laparoscopy has become the preferred technique for donor nephrectomy at most transplant centers due to the very well-described benefits of laparoscopic surgery with regard to operative morbidity, with equivalent complication risk.[14] As many donor volunteers are in younger patient cohorts, body image is a significant consideration leading to a preference for a laparoscopic approach.[15] Questions have been raised about the use of pneumoperitoneum and its potential impact on renal function. However, relative to open surgery there have been no demonstrable differences in allograft-related outcomes including delayed graft function, early graft loss, acute graft rejection, kidney function at 1 year, or graft loss at 1 year.[14] LESS donor nephrectomy has been employed in more recent years in an effort to further reduce surgical morbidity. Early results have suggested a possible shorter convalescence in these patients, although with longer operative and ischemia time.[16-18]

REFERENCES

1. Goldfarb DA, Matin SF, Braun WE, et al. Renal outcome 25 years after donor nephrectomy. J Urol 2001;166:43-2047. Epub 2001/11/07. PubMed PMID: 11696703.
2. Kasiske BL, Ma JZ, Louis TA, et al. Long-term effects of reduced renal mass in humans. Kidney Int 1995;48:814-9. Epub 1995/09/01. PubMed PMID: 7474669.
3. Hsu CY, McCulloch CE, Iribarren C, et al. Body mass index and risk for end-stage renal disease. Ann Intern Med 2006; 144:21-8. Epub 2006/01/04. PubMed PMID: 16389251.
4. Gelber RP, Kurth T, Kausz AT, et al. Association between body mass index and CKD in apparently healthy men. Am J Kidney Dis 2005; 46:871-80. Epub 2005/10/29. doi: 10.1053/j.ajkd.2005.08.015. PubMed PMID: 16253727.
5. Cuevas-Ramos D, Almeda-Valdes P, Arvizu M, et al. Association of the metabolic syndrome and long-term renal function in kidney donors. Transplant Proc 2011; 43:1601-6. Epub 2011/06/23. doi: 10.1016/j.transproceed.2011.02.058. PubMed PMID: 21693240.
6. Caliskan Y, Yildiz A. Evaluation of the medically complex living kidney donor. J Transplant 2012; 2012:450471. Epub 2012/06/02. doi: 10.1155/2012/450471. PubMed PMID: 22655169; PubMed Central PMCID: PMC3359716.
7. Reese PP, Feldman HI, McBride MA, et al. Substantial variation in the acceptance of medically complex live kidney donors across US renal transplant centers. Am J Transplant 2008; 8:2062-70. Epub 2008/08/30. doi: 10.1111/j.1600-6143.2008.02361.x. PubMed PMID: 18727695; PubMed Central PMCID: PMC2590588.
8. Matas AJ, Bartlett ST, Leichtman AB, et al. Morbidity and mortality after living kidney donation, 1999-2001: survey of United States transplant centers. Am J Transplant 2003; 3:830-4. Epub 2003/06/20. PubMed PMID: 12814474.
9. Segev DL, Muzaale AD, Caffo BS, et al. Perioperative mortality and long-term survival following live kidney donation. JAMA 2010; 303:959-66. Epub 2010/03/11. doi: 10.1001/jama.2010.237. PubMed PMID: 20215610.
10. Rees MA, Kopke JE, Pelletier RP, et al. A nonsimultaneous, extended, altruistic-donor chain. N Engl J Med 2009; 360(11):1096-101. Epub 2009/03/13. doi: 10.1056/NEJMoa0803645. PubMed PMID: 19279341.
11. Montgomery RA, Zachary AA, Ratner LE, et al. Clinical results from transplanting incompatible live kidney donor/recipient pairs using kidney paired donation. JAMA 2005; 294:1655-63. Epub 2005/10/06. doi: 10.1001/jama.294.13.1655. PubMed PMID: 16204665.
12. Takahashi K. Recent findings in ABO-incompatible kidney transplantation: classification and therapeutic strategy for acute antibody-mediated rejection due to ABO-blood-group-related antigens during the critical period preceding the establishment of accommodation. Clin Exp Nephrol 2007;11:128-41. Epub 2007/06/27. doi: 10.1007/s10157-007-0461-z. PubMed PMID: 17593512.
13. Richstone L, Seideman C, Baldinger L, et al. Conversion during laparoscopic surgery: frequency, indications and risk factors. J Urol 2008;180:855-9. doi: 10.1016/j.juro.2008.05.026. Epub 2008 Jul 17.
14. Wilson CH, Sanni A, Rix DA, et al. Laparoscopic versus open nephrectomy for live kidney donors. Cochrane Database Syst Rev. 2011(11):CD006124. Epub 2011/11/11. doi: 10.1002/14651858.CD006124.pub2. PubMed PMID: 22071829.
15. Kobayashi T, Terai A, Yoshimura K, et al. Assessment of body image alteration after renal surgery using a novel three-dimensional laser scanner. Urology 2004; 64:264-8. Epub 2004/08/11. doi: 10.1016/j.urology.2004.03.021. PubMed PMID: 15302475.
16. Afaneh C, Aull MJ, Gimenez E, et al. Comparison of laparoendoscopic single-site donor nephrectomy and conventional laparoscopic donor nephrectomy: donor and recipient outcomes. Urology 2011; 78:1332-7. Epub 2011/10/15. doi: 10.1016/j.urology.2011.04.077. PubMed PMID: 21996107.

17. Canes D, Berger A, Aron M, et al. Laparo-endoscopic single site (LESS) versus standard laparoscopic left donor nephrectomy: matched-pair comparison. Eur Urol 2010; 57:95–101. Epub 2009/08/12. doi: 10.1016/j.eururo.2009.07.023. PubMed PMID: 19664877.
18. Rais-Bahrami S, George AK, Montag S, et al. Laparoendoscopic single-site (LESS) partial nephrectomy short-term outcomes. BJU Int 2012. doi: 10.1111/j.1464-410X.2012.11374.x. [Epub ahead of print]
19. Golkar FC, Ross SB, Sperry S, et al. Patients' perceptions of laparoendoscopic single-site surgery: the cosmetic effect. Am J Surg 2012; 204:751–61. doi: 10.1016/j.amjsurg.2011.07.026.
20. Jacobs SC, Cho E, Foster C, et al. Laparoscopic donor nephrectomy: the University of Maryland 6-year experience. J Urol. 2004;171(1):47-51. PubMed PMID: 14665841.
21. Barry JM, Conlin M, Golconda M, et al. Strategies to increase living donor kidney transplants. Urology. 2005; 66(5 Suppl):43-6. PubMed PMID: 16194706.

CHAPTER 27

Avoiding and Managing Hazards During Live Donor Nephrectomies

Carlos E Marroquin

INTRODUCTION

The incidence of end-stage renal disease (ESRD) has increased steadily over the last several decades. As a result, the number of patients who require renal replacement therapy for ESRD has also increased; the majority of these patients receive renal replacement therapy in the form of dialysis. Alternatively, a growing number also receive renal replacement therapy in the form of transplantation. As the dialysis population increases, so does the number of patients waiting for a transplant. While our demand continues to increase, the organ supply has not changed appreciably over the last two decades. This disparity affects our renal population the most, since more patients are surviving to go onto dialysis and as a result, the percentage of patients who are eligible for a transplant also continues to increase. This huge disparity between organ supply and demand limits our ability to transplant every eligible patient. However, in terms of kidney disease, we do have a viable option in live donation. While it has been demonstrated that live donation is safe with an acceptable risk profile in well-selected patients, and while major complications are rare events, complications do occur. Our objectives should be to work toward a zero event occurrence. As such, we should consistently strive to avoid well-described hazards in live donors.

VISCERAL OR VASCULAR INJURIES DURING INSUFFLATION

Unless one is performing a modified laparoscopic technique, most donor surgeons utilize the Veress needle technique to insufflate the abdomen.

- Since most surgeons establish their pneumoperitoneum in the upper abdomen and since a distended, patulous stomach makes an easier target than a decompressed stomach, all patients should have a well-placed and functioning nasogastric or oralgastric tube prior to attempting a Veress needle insufflation
- The double-click test the hanging drop test, the aspiration test and the initial pressures at the time of insufflation are commonly used to evaluate the safety of establishing a pneumoperitoneum with the Veress needle
- Preinsufflation tests have poor sensitivity for evaluating proper Veress needle placement. The pressures after initial insufflation have the greatest sensitivity and strongest predictive value of a misplaced needle[1]
- Measuring the abdominal wall width on preoperative CT scans may provide a sense of the depth the Veress needle needs to travel to be within the peritoneum. Lifting the abdominal wall away from the viscera may also increase the margin of safety provided by knowing the expected depth beyond which one may expect visceral and vascular injuries
- Preperitoneal insufflation and omental emphysema are commonly encountered and of no consequence. However, hollow visceral and vascular injuries, on the other hand, are less commonly reported and more serious. Injuries are more common when multiple passes are required
- Hollow viscus injuries may or may not be identified immediately and are believed to occur < 1% of all cases.[2] After the exchange of the Veress needle for a trocar, one should inspect for signs of visceral injury.

These could include the presence of succus entericus or bile in the field. Commonly, the injury is not identified until one is well into the procedure or at its conclusion. Once identified, the injury should be inspected and a critical assessment of the ability to perform a proper repair should be made. Injuries that are easily identified will lend themselves to a laparoscopic repair in facile hands. However, those that are identified by the presence of spilled intraluminal contents tend to require an open approach to be sure the injury has been identified and no others exist. Because a reasonable number of hollow viscus injuries are not diagnosed at the initial laparoscopic procedure, one must have a high index of suspicion for such injuries in patients who are not making the usual and customary progress after a laparoscopic nephrectomy. These patients should be studied with an oral contrast CT scan once suspected as a delay in diagnosis compounds the morbidity and recovery

- Similarly, vascular injuries are infrequent (< 1%) and can involve any variety of vessels from omental vessels to the great vessels.[3] Injury to a large named vessel is usually characterized by hemodynamic instability. When an injury to a vascular structure is suspected, the procedure should be immediately converted to an open exploration of the region the needle penetrated. The initial reflex should be to apply pressure and allow anesthesia to catch up before attempting further inspection to repair the injury. In these cases, another experienced surgeon should be called to assist in a rapid and careful evaluation and management of the findings

AIR EMBOLUS DURING INSUFFLATION

- Air embolism can occur during insufflation for either a right or left donor nephrectomy
- On the right, it can occur by placement of the Veress needle into the vena cava or the liver
- On the left, it can occur by placement into the renal vein or a large mesenteric vein such as the superior mesenteric vein or primary tributary
- When CO_2 is introduced into the venous circulation, cardiac collapse occurs because of obstruction of the pulmonary outflow tract. This immediately decreases preload with resulting increase in central venous pressures and hemodynamic instability
- Confirming the diagnosis of CO_2 air embolism is difficult if not impossible. This can be masked by the rapid absorption of CO_2 from the circulation. As such, it is often a diagnosis of exclusion
- The temporal relationship of insufflation and hemodynamic compromise should provide a high index of suspicion. As such, the insufflation should be stopped immediately, and the potential donor placed in a steep left lateral decubitus
- Supportive care is critical and placement of a central line may be, theoretically, both diagnostic and therapeutic by allowing aspiration of air
- Ultimately, the diagnosis may be made intraoperatively by performing transesophageal echocardiography with the demonstration of air in the right ventricle and may show evidence of acute right ventricular dilation and pulmonary artery hypertension consistent with air embolism[4,5]

PNEUMOTHORAX DURING A LEFT DONOR NEPHRECTOMY

- The diaphragm drapes down into the retroperitoneum where it originates from the lumbocostal arches, and from the lumbar vertebrae forming two crura. During the course of mobilizing the kidney, it is entirely possible to violate these thin muscle fibers producing a pneumothorax. In one report that looked at all donor nephrectomies, including open nephrectomies, the incidence of pneumothorax approached 8%.[6] In a separate report of 200 donor nephrectomies, the incidence of a pneumothorax requiring a chest tube was 1%[7]
- Most pneumothoraces are incidentally diagnosed on a postoperative chest X-ray. In patients who develop high airway pressure, tachycardia or hypotension intraoperatively, one must consider a pneumothorax as part of the differential diagnosis. Once the diagnosis is made, management involves a chest tube if unstable. If diagnosed postoperatively and the pneumothorax is small and not symptomatic, conservative management is warranted as it should resolve since there has been no parenchymal injury and there is no positive pressure ventilation
- The key is to avoid injury to the leafs of the diaphragm. Mobilization of the kidney should be performed with clear visualization and a concerted effort should be made not to enter the psoas muscle posteriorly that extends into the region of the diaphragm as the dissection proceeds cephalad

STAPLER MALFUNCTION DURING DIVISION OF THE RENAL VESSELS

- The Food and Drug Administration (FDA) site on medical devices states that each year over the past 5 years there have been 8000 to 9000 adverse event reports related to surgical staplers and 90% of these reports involved malfunctions.[8] This underscores the magnitude of the risk involved in utilizing staplers and placing complete reliance on their fidelity
- While staplers are excellent instruments that have allowed surgical innovation, we need to think beyond the routine reliance on the staplers during these procedures
- It is critical to be prepared for a malfunction while dividing the vessels. The operating room team needs to understand the importance of being completely focused on the task during this portion of the procedure. Circulators need to be present in the room and ready to react. They need to have alternate staplers, cartridges, and laparotomy instruments at the ready. The scrub technician needs to have the preferred grasper selected and ready
- The surgeon needs to be ready to apply a laparoscopic clamp consisting of either a grasper or a paper clip immediately after firing a stapler if it misfires and bleeding results. In some cases, a stapler jams. In these instances, it is unclear whether the staples were deployed appropriately. While a malfunctioned stapler is removed, the surgeon and their team need to be prepared to react
- The stapler may be removed without consequence. In this instance, it is critical to verify whether the staple line was properly applied. If it is not clear whether the staple line is adequate, a second staple line should be applied. In this case, we would recommend placing a TA stapler to minimize loss of vessel length
- If the surgeon is unable to control the vessel upon removing the stapler and uncontrolled bleeding ensues, a cut Raytec should be inserted and used to apply direct pressure while an assistant opens the abdomen through a subcostal approach. Precious time should not be spent attempting to control the situation laparoscopically. Another senior surgeon should be called for assistance in control
- Stapler malfunction can occur due to stapler malpositioning when the stapler is placed on or around clips that were used to control and divide gonadal, adrenal, and lumbar veins.[9] As such, this is an avoidable hazard and requires attention while placing the stapler on the vessel being divided
- While not reported in donor nephrectomies, staplers have been reported to fail from a lack of a proximal staple line. As such, we would recommend pulling the intended cartridges and inspecting all cartridges and identifying preferred instruments for specific situations before embarking on the procedure. This type of "check-list" approach is key as once the procedure is on its way; we often forget to inspect the cartridge in the interest of completing the nephrectomy. Moreover, when the technician who is scrubbed knows which instruments are intended for each portion of the procedure; they are more reliably and consistently obtained in an appropriate time frame
- Finally, selection and close attention to the staple cartridge is also critical. The 2.5-mm stapler closes to 1.0-mm and the 2.0-mm staplers close to 0.75 mm. These are the only two cartridges that should be utilized to divide the renal vessels. In fact, pulsatile bleeding has been reported from the opposed edges of renal arteries after appropriate deployment of an endovascular stapler.[10] This likely occurs when the diameter of a deployed staple is greater than the width of an opposed vessel. This was and can be managed by careful application of a clip blow the staple line. Mass ligation should also be avoided as the initial purchase on more tissue than the vessel may result in a poorly applied staple line that subsequently slides off of the vessel of interest. Ensuring adequate dissection and exposure of the vessel with placement of the stapler only on the vessel of interest with clear visualization of the proximal and distal portions of the anvil will avoid these hazards

HEMOCLIPS

Hemoclips have been associated with donor mortality and have received a black box warning from the FDA for use in donor nephrectomies.

- While any method of controlling the renal artery and vein has been found to fail on occasion, the report of a survey of ASTS members by Freidman et al.[11] in 2006 concluded that life-threatening hemorrhage appears to be associated more frequently with surgical clips than with other methods of arterial and venous control. They also revealed the perception that transfixing or placing the suture or staple through the stump to be ligated and divided was safer than placing a device around the vessel such as a clip. They also discussed the importance of postoperative pain control as it relates to blood pressure and bleeding by relating the observation that a tie had become dislodged in one patient with increased blood pressure and as a result a delayed bleed

- While some groups, predominantly in urologic literature, have argued that hemoclips or self-locking clips are safe. It is reasonable to think the clinical setting is critical. In one setting, the clip is being applied to a long segment vascular cuff during a nephrectomy for indications other than live donation. In this setting, the clip has an abundant margin of safety and slipping is inconceivable. In the case of donor nephrectomies, the transplant procedure relies on the length of vessel obtained during the donor nephrectomy. As such, we work to deliver the longest possible vessel. This forces us to leave very short cuffs and it is not inconceivable that a clip may migrate with greater ease
- A follow-up report from the same group[10] indicates there have been at least nine known mortalities associated with the use of Hem-o-lok clips[16]
- Our recommendation is to avoid this real hazard by not using clips and become intimately familiar with the function of transfixing stapling devices

BLADDER INJURIES

Bladder injuries have been documented during the process of live donation.

- These injuries occur during the kidney extraction in patients who had previous pelvic surgeries that increase the risk of bladder injury.[12] Moreover, the extraction was performed via a Pfannenstiel incision in all patients who suffered bladder injury
- The presence of blood in the urine should raise one's index of suspicion of a possible bladder injury. Unfortunately, the diagnosis is most likely to be made during the postoperative recovery. The workup should include a retrograde cystogram or CT cystogram
- While management is relatively straightforward, when this injury is diagnosed early in the course of a donor nephrectomy, some variation in its management may be justified. Intraperitoneal injuries should be managed operatively with two-layer repair. This may be done open or laparoscopically depending on the local expertise. Retroperitoneal injuries should be managed with a Foley catheter and repeat cystogram after 2 weeks. Injuries between the bladder and the anterior abdominal wall with no peritoneal communication, which are a common location, present a special conundrum. While the accepted standard has been to manage these injuries conservatively with a Foley catheter or suprapubic catheter, the anterior location in a perfectly healthy, well-nourished donor lends itself to a surgical repair. In the interest of a rapid return to their premorbid, healthy state, one may argue for the more aggressive operative approach in a low risk donor
- Ideally, these injuries are prevented by avoiding a Pfannenstiel incision in patients with a known history of pelvic surgeries. These patients should be managed with an infraumbilical midline incision for kidney extraction

RENAL INJURIES

Renal injuries during extraction can result in degloving and parenchymal injuries.

- The delivery of an intact, uninjured kidney that will function immediately with reperfusion is a critical principle of live donor surgeries. This tenet is second only to donor safety. Unfortunately, traumatic injury to the potential renal allograft has been reported
- Extraction of a kidney with an Endo catch bag through an enlarged working port in the left iliac fossa resulted in complete detachment of the renal pelvis from the kidney.[13] Another report of a kidney, also removed with an Endo catch bag through a Pfannenstiel incision resulted in parenchymal transection[14]
- Kidneys have sustained degloving injury of the capsule during extraction through a suprapubic Pfannenstiel incision[15] that resulted in a urine leak. In this case, an initial capsular tear occurred during the dissection that extended to a complete degloving during the manual retrieval of the kidney through the hand-assisted device
- While all of these grafts were salvaged, considerable morbidity is associated with these injuries, even when the outcomes are positive. The objective should be to avoid these by methodic dissection and deliberate, careful retraction of the allograft. When it is time to proceed with extraction, one important maneuver is to ensure the kidney is completely within the Endo catch bag. If it is not completely placed within the bag, the rod, to which the bag is attached, can collapse around the kidney during extraction and inadvertently injure the kidney. Alternatively, once the kidney is within the bag, the bag detaches from the rod. At this point, one should control the string and divide it from the rod attachment and methodically remove the rod and subsequently remove the kidney in the bag. Another alternative is to remove the kidney by placing a hand through the incision and manually removing the kidney, eliminating the risk of the bag altogether

REFERENCES

1. Teoh B, Sen R, Abbott J. An evaluation of four tests used to ascertain Veress needle placement at closed laparoscopy. J Minim Invasive Gynecol 2005;12:153.
2. Wind J, Cremers J, van Berge Henegouwen M, et al. Medical liability insurance claims on entry-related complications in laparoscopy. Surg Endosc 2007;21:2094–99.
3. Pemberton RJ, Tolley DA, van Velthoven RF. Prevention and management of complications in urological laparoscopic port site placement. Eur Urol 2006;50:958–68.
4. Muth CM, Shank ES. Gas embolism. N Engl J Med 2000; 342:476.
5. Marcus RH, Weinert L, Neumann A et al. Venous air embolism: diagnosis by spontaneous right-sided contrast echocardiography. Chest 1991;99:784.
6. Stephen T, Bartlett, MD, Eugene J. Schweitzer MD. Laparoscopic living donor nephrectomy for kidney transplantation. Dial Transplant 1999;28:318–31.
7. David Shaffer MD, Anthony I, Sahyoun MD, et al. Two hundred one consecutive living-donor nephrectomies. Arch Surg 1998;133:426–31.
8. http://www.fda.gov/medicaldevices/products and medical procedures/general hospital devices and supplies/ surgical stapler information
9. Chan D, Bishoff JT, Ratner L, et al. Endovascular gastrointestinal stapler device malfunction during laparoscopic nephrectomy: early recognition and management. J Urol 2000;164:319–21.
10. Hsu TH, Su LM, Ratner LE, et al. Renovascular complications of laparoscopic donor nephrectomy. Urology 2002;60:811-5;discussion 815.
11. Friedman AL, Peters TG, Jones KW, et al. Fatal and nonfatal hemorrhagic complications of living kidney donation. Ann Surg 2006;243:126–30.
12. Metcalfe PD, Hickey L, Lawen JG. Bladder perforation during laparoscopic donor nephrectomy. Can J Urol 2004; 11:2456-8.
13. Rao MM, Russell CH, Padmakar NP, et al. Transection of the renal pelvis by endocatch bag during laparoscopic donor nephrectomy. Surg Laparosc Endosc Percutan Tech 2008;18: 429–32.
14. Mohamed HK, Lin A, Savage SJ, et al. Parenchymal transection of the kidney inflicted by endocatch bag entrapment during a laparoscopic donor nephrectomy. Am J Transplant 2006;6:232-5.
15. Mekeel KL, Mazur MJ, Reddy KS, et al. Diffuse parenchymal urine leak after kidney transplantation following degloving injury during donor nephrectomy. Am J Transplant 2007;7:2039–41. Epub 2007 Jun 18.
16. Friedman AL, Peters T, Ratner LE. Regulatory failure contributing to deaths of live kidney donors. Am J Trans 2012; 12:829–34.

CHAPTER 28

Deceased Donor Procurement

Ernesto P Molmenti and Collaborators

INCISION AND EXPOSURE (FIG. 1)

- We detail below the technique for abdominal multiorgan procurement
- Usually several surgical teams are involved in the procedure
- Coordination among all of those involved is essential for a successful outcome

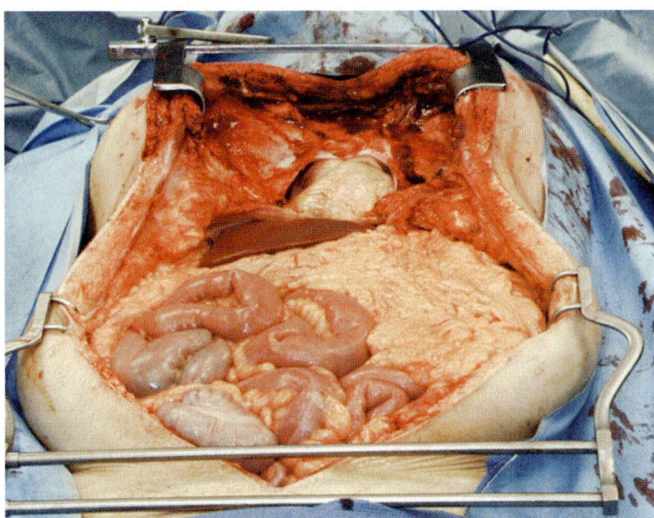

Fig. 1: After the brain dead donor has been correctly identified and all other requirements fulfilled as per the corresponding protocols, a midline incision from neck to pubis is undertaken. Retractors are used to achieve complete exposure of the chest and abdomen.

- In the case of donors after cardiac death (DCD), once the donor has been pronounced dead, a laparotomy is immediately performed. Aortic and inferior mesenteric veins cannulas are rapidly placed, the body is perfused with preservation fluid, and the organs covered with ice

DISSECTION OF THE AORTA (FIGS. 2 TO 4)

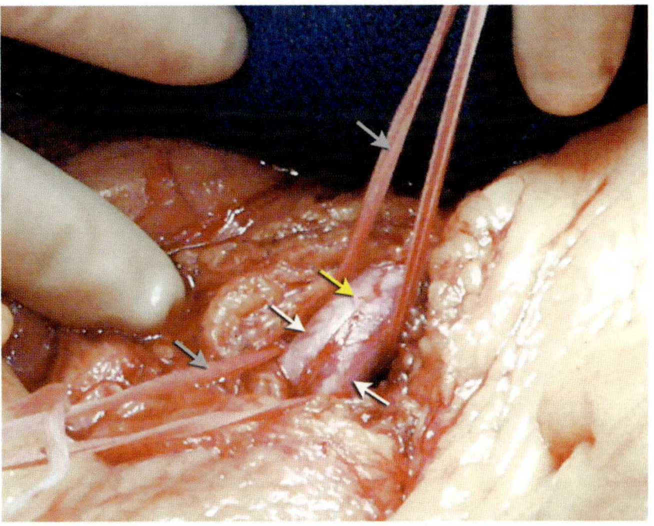

Fig. 2: The distal aorta (yellow arrow) and common iliac arteries (white arrows) are exposed. Umbilical tapes (gray arrows) are placed proximally and distally. We routinely identify these structures immediately after opening the body, since instances such as hemodynamic instability may require immediate cannulation and perfusion. COMMENTS: The procuring surgeon should always evaluate for the presence of horseshoe kidneys and prevent injuring them in the region of the inferior mesenteric artery. In the highly unlikely event that a previously transplanted kidney is being procured, cannulation should be at the contralateral common or external iliac artery, or otherwise at the ipsilateral femoral artery making sure the cannula is distal to the origin of the transplant renal artery.

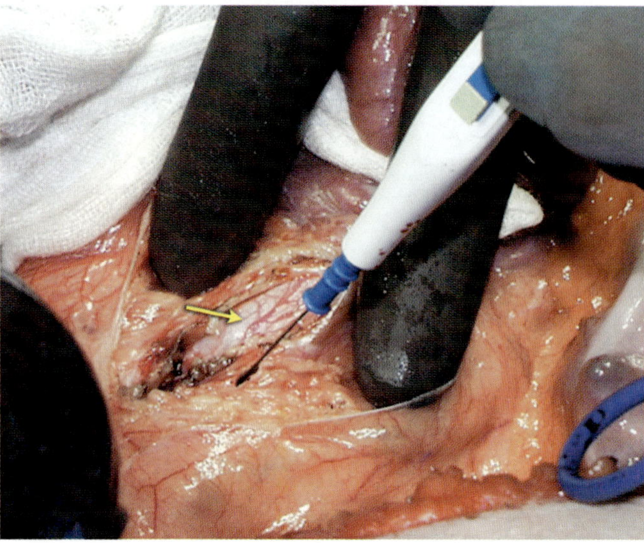

Fig. 3

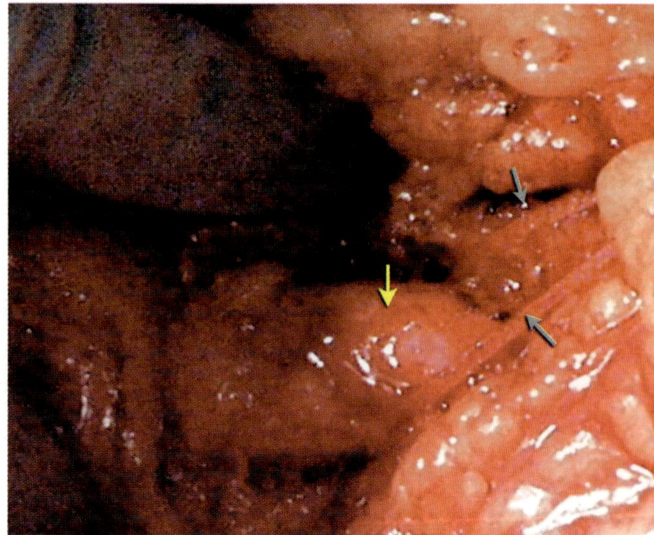

Fig. 4

Figs. 3 and 4: Alternatively, the aorta (yellow arrows) can also be dissected just proximal to its bifurcation into right and left common iliac arteries. As previously described, umbilical tapes (gray arrows) are placed around it. Irrespective of the approach chosen, care should be taken not to injure the lumbar branches or inferior mesenteric artery, since bleeding from these sites is fastidious to control and can create difficulties visualizing the operative site.

DISSECTION OF THE INFERIOR MESENTERIC VEIN (FIGS. 5 TO 7)

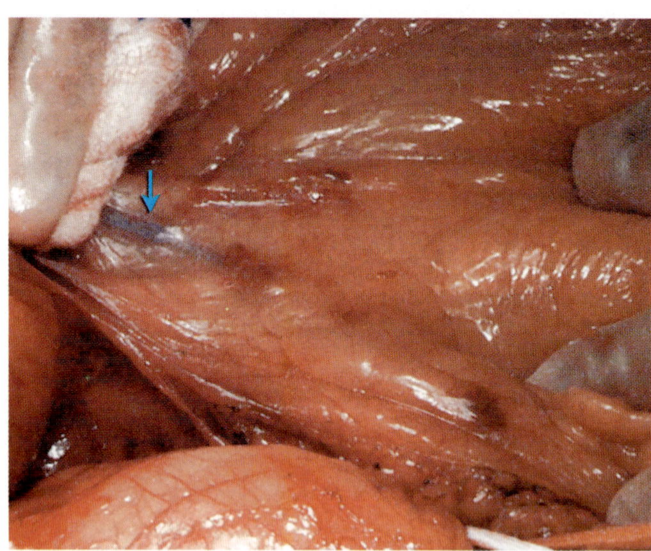

Fig. 5

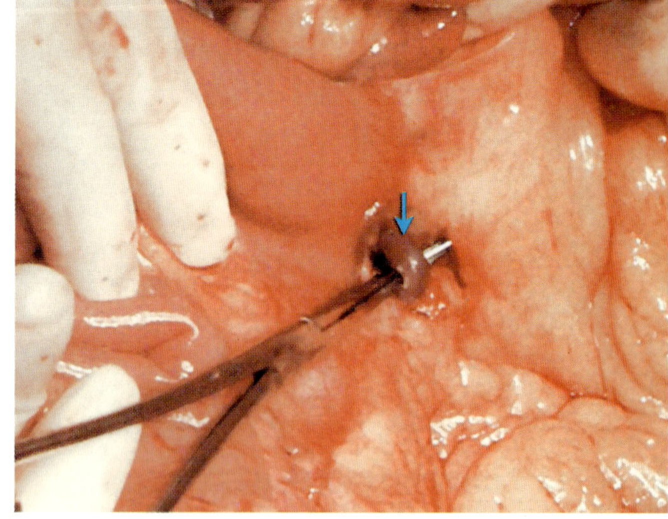

Fig. 6

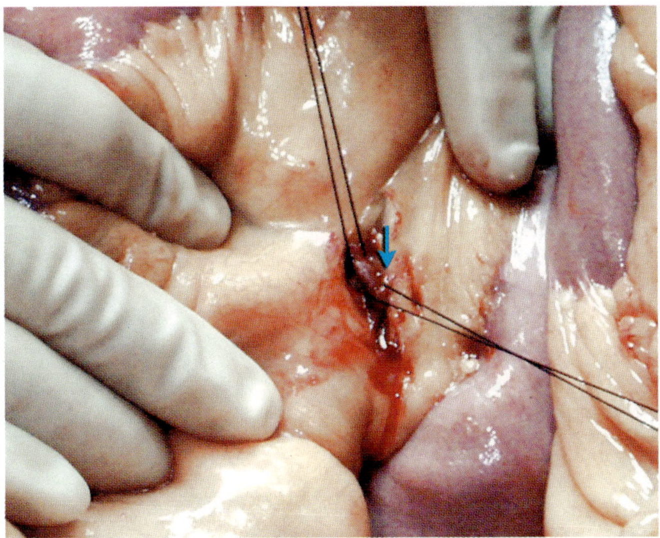

Fig. 7

Figs. 5 to 7: The inferior mesenteric vein (blue arrow) is also dissected for future cannulation. Ties are placed proximally and distally. Alternatively, in donors where the pancreas and/or small intestine is/are not procured, the superior mesenteric vein can be dissected at the root of the small bowel mesentery and used for perfusion.

MOBILIZATION OF THE RIGHT COLON (FIGS. 8 AND 9)

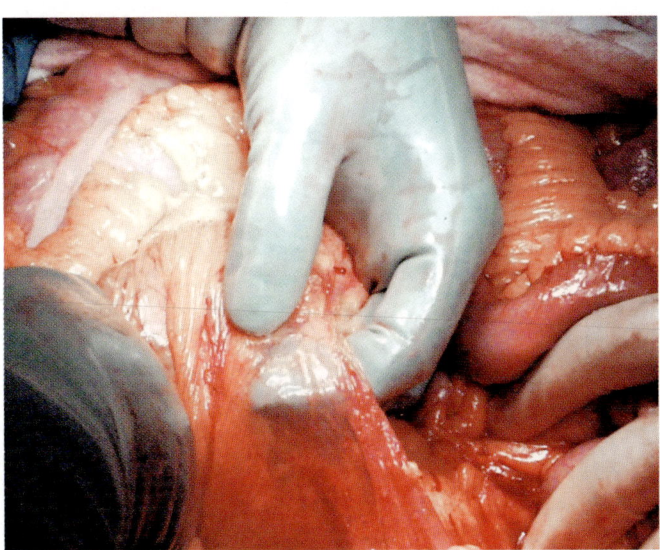

Fig. 8: The right (ascending) colon is mobilized along its avascular embryological plane of adhesion. Although the usual approach to this mobilization is starting distally at the cecum and proceeding proximally toward the hepatic flexure, we prefer to star the mobilization at the hepatic flexure and advance distally toward the cecum. This has the potential advantage of being associated with fewer ureteral injuries since if the correct plane of dissection is obtained the ureter will always remain dorsal to it.

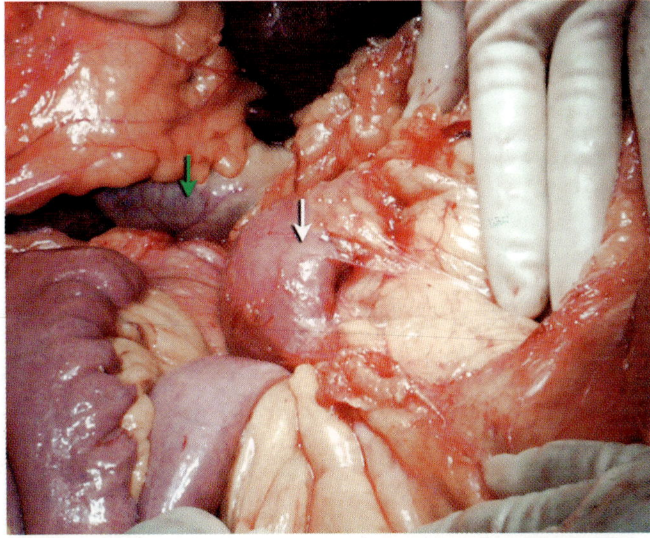

Fig. 9: The duodenum (white arrow) and gallbladder (green arrow) are easily seen and approached after the right colon is mobilized.

MOBILIZATION OF THE SMALL BOWEL MESENTERY (FIGS. 10 TO 13)

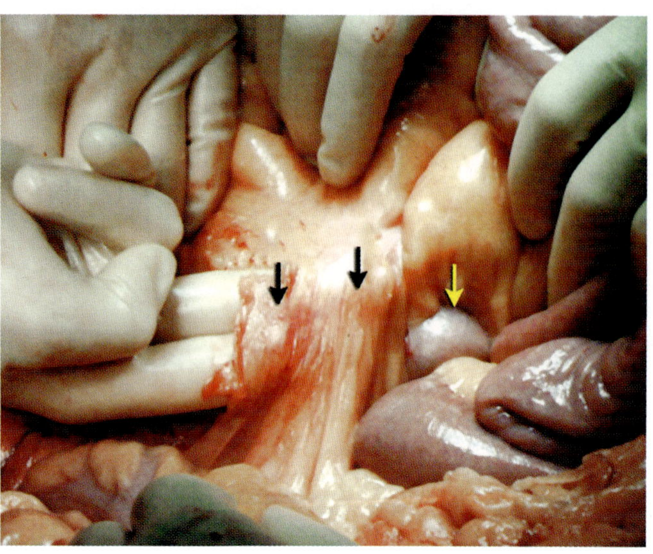

Fig. 10

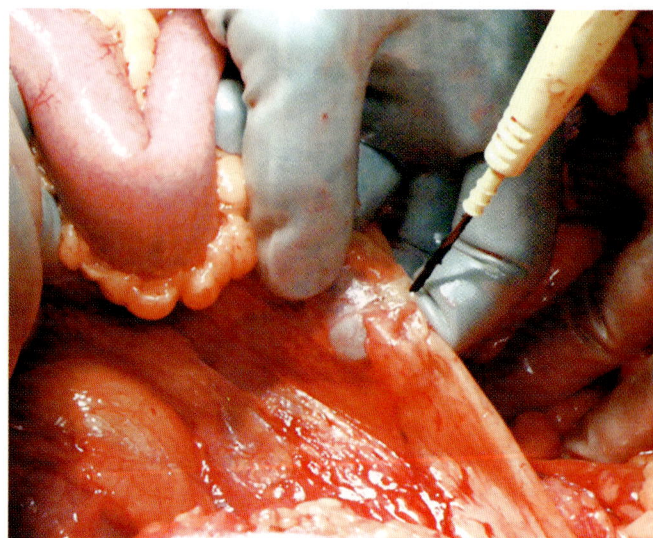

Fig. 11

Figs. 10 and 11: Subsequently the root of the small bowel mesentery is mobilized by transecting (black arrows) along its embryologic plane of adhesion from right lower quadrant (distal ileum) to left upper quadrant (duodenojejunal junction, yellow arrow).

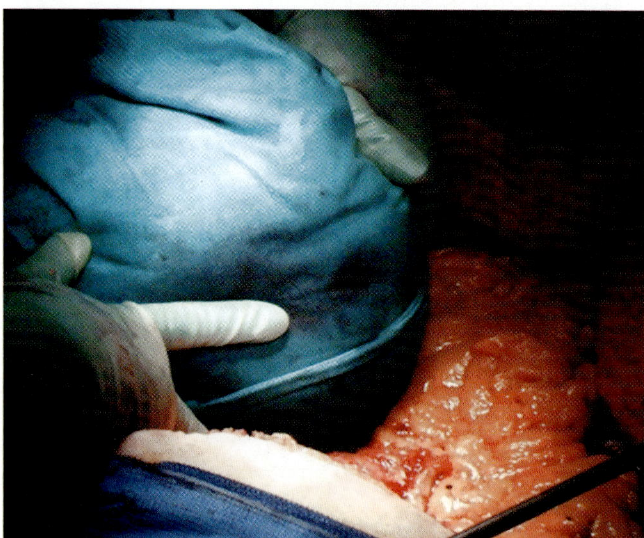

Fig. 12

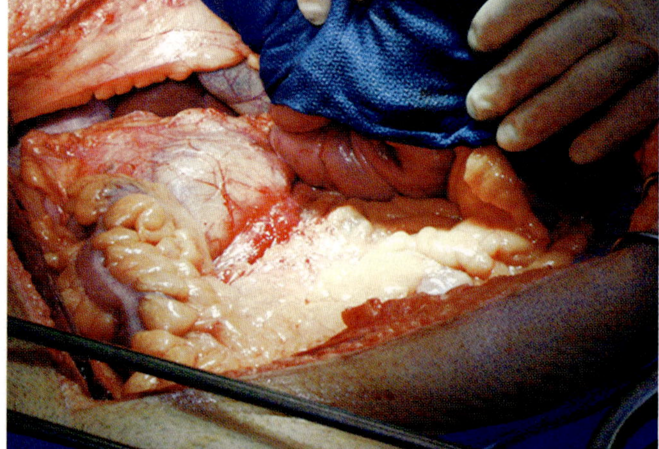

Fig. 13

Figs. 12 and 13: In order to handle the small bowel and colon in an organized fashion, we frequently wrap it in a towel (or sponge) soaked in warm saline. After the viscera have been mobilized, there is free access to the retroperitoneal area, as shown in the image on the right. The mobilization so far has not been associated with any irreversible step such as ligation of any vessels or transection of any organ.

MOBILIZATION OF THE RIGHT COLON AND LEFT COLON (FIGS. 14 TO 17)

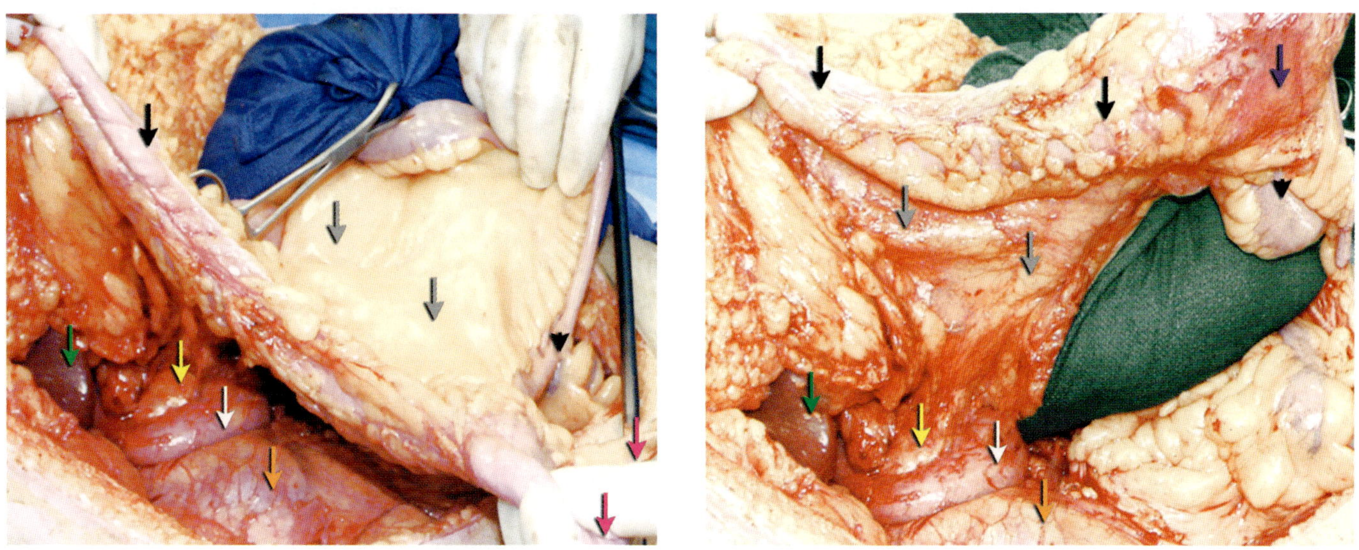

Fig. 14 Fig. 15

Figs. 14 and 15: View of the mobilized ascending colon (black arrows) and its mesentery (gray arrows). The small bowel has been wrapped in a warm soaked blue towel. Also visible are the duodenum (white arrows), right kidney (orange arrows), head of the pancreas (yellow arrows), liver (green arrows), cecum (purple arrow), appendix (pink arrows) and distal ileum (arrowhead).

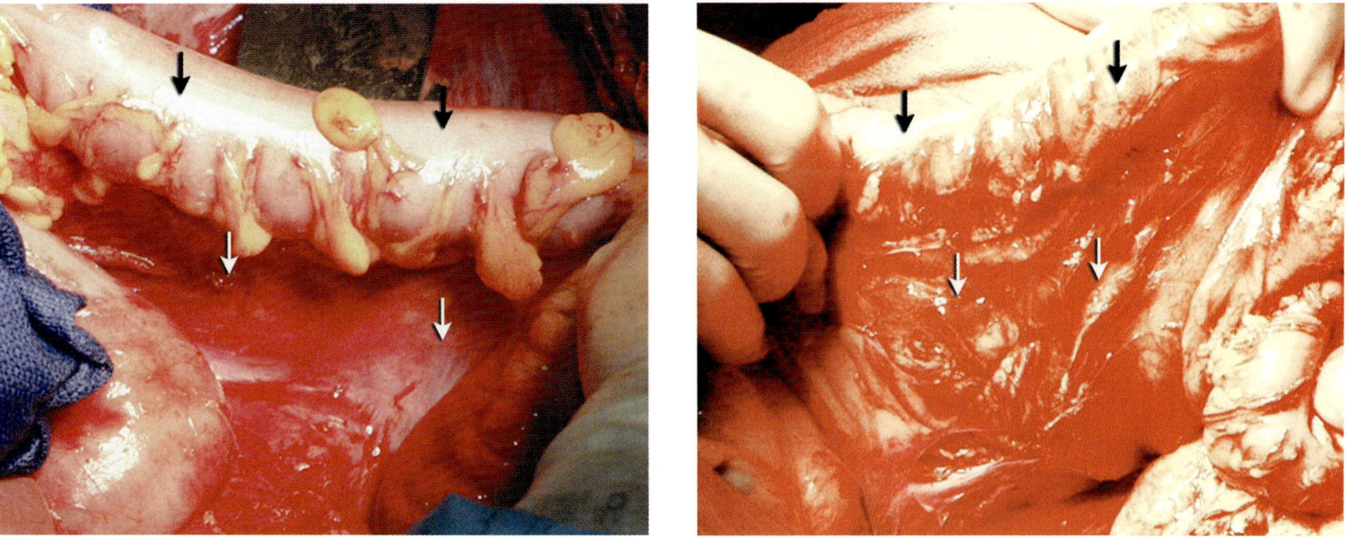

Fig. 16 Fig. 17

Figs. 16 and 17: The left colon is also mobilized. The black arrows show the descending colon. Its mesentery is shown by the white arrows. The image on the left is a view from the medial side while the image on the right represents a lateral view.

MOBILIZATION OF THE DUODENUM AND HEAD OF THE PANCREAS (FIGS. 18 TO 21)

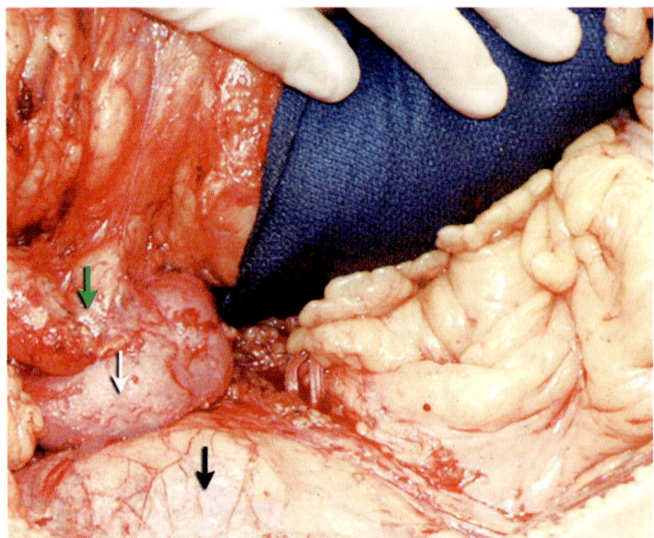

Fig. 18: After the ascending (right) colon is mobilized, the duodenum (white arrow), head of the pancreas (green arrow) and right kidney (black arrow) can be visualized.

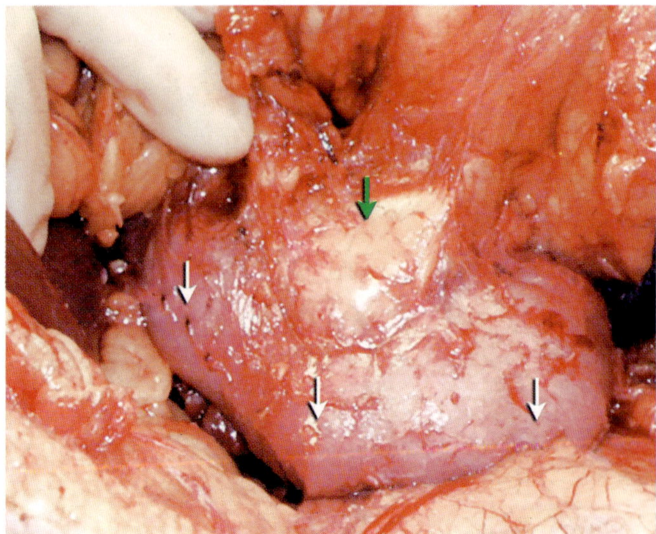

Fig. 19: The duodenum (white arrows) and head of the pancreas (green arrow) are addressed next.

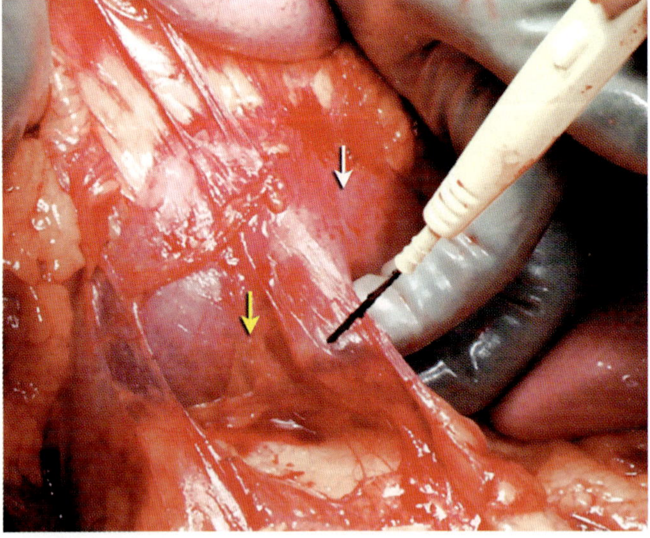

Fig. 20

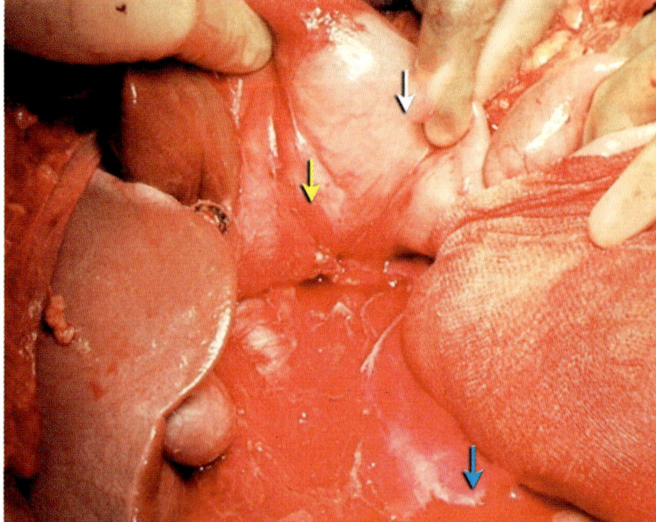

Fig. 21

Figs. 20 and 21: The duodenum (white arrows) and head of the pancreas (yellow arrows) are mobilized along an avascular plane of embryological adhesion. The distal inferior vena cava (IVC) can be seen (blue arrow).

SEPARATION OF THE TRANSVERSE COLON FROM THE GREATER OMENTUM
EXPOSURE OF THE ANTERIOR SURFACE OF THE PANCREAS
MOBILIZATION OF THE PANCREAS AND SPLEEN (FIGS. 22 TO 26)

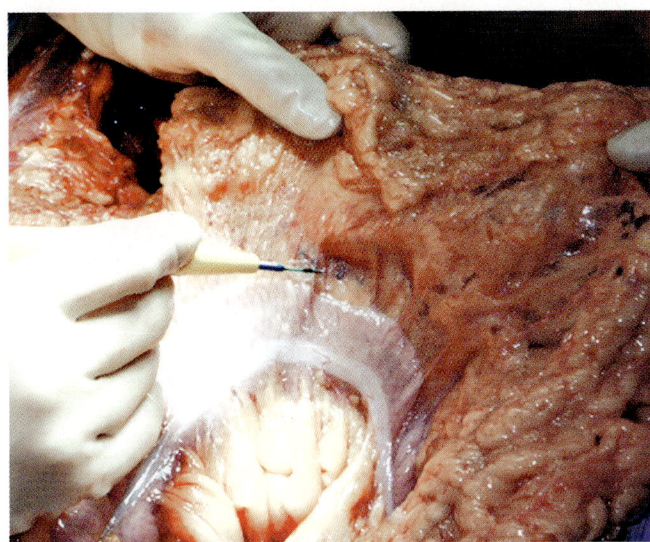

Fig. 22: Dissecting along the embryological plane of adhesion between transverse colon/mesocolon and greater omentum allows access to the pancreas.

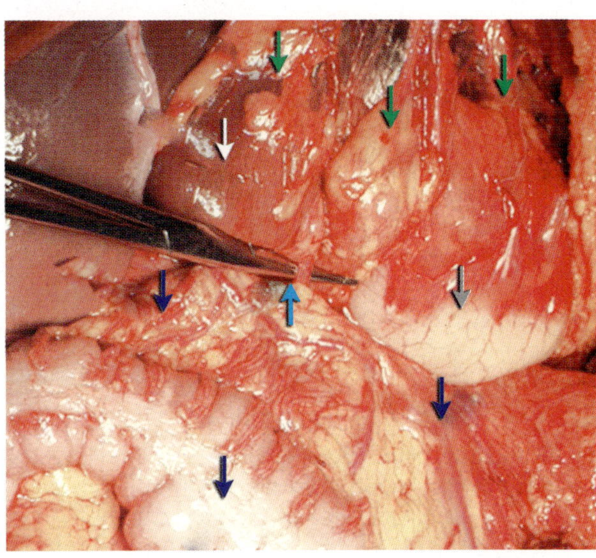

Fig. 23: This should be an avascular plane except for the presence of a single vein (light blue arrow) being shown on top of the clamp. Note the transverse colon and its mesentery (blue arrows) separate from the omentum (green arrows). The posterior surface of the stomach (gray arrow) and left lateral lobe of the liver (white arrow) can be seen covered by the omentum that has been retracted upward.

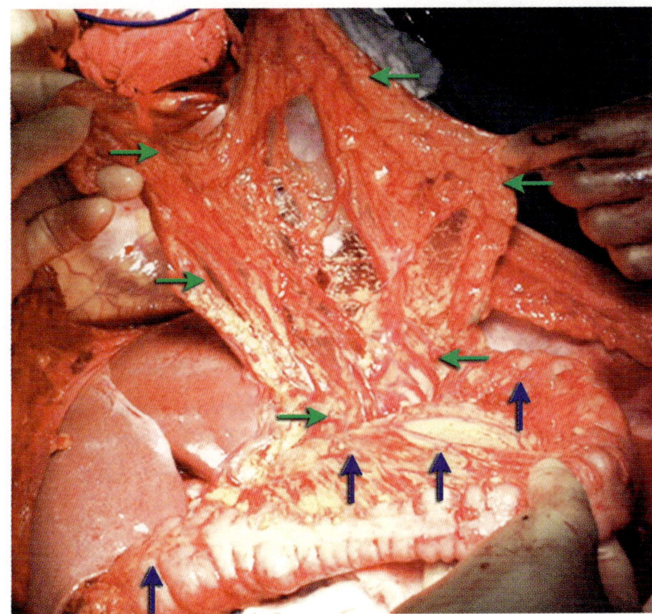

Fig. 24: Once the dissection is complete, the greater omentum (green arrows) is completely decolated from the transverse colon/ mesocolon (blue arrows).

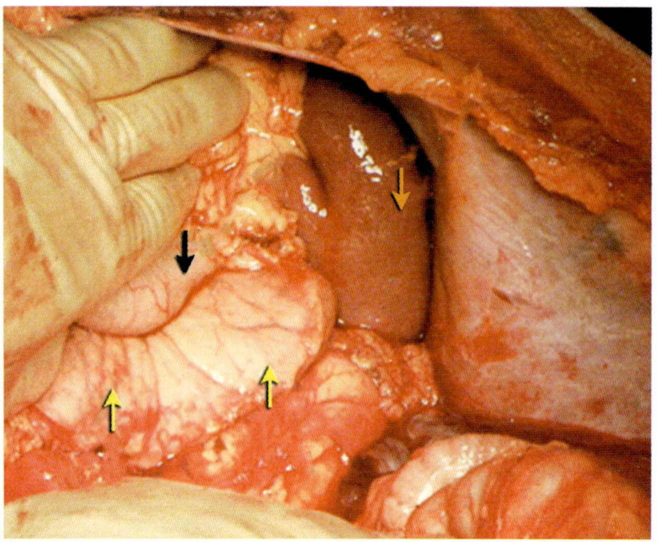

Fig. 25

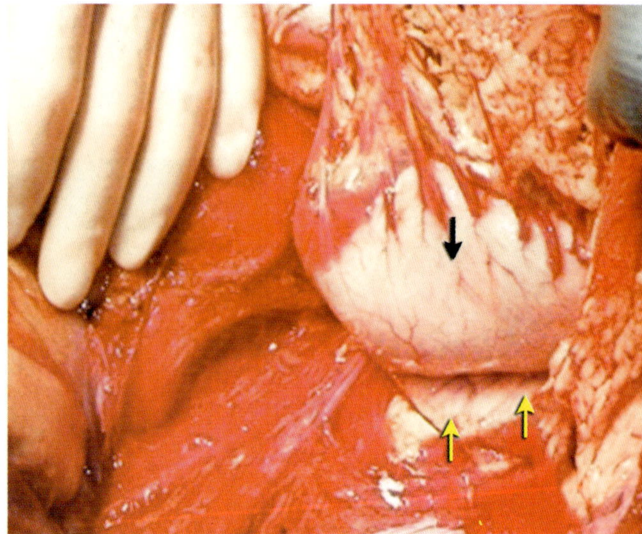

Fig. 26

Figs. 25 and 26: This maneuver allows exposure of the pancreas along its anterior surface (yellow arrows). Note also the spleen (orange arrow) and posterior aspect of the stomach (black arrows).

MOBILIZATION OF THE PANCREAS AND SPLEEN (FIGS. 27 TO 37)

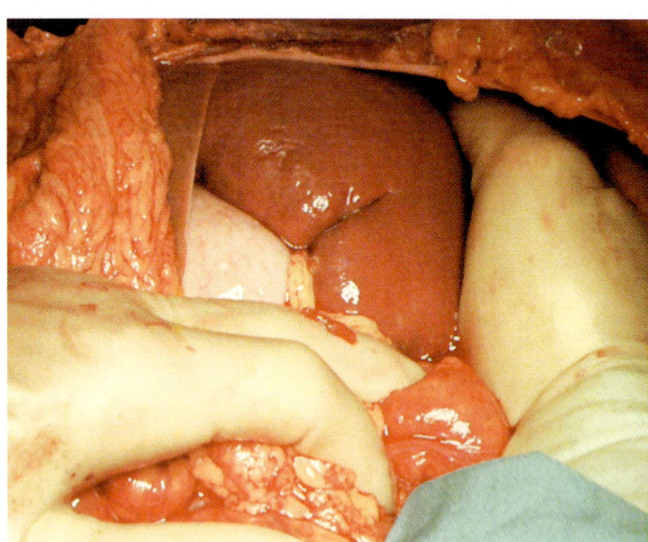

Fig. 27: Once the anterior surface of the pancreas has been exposed, we proceed to mobilize the spleen and pancreas.

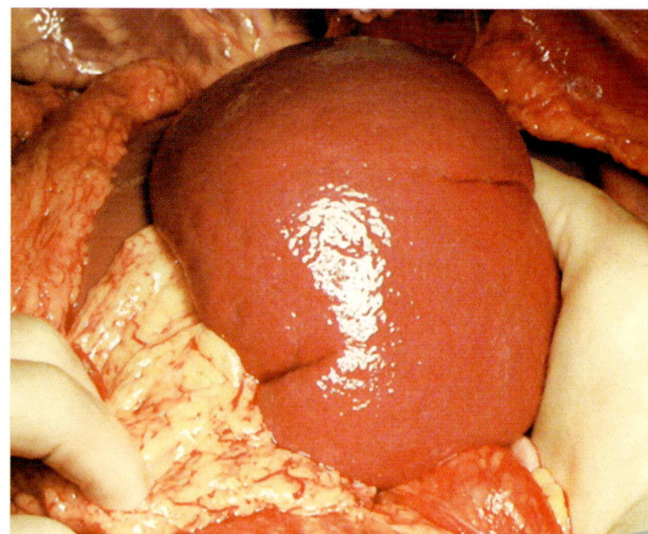

Fig. 28: The peritoneal reflexions on the lateral aspect of the spleen are transected.

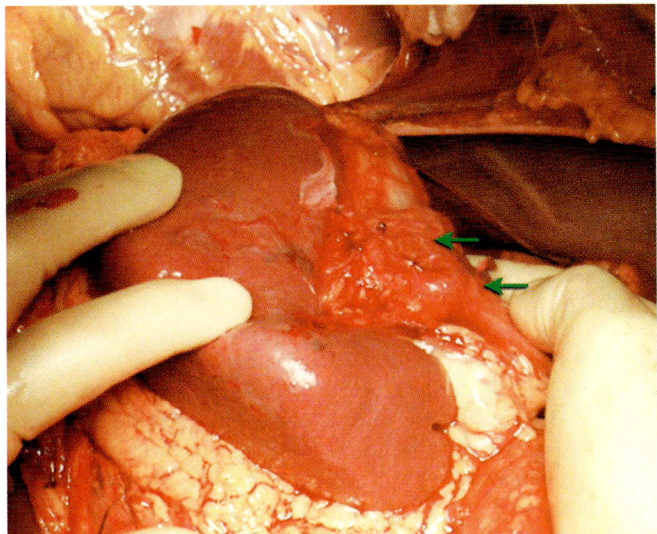

Fig. 29: The spleen and pancreas are mobilized in a lateral to medial fashion, exposing the dorsal surface of the pancreas (arrows). Care should be taken not to injure the spleen or splenic vein (located on the posterior aspect of the pancreas).

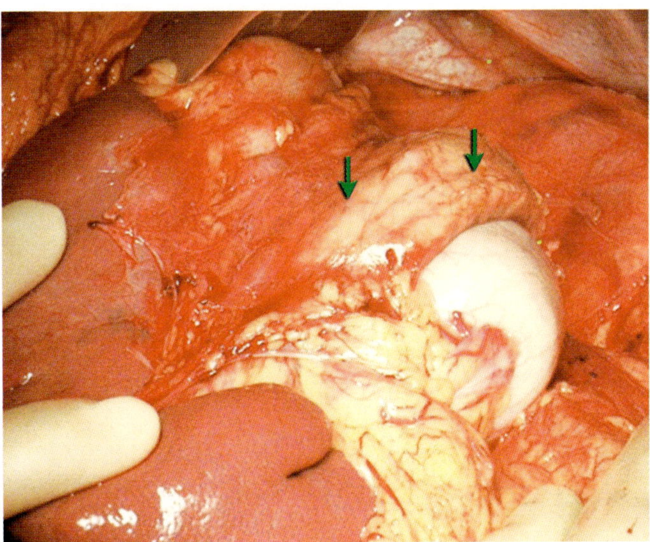

Fig. 30: The pancreas (arrows) can be mobilized up to the aorta and origin of the superior mesenteric artery (SMA). At this point, the pancreas is free of embryological planes of coalescence, since the lateral-to-medial mobilization maneuver reaches the previously performed Kocher maneuver that had mobilized the duodenum and head of the pancreas.

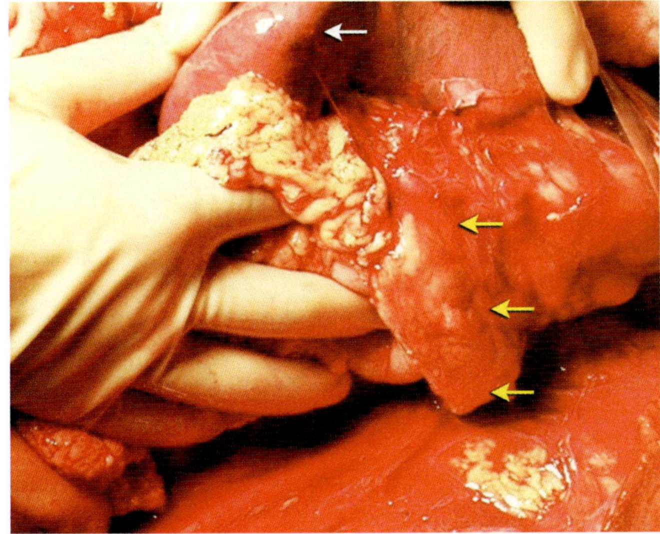

Fig. 31: This illustration further shows the medial-to-lateral mobilization maneuver of the spleen (white arrow) and pancreas (yellow arrows). This maneuver takes place along an avascular plane of embryological coalescence.

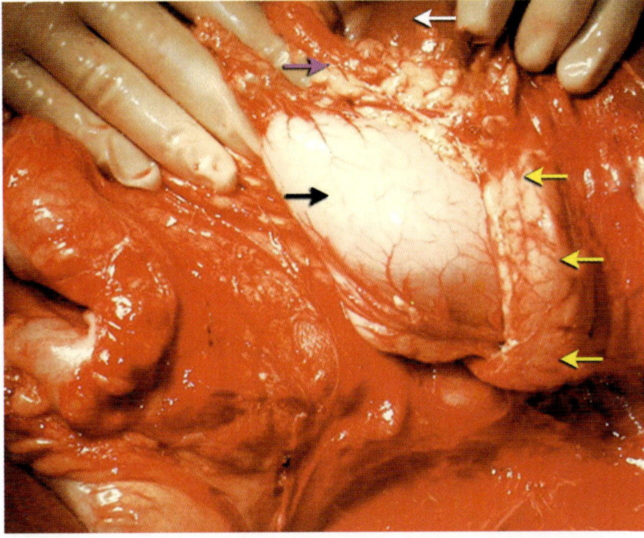

Fig. 32: The spleen (white arrow) and pancreas (yellow arrows) are free of surrounding tissues. The posterior surface of the stomach (black arrow) and omentum (purple arrow) are also visible.

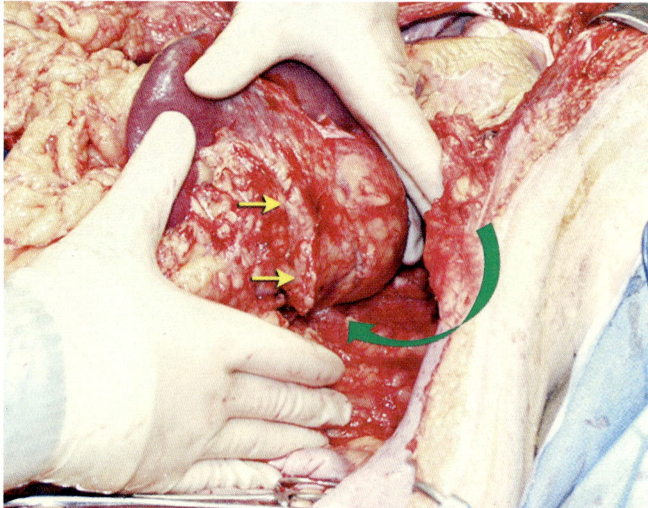

Fig. 33: As previously mentioned, the pancreas (yellow arrows) can be mobilized (green arrow) medially up to the aorta and superior mesenteric artery (SMA), where it reaches the previously performed mobilization plane of the duodenum and head of the pancreas. As viewed in the illustrations, there are no vessels along this plane.

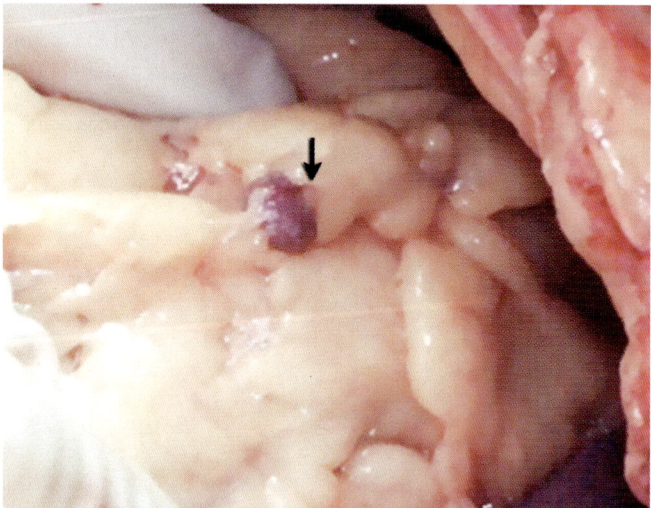

Fig. 34

Fig. 35

Figs. 34 and 35: Occasionally accessory spleens (black arrows) are encountered.

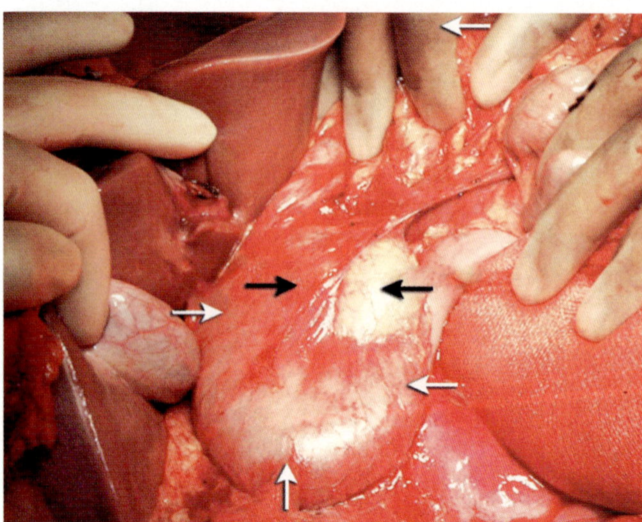

Fig. 36: The duodenum (white arrows) and head of the pancreas (black arrows) had been previously mobilized.

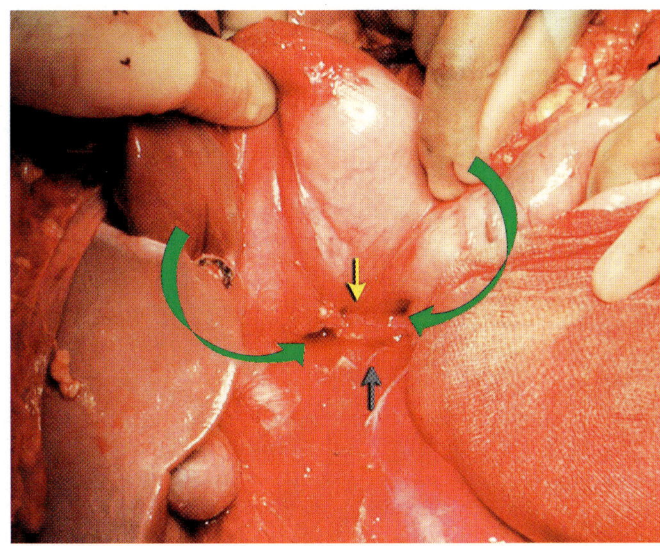

Fig. 37: The mobilization planes (green arrows) have freed pancreas from embryological coalescences. The area of origin of the superior mesenteric artery (SMA) is indicated by a yellow arrow. The aorta is indicated by a gray arrow.

MOBILIZATION OF THE LIVER

Lesser Omentum (Figs. 38 and 39)

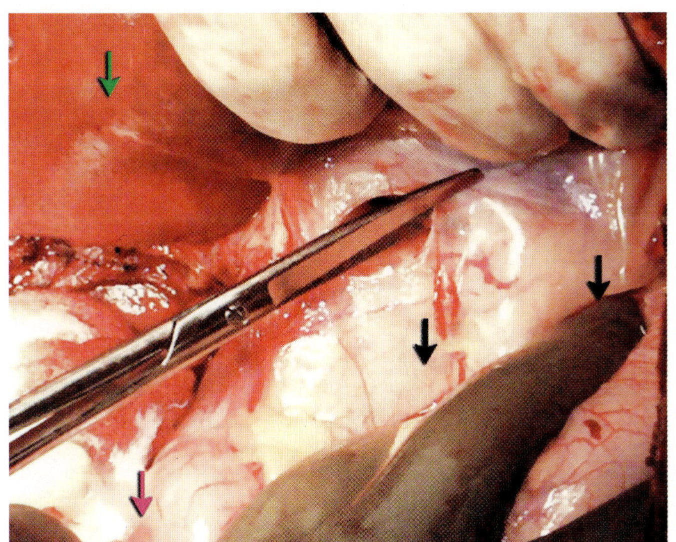

Fig. 38

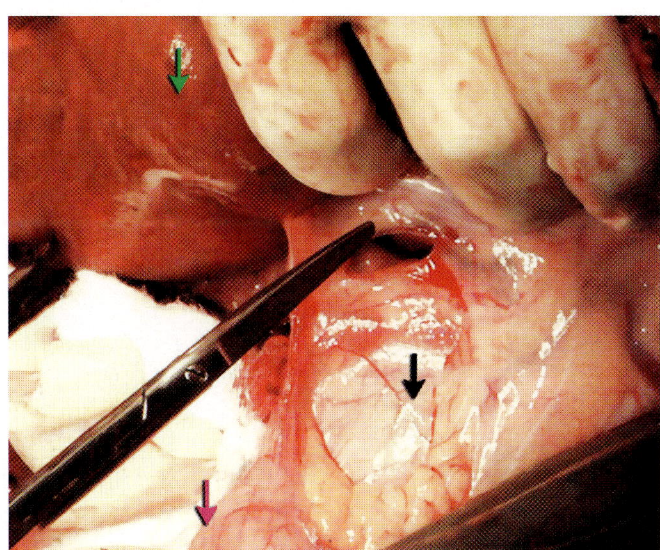

Fig. 39

Figs. 38 and 39: The lesser omentum is evaluated for the presence of replaced/accessory left hepatic arteries. If none are present (as in this case), the lesser omentum is incised as shown in this illustration. This will allow for further mobilization of the upper border of the pancreas and liver. Note the liver (green arrows), stomach (pink arrows) and pancreas (black arrows). In cases where there is a replaced/accessory left hepatic artery arising from the left gastric artery, the surgeon should preserve it in order to maintain the arterial supply of the liver intact.

Liver (Figs. 40 to 44)

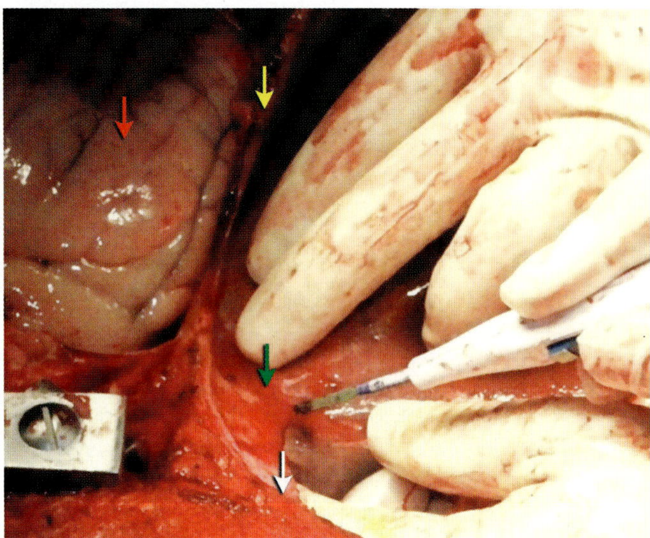

Fig. 40: The falciform ligament is transected all the way to the inferior vena cava (IVC). In addition to the falciform ligament (green arrow) being transected with electrocautery, the heart (red arrow), diaphragm (white arrow), central tendon of the diaphragm (yellow arrow) and chest retractor can also be seen.

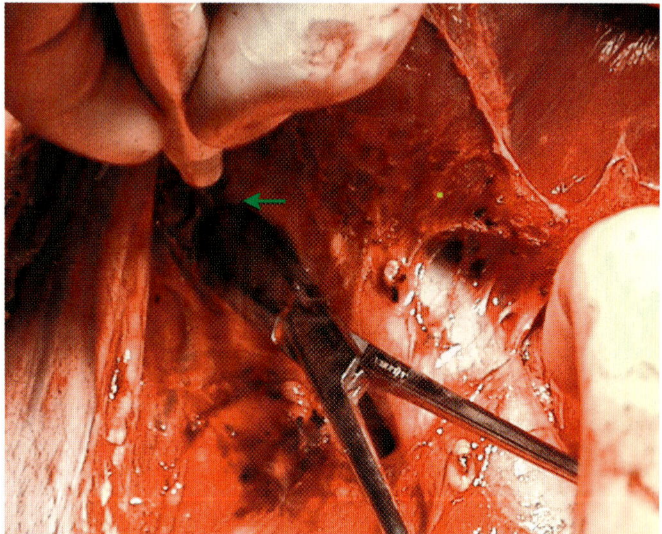

Fig. 41: The liver is further mobilized by transecting the coronary and triangular ligaments on the right (green arrow) and left sides. This dissection can reach up to the corresponding right and left hepatic veins. Otherwise, only a slight in situ mobilization can be undertaken, to be completed during the back table preparation.

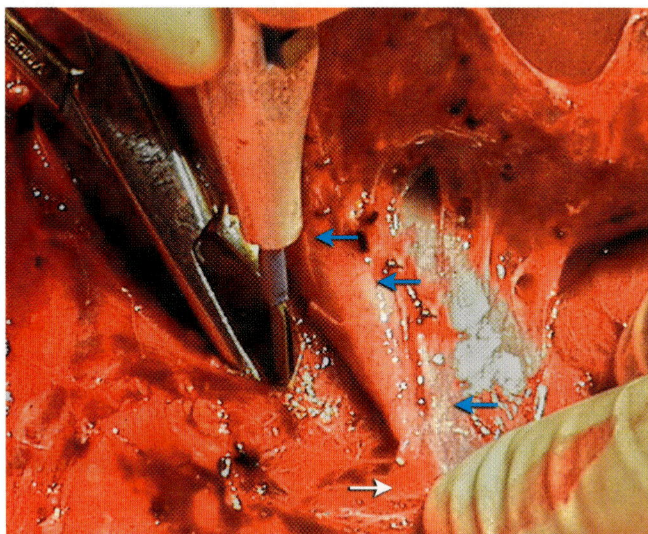

Fig. 42: The inferior vena cava (IVC) (blue arrows) is freed of surrounding tissues. The right adrenal vein (white arrow) can be tied and transected if necessary.

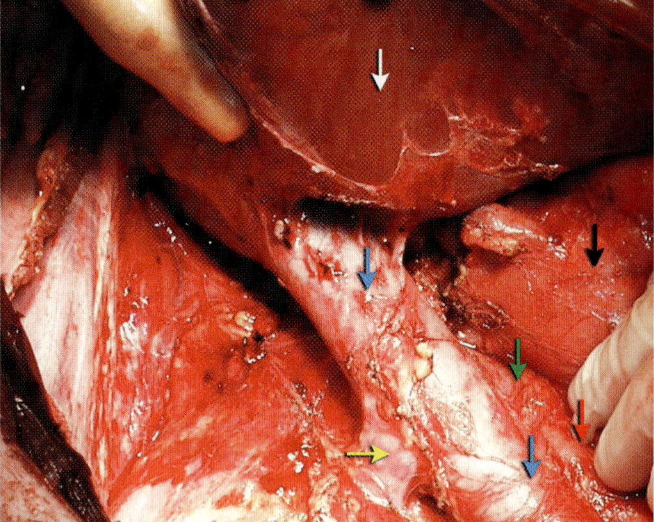

Fig. 43: The liver (white arrow) is now completely mobilized. In this illustration, it is rotated medially in order to visualize the retrohepatic area. Note the inferior vena cava (IVC) (blue arrows), right renal vein (yellow arrow), left renal vein (green arrow), aorta (red arrow) and the duodenum (black arrow). The liver and duodenum have been rotated medially.

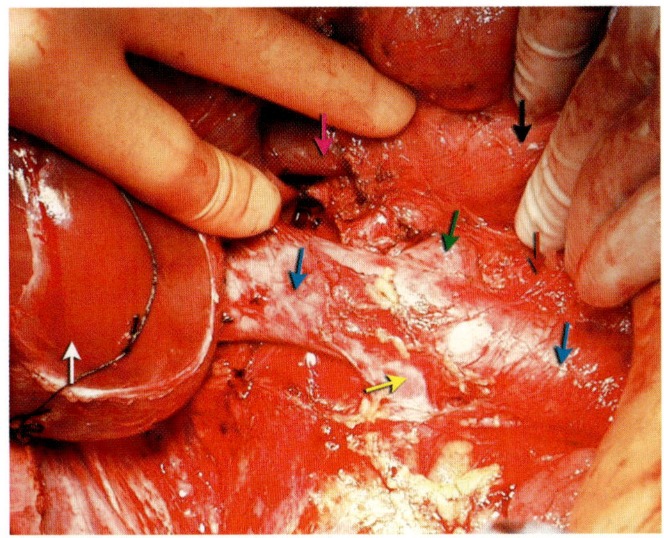

Fig. 44: In this illustration, the liver (white arrow) is in its nonrotated anatomical position. The duodenum (black arrow) is still rotated medially. Note the inferior vena cava (IVC) (blue arrows), right renal vein (yellow arrow), left renal vein (green arrow), the portal hepatis (pink arrow) and the aorta (red arrow, not fully dissected). The porta hepatis should be evaluated for the presence of accessory/replaced right hepatic arteries. If present, they should be preserved in order to maintain the arterial supply of the liver intact.

INCISION/RESECTION OF THE GALLBLADDER (FIGS. 45 TO 48)

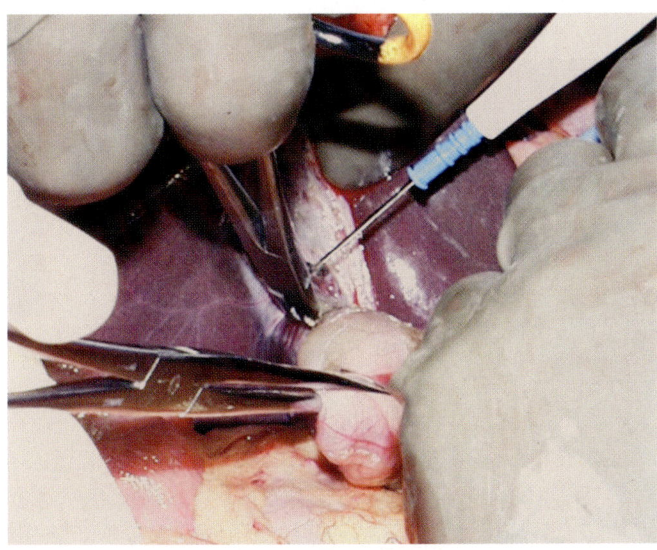

Fig. 45

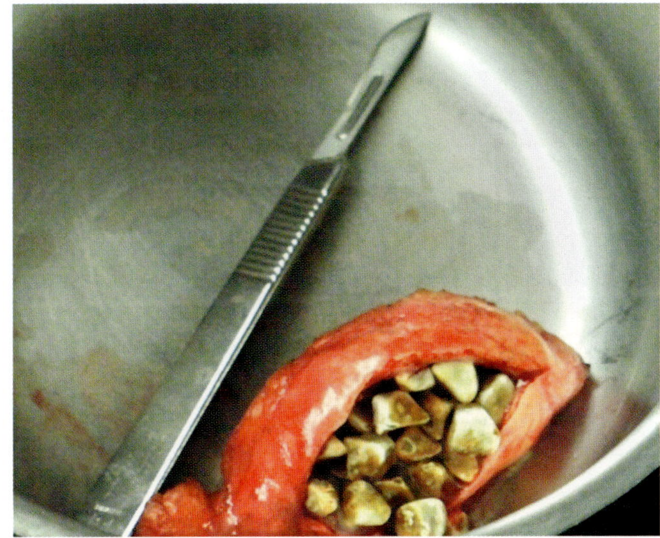

Fig. 46

Figs. 45 and 46: As shown in this case, we prefer to perform a cholecystectomy rather than incising, draining, and irrigating the gallbladder. We perform the cholecystectomy starting at the fundus and dissecting toward the neck in order to attempt to prevent bile duct injuries. In instances of procurement of both liver and pancreas, we also prefer to transect the common bile duct while separating the two organs in the back table (see Figures 47 and 48 for an alternate technique). In the donor illustrated in this picture, the gallbladder contained stones.

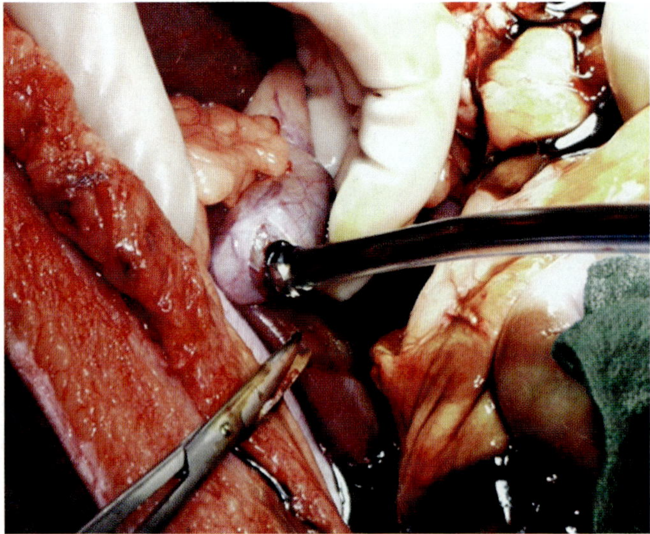

Fig. 47: The gallbladder may alternatively be incised and its contents drained.

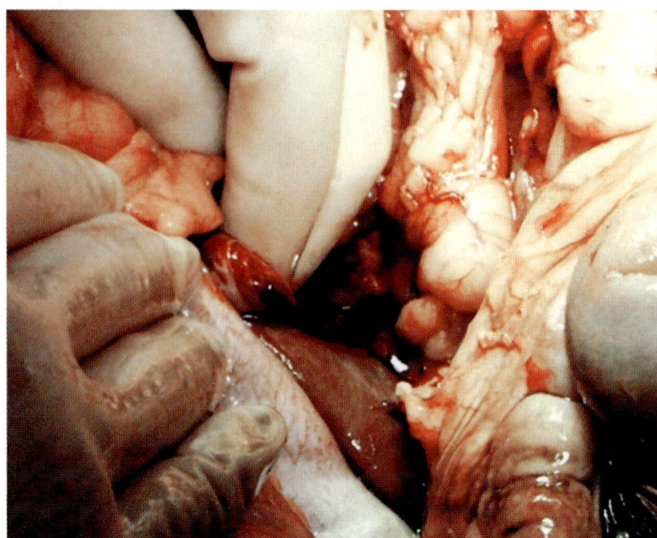

Fig. 48: The common bile duct is transected distally. The gallbladder is flushed with sterile saline.

INTERURETERIC FASCIA (FIGS. 49 TO 52)

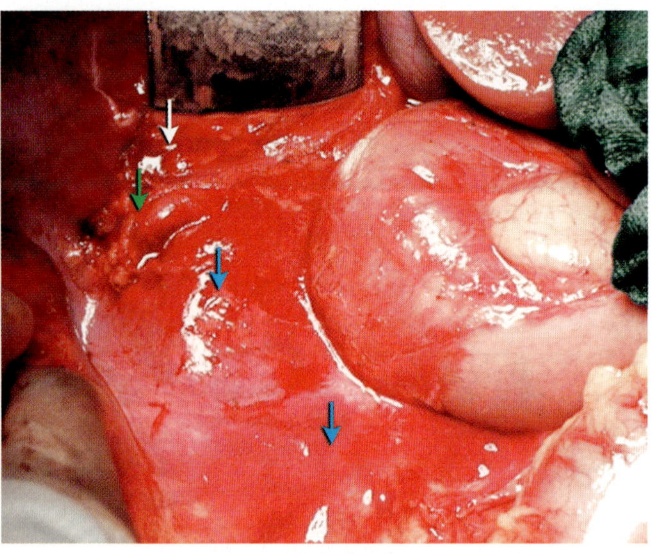

Fig. 49

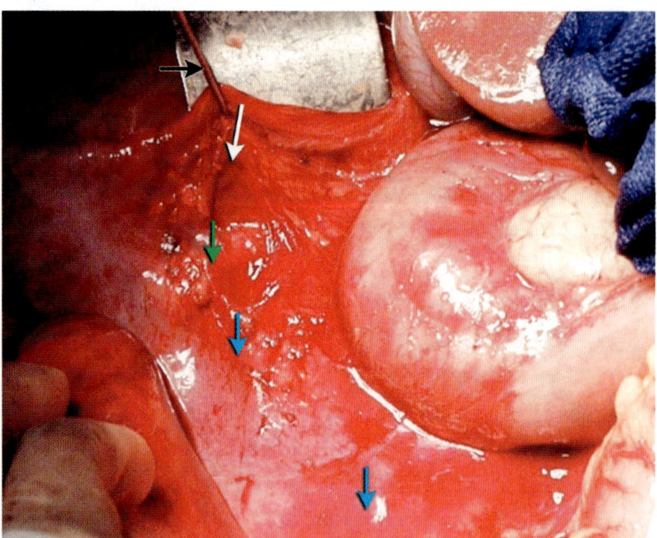

Fig. 50

Figs. 49 and 50: View of the right ureter (green arrow). The interureteric fascia is shown by the light blue arrows. A clamp (black arrow) is used to retract the right lateral extension of the fascia (white arrows). The right colon has been mobilized and retracted medially.

A fascia expanding from one ureter to the other (interureteric fascia) with lateral extensions and probably reaching to the inferior portion of the duodenum has been previously described (Albanese). This fascia is relevant to the ureter from a nutritious point of view. In the native environment, the ureter receives its blood supply from the renal, gonadal, and superior vesical arteries. The transplant ureter retains only the blood supply from the renal artery. It is important to preserve the fascia around the ureter in order to maintain its viability. Removing the tissues surrounding the ureter can be associated with postimplantation ischemia and/or necrosis, especially of the distal ureter.

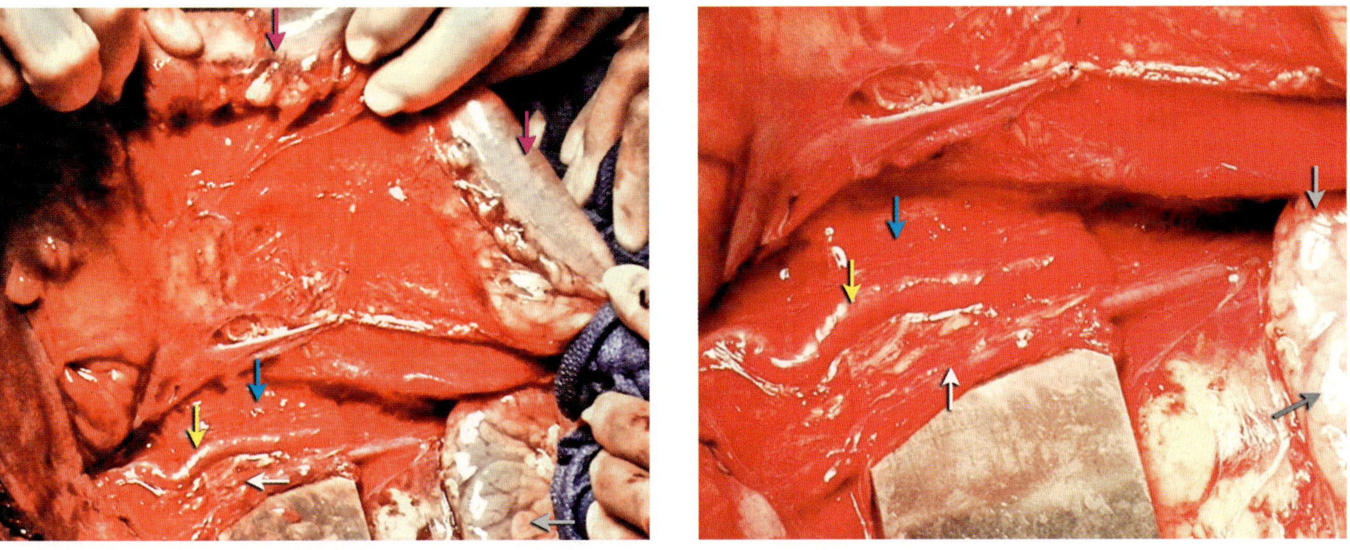

Fig. 51 Fig. 52

Figs. 51 and 52: View of the left ureter (yellow arrows) and the interureteric fascia (light blue arrows). The left colon (pink arrows) has been mobilized. The pancreas (gray arrows) is visible. A flat malleable retractor has been placed behind the fascia and its lateral extension (white arrows).

DISSECTION OF THE PYLORUS AND THE DUODENUM (FIGS. 53 AND 54)

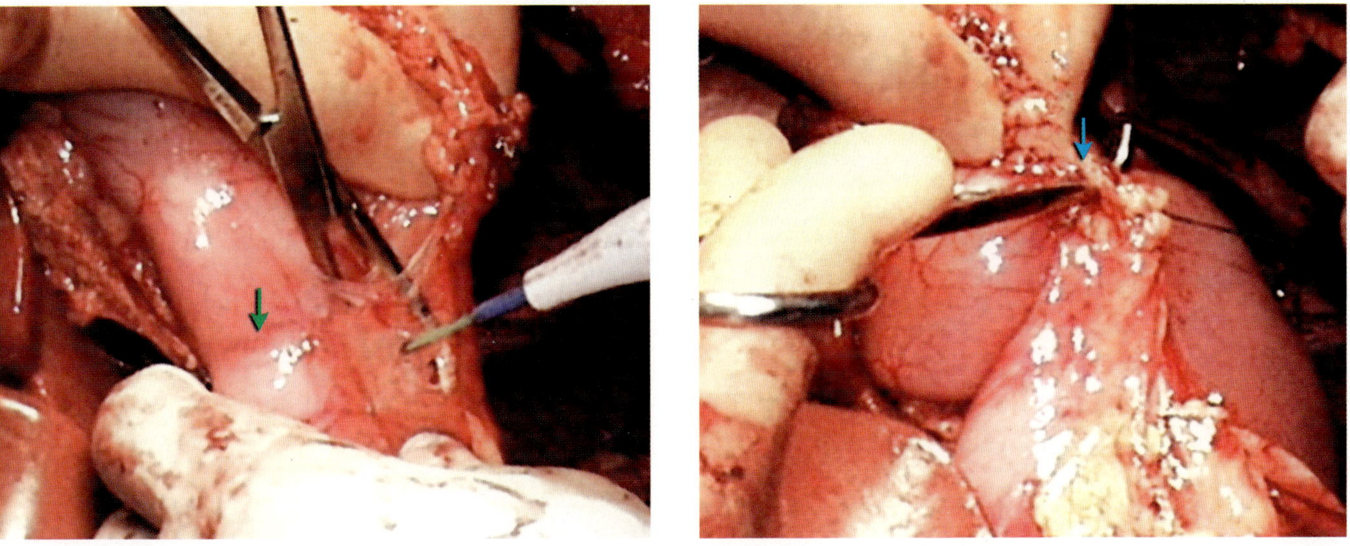

Fig. 53 Fig. 54

Figs. 53 and 54: The distal stomach, pylorus (green arrow), and proximal duodenum are freed of surrounding tissues. Vessels (blue arrow) are tied and transected. This will allow for better access when stapling across the first portion of the duodenum.

STAPLING OF THE DUODENUM (FIGS. 55 TO 58)

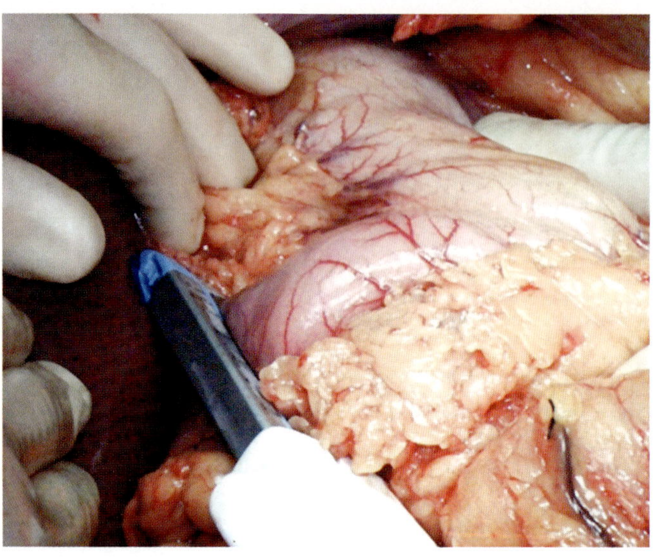

Fig. 55

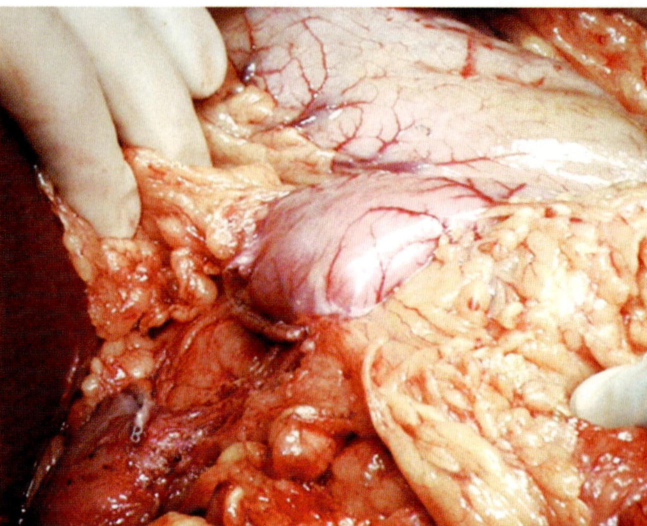

Fig. 56

Figs. 55 and 56: The first portion of the duodenum (that had been previously freed of surrounding tissues) is stapled. The pancreas graft is isolated (and subsequently implanted in the recipient) with the first, second, third (and sometimes fourth) portions of the donor duodenum. When stapling the first portion of the duodenum, care should be taken to make sure that any nasogastric tubes placed to empty the stomach are not within the staple line.

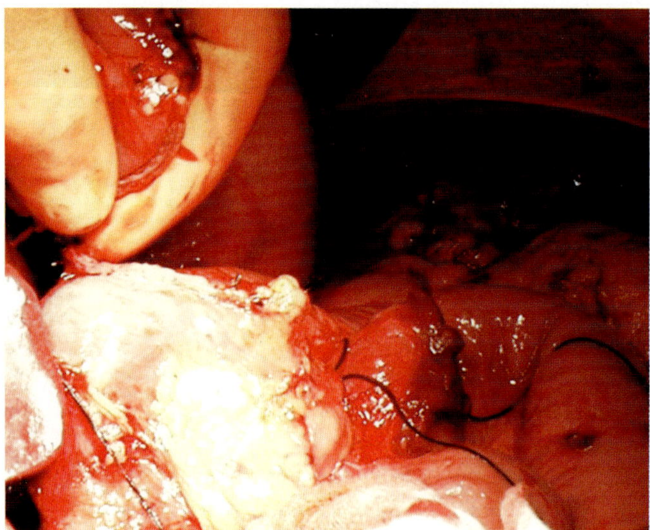

Fig. 57: The staple line is inspected.

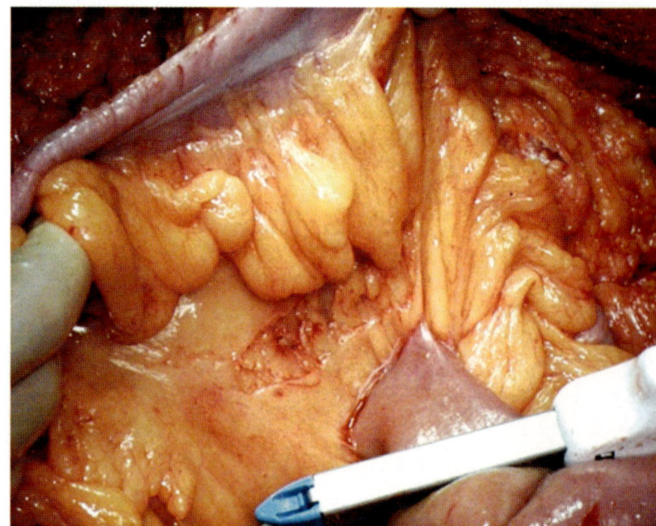

Fig. 58: Subsequently the distal duodenum/proximal jejunum is also stapled. This staple line will be addressed during the back table preparation of the pancreas allograft. At that time, the staple line is shifted to the third portion (sometimes fourth portion) of the duodenum.

SMALL BOWEL PROCUREMENT (FIGS. 59 TO 62)

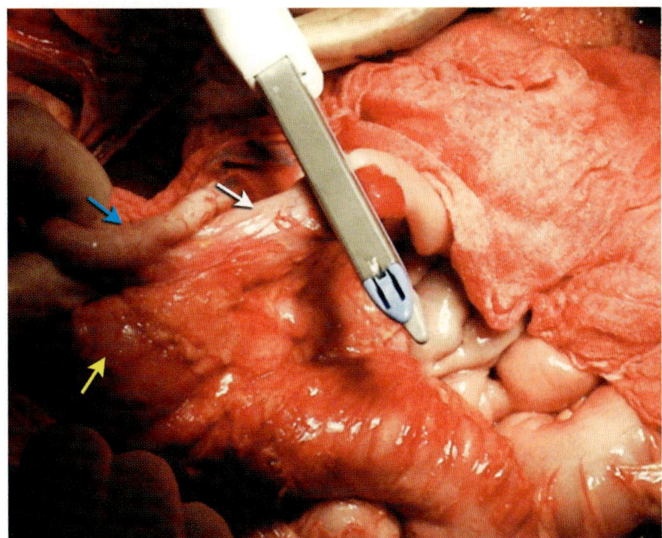

Fig. 59: In instances of small bowel graft procurement, the terminal ileum is stapled close to the ileocecal valve. Note the terminal ileum (white arrow), cecum (yellow arrow) and appendix (blue arrow).

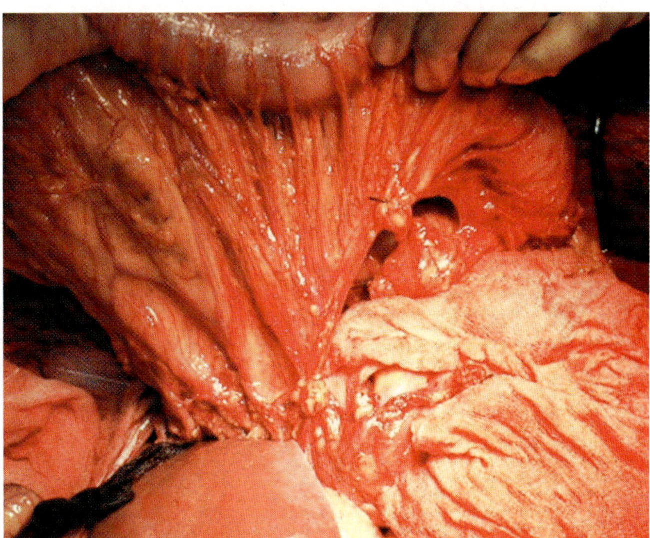

Fig. 60: Since the colon is not routinely part of the intestinal graft for transplantation, it is resected.

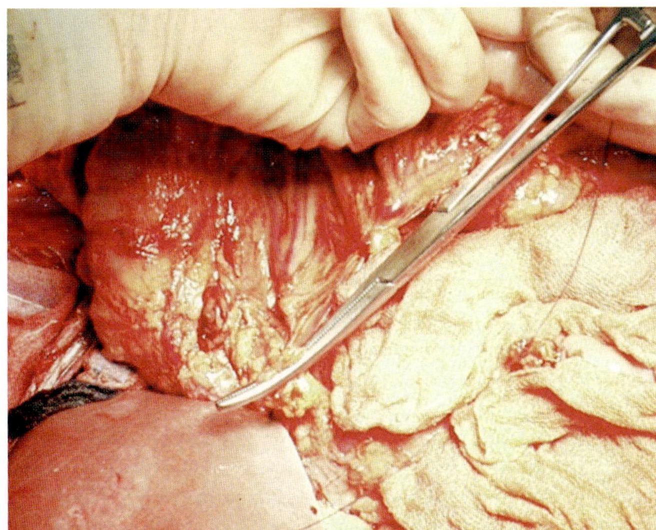

Fig. 61: The vessels in the ascending, transverse, and descending mesocolon are clamped, transected and tied.

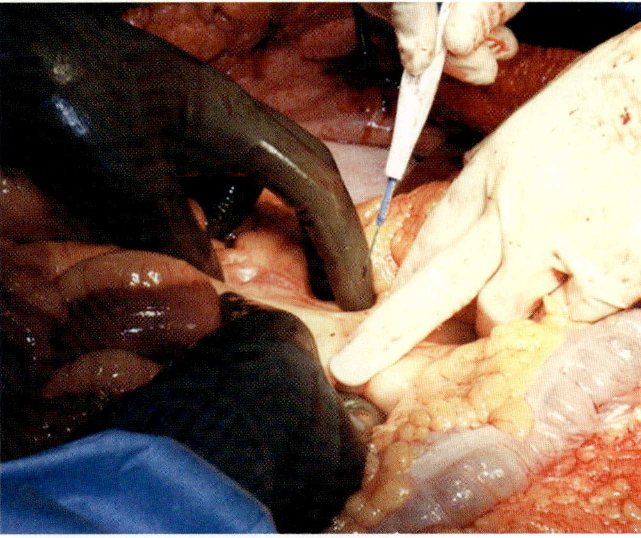

Fig. 62: The root of the mesentery is addressed, and the superior mesenteric vein and artery dissected.

CANNULATION OF THE AORTA AND INFERIOR MESENTERIC VEIN—PERFUSION WITH PRESERVATION FLUID (FIGS. 63 TO 65)

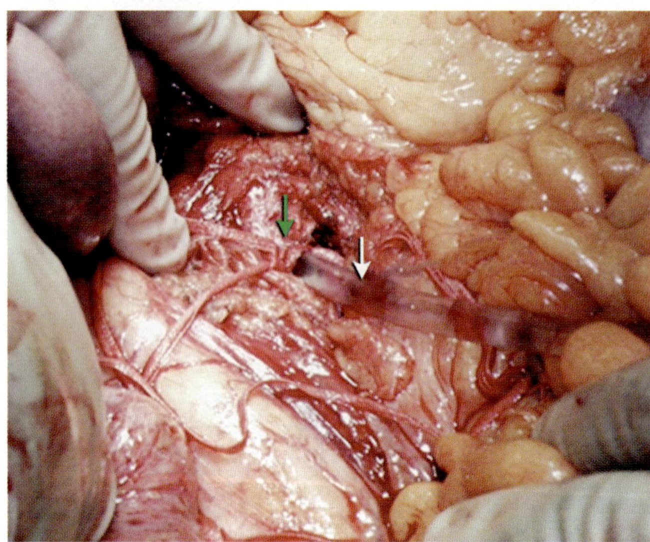

Fig. 63: The distal aortic umbilical tape is tied to prevent back-flow from the common iliac arteries. The aorta (green arrow) is incised along its anterior surface and cannulated (cannula shown with a white arrow) while the proximal umbilical tape placed at the beginning of the procurement is tied around the cannula.

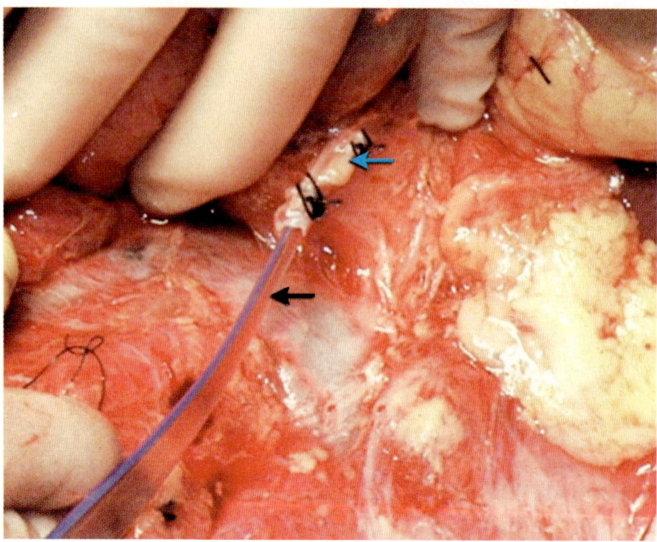

Fig. 64: The inferior mesenteric vein (light blue arrow) is also cannulated (cannula shown with black arrow) and secured in place with a tie. The distal end of the vein is tied to prevent bleeding.

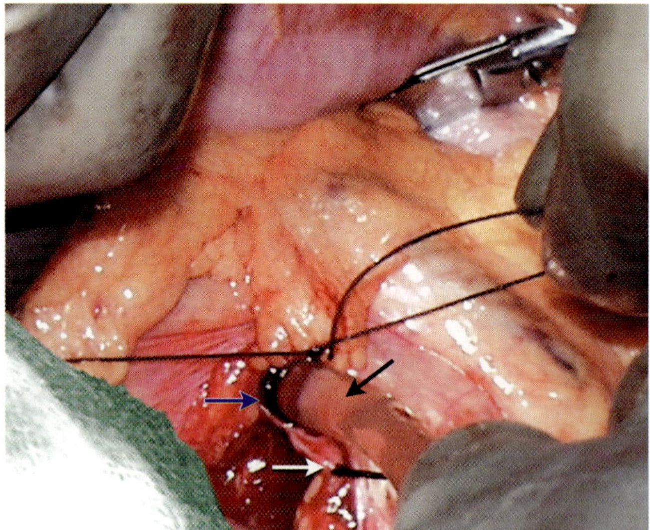

Fig. 65: In cases where the pancreas and small bowel are not procured, the liver can be perfused via a large cannula (black arrow) inserted into the superior mesenteric vein (blue arrow). The superior mesenteric vein is dissected at the root of the small bowel mesentery. Its proximal end is cannulated, while its distal end is tied (white arrow).

TRANSECTION OF THE ROOT OF THE SMALL BOWEL MESENTERY IN INSTANCES WHERE THE SMALL BOWEL IS NOT PROCURED (FIGS. 66 TO 69)

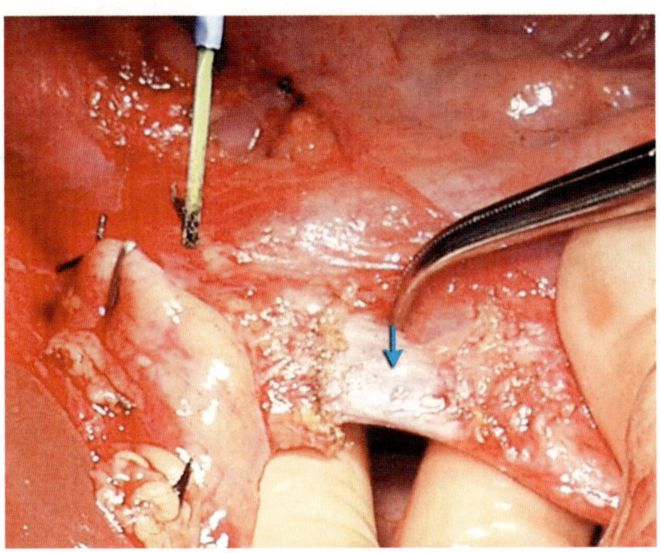

Fig. 66

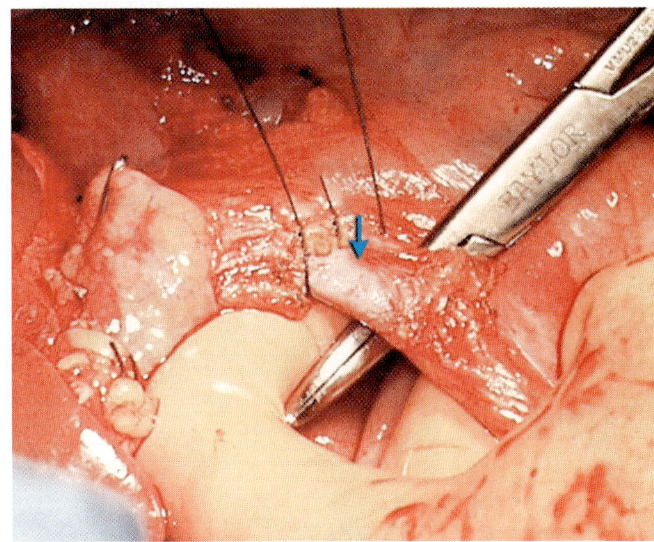

Fig. 67

Figs. 66 and 67: In instances where the small bowel is not procured, the root of the mesentery can be ligated (or stapled – and subsequently over-sewn as needed) below the pancreas. As shown in the two illustrations above, the superior mesenteric vein (blue arrows) is being dissected and circled with ligatures.

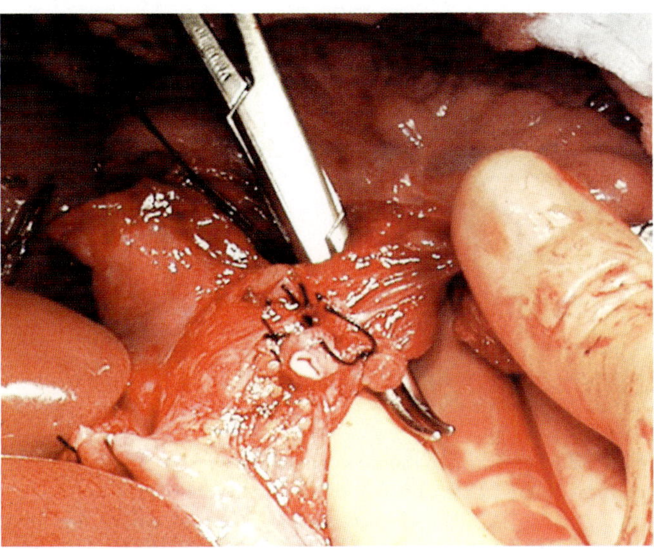

Fig. 68

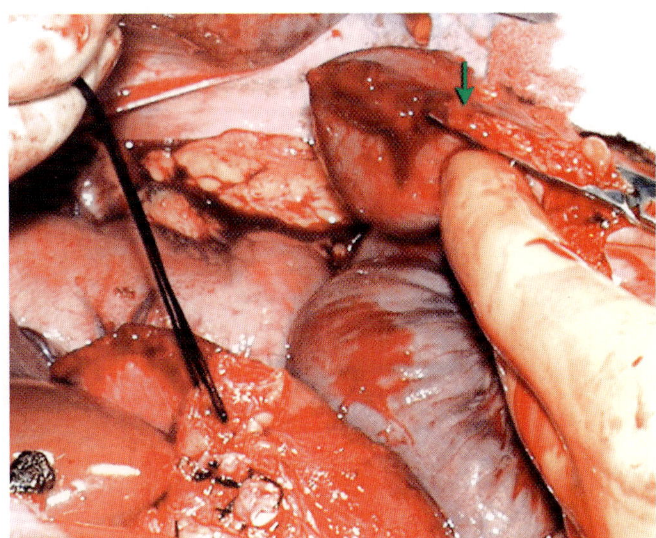

Fig. 69

Figs. 68 and 69: The superior mesenteric artery (SMA) and other structures within the small bowel mesentery are also tied and transected proximally. While the proximal ends of the superior mesenteric vessels need to be tied or stapled to prevent subsequent hemorrhage in the recipient, their distal ends can be clamped (green arrow).

CROSS-CLAMPING OF THE THORACIC AORTA (FIGS. 70 TO 72)

Prior to cross-clamping (at least 3 minutes in advance) a bolus of heparin is administered intravenously to prevent thrombosis within the organs being procured. The routine dose is approximately 3000 units of heparin/kg of body weight.

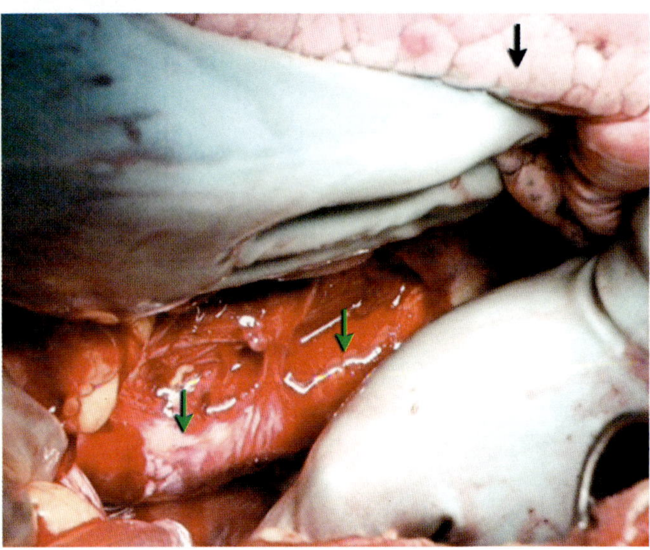

Fig. 70: In instances where the lungs are not procured, we routinely perform the cross-clamping of the aorta in the thorax. The right lung (black arrow) is retracted, and the aorta (green arrows) identified and exposed.

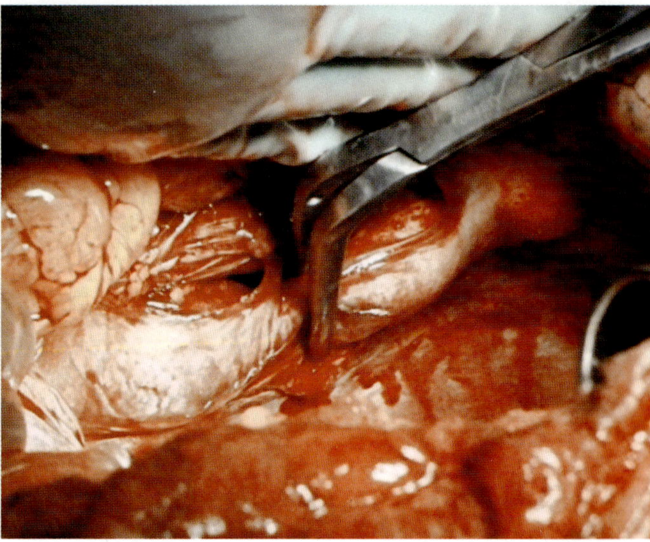

Fig. 71: Once all members of the procurement teams agree, the aorta is cross-clamped and the body perfused with cold preservation fluid via the distal aorta and inferior mesenteric vein.

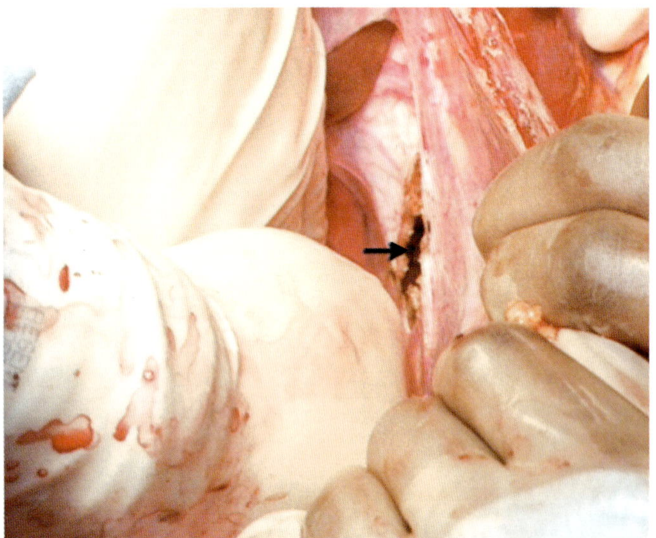

Fig. 72: Alternatively, the thoracic aorta can be accessed via an incision in the posteromedial aspect of the left diaphragm (black arrow) close to the vertebral bodies. In cases where the lungs are procured, the aorta is cross-clamped intra-abdominally after incising the left crus of the diaphragm.

INCISION OF THE RIGHT ATRIUM (FIGS. 73 TO 75)

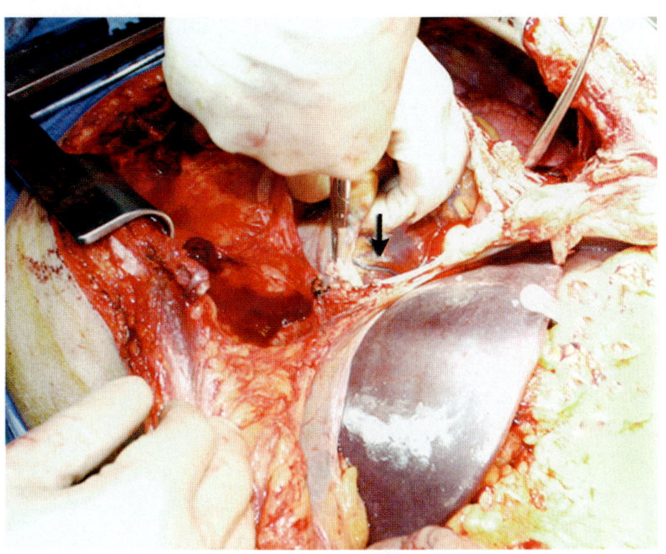

Fig. 73

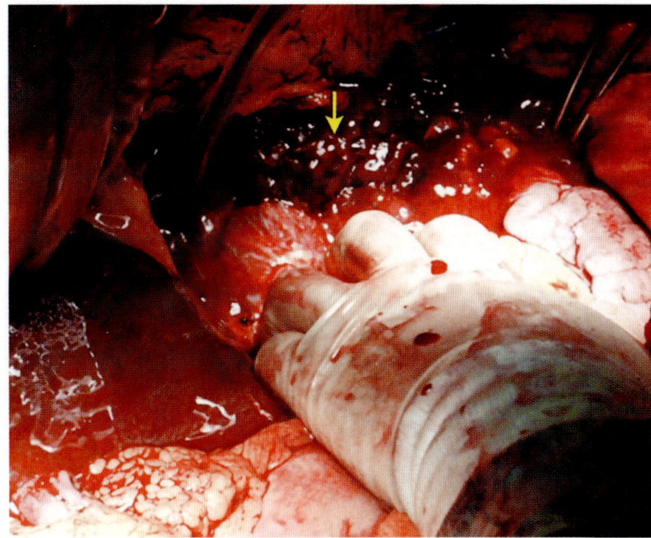

Fig. 74

Figs. 73 and 74: As the body is perfused with cold preservation fluid via the aortic and inferior mesenteric vein cannulas, the right atrium (black arrow) is incised in order to allow for the outflow of blood (yellow arrow) and subsequently of preservation fluid. In instances of cardiac procurements, the intrapericardial inferior vena cava (IVC) is incised at a site agreed upon with the cardiac team and sterile ice is placed surrounding all organs in order to achieve hypothermia and diminish the ischemic damage.

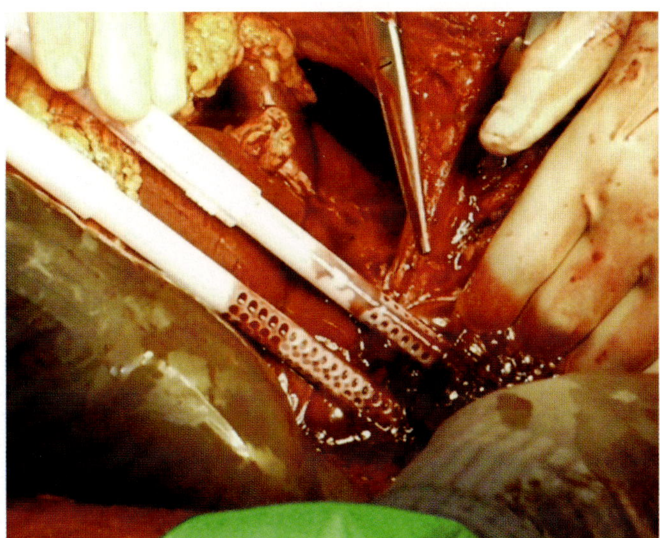

Fig. 75: Blood and preservation fluid are suctioned as they enter the left hemithorax.

PERFUSION AND COOLING OF ORGANS (FIGS. 76 TO 78)

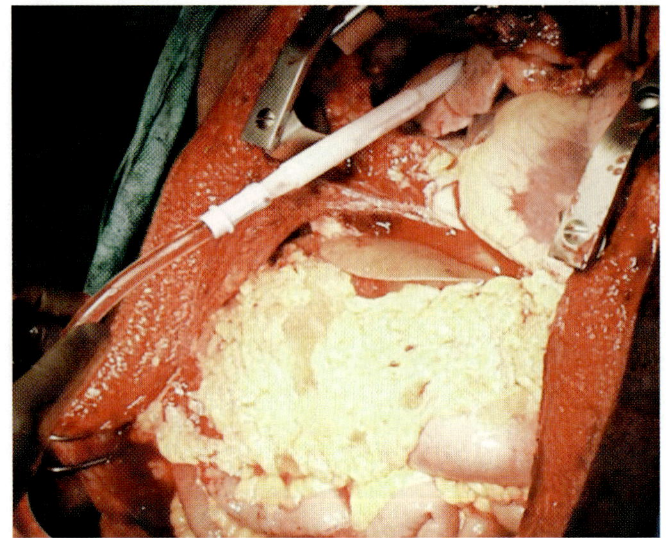

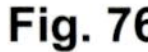

Fig. 76

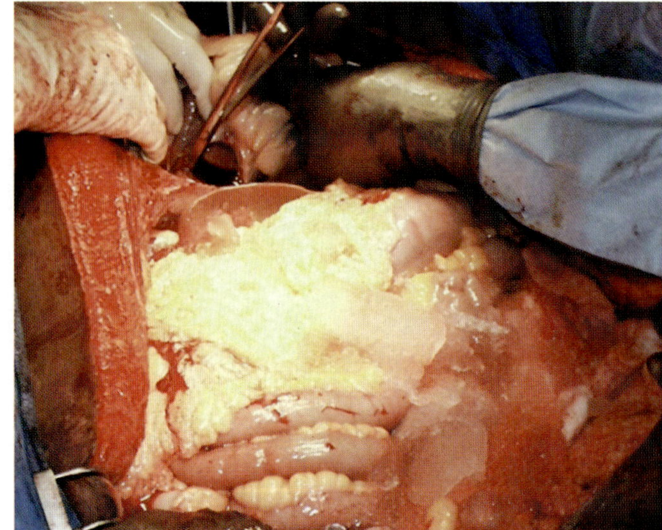

Fig. 77

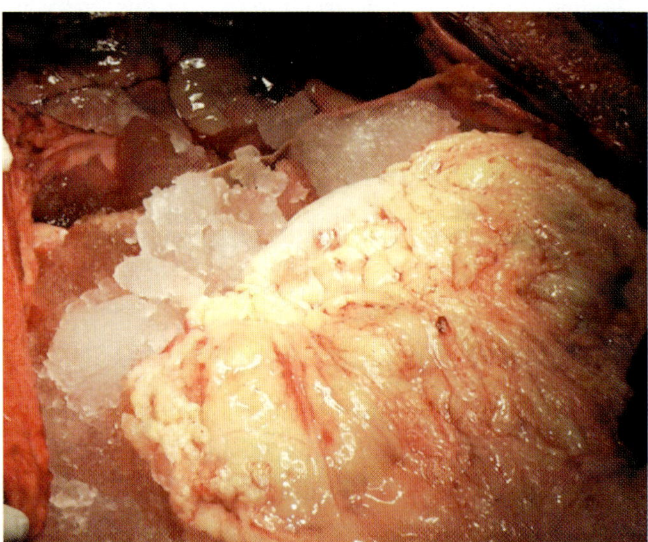

Fig. 78

Figs. 76 to 78: As the body is perfused and cold preservation fluid replaces the blood within the organs, ice is placed within the abdominal cavity to maintain the organs at a low temperature.

REMOVAL OF PANCREAS AND LIVER GRAFTS (FIGS. 79 TO 94)

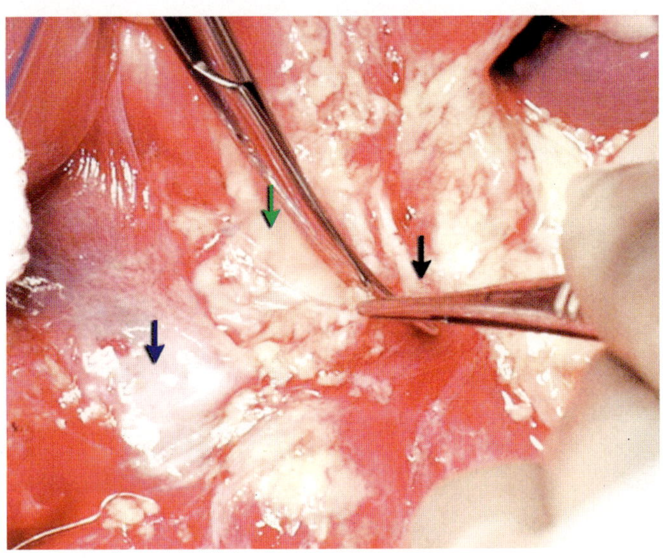

Fig. 79

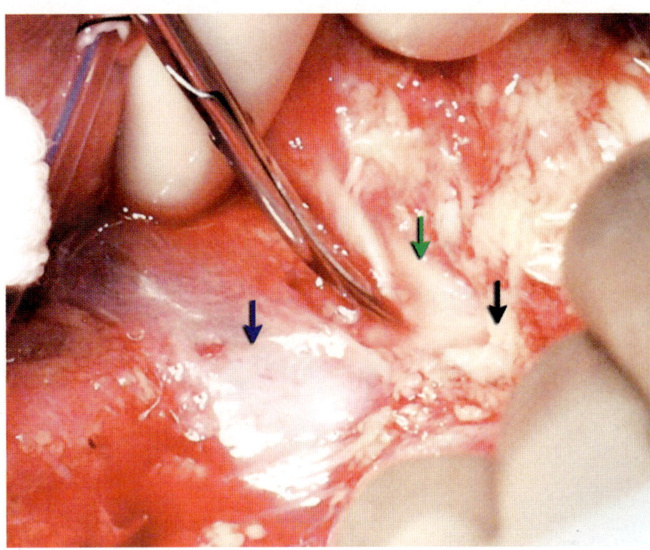

Fig. 80

Figs. 79 and 80: Once the organs have been perfused with the desired amount of preservation fluid, we proceed to remove them from the body. The heart is removed first, followed in specific order by the lungs, liver, pancreas, and kidneys. We usually procure the liver and pancreas en-bloc and subsequently separate them in the back table. As the celiac plexus (black arrows) on the left side is transected, the superior mesenteric artery (SMA, green arrows) is fully exposed. Note the left renal vain (blue arrows) as it crosses the aorta underneath the aortic-SMA angle.

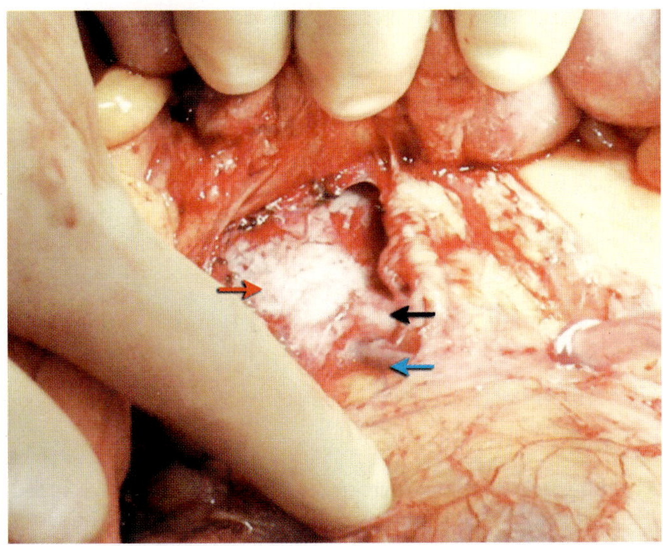

Fig. 81: On occasions, as in this illustration, the left renal vein follows a retro-aortic course (rather than crossing ventral to the aorta) prior to joining the inferior vena cava (IVC). Note the left renal artery (black arrow), left renal vein (blue arrow) and aorta (red arrow).

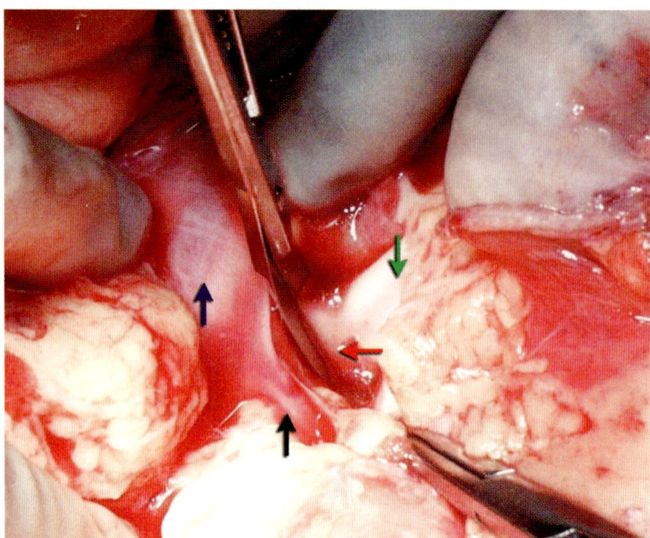

Fig. 82

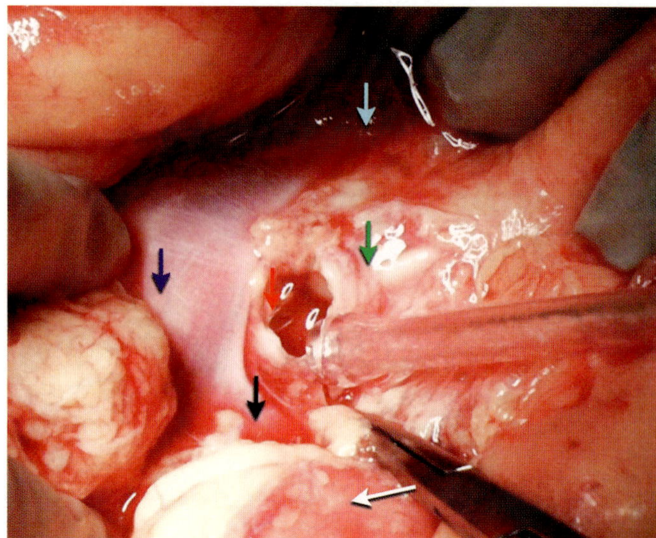

Fig. 83

Figs. 82 and 83: The aortic transection (red arrows) is undertaken at the lower end of the origin of the superior mesenteric artery (SMA) (green arrows). We routinely try to identify the left and right renal arteries in order to leave an aortic patch proximal to their origin. If the renal arteries cannot be clearly identified, we transect the aorta in an almost horizontal plane below the SMA. Also visible in these illustrations are the left renal vein (blue arrows), left adrenal vein (black arrows) the left kidney (white arrow), and the left lateral wall of the inferior vena cava (IVC) (Light blue arrow).

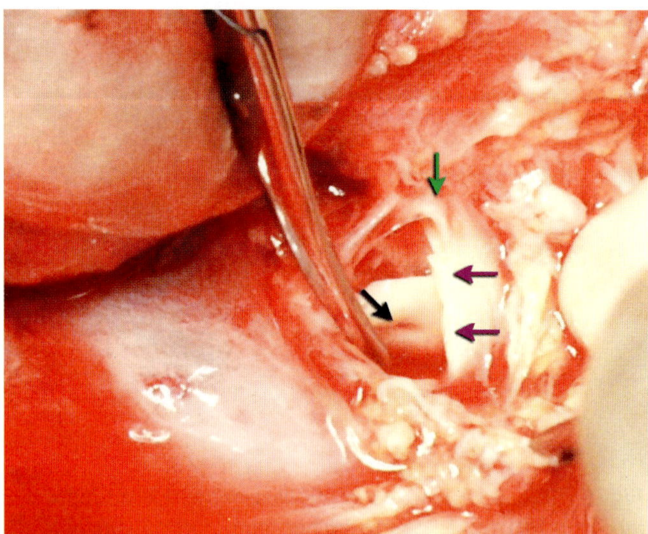

Fig. 84: The anterior aspect of the aorta is opened (purple arrows) just distal to the origin of the superior mesenteric artery (SMA) (green arrow). The ostium of the right renal artery is clearly identified (black arrow).

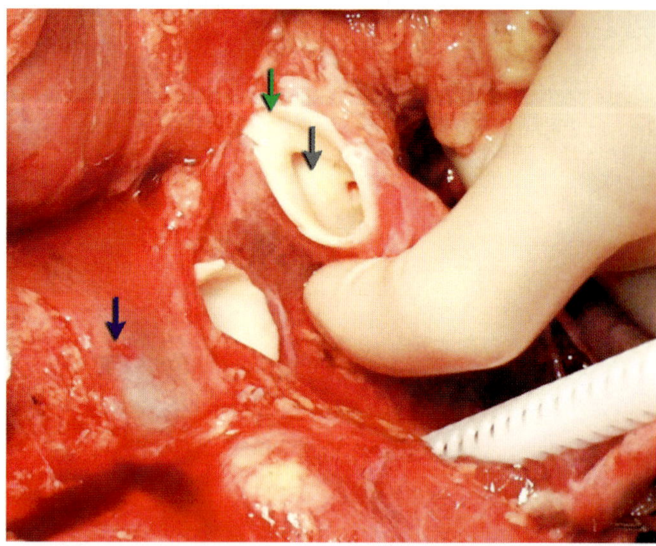

Fig. 85: Once the ostia of the renal arteries are clearly visualized, the aorta is completely transected, leaving space for an aortic patch around the renal arteries. Note the openings of the superior mesenteric artery (SMA) (green arrow) and celiac trunk (gray arrow). The left renal vein is shown with a blue arrow.

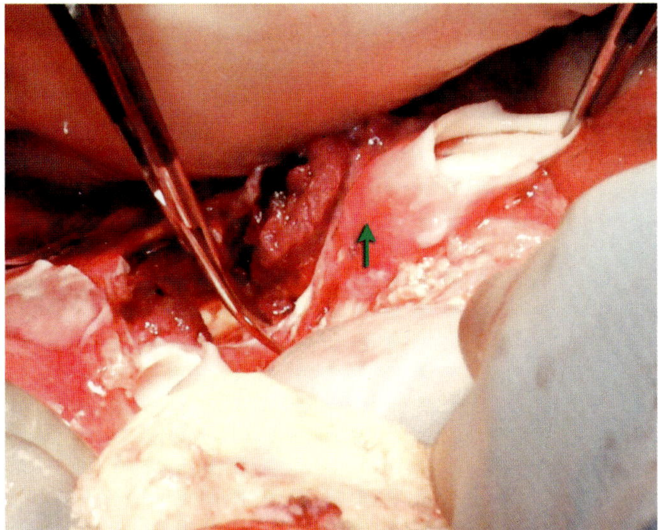

Fig. 86: The proximal aorta (green arrow) is subsequently dissected free and transected as far proximally as desired by the surgeon.

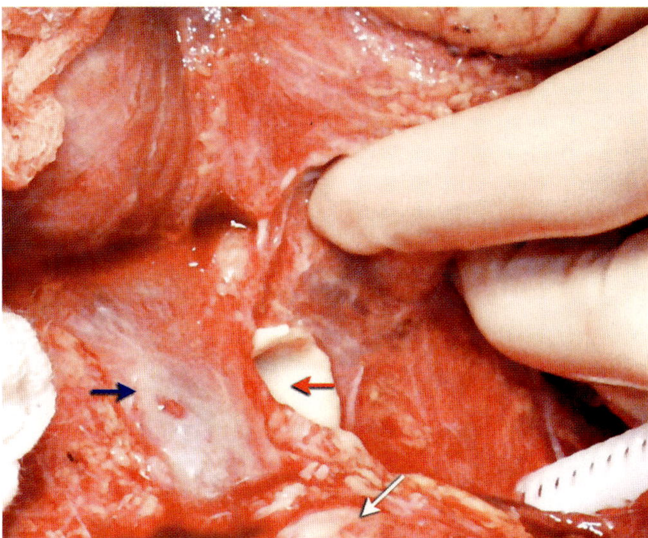

Fig. 87: The distal aorta (red arrow) and kidneys will be addressed after the liver and pancreas (and small bowel) are removed. Note the left renal vein (blue arrow) and the left kidney (white arrow).

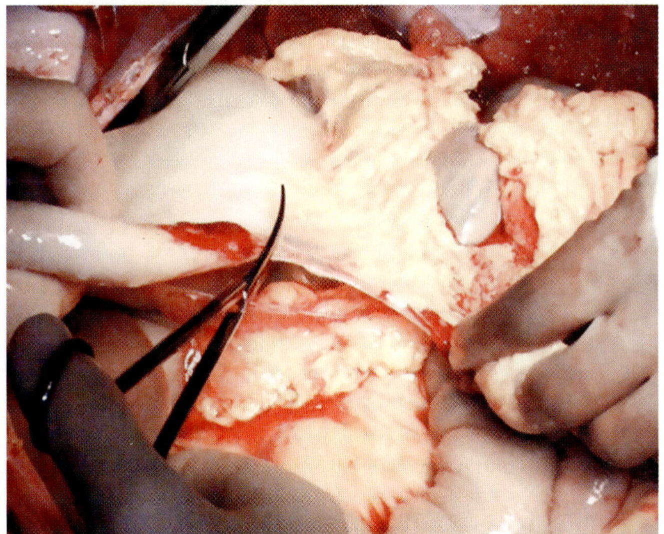

Fig. 88: The greater curve of the stomach can be freed from its associated tissues and structures in order to improve exposure.

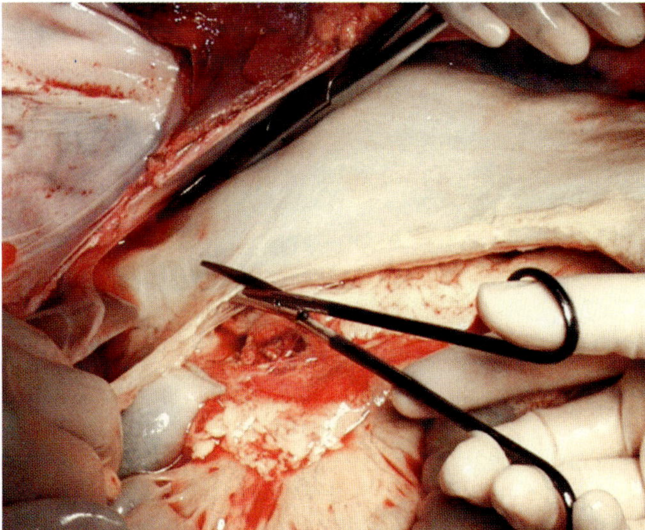

Fig. 89: The lesser omentum is freed from the lesser curve of the stomach. The esophagus is also freed from surrounding tissues and structures. Special care is taken in instances of accessory/replaced left hepatic arteries in order to preserve them with the liver free of injuries.

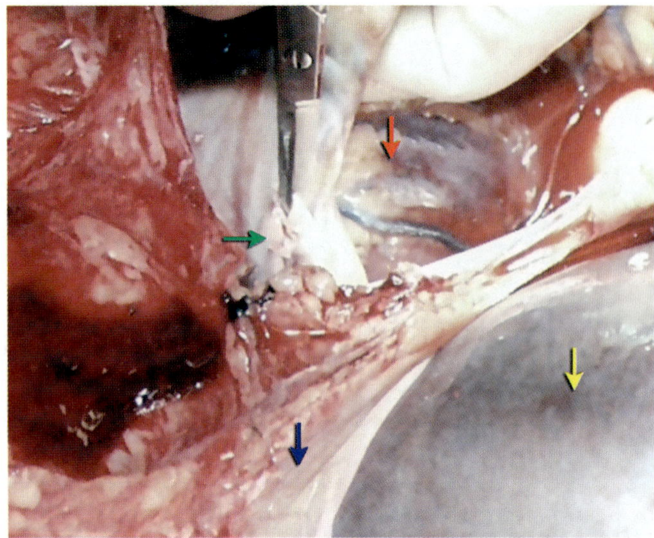

Fig. 90: The diaphragm (blue arrow), pericardium (green arrow), and other structures overlying the esophagus are cut. The diaphragm is transected around the inferior vena cava (IVC), aorta and liver. Note the heart (red arrow) that in this specific instance was not procured, and the right lobe of the liver (yellow arrow).

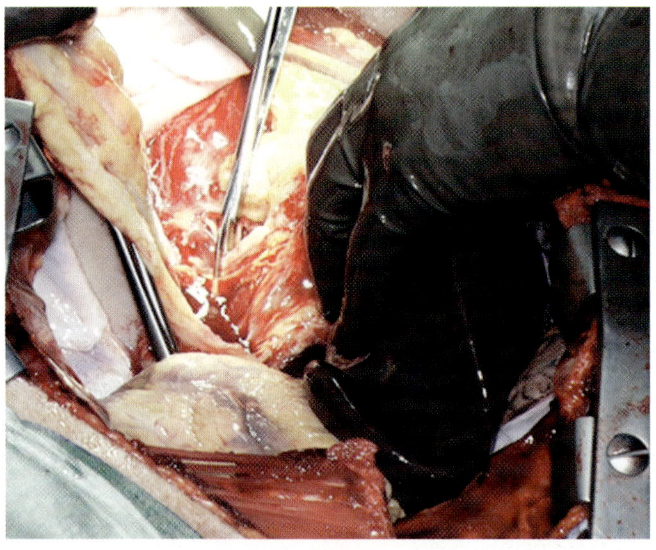

Fig. 91

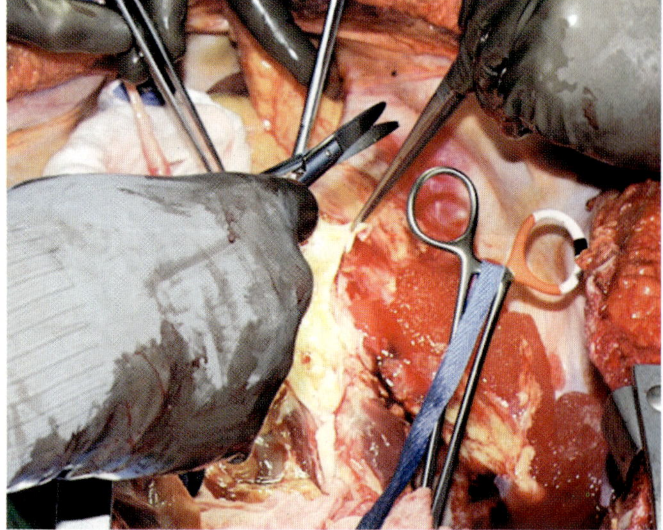

Fig. 92

Figs. 91 and 92: The aorta is detached along its dorsal aspect, transecting lumbar and intercostal branches. Care should be taken not to injure the celiac trunk or superior mesenteric artery (SMA).

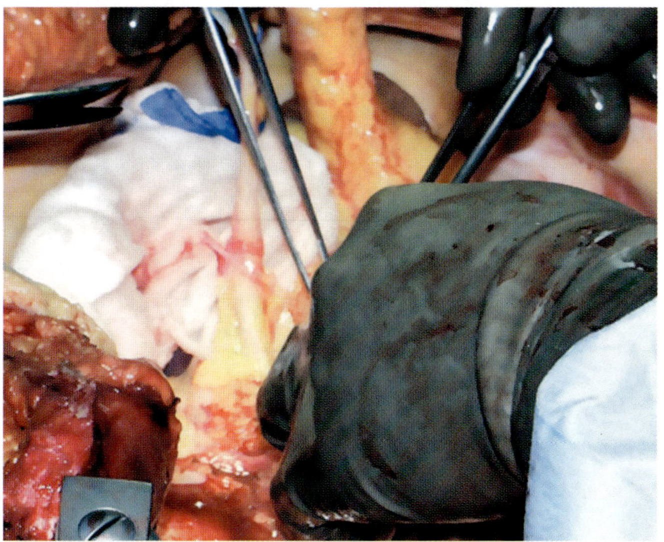

Fig. 93

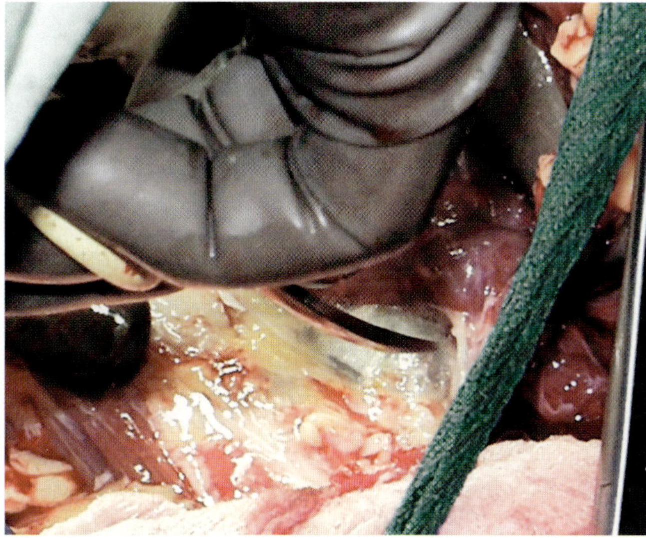

Fig. 94

Figs. 93 and 94: The liver-pancreas graft is completely freed by transecting the inferior vena cava (IVC) above the right renal vein, the intrapericardial IVC and diaphragm around it, the crura of the diaphragm, the prevertebral muscles and freeing the retrohepatic IVC. In cases where the small bowel is also procured, it is removed together with the liver and pancreas.

LIVER-PANCREAS GRAFT (FIG. 95)

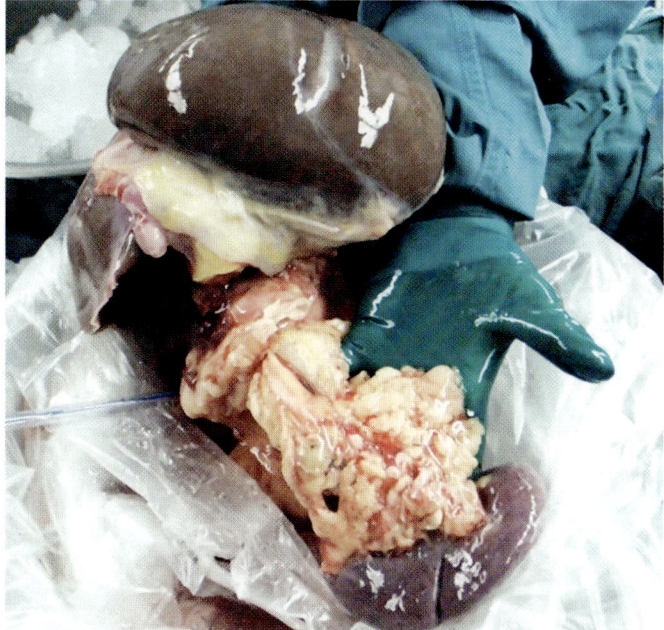

Fig. 95: In instances where the small bowel is not procured (such as in this illustration), the vessels at the root of the mesentery can be tied independently or stapled (and subsequently over-sewn if considered necessary) with a vascular device.

LIVER-PANCREAS–SMALL BOWEL GRAFT (FIG. 96)

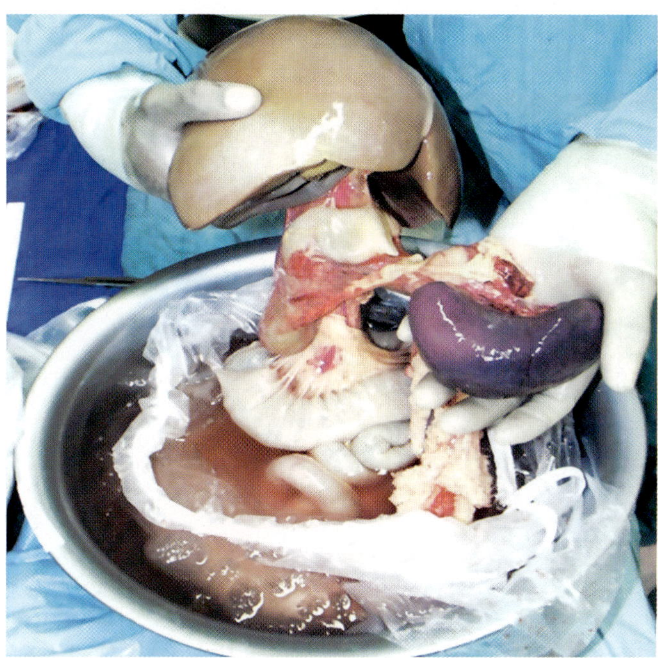

Fig. 96: In instances where the small bowel is procured, the mesentery is kept intact. Once in the back table, further dissection will be undertaken. The superior mesenteric artery (SMA) and vein will be dissected and transected in order to free the small bowel graft.

REMOVAL OF THE KIDNEYS (FIGS. 97 TO 104)

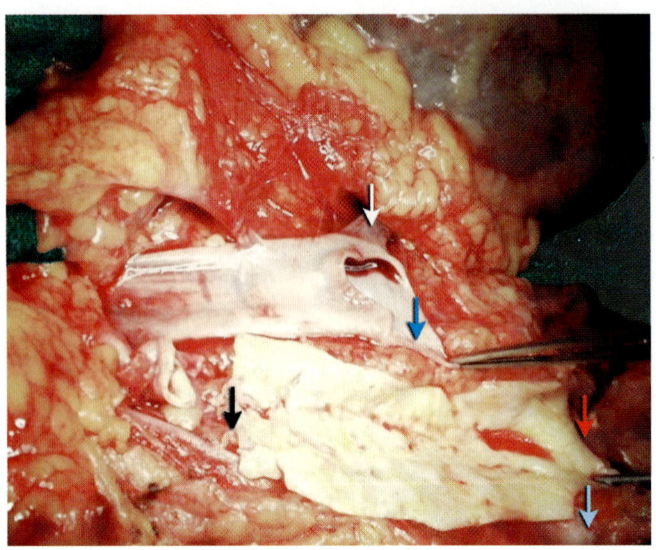

Fig. 97

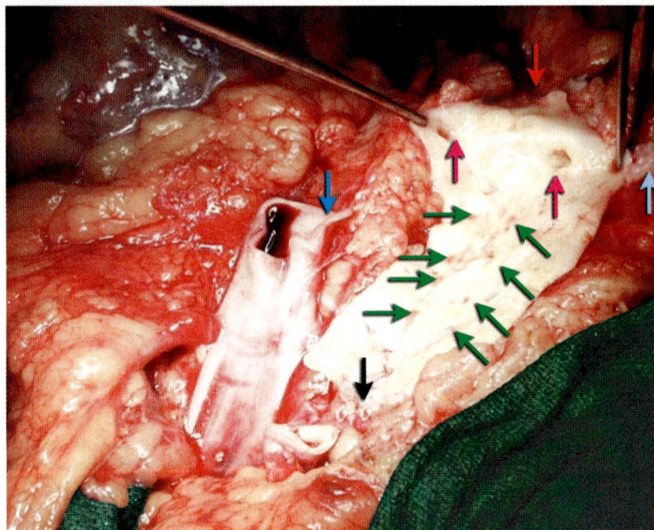

Fig. 98

Figs. 97 and 98: The distal aorta and kidneys are addressed next. The kidneys can be removed en block or independently. We prefer to remove them independently. The left renal vein (light blue arrows) has been transected at its confluence into the inferior vena cava (IVC) (light blue arrows). The aorta is incised longitudinally along its anterior midline from its proximal (red arrows) to its distal transection (black arrows) sites. Once we verify that there are no distal renal arteries (sometimes they may arise as distally as the iliac vessels) we transect the aorta at its bifurcation (black arrows) (or further distally if necessary). Note in the illustrations the ostia of the renal arteries (pink arrows) and the right renal vein (white arrow). The openings of the main and accessory (if any) renal arteries should not be confused with those of the lumbar arteries (green arrows).

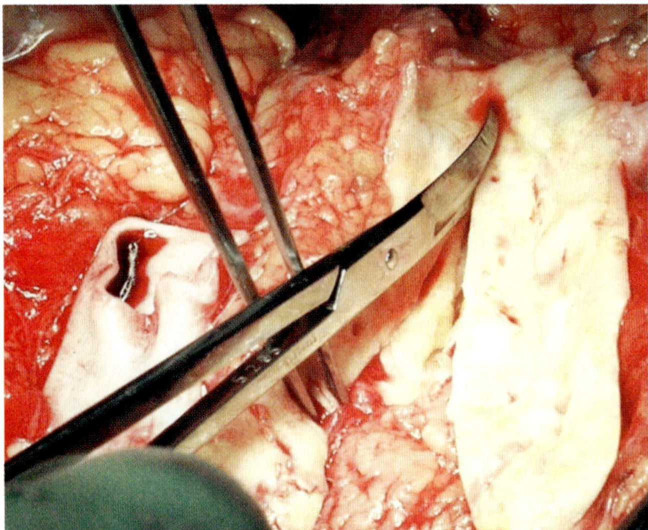

Fig. 99: The aorta is transected along its dorsal midline, in between the origins of the lumbar arteries.

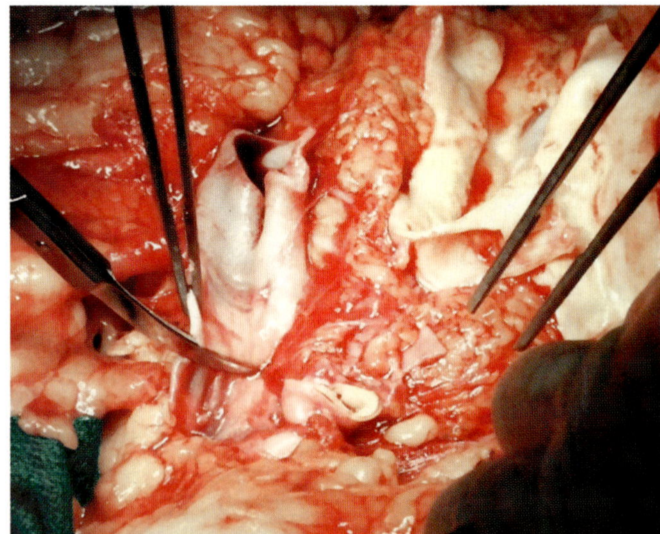

Fig. 100: The inferior vena cava (IVC) is transected just proximal to the origin of the common iliac veins.

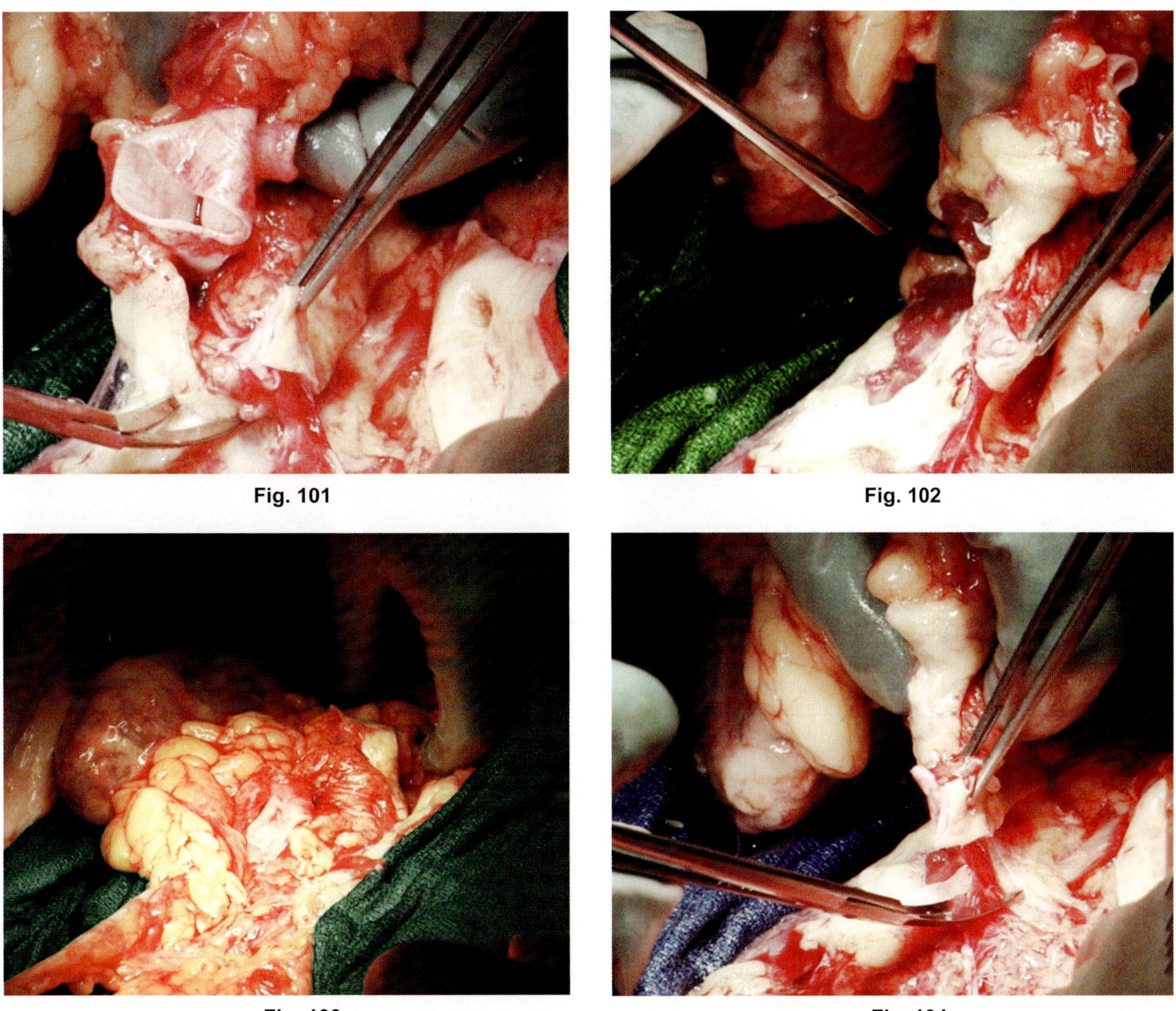

Fig. 101

Fig. 102

Fig. 103

Fig. 104

Figs. 101 to 104: The ureters are transected at their entrance into the urinary bladder, always preserving the tissues surrounding them. Each kidney is removed independently by incising along the retroperitoneal tissues as close as possible to the vertebral bodies.

ILIAC VESSELS (FIGS. 105 AND 106)

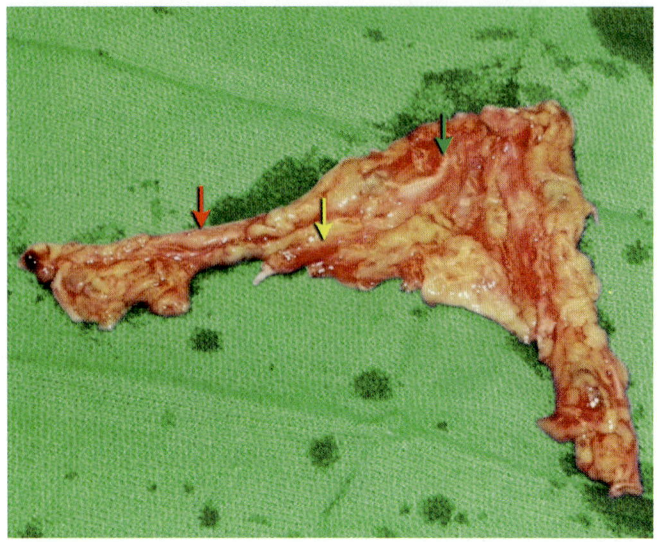

Fig. 105: The common (green arrow), external (red arrow) and as much of the internal (yellow arrow) iliac arteries and their corresponding veins are procured for further use. The arteries are used for the pancreatic arterial reconstruction in the back table. Some authors use the common iliac vein to elongate the portal vein in the pancreas graft. They can also be necessary for arterial and/or venous reconstructions when implanting the liver. As a general rule, the pancreas and liver teams each keep vessels from one side. In this specific example, the right and left sided iliac vessels have been procured en bloc.

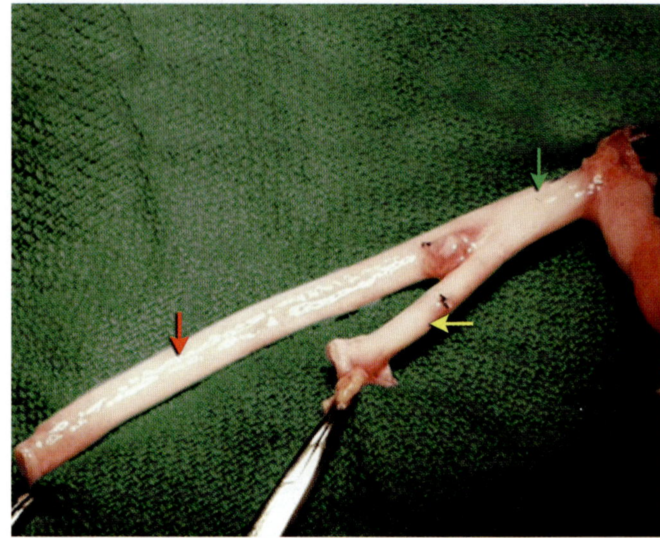

Fig. 106: These vessels are subsequently dissected and prepared for further use (common, external, and internal iliac arteries shown with green, red and yellow arrows respectively).

BACK TABLE SEPARATION OF ORGANS (FIGS. 107 TO 109)

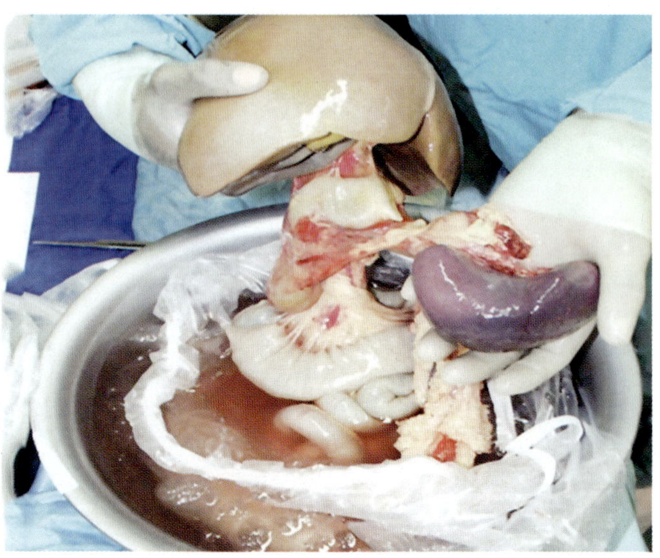

Fig. 107: The liver, pancreas, duodenum, spleen and small intestine are seen still attached in the back table.

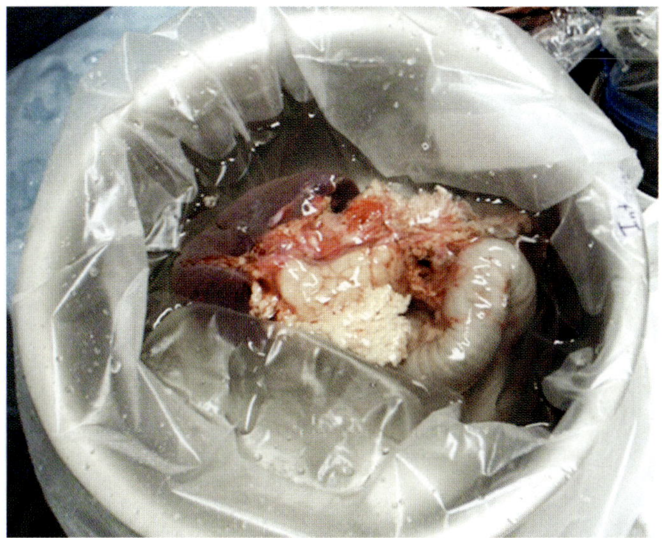

Fig. 108

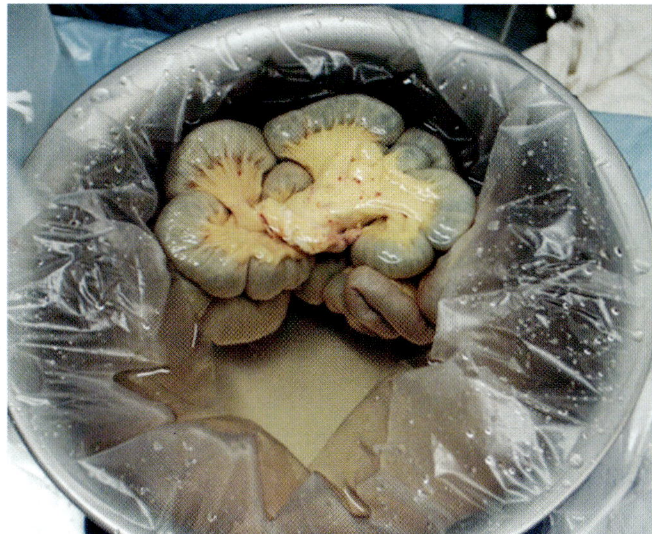

Fig. 109

Figs. 108 and 109: The small intestine graft is separated from the liver–pancreas graft by transecting the superior mesenteric vein and artery.

SEPARATION OF LIVER AND PANCREAS (FIGS. 110 TO 115)

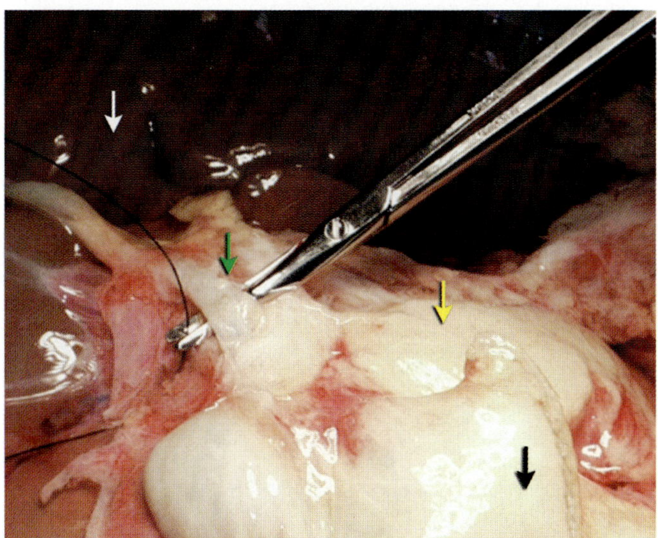

Fig. 110: The liver is being separated from the pancreas. The common bile duct (green arrow) is tied distally (in order to prevent leaks from the duodenum—black arrow) and transected. The pancreas is shown with a yellow arrow and the liver with a white arrow.

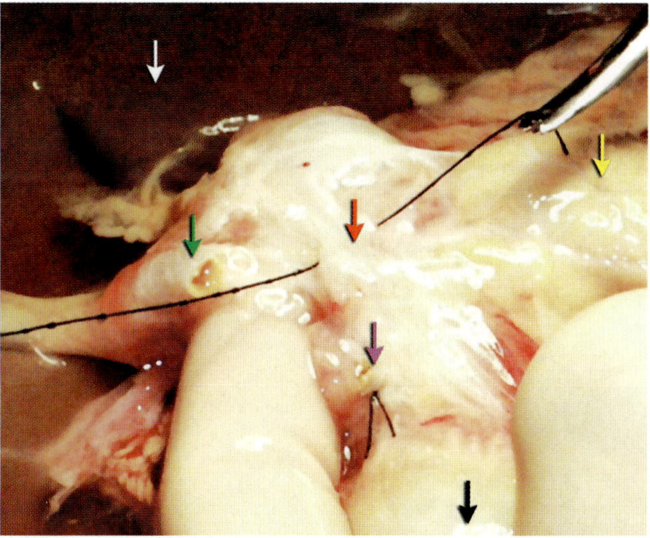

Fig. 111: The gastroduodenal artery (red arrow) is tied and transected. The splenic and superior mesenteric arteries are subsequently transected at their origin from the celiac trunk and aorta, respectively. The duodenum (black arrow), proximal transected common bile duct (green arrow), pancreas (yellow arrow), tied distal bile duct (purple arrow) and liver (white arrow) are also visible.

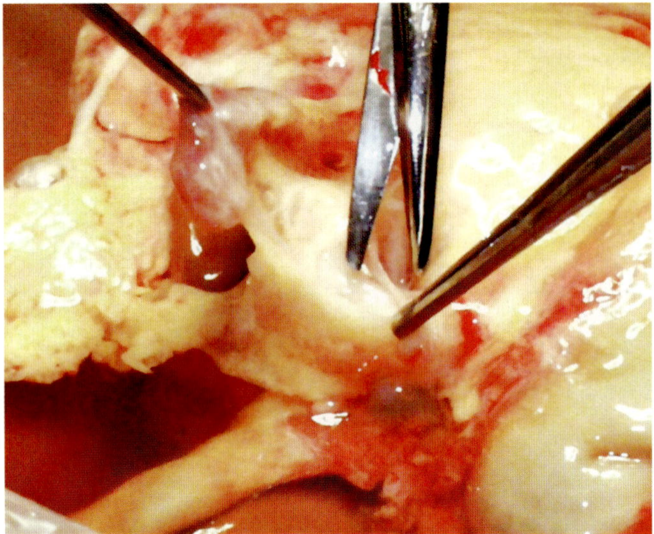

Fig. 112: The splenic artery can be located by dissecting along the superior border of the pancreas, as it originates at the celiac trunk. It is then transected. Its distal end is tagged for ease of identification during the subsequent back table reconstruction.

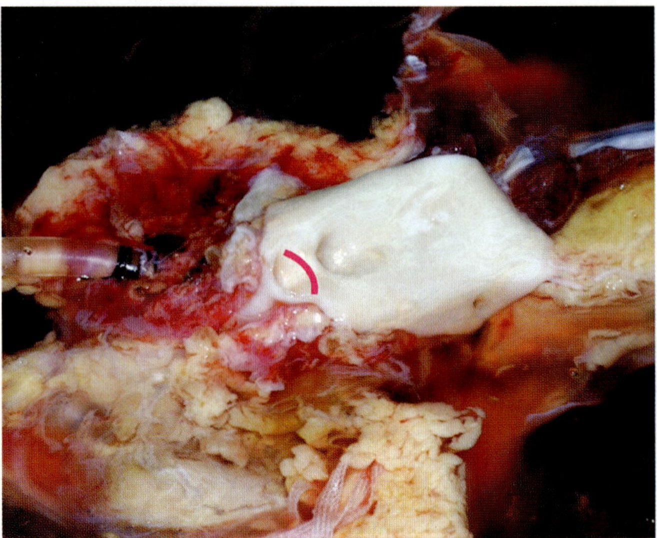

Fig. 113: In instances where there is no accessory/replaced right hepatic artery (RHA) originating from the SMA, the SMA and celiac trunk can be separated by transecting the aorta in between their ostia (pink line). In cases of an accessory/replaced right hepatic artery (RHA) originating from the SMA, the SMA should be transected distal to the origin of the replaced/accessory RHA so to allow for a more simple reconstruction.

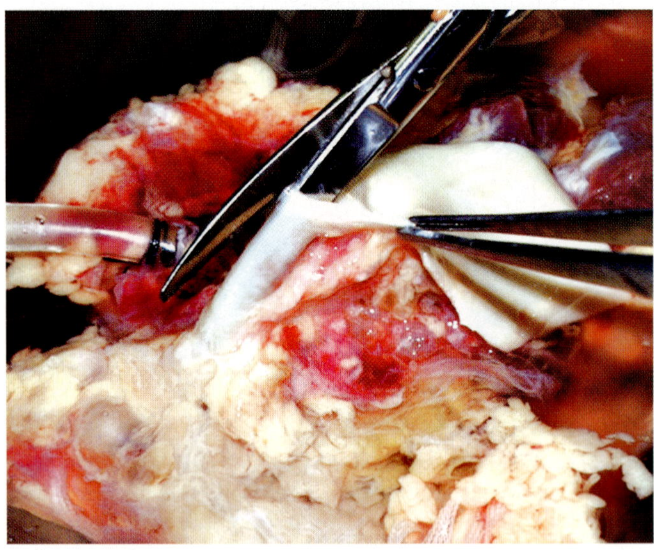

Fig. 114

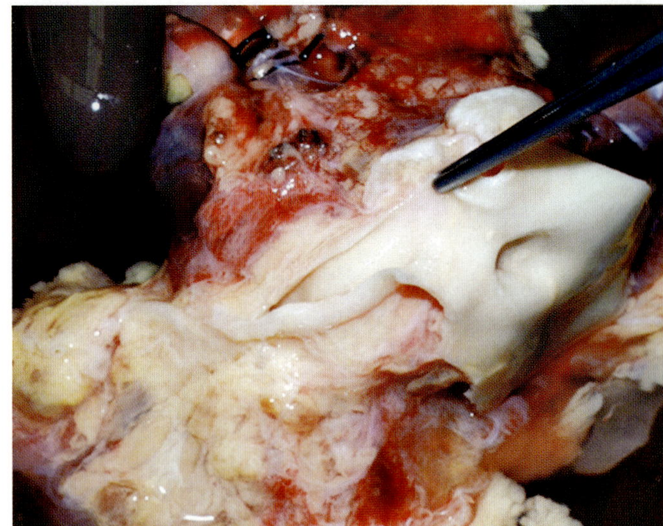

Fig. 115

Figs. 114 and 115: Alternatively, in instance where there is uncertainty about the presence of a replaced/accessory right hepatic artery from the SMA, the proximal SMA can be opened and its interior inspected for the origin of such accessory/replaced vessels.

PANCREAS ALLOGRAFT (FIGS. 116 AND 117)

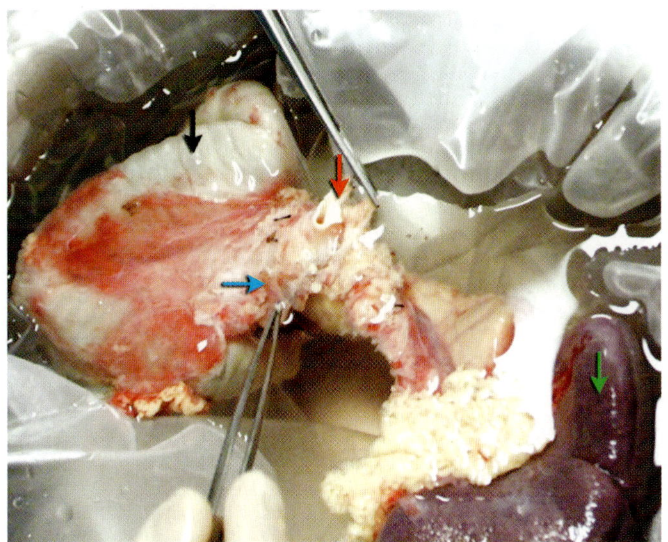

Fig. 116

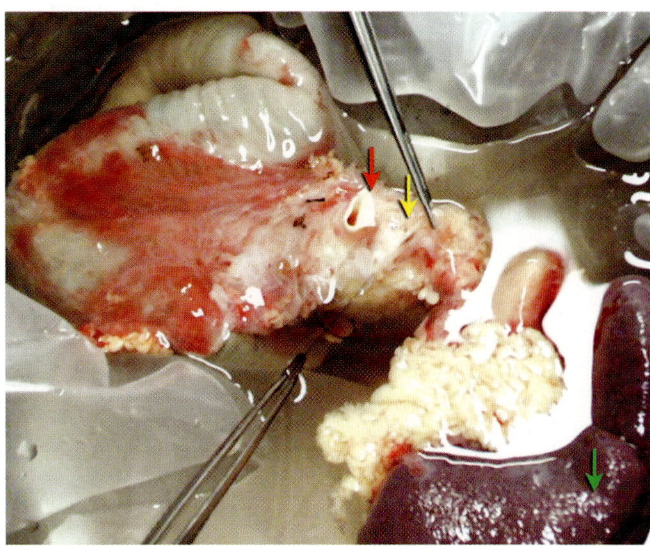

Fig. 117

Figs. 116 and 117: The pancreas graft inclusive of duodenum and spleen (the latter to be later removed) is ready for being packed. The superior mesenteric artery (SMA) (red arrows), splenic artery (yellow arrow), portal vein (blue arrow), spleen (green arrows) and duodenum (black arrows) can be appreciated.

LIVER ALLOGRAFT (FIGS. 118 AND 119)

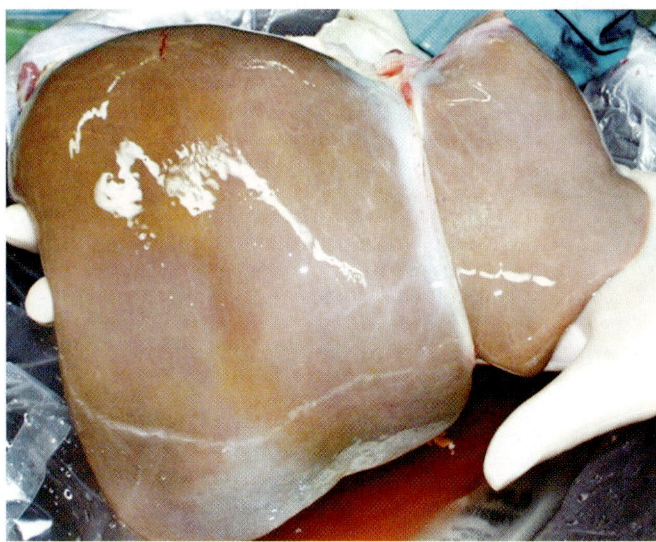

Fig. 118

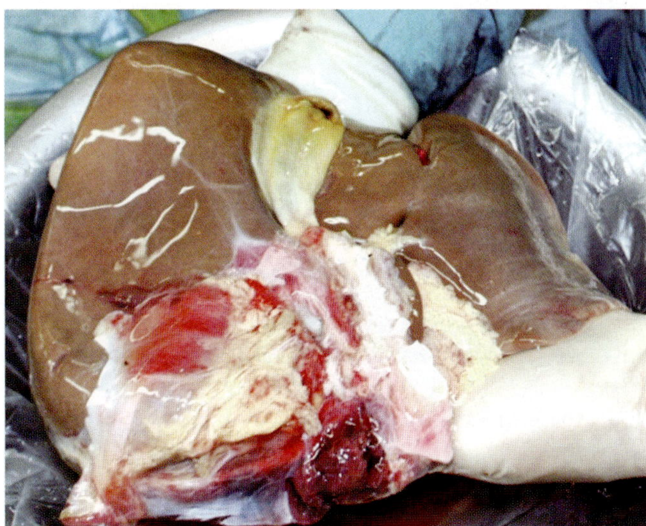

Fig. 119

Figs. 118 and 119: Anterior and posterior views of the liver.

KIDNEY ALLOGRAFTS (FIGS. 120 TO 128)

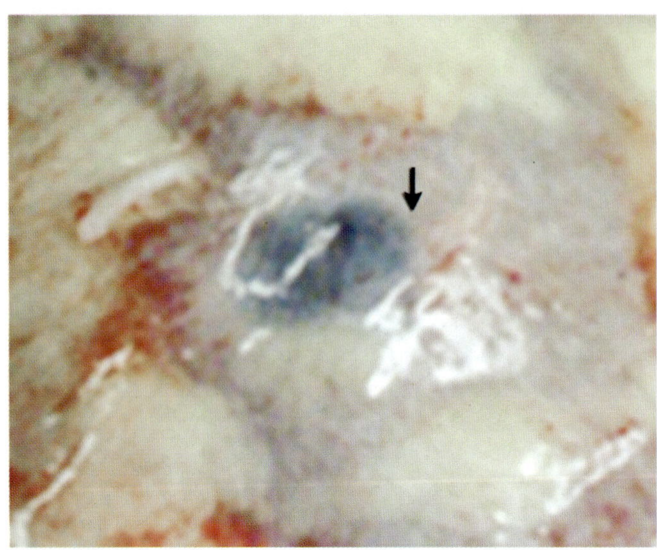

Fig. 120: The procured kidneys (including the ureters) are inspected for lesions and/or surgical damage. In this specific case, a simple cyst is shown by the arrow. Simple cysts are considered benign. Complex cysts and other lesions should always be evaluated for the possibility of malignancy.

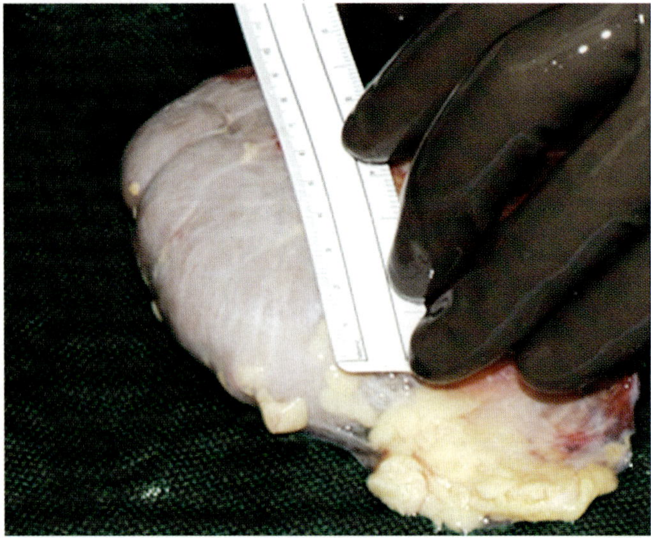

Fig. 121

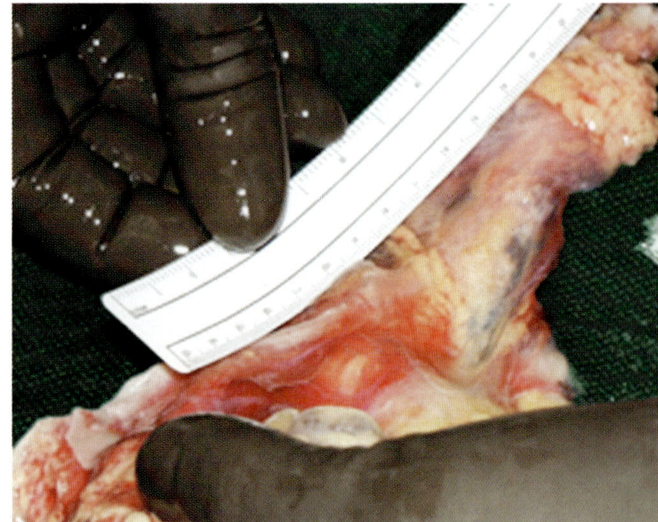

Fig. 122

Figs. 121 and 122: Measurements are obtained.

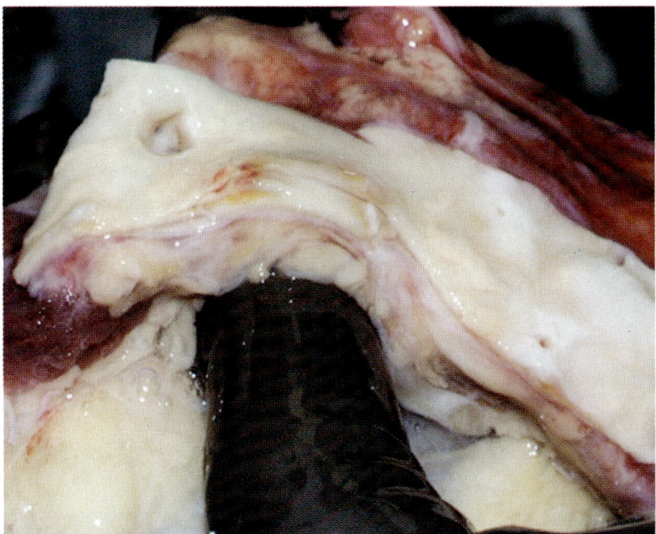

Fig. 123: The aortic segment is inspected for plaque.

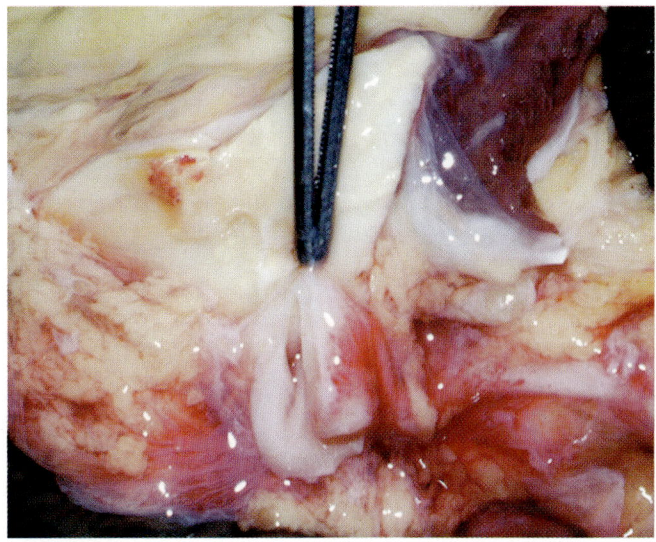

Fig. 124: The renal vein is evaluated (in this case of a left kidney, an inferior vena cava, patch is attached) and measured.

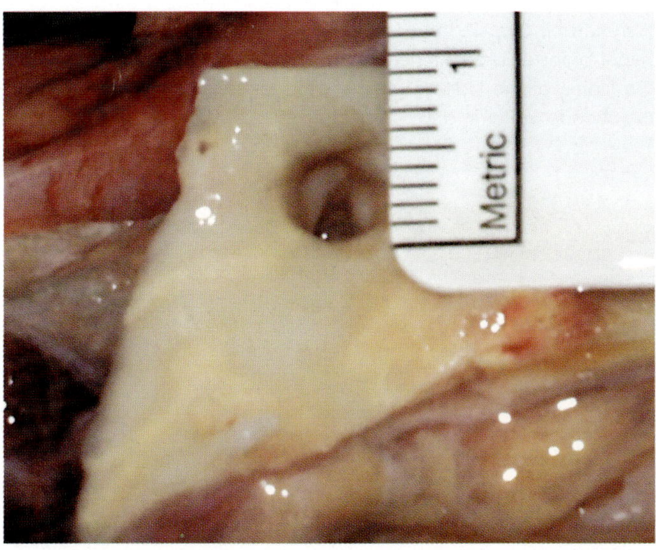

Fig. 125: The diameter and length of the renal artery is obtained. It is also inspected for the presence of plaque, other pathologies, or surgical lesions.

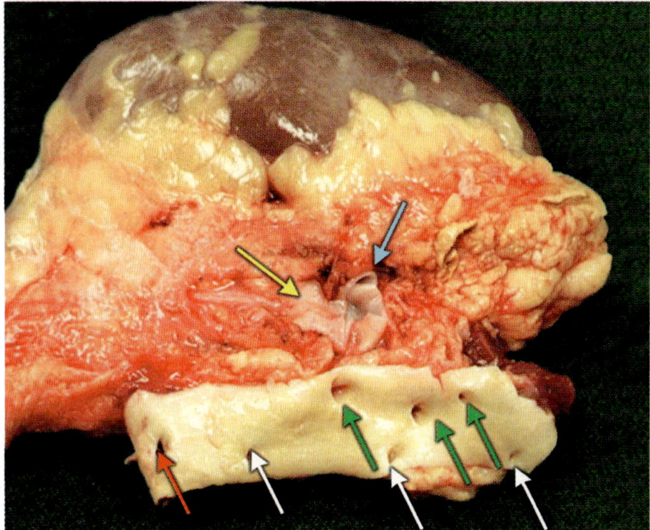

Fig. 126: The right kidney in this case has the inferior vena cava (IVC) (yellow arrow) attached to its renal vein (light blue arrow). The aortic patch contains the openings of three renal arteries (green arrows). They should not be confused with the ostia of the lumbar (white arrows) and inferior mesenteric (red arrow) arteries.

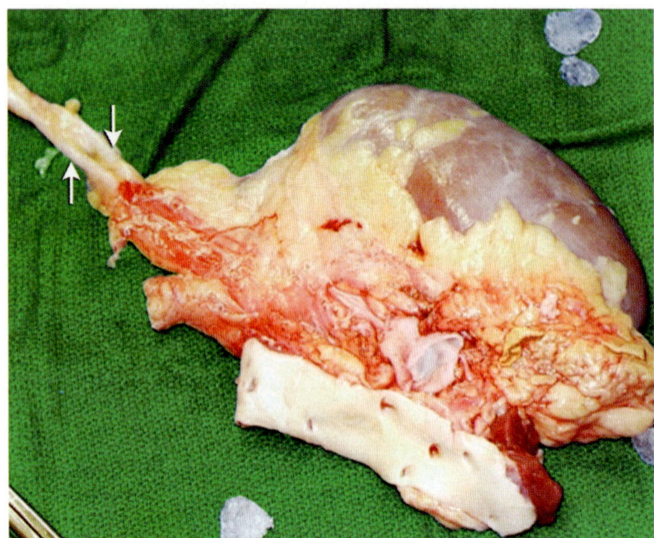

Fig. 127: Further inspection of the kidney shows a double ureter (arrows).

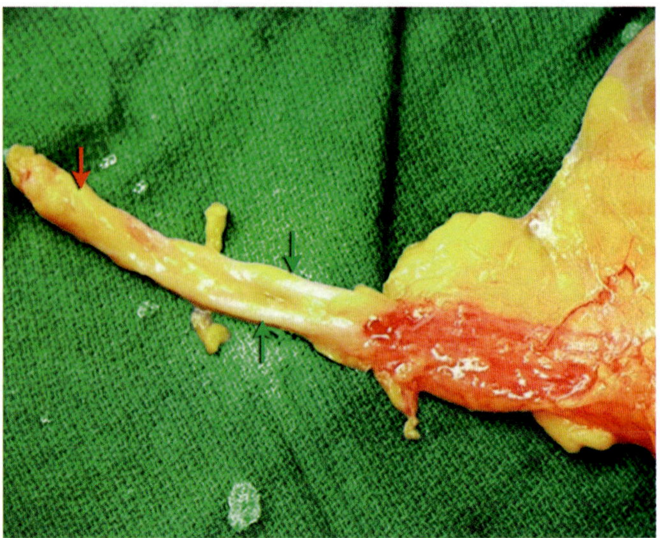

Fig. 128: Detailed view of the double ureters (green arrows). In this case, they join distally into a single ureter (red arrow). The perirenal fat should be removed in order to be able to identify potential masses, cysts, or other pathologies. In cases where a mass is found, it should be biopsied and evaluated immediately by frozen section. Renal biopsies are routinely requested by some centers to evaluate the status of the kidney. Care should be taken to preserve tissues around the ureter in order to avoid post-transplant ischemic injuries.

CHAPTER 29

Back Table Preparation

Ernesto P Molmenti and Collaborators

INTRODUCTION

- Back table entails the preparation of the organ to be transplanted
- Traditionally, it is performed in a back table in the recipient operating room (thus the adoption of the name)
- Correct identification of donor organs and intended recipients following established protocols is essential to prevent potentially fatal errors
- Sterility is maintained at all times
- All tissue specimens should preferably be sent for pathologic identification and evaluation

KIDNEYS RECEIVED IN PUMPS OR SHIPPING CONTAINERS (FIGS. 1 TO 3)

- The kidney is placed inside a bag containing cold preservation fluid within a basin with ice
- Renal parenchyma, ureter and vessels are inspected for injuries and/or abnormalities
- The artery and vein are prepared for implantation
  - The distal ends are freed of surrounding tissues
  - Venous branches (such as gonadal, suprarenal, lumbar, small branches to surrounding fatty tissues) are tied if not previously addressed during the procurement
  - Although we do not routinely reconstruct right renal veins some surgeons do it on a regular basis
    - We encountered no major problems implanting grafts with short veins
    - Alternatively, it is possible to reconstruct them (in order to achieve a greater length) with a donor inferior vena cava (IVC) segment or by means of other surgical techniques
  - In instances of multiple renal veins, it is generally safe to preserve only the dominant one for implantation
  - If multiple renal arteries are present, we prefer to reconstruct them into a single ostium
  - Alternatively, if not reconstructed into a common opening, each artery has to be implanted individually
- The native ureter receives its blood supply from the renal, gonadal, and superior vesical arteries through branches that travel in the periureteral tissues and fascia. Since after procurement only the renal artery is preserved, it is important to minimize ischemic changes by:
  - Maintaining and reconstructing lower pole arterial branches
  - Preserving periureteric fascia and tissues
- Perirenal fat is removed as necessary
- Dissection of the hilum should be kept to a minimum to avoid back table injuries
- The gonadal vessels should be preferably tied distally to prevent bleeding

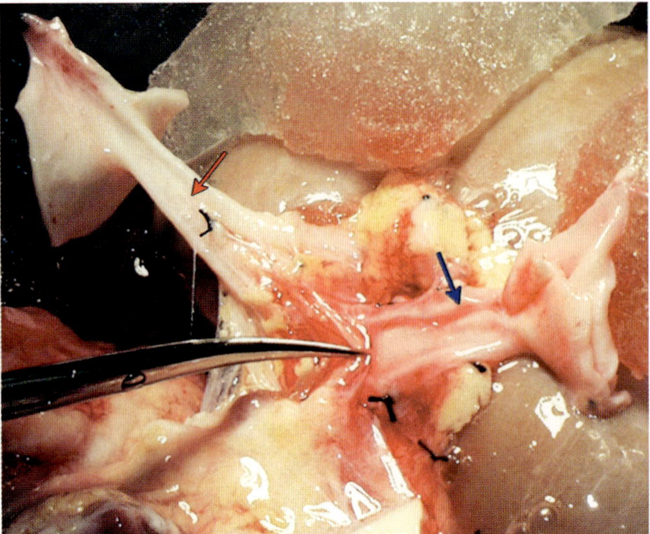

Fig. 1

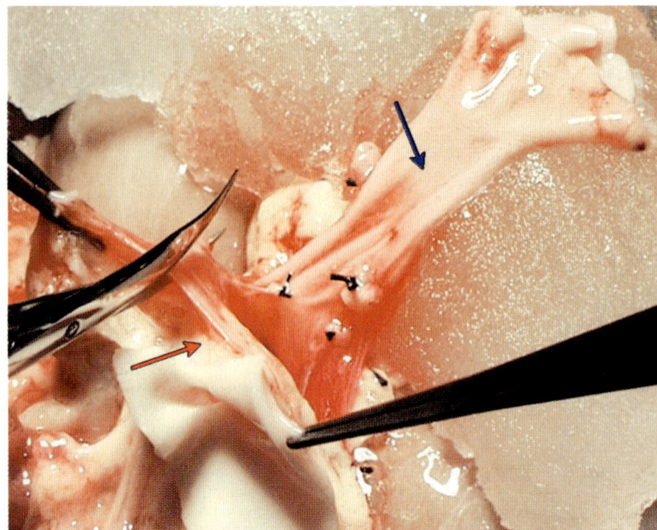

Fig. 2

Figs. 1 and 2: The kidney is kept in a cold bath of preservation fluid. As seen in the illustration, ice can be used to maintain it cold at sites not totally covered by fluid. The renal artery (red arrows) and vein (blue arrows) are dissected free of surrounding tissues. Perirenal tissues are removed. It is important to tie arterial and venous branches in order to prevent hemorrhage (especially at the hilum) that may be difficult to control after reperfusion. In this specific case, a left kidney is shown. The left renal vein, given its greater anatomical length, does not require venous reconstruction.

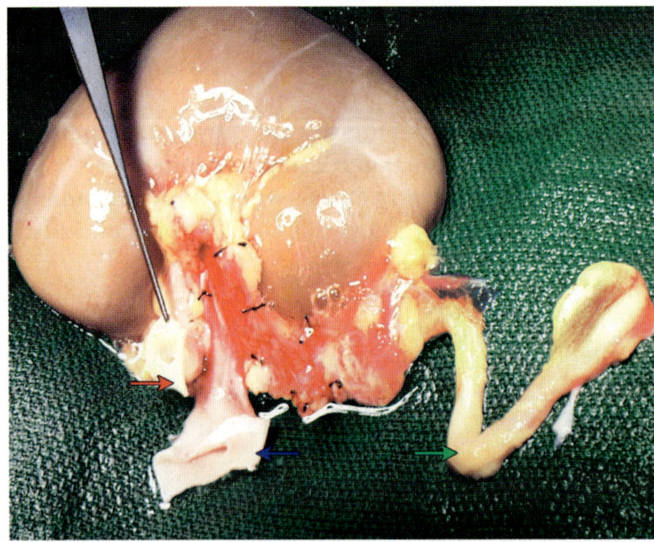

Fig. 3: The graft is ready for implantation. Note that it has no areas of blood discoloration, implying that it has been well perfused with preservation fluid. The renal artery with an aortic patch (red arrow), renal vein with an inferior vena cava (IVC) patch (blue arrow) and ureter (green arrow) can be seen.

KIDNEYS PROCURED FROM LIVE DONORS (FIGS. 4 TO 8)

- The kidney is placed inside a bag containing cold preservation fluid within a basin with ice
- Clips/staples are removed from the artery and vein
- Preservation fluid is perfused through the artery until the venous effluent is clear (usually 60–120 mL)
- Renal parenchyma, ureter, and vessels are inspected for injuries and/or abnormalities
- The artery and vein are prepared for implantation
  - The distal ends are freed of surrounding tissues
  - Venous branches (such as gonadal, suprarenal, lumbar, small branches to surrounding fatty tissues) are tied if not previously addressed during the procurement
  - We prefer to reconstruct multiple arteries (if present) so that a single ostium is implanted onto the recipient
  - Alternatively, if not reconstructed into a common opening, each artery has to be implanted individually
  - We implant right renal veins into the recipient without performing any type of reconstruction
- Perirenal fat is removed as necessary
- Dissection of the hilum should be kept to a minimum to avoid back table injuries
- The ureter should be kept with as much fascia and tissues surrounding it in order to prevent unnecessary devascularization. Since after procurement only the renal artery is preserved, it is important to minimize ischemic changes by:
  - Maintaining and reconstructing lower pole arterial branches
  - Preserving periureteric fascia and tissues
- The gonadal vessels should be preferably tied distally to prevent bleeding

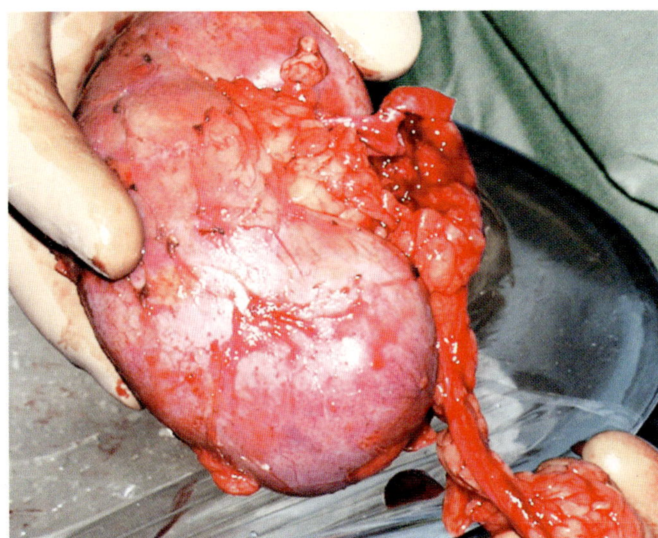

Fig. 4: After the kidney is procured laparoscopically, we proceed to rapidly inspect it for any gross damage. If a plastic bag is used to remove the kidney from the donor, the ureter should be carefully identified in order to prevent its transection or other injuries at the time of removal from the bag. Any staples present in the renal artery and vein are removed.

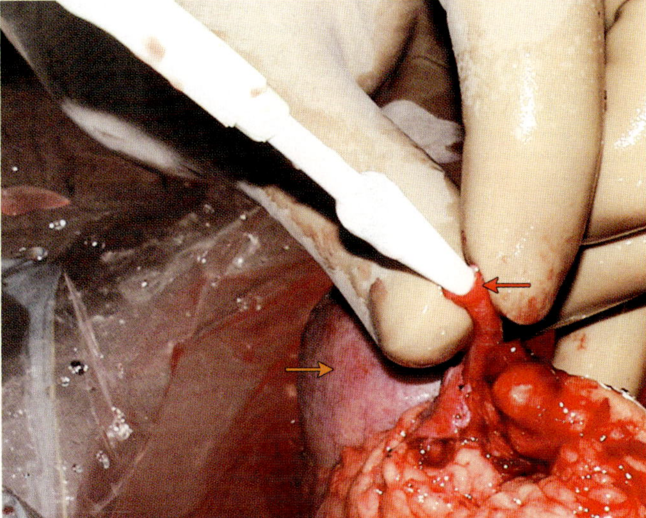

Fig. 5: Cold preservation fluid is instilled via the renal artery (red arrow). This can be done manually with a syringe (as shown in this illustration) or alternatively by gravity using a bag of preservation fluid hanging from an IV pole. Whatever method is chosen, care should be taken not to cause intimal dissections or other type of arterial injuries. The renal parenchyma (orange arrow) is still red, as blood has not been completely flushed yet.

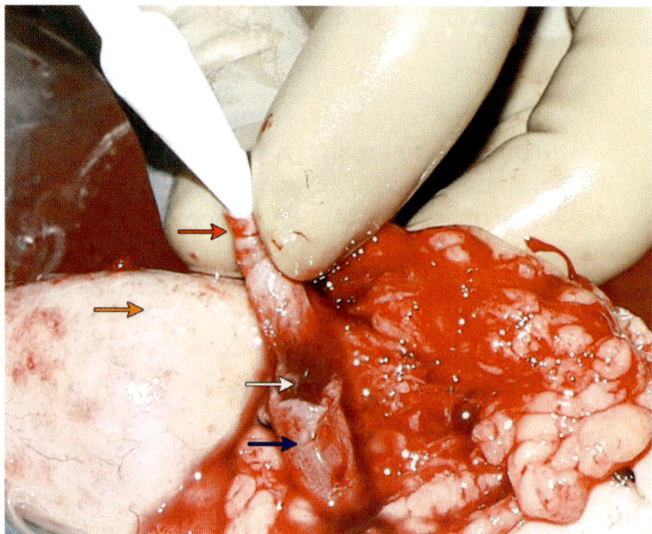

Fig. 6: The kidney is perfused with preservation fluid via the renal artery (red arrow). Blood and preservation fluid can be seen coming out (white arrow) at the renal vein (blue arrow). Note that the renal parenchyma (orange arrow) is changing color as the perfusion with preservation fluid turns it asanguineous.

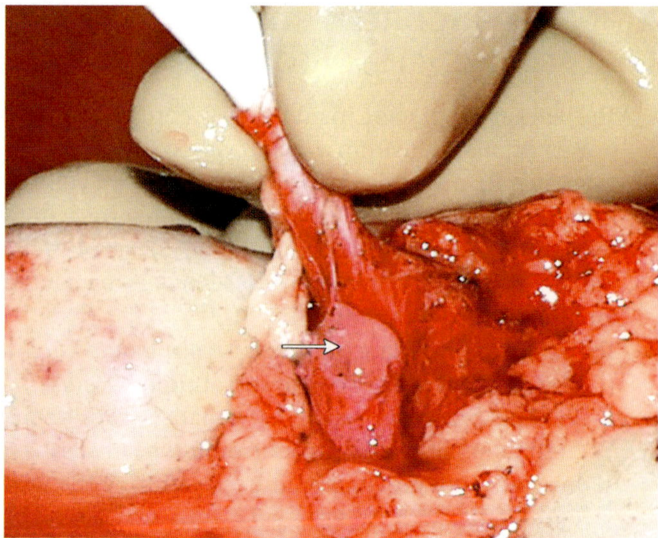

Fig. 7: We continue perfusion until the effluent from the renal vein is clear (white arrow).

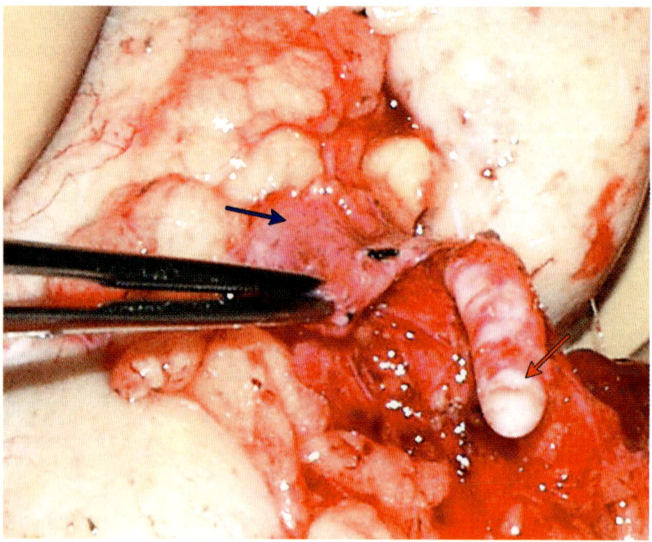

Fig. 8: We verify that the renal artery (red arrow) and vein (blue arrow) have no injuries and are ready for implantation.

RENAL ARTERY RECONSTRUCTION (FIGS. 9 TO 12)

- Our preferred reconstruction technique in instances of multiple renal arteries is to perform a fish mouth anastomosis (Figs. 9 and 10)
- Another possibility is to anastomose a smaller artery in an end-to-side fashion onto the main renal artery (Figs. 11 and 12)
- Other types of reconstructions can also be performed:
  - Each artery can be implanted independently into the recipient external (or common) iliac artery
  - In other instances, while the main renal artery is implanted onto the external (or common) iliac artery, an accessory renal artery can be implanted independently in an end-to-end fashion onto the internal iliac artery

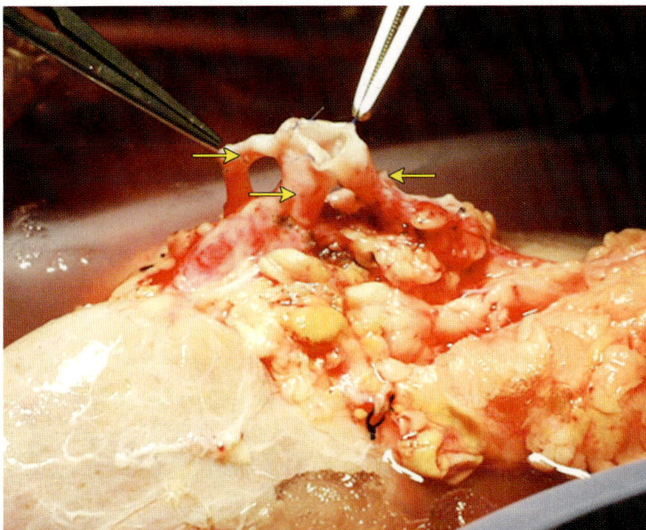

Fig. 9: Laparoscopically procured kidney from a live donor with three renal arteries (arrows). The three vessels were reconstructed by fishmouthing them into a common opening.

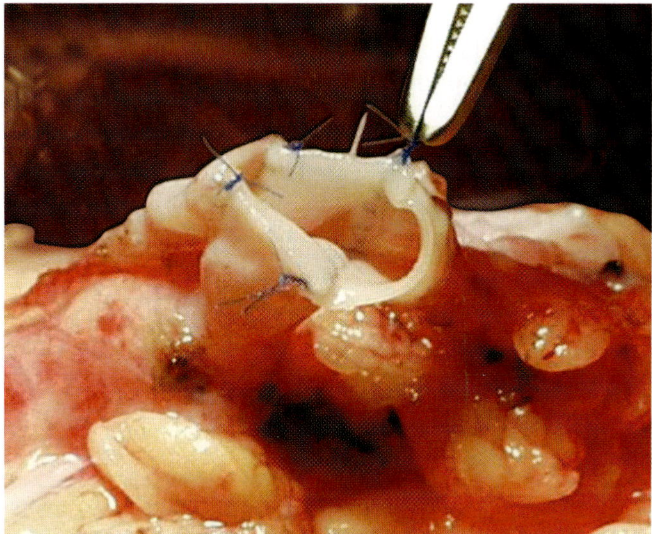

Fig. 10: Close-up view of the arterial reconstruction that allowed implantation of all three vessels as a single arterial ostium. When performing the implantation, it is important to make sure that the suture tails of the reconstruction do not lay within the lumen of the anastomosis.

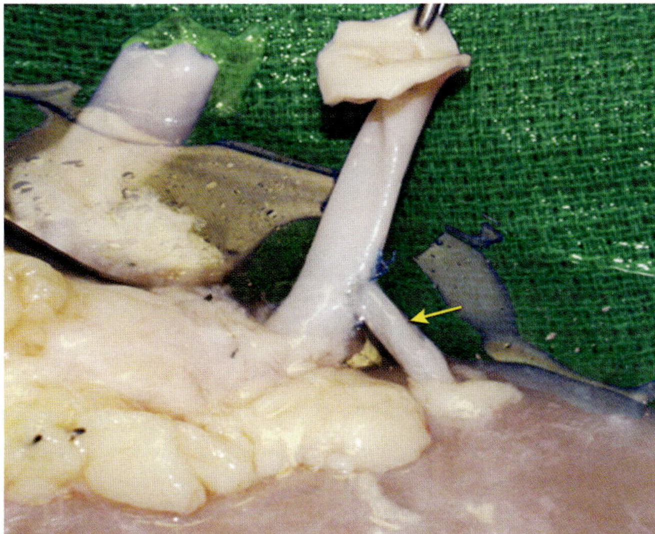

Fig. 11: Alternatively, accessory renal arteries (arrow) can be anastomosed in an end-to-side fashion onto the main renal artery.

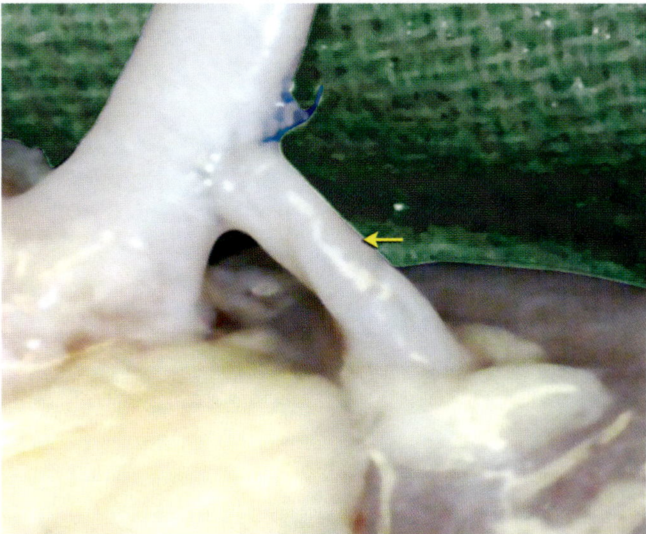

Fig. 12: Close-up view of such technique.

RENAL VEIN RECONSTRUCTION (FIGS. 13 TO 16)

- Renal vein reconstructions can be undertaken in right kidney allografts (where the renal vein is short), mostly in deceased donor kidneys
- Vessels (usually IVC, but sometimes common or external iliac vein) procured from the same donor are routinely used for this purpose
- This technique can be also undertaken in live donors with vein grafts procured from the live donor, the recipient, or commercially available cryopreserved vessels (given this option, live donors and their recipients should be made aware and consented for the possibility of vessels procurement)
- In instances of multiple renal veins, when the main renal vein is of sufficient diameter, accessory ones can be tied
- We do not routinely perform reconstructions of the renal vein. In instances of right kidneys (for both live and deceased donors), we anastomose the renal vein (with no reconstruction) onto the mobilized external iliac vein. Transposing the external iliac vein with respect to the external iliac artery may make the venous anastomosis easier. In these cases, to prevent arterial twists or kinks, we trim the renal artery to a length similar to that of the vein at the time of implantation

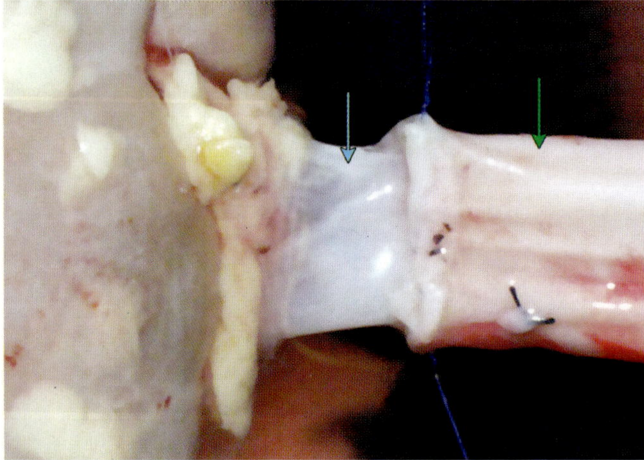

Fig. 13: Right kidneys have a shorter vein than left kidneys based on their anatomical configuration. This finding makes their implantation potentially more difficult. In order to facilitate this finding, the right renal vein can be reconstructed. In this specific example, the reconstruction was done with a segment of donor IVC (green arrow) sewn end-to-end to the renal vein (light blue arrow).

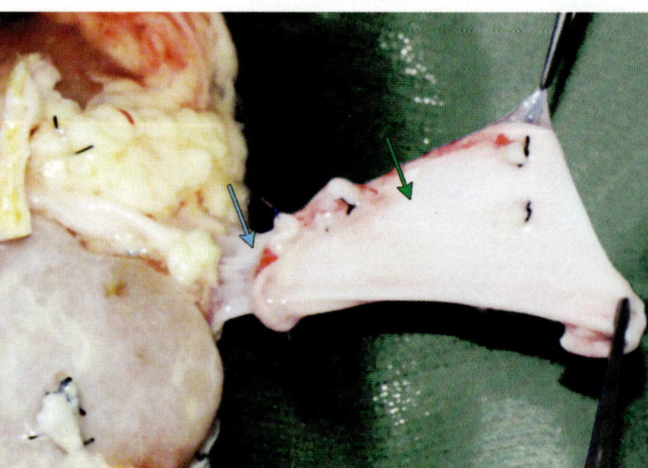

Fig. 14: The reconstructed vein is longer, and can be more easily implanted onto the recipient iliac vein. The IVC extension is shown with a green arrow, while the renal vein is indicated with a light blue arrow).

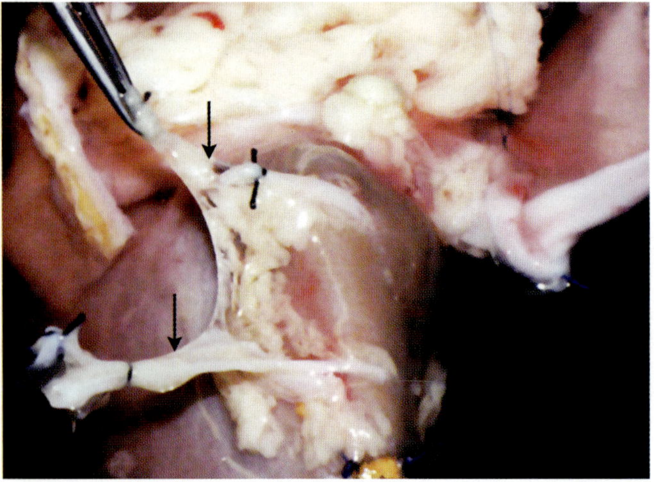

Fig. 15

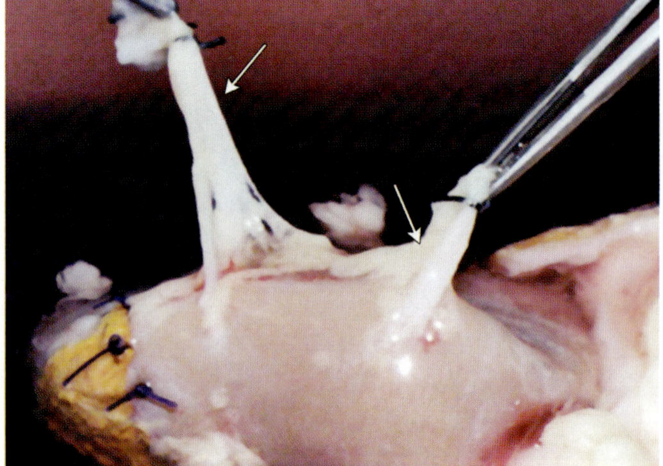

Fig. 16

Figs. 15 and 16: The main renal vein should always be kept intact. Smaller accessory veins such as the ones shown on the left illustrations (arrows) (that frequently are not preserved during procurement) entering the renal parenchyma peripherally (or even at the hilum) can be tied.

UNROOFING/RESECTION OF CYSTS (FIGS. 17 TO 20)

- We do not routinely unroof or resect simple cysts in the allograft
- Complex cysts or cysts considered to be potentially pathologic should be biopsied to exclude malignancy

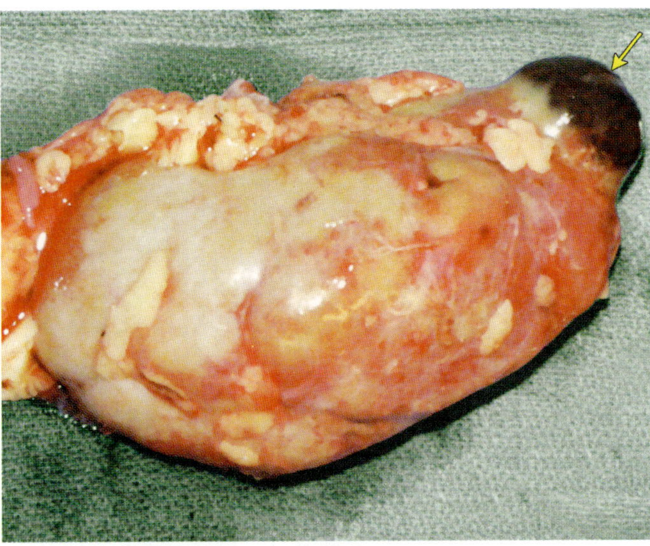

Fig. 17

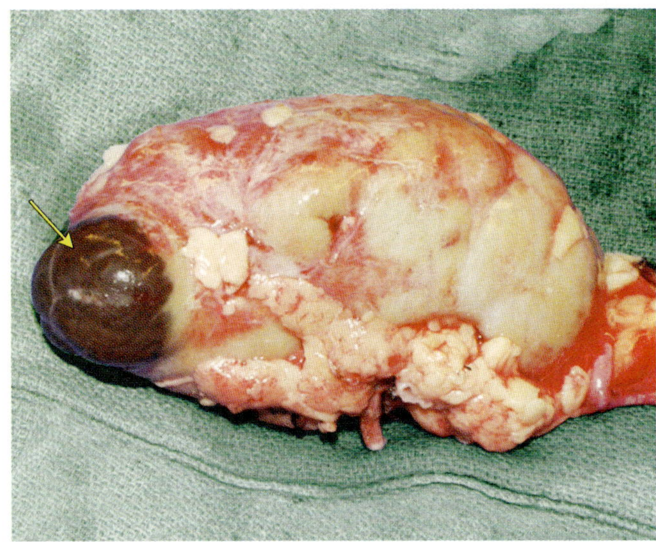

Fig. 18

Figs. 17 and 18: On occasions the procured allografts may contain one or more cysts (arrows). In this instance, the kidney had been procured laparoscopically from a live donor. We do not routinely unroof benign cysts. In instances, however, where the donor and/or recipient surgeons have questions about the nature of the cysts, we recommend that they be unroofed (or excised) and evaluated by microscopic examination prior to implantation in order to exclude malignancies.

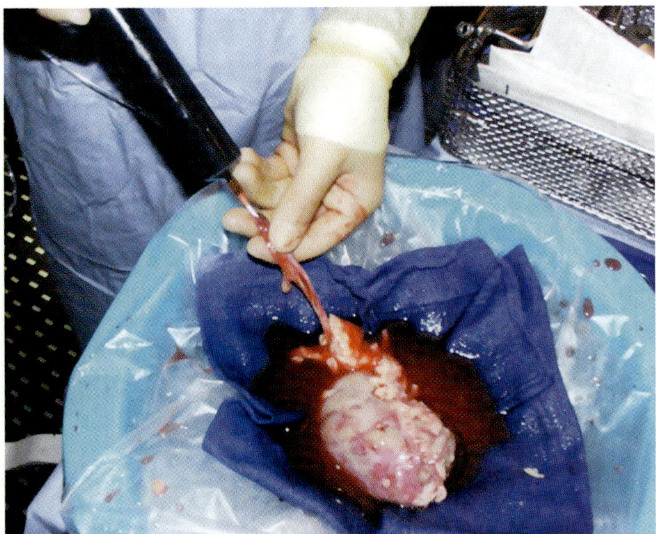

Fig. 19: After the cyst has been unroofed or resected, we usually instill a solution with a visible color (methylene blue in this case) via the ureter.

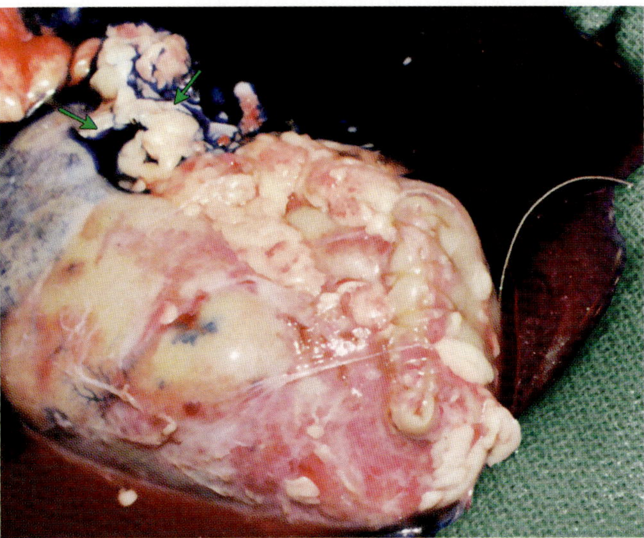

Fig. 20: As the dye is infused in a retrograde fashion via the ureter, we look for extravasation (arrows) at the site of the unroofed/resected cyst. We try to repair these defects in order to avoid urinary leaks after implantation.

HORSESHOE KIDNEYS (FIGS. 21 TO 24)

- Horseshoe kidneys can be transplanted en bloc or independently
- Separation is accomplished by transecting the isthmus (or addressing the isthmus already accidentally transected at the time of procurement) and oversewing the vascular, calyceal, and parenchymal cut surfaces
- Special attention should be given to the almost certain presence of vascular variations as well as the short ureters at the time of implantation

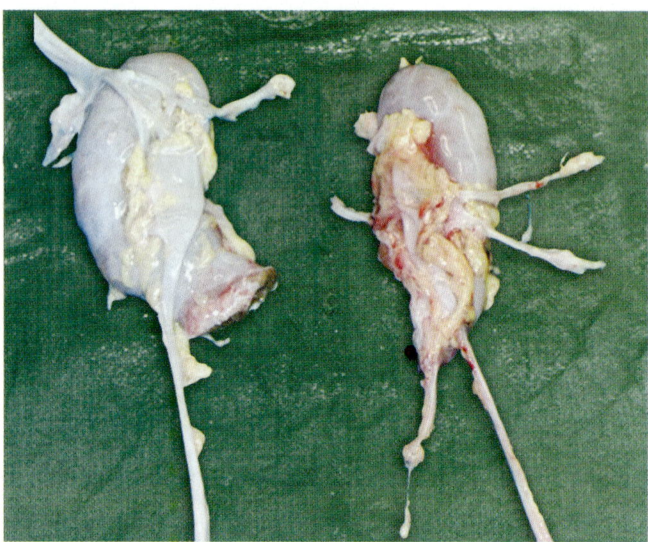

Fig. 21

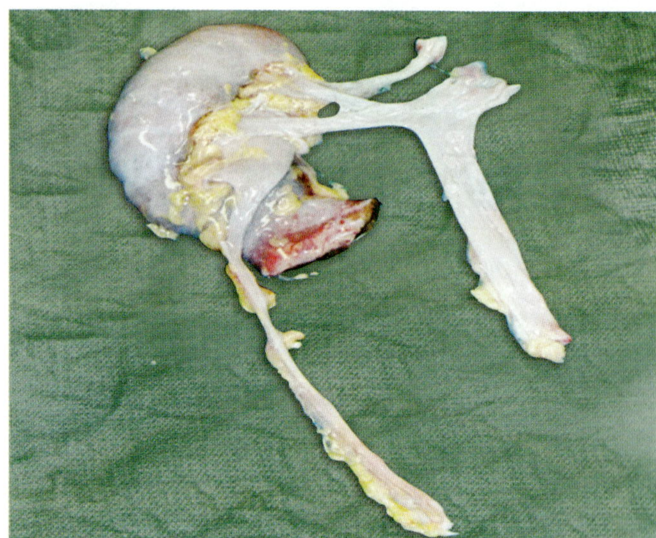

Fig. 22

Figs. 21 and 22: Horseshoe kidney with transection of the parenchyma at the time of procurement. The unexpected presence of a horseshoe kidney can be associated with procurement injuries encountered even at the time of cannulation of the aorta (such kidneys usually have an isthmus at the inferior mesenteric artery). Vascular and ureteral variants are frequent. Arterial cannulation and perfusion via the iliac artery (with clamping of the contralateral one) can avoid many of such injuries.

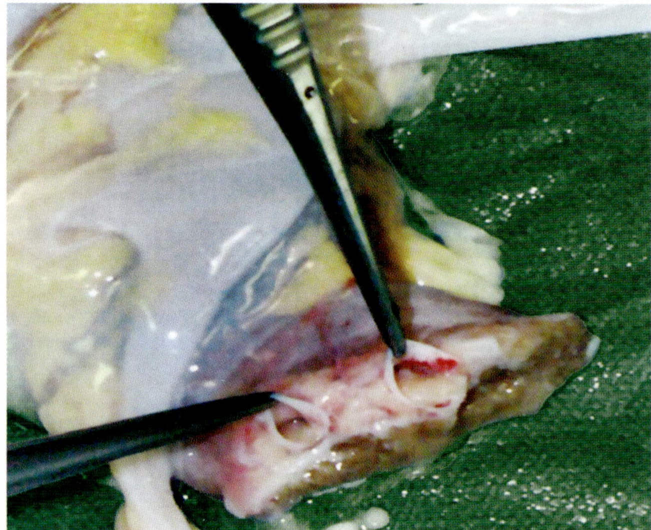

Fig. 23: Further inspection of the injured site revealed a transected collecting system.

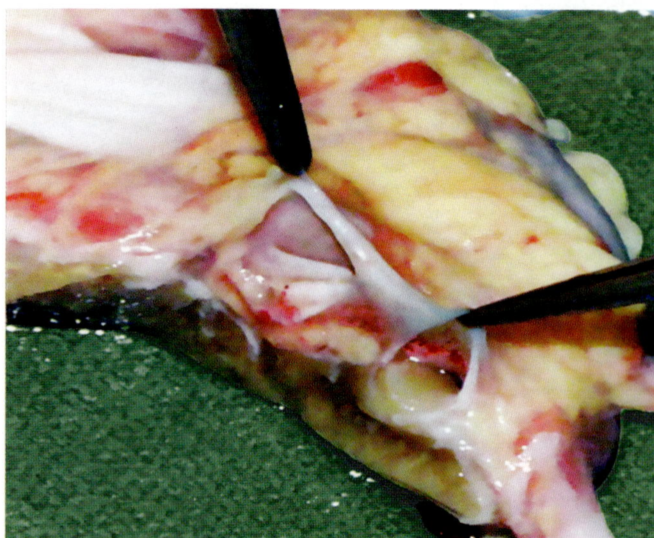

Fig. 24: Close-up view of the contralateral structures.

CHAPTER 30

Implantation

Ernesto P Molmenti and Collaborators

PREOPERATIVE CONSIDERATIONS

- Complete blood count, electrolytes, and all other preoperative requirements are addressed
- We routinely meet with the patient immediately prior to the procedure to address any pending questions
- The kidney can be implanted onto the right or the left lower quadrant
- Right or left side is based on
  - Surgeon preference
  - Vascular disease involvement of the iliac vessels
  - Previous surgeries (transplants, ostomies, scars)
  - Other factors
- Prior to starting the procedure we always make certain that the correct allograft is available or will be available at the time of implantation
- The recipient should have adequate venous access—at least two large bore peripheral IV
- We do NOT routinely insert central venous lines
- Arterial lines ONLY if needed based on recipient characteristics
- Urinary catheter ALWAYS placed
- We routinely administer oral aspirin prior to and after the procedure
- It is also our practice NOT to discontinue medications that recipients may have been taking on a routine basis such as clopidogrel and oral anticoagulants given the high risk of cardiovascular complications faced by most of our patients
- We routinely administer 2–4 L of isotonic crystalloids during the entire procedure
  - We prefer normal saline
  - Lactated Ringer's solution is preferred by some. If used, potassium levels should be monitored very closely
  - Adding potassium to IV fluids is discouraged
- We routinely administer subcutaneous heparin (unless therapeutically anti-coagulated) immediately prior to the case, and maintain sequential compression devices on both lower extremities during the entire case to diminish the incidence of deep venous thromboses

TIMEOUT

- Performed immediately prior to incision after the abdomen has been painted and draped
- Review all medications given preoperatively
- IVs antibiotics administered (assuring that they are received within minutes of incision)
- Other medications administered
  - Induction agents
  - 500 mg Solu Medrol (or other desired dosage)
  - 25 g mannitol
  - 100 mg of furosemide
  - (alternatively, diuretics can be administered prior to reperfusion)

OPENING OF THE ABDOMEN AND DISSECTION OF THE ILIAC VESSELS

- Curvilinear right (or left) lower quadrant incision
- Subcutaneous tissues and muscles transected with electrocautery
- Extraperitoneal dissection exposes the retroperitoneum
  - If peritoneum entered, it can be repaired in order to prevent hernias through the defect
    - Some surgeons prefer to purposefully open the peritoneum and subsequently close it in order to allow for the intraperitoneal drainage of potential seromas or lymphoceles (beware, because in instances of urinary leaks, an opening in the

peritoneum would allow for the urine to drain into the peritoneal cavity rather than forming a localized collection)

- External iliac vessels exposed and dissected free of surrounding tissues
- In instances of kidneys with short renal veins (such as with right kidneys)
  - The entire length of the external iliac vessels should be dissected to allow for greater mobility
- Hemostasis should be addressed and verified throughout the entire procedure
- Lymphatic tissues surrounding the iliac vessels can be transected with electrocautery—or alternatively tied and transected

VASCULAR IMPLANTATION

- Verify that donor kidney and recipient are correctly identified
- Kidney allograft—already prepared in the back table—is brought onto the operative field
- Our preference is to wrap it in a gauze with ice slush
  - Renal artery and vein exteriorized through an opening to allow for their anastomosis
  - Upper and lower poles of the kidney clearly identified to prevent implantation mistakes
- Both anastomoses are constructed with nonabsorbable monofilament sutures (our preference is 6–0 polypropylene)
- The venous anastomosis is performed first—order can be altered based on surgeon preference
  - A semicircular clamp is placed on the external iliac vein
  - The vein is incised
  - The transplant renal vein is anastomosed end-to-side onto the recipient external iliac vein
    - Alternatively, it can be anastomosed end-to-side onto the common iliac vein (or potentially the inferior vena cava, IVC)
  - We routinely construct it with a continuous suture
  - After completion of the anastomosis, a bulldog clamp is placed on the renal vein and the semicircular clamp on the iliac vein is partially released
    - This allows for verification of hemostasis
  - The clamp on the iliac vein is subsequently released completely, allowing for continued venous flow from the lower extremity
- The arterial anastomosis is subsequently addressed
  - The semicircular clamp previously used for the vein is now placed on the external iliac artery
  - The artery is incised
    - The arterial opening can be made round with an aortic hole puncher
  - The transplant renal artery is anastomosed end-to-side onto the recipient external iliac artery
    - Alternatively, the transplant renal artery can be anastomosed
    - End-to-end onto the recipient internal iliac artery
    - End-to-side onto the recipient common iliac artery
  - We routinely perform the arterial anastomosis (as was the case with the venous anastomosis) with a continuous suture
  - After completion of the anastomosis, hemostasis is verified by gently clamping the renal artery, while the semicircular clamp on the iliac artery is partially released. Once this has been done, the iliac artery is reclamped
- Prior to reperfusion of the kidney, we verify that the recipient has:
  - Received at least 2-3 L of IV fluids
  - A systolic blood pressure of 120 mm Hg or higher
    - If this pressure is not achieved, options include
      - Additional IV fluids
      - Use of pressors (usually dopamine)
    - Hypotension can be an indicator of acute cardiac events
- Cardiac arrest at the time of reperfusion should be attributed to hyperkalemia until proven otherwise. All necessary treating agents (such as calcium chloride, calcium gluconate, insulin with glucose) should be readily available
- The kidney is reperfused
  - The semicircular clamp on the iliac artery and the bulldog clamp on the renal vein are released
- If reperfusion is slow or poor
  - Evaluate for vascular problems
    - Kinks/twists
    - Defective anastomosis
    - Poor inflow/outflow involving native vessels
- If there are isolated areas of poor or no perfusion
  - Evaluate for inadvertent transection of polar or small branching arteries that could have been missed at the time of procurement.
  - Poor perfusion of the lower pole can be associated with poor perfusion and subsequent ischemia of the ureter
- A kidney biopsy is obtained to
  - Evaluate the reperfused organ
  - Have as a baseline for comparison of future biopsies

- Place the kidney in a position that allows for the vessels to lie in a comfortable way with no kinks or twists
- Perform a Doppler evaluation of the
  - Renal artery
  - Renal vein
  - External iliac artery both proximal and distal with respect to the anastomosis
  - External iliac vein both proximal and distal with respect to the anastomosis
  - Renal parenchyma

URETERAL IMPLANTATION

- The urinary catheter is clamped, and approximately 120 mL of an iodine (or antibiotic) containing solution are instilled in the urinary bladder
  - This distends the bladder and makes it easier to identify
  - If in doubt, a syringe with a fine needle can be used to sample fluid from the bladder
  - The bladder is located in a position posterior to the pubic ramus
  - If still in doubt, the peritoneum can be opened and the bladder located by a combined intra and extraperitoneal palpation
- The bladder is incised at a site where the anastomosis to the ureter can be comfortably constructed
- The ureter is trimmed to an adequate length and spatulated
  - The vessels in the ureteric fascia are tied to prevent bleeding
  - The spatulation allows for an anastomosis with a greater surface area
  - In order to minimize positional strictures, we incise the periureteric fascia along the spatulated end of the ureter for a distance of approximately 2 cm
- We routinely perform the ureter to bladder anastomosis with:
  - Delicate full-thickness bites of ureter
  - Generous full-thickness bites of bladder
  - In a continuous running fashion
  - Using resorbable (to prevent stone formation) monofilament sutures (our preference is 5-0)
  - In a tension free manner
  - The ureter should be kept
    - Short enough to minimize the possibility of distal ischemia
    - Long enough if a revision is required
    - This can be achieved by allowing it to form a mild curve
    - With as much surrounding tissues in order to prevent devascularization and ischemia
- Prior to completing the anastomosis, with a right angle clamp we verify that there is adequate patency from ureter to bladder
  - If we are not satisfied with the patency, we redo the anastomosis
  - Once the patency has been verified, we place a ureteral stent into the donor ureter with its distal end in the bladder. Please note that some surgeons do not use ureteral stents
- We do not routinely construct antireflux mechanisms (such as nipple valves) since they can potentially be associated with urinary obstruction
- The presence of ureteral peristalsis is usually an indicator of renal function
  - Absent peristalsis is frequently indicative of delayed graft function

ABDOMINAL CLOSURE

- Hemostasis is verified
- Muscles and fascia are closed as a single layer with interrupted nonabsorbable figure-of-8 stitches
- We do not close the subcutaneous tissues
- The skin is closed with widely spaced interrupted simple 2-0 nylon stitches
  - In our experience this closure
    - Is associated with a lower incidence of infections
    - Avoids the use of drains
    - Provides satisfactory cosmetic results

IMMEDIATE POSTOPERATIVE CONSIDERATIONS

- We routinely obtain a duplex Doppler ultrasound imaging study of the transplanted kidney in the post-anesthesia care unit to document:
  - Adequate arterial and venous flow
  - Absence of hydronephrosis
  - Absence of bladder distension
  - Presence or absence of fluid collections
  - Baseline findings for future studies
- Although infrequent, positional changes at the time of closure can lead to poor allograft perfusion. If detected early, they can be addressed with limited or no renal injury. Absent or severely compromised flow by duplex Doppler ultrasound in the immediate postoperative period is an indication for immediate re-exploration

- Cardiology evaluations are obtained routinely in the immediate postoperative period
- We prefer to meet with family members/friends/others at the recipient's bedside to inform them of their outcome
  - In most instances, we have been updating them from the operating room as the case evolved
  - They should be reminded that no guarantees can be provided
- All recipients are followed by the multidisciplinary transplant team
- Referring physicians are welcome to participate in the immediate postoperative period as well
- It is not infrequent for recipients to experience, to a greater or lesser extent, some type of sensory disturbance on the upper (usually lateral) area of the thigh
  - This finding is usually temporary (may last weeks or a few months), and results from trauma to the lateral femoral cutaneous nerve of the thigh at the time of surgery
- We continue with deep venous thrombosis prophylaxis (subcutaneous heparin and sequential compression devices) immediately after the procedure and throughout the entire hospital stay (except in recipients therapeutically anticoagulated)
- It is our preference to have computerized (or preprinted) order sets and protocols in order to decrease the incidence of mistakes and errors

CLOSURE OF THE WOUND

- We do not routinely leave drains
- The abdominal wall and fascia are subsequently closed with interrupted figure-of-8 stitches of #5 nonabsorbable braided sutures
- The skin is closed with widely spaced (3–5 cm apart) simple interrupted 2-0 nylon sutures. We have observed that such closure decreases the incidence of fluid collections and wound infections
- Patients are routinely extubated intraoperatively and maintained in the recovery room until fully awake and alert. They are subsequently transferred to a transplant-specialized ward

KIDNEY IMPLANTATION—ABDOMINAL INCISION AND DISSECTION OF EXTERNAL ILIAC VESSELS (FIGS. 1 TO 10)

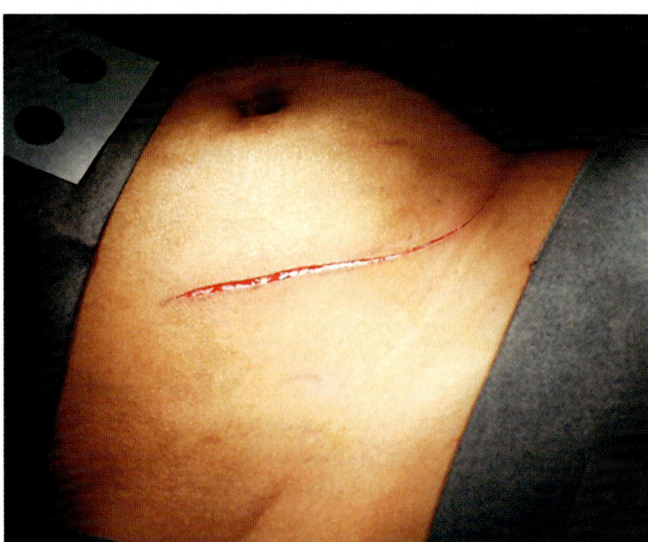

Fig. 1: After the patient is under general anesthesia and in the supine position, the abdomen is painted with an antiseptic solution and draped. We do not clip or shave hairs in the operative site. Once a timeout has been satisfactorily completed, a right lower quadrant curvilinear incision is undertaken.

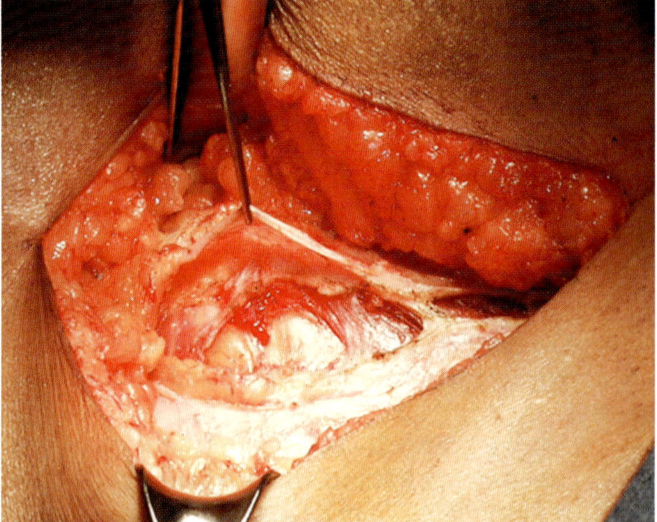

Fig. 2: The subcutaneous tissues are incised with electrocautery, and the abdominal muscles and fascia are reached. They are also incised with electrocautery. The peritoneum is usually not entered. In males, the spermatic cord and its structures should be kept intact. In females, the round ligament may be transected after verifying that there are no structures (such as an ovary) associated with it. The inferior epigastric vessels, if necessary, can be tied and transected. Care should be taken in individuals where these vessels are irrigating flaps or in those with prior ipsilateral subcostal incisions (such as in open cholecystectomies or liver transplants) where necrosis can occur.

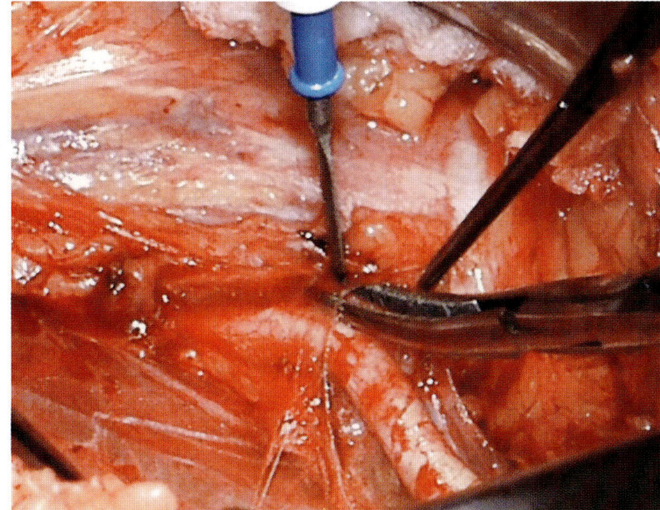

Fig. 3: After having gained access to the retroperitoneum, the external iliac artery and vein are identified.

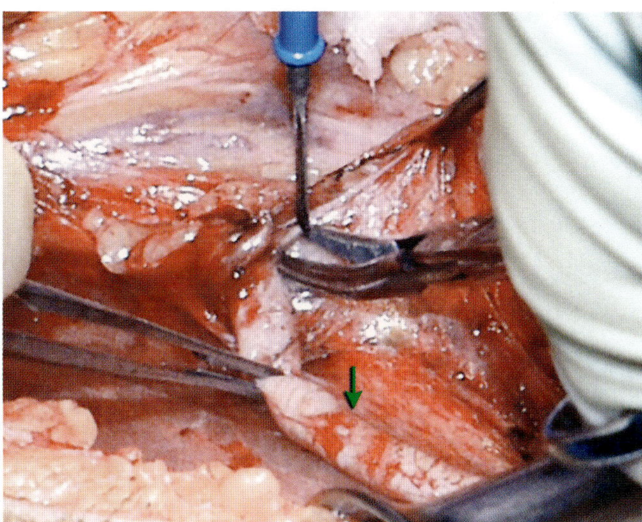

Fig. 4: The artery (green arrow), that usually lies lateral and ventral with respect to the vein, is dissected free of surrounding tissues.

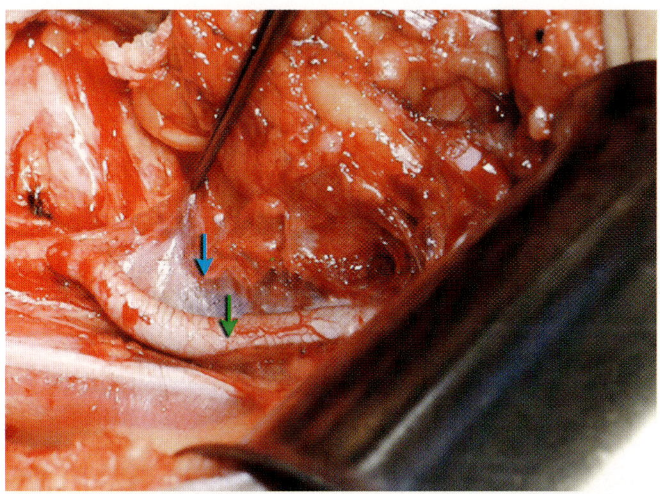

Fig. 5: The external iliac artery (green arrow) is now ready for implantation. We routinely dissect only the length of artery necessary for our surgical needs. Performing unnecessary extensive dissections can be associated with unwanted complications. The blue arrow shows the external iliac vein.

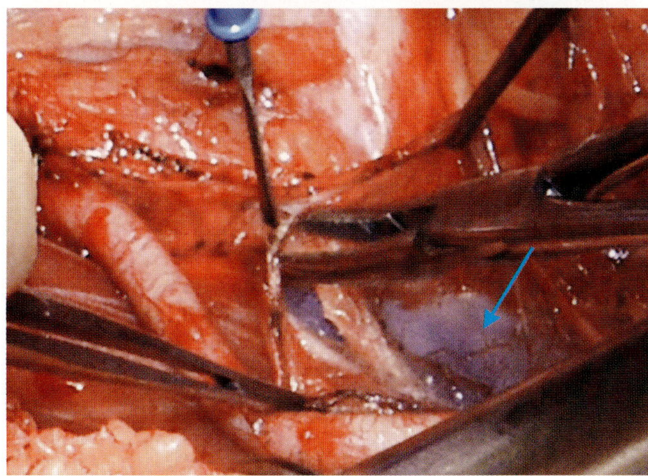

Fig. 6

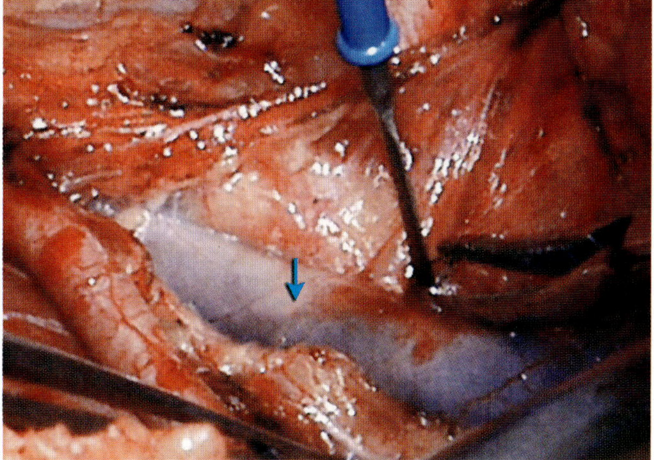

Fig. 7

Figs. 6 and 7: The vein (blue arrows) is subsequently dissected free of surrounding tissues. As was the case with the artery, the dissection should not be more extensive than necessary.

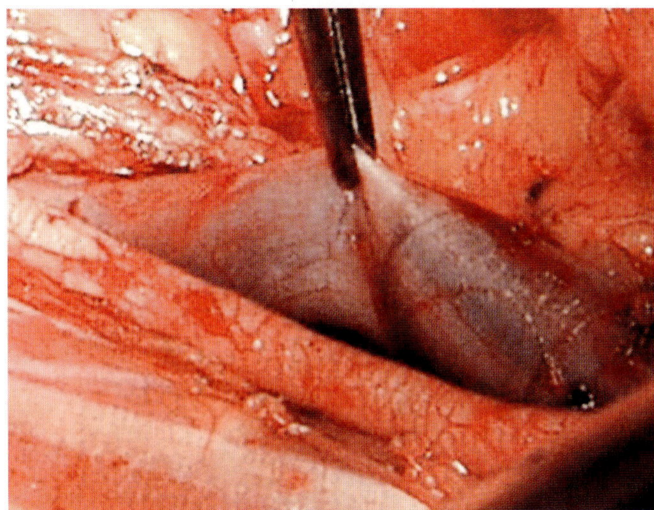

Fig. 8: As the vein is dissected, care should be taken not to avulse any of its branches. Such injuries can be associated with prominent blood loss. Furthermore, identification, control and hemostasis of avulsed branches that retract into the pelvic tissues can be very difficult.

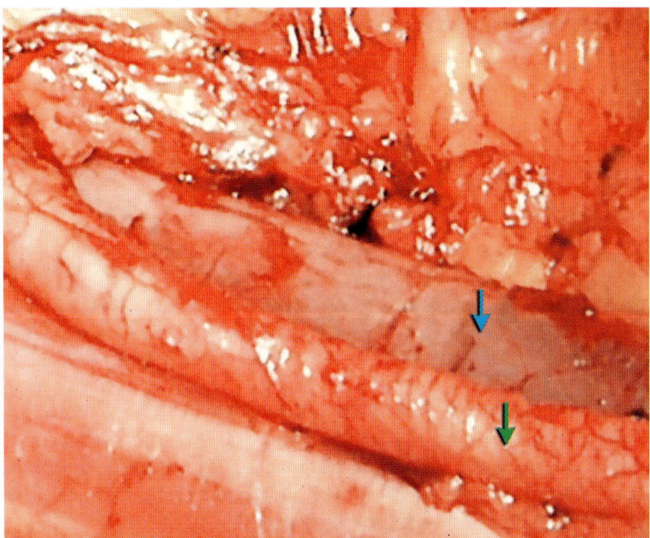

Fig. 9: External iliac vessels (artery green arrow, vein blue arrow) lying in their retroperitoneal location. We routinely use self-retaining retractors in order to prevent human fatigue that can be associated with unnecessary complications. In many instances, the external iliac artery and vein are of similar lengths.

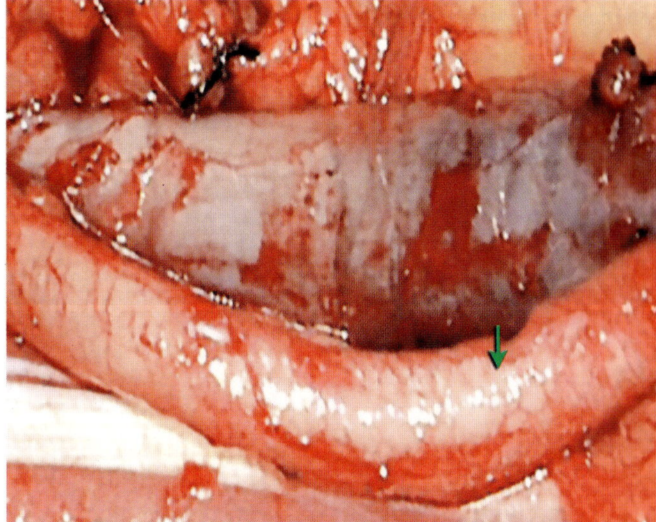

Fig. 10: On other occasions such as this one, the artery (green arrow) may be convoluted. Although this may pose a problem, we have observed that it can be of use in the implantation of allografts with short veins, where the external iliac vessels can be transposed. In this maneuver, the anastomoses are constructed so that the external iliac vein is brought laterally with respect to the corresponding artery.

KIDNEY IMPLANTATION—WRAPPING OF KIDNEY IN ICE BLANKET (FIGS. 11 TO 13)

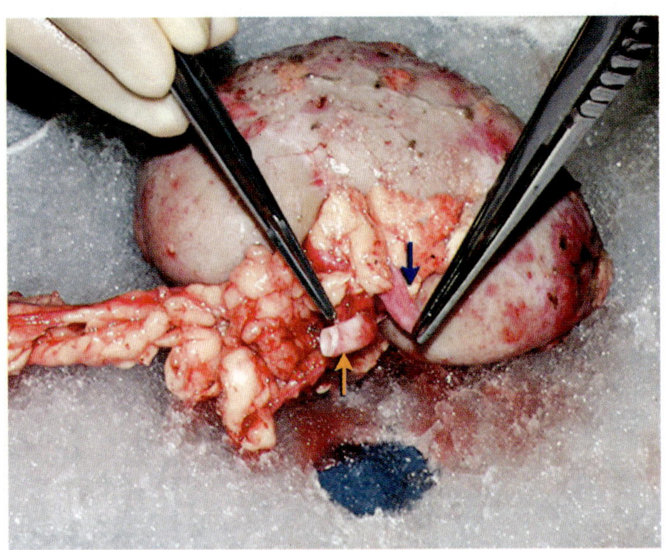

Fig. 11

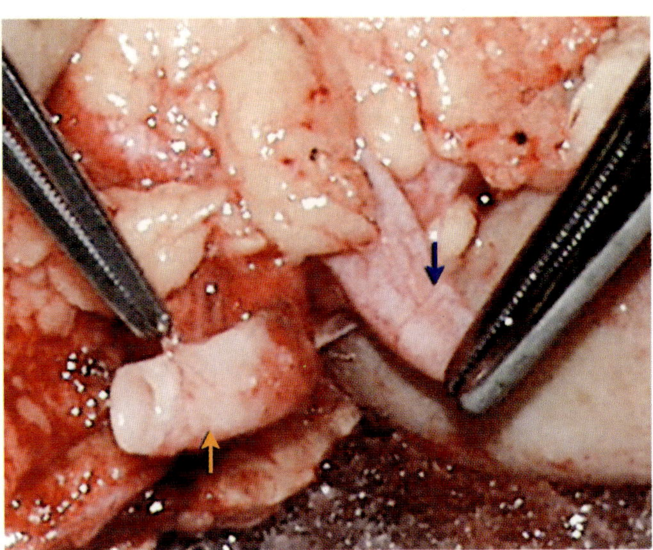

Fig. 12

Figs. 11 and 12: After the back table preparation of the kidney is finalized, the kidney is wrapped in a gauze coated with sterile fine ice. It is important to keep the orientation of the kidney in order not to lose track of the upper and lower poles at the time of the anastomosis. The artery (orange arrows) and vein (blue arrows) are clearly identified and ready for implantation.

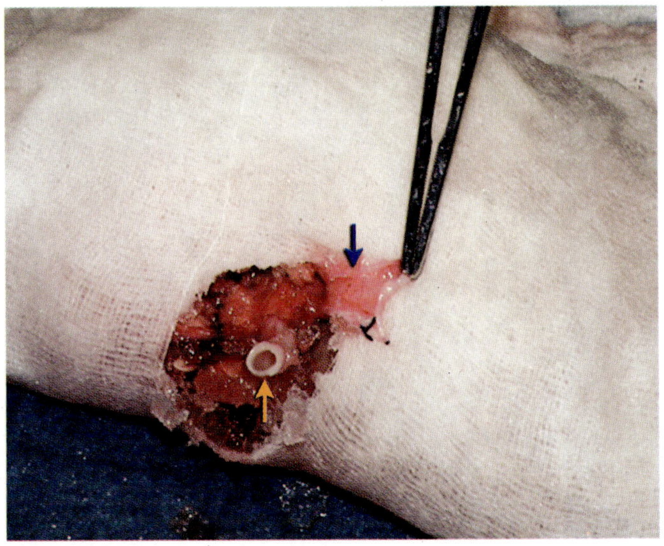

Fig. 13: As shown in the illustration, the artery (orange arrow) and vein (blue arrow) can be brought out through a circular opening in the gauze. Alternatively, a gauze with ice can be folded around the kidney, leaving a space for the vessels to exit.

KIDNEY IMPLANTATION—VENOUS ANASTOMOSIS (FIGS. 14 TO 28)

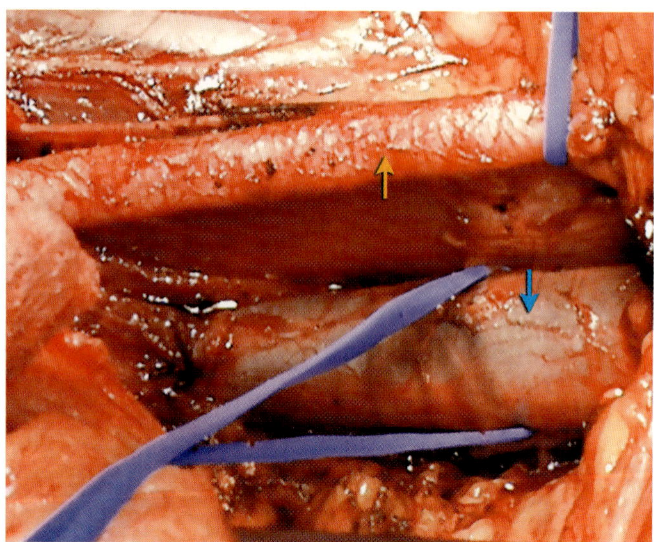

Fig. 14: The external iliac artery (orange arrow) and vein (blue arrow) are clearly identified.

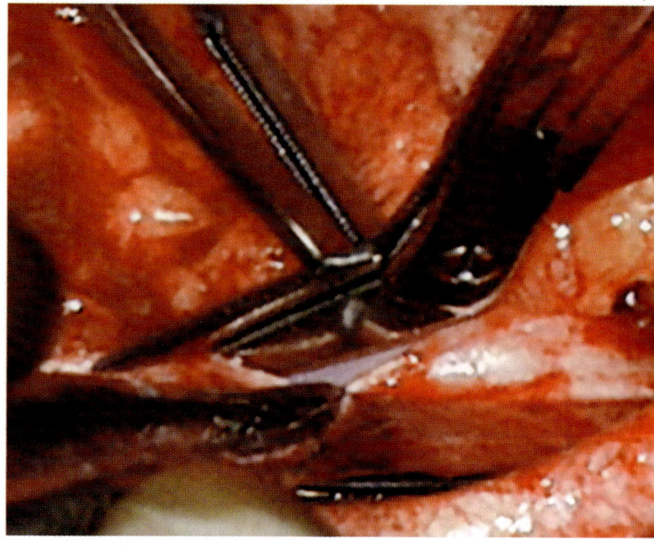

Fig. 15: The external iliac vein is clamped with a semicircular clamp in order to isolate the site of the future anastomosis. With fine scissors (as in this case) or alternatively with a sharp knife, the vein is incised.

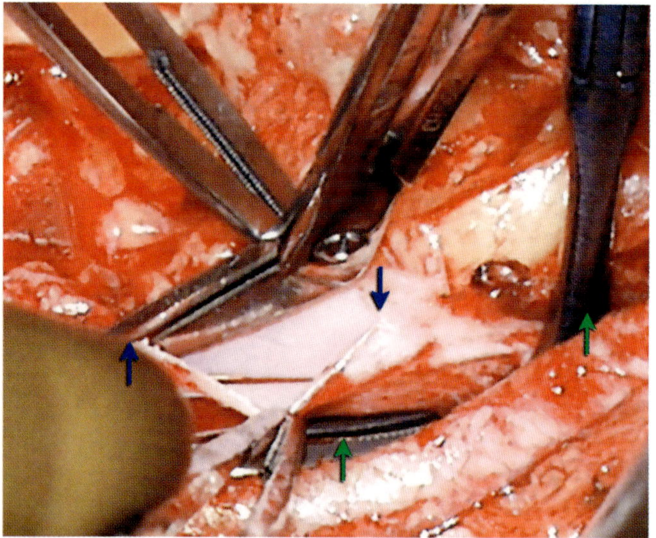

Fig. 16: The incision in the recipient external iliac vein (blue arrows) should be equivalent to the width of the donor renal vein. The surgeon and assistant should take special care not to disturb the semicircular clamp (green arrows) on the recipient external iliac vein.

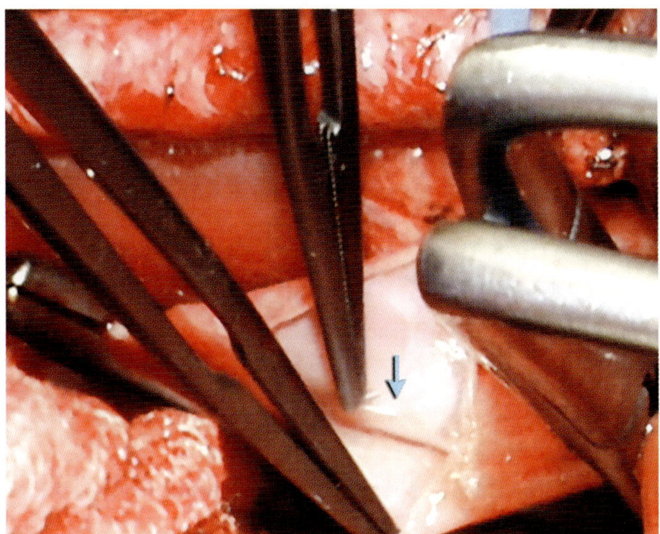

Fig. 17

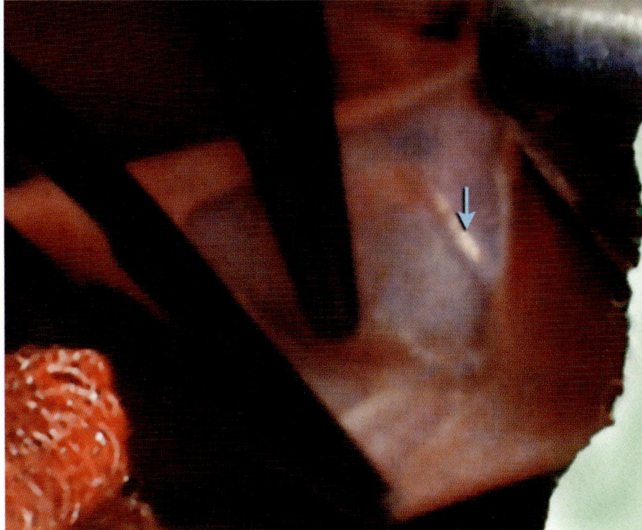

Fig. 18

Figs. 17 and 18: After the external iliac vein is clamped with a semicircular clamp and incised with a sharp scalpel or fine scissors, we inspect its intimal surface. As opposed to classic descriptions, in our experience we have not infrequently encountered valves (light blue arrows) in the external iliac vein. We transect the leaflets in instances where we consider that the presence of such valves can potentially impede outflow from the allograft. When we believe that there is no outflow risk, we leave the valve leaflets intact.

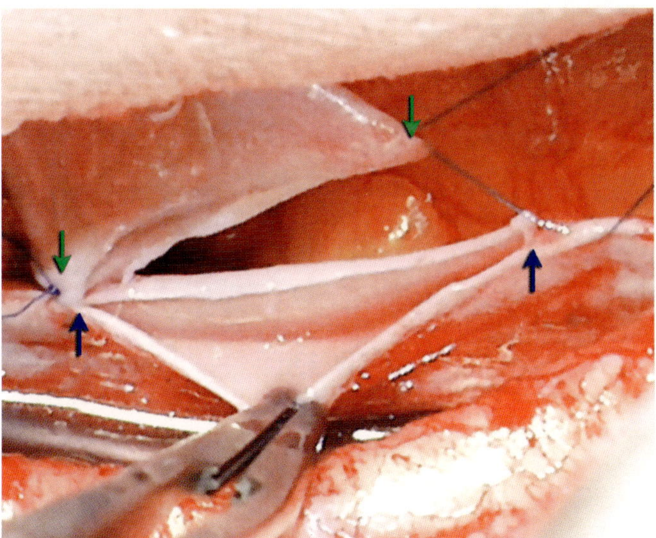

Fig. 19: With the allograft kidney wrapped in the ice blanket, we place 6-0 monofilament nonresorbable stitches at both ends of the opening in the recipient external iliac vein (blue arrows) and the transplant renal vein (green arrows). We routinely tie only one of the stitches (left up to the preference of the surgeon which end to tie).

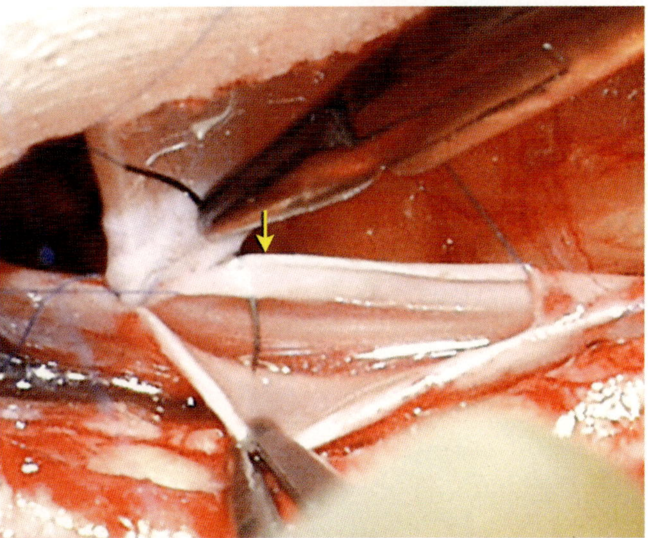

Fig. 20: When tying the corner stitch, we leave one of the arms much longer than the other one in order to run the entire anastomosis. Since the knots are on the outside surface of the anastomosis, the first stich should be at the corner, from outside to inside. As shown in the illustration, we run the back wall of the anastomosis from its inner aspect, everting the edges of the veins (yellow arrow) (whenever possible) in order to assure intima-to-intima apposition of the donor and recipient surfaces. Alternatively, rather than the surgeon sewing the back wall from the inside, the first assistant can sew his/her side of the anastomosis.

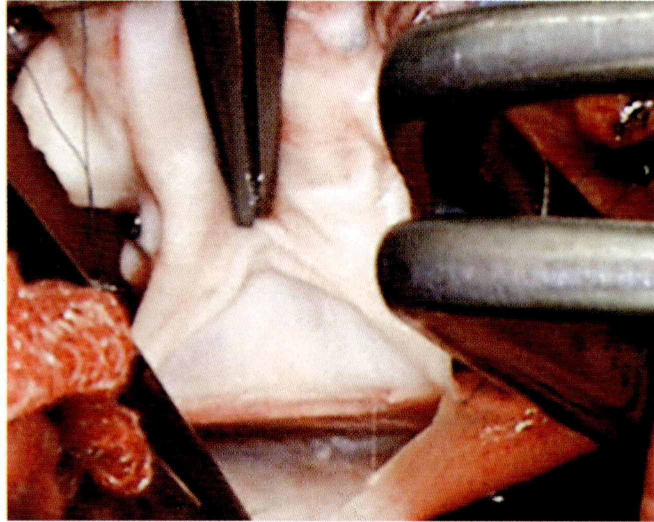

Fig. 21: View of the completed back wall of the venous anastomosis.

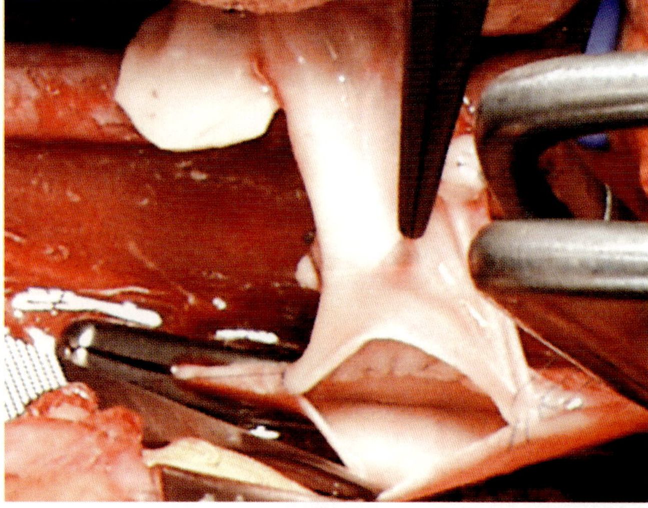

Fig. 22

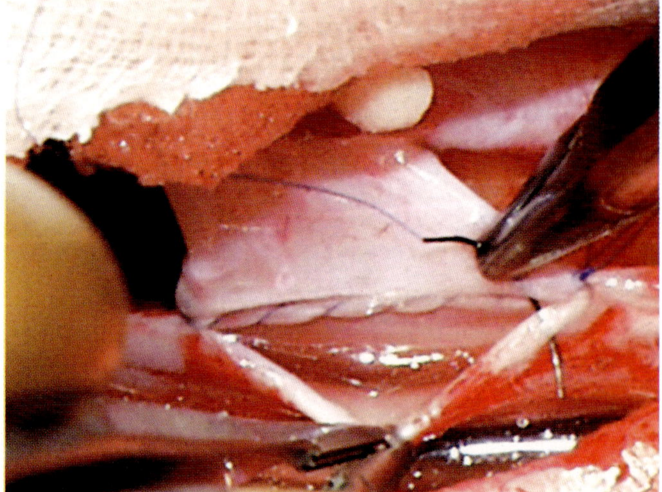

Fig. 23

Figs. 22 and 23: The anterior wall of the anastomosis is subsequently completed.

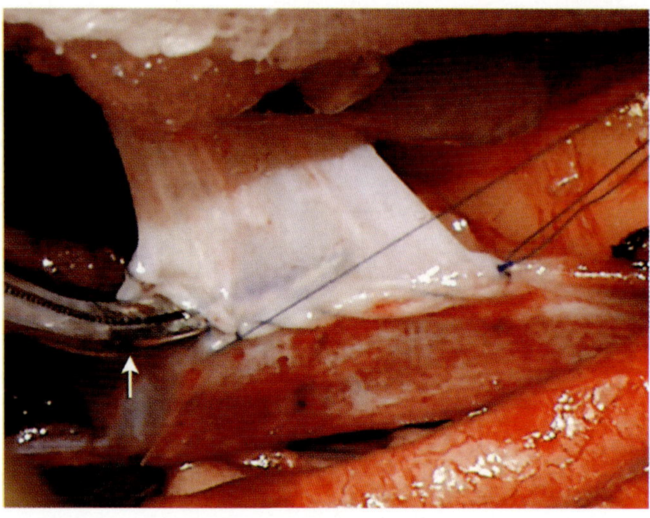

Fig. 24: Prior to finalizing the anastomosis, as a safety precaution, we sometimes verify with a right angle (white arrow) clamp that there is no back walling.

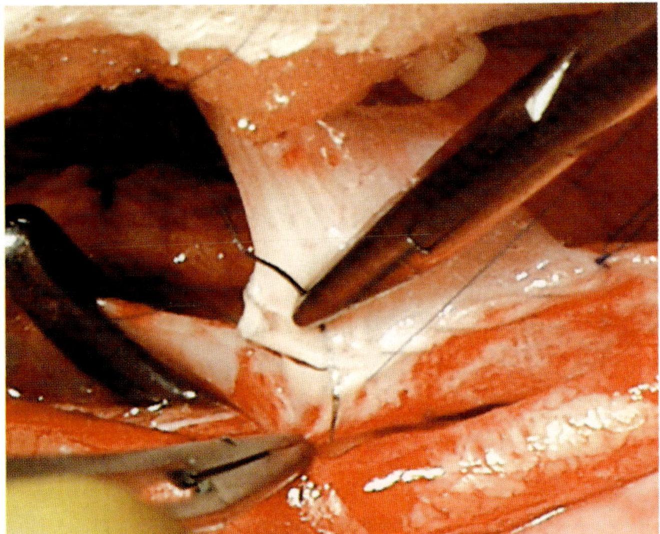

Fig. 25: The anastomosis is then completed and the other corner stitch tied.

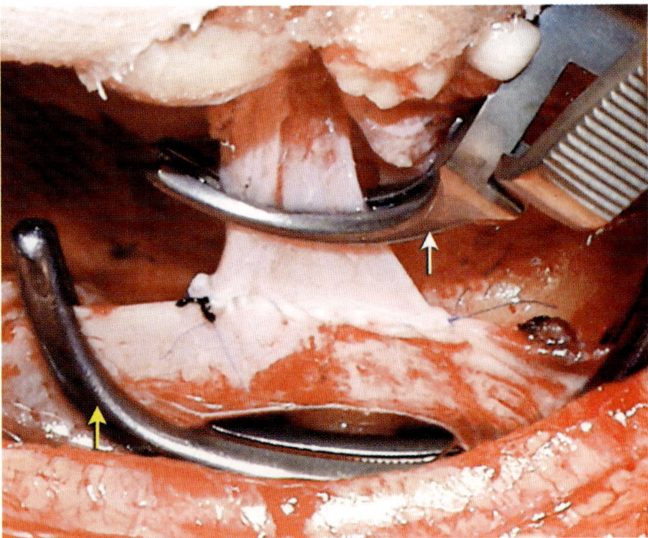

Fig. 26: A bulldog clamp (white arrow) is placed on the transplant renal vein. The semicircular clamp (yellow arrow) is still in place on the recipient external iliac vein.

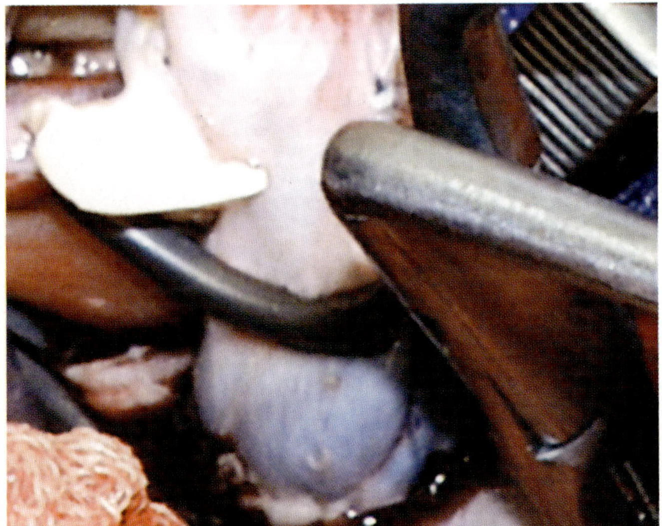

Fig. 27: The semicircular clamp is subsequently released, re-establishing the circulation in the external iliac vein and allowing for blood to reach the anastomosis. The bulldog clamp prevents blood from entering the kidney in a retrograde fashion.

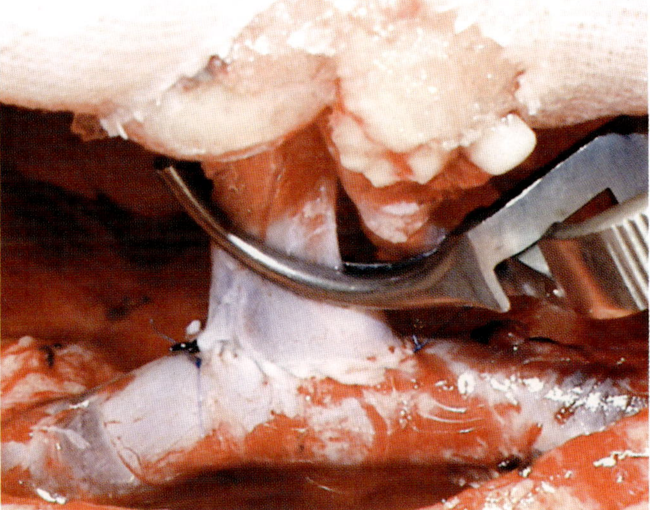

Fig. 28: We verify that there is adequate hemostasis at the anastomosis. If necessary, additional interrupted stitches can be placed to reinforce any bleeding sites. Small oozing points usually stop on their own. Re-establishing the venous circulation of the lower extremity prevents congestion and potentially deep venous thromboses.

KIDNEY IMPLANTATION—ARTERIAL ANASTOMOSIS (FIGS. 29 TO 42)

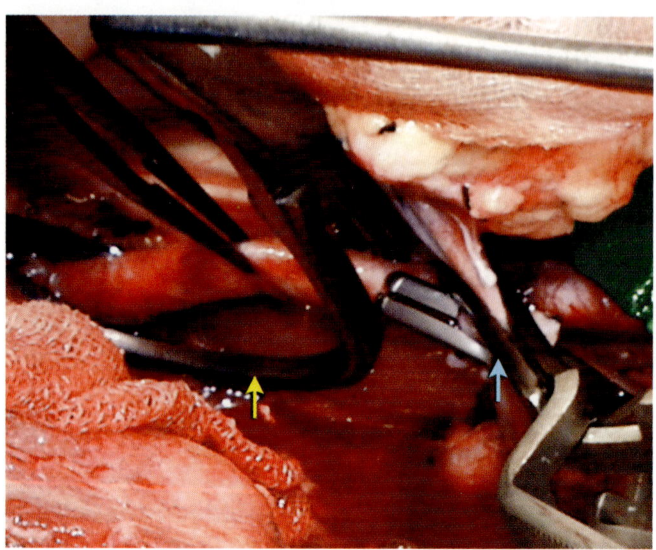

Fig. 29: After completion of the venous anastomosis, we place the semicircular clamp (yellow arrow) on the external iliac artery at the future site of the anastomosis. The transplant renal vein remains clamped (light blue arrow).

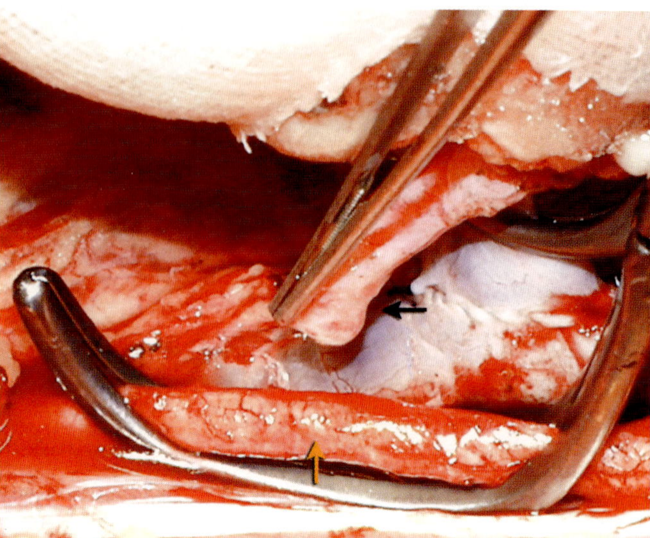

Fig. 30: After the external iliac artery (orange arrow) is clamped, prior to making any incisions we once again corroborate that the site is adequate by grasping the transplant renal artery (black arrow) with a forceps and ensuring that it will not be kinked, twisted, or under any tension once the anastomosis is completed.

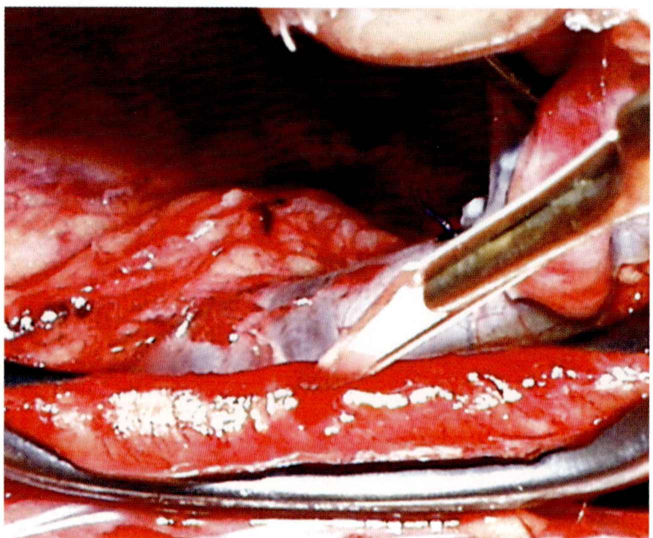

Fig. 31: The artery is incised with a sharp blade.

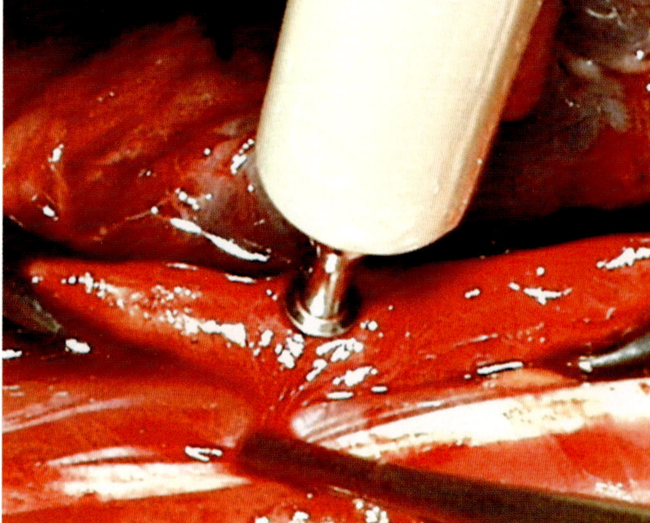

Fig. 32: We sometimes use an aortic hole puncher to make the arteriotomy round. If the donor renal artery is of large diameter, the opening in the recipient external iliac artery can be enlarged by further incising with a knife.

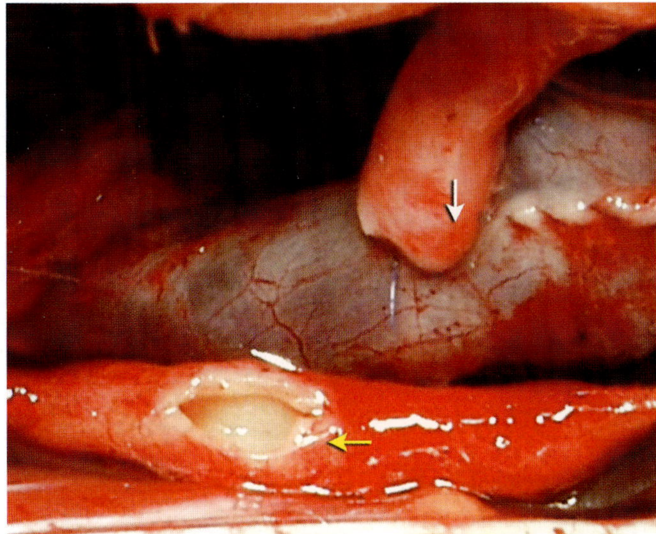

Fig. 33: The resulting opening in the recipient external iliac artery (yellow arrow) matches the diameter of the donor renal artery (white arrow).

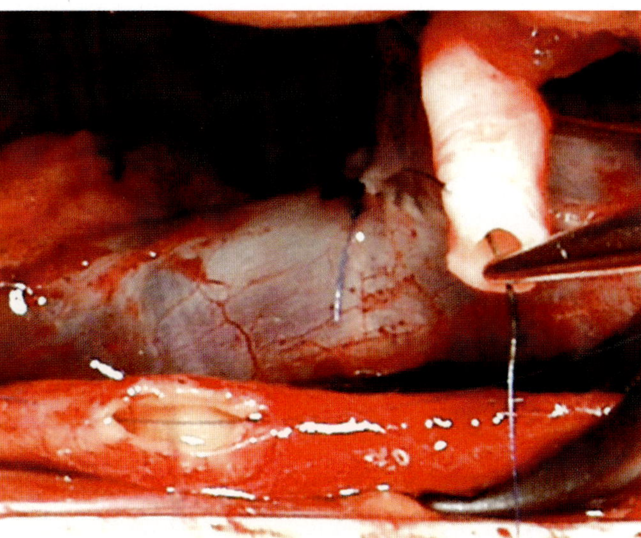

Fig. 34: A corner stitch is placed by obtaining full-thickness bites of the donor and recipient arteries.

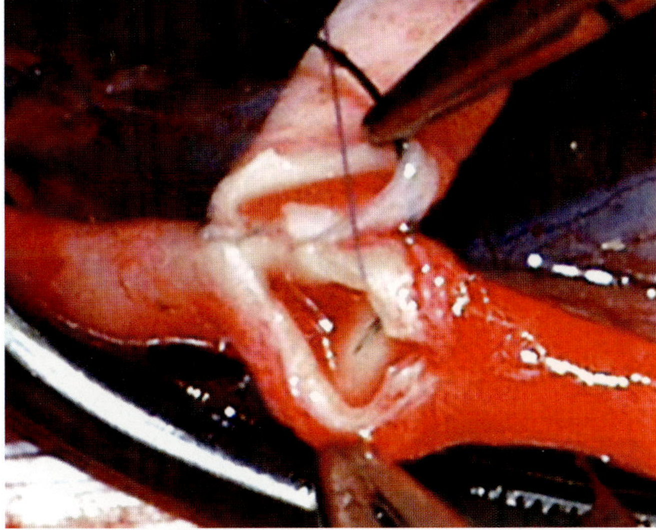

Fig. 35: The corner stitch is tied with the knots on the outside, leaving one limb much longer so to run the entire anastomosis. We routinely use 6-0 monofilament nonabsorbable. We sew the back wall of the anastomosis from the inside. Alternatively, the first assistant can sew it from his/her side.

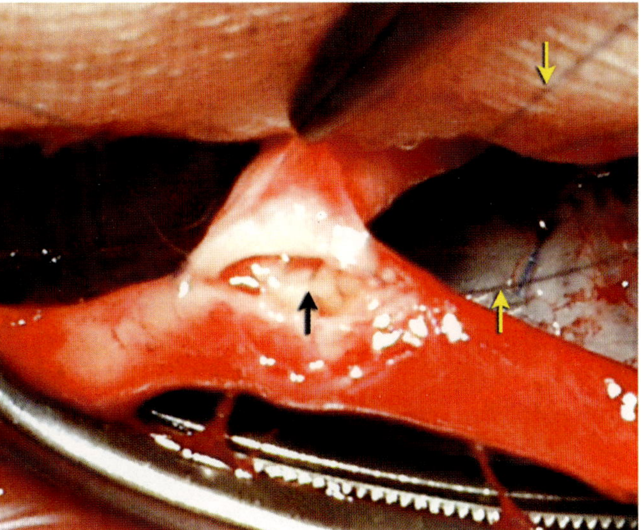

Fig. 36: When the back wall (black arrow) is completed, we place the second corner stitch (yellow arrows).

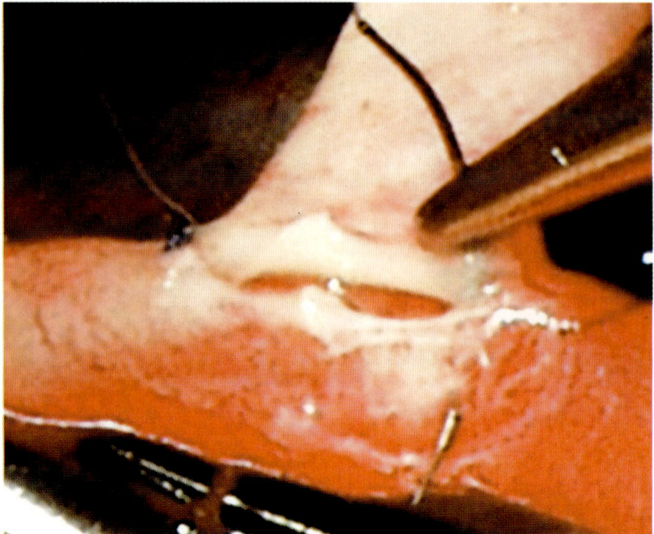

Fig. 37: The anterior wall is then addressed. These images represent a case of a kidney from a live donor, where the renal artery had no aortic patch.

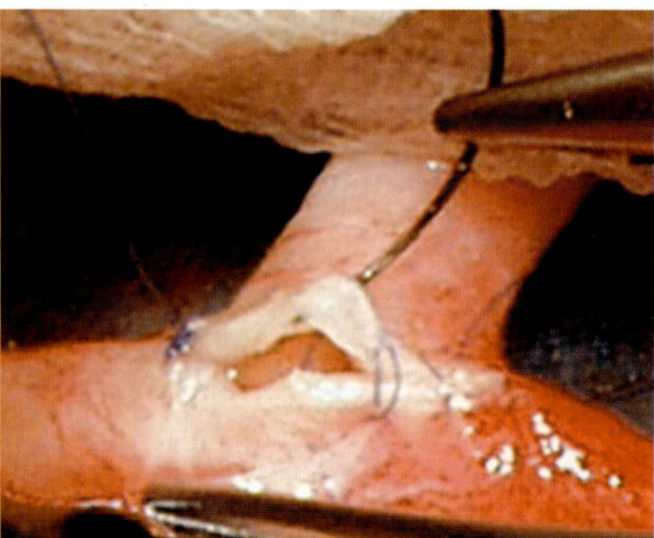

Fig. 38: We pay special attention not to back wall any part of the anastomosis.

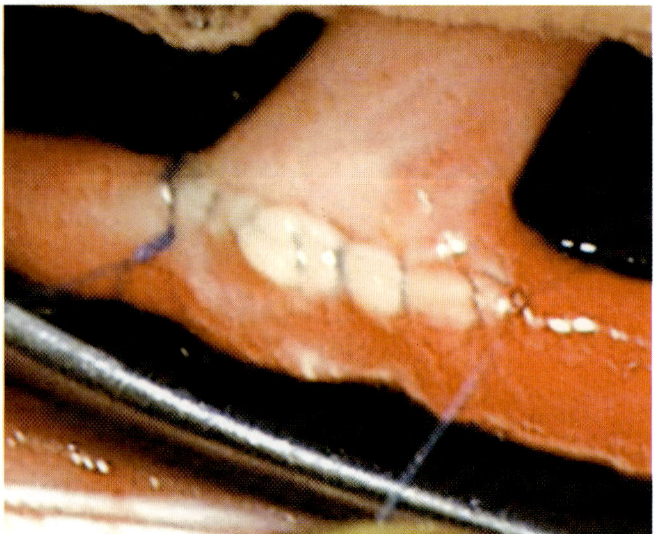

Fig. 39: After the anastomosis is completed, we tie the second corner stitch.

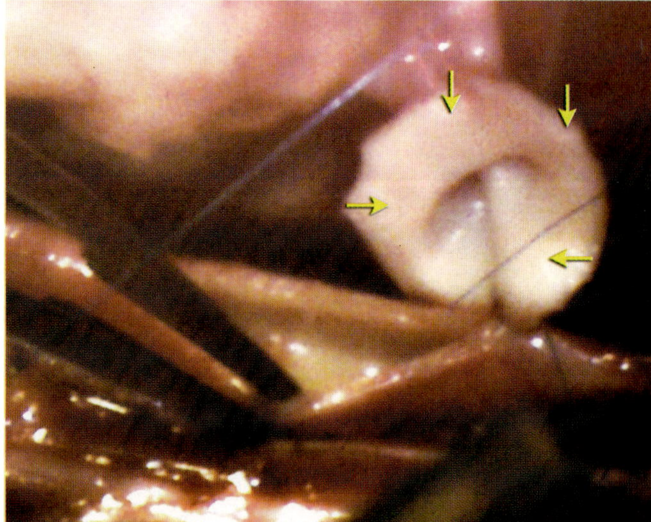

Fig. 40: This sequence of illustrations represents a graft from a deceased donor, where the renal artery has attached a patch of aorta (yellow arrows). As we had previously described, a corner stitch is placed first.

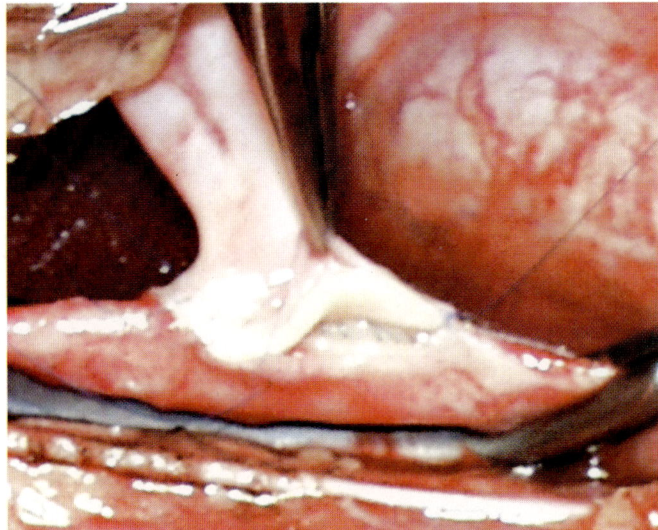

Fig. 41: The anastomosis is constructed with 6-0 monofilament nonresorbable sutures in a continuous fashion. The presence of an aortic patch allows for a broader anastomosis.

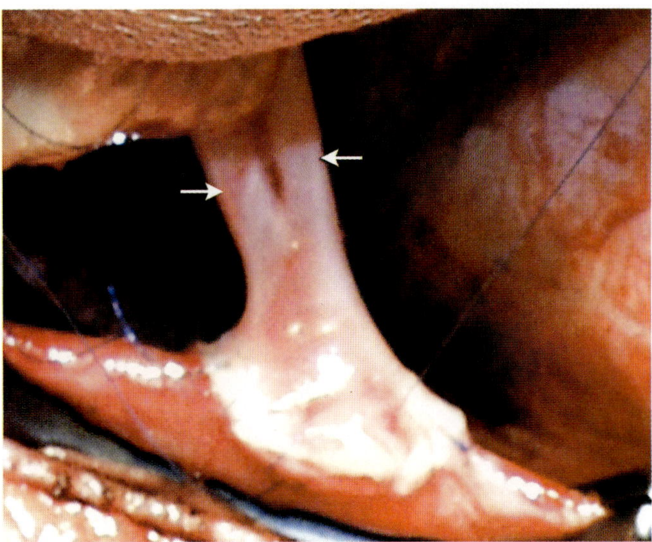

Fig. 42: The anastomosis is finally completed. Note the early bifurcation (arrows) of the renal artery.

KIDNEY IMPLANTATION—REPERFUSION (FIGS. 43 TO 47)

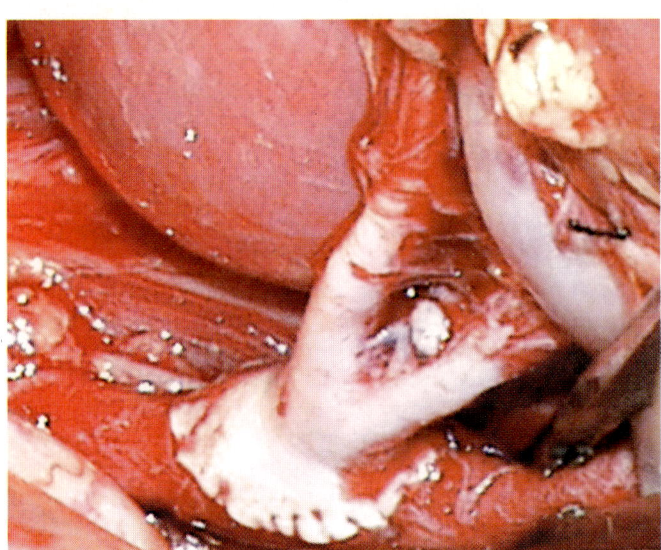

Fig. 43

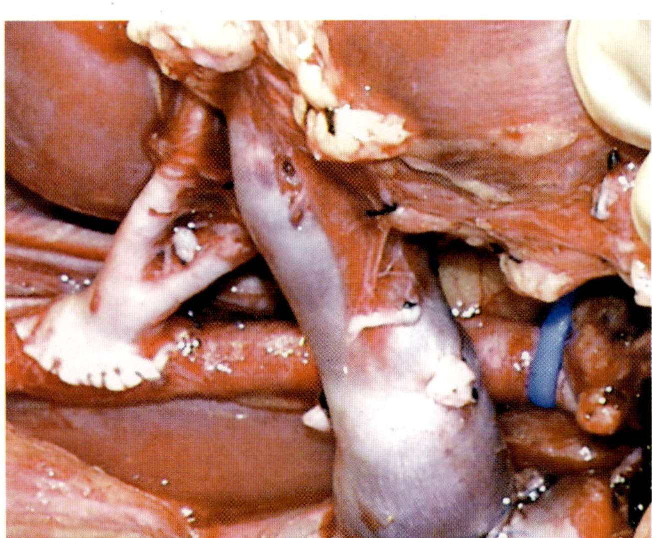

Fig. 44

Figs. 43 and 44: While clamping the renal artery, the semicircular clamp in the external iliac artery is partially released and hemostasis verified. If there are no sites of bleeding, the semicircular clamp in the artery and the bulldog clamp in the renal vein are removed and blood allowed to flow into the kidney reperfusing it. The kidney should turn pink rapidly without any evidence of ischemia (as in the illustration above). Its turgor should also improve. In instances where these events do not occur, the surgeon should immediately search for the cause of the abnormal reperfusion, and attempt to correct it rapidly. We also recheck for adequate hemostasis and routinely evaluate by means of Doppler the transplant renal artery and vein as well as the external iliac artery and vein. Note that this is a case of a deceased donor graft with an aortic patch.

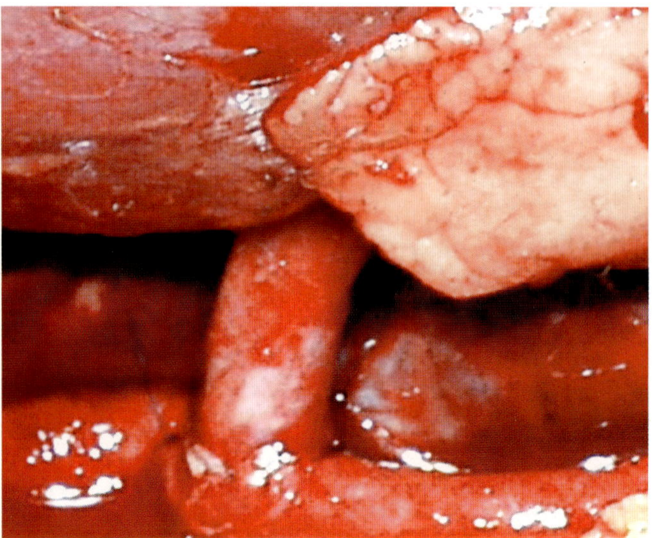

Fig. 45

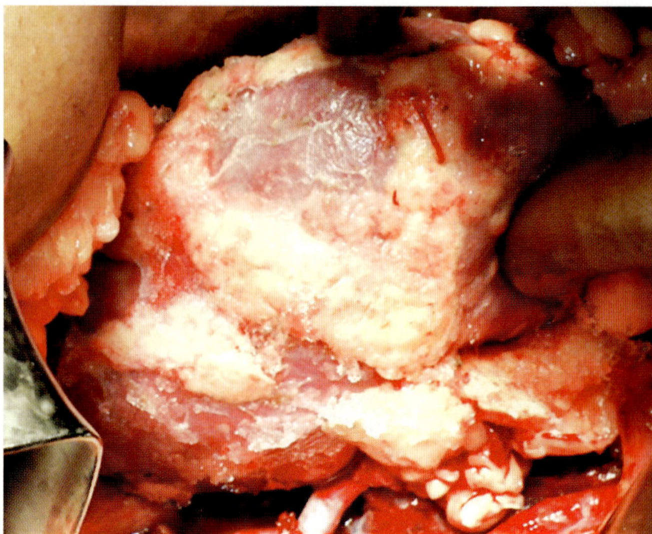

Fig. 46

Figs. 45 and 46: In cases of live donor grafts, there is no aortic patch as shown in Figure 45. The kidney should always look pink (as illustrated on both images) by the time of abdominal closure. In all instances, we obtain a routine duplex Doppler study of the transplanted kidney in the recovery room immediately after completing the surgery to verify that there is adequate perfusion of the organ and no hydronephrosis. If this evaluation shows compromised blood flow, we proceed to immediately re-explore the patient. Etiologies of abnormal blood flow include arterial or venous thromboses, malpositioning of the kidney associated with closure of the abdomen, twisting or kinking of the vessels, among others. We routinely obtain a biopsy of the transplanted kidney after reperfusion. This serves both as a baseline reference as well as a comparison for future biopsies.

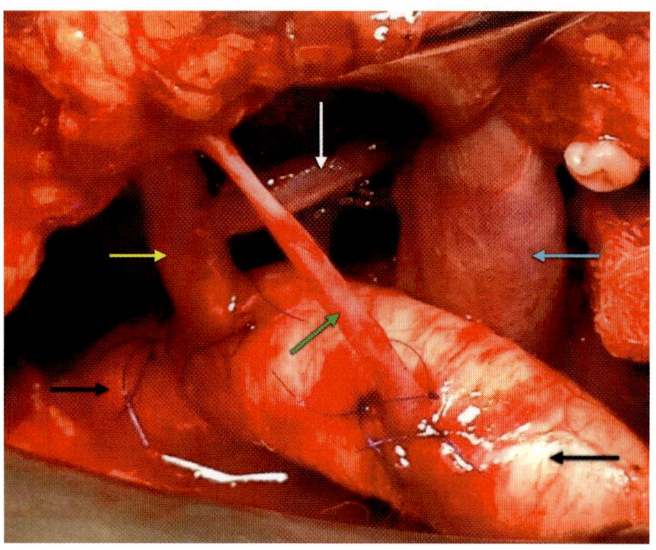

Fig. 47: On occasions, we perform additional anastomoses as considered necessary based on clinical findings. The case illustrated here is of a live donor kidney with 3 arteries originating independently from the aorta. An accessory lower pole artery (white arrow) was reconstructed in an end-to-side fashion onto the main renal artery (yellow arrow) during the back table preparation. A third small accessory renal artery had not been reconstructed since it was determined that it likely did not irrigate a large territory. However, after reperfusion the renal parenchyma showed a limited area of diminished blood flow. It was then decided to anastomose this small accessory vessel (green arrow) individually onto the recipient external iliac artery (black arrows) at a point distal to the anastomosis of the main renal artery (in order to avoid any interruption of flow to the kidney). Note also the transplant renal vein (blue arrow) being retracted sideways.

KIDNEY IMPLANTATION—IMPLANTATION OF THE URETER (FIGS. 48 AND 49)

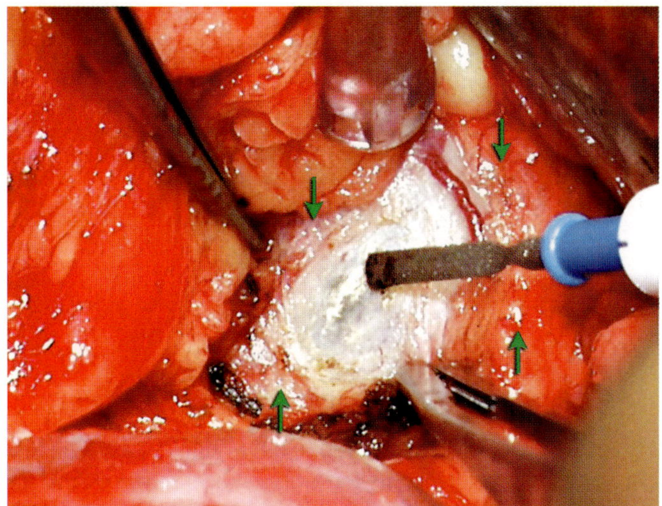

Fig. 48: After the transplanted kidney is reperfused, the urinary catheter is clamped and the bladder filled with an antibiotic (or iodine) containing solution in order to distend it and facilitate its identification. Once the bladder has been identified with certainty, the fatty tissues and detrusor muscle at the site of the future ureteral implantation site are cleared (green arrows), leaving only mucosa.

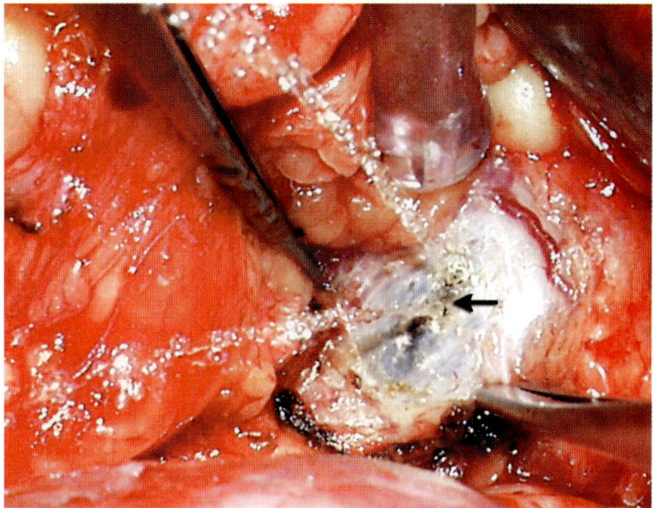

Fig. 49: The bladder mucosa is then incised with electrocautery. The instilled solution flows out (black arrow). The incision should be of an adequate size for the implantation of the ureter. When the incision is too large, the implantation becomes difficult and the likelihood of complications increases. In instances where the bladder cannot be identified with certainty, the surgeon can incise the peritoneum and palpate it from within the peritoneal cavity.

KIDNEY IMPLANTATION—IMPLANTATION OF THE URETER IN A SIMULTANEOUS PANCREAS TRANSPLANT WITH PORTAL VENOUS DRAINAGE (FIGS. 50 AND 51)

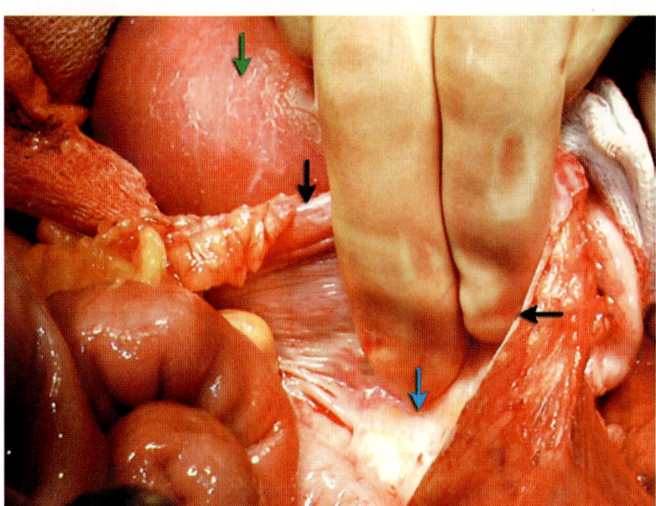

Fig. 50

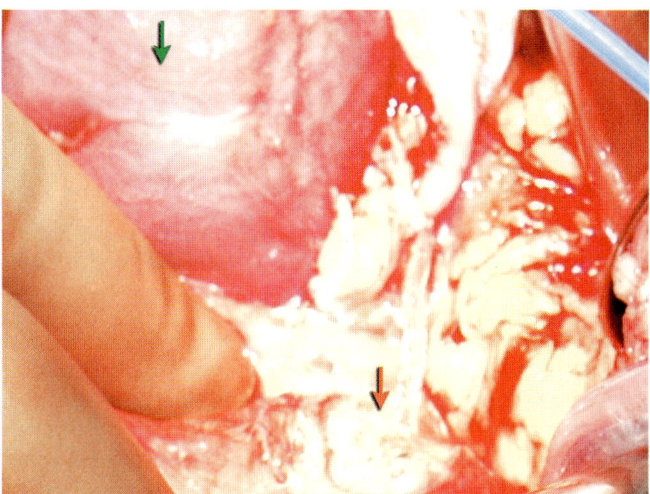

Fig. 51

Figs. 50 and 51: The kidney (green arrows) has been implanted in a retroperitoneal location by separating the peritoneum (black arrows) from the overlying muscles and fascia via the midline incision. After reperfusion of the renal allograft, we clamp the urinary catheter and fill the bladder with an antibiotic (or iodine) containing solution in order to distend it for better identification. The midline incision allows for palpation of the bladder from within the peritoneal cavity (blue arrow). The bladder is subsequently incised (orange arrow) with outflow of the previously instilled solution.

KIDNEY IMPLANTATION—IMPLANTATION OF THE URETER (FIGS. 52 TO 66)

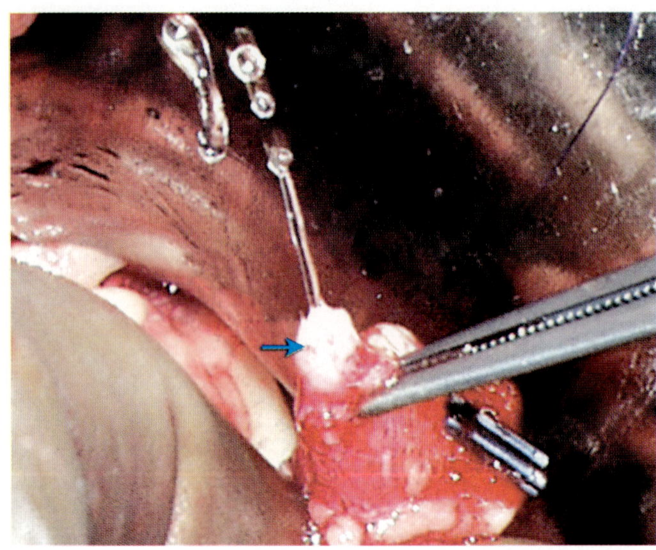

Fig. 52: As shown in this illustration, urine can be produced and seen coming out of the ureter (arrow) soon after reperfusion of the allograft. This is encountered more frequently with live rather than with deceased donors.

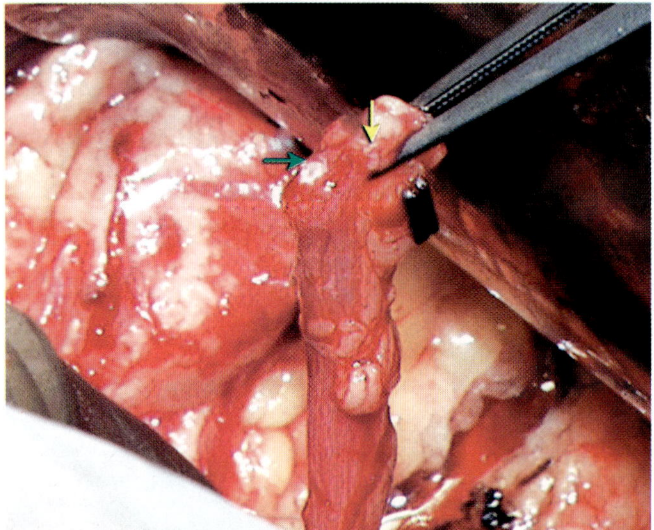

Fig. 53

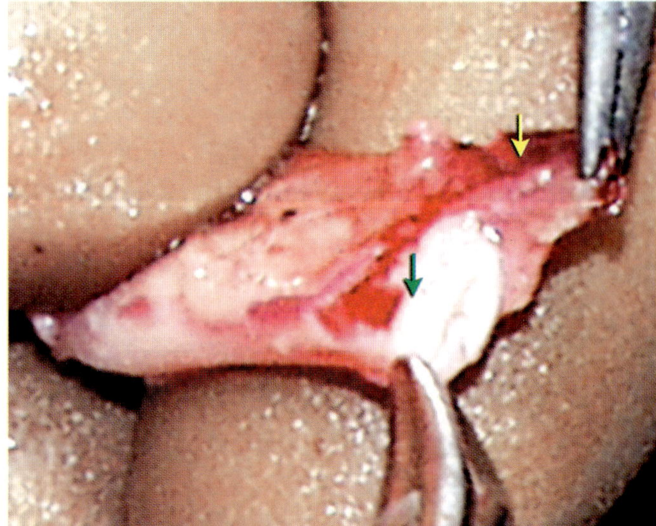

Fig. 54

Figs. 53 and 54: Prior to implantation of the ureter onto the bladder, the ureter (green arrows) is trimmed to an adequate length. Since the only blood supply to the ureter is from the transplant renal artery (its blood supply from the gonadal and superior vesical arteries is lost at the time of procurement), the ureter should have enough length to allow for an anastomosis with no tension, but as short as possible so to prevent distal ischemic changes. The tissue surrounding the ureter (yellow arrows), that contain nutritious vessels as well as remnants of the gonadal vessels, should be tied to prevent immediate and/or delayed bleeding.

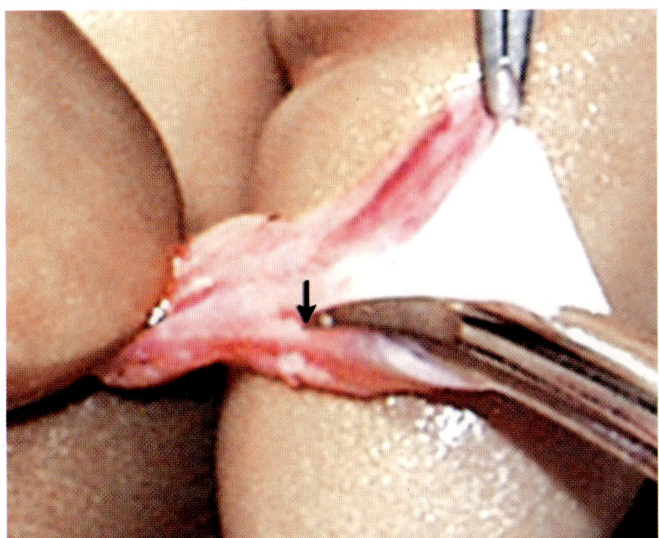

Fig. 55: After the ureter is trimmed to an adequate length, it is spatulated. The process of spatulation entails incising the ureter (black arrow) in order to allow for a more ample anastomosis.

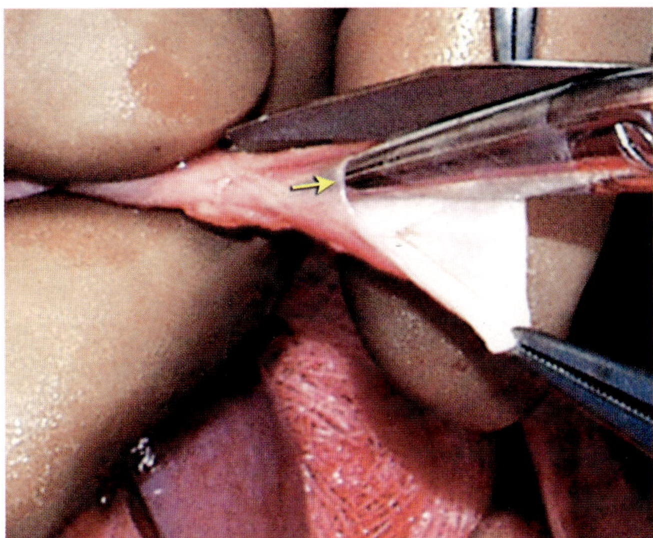

Fig. 56: After incising the ureter, we also incise the tissues surrounding it (yellow arrow). This prevents potential positional strictures after implantation.

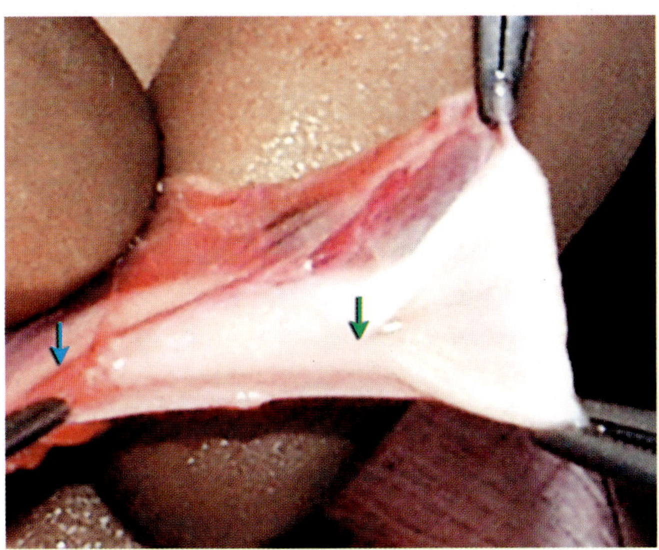

Fig. 57: The incision of the periureteral tissues (blue arrow) should be more extensive than the incision on the ureter itself (green arrow). Hemostasis should always be verified, since delayed bleeding from nutritious vessels along the tissues surrounding the ureter can be a cause of hemorrhage leading to reinterventions.

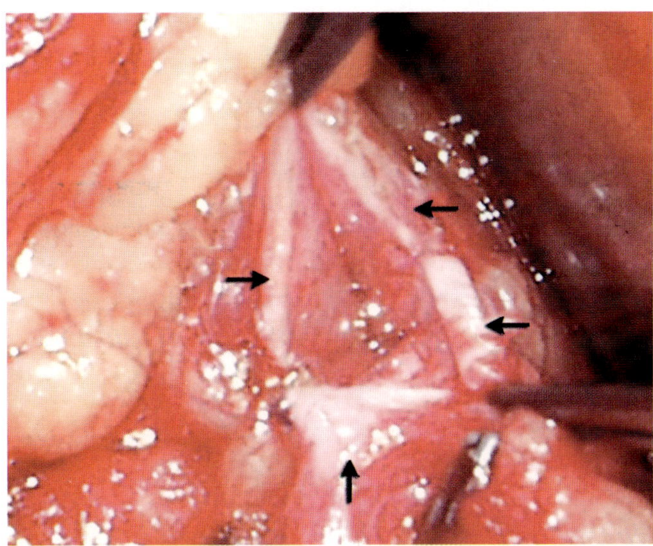

Fig. 58: The opening in the bladder is identified (black arrows).

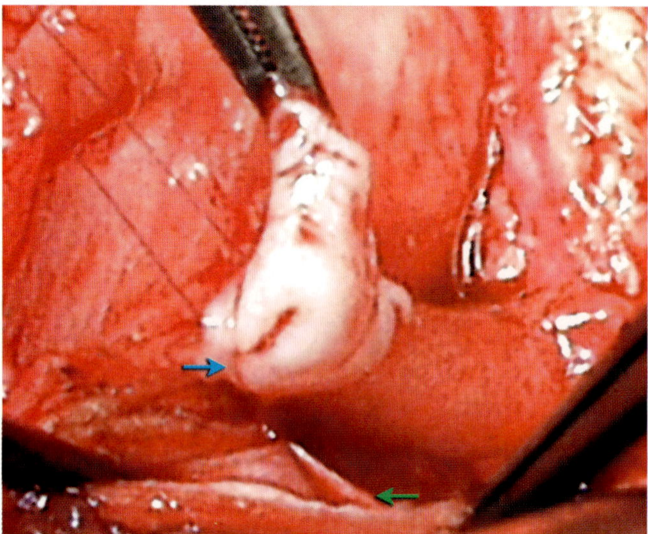

Fig. 59: The spatulated ureter is sewn onto the bladder with running resorbable sutures with full-thickness bites of both bladder and ureter. An initial stitch is placed at the heel of the spatulated ureter (blue arrow) and a distal point in the bladder (green arrow).

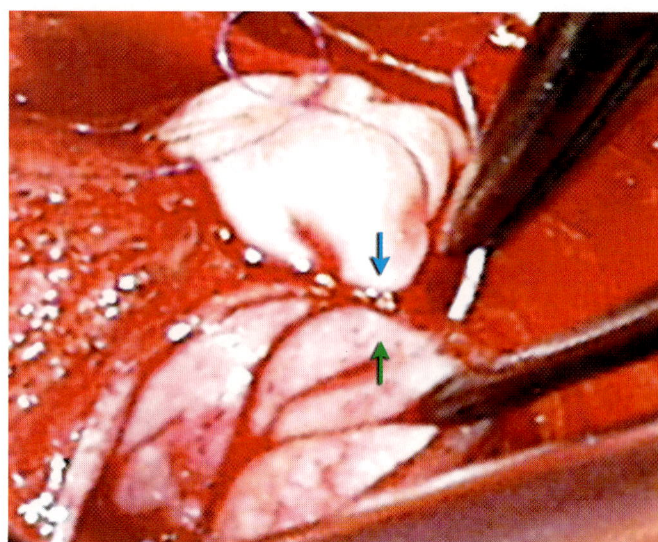

Fig. 60: The ureter (blue arrow) to bladder (green arrow) anastomosis is fashioned with delicate full-thickness bites of the muscular ureter in order to prevent strictures, especially near the heel of the spatulated ureter.

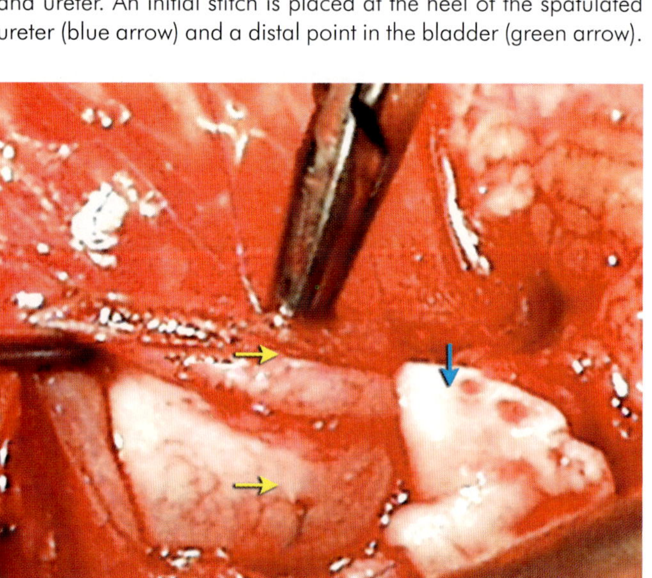

Fig. 61: The full-thickness bites of the bladder (yellow arrows) should be more encompassing than those of the ureter (blue arrow) in order to prevent disruptions of the suture line.

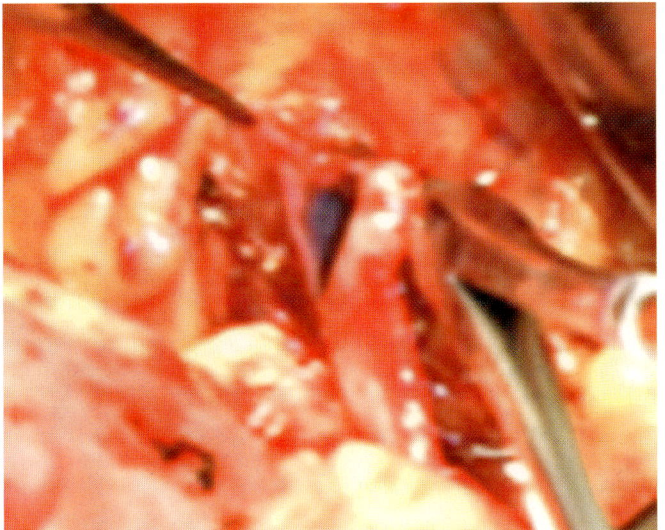

Fig. 62

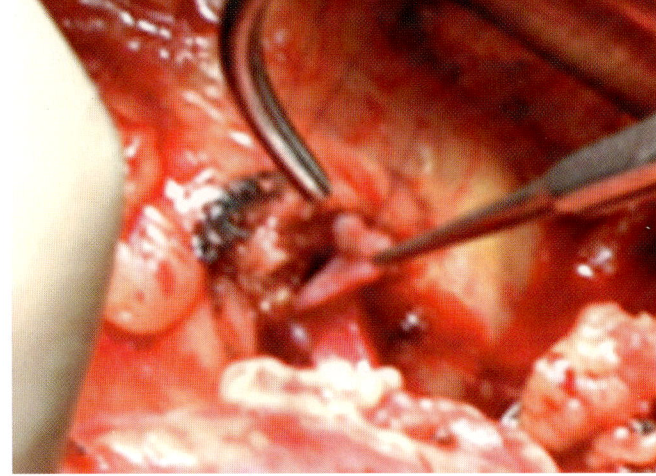

Fig. 63

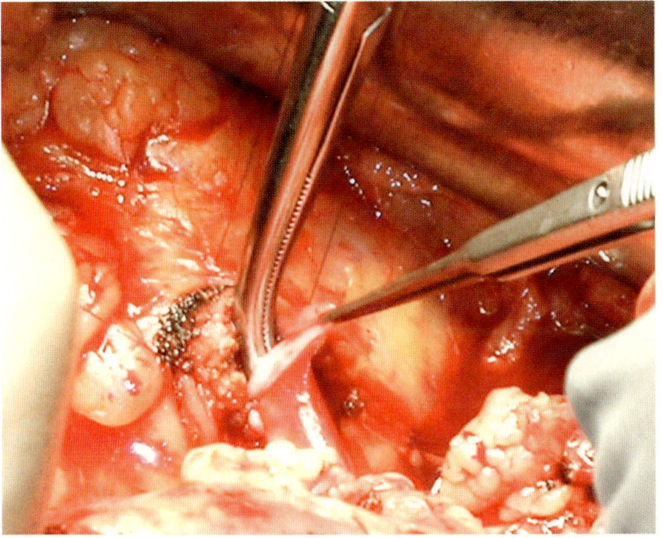

Fig. 64

Figs. 62 to 64: In order to prevent strictures, prior to completing the anastomosis (Fig. 62), with a right angle clamp (Fig. 63) we test for patency between ureter and bladder (Fig. 64). If we are not satisfied by the patency, we take down the anastomosis and re-do it, making sure we take delicate bites of the ureter to prevent strictures. Even minor stenoses may become temporarily relevant because of edema (that resolves after a few days/weeks) in the immediate postoperative period. At this point, we place a stent in the donor ureter, going into the bladder. This stent is usually removed six weeks later.

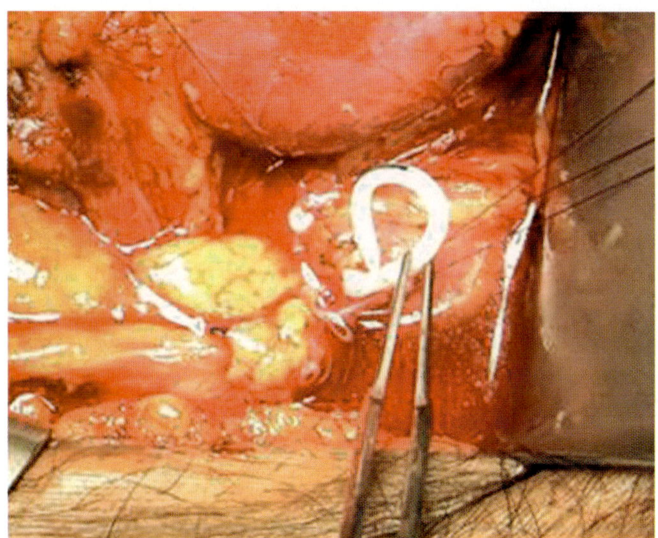

Fig. 65: Stent being placed.

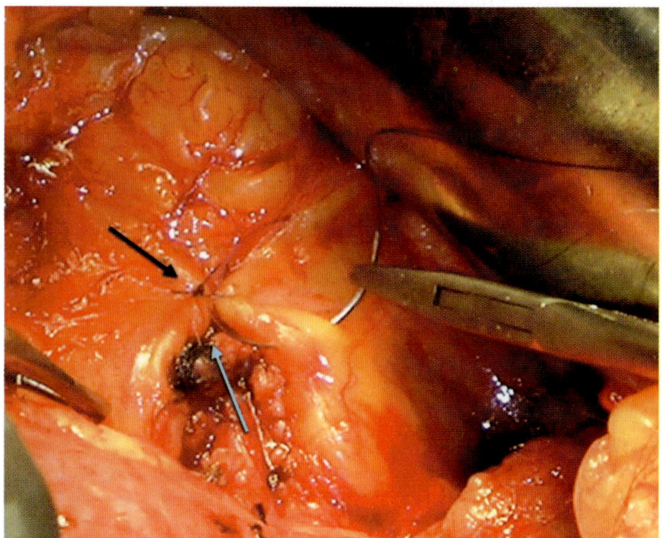

Fig. 66: Once the anastomosis has been completed, on very rare occasions we may fashion an antireflux nipple-valve mechanism with one or two interrupted 4–0 absorbable stitches (black arrow) of the bladder wall in the region of the toe (blue arrow) of the ureter-to-bladder anastomosis. Special care should be taken not to cause a ureteral obstruction with a very tight antireflux mechanism.

CHAPTER 31

Minimally Invasive Kidney Transplantation

Pranjal Modi, Akshay Sood, Wooju Jeong, Mahendra Bhandari, Rajesh Ahlawat, Ramesh Kumar, Mani Menon

INTRODUCTION

- Minimally invasive surgery reduces perioperative morbidity. Benefits include, but are not limited to, smaller incision, lesser surgical site infection, blood loss and postoperative pain, shorter hospital stay and convalescence period, and better cosmesis[1-5]
- Indeed, the role of minimally invasive surgery in donor nephrectomy has been well established;[6] however, its utility for recipient surgery has not been rigorously evaluated
- Being fragile and immunocompromised, patients undergoing kidney transplantation (KT) are at a higher risk for developing perioperative complications than the renal donor. Complications affect not only short-term patient convalescence adversely but also compromise long-term graft and patient survival.[7-10] Thus, transplant recipients may benefit substantially from minimally invasive surgery
- Minimally invasive approaches to KT have been described recently
  - In 2010, Modi et al. introduced the technique of laparoscopic KT,[11] and Giulianotti et al. described their technique of robotic KT (RKT)[12]
  - Both groups noted a slightly slower return of graft function.[13,14] These studies were performed without renal cooling
  - We reasoned that warm ischemia may have played a role in the slight delay in recovery of graft function and sought to develop a technique for RKT that eliminated warm ischemia during the recipient surgery
- Here, we describe our novel technique of RKT with regional hypothermia

PATIENT SELECTION

Patients were inducted into the study if they expressed the desire to undergo minimally invasive surgery. Patient selection criteria are detailed below (informed consent was obtained in each case):[15,16]

- Inclusion criteria:
  - Irreversible renal disease, defined as end-stage renal disease (ESRD) or anticipated ESRD within the next 12 months (pre-emptive transplant)
  - Matched living donor
- Exclusion criteria:
  - Previous major abdominal surgery with a high suspicion for intra-abdominal adhesions
  - Significant atherosclerotic disease of the iliac vessels (> 30% blockage)
  - Immunologically high-risk transplant
  - Second transplant
  - Simultaneous dual/multiple organ transplant

INSTRUMENTS

Robotic Instruments and Ports

- Robotic 8 mm ports × 3
- Robotic Maryland bipolar grasper
- Robotic monopolar curved scissors
  - Cover-tip accessory
- Robotic Black Diamond micro forceps
- Robotic large needle driver

- Robotic Hem-o-Lok applier
- Robotic ProGrasp forceps (on the 4th arm)

Laparoscopic Instruments

- Microfrance laparoscopic grasper
- Suture passer
- Hem-o-Lok applier (5 mm, 10 mm, 12 mm)
  - Weck clips: 5 mm, 10 mm, 12 mm
- Bulldog clamps with appliers (Scanlan International, Saint Paul, MN)

Disposables

- GelPOINT platform × 1 (Applied Medical Corp, Rancho Santa Margarita, CA)
- 12 mm camera port × 1 and 12 mm assistant port × 1
- 5-F ureteric catheter for flushing
- Sutures:
  - 5-0 CV-6 ePTFE (Gore-Tex; W L Gore & Associates Inc, Flagstaff, AZ)
  - 4-0 PDS/3-0 V-Loc CV23 6″ (Covidien Inc, New Haven, CT, USA)

Other

- Ice slush machine (OR Solutions Model: ORS-1075 H5)
- Slush machine drape (OR Solutions Model: ORS-321)
- Toomey syringes (modified)
- 3.6 mm aortic punch (Teleflex-Medical Inc, Research Triangle Park, NC)

SURGICAL TECHNIQUE

Preparation of the GelPOINT

- The GelPOINT device is a hand-access platform that allows easy introduction of the ice slush and the graft
- The GelPOINT platform consists of two parts: a GelSeal cap and an access port. A 12 mm camera port and a 5 mm suction port are placed into the GelSeal cap ahead of time (Fig. 1A)

Patient Position and Port Placement

- Patient positioning and placement of the GelPOINT device followed the standard template used for the Vattikuti Institute prostatectomy (VIP) technique of robotic radical prostatectomy[17,18]
- With the patient in supine position, a 4–5 cm vertical incision is made in the periumbilical region. The access port is inserted through the incision and the prepared GelSeal cap is secured to the access port. Other ports, including three 8 mm robotic ports and one 12 mm assistant port are placed as shown (Fig. 1B)

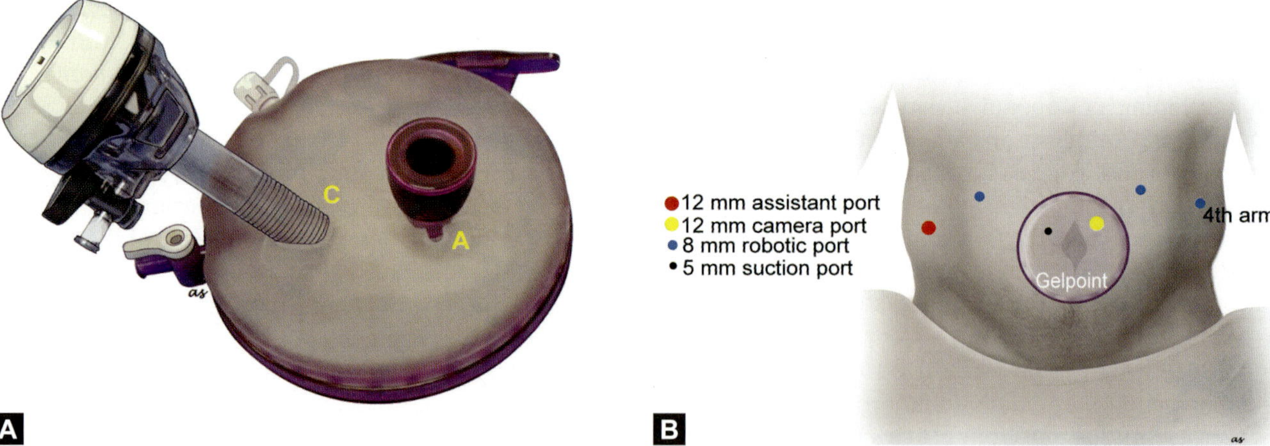

Figs. 1A and B: (A) GelSeal cap with a 12 mm camera port (C) and a 10 mm assistant port, for the 5 mm suction (A); (B) Diagrammatic illustration of port placement for robotic kidney transplantation with regional hypothermia.

Source: Illustrations reproduced with permission from Elsevier Inc: Menon M, Sood A, Bhandari M, et al. Robotic kidney transplantation with regional hypothermia: a step-by-step description of the Vattikuti Urology Institute-Medanta Technique (IDEAL Phase 2a). Eur Urol. 2014;65(5):991-1000.

- The patient is then moved to lithotomy position with a 15–20° Trendelenburg tilt, and the da Vinci robot is docked between the legs (Fig. 2)

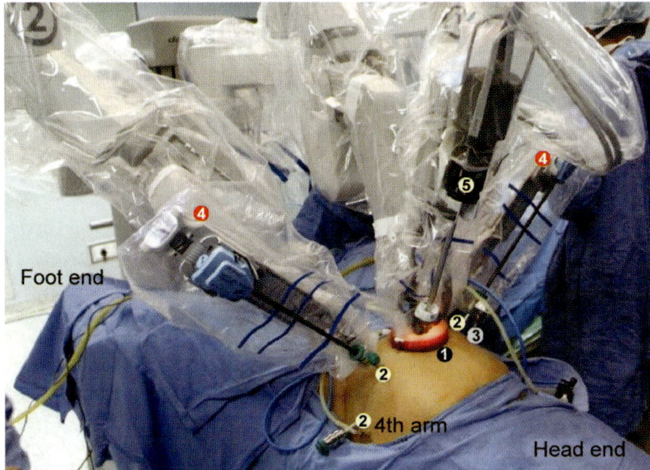

Fig. 2: Robot docked in between the legs of the patient, in a manner typical for robotic radical prostatectomy. Patient position and Robot dock position [(1) GelPOINT™; (2) 8 mm robotic ports; (3) 12 mm assistant port; (4) Robotic arms; (5) Camera arm].
Source: Illustrations reproduced with permission from Elsevier Inc: Menon M, Sood A, Bhandari M, et al. Robotic kidney transplantation with regional hypothermia: a step-by-step description of the Vattikuti Urology Institute-Medanta Technique (IDEAL Phase 2a). Eur Urol. 2014;65(5):991-1000.

Preparation of the Vascular Bed and Bladder

- With the camera lens in the 30° up position, the bladder is taken down. The camera is then changed to the 30° down position, and the external iliac vessels are skeletonized (Fig. 3A)
- Next, a transverse incision is made 2–3 cm caudal to the cecum and peritoneal flaps are raised on both sides over the psoas muscle, to be utilized later for retroperitonealizing the kidney
- The bladder is then distended with 240 mL of normal saline and bladder is prepared for a modified Lich-Gregoir ureteroneocystostomy (Fig. 3B)

Preparation of the Donor Graft

- While the recipient is being readied, the graft kidney is harvested laparoscopically in an adjacent operating room. The donor organ is defatted and perfused with cold Ringer's lactate as for conventional KT
- The graft kidney is wrapped in a gauze jacket filled with ice slush with an opening to allow egress of the hilar structures (Fig. 4B). The upper pole of the kidney is marked with a long silk-tie tail. The ice jacket serves two functions:
  1. Cooling the kidney, and
  2. Facilitating atraumatic handling during the anastomoses.

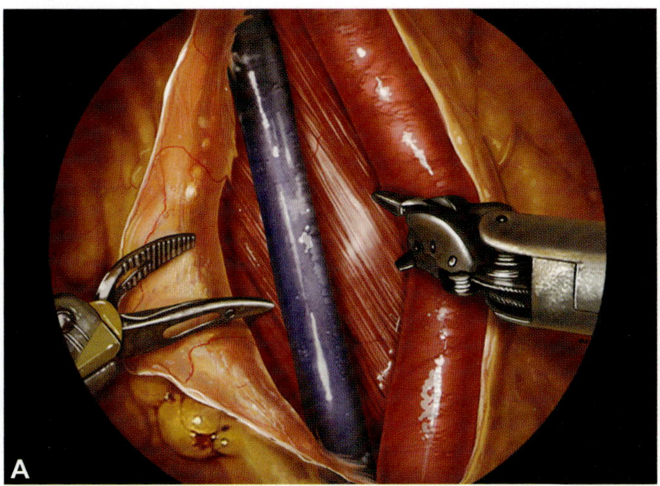
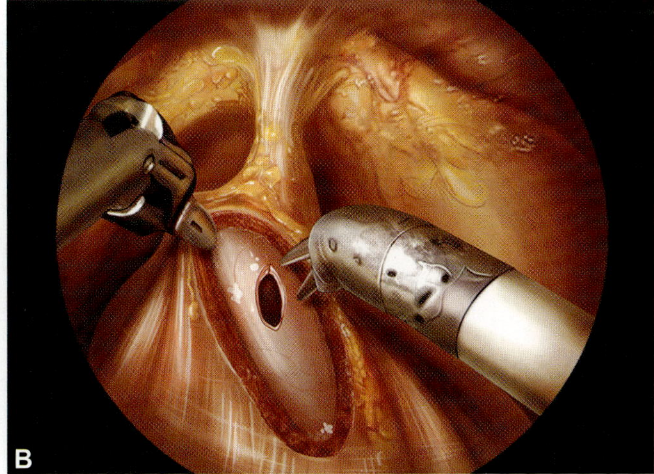

Figs. 3A and B: (A) Skeletonized iliac vessel bed; (B) Bladder preparation: detrusor flaps created for subsequent ureteroneocystostomy (modified Lich-Gregoir technique).
Source: Illustrations reproduced with permission from Elsevier Inc: Menon M, Sood A, Bhandari M, et al. Robotic kidney transplantation with regional hypothermia: a step-by-step description of the Vattikuti Urology Institute-Medanta Technique (IDEAL Phase 2a). Eur Urol. 2014;65(5):991-1000.

Introduction of the Graft and Cooling

- The pelvic bed is cooled to 18–20°C with the introduction of 180–240 mL ice slush (Fig. 4C) via modified Toomey syringes (the nozzle is cut off) (Fig. 4A)
- The robotic camera arm and the GelSeal cap are removed and the graft in its ice jacket is inserted effortlessly though the access port. It is important to orient the lower pole towards the feet of the recipient and the hilum towards the external iliac vessels
- More ice slush is added (Fig. 4D) to achieve uniform and effective regional hypothermia

Venous Anastomosis

- The external iliac vein (EIV) is clamped using robotic bulldog clamps (Fig. 5A)
- A venotomy is made using cold scissors. The graft renal vein is anastomosed in an end-to-side continuous fashion to the EIV (Fig. 5B) using an ePTFE suture
- The large needle holder is used in the dominant hand (to pass the stitch) and the Black Diamond micro forceps are used in the nondominant to atraumatically hold the vein open and to pull the stitch through
- Just prior to completing the venous anastomosis, the lumen is flushed with heparinized saline via a 5F ureteric catheter introduced through the assistant port
- The graft renal vein is occluded using a bulldog clamp and the EIV is unclamped. Additional ice slush is introduced as and if required (if the anastomosis is taking long to be completed)

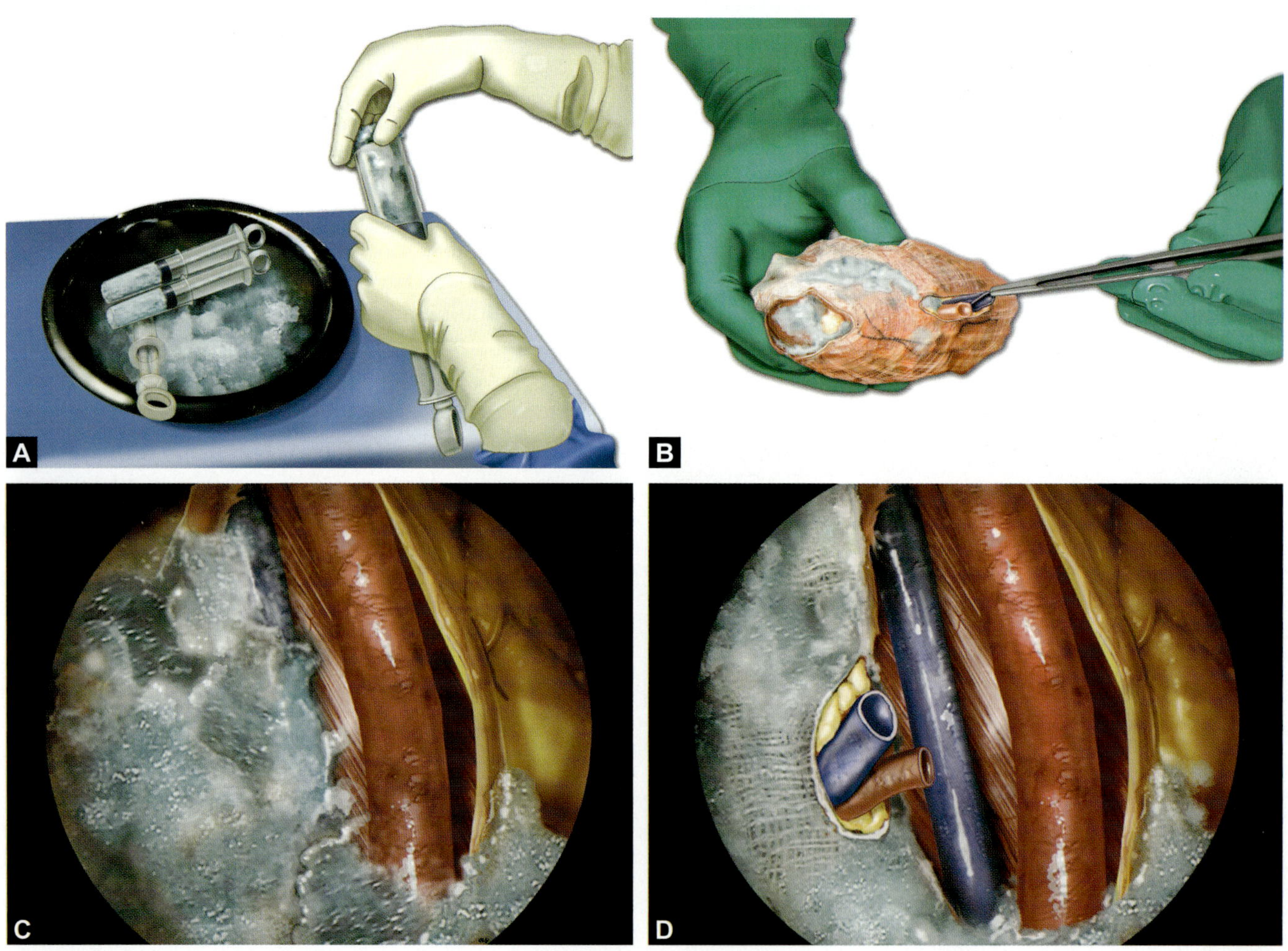

Figs. 4A to D: (A) Multiple modified Toomey syringes (nozzles cut off) being readied for rapid delivery of ice slush; (B) Graft kidney wrapped in a gauze jacket filled with ice slush; (C) Pelvic bed lined with ice slush to achieve pelvic-bed cooling before introduction of the graft kidney; (D) Additional ice slush delivered onto the graft kidney immediately after its introduction, to achieve uniform cooling.
Source: Illustrations reproduced with permission from Elsevier Inc: Menon M, Sood A, Bhandari M, et al. Robotic kidney transplantation with regional hypothermia: a step-by-step description of the Vattikuti Urology Institute-Medanta Technique (IDEAL Phase 2a). Eur Urol. 2014; 65(5):991-1000.

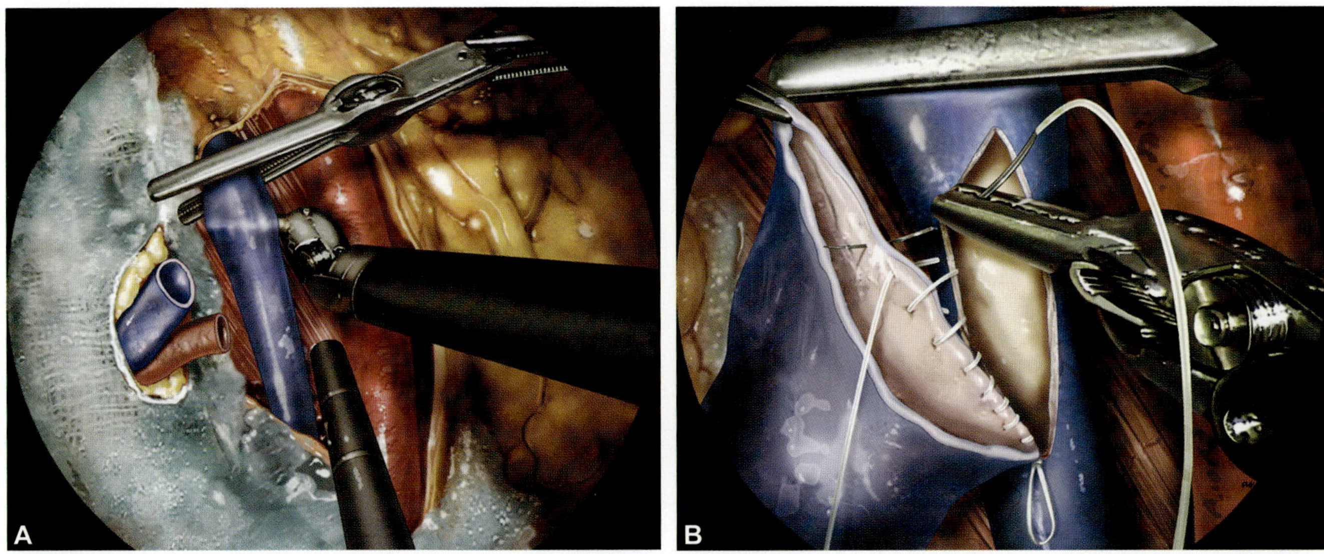

Figs. 5A and B: (A) External iliac vein clamped with a robotic bulldog clamp; (B) End-to-side venous anastomosis.
Source: Illustrations reproduced with permission from Elsevier Inc: Menon M, Sood A, Bhandari M, et al. Robotic kidney transplantation with regional hypothermia: a step-by-step description of the Vattikuti Urology Institute-Medanta Technique (IDEAL Phase 2a). Eur Urol. 2014;65(5):991-1000.

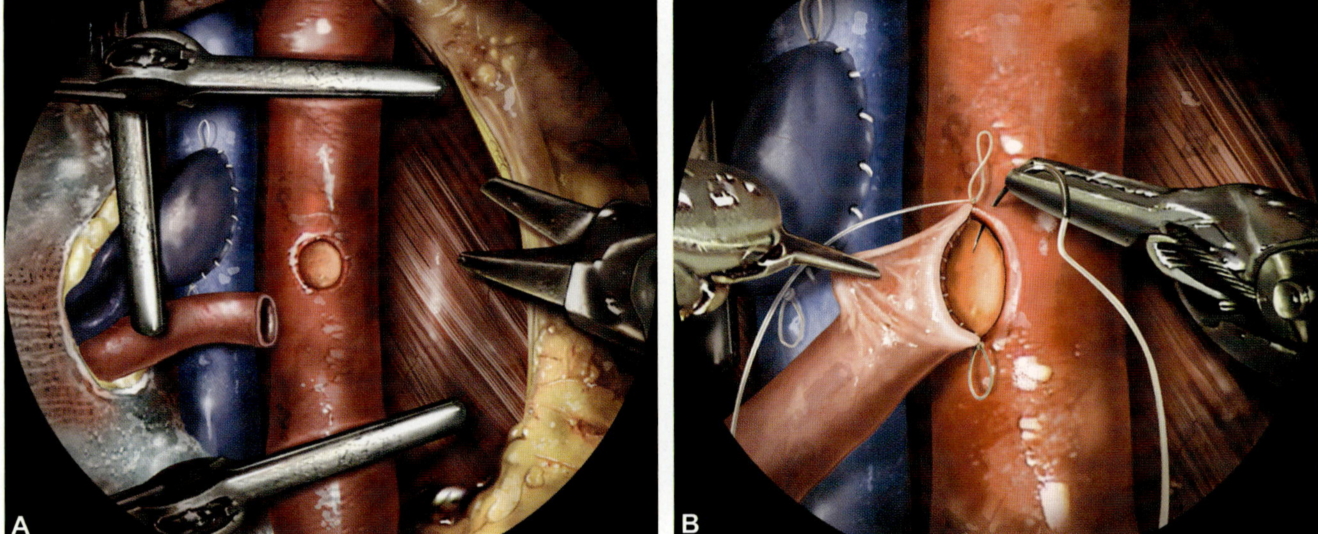

Figs. 6A and B: (A) Linear arteriotomy converted to circular arteriotomy using a 3.6 mm aortic punch; (B) End-to-side arterial anastomosis.
Source: Illustrations reproduced with permission from Elsevier Inc: Menon M, Sood A, Bhandari M, et al. Robotic kidney transplantation with regional hypothermia: a step-by-step description of the Vattikuti Urology Institute-Medanta Technique (IDEAL Phase 2a). Eur Urol. 2014;65(5):991-1000.

Arterial Anastomosis

- Next, the external iliac artery (EIA) is clamped
- A linear arteriotomy is made using the monopolar scissors. This is converted to a circular arteriotomy (Fig. 6A) using a 3.6 mm aortic punch introduced through the GelPOINT
- The renal artery is anastomosed in an end-to-side continuous fashion to the EIA using the Gore-Tex CV-6 suture (Fig. 6B)
- After flushing and testing the integrity of the anastomosis, the donor renal artery is clamped temporarily and the EIA is unclamped. If the anastomosis is secure, the renal artery and vein clamps are removed and the gauze jacket is cut away
- The graft kidney is visually inspected for color, turgor, and on-table diuresis
- Then the kidney may be retroperitonealized by approximating the peritoneal flaps prepared previously

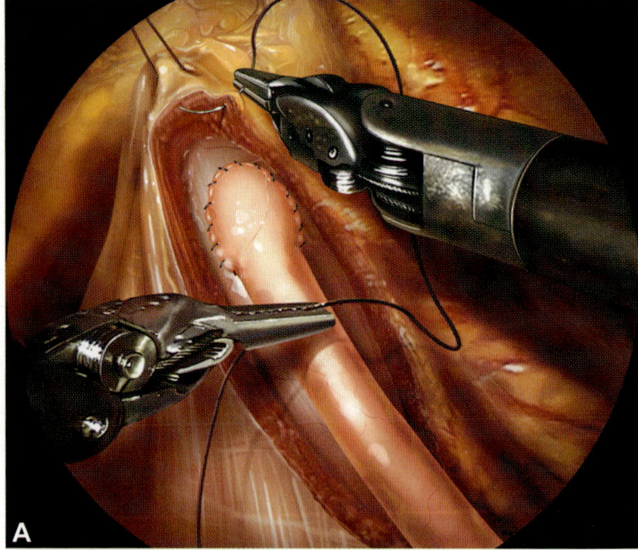

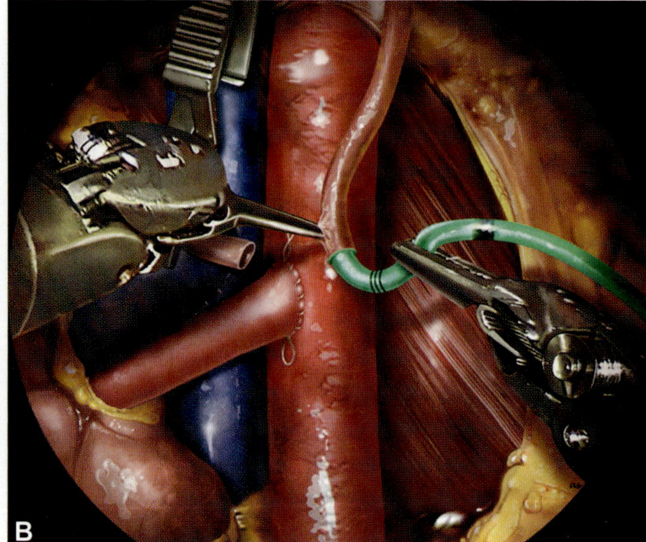

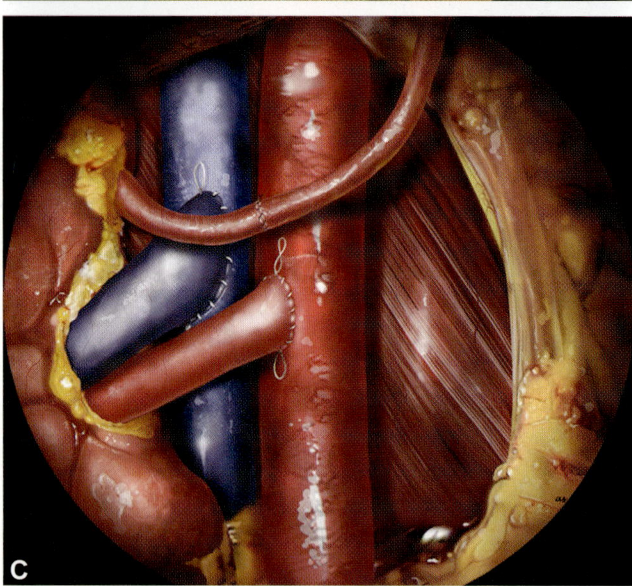

Figs. 7A to C: (A) Ureteroneocystostomy; (B) Inferior epigastric artery being flushed with heparinized saline using a 5F ureteric catheter; (C) Lower-pole accessory artery anastomosis to the inferior epigastric artery using 6-0 prolene sutures.

Source: Illustrations reproduced with permission from Elsevier Inc: Menon M, Sood A, Bhandari M, et al. Robotic kidney transplantation with regional hypothermia: a step-by-step description of the Vattikuti Urology Institute-Medanta Technique (IDEAL Phase 2a). Eur Urol. 2014;65(5):991-1000.

- The pneumoperitoneum pressure is dropped to 8 mm Hg and an intravenous bolus of 100 mg furosemide is given

Ureteroneocystostomy

- Using the modified Lich-Gregoir technique, the ureter is approximated to the bladder mucosa in a continuous fashion using a 4-0 polydiaxone suture. A 6F, 16 cm double-J stent, introduced through the 12 mm assistant port, is inserted into the ureter after completing the posterior part of the anastomosis
- The detrusor muscle is closed in a continuous fashion using 6-in V-Loc 3-0 CV23 (Fig. 7A), creating an antirefluxing mechanism
- We perform the retroperitonealization prior to ureteroneocystostomy, as it gives us time to observe the graft for any potential kinking or compression of the vessels that might occur during retroperitonealization

Accessory Vessels

- In four of the 50 cases, the graft kidney had an accessory lower pole artery measuring 1.2–1.6 mm in diameter, perfusing greater than 10% of the parenchyma. These were considered unsuitable for bench reconstruction
- Thus, we decided to anastomose the lower pole artery to the recipient inferior epigastric artery (IEA). The recipient IEA is prepared for anastomosis prior to introduction of the kidney. A laparoscopic bulldog clamp is used to occlude the stump, and the distal end is secured (Fig. 7B). The lower pole artery is anastomosed to the IEA using 7-0 or 6-0 prolene sutures (Fig. 7C)

INDICATIONS TO CONVERT TO OPEN PROCEDURE

- Failure to progress
- Inability to maintain graft hypothermia
- Poor quality of vascular anastomoses
- Concerns regarding safety and quality
- Other factors

It must be noted that in none of the patients (n = 50) there arose a need to convert to an open setting[15,16]

EARLY OUTCOMES

- We have reported in detail the outcomes in patients undergoing RKT with regional hypothermia, previously[15,16,19]
- Briefly, in the first of the series of 2 papers, we established the feasibility, safety and reproducibility of the technique and worked out small nuances that made the procedure more efficient[15]
  - With our approach, the kidney is introduced in its ice jacket, lying naturally on the bladder, which provides support, thereby minimizing renal manipulation. And, the close approximation of the graft to the external iliac vessels allows the vessel length for the donor vessels to be shorter than for open KT (OKT), eliminating the need for a vena caval cuff
  - The whole procedure could be performed without the need to reposition the patient side cart, in contrast to the technique described by Giulianotti et al.[12]
  - The magnification and stability provided by the robotic platform allows the performance of precise anastomoses of vessels
  - Graft kidney could be reproducibly cooled to 18–20°C
- Subsequently, in the second paper, we reported that the technical and functional outcomes in patients undergoing RKT with regional hypothermia were similar to those reported in the literature for patients undergoing OKT[16]
  - None of the patients (n = 25) needed dialysis
  - Mean serum creatinine at time of discharge, 1 month and 6 months postoperatively was 1.3, 1.1 and 1.1 mg/dL, respectively
  - No patient developed anastomotic leaks (vascular or urinary), wound complications, or wound infections
  - Two patients underwent re-exploration and one patient died of congestive heart failure (1.5 months postoperatively) due to prior underlying cardiac condition
- Here, for the first time, we present the comparative data from our study
  - We show that early outcomes in the RKT group are equivalent to OKT; with a propensity towards lower complications (Tables 1 and 2), lesser blood loss and postoperative pain (Fig. 8A), quicker graft function recovery (Fig. 8B) and shorter patient convalescence
  - Operative times are longer in the RKT patients.
  - Lymphocele occurrence is significantly reduced in RKT patients (Table 1)
  - In our series, the patients undergoing RKT with regional hypothermia did not experience slower return of graft function (Fig. 8B), in contrast to what was observed by Oberholzer et al. and Modi et al. in their series[13,14]

CONCLUSIONS

The principles of recipient surgery are consistent regardless of whether open, laparoscopic or robotic approach is utilized. The goal is first and foremost the safety of the patient, and second to achieve optimal graft function.

Our initial results are very encouraging. Results from our group and others suggest that the early outcomes achieved with RKT are at par with the outcomes achieved with the conventional open technique, with a propensity towards reduced complications and lower morbidity.

Table 1: Intraoperative outcomes in patients undergoing robotic kidney transplantation with regional hypothermia or traditional open kidney transplantation

Operative parameters	Robotic KT (n = 25)	Open KT (n = 41)	P
Operative time: incision closure (min), mean (SD)	214.1 (39.8)	166.6 (40.1)	< 0.001
Intracorporeal kidney cooling			
Surface temp. (before unclamping; °C), mean (SD)	20.3 (2.9)	18.9 (1.3)	0.009
Blood loss (mL), mean (SD)	151.7 (103.5)	296.8 (183.2)	< 0.001
Intraoperative vascular injuries (Yes: No), No. (%)	0 (0)	0 (0)	1.00
Incision length (cm), mean (SD) [range]	6.1 (0.5) [7.1–5.4]	15.6 (1.1) [17.2–13.4]	< 0.001
Conversion to open, No. (%)	0 (0)	NA	NA

Table 2: Peri- and postoperative outcomes in patients undergoing robotic kidney transplantation with regional hypothermia or traditional open kidney transplantation

Peri- and postoperative parameters	Robotic KT (n = 25)	Open KT (n = 41)	P
Need for dialysis, No. (%)	0 (0)	2 (4.8)	0.52
*Composite complication score, No. (%)**	4 (16.0)	15 (36.6)	0.09
Complications (detail)			
Delayed graft function, No. (%)	0 (0)	0 (0)	1.00
Graft biopsy, No. (%)	4 (16)	8 (19.5)	0.73
Graft vascular thrombosis/stenosis, No. (%)	0 (0)	2 (4.8)	0.52
Rejection episodes			
ACR, No. (%)	1 (4)	3 (7.3)	0.99
AMR, No. (%)	0 (0)	0 (0)	1.00
ACR + AMR, No. (%)	0 (0)	0 (0)	1.00
Wound complications/infections, No. (%)	0 (0)	2 (4.8)	0.52
Re-explorations, No. (%)	2 (8)	3 (7.3)	0.99
NCCT findings at 3 months			
Evidence of lymphocele (perigraft collection), No. (%)	0 (0)	5 (23.8)	0.05
Change in graft position/evidence of torsion, No. (%)	0 (0)	0 (0)	1.00
Graft survival at latest follow-up (6 mo), No. (%)	24 (100)	40 (96)	0.99
Patient survival at latest follow-up (6 mo), No. (%)	24 (96)	41 (100)	0.38

*Composite complication score was calculated based on delayed graft function, graft biopsy, graft vascular thrombosis, rejection incident, wound complication/infections, re-exploration and incidence of lymphocele.

(ACR: Acute cellular rejection; AMR: Antibody mediated rejection; NCCT: Noncontrast computerized tomography; KT: Kidney transplantation)

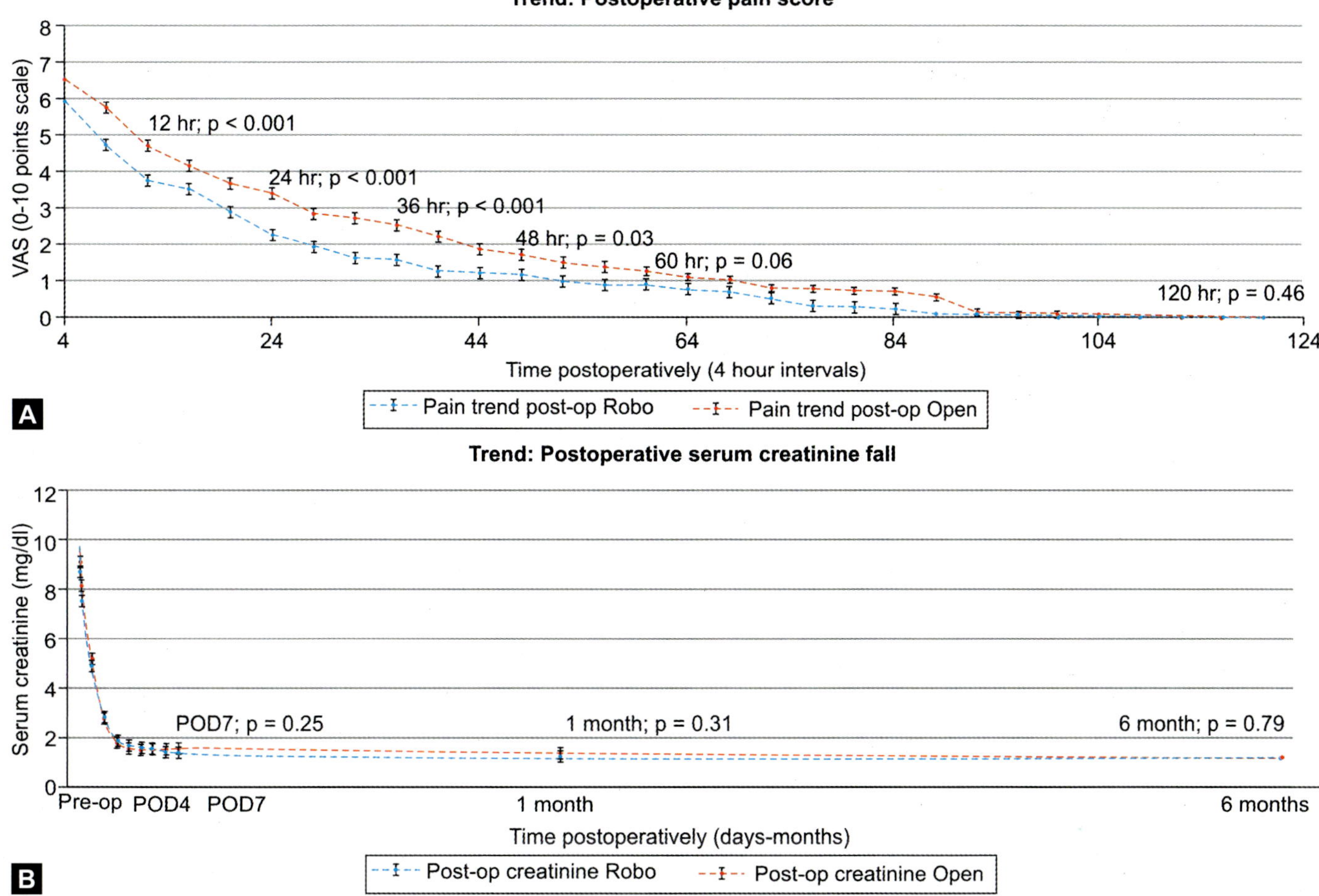

Figs. 8A and B: Trends (A) Postoperative pain; (B) Postoperative creatinine fall.

REFERENCES

1. Trinh QD, Sammon J, Sun M, et al. Perioperative outcomes of robot-assisted radical prostatectomy compared with open radical prostatectomy: results from the nationwide inpatient sample. Eur Urol. 2012;61(4):679-85.
2. Nguyen NT, Goldman C, Rosenquist CJ, et al. Laparoscopic versus open gastric bypass: a randomized study of outcomes, quality of life, and costs. Ann Surg. 2001; 234(3):279-89; discussion 289-91.
3. Park A, Birch DW, Lovrics P. Laparoscopic and open incisional hernia repair: a comparison study. Surgery. 1998;124(4):816-21; discussion 821-2.
4. Park Y, Ha JW. Comparison of one-level posterior lumbar interbody fusion performed with a minimally invasive approach or a traditional open approach. Spine. 2007;32(5):537-43.
5. Romy S, Eisenring MC, Bettschart V, et al. Laparoscope use and surgical site infections in digestive surgery. Ann Surg. 2008;247(4):627-32.
6. Fabrizio MD, Ratner LE, Montgomery RA, et al. Laparoscopic live donor nephrectomy. Urol Clin North Am. 1999;26(1):247-56.
7. Giral-Classe M, Hourmant M, Cantarovich D, et al. Delayed graft function of more than six days strongly decreases long-term survival of transplanted kidneys. Kidney Int. 1998;54(3):972-8.
8. Lynch RJ, Ranney DN, Shijie C, et al. Obesity, surgical site infection, and outcome following renal transplantation. Ann Surg. 2009;250(6):1014-20.
9. Matas AJ, Gillingham KJ, Payne WD, et al. The impact of an acute rejection episode on long-term renal allograft survival (t1/2). Transplantation. 1994;57(6):857-9.
10. Osman Y, Shokeir A, Ali-el-Dein B, et al. Vascular complications after live donor renal transplantation: study of risk factors and effects on graft and patient survival. J Urol. 2003;169(3):859-62.
11. Modi P, Rizvi J, Pal B, et al. Laparoscopic kidney transplantation: an initial experience. Am J Transplant. 2011; 11(6):1320-4.
12. Giulianotti P, Gorodner V, Sbrana F, et al. Robotic transabdominal kidney transplantation in a morbidly obese patient. Am J Transplant. 2010;10(6):1478-82.
13. Modi P, Pal B, Modi J, et al. Retroperitoneoscopic living-donor nephrectomy and laparoscopic kidney transplantation: experience of initial 72 cases. Transplantation. 2013;95(1):100-5.

14. Oberholzer J, Giulianotti P, Danielson KK, et al. Minimally invasive robotic kidney transplantation for obese patients previously denied access to transplantation. Am J Transplant. 2013;13(3):721-8.
15. Menon M, Abaza R, Sood A, et al. Robotic kidney transplantation with regional hypothermia: evolution of a novel procedure utilizing the IDEAL Guidelines (IDEAL Phase 0 and 1). Eur Urol. 2014;65(5):1001-9.
16. Menon M, Sood A, Bhandari M, et al. Robotic kidney transplantation with regional hypothermia: a step-by-step description of the Vattikuti Urology Institute-Medanta Technique (IDEAL Phase 2a). Eur Urol. 2014; 65(5):991-1000.
17. Jeong W, Sood A, Ghani KR, et al. Bimanual examination of the retrieved specimen and regional hypothermia during robot-assisted radical prostatectomy: a novel technique for reducing positive surgical margin and achieving pelvic cooling. BJU Int. 2013.
18. Menon M, Shrivastava A, Kaul S, et al. Vattikuti Institute prostatectomy: contemporary technique and analysis of results. Eur Urol. 2007;51(3):648-57; discussion 657-8.
19. Sood A, Ghani KR, Ahlawat R, et al. Application of the statistical process control method for prospective patient safety monitoring during the learning phase: robotic kidney transplantation with regional hypothermia (IDEAL Phase 2a-b). Eur Urol. 2014;65(6).

CHAPTER 32

Implantation—Ureteroneocystostomy Techniques

Liise Kayler, Ernesto P Molmenti, Stuart Greenstein

LEADBETTER–POLITANO URETERONEOCYSTOSTOMY[1] (FIG. 1)

This *intravesical* technique utilizes one cystostomy to access the interior of the bladder and another cystostomy to recreate a new ureteric orifice in a normal anatomic position. Technique is described as follows:

- Make a 4-cm full-thickness opening in the anterior aspect of the bladder
- Insert a right angle clamp through the opening into the cavity of the bladder and through the superior posterior wall of the bladder. Grasp the transplant ureter with the clamp and pull it into the bladder through the posterior wall hole making sure the ureter has not twisted
- At the site of the posterior wall opening, insinuate a right angle clamp in the submucosal plane posteriorly for a distance of 2–3 cm. Bovie or cut the mucosa over the right angle clamp to make a hole. Use another clamp to backtrack through the submucosal plane, grasp the ureter, and pull it through the submucosal tunnel out the new hole
- Pass a double J stent through the ureter into the renal pelvis
- The button of the ureter is secured with a 4-0 Vicryl interrupted sutures placed in four corners of full-thickness ureter to bladder mucosa/muscularis (additional stitches can be placed if so desired by the surgeon)

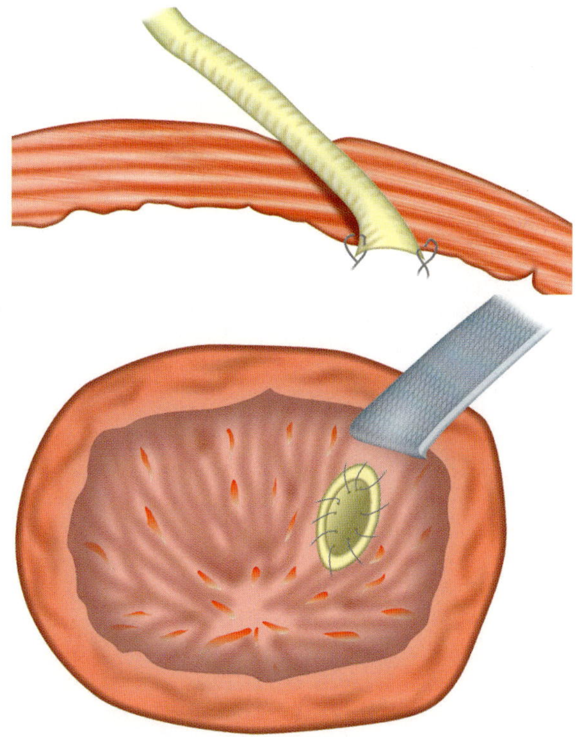

Fig. 1: Politano–Leadbetter intravesical technique:[13] An anterior cystostomy is performed to visualize the interior of the bladder. A retractor is used to flatten the trigone and a circumferential incision is made around the ureteral orifice. A neohiatus is made into which the transplanted ureter is inserted and a submucosal tunnel created. The distal ureter is sutured in place with absorbable sutures and the bladder is closed in two layers.

- At the posterior wall opening, close the bladder mucosa over the ureter (internal aspect) and where the ureter has entered (external aspect), place a single 4-0 Vicryl interrupted full-thickness bladder suture to tighten the opening that the ureter is going through being sure not to constrict the ureter. Usually only one stitch is required
- Close the anterior bladder opening with 3-0 Vicryl running full-thickness bladder sutures

LICH–GREGOIR URETERONEOCYSTOSTOMY[2–4] (FIG. 2)

This *extravesical* technique consists of an anastomosis of the distal ureter to the bladder mucosa that is then buried in a muscular tunnel intended to provide a valve effect. Technique is described as follows:

- Incise the bladder wall musculature at the dome of the bladder for a distance of 2–3 cm to expose the bladder wall mucosa. Make a small incision in the distal mucosa. Trim the ureter to an appropriate length and cut it at an angle (spatulate). With 5-0 absorbable suture, anastomose the full thickness of the ureter to the bladder mucosa in a running or interrupted fashion. Approximate the bladder muscle layer over the ureter for a short distance, enough to create a submucosal tunnel but not so long as to constrict the ureter

Several variations in the Lich–Gregoir implantation have been described, such as the use of running instead of interrupted sutures to create the ureteral mucosal anastomosis,[5–8] performance of a tunnel by submucosal blunt dissection instead of muscular imbrication,[9] placement of a single horizontal Halsted stitch at the proximal apex of the bladder incision to the ureter to prevent

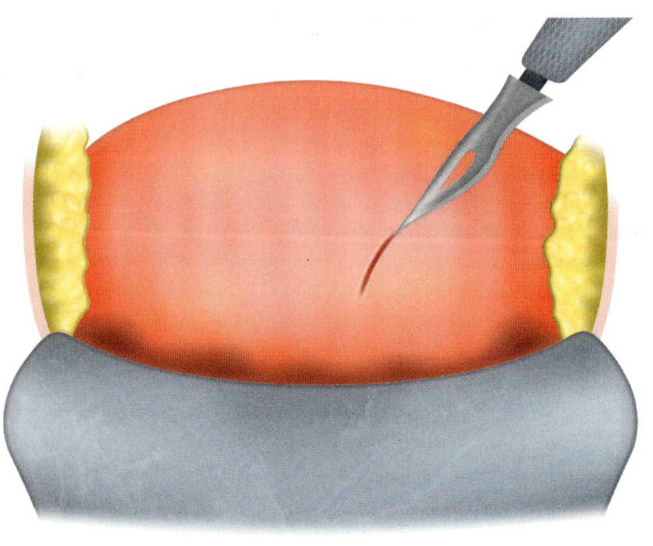

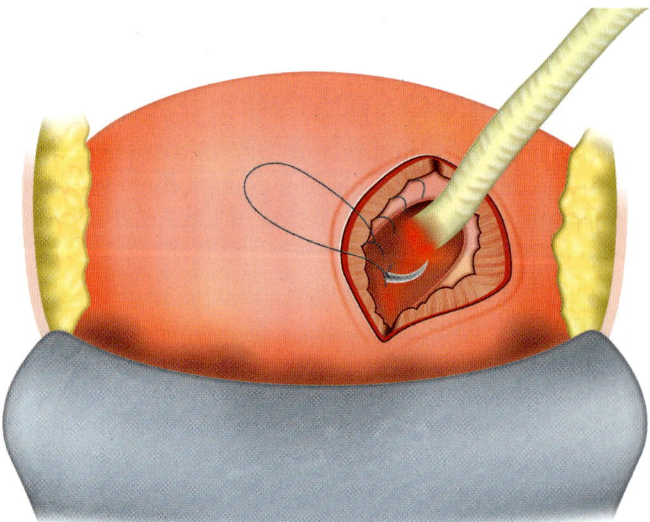

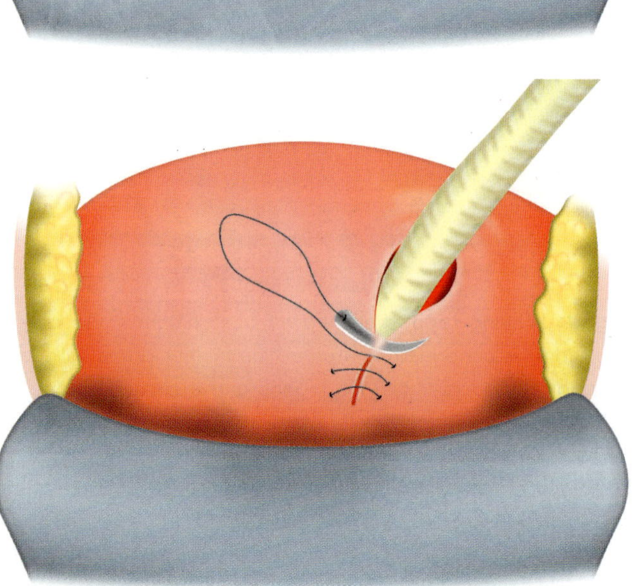

Fig. 2: Lich–Gregoir extravesical technique[16]: An incision is made in the bladder wall musculature at the dome for 2–3 cm to expose mucosa of the bladder wall. A small incision is made in the mucosa. The mucosa of the bladder is then sutured to the ureteral end with interrupted absorbable sutures. The detrusor muscle is then closed over the anastomosis to create a submucosal tunnel with an antireflux mechanism.

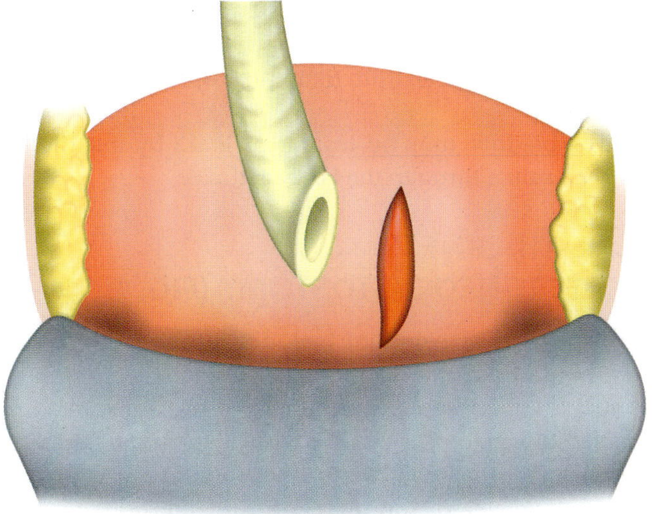

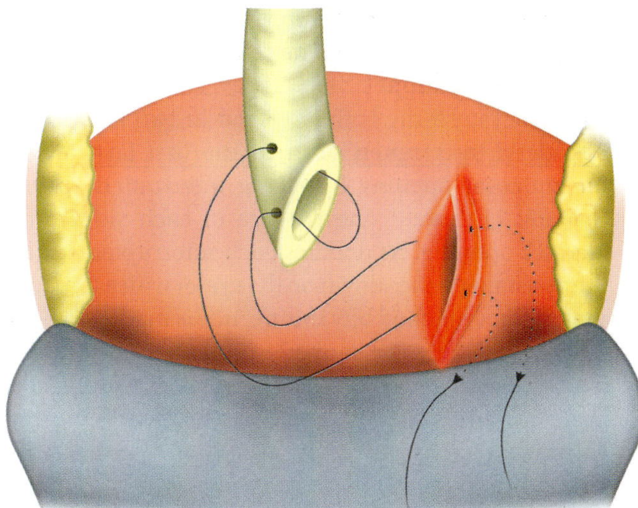

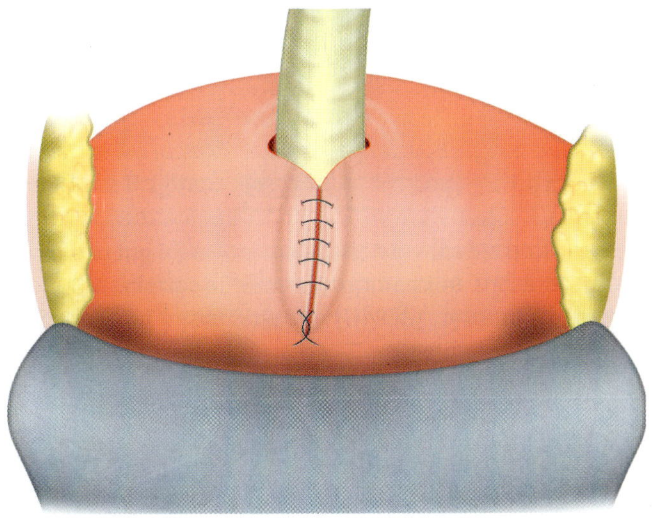

Fig. 3: U stitch technique An incision is made in the bladder wall musculature at the dome for 2–3 cm to expose the mucosa of the bladder wall. An absorbable U stitch is placed on the anterior aspect of the ureter so that each thread comes out into the ureteral lumen. An incision is made in the bladder mucosa. The ureteral end is then brought through the bladder mucosa after each thread is passed through and taken out through the bladder 2 cm distal to the caudal edge of the ureteral orifice. The U stitch is then tied, anchoring the ureteral end against the inside of the bladder. The detrusor muscle is then closed over the anastomosis to create a submucosal tunnel with an anti-reflux mechanism.

tension at the acute angle of the anastomosis,[8] placement of an anchor stitch on the distal ureteral tip to the full of the bladder,[10] folding back the tip of the ureter to make a "terminal cuff,"[11] and incorporation of the muscular layer with the mucosal layer of the bladder in the anastomosis.[9,12]

THE U STITCH URETERONEOCYSTOSTOMY (FIG. 3)

This extravesical technique was described separately by Shanfield[13] and Taguchi[14]: The ureter is spatulated, passed through the bladder opening, and the sutures taken out through the anterior bladder wall so that the ureteral end is anchored to the inner bladder wall (Fig. 3). The technique described by Shanfield uses only one stitch for the bladder attachment placed at the distal aspect of the ureter; whereas that described by Taguchi uses two stitches at the distal aspect of the ureter. Description of technique is as follows:

- Make an opening on the anterior surface of the bladder not more than 1 cm in size
- Shorten and spatulate the ureter (approximately 1 cm spatulation) and place a 2-0 double arm absorbable suture. Drive one needle inside-out near the tip of the spatulation. Drive the other needle inside-out near the posterior crux (pulling up on the sutures will result in a rose petal)
- Drive both needles separately through the cavity of bladder, inside-out of the bladder wall 1.5 cm from the opening and 3 mm apart. To assist in driving the needles through the bladder, grasp the free wall of bladder at the level of the opening with an Alice clamp to put tension on the bladder

- The two ends of this suture are then pulled up and tied, and a clamp is left on the tie to act a marker for later creation of the tunnel
- The neocystostomy is then closed in two layers with 3-0 Vicryl interrupted sutures. The first layer closes the mucosal opening by taking interrupted sutures (usually 2) through the mucosa of each side of the bladder opening. As one ties each interrupted suture, the assistant pushes down on the ureter with a forcep so that it is not pinched buy this tie, nor is made too tight. The second layer is also made using 3-0 Vicryl suture placing interrupted Lembert stitches (seromuscular layer of the bladder) to cover the original 2-0 Vicryl suture marked by the clamp (which is removed at this point) and to cover the bladder mucosa. Again care is taken not to tighten too much close to the ureter too prevent stenosis. A double J stent may be placed into the ureter prior to pulling it inside the bladder to aid in preventing one from tightening up too much on the ureter
- The bladder may be tested for leaks by insufflating with saline through the Foley catheter

FULL-THICKNESS URETERONEOCYSTOSTOMY (FIG. 4)

This extravesical technique includes suturing the spatulated ureter directly to the bladder without any attempt to tunnel it.[15-18] Lucas et al.[16] and Woodruff et al.[15] separately performed this method as an intravesical technique utilizing parallel incisions and performance of the ureterovesical anastomosis of the ureter to the "muscularis" from

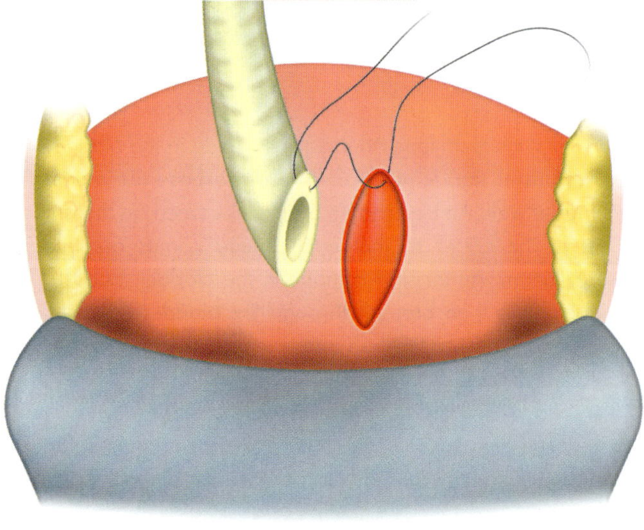

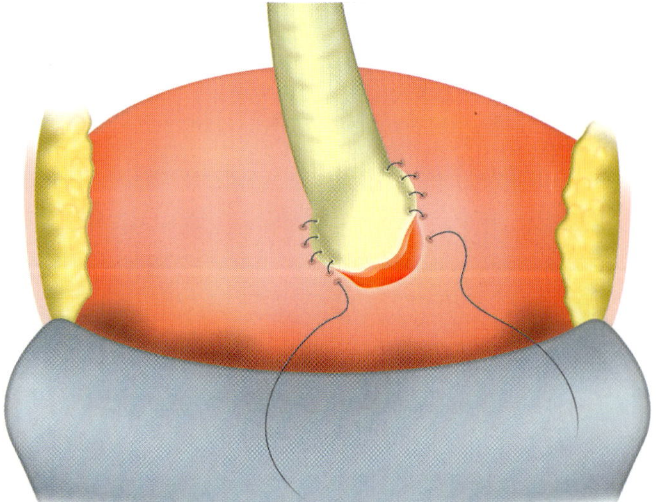

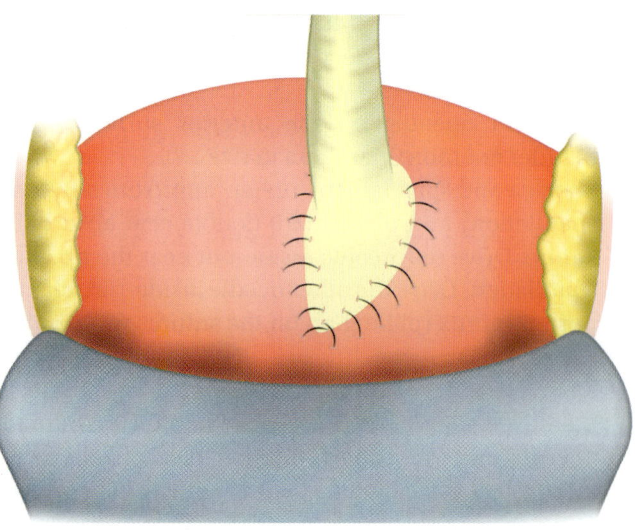

Fig. 4: Full-thickness technique (Molmenti–Kayler). A cystostomy is made through all layers of the bladder. The spatulated ureter is continuously sutured to the full-thickness of the bladder (mucosa, musculature and serosa) using absorbable suture. There is no additional closure of the bladder muscle layer over the anastomosis.

inside the bladder. Starzl[17] took a more direct approach through a single cystostomy and sutured the ureteral mucosa to the bladder mucosa. Molmenti and Kayler[18-20] described a simple approach of suturing the ureter to the full thickness of the bladder and that technique is described herein:

- Make a 1-cm full-thickness incision in the anterior aspect of the bladder
- Shorten and spatulate the ureter
- Place 5-0 polyglyconate sutures at the corners of the ureter and bladder and tie down the sutures
- Anastomose the full thickness of the ureter using 2–3 mm bites to the full thickness of the bladder making sure to incorporate bladder mucosa into each bite

REFERENCES

1. Politano VA, Leadbetter WF. An operative technique for the correction of vesicoureteral reflux. J Urol 1958; 79:932.
2. Witzel O. Extraperitoneale ureterocystostomie mit Schragkanalbildung. Zentralbl Gynakol 1986; 11:289–93.
3. Gregoir W. Le reflux vesico-ureteral congenital. Acta urol Belg 1962; 30:286.
4. Lich R, Hoverton LW, Davis LA. Recurrent urosepsis in children. J Urol 1961; 86:554–8.
5. Veale JL, Yew J, Gjertson DW, et al. Long-term comparative outcomes between 2 common ureteroneocystostomy techniques for renal transplantation. J Urol 2007; 177: 632–6.
6. Secin FP, Rovegno AR, Marrugat RE, et al. Comparing Taguchi and Lich-Gregoir ureterovesical reimplantation techniques for kidney transplants. J Urol 2002; 168: 926–30.
7. Woodruff M, Robson JS, Nolan B, et al. Renal transplantation in man. Lancet 1969; 1:6–12.
8. McDonald JC, Rohr MS, Frentz GD. External ureterocystostomy and ureteroureterostomy in renal transplantation. Ann Surg 1979; 190:663–7.
9. Barry JM. Unstented extravesical ureteroneocystostomy in kidney transplantation. J Urol 1983; 129:918–9.
10. Cos Lr, Light JA, Stutzman RE. External ureteroneocystostomy in renal transplantation. Urology 1985; 26:362.
11. Paquin AJ Jr. Ureterovesical anastomosis: the description and evaluation of a technique. J Urol 1959; 82:573–83.
12. Konnak JW, Herwig KR, Finkbeiner A, et al. Extravesical ureteroneocystostomy in 170 renal transplant patients. J Urol 1975; 113:299–301.
13. Schanfield I. New experimental methods for implantation of the ureter in bladder and conduit. Transplant Proc 1972; 4:637–8.
14. MacKinnon KJ, Oliver JA, Morehouse DD, et al. Cadaver renal transplantation: emphasis on urological aspects. J Urol 1968; 99:486.
15. Lucas BA, McRoberts JW, Curtis JJ, et al. Controversy in renal transplantation: antireflux versus non-antireflux ureteroneocystostomy. J Urol 1979;121:156.
16. Woodruff MW, Bachrach P, Corica A, et al. Ureteroneocystostomy in renal transplantation. Urology 1973; 1:414.
17. Starzl TE, Shapiro R, Tzakis A, et al. A new technique of extravesical ureteroneocystostomy for renal transplantation. Transplant Proc 1989; 21:3856–8.
18. Kayler LK, Zendejas I, Molmenti E, et al. Kidney transplant ureteroneocystostomy: comparison of full-thickness vs. Lich-Gregoir techniques. Clin Transplant 2012; 26:E372–80.
19. Glazer ES, Benedict K, Akhavanheidari M, et al. Living donor renal transplant recipients tolerate early removal of bladder catheters. Int J Angiol 2009; 18:67–8.
20. Glazer ES, Akhavanheidari M, Benedict K, et al. Cadaveric renal transplant recipients can safely tolerate removal of bladder catheters within 48 h of transplant. Int J Angiol 2009; 18:69–70.

CHAPTER 33

Implantation—Ureteroureterostomy and Ureteropyelostomy

Liise Kayler, Ernesto P Molmenti, Stuart Greenstein

- Both of these approaches are carried out:
  - In instances of
    - Ureteral strictures
    - Urinary leaks
  - Preferably in an ipsilateral fashion
  - In recipients with healthy native ureters
  - Significant properative reflux must be ruled out in the native ureter
- The choice of Ureteroureterostomy (UU) or Ureteropyelostomy (UP) is based on the level of ureteral involvement:
  - UU is an option for lower or mid ureter disease
  - UP is an option for any level of disease
- Prior to starting the procedure, some surgeons perform a cystoscopy with placement of a stent in the native ureter
- This ensures patency and easier intraoperative access of the native ureter
- In most cases, the transplanted kidney has a percutaneous nephrostomy (and potentially a stent) in place
  - This allows for easier identification of the transplant renal pelvis and ureter
- The peritoneum is entered via:
  - Reopening the transplant incision
  - A lower midline incision
- The native ureter is adherent to the posterior peritoneum and can be identified as it crosses the iliac vessels
  - It should be mobilized as far proximally as possible so to create a tension-free anastomosis (may require mobilization of the colon)
  - The fascia and tissues surrounding it should be preserved to prevent ischemia
- The injured donor ureter is carefully identified and dissected, making sure not to denude it
- Once the native ureter has been mobilized proximally enough, it is transected and its end toward the native nonfunctioning kidney tied
- In instances where the native ureter is considered not satisfactory for the reconstruction (such as when it is not patent or not viable), the contralateral ureter can be used
- The transplant kidney can be mobilized if necessary:
  - Left donor kidneys transplanted to the right iliac fossa and right kidneys transplanted to the left iliac fossa have their pelvises exposed medially and require minimal mobilization
  - Right kidneys transplanted to the right iliac fossa and left kidneys transplanted to left iliac fossa have laterally located pelvises and usually require some mobilization to expose their pelvises or ureteropelvic junctions
- The site for the UU or UP anastomosis can be identified as follows:
  - Hydronephrotic kidneys with medially located renal pelvises can usually be easily identified
  - In instances where a percutaneous nephrostomy is within the renal pelvis, saline can be infused via the nephrostomy tube to cause the pelvis to bulge
  - A syringe with a small needle (preferably a TB needle) can be used to aspirate the bulging area and ensure that the urinary system is accessed without injuring the surrounding hilar vessels

- After transecting the diseased transplant ureter (and tying the distal end), a probe (such as a coronary dilator) can be inserted into the proximal ureter and followed by palpation to the desired location
- Identification of the ureter is easier in the early post-transplantation when adhesions are soft. With time, adhesions become firmer and identification usually requires a combination of blunt and sharp dissection

- Once the site of the anastomosis has been identified and exposed, the native ureter is brought next to the transplant ureter or pelvis making certain that there is mobility and no tension

UP ANASTOMOSIS (FIG. 1)

- The native ureter is spatulated and anastomosed in an end-to-side fashion onto a 5–6 mm incision on the transplant renal pelvis with running (or alternatively interrupted) 5-0 synthetic absorbable sutures
- The back wall is sutured first
- A double-J stent can be placed if desired by the surgeon or if recommended based on the specific case
- The front wall is subsequently completed

UU ANASTOMOSIS (FIG. 2)

- The native and donor ureters are spatulated for approximately 5–6 mm
- The spatulated ureteral ends are anastomosed by first placing a 6-0 synthetic absorbable suture through the corner of one ureteral segment and the apex of the other, tying on the outside of the lumen
- A second suture is placed in the opposite corner and apex and also tied outside of the lumen
- The anastomosis is completed by running the two sutures and tying them to each other
  - Alternatively, it can be done with interrupted sutures
- A double-J stent can be placed if desired by the surgeon or if recommended based on the specific case
- The abdomen is then closed
- A drain can be left in place
- Postoperatively the native kidney (if still functional) can become somewhat hydronephrotic. This is usually self-limiting

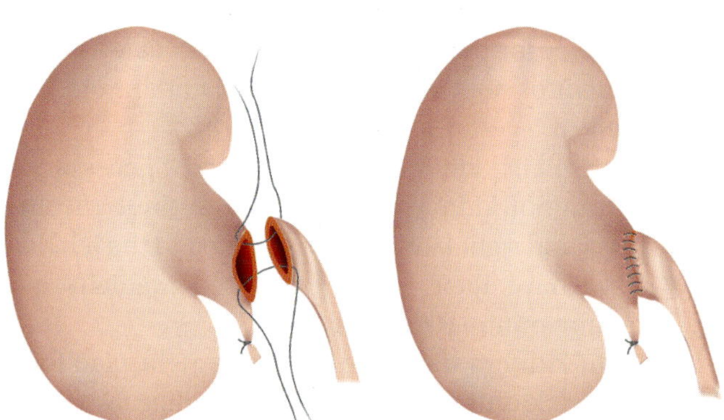

Fig. 1: Anastomosis between the transplant renal pelvis and the recipient native ureter—Ureteropyelostomy technique.

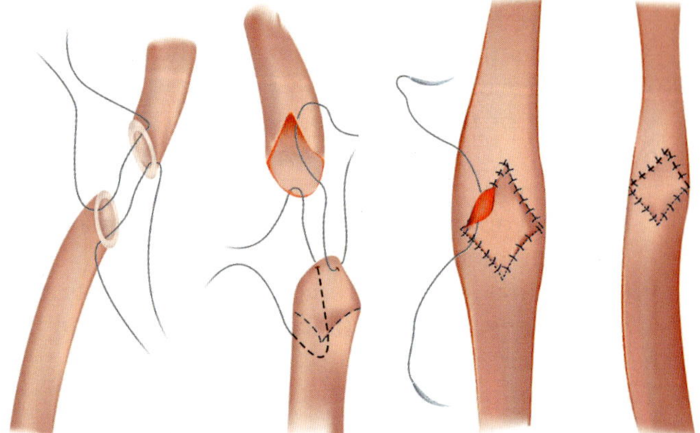

Fig. 2: Anastomosis between the transplant ureter and the recipient native ureter—Ureteroureterostomy technique.

CHAPTER 34

Implantation—Unilateral Dual Kidney Transplantation Technique

Liise Kayler

INTRODUCTION

- This technique is usually employed in cases of severe atherosclerosis of the recipient vessels
- It requires only one anastomotic site

EN BLOC TECHNIQUE

- This technique requires the kidneys to be preserved en bloc (not separated) at the time of procurement
- In addition to the usual back table preparation, the nonrenal branches of the inferior vena cava (IVC) and aorta are tied
- The suprarenal IVC and aorta are stapled or oversewn
- The inferior orifices of the IVC and aorta are anastomosed end-to-side to the external iliac vein and artery
- After perfusion, the kidneys are positioned facing each other

COMBINATION TECHNIQUE (FIG. 1)

- This technique is useful in cases where the en bloc technique is not feasible (due to prior separation of the kidneys or inadequate aortic or IVC conduit), yet a single arterial and/or venous anastomoses is desirable
- The location of the anastomoses is determined based on the status of the recipient vessels and the type of donor renal vessels available to perform the vascular reconstruction
- An arterial Y-graft and a venous graft are prepared with the donor iliac artery and vein
- The right donor renal artery is anastomosed in the back table to the internal iliac artery of the Y-graft in an end-to-end fashion
- The right donor renal vein is anastomosed in an end-to-side fashion onto the mid portion of the donor venous graft
- The left donor renal artery is subsequently anastomosed in an end-to-end fashion onto the external iliac artery of the Y-graft
- The left donor renal vein is anastomosed in an end-to-end fashion onto the end of the venous graft

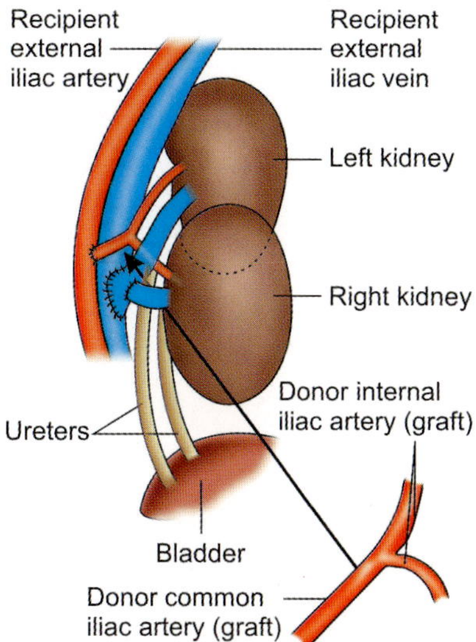

Fig. 1: Unilateral dual kidney transplantation with single recipient arterial and venous anastomoses.

- The common iliac artery and vein grafts (with both kidneys attached to them) are anastomosed onto the recipient iliac artery and vein
- Ureteroneocystostomies can be performed separately (right ureter lateral to left) or together

FURTHER READING

1. Kayler LK, Shapiro R, Molmenti E. Transplantation of dual adult kidneys into a recipient with minimal abdominal vascular access. Transplantation 2007; 83:827–8.

CHAPTER 35

Implantation—Other Variants

Ernesto P Molmenti and Collaborators

INTRODUCTION

- Sometimes factors associated with donors and/or recipients require variations technical
- Below are some examples
- It is up to the transplant team to determine the best approach

EXTERNAL ILIAC ARTERY AND VEIN INTERPOSITION (FIGS. 1 TO 4)

This technique is useful in instances where there is a short transplant renal vein, such as in right kidney grafts from live donors, right kidney grafts from deceased donors where a reconstruction is not desired or possible, or organs with arterial or venous injuries that cannot be reconstructed.

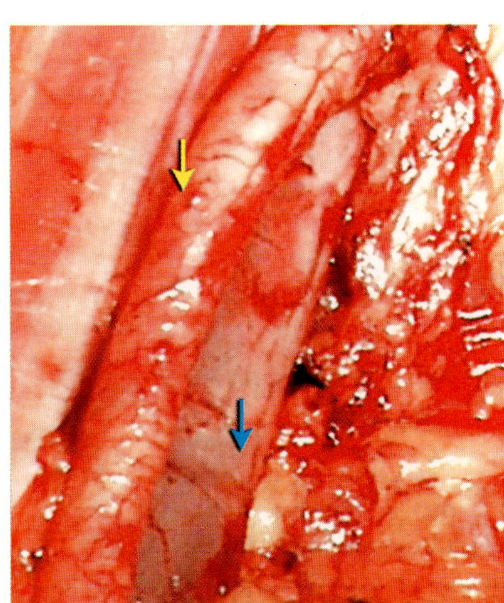

Fig. 1: The external iliac vessels are dissected in their entire length. In this specific example, it is possible to view the right external iliac artery (yellow arrow) and vein (blue arrow) of the recipient in their usual position, with the artery lateral and ventral with respect to the vein.

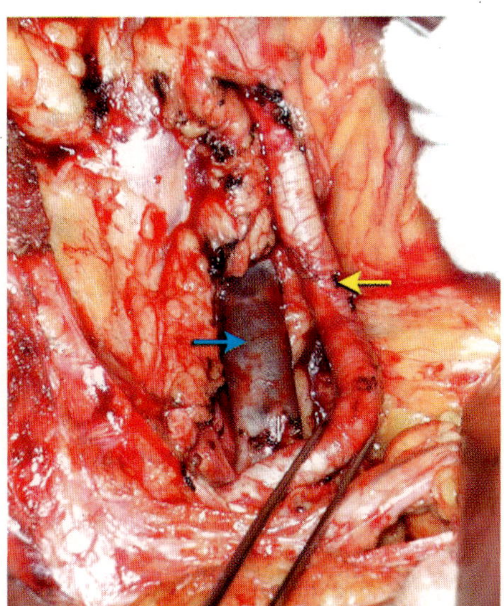

Fig. 2: Once the vessels have been dissected and mobility achieved, the external iliac artery (yellow arrow) is interposed medial to the external iliac vein (light blue arrow). If this is not possible, the internal iliac vein can be ligated and transected in order to obtain further length and mobility.

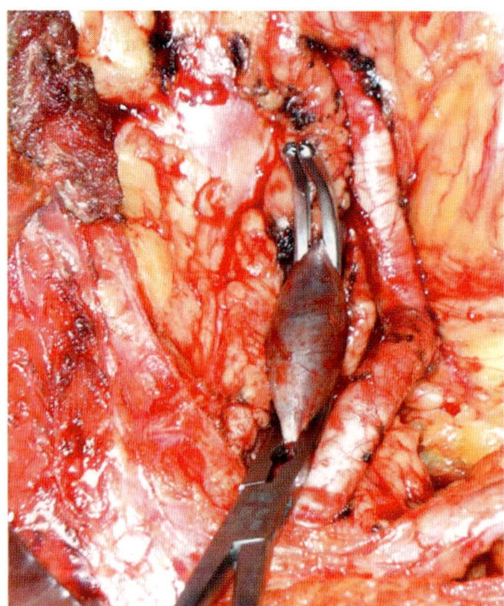

Fig. 3: The implantation technique is subsequently undertaken.

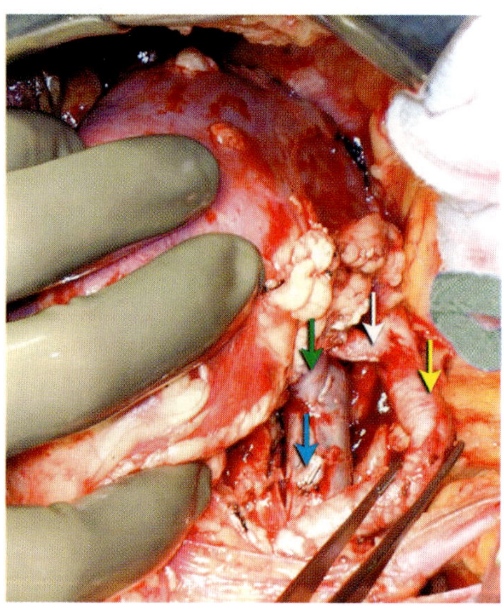

Fig. 4: After the kidney is reperfused, all vessels lie in a comfortable position. Note the external iliac artery (yellow arrow) and vein (blue arrow), as well as the transplant renal artery (white arrow) and vein (green arrow). As in all transplants, the kidney should be positioned in such a way so that the vessels and ureter lie in a comfortable position, without any twist, kinks, or compressions.

IMPLANTATION OF THE TRANSPLANT RENAL VEIN ONTO THE RECIPIENT IVC (FIGS. 5 AND 6)

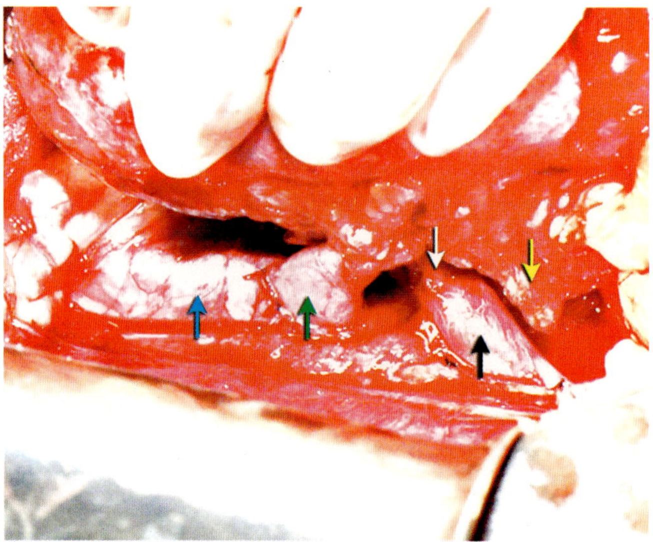

Fig. 5: Note in this right-sided view the inferior vena cava (IVC) (blue arrow), transplant renal vein (green arrow), transplant renal artery (white arrow), recipient iliac artery (black arrow) and periureteral tissues (yellow arrow).

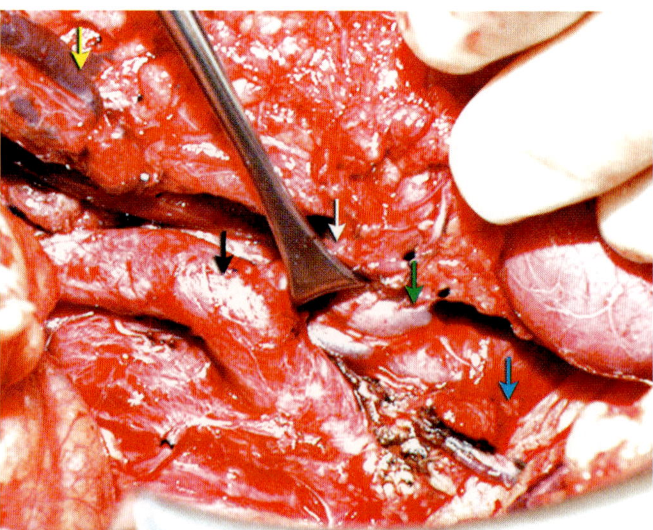

Fig. 6: In this view from the left side of the recipient, note the inferior vena cava (IVC) (blue arrow), transplant renal vein (green arrow), transplant renal artery (white arrow), recipient iliac artery (black arrow) and periureteral tissues (yellow arrow), where the donor gonadal vessels can also be seen.

In instances where the renal vein is very short (and no venous graft is desired or available), implantation of the kidney may be facilitated by anastomosing the renal vein onto the recipient inferior vena cava (IVC).

TWO FOR ONE KIDNEYS—IMPLANTATION OF TWO DONOR KIDNEYS (FIGS. 7 TO 13)

In instances where two kidneys are transplanted (such as in cases where a single kidney is not considered to provide adequate function), the surgeon must decide whether to implant them ipsilaterally or contralaterally.

- Ipsilateral Implantation (Figs. 7 to 10)
  - In instances of ipsilateral placement, both kidneys are attached onto the external iliac artery and

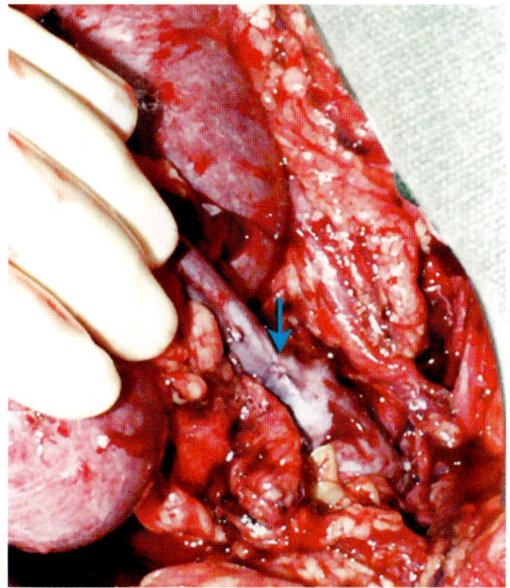

Fig. 7: View of the distal kidney allograft being held by the surgeon. The blue arrow shows the donor renal vein.

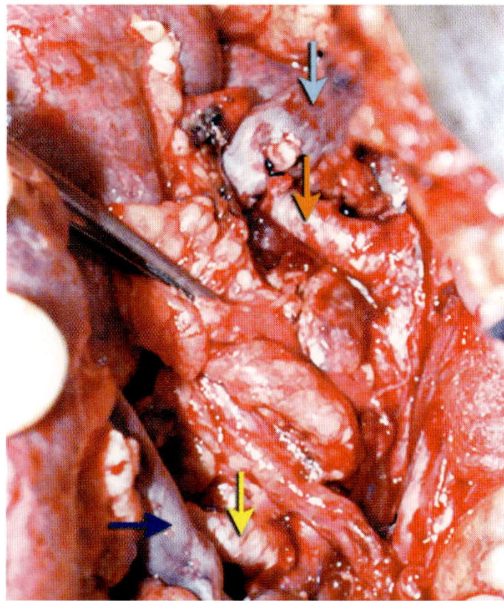

Fig. 8: View of the anastomoses of both allografts. The orange and light blue arrows show the renal artery and vein of the proximal allograft. The corresponding vessels of the distal allograft (that was implanted after the proximal one) are shown with yellow and dark blue arrows.

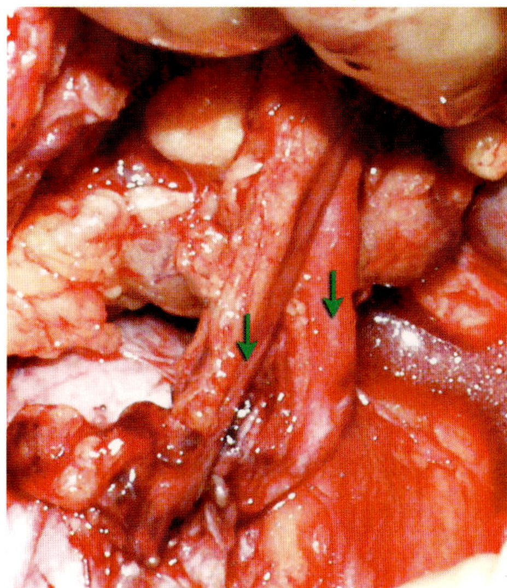

Fig. 9: The two ureters (arrows) are implanted independently onto the bladder. Alternatively, they can be joined distally and implanted onto a common opening in the bladder.

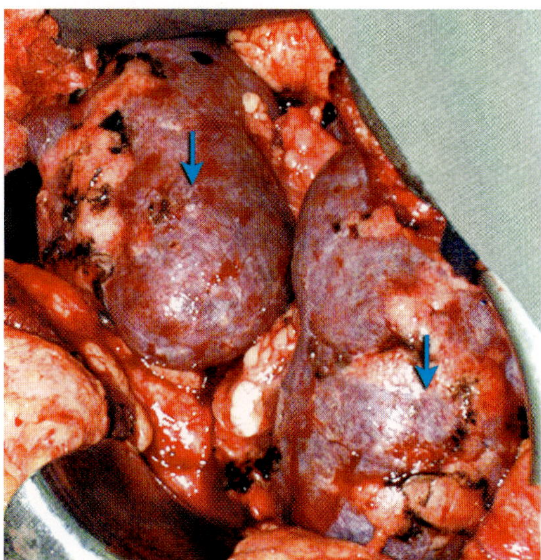

Fig. 10: Both kidneys (arrows) can be seen lying in the iliac fossa. The allografts are positioned in order for the blood vessels and ureters to lie in a comfortable position without kinks or twists. As in all transplants, we routinely obtain a Doppler-duplex ultrasound examination in the recovery room immediately after the surgery in order to verify that there is adequate flow and no evidence of hydronephrosis.

external iliac vein of the chosen side. The proximal kidney should be implanted and reperfused first. Once this is done, the distal one can be implanted. This sequence will prevent ischemia of either allograft, since the clamping of the external iliac artery when performing the distal arterial anastomosis will not affect the previously implanted allograft

- Contralateral Implantation (Figs. 11 to 13)
  - The kidneys are implanted onto the right and left lower quadrants, one on each side

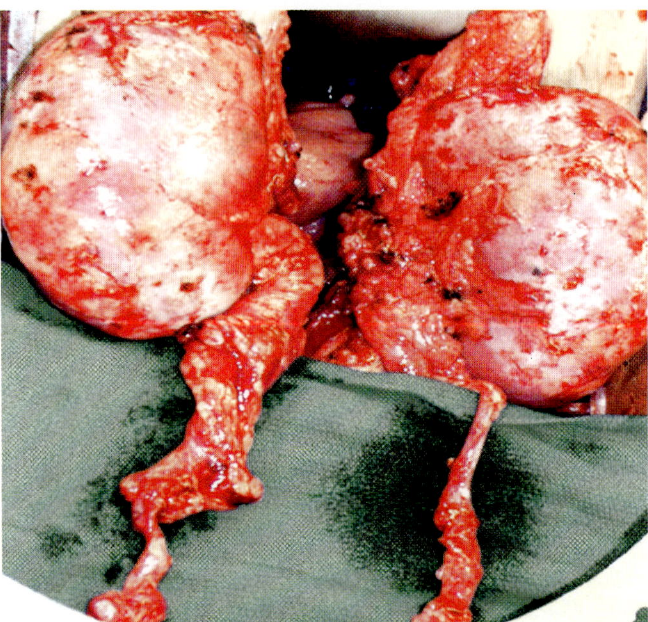

Fig. 11: A midline incision allowed for the intra-abdominal placement of both kidneys. Alternatively, two separate lower quadrant incisions can be undertaken in order to allow the retroperitoneal placement of the allografts. The ureters are implanted onto the bladder, either independently or as a common conduit.

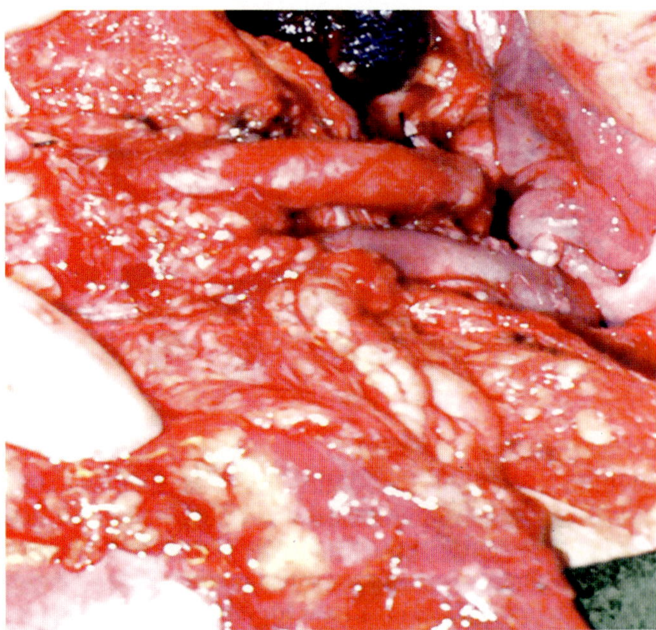

Fig. 12: View of the renal allograft vessels implanted onto the right external iliac vessels.

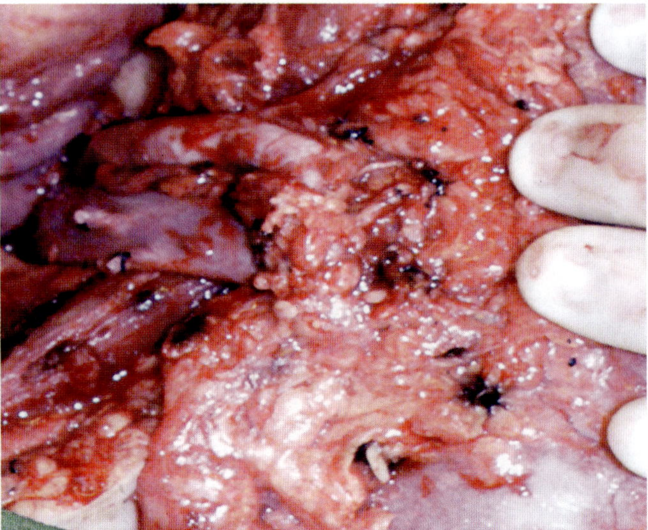

Fig. 13: View of the renal allograft vessels implanted onto the left external iliac vessels.

DOUBLE URETER—IMPLANTATION (FIGS. 14 TO 22)

- A double ureter in the donor can be addressed in a variety of ways

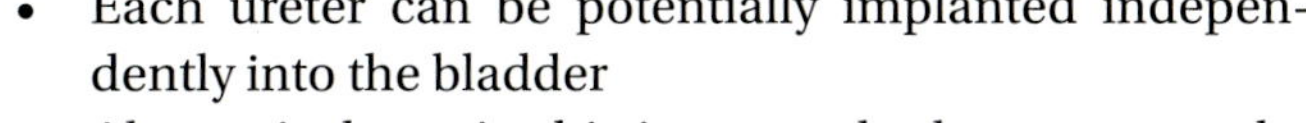

- Each ureter can be potentially implanted independently into the bladder

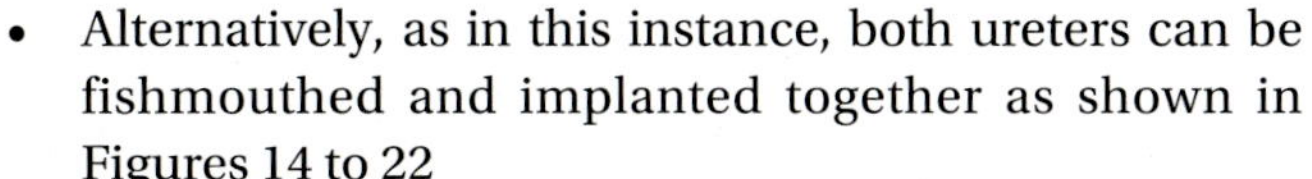

- Alternatively, as in this instance, both ureters can be fishmouthed and implanted together as shown in Figures 14 to 22

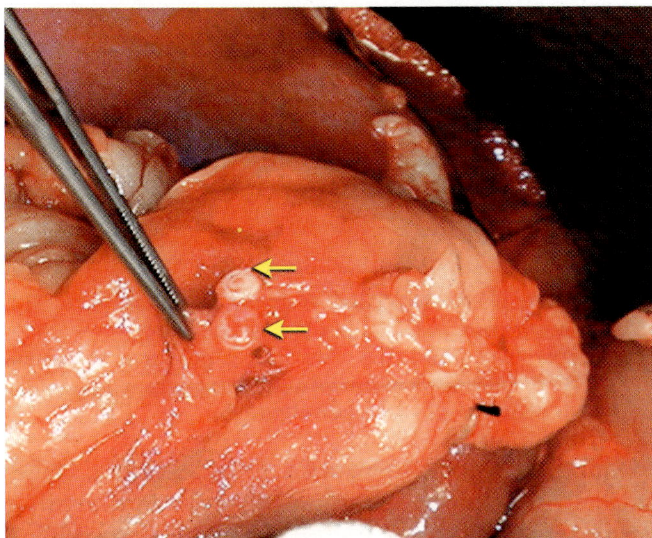

Fig. 14: A double ureter (arrows) is identified in the donor kidney.

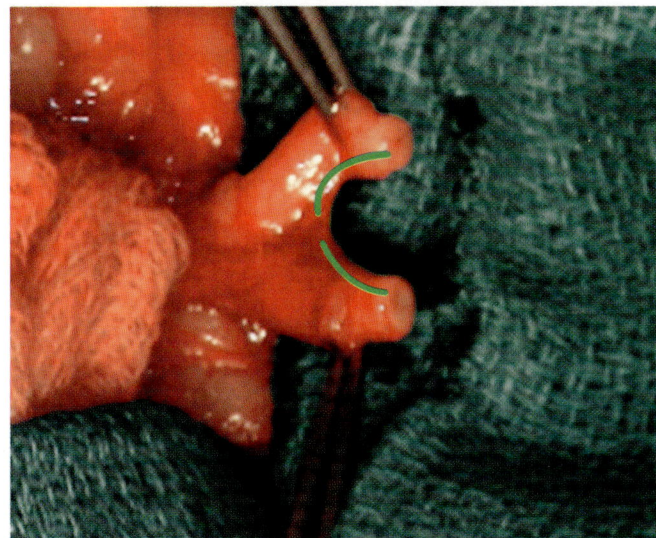

Fig. 15: The ureters are minimally dissected and separated only enough to allow for the anastomosis of their distal ends. Subsequently, they will be incised along their internal borders for a distance of a few millimeters (markings).

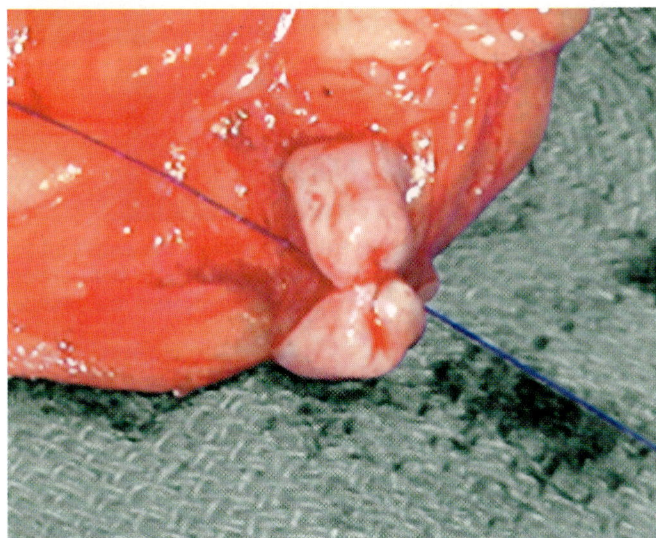

Fig. 16: A corner stitch is placed at the base of the incision with full-thickness bites of both ureters. We routinely use a 5-0 absorbable monofilament suture material.

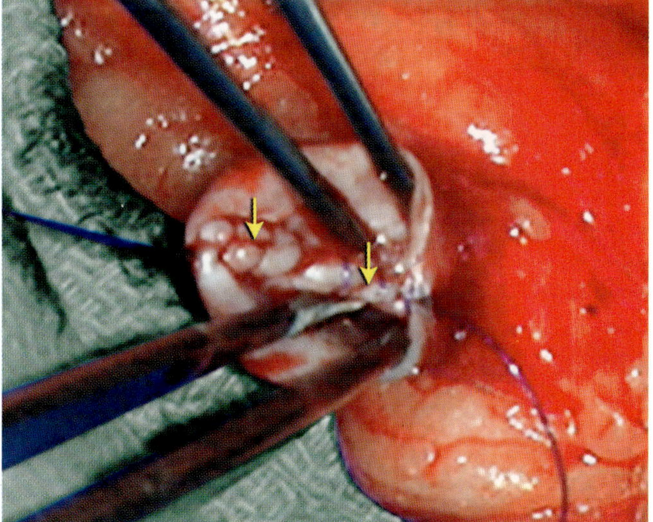

Fig. 17: A fishmouth anastomosis (arrows) is subsequently constructed with running (or interrupted) sutures, creating a common opening for both ureters.

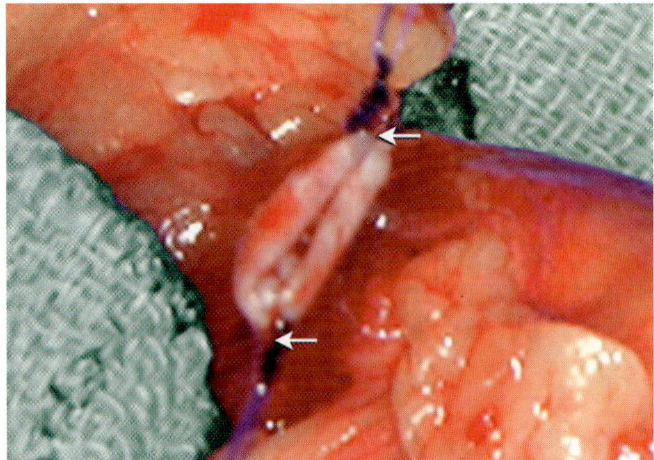

Fig. 18: The anastomosed ureters are ready for implantation. We preserve the corner stitches (arrows) in order to maneuver the graft and as a way to maintain an orientation and minimize the risk of kinks and twists.

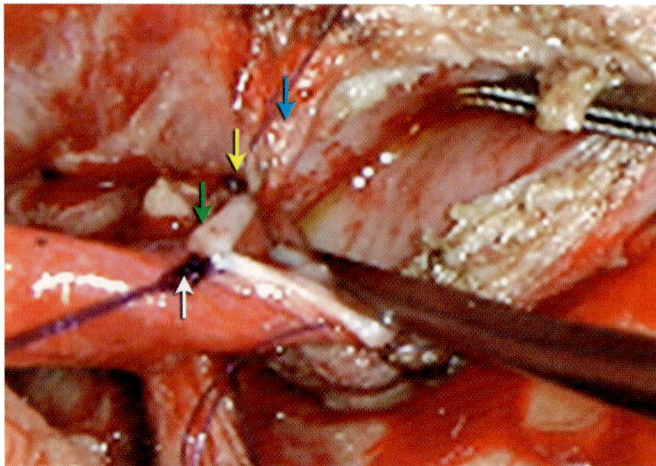

Fig. 19: The bladder is incised. A corner stitch (yellow arrow) is placed encompassing full-thickness bites of both ureter (green arrow) and bladder (blue arrow). The ureter stitch is positioned so to leave the previous sutures (white arrow)—used to perform the ureteral fishmouth anastomosis—in a lateral position.

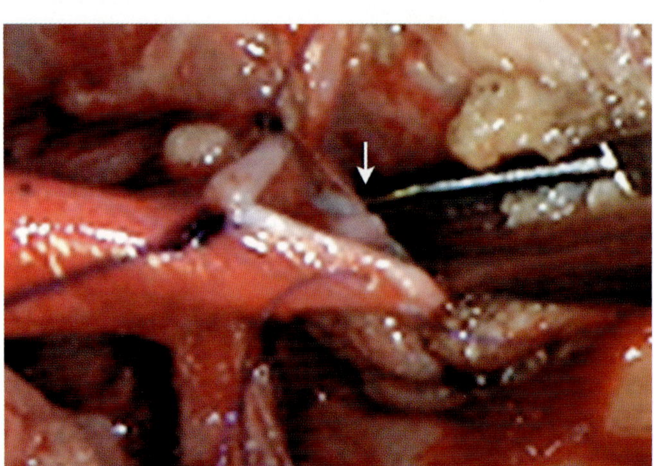

Fig. 20: One side of the anastomosis (white arrow) is completed.

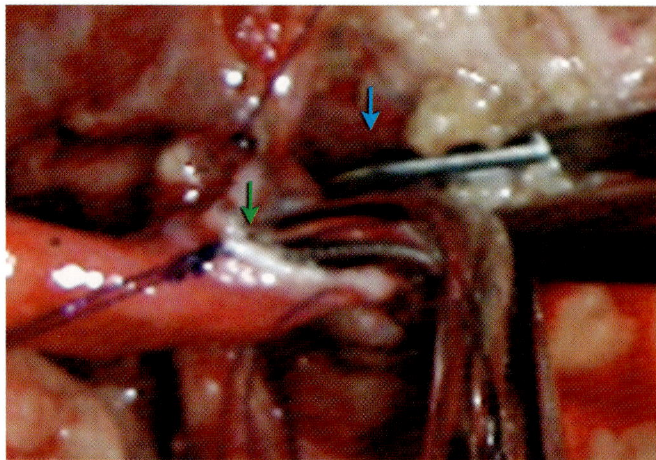

Fig. 21: Prior to constructing the other side of the anastomosis, with a right angled clamp we verify for patency in both ureters (green arrow), while with a forceps we verify that the bladder entrance is patent (blue arrow).

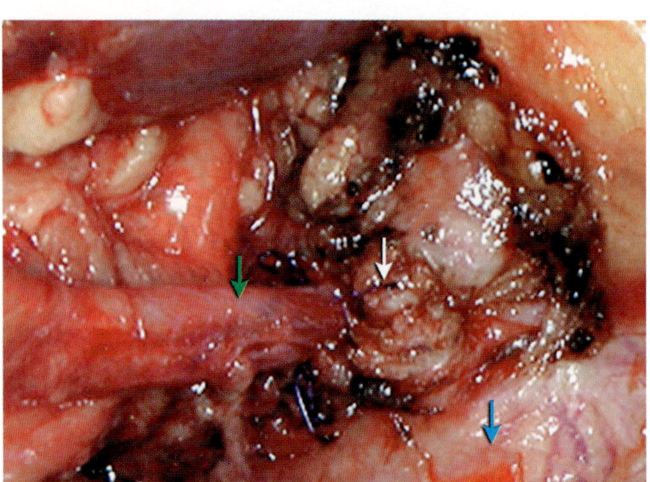

Fig. 22: The anastomosis (white arrow) is finalized. A separate stent can be placed in each of the two ureters. In order to prevent any strictures or unwanted kinks, we do not construct an antireflux mechanism. The ureter (green arrow) and bladder (blue arrow) show no gross signs of pathology.

IMPLANTATION OF THE URETER ONTO AN AUGMENTED BLADDER (FIGS. 23 TO 26)

Recipients on occasions have undergone bladder augmentation procedures in the past

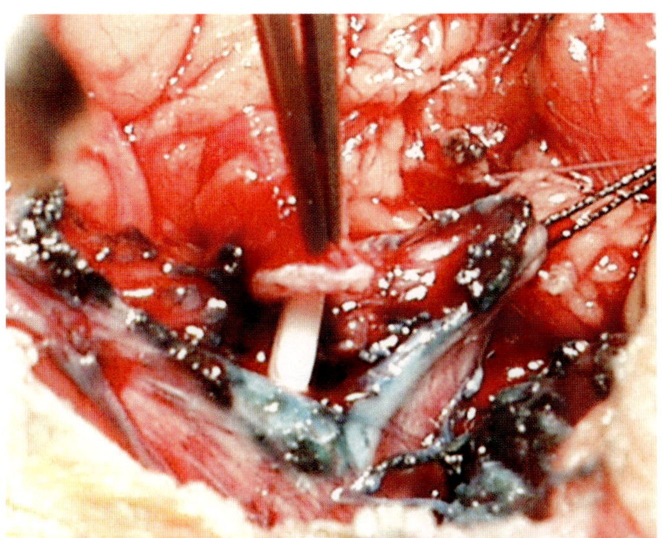

Fig. 23

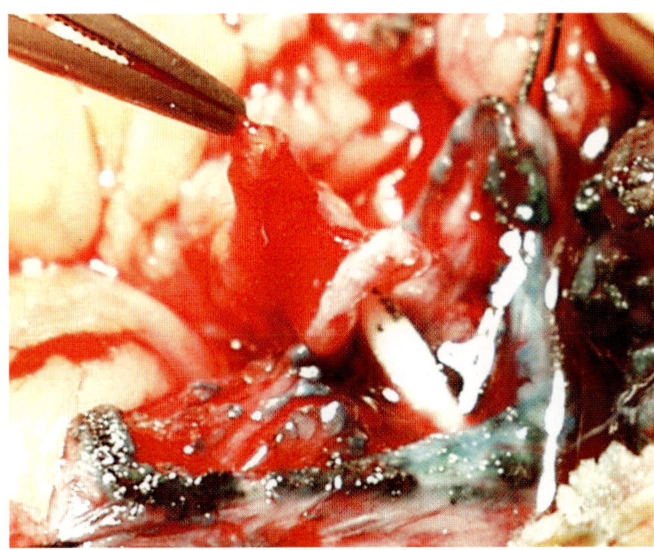

Fig. 24

Figs. 23 and 24: In this specific case, the bladder had been augmented with colon. Methylene blue had been infused into the bladder in order to aid in its identification. The augmenting colonic tissue of the bladder was then incised. The ureter was trimmed to an adequate length and slightly spatulated. A stent was placed into the transplant ureter going into the bladder.

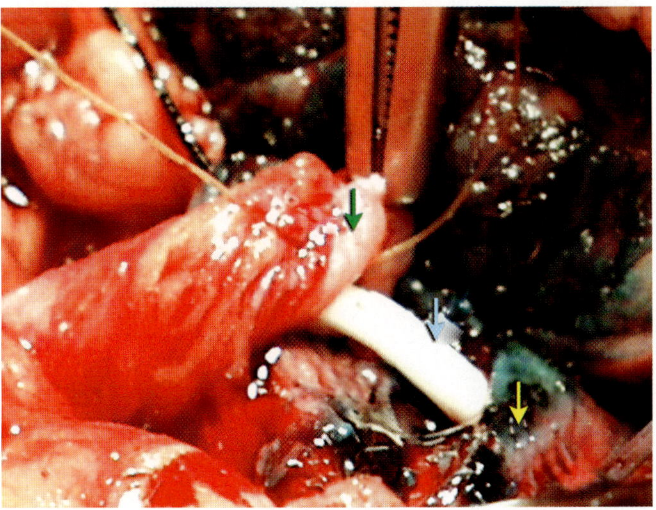

Fig. 25

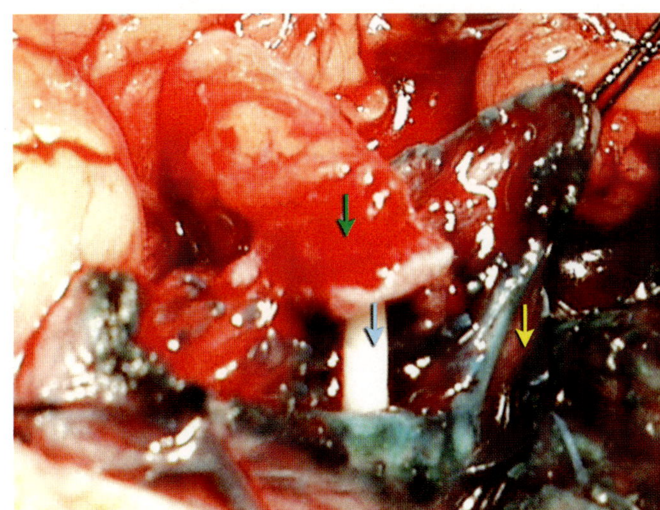

Fig. 26

Figs. 25 and 26: With the assistance of the Urology Service, the ureter (green arrows) was implanted into the augmenting colonic tissue (yellow arrows). A ureteral stent (blue arrows) was used in the reconstruction. Using resorbable sutures, the ureter was anastomosed onto the augmented bladder. The ureter was subsequently removed 6 weeks later by cystoscopy.

POLYCYSTIC KIDNEYS (FIGS. 27 AND 28)

Polycystic kidney disease is a cause of renal failure leading to transplantation. On occasions, the kidneys reach large size, as the ones shown in the nephrectomy specimens of Figures 27 and 28. Kidney transplant recipients with a history of polycystic kidney disease tend to do better than recipients with other etiologies of kidney failure. We evaluate all candidates with polycystic kidney disease for intracranial aneurysms given the reported higher incidence in this population. Polycystic kidney disease is usually transmitted as an autosomal dominant disease, although an autosomal recessive form (usually encountered in children) also exists. The presence of polycystic kidney disease should be excluded in all relatives willing to donate. The liver as well as other organs can also exhibit polycystic changes. The size of polycystic kidneys is usually impressive. We do not routinely perform native nephrectomies at the time of transplantation. Unnecessary additions to the transplant procedure can lead to complications that in turn could affect the outcome of the allograft. We have not encountered so far an instance in which the size of the native polycystic kidneys prevented us from implanting the allograft.

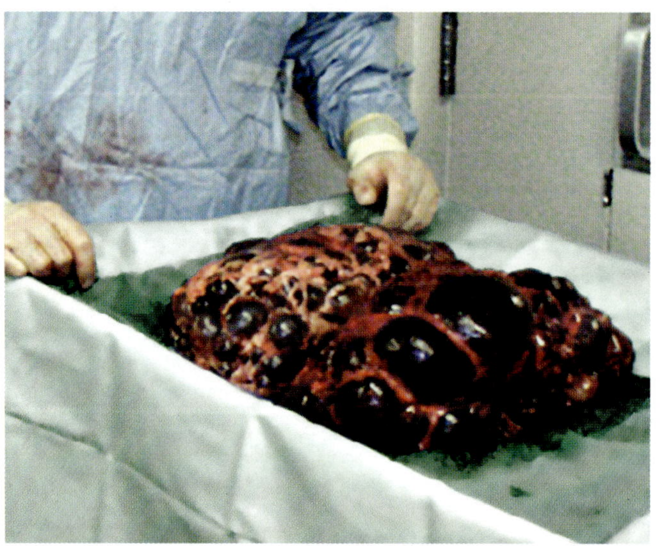

Fig. 27

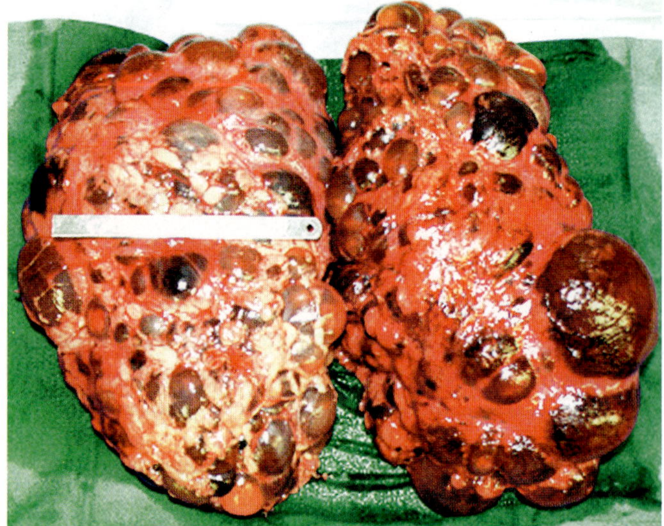

Fig. 28

Figs. 27 and 28: Images of polycystic kidneys. In instances where recipients wish to have the kidneys removed, we routinely recommend the nephrectomy either prior to transplantation or once the allograft has stable function.

CHAPTER 36

Implantation—En Bloc Kidneys

Benjamin Philosophe, Alicia Eubanks, Amit Basu, Ernesto P Molmenti

PROCUREMENT AND BACK TABLE PREPARATION

- The decision when to split pediatric kidneys or use them en bloc remains controversial. Traditionally, kidneys from donors less than 2 years or under 15 kg are split, but recent publications have shown good results with split kidneys at a much younger age or lesser weight
- En bloc kidneys are procured making sure that as much inferior vena cava (IVC) and aorta are retained both proximally and distally (Fig. 1)
- In the back table preparation, the proximal IVC and aortic openings are sutured close taking care not to compromise orifices of renal arteries or veins (Figs. 2 and 3)

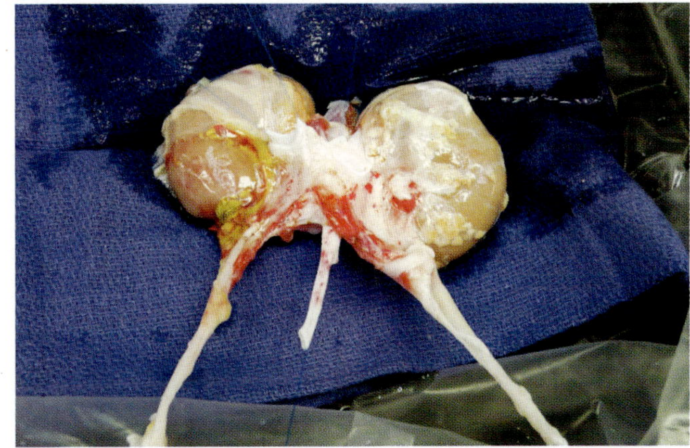

Fig. 2: The kidneys are dissected and prepared for implantation. It is important to closely inspect for injuries. In this specific case, the right renal artery was found to have sustained a laceration during procurement.

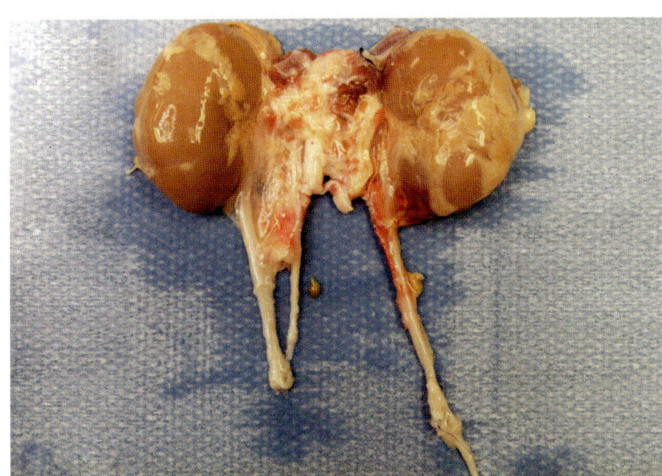

Fig. 1: En bloc kidneys as seen prior to back table work.

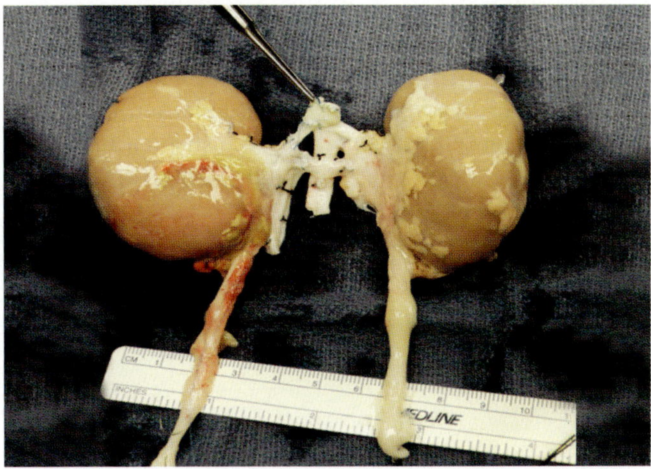

Fig. 3: En bloc kidneys ready for implantation. Note the repaired right renal artery.

- Small collaterals as well as lumbar vessels are identified and tied in order to prevent post-implantation bleeding
- Some surgeons prefer not to remove the adrenal glands, and leave them in place

IMPLANTATION

- Low dose intravenous heparin (300-500 u/hr) is usually started to decrease the risk of thrombosis
- A lower quadrant abdominal incision is undertaken
- The right lower quadrant is usually preferred, although the left lower quadrant can be alternatively used
- We perform an extraperitoneal implantation
- The external iliac artery and vein are dissected free of surrounding structures
- The en bloc kidneys are wrapped in a sponge with ice and brought onto the operative field
- Care must be taken during the entire procedure to avoid any twisting or kinking of the blood vessels to and from the kidneys
- The external iliac vein is clamped and incised
- The distal end of the donor IVC is anastomosed onto the recipient external iliac vein in an end-to-side fashion with 6-0 or 7-0 nonabsorbable sutures. The anastomosis can be constructed with running or with interrupted sutures
- A delicate clamp is placed on the donor IVC distal to the kidneys and the clamp on the recipient iliac vein released
- Hemostasis is verified—and additional sutures placed if necessary
- The external iliac artery is clamped
- The distal end of the donor aorta is anastomosed in an end-to-side fashion onto the external iliac artery of the recipient. 6-0 nonabsorbable running or interrupted sutures are used for this anastomosis
- Hemostasis is verified—and additional sutures placed if necessary
- With a Doppler probe we evaluate for adequate flow in both donor and recipient vessels
- The ureter to bladder anastomosis can be fashioned in a variety of ways:
  - Both ureters can be anastomosed to each other and subsequently implanted as a single opening into the bladder
  - Each of the two ureters can be implanted independently into the bladder
  - Absorbable sutures are used for this anastomosis. It is recommended to stent the ureters with size 4.8 F stents
  - The use of pediatric double J ureteral stents is very common given the high rate of ureteral complications or leaks (usually size 4.8 F stents)
- The abdominal wall muscles and fascia can be closed with interrupted sutures
- The skin is closed with widely spaced sutures to decrease the incidence of infections

FOLLOW-UP

We routinely obtain a duplex-Doppler ultrasound evaluation in the immediate postoperative period to verify that there is adequate flow and no vascular compromise has occurred at the time of closing. Blood pressure control in the recipients is crucial to prevent hyperperfusion injury. Recipients can be converted from intravenous heparin to full dose aspirin prior to discharge.

FURTHER READING

1. Balachandran VP, Aull MJ, Goris M, et al. Successful transplantation of single kidneys from pediatric donors weighing less than or equal to 10 kg into standard weight adult recipients. Transplantation. 2010;90(5):518-22. doi: 10.1097/TP.0b013e3181e98d35
2. Mohanka R, Basu A, Shapiro R Kayler LK. Single versus en bloc kidney transplantation from pediatric donors less than or equal to 15 kg. Transplantation. 2008;86(2):264-8. doi:10.1097/TP.0b013e318177894e. PMID:18645489 [PubMed-indexed for MEDLINE]
3. Pelletier SJ, Guidinger MK, Merion RM, et al. Recovery and utilization of deceased donor kidneys from small pediatric donors. Am J Transplant. 2006;6(7):1646-52.
4. Ratner LE, Cigarroa FG, Bender JS, et al. Transplantation of single and paired pediatric kidneys into adult recipients. J Am Coll Surg. 1997;185(5):437-45.
5. Satterthwaite R, Aswad S, Sunga V, et al. Outcome of en bloc and single kidney transplantation from very young cadaveric donors. Transplantation. 1997;63(10):1405-10.

CHAPTER 37

Implantation—Complications

Ernesto P Molmenti and Collaborators

KINKS OR MILD TORSIONS—RENAL ARTERY AND/OR RENAL VEIN

- Mild kinks are usually associated with uneven vessel lengths at the time of implantation
- Repositioning the kidney in a way that allows the vessels to lie in a comfortable way may be of help in instances of mild twists and kinks (Figs. 1 to 3)
- Placing a fat pad (obtained from the retroperitoneal tissues of the recipient, from the back table preparation of the donor, or alternatively from other sites such as the recipient omentum) at the site of the kink may help maintain a gentle curve that allows for adequate blood flow
- In instances where the kink or torsion cannot be repaired in a satisfactory fashion, it may be necessary to redo the anastomosis

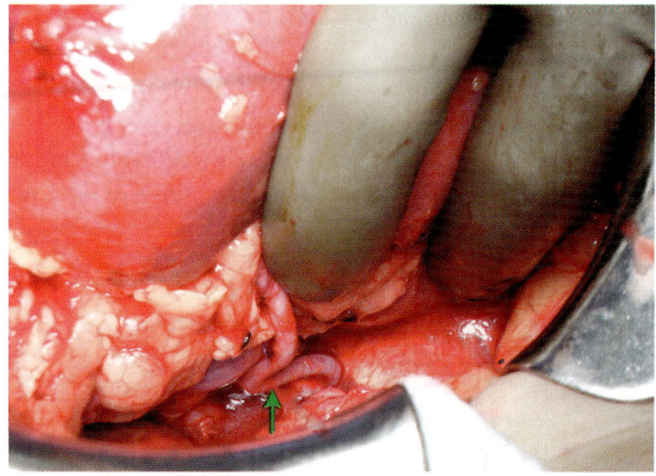

Fig. 1: Prior to closure, it is necessary to inspect the transplant kidney for any evidence of correctable problems. In this specific instance, there is a twist in an accessory renal artery (green arrow).

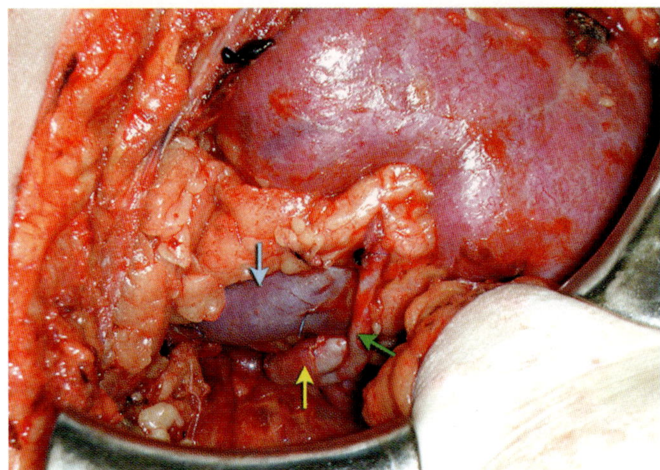

Fig. 2

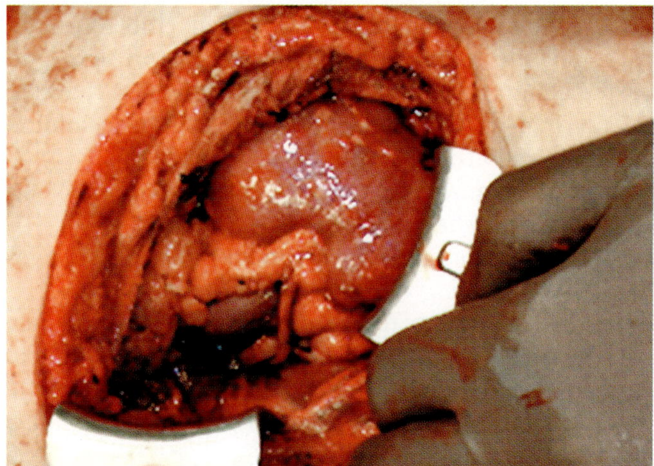

Fig. 3

Figs. 2 and 3: Repositioning the kidney allowed for all vessels (main renal artery-yellow arrow, accessory renal artery-green arrow, renal vein-blue arrow) to lie in a comfortable way without any impaired flow. The abdomen could subsequently be closed. In instances where repositioning the allograft will not allow for a comfortable positioning of the vessels, alternative techniques (such as placing a fat pad in order to maintain a comfortable curvature) may be necessary.

IMPLANTATION OF THE KIDNEY IN AN INVERTED (UPWARD-DOWN) POSITION

- Usually identified after reperfusion once the vascular anastomoses are complete
- Should not constitute an impediment to adequate renal function
- In order to prevent any ureteral kinks (since the ureter is oriented cephalad)
  - Special care should be taken when implanting the ureter into the bladder
  - The native ureter can be mobilized and a ureter-to-ureter anastomosis performed
- Some centers purposefully implant renal allografts in this fashion so to allow for alignment of the recipient iliac and donor renal vessels[1]

INFARCTS AT REPERFUSION

- If small (Fig. 4), no further action is required
- If large or expanding, an immediate re-evaluation is required to exclude an ongoing thrombosis or embolization

THROMBOSIS—RENAL VEIN AND/OR RENAL ARTERY—AT REPERFUSION OR SOON THEREAFTER

- Requires immediate attention and treatment
- Once the thrombosis is detected, the cause should be determined
- The most effective approach is to place clamps on the recipient artery and vein, and rapidly remove the kidney by taking down the recently constructed anastomoses
- As soon as the allograft is removed, all visible thrombi should be removed from the artery and vein and the allograft flushed with cold preservation fluid (or alternatively with cold crystalloid solution) avoiding embolization of thrombi
- Thrombectomy of the vein and/or artery with a balloon catheter may be necessary
- Thrombosis of the entire organ may not be a salvageable condition
- Both the donor and recipient vessels should be carefully evaluated for the presence of pathologies (technical complications such as back walling or stenosis of the anastomosis, thrombi, dissections, obstructing plaque, clamp injuries, other)
- Hyperacute rejection can be a causative factor
- If the allograft is found to be viable and there are no recipient contraindications, it can be reimplanted
- In cases where the kidney is reimplanted at a different site (such as the contralateral iliac vessels), a venous or synthetic patch may be required to maintain the diameter of the vessels originally used

URETER—TOO SHORT OR DEVASCULARIZED

- It is essential to ensure that the distal ureter is adequately perfused
- If necrotic, the ureter should be trimmed until a viable zone is reached
- The bladder can be mobilized to allow for a more proximal anastomosis
  - A ureter-to-bladder anastomosis that is under tension or involves a poorly vascularized ureter is prone to breakdown and should be avoided
- A ureter-to-ureter anastomosis is our next choice
  - Ipsilateral ureter preferred given its proximity
  - Contralateral ureter is also a possibility

KIDNEY—TOO BIG-DOES NOT FIT WITHIN THE RETROPERITONEAL SPACE

- Trying to accommodate the kidney within an inadequate space can lead to vascular kinks and subsequent thrombosis
- The initial step is to try to find additional space on top of the psoas muscle

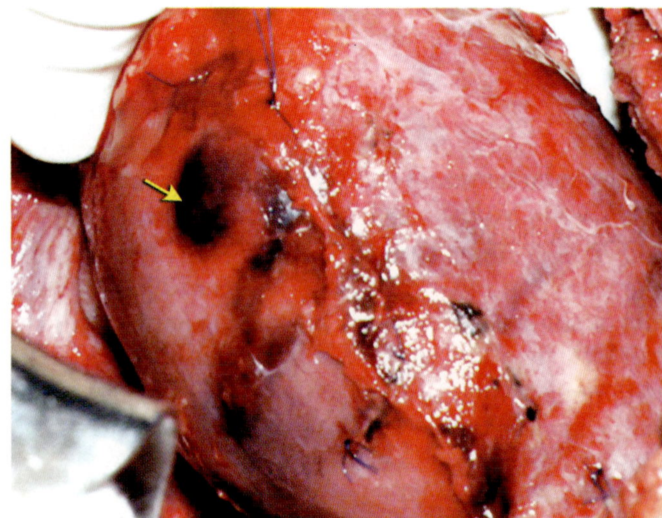

Fig. 4: Small infarcts (arrow) can be seen sometimes on the surface at the time of implantation. These findings can be due to a variety of factors, including accidental transection of branches of the renal artery or embolic phenomena.

- A relaxing incision of the rectus muscle may also be of help
- However, in many instances these maneuvers do not suffice
- When such situations arise, we prefer to open the peritoneum and accommodate the kidney in an intraperitoneal position
- In these cases, we always make sure that the vessels are not bent, rotated, or twisted, and that the kidney is as close to the body wall in order to allow for future biopsies

FURTHER READING

1. Shapiro R, Simmons R, Starzl T. Renal Transplantation. Appleton and Lange. 1997.

REFERENCE

1. Simforoosh N, Aminsharifi A, Tabibi A, et al. Right laparoscopic donor nephrectomy and the use of inverted kidney transplantation: an alternative technique. BJU Int 2007; 100:1347–50. Epub 2007 Sep 10. PMID: 17850376

CHAPTER 38

Postoperative Guidelines

Ernesto P Molmenti and Collaborators

- Health-care personnel caring for transplant patients should be familiar with the care of such patients. In many instances, specific requirements may have to be fulfilled
- Postoperatively, we observe recipients in the post-anesthesia care unit until stable to be transferred to the designated transplant floor
- Recipients who require thorough monitoring and management are admitted to the intensive care unit
- Recipients are under the continuous care of our multidisciplinary transplant team
- Urinary output is replaced with an equivalent volume of intravenous (IV) fluids (routinely normal saline) for the first 24 hours after transplantation
  - Warming IV fluids postoperatively helps maintain a normal body temperature, especially in patients with high urine outputs
  - In cases where the recipient has adequate oral intake, IV fluids are discontinued after the first 24 hours
  - Recipients with marginal oral intake remain on maintenance IV fluids (routinely 100 mL/hour) until able to tolerate an adequate oral intake
- Urinary catheters are routinely removed 24 hours after transplantation
  - They may be kept in place for longer periods of time based on specific clinical indications that should be clearly documented
- We advance intake to a solid diet as tolerated immediately after transplantation once the recipient is fully awake
  - In instance of adequate renal function, we eliminate any renal diet restrictions immediately after surgery
- Constipation is a frequent finding in the end-stage renal disease population. It is worsened by pain and discomfort associated with the surgery
  - We routinely administered oral agents (such as magnesium citrate or lactulose) as well as enemas and suppositories in order to achieve bowel function within the first 24 hours after transplantation
- Patients are encouraged to ambulate as soon as tolerated
  - Although this occurs usually the day after transplantation, earlier ambulation is not discouraged
- Wound sutures are usually removed 4–6 weeks after transplantation
- Ureteral stents are routinely removed 6 weeks after transplantation in cases with no complications

TRANSFER OF CARE FROM INPATIENT TO OUTPATIENT

- In many recipients with immediate graft function, a safe transfer of care from inpatient to outpatient can be achieved as early as 48 hours after transplantation. Early discharge criteria include but is not limited to:
  - Hemodynamic stability
  - Adequate urine output
  - No urinary catheters
  - Satisfactory oral intake

- No IV fluids
- Decreasing creatinine
- Adequate social support
- Ability to take immunosuppression
- No major complications
- Controlled co-morbidities
- Outpatient follow-up within the next 24–48 hours

- We believe that transplantation is a multidisciplinary concept. As such, we engage recipients and their families in decisions affecting their care

CHAPTER 39

Allograft Function

Kellie Calderon

EARLY ALLOGRAFT FUNCTION

- Most transplant allografts with short cold ischemic time begin to produce urine in the operating room or soon thereafter
- We monitor graft function in the first 24 hours by
  - Hourly urine output
    - Since polyuria is common during this time period, we maintain volume status with a combination of maintenance crystalloid (usually normal saline) at 1 mL/kg/hour and a replacement crystalloid (usually normal saline) measured 1 ml :1 ml for hourly urine output
    - In cases of very high urine output, a fluid warmer is useful to maintain body temperature
    - Close and continuous nursing monitoring helps to detect potential complications within the first 24 hours
    - Vital signs: The newly created vascular bed is susceptible to hypotension, which is relative in patients with long-standing CKD who often have concomitant hypertension. For this reason, we aim for systolic blood pressure > 120 mm Hg during this time period (we prefer to follow systolic rather than mean pressures)
    - If urine output declines abruptly:
      - Irrigate the urinary catheter to assure patency and verify that it is correctly placed in the bladder: Hematuria is common after surgery and if significant, blood clots are possible. It is also important to confirm the correct placement of the catheter, since twists, kinks, and the lack of drainage by a partially inflated balloon or residue from the bladder may account for the lack of drainage. If in doubt, replace the urinary catheter with a new one (disruption of a fresh anastomosis is unusual with such replacement)
      - Urgent renal ultrasound (US) with arterial and venous duplex Doppler studies to evaluate for surgical complications including
        - Vascular thrombosis
        - Mechanical or functional obstruction
        - Extravasation of blood and/or urine
        - Extravasation tends to occur earlier in the post-transplant course than does obstruction
        - Renal US can detect perinephric fluid collections. Differential diagnoses includes:
          - Hematoma
          - Lymphocele
          - Urinoma
        - Fluid from wound drainage or the aspiration of a collection can be evaluated for creatinine concentration to differentiate between a urinoma or lymphocele. In urinomas, the creatinine concentration is similar to that in urine. In nonurinoma collections, the fluid creatinine resembles that in serum
        - For this reason, in such cases it is important to measure simultaneously the creatinine concentrations of serum, urine, and fluid specimen
      - Urgent electrolyte and complete blood count (CBC). Hyponatremia and/or hyperkalemia may be early signs of obstruction or urinary leaks

- Graft function postoperative day one:
  - Hourly urine output and daily weights
    - Once the patient is ambulatory, we discontinue the Foley catheter
      - In order to minimize pressure at the ureteral anastomosis, the patient is instructed to empty his/her bladder every 60 minutes on POD#1
      - If after a 1–3 hour trial of voiding the patient is unable to void, an initial bladder catheterization is undertaken. This procedure may be repeated from one to three occasions. After such attempts, a urinary catheter can be replaced
        - In instances of recipients with known severe benign prostatic hypertrophy, the urinary catheter can be placed earlier, the patient sent home on appropriate agents, and followed up as an outpatient medications (to address the prostatic hypertrophy) with the urinary catheter in place
      - Constipation is aggressively managed to avoid straining. We routinely administer oral magnesium citrate or lactulose on the first postoperative day. Enemas and suppositories are also used if necessary
    - Crystalloid management:
      - We discontinue urinary replacement fluids on POD#1
      - We discontinue maintenance fluids when the patient resumes a regular diet, usually also on POD#1
  - Serum chemistry is usually evaluated twice on POD#1, largely to monitor for electrolyte abnormalities which are common in the polyuric phase
  - Calcineurin inhibitor trough levels during the first 3 months:
    - In low immunologic risk patients, we aim for tacrolimus levels 8–10 ng/dL
    - In high immunologic risk patients, we aim for tacrolimus levels 10–13 ng/dL
      - Generally, dose adjustments are made only after four pharmacologic half lives when steady state is achieved
  - Evaluation of decreased urine output or a lack of decline in the serum creatinine is undertaken in a way similar to that in the immediate postoperative period as described above
  - Urinalysis
    - We monitor daily urinalysis with special attention to patients with underlying glomerular disease for early recurrence, particularly in patients with native kidney focal segmental glomerulosclerosis (FSGS)
- Graft function for the remainder of inpatient stay:
  - Daily serum chemistry, CBC, urine output measurement, daily weights
  - If the serum creatinine does not decline appropriately, we investigate with:
    - Renal US with duplex Doppler study to evaluate for possible surgical complications as described above
    - Calcineurin inhibitor (CN-I) trough/medication review: Early toxicity of CN-I may include thrombotic microangiopathy. Concomitantly evaluate for anemia, thrombocytopenia and intravascular hemolysis. Patients with supratherapeutic CN-I levels are also often hypertensive
    - Centrifuged urine sediment microscopic examination may be helpful to evaluate suspected acute tubular necrosis. Classic "muddy brown casts" may be numerous. In this case, continue supportive care and immunotherapy
    - In high immunologic risk patients, we consider evaluating for donor-specific antibodies at this time and/or biopsy
    - Evaluate for nosocomial infections, particularly urinary tract infections

OUTPATIENT GRAFT MONITORING

- Twice weekly outpatient office visits for the first 2 weeks
- Weekly outpatient office visits for the second 2 weeks
- Tapered office visits subsequently as condition warrants
  - Urinalysis with total protein: creatinine calculation and serum creatinine each visit
  - Evidence of hematuria generates an investigation for:
    - Intrarenal generation of hematuria (dysmorphic RBC):
      - Recurrent or de novo glomerulonephritis
      - Viral nephropathy (e.g., BKV or adenovirus)
    - Extrarenal generation of hematuria (normal morphologic RBC):
      - Stone formation
      - Malignancy
      - Trauma
      - Other (more unusual pathologies such as a fungal bezoar)

Table 1: Approach to allograft screening and investigation of dysfunction

Immunologic injury

Screening:

- CNI trough

Investigation:

- CN-I trough trend review
- Donor-specific antibody testing
- Renal duplex Doppler US including intraparenchymal resistive indices

Calcineurin inhibitor toxicity

Screening:

- 12-hour trough monitoring

Investigation:

- Trough trend review
- Blood pressure review
- Evaluation of thrombotic microangiopathy

Other medication toxicity

- Urine and peripheral blood evaluation of eosinophils, skin exam for rash, and medication review with patient
- Urine microscopy evaluation, muddy brown casts or WBC casts

Diabetes evaluation

Screening:

- Urinary protein measurement
- Home glucometer reading review
- Serum glycosylated hemoglobin

Obstruction

- Renal US
- Stone, ureteral stricture, bladder outlet obstruction, fungal bezoar.

Viral-related nephropathy

Screening:

- BKV prophylaxis is every other week for first three months; then monthly for the first twelve months. It is done three monthly in second and third years and thereafter six monthly till five years
- CMV PCR is done monthly after the first 6 months (once Valganciclovir prophylaxis is stopped) for the second half of the first year. Every 2 months for the second year post-transplant. Every 3 months for the third year. As indicated after that
- CMV, BKV PCR every 3 months during the first year post-transplant, yearly thereafter

Investigation:

- May present with AKI, proteinuria, or hematuria
- Hepatitis B/C, HIV, and EBV (as PTLD) may also cause allograft dysfunction but are not routinely screened post-transplant

Malignancy evaluation

Screening:

- Age-related cancer screening
- Yearly US of native kidneys

Investigation:

- When PTLD is suspected, we investigate with serum protein electrophoresis, immunofixation, quantification of serum free light chains and EBV PCR, and possible CT to search for lymphadenopathy
- Renal US may show enlarged kidneys from infiltrative process
- Thorough review of systems is key

- Evaluation of proteinuria:
  - Early postoperative:
    - Glomerulonephritis, either de novo or recurrent, particularly if native kidney disease was FSGS
    - Acute immunologic injury
    - Post-transplant lymphoproliferative disorder
    - UTI/Pyelonephritis
  - Late postoperative:
    - In addition to those listed in the early period:
    - Diabetic nephropathy
    - Chronic immunologic injury
- Renal insufficiency with little or no proteinuria
  - Early postoperative:
    - Acute immunologic injury
    - Acute tubular necrosis
    - Acute calcineurin inhibitor toxicity
    - Obstruction
    - Viral infection
    - Medication-induced acute interstitial nephritis
  - Late postoperative: (in addition the early causes)
    - Chronic immunologic injury
    - Chronic CN-I toxicity
    - Recurrent or de novo glomerulonephritis
    - Hypertensive nephropathy

Table 1 summarizes our approach to the evaluation of renal allograft dysfunction.

CHAPTER 40

Critical Care Considerations in the Management of Renal Transplant Patients

Richard Barnett, Rose Marie Pasmantier, Asha Alex, Narendra Singh, Jeffrey Nicastro

INTRODUCTION

The purpose of this section is to review the management of adult renal transplant patients, which may warrant critical care intervention. Critical care specialists are expected to work closely with the transplant team in a variety of settings, including the emergency department, PACU, MICU, SICU, and CCU. We will initially focus on issues that are peculiar to these patients in the postoperative period, which reflect patient selection, nature of the surgery, and adverse consequences of immunosuppression. Many of the metabolic concerns have already been reviewed in the chapter on "Fluid and Electrolyte Considerations in Renal Transplant Patients." The remainder of this chapter will discuss the critical care challenges posed particularly during the first year of transplantation and beyond with an emphasis on:

A. Immediate PACU postoperative considerations
B. Immediate ICU postoperative considerations
C. Late ICU postoperative considerations

POSTOPERATIVE PERIOD

Following transplantation, the immediate care is typically rendered in the PACU with emphasis on optimizing respiratory and hemodynamic performance.

- Goals:
  - Expedite the transfer of the patient to a specialized renal transplant unit (typically geographically aggregated med-surg floor beds)
  - Management of immunosuppression
  - Renal replacement therapy when required
  - Observation for potential infections, urinary obstruction, complications of the graft

Immediate PACU Postoperative Considerations

Major limiting factors in timely transfer to the specialty renal transplant unit include:

- Persistent respiratory compromise
- Respiratory alkalosis
- Hemodynamic instability
- Cardiovascular problems
- Severe hypertension
- Uncontrolled hyperglycemia (including DKA)

Persistent Respiratory Compromise

- Delayed metabolism of anesthetics and sedatives in these patients with renal insufficiency may result in prolonged respiratory and cognitive depression
- Body habitus, preexisting cardiac and medical conditions may complicate extubation
- Despite these factors, most patients under careful observation are discharged from the PACU without major ventilatory support within a few hours
- Persistent hypoxemia with ventimask, signs of airway obstruction, significant respiratory acidosis and neurologic depression may require longer PACU admission or consideration for transfer to a critical care unit, usually the SICU

- Management: Noninvasive positive pressure ventilation in extubated patients may be required before transition to supplemental oxygen either by mask or nasal cannula
- The decision to transfer the patient to the critical care unit should be made collaboratively by the transplant, PACU and SICU teams with the knowledge that the major advantages of a higher level of care may be offset by delay in placing the patient in a care setting optimized by experience and protocol for post-transplant rehabilitation

Certain conditions, if persistent, may warrant further management in the critical care unit.

Respiratory Alkalosis

- Causes:
  - Usually results from pain and discomfort and rarely from significant hemorrhage
  - If associated with a widened A-a gradient, could indicate volume overload, aspiration, pneumonia and infrequently systemic infection, pulmonary embolus or acute MI
- Management: Careful monitoring of standard clinical parameters: O_2 saturation, ABGs, routine EKG and CXR when indicated
- Consultation: In doubtful cases, the input of a pulmonary critical care specialist may be invaluable

Hemodynamic Instability Manifested by Hypotension

- Common cause of delayed PACU transfer
- Cause of hypotension should always be vigorously sought and never attributed solely to prolonged effects of perioperative drugs with vasorelaxant effects
- Persistent, high-level pressor support is a strong indicator for monitoring in a critical care setting but different transplant units may have established protocols permitting lower level administration
- Management: Most patients are responsive to volume resuscitation
  - Urine output as a guide to end-organ perfusion may be misleading because of early renal tubular dysfunction, hyperglycemia, or loop diuretic administration

Cardiovascular Problems

- Although all transplant recipients are screened preoperatively for the presence of coronary artery disease,[1] the "stress test" of transplantation may uncover disease in this group of patients with a high incidence of diabetic and vascular complications
- Evaluation:
  - EKG and continuous rhythm monitoring provide invaluable clues to evolving ischemic disease or significant arrhythmias
  - Echocardiography to assess wall motion abnormalities and estimates of central filling pressures previously obtained with invasive central monitoring
- Consultation: Input from the cardiology consultation service

Severe Hypertension

- Management: Almost invariably responds to combination of intravenous (IV) and oral medications including diuretics
  - Ultrafiltration is an additional option but requirement for continuous IV administration of antihypertensive agents is best accomplished in the critical care setting

Uncontrolled Hyperglycemia including DKA

- Warrants serious ICU attention
- Causes:
  - High-dose steroids, calcineurin inhibitors,[2] Sirolimus,[3] and postoperative stress routinely contribute to insulin resistance
  - Must address additional factors such as infection, cardiorespiratory compromise, and hemorrhage
- Management: Improve patient and graft survival with tighter glycemic control.[4] However, continuous insulin infusion to maintain glucoses 70–110 mg% in renal transplant patients may be associated with worse outcomes[5]

Immediate ICU Postoperative Considerations

Historically, renal transplant patients were routinely admitted to the SICU for a "period of observation." Specialized renal transplant floor teams were created to drive better outcomes and shorter lengths of stay. The major challenge to optimal care of the renal transplant patient in the ICU is close coordination between the renal transplant and ICU teams. Communication is key but because of the frenetic schedules of these groups, optimal care may be thwarted. Intensivists are dependent on the transplant team to guide dosing and route of medications, timing, and type of renal replacement therapy as well as diagnosis and treatment of ARF including rejection. Conversely, the transplant team will benefit from the intensivist experience in volume assessment and management, impact of volume overload on ventilator weaning status, and assessment of postoperative complications.

Postoperative Considerations the ICU include

- Hemorrhage
- Respiratory failure
- Hypotension
- Renal failure
- Infections
- Metabolic abnormalities

Hemorrhage

- Most patients undergoing transplant manifest anemia postoperatively
  - Preoperative optimization: Current routine use of erythropoietin stimulating agents in advanced chronic kidney disease typically has limited its magnitude
  - Hemodilution sustained by significant crystalloid administration can complicate interpretation of the initial CBC, which acutely may not reflect the magnitude of a significant hemorrhage
- Evaluation: Renal transplant ultrasound is invaluable in the initial assessment, and some centers perform this routinely
  - Small perirenal hematomas are common
  - It is somewhat surprising that larger collections are not observed more frequently given the wide use of anticoagulant and/or antiplatelet agents to enhance graft viability
    - May reflect the technical skill of modern transplant surgeons who have a low threshold for re-exploring the graft in doubtful cases
- Management:
  - Anticoagulant and/or antiplatelet drugs should be held in severe bleeding and standard methods to reverse their effects employed
  - Additional measures to enhance clotting in the setting of renal failure include IV DDAVP administered q24h as needed
- Other sources of hemorrhage such as the GI tract are less common and require a high index of suspicion
  - IV conjugated estrogens may be especially useful in such cases where a disproportionate number of patients manifest angiodysplasia
  - GI consultation should be obtained in such patients
- The risk to renal function of radiocontrast angiography in severe hemorrhage of uncertain origin may be weighed against the benefit of salvaging the patient, and the input from an experienced interventional radiology group can be invaluable
- Management with transfusion:
  - Determining when to transfuse the patient is among the most common issues confronting the transplant and ICU teams
  - The risk of sensitization has traditionally fostered a high threshold for blood product administration by the transplant team
  - Recent multicenter ICU trials has supported a benefit to limiting transfusion in a wide range of patients with hemoglobin > 7 gm%[6]
  - The decision to transfuse transplant patients with hemoglobin < 7 gm% should be individualized jointly by the ICU and transplant services
  - Leukocyte depleted, irradiated PRBCs are preferred when required
  - Absolute indication: Acute, hemodynamically significant hemorrhage
  - Cardiac ischemia may require hemoglobin as high as 10 gm% to optimize oxygen carrying capacity

Respiratory Failure

- Goals of therapy:
  - Limit the duration of invasive ventilation[7] in order to minimize ventilator-associated pneumonia,[8] which can be particularly challenging in these immunocompromised individuals
  - Minimizing lung injury from barotrauma and oxygen toxicity is routine. It is beyond the scope of this section to review the major principles of ventilator management, which apply to most postoperative patients
  - Identify reversible causes:
    - Reversible noncardiogenic pulmonary edema may be consequent to drugs used to treat acute rejection
    - The treatment of aspiration and postoperative pneumonia is determined by the ICU team with appropriate input regarding interval and dosing of antibiotics when required from the transplant service
      - Fortunately the opportunistic organisms observed later in the first year after engraftment are seldom observed initially
      - Attention directed at minimizing secretions and treating bronchospasm is routine

  - Hypokalemia and hypocalcemia may contribute to respiratory muscle weakness
  - Hypophosphatemia alters muscle strength and limits oxygen delivery by adverse effects on the oxygen dissociation curve
  - Nutritional deficits may limit weaning
  - Carbohydrate limited formulations decrease CO_2 generation and lessen ventilation requirements
  - Volume overload with pulmonary congestion is a frequent contributor
    - Aggressive diuresis, plasma ultrafiltration, and dialysis may decrease preload and improve pulmonary compliance sufficiently to decrease ventilator dependence
- Ischemic heart disease may be an important factor in failure to wean particularly in severely anemic patients

Hypotension

- Persistent hypotension unresponsive to volume resuscitation is a major cause for transfer of new transplant patients to the ICU
- Etiology: Evaluate postoperative third spacing, hemorrhage, cardiac compromise, and evolving infection
- Management:
  - Achieving optimal mean arterial pressure is key in maintaining renal perfusion, thereby improving kidney function or diminishing duration of ARF
  - The appropriate mix of volume expansion and vasopressors is usually ascertained empirically; rarely requires invasive central monitoring
  - Swan-Ganz catheterization is always an option, but its benefit in ICU patient survival is lacking.[9] May still be useful in ascertaining etiologies and potential therapy in individuals with concomitant respiratory failure

Renal Failure

- Isolated renal failure is usually managed successfully on the renal transplant floor unit
- Etiology: Distinguishing the myriad causes of ARF in the early transplant setting including obstruction and rejection have been discussed extensively in other sections
- Persistent or ARF frequently complicates the course of transplant patients admitted to the ICU
  - The hemodynamic derangements resulting from impaired cardiac function, infection, and respiratory failure impact adversely on renal perfusion and function
- Management:
  - A conservative, expectant approach to renal failure is often insufficient to adequately manage these complex patients in the ICU setting
  - Standard hemodialysis for those requiring renal replacement therapy
    - Benefits: Hemodialysis ameliorates the metabolic derangements and may achieve fluid balance sufficient to decrease or eliminate invasive ventilator support
    - The patient's preexisting AV access when available is a preferred route
    - Femoral catheterization should generally be avoided because of inferior flows and clearances as well as higher risk of blood borne infections.[10] All catheters should be placed under sonographic guidance
  - Continuous dialysis, typically CVVHDF, has been used preferentially to treat hypotensive patients, especially those with acidemia requiring pressor support
    - In these individuals, we recommend a citrate-based protocol to minimize clotting of the hemofilter[11]
    - Alkalemia resulting from citrate metabolism to bicarbonate is observed occasionally but usually does not require specific therapy
    - CVVHDF has not been demonstrated to have an overwhelming patient or renal survival advantage compared with HD[12]
    - Antibiotic therapy:
      - Appropriate antibiotic dosing is particularly challenging using this technique because of the range of clearances achieved by variably adjusting ultrafiltration or dialysis flow rates
      - Vancomycin is cleared by continuous dialysis but drug levels should guide redosing
      - Conversely, it may be misleading to rely on drug levels to manage IV calcineurin inhibitors, which are typically administered as a continuous infusion using one-third the estimated total daily PO dose. They are not however removed significantly by dialysis
- Ultimately selection of dialysis modality usually reflects center experience, staff preference, and patient hemodynamics

Infections

- Etiology:
  - Common bacterial pathogens should be considered in the immediate post-transplant period[13]

- Clostridium difficile colitis:
  - Not infrequently encountered; may, in combination with mycophenolate-associated diarrhea, promote profound volume depletion requiring treatment in the ICU
- Cytomegalovirus (CMV) colitis—very rare in this setting

- Management:
  - Early removal of indwelling urinary catheters and IV/central lines will decrease the risk of endovascular and urinary tract infections
  - Low-grade pulmonary infections:
    - Usually respond to noninvasive oxygen supplementation, respiratory therapy, and standard antibiotics when indicated
  - Treatment of ventilator-associated pneumonia: far more challenging; provides an incentive to evaluate and treat early to minimize subsequent invasive support

Metabolic Abnormalities

- The management of electrolyte derangements observed in transplant patients has been reviewed in the chapter on fluid and electrolytes and except in severe hyperkalemia seldom requires ICU management
- Severe, uncontrolled diabetes mellitus:
  - Is frequently encountered in the early post-transplant period
  - Can be precipitated by combination of perioperative stress, immunosuppressives,[2,3] and high-dose steroids
  - Severe hyperglycemia and DKA should not be solely attributed to high-dose steroids and other agents employed in most induction immunosuppression regimens
    - Conditions associated with elaboration of counterregulatory factors promoting insulin resistance include infection, cardiac ischemia, hemorrhage, and respiratory decompensation
  - Management:
    - Optimal level of glycemic control in renal transplant patients has not been firmly established, but improved outcomes and decreased risk of infection in other surgical and critical patients have been extensively reported. However, the very tight control initially recommended for SICU patients[4] may have worse outcomes for transplant recipients including a higher rate of rejection[5]
    - Reasonable to provide continuous insulin therapy to those patients whose postoperative glucose levels consistently exceed 180mg%, and in many centers this approach may require an ICU venue
    - Levels of 70–180 mg% that can be achieved with subcutaneous therapy seem reasonable
  - Diabetic ketoacidosis:
    - Management in critical care unit
    - Consultation with an endocrinologist is strongly encouraged

Late ICU Postoperative Considerations

The management of transplant patients in the ICU more than a month after surgery can be especially challenging. The following should be considered:

- Postsurgical complications
- Steroid withdrawal
- Infections
- Encephalopathy

Postsurgical Complications

- Abscess formation, ureteral stenosis, and narrowing of the renal artery
  - Management:
    - Previously required surgery and general anesthesia
    - Are now increasingly handled in the interventional radiology suite—this has decreased post-procedure SICU requirements

Steroid Withdrawal

- Wide employment of glucocorticoid-sparing immunosuppression regimens in the past decade has dramatically limited the incidence of steroid withdrawal
  - This approach has paralleled a transition toward tacrolimus as the predominant calcineurin inhibitor
- Most individuals on cyclosporine are concurrently maintained on chronic low-dose steroids
    - Nonetheless, established patients with an unclear history of chronic prednisone use presenting with constitutional symptoms, mental status changes, and hypotension may benefit from a trial of "stress dose" IV hydrocortisone 100 mg intravenous three times daily or equivalent
  - Conditions provoking this increase in steroid requirements include surgery, cardiac ischemia, and infection

Infections

- The spectrum of infections shifts dramatically following the first weeks after renal transplantation[13]
- Is the leading cause of mortality during the first year of transplantation
  - The decline in immunocompetence persisting up to a year or greater is reflected in the types of opportunistic infections afflicting these individuals and have been reviewed elsewhere
- Etiology:
  - From the viewpoint of the intensivist, the differential for sepsis and pneumonia is substantially broadened. The degree and time span of this severely immunocompromised state are increased in patients treated for one or more episodes of acute rejection
  - Pre-transplant immunomodulating viruses such as HIV, hepatitis B, and C may render these patients even more susceptible to unusual pathogens
  - Typical bacterial diseases are still more common but pseudomonas, fungi, viruses, and respiratory failure resulting from opportunistic pathogens may need to be considered
- Evaluation:
  - The consulting staffs from the pulmonary and infectious disease services are invaluable in sorting the myriad possibilities
  - Transbronchial evaluation is occasionally needed for demonstrating PCP, but larger sampling requiring the expertise of thoracic surgery may be required for the diagnosis of Aspergillus, Nocardia, and CMV
- Management:
  - Medication regimens at most centers include prophylaxis for *Pneumocystis* (Bactrim has activity for *Nocardia*, *Listeria*, and *Toxoplasma*) and CMV. The incidence of PCP[14] and CMV has fallen dramatically as a result of routine prophylaxis
  - Failure of severe CMV infections to respond to Ganciclovir should lead to assessment of viral resistance and use of alternative but more toxic therapies
  - Decisions to reduce immunosuppression in the setting of infection should be made collaboratively among the transplant, critical care, and ID consult services

Encephalopathy in Transplant Patients

- Transplant patients exhibiting severe mental status changes are frequently referred to the critical care units for evaluation and management
- Evaluation of acute encephalopathy:
  - Head CT scan to exclude significant structural problems either in the emergency department or acute hospital
  - Team care by the intensivist and renal transplant services
- Causes of acute encephalopathy:
  - "ICU psychosis"
    - A diagnosis of exclusion observed most commonly in patients requiring prolonged invasive ventilatory support
  - Medication side effects:
    - Glucocorticoids:
      - Induction level doses may contribute to acute encephalopathy in the early transplant period, exacerbated by electrolyte disturbances and uremia
    - Calcineurin inhibitors:
      - Commonly induce tremor (especially at high levels)
      - Can cause encephalopathy (rarely)
      - Occasionally cause the development of a thrombotic microangiopathy manifested by encephalopathy and ARF[15]
    - Antiplatelet drugs used in some transplant protocols may also be implicated. This TTP-HUS syndrome can be devastating, but usually responds to discontinuing the offending agent(s) and/or plasma exchange with plasmapheresis
  - CNS infections:
    - Concerns for opportunistic CNS infections are greatest after the first month of transplant and diminish substantially during the subsequent 6 months to 1 year
    - Etiology:
      - In addition to the usual bacterial culprits of meningitis, *Listeria* and fungi, including *Cryptococcus*, should also be considered
      - CNS Mucor infections usually arise from mucocutaneous spread, especially in poorly controlled diabetes
      - Encephalitis from latent varicella zoster, HHV-6, and new infections by influenza, West Nile,[16] and other viruses have been reported

- CVA
- Vasculitis
- Electrolyte disturbances:
  - Abnormalities in sodium, potassium, magnesium, calcium, and phosphorus have been implicated in acute toxic metabolic encephalopathy and are usually easily addressed
- Liver failure
- Uremia:
  - Delayed graft function, rejection, and chronic allograft nephropathy may limit patient clearance of uremic toxins
  - A trial of dialysis may resolve the etiology of encephalopathy in borderline cases

FURTHER READING

1. Danovitch GM. Handbook of kidney transplantation. 5th edition. Philadelphia. Lippincott Williams and Wilkins, 2007.
2. Parillo JE, Dellinger RP. Critical care medicine: principles of diagnosis and management in the adult. 3rd edition. Philadelphia, Mosby Elsevier, 2008.
3. Rose BD, Post TW. Clinical physiology of acid-base and electrolyte disorders. 5th edition. New York: McGraw Hill, 2001.
4. Taal MW, Chertow GW, Marsden PA, et al. Brenner and Rector's the kidney. 9th edition. Philadelphia: Saunders, 2010.

REFERENCES

1. Ojo AO, Hanson JA, Wolfe RA, et al. Long term survival in renal transplant recipients with graft function. Kidney Int 2000;57:307.
2. Bloom RD, Crutchlow MF. New onset diabetes mellitus in the kidney recipient: diagnosis and management strategies. Clin J Am Soc Nephrol 2008;3:538.
3. Johnston O, Rose CL, Webster AG, et al. Sirolimus is associated with new onset diabetes in kidney transplant recipients. J Am Soc Nephrol 2008;19:1411.
4. Van den Berghe G, Wouters P, Weekers F, et al. Intensive insulin therapy in critically ill patients. N Eng J Med 2001; 345:1359.
5. Hermayer KL, Egidi MF, Finch NJ, et al. A randomized controlled trial to evaluate the effect glycemic control on renal transplantation. J Clin Endo Metab 2012;97:4399.
6. Carson JL, Grossman BJ, Kleinman S, et al. Red blood cell transfusion: a clinical practice guideline from the AABB. Ann Int Med 2012;157:49.
7. Girard TD, Kress JP, Fuchs BD, et al. Efficacy and safety of a paired sedation and ventilator weaning protocol for mechanically ventilated patients in intensive care. Lancet 2008;371:126.
8. American Thoracic Society, Infectious Diseases Society of America. Guidelines for the management of adults with hospital acquired, ventilator associated, and healthcare associated pneumonia. Am J Resp Crit Care Med 2005; 171:388.
9. Sandham JD, Hull RD, Brant RF, et al. A randomized, controlled trial of the use of pulmonary artery catheters in high risk surgical patients. N Eng J Med 2003;31:2734.
10. Merrer J, De Jonghe B, Golliot F, et al. Complications of femoral and subclavian catheters in critically ill patients: a randomized controlled trial. JAMA 2007;286:700.
11. Kutsogiannis DJ, Gibney RT, Stollery D, et al. Regional citrate versus systemic heparin anticoagulation for continuous renal replacement in critically ill patients. Kidney Int 2005;67:2361.
12. Van Wert R, Scales DC, Friedrich JO, et al. High-dose renal replacement therapy for acute kidney injury: systematic review and meta-analysis. Crit Care Med 2010;38:1360.
13. Fishman JA, Issa NC. Infection in organ transplantation: risk factors and evolving patterns of infection. Infect Dis Clin North Am 2010; 24:273-83.
14. Fishman JA, Issa NC. Prevention of infection caused by Pneumocystis carinii in transplant recipients. Clin Infect Dis 2001;33:1397.
15. Zarifian A, Meleg-Smith A, O'Donovan R, et al. Cyclosporine associated thrombotic microangiopathy in renal allografts. Kidney Int 1999;5:2457.
16. Kleinschmidt-DeMasters BK, Marder B, Levi M, et al. Naturally acquired West Nile virus encephalomyelitis in transplant recipients: clinical, laboratory, diagnostic and neuropathological features. Arch Neurol 2004;61:2010.

CHAPTER 41

Rejection

Ezra Israel, Edward Kraus

OVERVIEW

- Definition: A recipient's immune response to foreign antigens expressed by the donor that if unresolved will lead to graft loss
- Incidence: (SRTR 2010 Annual Report) approximately 10–12% at 1 year (15–20% by 6 years)
- Significance:
  - Approximately 12% of grafts that are lost over 10 years are due to direct consequences of an acute rejection. Acute rejection accounts for another 10–30% of graft loss by 10 years following transplantation, since progressive chronic injury is linked in many instances to persistent low-level immune injury causing both interstitial fibrosis with tubular atrophy and/or transplant glomerulopathy[1]
  - GFR can be lower post episode(s) of acute cellular rejection:
    - Decreased GFR leads to increased medical co-morbidities and increased risk of death
    - Patients returning to dialysis have poorer survival than patients never transplanted or having functioning allografts[2]

TYPES OF ACUTE REJECTION

Classification is based on pathology and concurrent antibody data—Banff classification (Banff Meeting Reports).[3,5]

- Hyperacute—Rare event due to antibodies targeting HLA, blood group, and/or other endothelial antigens leading to rapid complement activated thrombotic microangiopathy with extensive hemorrhage and infarction
- Cellular—Pathology reflects lymphocyte migration, inflammation, and injury at sites of antigen expression on tubular epithelium and vascular endothelium
  - Banff 1A—Significant interstitial inflammation (> 25% of parenchyma affected, i2 or i3) and focal moderate tubulitis (t2)
  - Banff 1B—Significant interstitial inflammation (> 25% of parenchyma affected, i2 or i3) and severe tubulitis (t3)
  - Banff 2A—Mild-to-moderate arteritis (v1)
  - Banff 2B—Severe arteritis, which is associated with > 25% loss of the luminal area (v2)
  - Banff 3—Transmural arteritis, and/or arterial fibrinoid alterations, and necrosis of medial smooth muscle cells occurring in association with lymphocytic inflammation of the vessel (v3)
- Antibody mediated rejection (injury) requires the presence of antibody and indirect evidence of active endothelial injury by demonstration of complement activation (in the near future endothelial gene activation might be an alternate marker). It is defined by three criteria:
  i. Pathology (one or more of the following)
    - Most common sign will be "capillaritis"—leukocytes present in peritubular and glomerular capillaries
    - Thrombotic microangiopathy with or without capillaritis
    - Isolated (no tubulointerstitial inflammation) vascular rejection may be a sign of antibody-mediated rejection
    - Acute tubular injury without "capillaritis" has been defined as suspicious for the presence of antibody-mediated injury

ii. Evidence of complement activation reflected by C4d deposition on peritubular capillaries (This may be absent in some instances-incidence of C4d negative antibody-mediated rejection is still being defined but may be as high as 30% or more. In those cases there should be moderate–severe capillaritis)
iii. De novo or increasing strength of antibody targeting donor-derived antigen(s)
iv. If only two of the three (i, ii or ii) criteria above are present then biopsies can be considered "suspicious" for antibody mediated rejection[4,5]

- Mixed—Pathology demonstrates findings of cellular and antibody-mediated rejection

PRESENTATION

- Clinical
  - Symptoms—Prior to the introduction of calcineurin inhibitor therapy, patients developing acute rejection would often experience low-grade fever, tenderness over their allograft, and decreasing urine output. Since the advent of calcineurin inhibitor therapy in 1984, patients rarely have any symptoms at the time they develop rejection
  - Signs—Since clinical symptoms rarely occur with development of acute rejection, the main sign of a rejection episode is acute kidney failure. A rise of a patient's serum creatinine of 15–20% over their baseline should prompt an immediate evaluation for this
- Subclinical
  - When biopsies are performed per monitoring protocol during the first year following transplantation for patients who are not at high immunologic risk and who have received antibody induction with maintenance immunosuppression consisting of tacrolimus and mycophenolate, there is a 3–5% frequency of finding pathology consistent with a cellular rejection despite stable kidney function. This is termed subclinical rejection
  - For patients at high immunologic risk (blood group-incompatible donor recipient pairs or recipients who have anti-HLA donor-specific antibody (DSA) at the time of transplantation), the incidence of subclinical rejection at 1, 3, 6, and 12 months can be as high as 20–30%
  - Whether intervention for subclinical rejection changes long-term outcome or not, remains to be clarified

EVALUATION

- DDx:
  - The approach to determining if an acute rejection is occurring requires a history and exam to rule out:
    - Obstructive uropathy—Suggested by urinary symptoms such as changing stream, hesitancy, frequency, urgency and/or a patients reporting decreasing urine volume and confirmed by the finding of hydronephrosis by ultrasound
    - Prerenal factors:
      - History and exam consistent with either volume depletion or congestive heart failure
      - Physical findings suggestive of renal or iliac artery stenosis (bruits) in setting of worsening hypertension and edema ± recent addition of agents such as ACE inhibitors and ARB
      - Sudden increase of calcineurin inhibitor levels that can cause intrarenal vasoconstriction
    - Intrinsic kidney disease:
      - Drug effects causing acute interstitial nephritis
      - Infection—Screen for BK viremia
      - Role of biopsy:
        - In the end if there is no obvious cause by history and physical exam, a biopsy is necessary to determine if acute rejection is present. The ultrasound at the time of the biopsy can first be used to screen for obstructive uropathy and renal vascular disease. If present the biopsy can be postponed
        - In rare instances when the risk of biopsy is too high due to a bleeding diathesis or anatomic barriers, patients can be treated empirically for rejection. A detailed history and exam is imperative to avoid treating in clinical settings where acute kidney failure can be clearly linked to altered volume status, infection, obstruction and infection. Once these factors are excluded or adequately managed, if kidney function does not improve empiric therapy can be considered

MANAGEMENT

- Therapy
  - Cellular rejections:
    - For mild tubulointerstitial (Banff 1A) and vascular (Banff 2A) rejections, therapy is usually initiated with intravenous (IV) bolus steroids (Solu medrol 500 mg or dexamethasone 100 mg)

daily for 3 days with a reduction in the dose over the next 3–4 days (Solumedrol 250 mg, 125 mg then 75 mg; dexamethasone 75 mg, 50 mg, 25 mg) followed by an oral prednisone taper (60 mg for several days, 40 mg for several days, 30 mg for several days and then 20 mg for several weeks) or an oral prednisone taper beginning after the first 3 days of IV steroids

    - For moderate-to-severe tubulointerstitial (Banff 1B) and vascular (Banff 2B and 3) rejections, T-cell depletional therapy is usually prescribed. The most commonly used agent is Thymoglobulin 1.5 mg/kg/day for cumulative dose of 10–15 mg/kg
    - A Banff 2a vascular rejection with moderate-to-severe tubulitis and interstitial inflammation, which would have classified the rejection as 1b, if the vascular component was not present, is usually managed with T-cell depletional therapy
  - Antibody-mediated rejections—There is no definitive therapy for this:
    - In most programs, this is treated with plasmapheresis with infusion of intravenous immunoglobulin (IVIg) 100 mg/kg following each session. Plasmapheresis is performed three to four times a week on an every other day basis but sometimes initially on a daily basis dependent on the strength of DSA. Duration of therapy is guided by the change of strength of DSA. In many instances, this will not completely clear but fall and then plateau at a low level
    - If strength of DSA does not trend down over several sessions, many programs will administer anti-CD20 antibody to deplete circulating B cells. This will be dosed after a plasmapheresis session or at the end of all plasmapheresis sessions. If plasmapheresis is continued, it is advisable to wait about 36 hours before the next session to avoid clearance of the agent. About 5–6 days later a CD19 cell count should be obtained. If the CD19 count has not decreased to < 2–3%, another infusion of anti-CD19 antibody should be considered
    - Antibody-mediated rejection when severe can present with acute oligoanuric kidney failure. This usually occurs around 5–7 days post-surgery. Pathology can reveal thrombotic microangiopathy with interstitial hemorrhage, neutrophils in glomeruli, and peritubular capillaries and acute tubular injury. Emergency splenectomy has been demonstrated to resolve this. Complement inhibitors (C5 inhibitor—eculizumab) may be effective as well, but clinical evidence is only now being obtained
    - Bortezomib (Velcade) is being used for patients with persistent high levels of DSA ± persistent pathologic findings of ongoing acute antibody injury (persistent capillaritis). The jury is out about the efficacy of this agent and appropriate dosing strategies
    - It may be important to document the occurrence of "sensitizing events" (transfusions, pregnancy, infections especially viral and surgery) prior to the discovery of de novo DSA and a biopsy that is felt consistent with acute antibody-mediated injury. Although theoretical, therapies for acute antibody-mediated injury may be more effective if this is linked to a sensitizing event that occurred during the few months prior to diagnosis than if de novo DSA is found with a corroborating biopsy for AMR for a patient who has been clinically stable for years
    - High-dose IVIg (2 g/kg infused in 4 doses over 4 days) has been used. The jury is out about the effectiveness of this therapy
    - Therapy should be tempered if biopsies demonstrate advanced chronic changes (marked glomerular sclerosis and/or transplant glomerulonephritis) and/or marked tubulointerstitial scarring with tubular atrophy. Therapy might place a patient at high risk of complications with little hope of salvage of allograft function. The best option for care might in that instance be evaluation for another transplant. This option is increasing even for sensitized patients given widening donor pools through paired kidney exchanges and chains
  - Mixed rejections—These are managed with both steroids ± T-cell depletional therapy and plasmapheresis and low-dose IVIg
- Follow-up
  - Biopsy—If serum creatinine does not decrease to a patient's baseline at the end of the course of therapy, a follow-up biopsy may be useful to determine if further intervention is required
    - Allograft function might improve slowly due to unresolved acute tubular injury
    - For cellular rejections, this may be the addition of T-cell depletional therapy if only a course of steroids was administered or further T-cell depletional therapy mindful of limits of the cumulative dosage given increasing risks of malignancy

    - For persistent antibody-mediated injury, further plasmapheresis may considered or based on pathology addition of anti-CD20 antibody, high-dose IVIg, and/or bortezomib
  - Lab
    - Close monitoring of serum creatinine during the months following a rejection is important since incompletely treated rejection may flare
    - Serial monitoring of antibody strength during the few months following therapy is important to assess adequacy of therapy
    - BK viremia might occur post therapy. It is advisable to screen periodically during the 6–12 months following therapy for development of this
  - Maintenance immunosuppression—There is no consensus about whether to initiate higher calcineurin inhibitor and mycophenolate exposure following treatment. If there is a sense from follow-up biopsies that there is lingering inflammation then this may be advisable

FUTURE DIRECTIONS

- Screening
  - Monitoring of rejection currently is reactive rather than proactive. Evaluation is initiated based on changing kidney function determined by a rise of serum creatinine
  - More sensitive noninvasive biomarkers of rejection that might be indicative of rejection prior to a rise of serum creatinine include blood and urinary screens for inflammatory cytokines and enzymes associated with T and B cell activation (IL2, interferon, chemokines, caspase, perforin, granzyme A and B)
  - Different patterns of gene activation are now being associated with rejection, infection, and drug toxicity. Individualized care in the future might consist of monitoring patterns of gene expression rather than or in addition to therapeutic drug levels to adjust immunosuppressive therapy and predict risk of rejection as well as response to treatment

REFERENCES

1. El-Zoghby ZM, Stegall MD, Lager DJ, et al. Identifying specific causes of kidney allograft loss. Am J Transplant 2009;9:527–35. doi:10.1111/j.1600-6143.2008.02519.x. Epub 2008 Feb 3.
2. Ho J, Wiebe C, Gibson IW, et al. Immune monitoring of kidney allografts. Am J Kidney Dis 2012; 60:629–40. doi: 10.1053/j.ajkd.2012.01.028. Epub 2012 Apr 26.
3. Nankivell BJ, Alexander SI. Rejection of the kidney allograft. N Engl J Med 2010;363:1451–62. doi:10.1056/NEJMra 0902927.
4. Mengel M, Sis B, Haas M, et al. Banff Meeting Report Writing Committee. Banff 2011 Meeting report: new concepts in antibody-mediated rejection. Am J Transplant 2012;12:563–70. doi: 10.1111/j.1600-6143.2011.03926.x. Epub 2012 Feb 2. PMID: 22300494
5. Haas M, Sis B, Racusen LC, et al. As the Banff meeting report writing committee. Banff 2013 meeting report: inclusion of c4d-negative antibody-mediated rejection and antibody-associated arterial lesions. Am J Transplant. 2014;14(2):272-83. doi: 10.1111/ajt.12590. PMID: 24472190

CHAPTER 42

Recurrent Glomerular Diseases after Kidney Transplantation

Divya Monga, Hitesh H Shah

INTRODUCTION

- Glomerulonephritis (GN) is the primary cause of end-stage renal disease (ESRD) in a large percent of kidney transplant recipients
- Recurrence of the initial disease, that is, the disease that affected the native kidney, in the transplanted kidney significantly affects long-term allograft survival
- In this chapter, we review the important recurrent glomerular diseases seen after kidney transplantation

RECURRENT PRIMARY GLOMERULAR DISEASES

Focal Segmental Glomerulosclerosis (FSGS)

Recurrence rate: 20–40% of renal transplant recipients.

Risk factors: Childhood onset, rapid progression within 3 years from diagnosis to ESRD, diffuse mesangial hypercellularity in the native kidney, and recurrence of FSGS in previous allograft. Recently, serum-soluble urokinase receptor (suPAR) has been identified as a potential cause of primary FSGS.

Clinical features: Nephrotic range proteinuria within weeks of the transplant, hypertension, hematuria, and acute graft dysfunction.

Treatment: Plasmapheresis (based on the assumption that a circulating factor exists), cyclosporine, tacrolimus, cyclophosphamide, rituximab, and immunoadsorption.

Allograft prognosis: 20% of transplant recipients experience recurrence-related graft loss after 5–10 years.

Membranous Nephropathy (MN)

Recurrence rate: 10–30%.

Risk factors: No reliable predictors of recurrence, occurs earlier in recipient of live donor allograft.

Clinical features: Occurs mostly within the first 2 years post-transplant, proteinuria mostly in nephrotic range.

Treatment: Symptomatic treatment with diuretics, angiotensin-converting enzyme (ACE) inhibitors, angiotensin II receptor blockers (ARB), hypolipidemic agents. Rituximab has shown promising effects.

Allograft prognosis: 50% of transplant recipients experience recurrence-related graft loss after 5–10 years.

Membranoproliferative Glomerulonephritis (MPGN)

Recurrence rate:

- MPGN type I (idiopathic/secondary): 27–65%
- MPGN type II (dense deposit disease, DDD): 90%

Risk factors: Higher in live-related donors, hypocomplementemia and/or isolated C3 deposits suggesting DDD in a native kidney biopsy, younger age at initial diagnosis, and presence of crescents in original biopsy.

Clinical features: Hematuria, heavy proteinuria with slowly declining renal function.

Treatment:

Type I: Cyclophosphamide or high-dose MMF.

Type II: Steroids, cyclophosphamide and plasma exchange may be tried.

Allograft prognosis:

Type I: High rate of graft loss.

Type II: 34–66% graft loss after 5–10 years.

IgA Nephropathy

Recurrence rate: Most common recurrent GN, 9–61% patients.

Risk factors: Younger patients, rapid progression of original disease, zero HLA mismatched living donor grafts.

Clinical features: Hematuria, low-grade proteinuria.

Treatment: Optimal BP control, steroids, cyclophosphamide, tonsillectomy suggested by Japanese investigators.

Allograft prognosis: 3-16% of transplant recipients experience recurrence-related graft loss after 5-10 years.

Minimal Change Nephropathy (MCD)

MCD is rarely seen to recur after kidney transplantation. Hence, recurrence, risk factors, and allograft prognosis is not known.

RECURRENT SECONDARY GLOMERULAR DISEASES

Lupus Nephritis

Recurrence: Variable rates of recurrence in various studies. Some studies report about 10% of recurrence.

Risk factors: African American, non-Hispanic ancestry, female gender, young age. Other risk factors include patients with antiphospholipid antibody and those receiving kidneys from a living donor.

Clinical features: Mild proteinuria, microscopic hematuria, rarely arthralgias, or cutaneous rash.

Treatment: Intensification of immunosuppression should be reserved for the exceptional cases with severe lupus flare up.

Allograft prognosis: Graft loss in about 7% patients at 10 years.

Pauci Immune Anti-Neutrophil Cytoplasmic Antibody (ANCA) Vasculitis

Recurrence rate: 0–20%.

Risk factors: No predictable factors identified.

Clinical features: Microscopic hematuria, proteinuria, rapid rise in serum creatinine with active urine sediment with or without symptoms of vasculitis involving other organs.

Treatment: Cyclophosphamide, steroids, plasmapheresis, rituximab, IVIg for recurrence with high ANCA titers and cellular crescents on renal biopsy.

Allograft prognosis: 8% of transplant recipients experience recurrence-related graft loss after 5-10 years.

Antiglomerular Basement Membrane (AntiGBM) Disease

Recurrence rate: Rare, < 5% cases. Transplant is usually delayed until patient has been negative for serum anti-GBM antibody for at least 12 months.

Risk factors: Unclear.

Clinical features: Acute kidney allograft dysfunction, progressive GN.

Treatment: Plasma exchange, steroid pulses, and cyclophosphamide.

Allograft prognosis: Graft loss can occur.

Diabetic Nephropathy

Recurrence: Difficult to estimate.

Risk factors: Associated with autoantibodies and appearance of CD4T cells capable of mediating beta cell destruction.

Clinical features: Microalbuminuria, proteinuria, nephrotic syndrome, and progressive renal failure.

Treatment: Strict glycemic control, early use of ACE inhibitors.

Allograft prognosis: 1.8% graft loss.

Henoch–Schönlein Nephritis

Recurrence: 35% recipients.

Risk factors: Less studied, more frequent in patients who had rapidly progressive course and necrotizing/crescentic GN in native kidneys.

Clinical features: Hematuria, moderate proteinuria, and hypertension.

Treatment: Role of pulse steroids, cytotoxic drugs, and plasmapheresis unclear.

Allograft prognosis: Graft failure in 10% of patients with recurrence.

AA Amyloidosis

Recurrence: 20–30% of the recipients.

Risk factors: Risk of recurrence depends on the type and activity of original disease and older age of the recipient.

Clinical features: Varying degree of proteinuria and graft failure.

Treatment: Graft survival can be improved with better immunosuppression.

Allograft prognosis: Almost one-third of recurrent patients progress to graft loss.

Light Chain Deposition Disease (LCDD)

Recurrence: Very high recurrence, around 50% recipients.

Risk factors: Not well known.

Clinical features: Proteinuria, hematuria, progressive renal failure.

Treatment: Bortezomib and rituximab have been used; however, more long-term studies are needed for better understanding.

Allograft prognosis: Very poor prognosis.

Hemolytic Uremic Syndrome (HUS)

Recurrence: Nondiarrheal (D-) HUS recurs in 33–82% of recipients.

Risk factors: Complement factor H or factor I deficiency.

Clinical features: Hemolytic anemia, thrombocytopenia, and renal failure.

Treatment: Avoid calcineurin inhibitors, and mTOR antagonists in renal transplant recipients with (D-) HUS.

Allograft prognosis: 90% of transplant recipients experience recurrence-related graft loss after 5-10 years.

FURTHER READING

1. Canaud G, Audard V, Kofman T, et al. Recurrence from primary and secondary glomerulopathy after renal transplant. Transpl Int 2012;25:812–24.
2. Ivanyi B. A primer on recurrent and de novo glomerulonephritis in renal allografts. Nat Clin Pract Nephrol 2008;4:446–57.
3. Jan CI, Chen A, Sun GH, et al. Recurrent minimal change disease post-allograft renal transplant. Transplant Proc 2003; 35:2888–90.
4. Joshi K, Nada R, Minz M, et al. Recurrent glomerulopathy in the renal allograft. Transplant Proc 2007; 39:734–6.
5. Lorenz EC, Sethi S, Leung N, et al. Recurrent membranoproliferative glomerulonephritis after kidney transplantation. Kidney Int 2010; 77:721–8.
6. Ponticelli C, Glassock RJ. Posttransplant recurrence of primary glomerulonephritis. Clin J Am Soc Nephrol 2010; 5:2363–72.
7. Ponticelli C, Moroni G, Glassock RJ. Recurrence of secondary glomerular disease after renal transplantation. Clin J Am Soc Nephrol 2011; 6:1214–21.
8. Rodriguez EF, Cosio FG, Nasr SH, et al. The pathology and clinical features of early recurrent membranous glomerulonephritis. Am J Transplant 2012; 12:1029–38.
9. Shimizu A, Higo S, Fujita E, et al. Focal segmental glomerulosclerosis after renal transplantation. Clin Transplant 2011;23:6–14.

CHAPTER 43

De Novo Glomerular Diseases Post-Transplantation

Kenar D Jhaveri, Mohini Alexander, Surya V Seshan

INTRODUCTION

Novo (new-onset) glomerulonephritis is that which occurs in a transplant recipient whose original kidney disease was either not glomerular or was of a different pathological type. Typically, most appear a year after the kidney transplantation. De novo post-transplant glomerular diseases have the same pathological features as native diseases of that glomerular type when fully developed or sometimes modified by the immunosuppressive therapy. This may occur with or without other post-transplant pathologic findings including a component of acute or chronic rejection. Obtaining information about the original renal disease is useful to determine de novo or recurrent status of the glomerular disease in the renal allograft. The most common de novo glomerular diseases are membranous glomerulopathy, focal segmental glomerulosclerosis (FSGS), antiglomerular basement membrane (anti-GBM) disease, and drug-induced thrombotic microangiopathy (TMA).

A definitive diagnosis is made following a systematic examination of the renal biopsy for light, immunofluorescence, and electron microscopy.

FOCAL SEGMENTAL GLOMERULOSCLEROSIS (FSGS) (FIG. 1)

Incidence: 10–20% of renal allografts.

Risk factors: Long-standing chronic vascular damage, size-mismatched kidney grafts, grafts with severe vascular disease, grafts with chronic transplant glomerulopathy, chronic calcineurin inhibitor-induced glomerulopathy

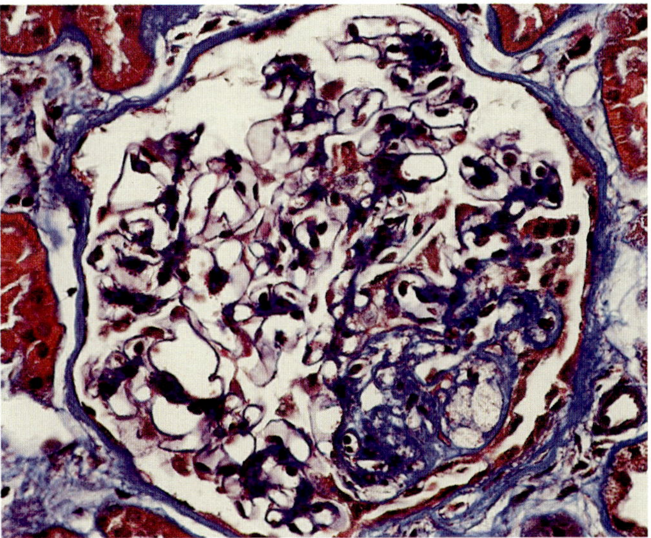

Fig. 1: Focal segmental glomerulosclerosis. Glomerulus showing a segmental scar/sclerosis with capsular adhesion and intracapillary foam cells, covered by hyperplastic podocytes. The rest of the glomerulus appears normal with thin capillary walls and patent lumina. There is diffuse foot process effacement by electron microscopy. ×400, Trichrome stain.

and viral infections such as hepatitis B virus (HBV), hepatitis C virus (HCV), parvovirus B19, EBV, and CMV. Medications such as mTOR inhibitors can also cause FSGS. If all secondary causes are excluded, the diagnosis of idiopathic FSGS occurring in the renal transplant is made, which is extremely rare.

Clinical features: 80% develop nephrotic range proteinuria or they present with hypertension, hematuria, and acute allograft dysfunction.

Treatment:

- Consider and treat secondary cause
- All receive antiproteinuric agents and antihypertensive medication
- If idiopathic, first line of treatment is high-dose steroids and cyclophosphamide (replacing the antimetabolite from the transplant regimen), followed by intravenous immunoglobulin (IVIg) and plasmapheresis. Second line is cyclosporine, rituximab, and galactose.

Allograft prognosis: The recipients with de novo FSGS and "chronic allograft parenchymal changes" had a graft survival rate of 40% at 5 years after diagnosis.

COLLAPSING GLOMERULOPATHY (FIG. 2)

Incidence: 0.6% of renal allografts

Risk factors: HIV-infected individuals, parvovirus B19, mTOR inhibitors, HTLV-1 virus, pamidronate use, or as an ischemic/adaptive form of podocytopathy leading to FSGS.

Clinical features: Nephrotic range proteinuria, severe hypertension and progressive allograft dysfunction 2–24 months after diagnosis, and rapid evolution to end-stage renal disease.

Treatment:

- Rule out and treat secondary cause
- All receive antiproteinuric agents and antihypertensive agents
- If idiopathic, first line of treatment is high-dose steroids and cyclophosphamide (replacing the antimetabolite from the transplant regimen), followed by IVIg and plasmapheresis. Second line is cyclosporine, rituximab, and galactose.

Allograft prognosis: 50% graft loss and median graft survival in the largest series if 38 weeks from time of biopsy.

MEMBRANOUS GLOMERULONEPHRITIS (MGN) (FIG. 3)

Incidence: 1.5–2% of renal allografts.

Risk factors: Time after transplantation, de novo membranous nephropathy in a first graft and HCV infection, and HBV infection and recipients of horse antithymocyte globulin. It is associated with transplant glomerulopathy and the renal biopsy often shows evidence of both rejection and the classic findings of MGN with immune complex deposits.

Clinical features: Varying degrees of proteinuria and graft dysfunction. Serum anti-PLAR2 and staining in the renal biopsy may be useful in making this diagnosis.

Treatment: Nonimmunosuppressive therapies including angiotensin inhibition, rigorous blood pressure control, and control of hyperlipidemia. Protein excretion < 4 g/day and stable renal function are treated with an increase in the maintenance dose of one or more components of the immunosuppressive regimen and those with protein excretion ≥ 4 g/day or deteriorating renal function are

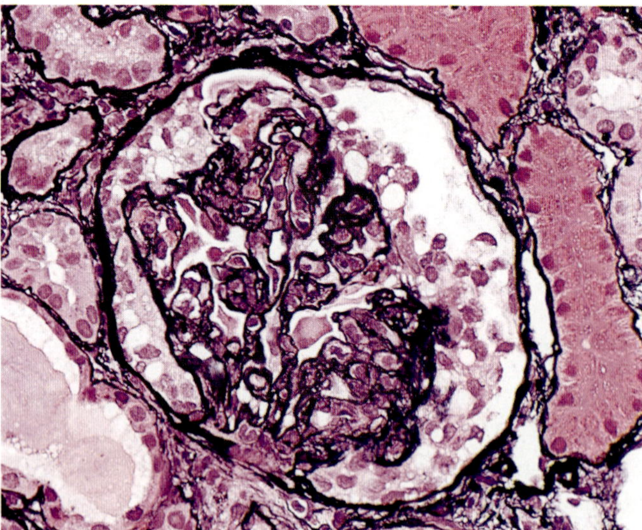

Fig. 2: Collapsing glomerulopathy. Glomerulus showing global collapse of the capillary tufts with occlusion of the capillaries and covered by hyperplastic and vacuolated epithelial cells partly filling the Bowman space. ×400, Jones Silver methenamine stain.

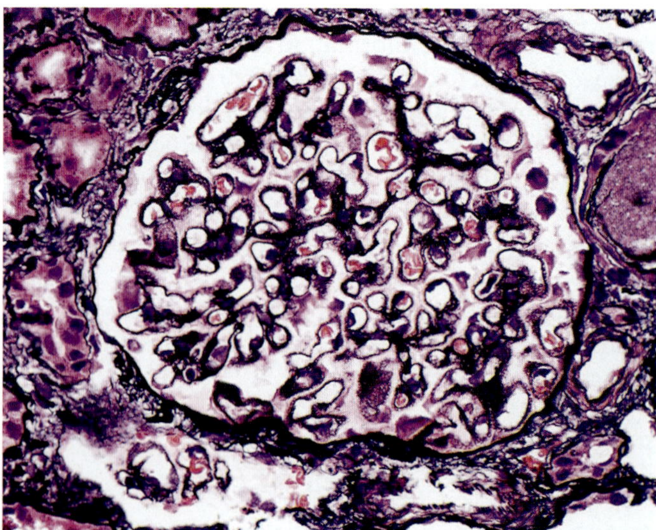

Fig. 3: Membranous glomerulonephritis. Glomerulus showing global, irregular thickening of the peripheral capillary walls with frequent spikes and lucencies on the outer aspect. No intraglomerular proliferation or inflammatory cell infiltration is noted. Numerous subepithelial immune deposits are noted by electron microscopy. ×400, Jones Silver methenamine stain.

treated with rituximab. Patients who do not respond to rituximab are given cyclophosphamide or high-dose glucocorticoids. Plasmapheresis may be considered among patients who have features of chronic rejection.

Allograft prognosis: 50% graft loss.

MEMBRANOPROLIFERATIVE GLOMERULONEPHRITIS (MPGN) (FIG. 4)

Incidence: limited information, infrequent.

Risk factors: Secondary causes have to be considered highly: Hepatitis C, medications, mixed cryoglobulinemia, malignancy, and chronic TMA. Transplant glomerulopathy can have similar morphologic appearance in the renal biopsy. Immunofluorescence and electron microscopy are essential in the differential diagnosis, since immune deposits are not present in chronic TMA and transplant glomerulopathy.

Clinical features: Varying degrees of proteinuria, hematuria, and graft dysfunction.

Treatment: Rituximab may be useful in this setting if it is an immunological cause and control of the underlying etiology if known. Data is limited on treatment.

Allograft prognosis: Not available.

THROMBOTIC MICROANGIOPATHY (FIG. 5)

Incidence: 0.8–14% with mean of 3.5%.

Risk factors: Vascular toxicity due to calcineurin inhibitors and mTOR antagonists, viral infections and/or graft rejection, younger recipient age, older donor age, and female recipient.

Clinical features: The majority of patients present with the symptoms of renal failure, hemolytic anemia, schistocytes, and thrombocytopenia that reflect the systemic TMA of HUS. Others exhibit TMA localized to the allograft; these individuals present with progressive or delayed graft dysfunction, which is often associated with arterial hypertension, and they lack thrombocytopenia and evidence of hemolysis.

Treatment: Withdrawal of the offending agent. Treatment with a drug that was the cause of a previous TMA episode should be avoided. Modification of the immunosuppressive regimen may be needed. Plasmapheresis may not be helpful.

Allograft prognosis: Graft survival rate after TMA is approximately 50% at 3 years.

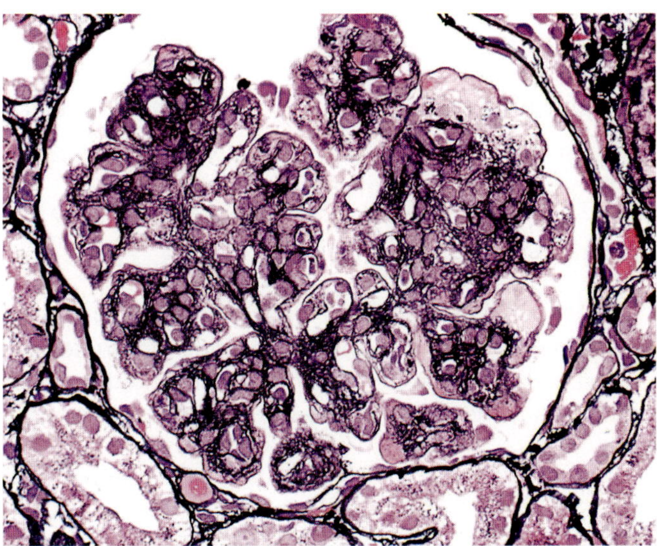

Fig. 4: Membranoproliferative glomerulonephritis. Glomerulus showing lobular accentuation, mesangial proliferation, global irregular thickening of the capillary walls with double contours and cellular interposition, leading to narrowing or occlusion of the lumina. Note focal subendothelial eosinophilic immune deposits. Abundant subendothelial and mesangial immune deposits along with new basement membrane formation are seen by electron microscopy. ×400, Jones Silver methenamine stain.

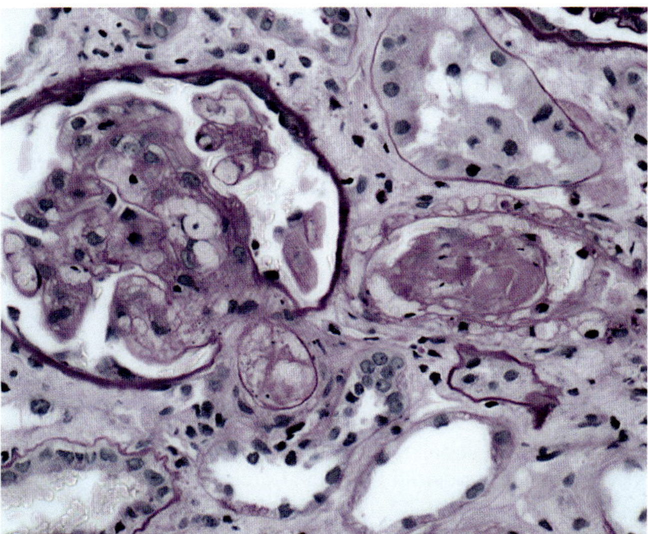

Fig. 5: Thrombotic microangiopathy due to CNI toxicity. Glomerulus showing endothelial injury, swelling and mesangiolysis causing occlusion of the capillary lumina. Note adjacent hilar arteriole and small artery with marked subendothelial swelling and luminal occlusion due to thrombosis. ×275, Periodic acid Schiff stain.

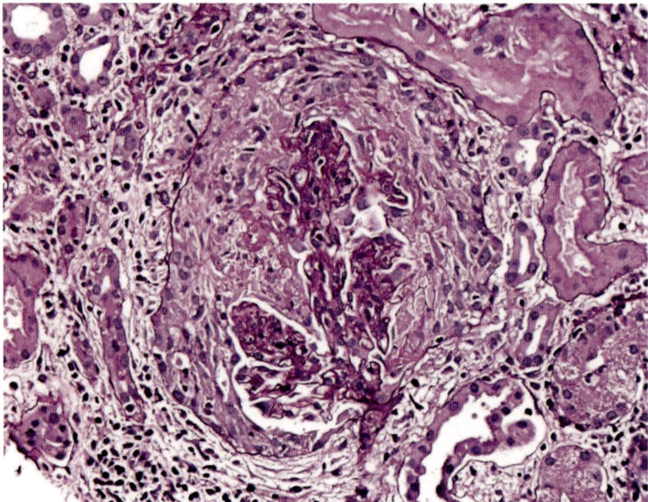

Fig. 6: Antiglomerular basement membrane glomerulonephritis. Glomerulus showing a large circumferential cellular crescent, mostly compressing the underlying normal appearing glomerular capillary tuft with a focus of fibrinoid necrosis, accompanied by active periglomerular inflammation. Global linear IgG staining is noted along the glomerular capillary walls by immunofluorescence microscopy ×400, Periodic acid Schiff stain.

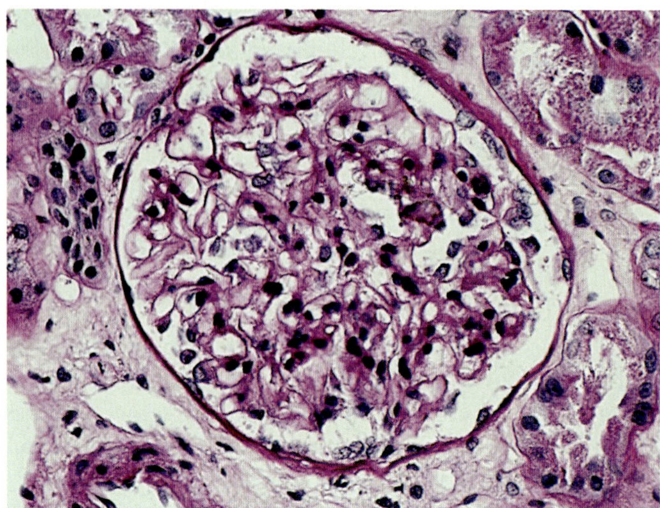

Fig. 7: Minimal change nephrotic syndrome. Glomerulus showing preserved architecture and patent capillary lumina without inflammatory or proliferative changes, but have electron microscopic findings of diffuse foot process effacement. ×400, Periodic acid Schiff stain.

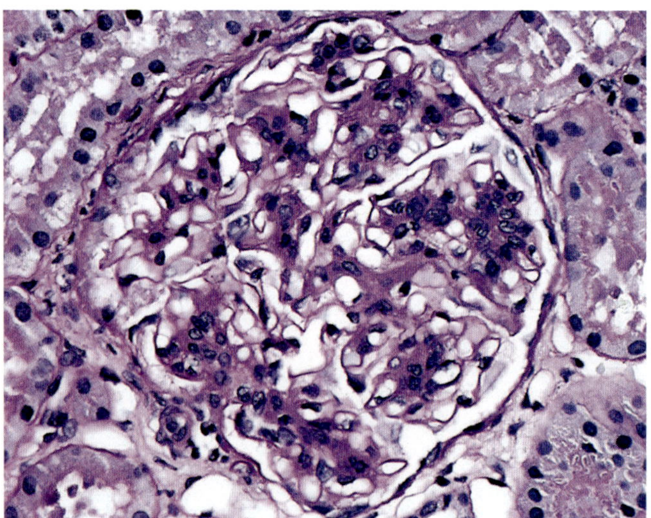

Fig. 8: Immunoglobulin A (IgA) nephropathy. Glomerulus shows global, mild-to-moderate mesangial proliferation and increased matrix, partly encroaching on the peripheral capillary lumina. The capillary walls are normal in thickness with a normal patency. Mesangial IgA immune deposits are localized by immunofluorescence and electron microscopy. ×400, Periodic acid Schiff stain.

ANTIGLOMERULAR BASEMENT MEMBRANE ANTIBODY GLOMERULONEPHRITIS (FIG. 6)

Incidence: Approximately 5% of patients with Alport syndrome who undergo transplantation develop anti-GBM nephritis due to de novo antibodies developed in the recipient against donor type IV collagen antigens.

Clinical features: The clinical presentation is commonly rapidly progressive glomerulonephritis in a few weeks to a few months and occasionally, delayed graft function.

Treatment: Anti-T-cell therapy, pulse methylprednisolone, and cyclophosphamide, longer-term plasmapheresis or mycophenolate mofetil have been of only limited benefit.

Allograft prognosis: Graft failure usually develops within a few weeks or months of diagnosis.

MINIMAL CHANGE DISEASE (FIG. 7)

Incidence: Inadequate data, but very rare.

Clinical features: Sudden onset nephrotic syndrome, rule out secondary causes such as malignancy and medications, exclude recurrent FSGS early in the post-transplant period.

Treatment: High-dose steroids.

Allograft prognosis: The glomerular disease had no meaningful long-term adverse effect on the renal allograft, when promptly treated.

IgA NEPHROPATHY (FIG. 8)

Incidence: Paucity of data, but very rare.

Clinical features: Hematuria, acute renal dysfunction, secondary causes such as infections and liver disease should be excluded

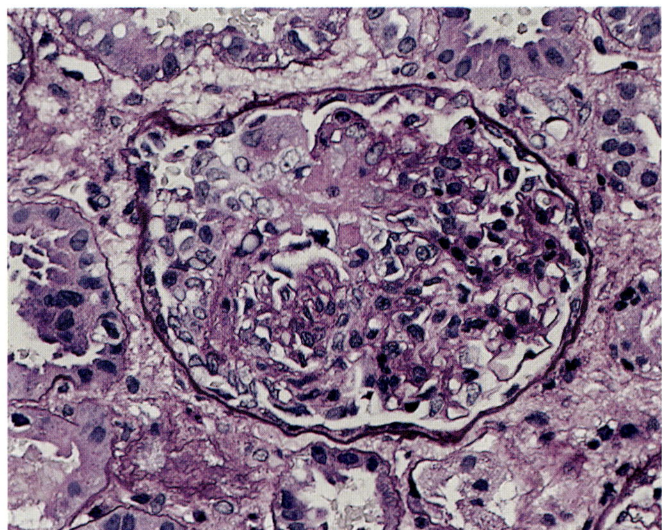

Fig. 9: ANCA-associated Pauci-immune crescentic glomerulonephritis. Glomerulus showing segmental fibrinoid necrosis and a cellular crescent in the Bowman space. The rest of the glomerulus is unremarkable. No glomerular immune deposits are identified by immunofluorescence and electron microscopy. ×400, Periodic acid Schiff stain.

Treatment: Steroids, alternative immunosuppressive agents

Allograft prognosis: Data not available.

PAUCI IMMUNE ANCA VASCULITIS/ CRESCENTIC GLOMERULONEPHRITIS (FIG. 9)

Incidence: Only anecdotal reports, but very rare.

Clinical features: Subacute renal insufficiency, proteinuria, hematuria, p-ANCA, or c-ANCA positivity.

Treatment: High-dose steroids, IV, or PO cyclophosphamide, plasmapheresis, or rituximab.

Allograft prognosis: Data not available.

POSTINFECTIOUS GLOMERULONEPHRITIS (FIG. 10)

Incidence: Not known, occasionally encountered.

Risk factors: Increased susceptibility of transplant recipients on immunosuppression for infections, commonly bacterial, viral, and fungal.

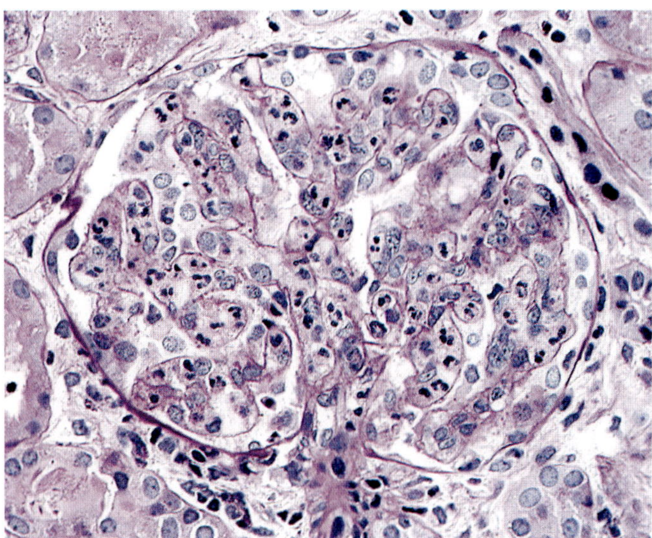

Fig. 10: Postinfectious glomerulonephritis secondary to bacterial infection. Glomerulus showing cell proliferation, endothelial swelling and marked infiltration of neutrophils within the capillaries, leading to narrowing or occlusion of the lumina. Immunofluorescence and electron microscopy display IgG and C3 positive subepithelial hump-like deposits on the basement membranes. ×400, Periodic acid Schiff stain.

Clinical features: Hematuria, proteinuria, acute renal failure, low serum complement levels, and new onset hypertension.

Treatment: Elimination or treatment of underlying infections and supportive therapy.

Allograft prognosis: Data not available.

FURTHER READING

1. Chailimpamontree W, Dmitrienko S, Li G, et al. Probability, predictors, and prognosis of post transplantation glomerulonephritis. J Am Soc Nephrol 2009; 20: 843–51.
2. Golgert W, Appel G, Hariharan S. Recurrent glomerulonephritis after renal transplantation: an unsolved problem. Clin J Am Soc Nephrol 2008; 3:800–7.
3. Ivanyi B. A primer on recurrent and de novo glomerulonephritis in renal allografts. Nat Clin Pract Nephrol 2008; 4:446–57.
4. Liapis H, Koch MJ, Mengel M. Kidney. In: Liapis H & Wang HL (eds), Pathology of solid organ transplantation. 1st edn. New York, NY: Springer, 2011:77–169.

CHAPTER 44

Neurologic Evaluation

Gabriel Pantol

Neurological Complications

- Frequently seen in the early postoperative period
- Can have a wide range of etiologies such as
  - Imbalances of glucose, electrolytes
  - Sleep deprivation
  - Psychological (i.e. guilt for receiving an organ)
  - Pharmacological agents
    - Corticosteroids
    - Sedatives
    - Calcineurin inhibitors
    - Other
- Symptoms include but are not limited to
  - Agitation
  - Anxiety
  - Coma
  - Delirium
  - Hallucinations
  - Headaches
  - Insomnia
  - Motor deficits
  - Seizures
  - Sensory deficits
  - Somnolence
  - Speech disturbances
  - Tremors
  - Visual deficits

Calcineurin Inhibitors

- Can produce acute neurotoxicity initially manifested as
  - Tremors
  - Hallucinations
  - Speech disturbances
- More severe presentations may include
  - Headaches
  - Seizures
  - Visual disturbances including cortical blindness known as PRES (posterior reversible leukoencephalopathy syndrome)
    - Brain MRI is usually characteristic with T2 posterior circulation white matter disease, but can also affect the anterior circulation territory and involve the frontal lobes (Fig. 1)
    - Associated with disruption of the blood-brain barrier and resultant vasogenic edema

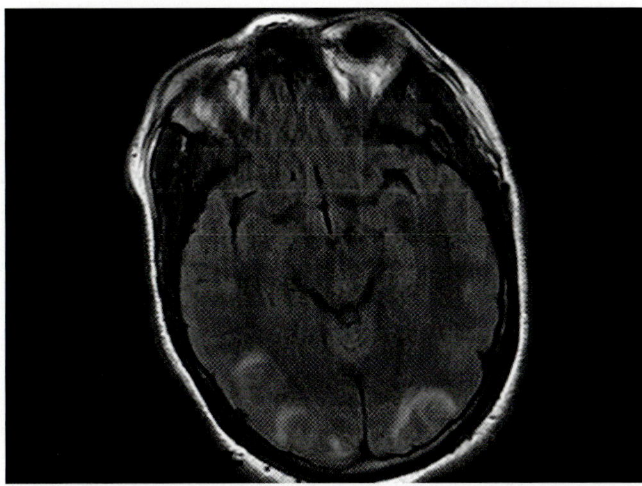

Fig. 1: PRES (posterior reversible leukoencephalopathy syndrome). T2 FLAIR sequence. Hyperintensities can be observed in the posterior circulation, mostly in the occipital lobes. The other lobes can also be involved, but to a lesser degree.

    - Can be prevented by slower drug administration or the use of alternative immunosuppressive agents
    - Symptoms may persist despite the description as a "reversible syndrome"

Corticosteroids

- Often produce agitation and insomnia when used in large doses
- In older patients may lead to mania
- The use of antipsychotics to treat agitation can precipitate a neuroleptic malignant syndrome, parkinsonism, or simply exacerbate tremors in those with yet undiagnosed Parkinson's disease

Seizures

- Can present de novo or as exacerbations of prior ictal disorders
- Focal seizures likely reflect organic lesions such as
  - Strokes
  - Abscesses
  - Bleeds
- Generalized tonic-clonic seizures suggest global processes such as
  - Meningitis
  - Electrolyte imbalances
  - Substance withdrawal (alcohol or short-acting benzodiazepines)
  - Side effects of medications that lower the seizure threshold
  - Haloperidol
  - β-Lactams (penicillin, imipenem)
  - Calcineurin inhibitors
- Nonconvulsive status epilepticus should be ruled out in all instances of
  - Failure to regain consciousness after a seizure
  - Prolonged post-ictal periods

Osmotic Myelinolysis

- Encountered as a complication of rapid correction of hyponatremia, and less likely hypernatremia
- *Central pontine myelinolysis* refers to this phenomenon within the central basis pontis, involved in about 90% of patients
- 10% of cases involve an extrapontine location
- History of alcohol abuse may be a predisposing factor
- Clinical presentation includes
  - Quadriparesis
  - Ophthalmoparesis
  - Behavior abnormalities
  - Seizures and coma may be present

Cerebrovascular Events

- Frequent among transplant recipients
- Should be suspected in the setting of acute neurologic changes associated with focal findings such as
  - Aphasia
  - Dysarthria
  - Weakness
  - Visual complaints
- 10-year risk around 8%
  - Most occurring within the first 5 years
- Predisposing factors include
  - Hypertension
  - Diabetes mellitus
  - Tobacco use
  - Hyperlipidemia
  - Polycystic kidney disease
  - Length of time on dialysis
- Two-third of strokes are
  - Ischemic
    - Likely due to occlusion of small perforating arteries (lacunes)
  - Embolic
    - From thrombi originating within the heart, valves, aorta, its arch or the carotids
- One-third of strokes are hemorrhagic
  - Often related to
    - Uncontrolled hypertension
    - Anticoagulation
- Subarachnoid hemorrhages are somewhat rare and associated with aneurysm rupture, most commonly in patients with polycystic kidney disease

Central Nervous System Infections

During the first weeks after transplant usually associated with

- Surgical complications
- Prolonged hospitalization

Bacterial Meningitis

- Presents with
  - Headaches
  - Neck stiffness
  - Fever
  - Encephalopathy
- May occur in patients with no prior history of sepsis

- Causative agents, encountered on cultures usually include
  - Staphylococci
  - Gram-negatives

Other Infections

- Atypical infections, including opportunistic entities, reactivation of dormant organis ms, and infection acquired from the organ donor
- Most common pathogens include
  - Viruses (HSV, CMV, VZV)
  - Mycobacteria
  - Fungi (*Candida, Cryptococcus, Aspergillus*)
- Neutropenic patients are most at risk and may not be able to mount a febrile response
- Any change in mental status, new focal symptoms, fever, or seizures in a post-transplant patient should prompt a battery of tests including
  - Blood cultures (bacterial, fungal, mycobacteria)
  - Viral serologies (including seasonal infections such as West Nile virus)
  - Chest X-ray
  - Lumbar puncture
  - Brain imaging (preferable MRI)

Acute Mononeuropathies

- Frequently caused by trauma or positioning during surgery
- The most common neuropathy involves the femoral nerve, caused by either direct trauma along its course anterior to the iliopsoas muscle or by the development of a retroperitoneal hematoma
- Presentation is usually weakness in a length-dependent fashion
- In femoral neuropathy, the first manifestation will be a quadriceps femoris weakness
- Acute generalized weakness may be due to problems involving
  - Multiple nerves (polyneuropathy)
  - The neuromuscular junction (such as myasthenia gravis), although this is less frequent and can be exacerbated by stress or medications such as aminoglycosides
  - The muscle itself

Critical Care Myopathy

- Encountered more frequently in intubated patients—not uncommonly diagnosed after failed ventilator weaning trials
- Risk factors include sepsis, the use of high dose steroids and paralytic agents
- Other common causes of acute and subacute myopathy are statins, colchicine, steroids, electrolyte imbalances or simply deconditioning

Subacute or Chronic Neuropathies

- Caused by exacerbation of prior conditions (such as uremia and alcoholism) or by medications such as tacrolimus or etoposide
- There are reports of acute inflammatory demyelinating polyradiculoneuropathy (AIDP, also known as Guillain–Barre syndrome) encountered months after transplantation that may be associated with CMV or host versus graft disease
- Whether acute, subacute, or chronic, all of these conditions share lower motor neuron disease characteristics that include
  - Hyporeflexia
  - Decreased tone
  - Weakness
  - Sensory deficits
  - Atrophy

Management

- Once *airway, breathing and circulation* are addressed, the first step in management includes evaluation of vital signs, obtaining a proper history inclusive of the patient's complaints (if able to verbalize them), and performing a physical examination
- In instances of *altered mental status,* blood work and brain imaging should be obtained STAT
- CBC with differential will help to diagnose acute anemia or infection
- Metabolic panel will reveal electrolytic and other imbalances (such as sodium, glucose and calcium disorders)
- *Hypo- or hyperkalemia and hypomagnesemia* will present with generalized weakness, EKG changes, and even cardiac arrhythmias
- Blood cultures should be ordered if an infection is suspected, even in the absence of fever
- Noncontrast head CT is recommended to rule out bleeds, acute strokes and to evaluate any pathologies that would contraindicate lumbar puncture
- If *meningoencephalitis* is suspected, treatment should be empiric and immediate. Antibiotic therapy should NOT be delaying while waiting for imaging or lumbar puncture results

- Medications administered recently as well as within the past 24–48 hours should be always addressed
- If a *benzodiazepine overdose* is suspected, administer flumazenil, giving 0.2 mg IV pushes every minute, up to five times
  - It is important to be aware that a possible and alarming side effect includes the onset of seizures
- Whenever *opiate overdose* is suspected (altered mental status seen in combination with bilateral miosis), naloxone 0.4–2 mg IV can be given
- In instances of suspected prior history of alcohol abuse, (clinically evident nystagmus, ophthalmoparesis, and ataxia), always give IV thiamine prior to the administration of glucose, given the likelihood of *Wernicke's encephalopathy*
- In general, older patients with history of dementia or mild cognitive impairment are more prone to *medication side effects*
- As stated earlier, *calcineurin inhibitors* can be neurotoxic, both immediately during the period of administration as well as beyond it. Sometimes, simply decreasing the dosage or switching to a different agent can lead to improvements in mental status. If symptoms persist, the immunosuppressive medication regimen should be reconsidered
- *Once all the above etiologies have been ruled out*, sleep deprivation or sundown phenomenon may be considered
  - Reassurance, providing visual cues regarding orientation in time and space, and establishing a circadian rhythm is extremely important
  - Overuse of antipsychotic medications in this setting will create a new dilemma, namely lethargy. If necessary a hypnotic like zolpidem 5–10 mg can be used
- If an *acute stroke* is suspected, the Neurology or Stroke team should be consulted immediately
  - A STAT head CT and blood work inclusive of a recent coagulation profile should be obtained
  - Most patients will not qualify for IV thrombolysis if surgery was recently performed
  - A normal head CT does not exclude an acute stroke but is very sensitive for intracranial hemorrhages and will prompt a different type of care
- For *seizures*, administer lorazepam 2 mg IV push
  - If patient has a history of *epilepsy*, add anticonvulsant levels to the routine blood work and (imaging testing)
  - If seizures continue for longer than 5 minutes, the patient is likely to develop *status epilepticus*—a neurological emergency
  - If the patient fails to awake in a timely fashion manner, order continuous EEG monitoring to rule out *nonconvulsive status epilepticus*
  - EEG might also help distinguishing other causes of encephalopathy
  - Generalized background slowing usually implies a *toxic or metabolic* cause and periodic lateralized epileptiform discharges can be seen with *herpes encephalitis* or other focal process
- *Brain MRI* is an important tool, though it may not be readily available in all settings
  - It is more sensitive than head CT in the diagnosis of PRES, acute stroke, abscess, encephalitis and other neurological conditions
  - The use of gadolinium may be limited depending on the patient's renal function secondary to an increased risk of developing nephrogenic systemic fibrosis especially in patients with a GFR (glomerular filtration rate < 30)
    - In some cases, immediate dialysis must be arranged following contrast administration
- For *peripheral nervous system presentations*, EMG, and NCS, along with muscle enzymes will help in diagnosis
- In cases of suspected *AIDP*, CSF should be obtain for analysis and will show increased protein
  - Patients with AIDP should be monitored in the intensive care unit setting given the risk of respiratory insufficiency and autonomic failure
  - Symptoms may include extremes in blood pressure (both low and high), arrhythmias, anhidrosis and gastroparesis

FURTHER READING

1. Amato AA, Barohn RJ, Sahenk Z, et al. Polyneuropathy complicating bone marrow and solid organ transplantation. Neurology 1993;43:1513–8.
2. Buis CI, Wijdicks EF. Serial magnetic imaging of central pontine myelinolysis. Liver Transpl 2002;8:643–5.
3. Bulsara KR, Baron PW, Tuttle-Newhall JE, et al. Guillain-Barré syndrome in organ and bone marrow transplant patients. Transplantation 2001;71:1169–72.
4. Eaton JM. A reversible posterior leukoencephalopathy syndrome. N Engl J Med 1996;334:1744.

5. Lanzino G, Cloft H, Hemstreet MK, et al. Reversible posterior leukoencephalopathy following organ transplantation. Description of two cases. Clin Neurol Neurosurg 1997;99:222.
6. Oliveras A, Roquer J, Puig JM, et al. Stroke in renal transplant recipients: epidemiology, predictive risk factors and outcome. Clin Transplant 2003;17:1–8.
7. Patchell RA. Neurological complications of organ transplantation. Ann Neurol 1994; 36:688–703. This is a review of the toxicity of immunosuppressive agents, CNS infections, and causes of encephalopathy in organ transplant recipients
8. Sharma KR, Cross J, Santiago F, et al. Incidence of acute femoral neuropathy following renal transplantation. Arch Neurol 2002;59:541–5.

CHAPTER 45

Vascular Complications

Ernesto P Molmenti and Collaborators

Intraoperative Doppler

- We routinely obtain an intraoperative Doppler evaluation of the transplant renal vessels as well as of the recipient vessels used for implantation (usually the external iliac artery and vein) both proximal and distal with respect to the anastomoses, to document satisfactory flow after the kidney has been placed in the position where it will lay after closure of the abdomen
- If flow is not satisfactory, consider
  - Malpositioning of the allograft
    - The kidney should be repositioned so that the renal artery and vein lie in a comfortable way with no kinks or twists
  - Anastomotic defects
    - Redoing the arterial or venous anastomosis entails a delicate process that includes additional ischemic time
  - Pathologies in the recipient native vessels such as dissections, atherosclerotic lesions, strictures, and thrombi
  - Pathologies in the donor vessels such as dissections, atherosclerotic lesions, strictures, or thrombi
  - External compression

Duplex Doppler Ultrasound Evaluation

We routinely obtain a duplex Doppler ultrasound imaging study of the transplant kidney in the recovery room immediately after transplantation to document:

- Adequate arterial and venous flow in the transplant renal vessels (both intra- and extraparenchymal)
- Flow at the anastomoses
- Absence of hydronephrosis in the transplant kidney
- Adequate arterial and venous flow in the recipient vessels used for implantation of the allograft
- Collections (absent, present, actively expanding)
- Baseline findings that can serve for comparison with future studies

Arterial Flow Velocities

- Immediate postoperative period
  - Usually elevated (especially at the renal artery anastomosis)
    - In the absence of clinical findings suggestive of allograft dysfunction, they can usually be managed by clinical observation and follow up studies
    - In cases of impaired function, additional diagnostic studies such as angiography with pressure measurements (or MR or CT) are indicated
- Short, intermediate, and long-term postoperative period
  - If elevated, suspect arterial stenosis
    - Proceed with additional studies (angiogram, pressure measurements, CT, MR) to further evaluate

Resistive Index

- RI = (Peak systolic velocity-End diastolic velocity)/ Peak systolic velocity
- RI range: 0–1 (or 0–100%) (Values >1 or >100% are associated with reversal of diastolic flow and should be immediately evaluated to determine their etiology)
- Normal arterial RI: 0.5–0.8
- Low arterial RI (< 0.5) suggestive of
  - Impaired flow (arterial strictures, kinks, twists, thromboses, external arterial compression)
    - Characterized by diminished peak systolic velocity
  - Arteriovenous fistulae
    - Characterized by elevated peak diastolic velocity

- Elevated arterial RI (> 0.8) suggestive of
  - Increased parenchymal resistance (ATN, rejection, edema)
  - Impaired outflow (venous thromboses external venous compression)
    - Characterized by reversal of diastolic flow with RI > 1.0

Absent or Severely Impaired Flow to the Transplanted Kidney

- Constitutes an emergency
- Can result from:
  - Thrombosis of the organ
  - Twists or kinks in the vessels
  - Anastomotic defects
  - Impaired flow in the native vessels used for implantation
  - External compression
- Parenchymal viability in the setting of absent or severely impaired flow is limited to a short time span
- Although in some instances an angiogram could be performed, absent or severely impaired flow documented by duplex Doppler ultrasound in the immediate postoperative period is an indication for emergency surgical re-exploration

Reimplantation of the Kidney

- Complex procedure
- Required in instances of defective arterial and/or venous anastomoses leading to inadequate allograft vascular inflow and/or outflow intraoperatively or immediately postoperatively
- Requires reclamping of recipient iliac vessels
- Perfusion with cold preservation fluid or crystalloid is required in instances where the anastomosis cannot be taken down and redone in a rapid fashion
- A basin with ice should always be available to allow for the kidney to be removed and perfused with cold preservation fluid or crystalloid and kept in a hypothermic environment until the operative field is prepared for the reimplantation

Renal Artery Stenosis

Presentation

- Allograft dysfunction
- Uncontrollable hypertension
- Location
  - Anastomosis (most frequent)
  - Transplant renal artery

Etiology

- Technical complications
- External compression
- Kinking or twisting of the artery
- Donor atherosclerotic disease
- Acquired atherosclerotic disease
- Ischemia
- Rejection
- Infection
- Injuries (surgical instruments at implantation, procurement damage)

Diagnosis

- Duplex Doppler ultrasound examination shows post-stenotic turbulence, elevated velocities, and decreased resistive indices
- Angiography and other imaging studies (CT, MR)
- Decreased function on "captopril scans"

Treatment

Immediate postoperative period:

- In the immediate postoperative period (such as evidenced by a Duplex Doppler study obtained in the recovery room), impaired flow can be due to malpositioning of the kidney at the time of abdominal closure. In such instances, our policy is to return immediately to the operating room (without any further studies). In some instances in which the impaired flow is due to malpositioning of the allograft or small arterial or venous kinks or twists it may be possible to treat by placing the kidney in a way in which the vessels lie in a comfortable position without having to redo the anastomoses. Prompt treatment is required in order to minimize damage to the allograft
- Other etiologies (such as back-walling of the anastomosis or intimal dissections) should always be considered in the differential diagnosis. In these cases, the underlying problem should be identified and corrected

Delayed Fashion

- Percutaneous pressure gradient measurements provide evidence of the severity of the stricture
- Percutaneous angioplasty can lead to temporary improvement—repeat dilatations are frequently required
- Percutaneous stent placement is usually successful
  - May not be possible in instances of very recent anastomoses where it could lead to disruption of the anastomosis
- Surgical repair is usually reserved for cases that have failed or are not amenable to percutaneous correction (Figs. 1 to 4)

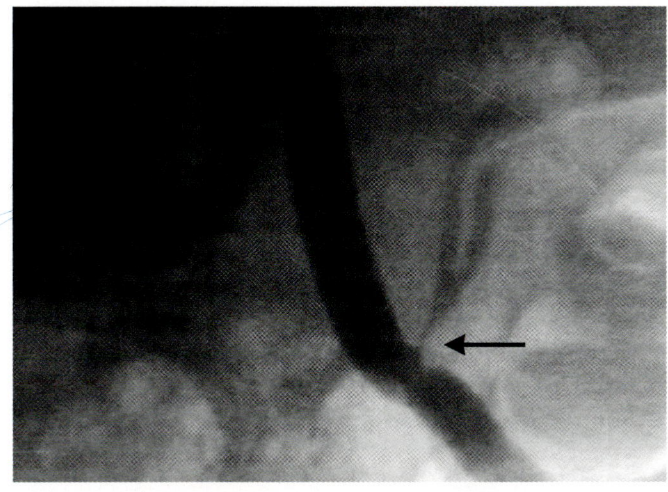

Fig. 1: Renal transplant recipient who presented with uncontrollable hypertension. Patient initially underwent percutaneous angioplasty that eventually restenosed (arrow).

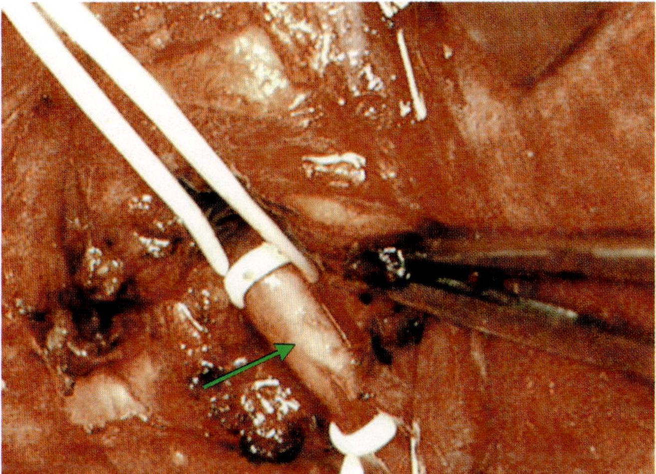

Fig. 2

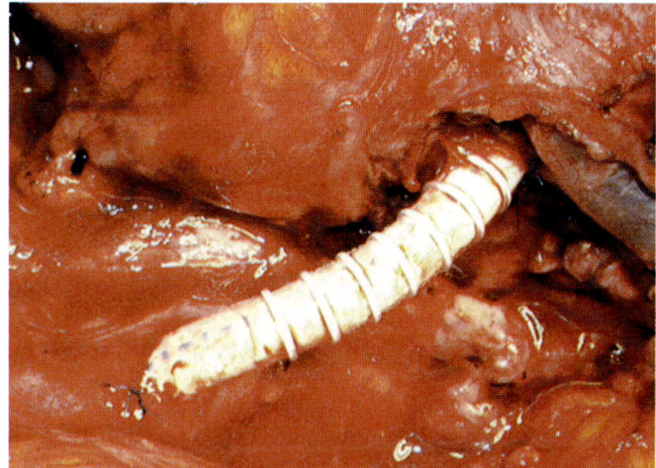

Fig. 3

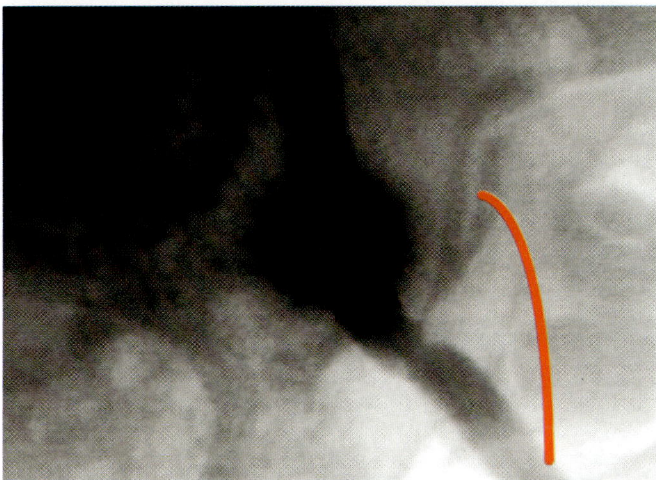

Fig. 4

Figs. 2 to 4: Surgical repair was undertaken with a prosthetic graft that bridged the iliac artery (distal to the site of implantation, green arrow) to one of the bifurcation branches of the transplant renal artery (as shown by the red line). This maneuver allowed for continuous perfusion of the allograft during the vascular repair.

Renal Artery Thrombosis

Presentation

- Sudden allograft failure

Etiology

- Technical complications
- Hypercoagulability
- External compression
- Kinking or twisting of the artery
- Hyperacute rejection
- Hypotension
- Injuries (surgical instruments at implantation, procurement damage)

Diagnosis

- Duplex Doppler ultrasound examination shows no flow
- Angiography and other imaging studies (CT, MR)
- Radionuclide studies show no perfusion

Treatment

- Immediate thrombectomy and revascularization has been successful in only a few instances
- Allograft nephrectomy, when indicated (Figs. 5 and 6)

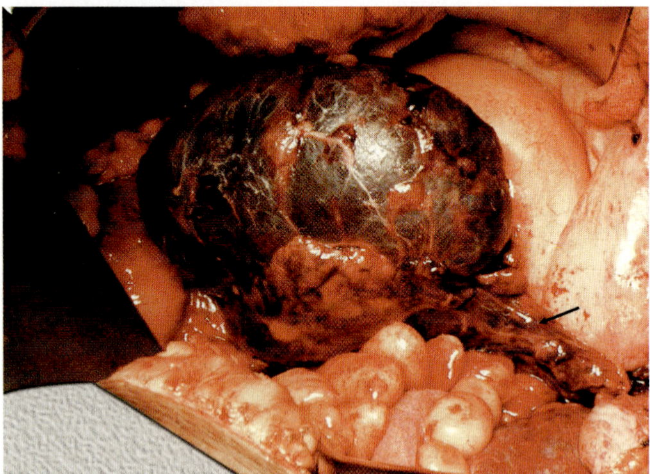

Fig. 5: Renal artery thrombosis with infarction and necrosis of the renal allograft. This usually happens at the time of the surgery or soon thereafter. Other potential causative agents of renal infarction include but are not limited to hyperacute rejection, malpositioning of the kidney, hypotension, torsion of the vessels, incorrectly placed sutures, and idiopathic causes. Note the associated necrosis of the ureter (arrow).

Segmental Renal Artery Thrombosis

Presentation

- Variable allograft dysfunction based on the extent of involvement

Etiology

- Technical complications
- Hypercoagulability
- External compression
- Kinking or twisting of an arterial branch
- Embolic
- Injuries (surgical instruments at implantation, procurement damage)

Diagnosis

- Usually discovered incidentally
- Duplex Doppler ultrasound examination shows no flow in the region/s involved
- Angiography and other imaging studies (CT, MR)
- Radionuclide studies show no perfusion of the involved areas ("cold spots")

Treatment

- Correction of predisposing factors (if present)
- Further treatment based on the extent of involvement and clinical findings

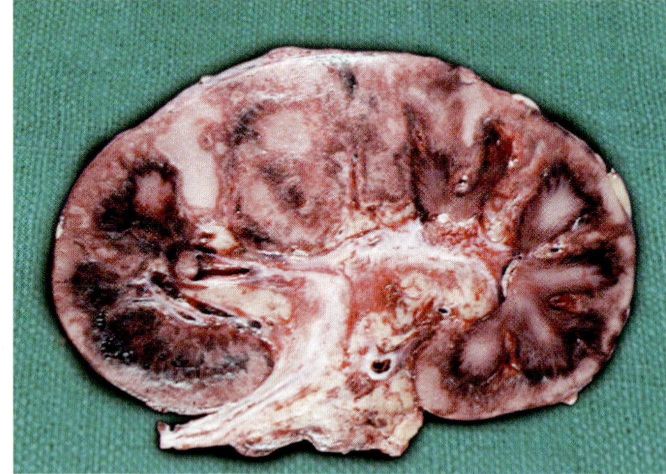

Fig. 6: Transected gross specimen of the resected thrombosed allograft.

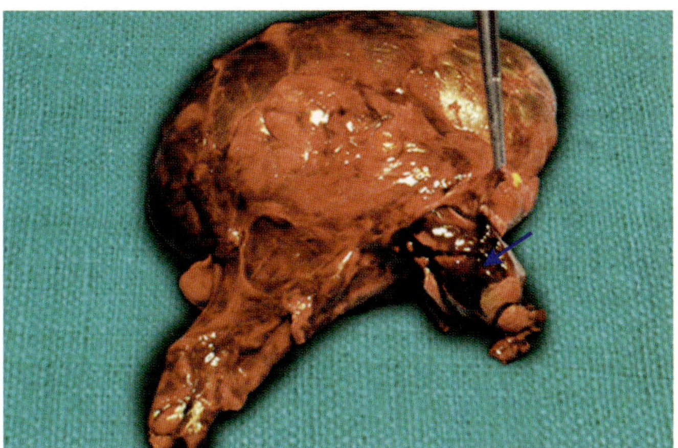

Fig. 7: Thrombosed renal vein (shown by an arrow) that resulted in allograft thrombosis.

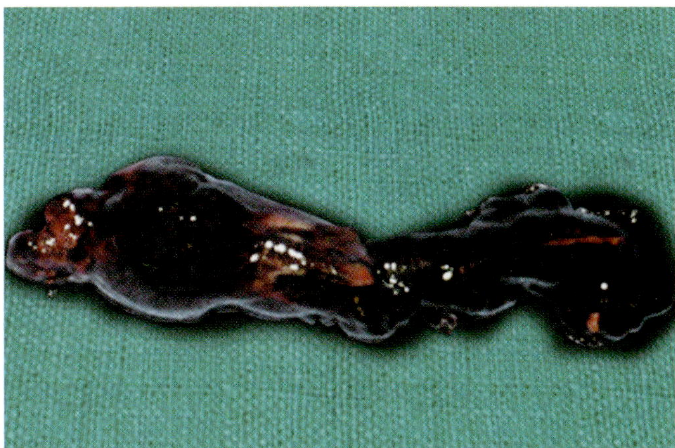

Fig. 8: Thrombus after it was removed from the renal vein.

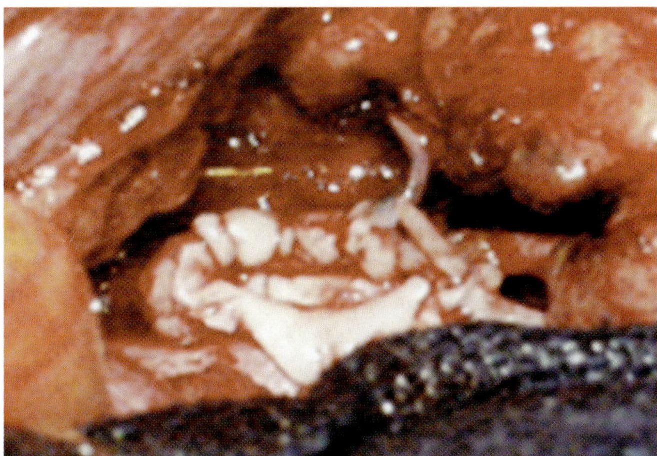

Fig. 9: It is useful (although of no clinical benefit) to evaluate the site of the venous anastomosis to determine whether a technical problem (such as back walling of the anastomosis) was accountable for the complication.

Renal Vein Stenosis

Presentation

- Allograft dysfunction (acute setting)
- Insidious presentation (chronic setting)

Etiology

- Technical complications
- External compression
- Kinking or twisting of the vein
- Fibrosis

Diagnosis

- Duplex Doppler ultrasound examination shows increased poststenotic venous velocities
- Angiography and other imaging studies (CT, MR)
- Radionuclide studies may show decreased perfusion and function depending on the severity of the stricture

Treatment

Correction of the stricture or its causative factors (such as external compression) in instances of clinical relevance and/or potential predisposition to venous thrombosis

Renal Vein Thrombosis

Presentation

- Allograft dysfunction (acute setting)
- Insidious presentation (chronic setting)

Etiology

- Technical complications
- External compression
- Kinking or twisting of the vein
- Thrombosis of the recipient iliac vein
- Nephrotic syndrome
- Recipient factors (hypercoagulable conditions, malignancies, pregnancy, hypovolemia, trauma)

Diagnosis

- Duplex Doppler ultrasound examination shows absent venous flow and reversal of arterial diastolic flow
- Angiography and other imaging studies (CT, MR)

Treatment

- Acute thrombosis:
  - Emergent exploration with potential thrombectomy in the absence of parenchymal thrombosis
  - Allograft nephrectomy in the presence of parenchymal thrombosis (Figs. 7 to 9)

- Chronic thrombosis:
  - Percutaneous lysis of thrombus, when clinically indicated
  - Surgical intervention, an unlikely consideration
  - Serial observation
- Correction of predisposing factors
  - Hypercoagulability
  - Kinks and twists
  - External compression
  - Technical complications
  - Other (such as vessel size discrepancy between donor and recipient)
- Impaired flow in the recipient vein (such as seen with DVT) may mimic renal vein thrombosis. In such instances, every effort should be directed to correct the underlying impairment in order to prevent thrombosis of the transplant renal vein

Intrarenal Pseudoaneurysms and Arteriovenous Fistulas

Presentation

- Usually asymptomatic (except in instances of rupture or steal syndrome)
- Hematuria
- Graft dysfunction associated with shunting

Etiology

Almost always secondary to needle renal biopsies.

Diagnosis

- Usually discovered accidentally
- Duplex Doppler ultrasound:
  - Pseudoaneurysms:
    - Turbulent "to-and-fro" pattern with a tight neck (entrance)
  - Arteriovenous fistulas
    - High velocity
    - Low resistive index
    - Arterialized venous waveform
- Angiography/CT/MR
- Radionuclide imaging
  - Pseudoaneurysms
    - Areas of isotope accumulation ("hot spots")
  - Arteriovenous fistulas
    - Premature venous isotope activity

Treatment

- Symptomatic or large:
  - Percutaneous embolization

Extrarenal Pseudoaneurysms and Arteriovenous Fistulas

Presentation

- Usually asymptomatic, (Except when ruptured or associated with steal syndrome)
- Sepsis, if infected
- Massive exsanguination and hemodynamic instability, if ruptured

Etiology

- Technical complications at the time of transplantation, most frequent
- Infectious
- Secondary to needle renal biopsies

Diagnosis

- Usually discovered incidentally, if not ruptured
- High degree of clinical suspicion in the setting of exsanguination, if ruptured
- Duplex Doppler ultrasound:
  - Pseudoaneurysms:
    - Turbulent "to-and-fro" pattern with a tight neck (entrance)
  - Arteriovenous fistulas:
    - High velocity
    - Low resistive index
    - Arterialized venous waveform
- Angiography/CT/MR
- Radionuclide imaging
  - Pseudoaneurysms
    - Areas of isotope accumulation ("hot spots")
  - Arteriovenous fistulas
    - Premature venous isotope activity

TREATMENT

- Repair
  - Surgical
  - Percutaneous
- If infected:
  - Nephrectomy with resection of involved vessels and vascular reconstruction (Reimplantation of the allograft at a different site could potentially be considered based on individual specific circumstances)

FURTHER READING

1. Shapiro R, Simmons R, Starzl T. Renal transplantation. Appleton and Lange, 1997.

CHAPTER 46

Allograft Nephrectomy

Ernesto P Molmenti and Collaborators

- In instances of failed allografts that require removal, several surgical approaches are possible
- When a nephrectomy is performed within a short time after transplantation, the incision can be reopened and the kidney removed
- In cases where the allograft has been in place for a prolonged time, the allograft can be removed in an open way or laparoscopically
- Open approach (Figs. 1 to 6) entails:
  - Subcapsular dissection and mobilization of the allograft
  - Clamping and subsequent transection of the hilar structures (transplant renal artery, transplant renal vein, ureter)
  - Removal of the allograft
  - Oversewing of the hilar structures (making sure that the native vessels, bladder, and surrounding structures are not injured)
  - Closure of the abdominal wall muscles, fascia, and skin
  - Optional placement of a drain

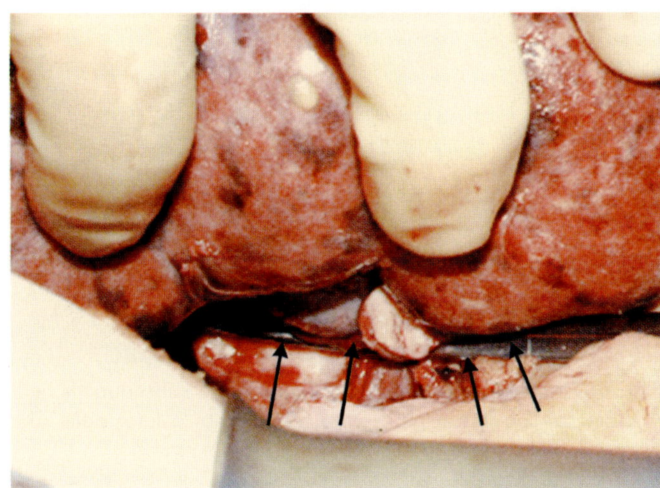

Fig. 1: We gain access by making an incision following the original one. After the abdominal wall muscles have been transected (taking care not to injure any viscera), we proceed to perform a subcapsular blunt dissection of the kidney. This maneuver will free the allograft up to its hilar area. The hilum is identified, and a clamp (arrows) placed encompassing the transplant renal artery, vein, and ureter. It is very important when doing this not to injure the recipient iliac vessels.

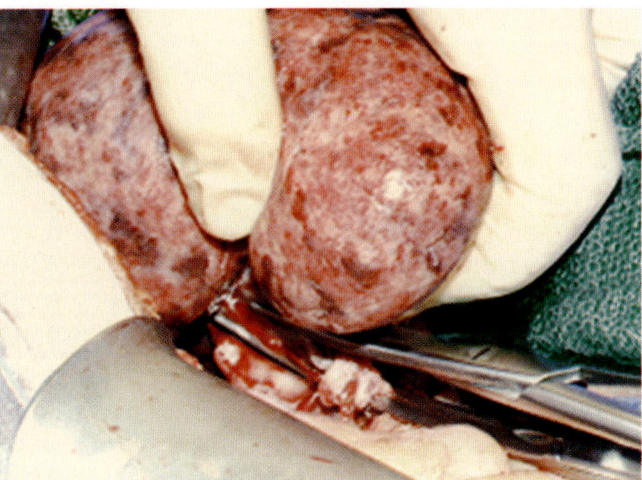

Fig. 2: Once the hilar structures have been securely clamped, they are transected as close as possible to the renal parenchyma.

- Fluid collections are almost the norm at the site of the nephrectomy
- In such instances it is important to ensure that these collections
  - Are not infected
  - Are not associated with ongoing hemorrhage
- As little as possible, tissue from the allograft vessels should be left in place to prevent a potential rejection (after withdrawal of immunosuppression) that could lead to pseudoaneurysms or ruptures
- Although apparently a simple procedure, allograft nephrectomy can be associated with major complications that should not be underestimated

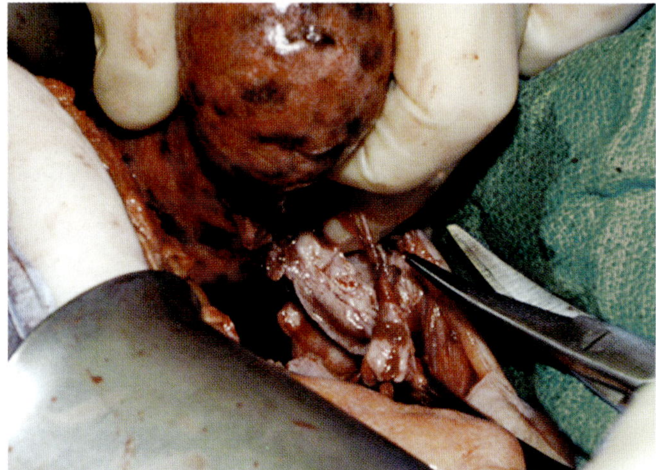

Fig. 3: The hilar structures are transected.

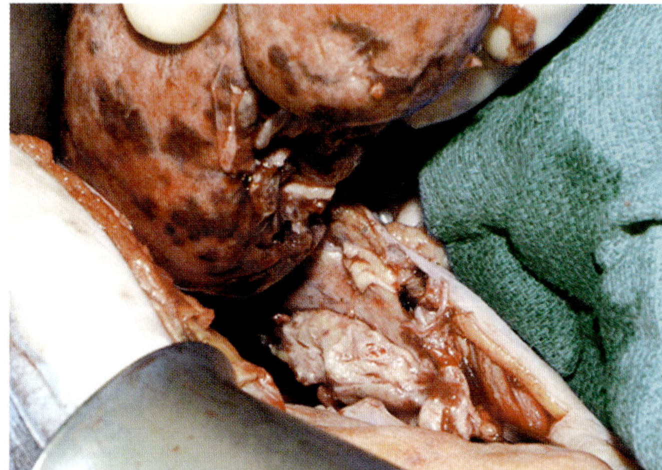

Fig. 4: The allograft is removed.

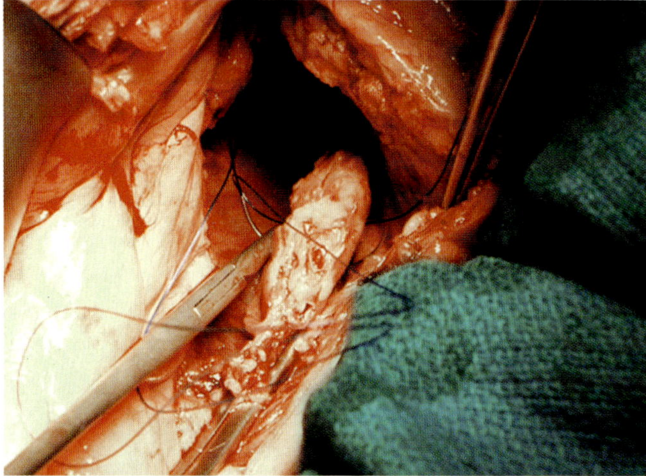

Fig. 5: The hilar stump is oversewn. We prefer to do this with a continuous suture of nonabsorbable material (such as 2-0 monofilament polypropylene).

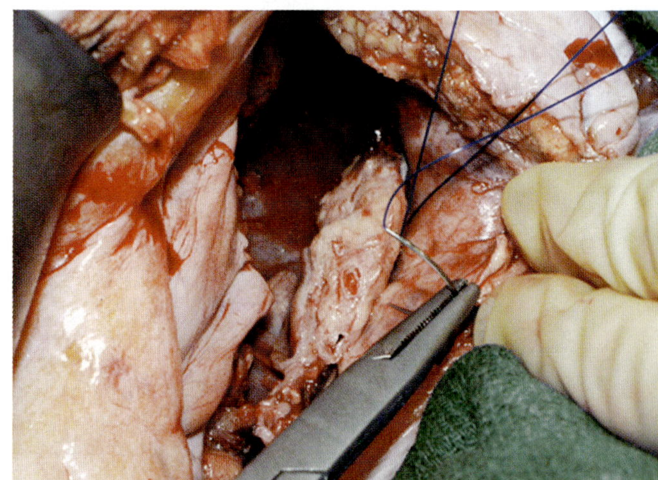

Fig. 6: The suture is run back and forth, and subsequently tied. A drain can be left in place and removed at a later date. The overlying muscle layer is sutured, and the skin closed.

CHAPTER 47

Urologic Complications and Fluid Collections

Ernesto P Molmenti and Collaborators

BLOOD SUPPLY OF THE URETER

The native ureter receives its blood supply from three different arterial sources:

- Renal artery
- Gonadal artery
- Superior vesical artery

The transplant ureter receives its arterial supply solely from the

- Renal artery

This is especially important in instances of accessory arteries to the lower pole of the kidney. In such cases, the lower pole artery may constitute the main (or only) arterial supply to the ureter. Failure to reconstruct these lower pole arteries may lead to ureteral necrosis. Furthermore, the ureter should not be skeletonized, since the periureteral tissues and fascia help preserve its irrigation and viability.

Figures 1 to 4 illustrate various findings in procured kidneys.

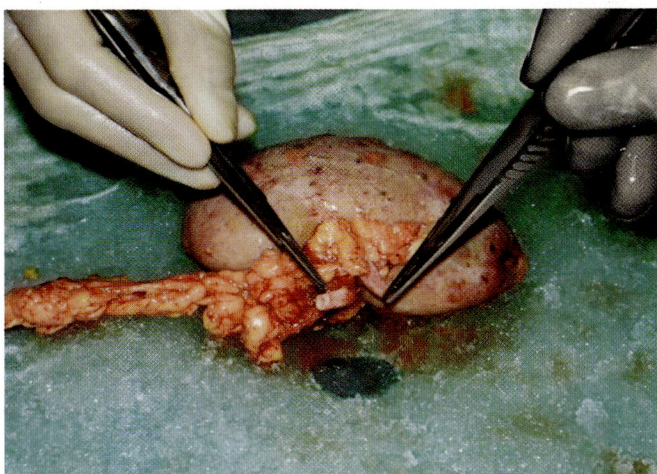

Fig. 1: The surrounding fascia and tissues of the ureter are essential components in preserving its blood supply.

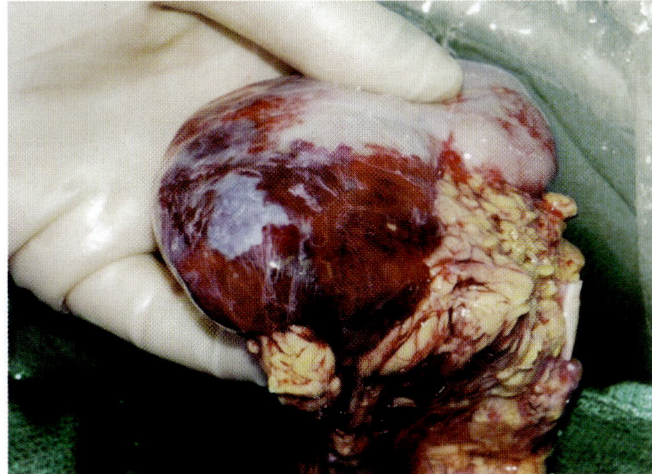

Fig. 2: In this specific instance, there is a hematoma and the lower pole of the kidney has not flushed like the remaining parenchyma. This finding should be of concern, since it raises the possibility of an injury to an accessory lower pole artery and a potential devascularization of the ureter. Although at the time of transplantation such findings may not be of major concern (the majority of the renal parenchyma will be well perfused), delayed ischemic ureteral injuries are a frequent corollary.

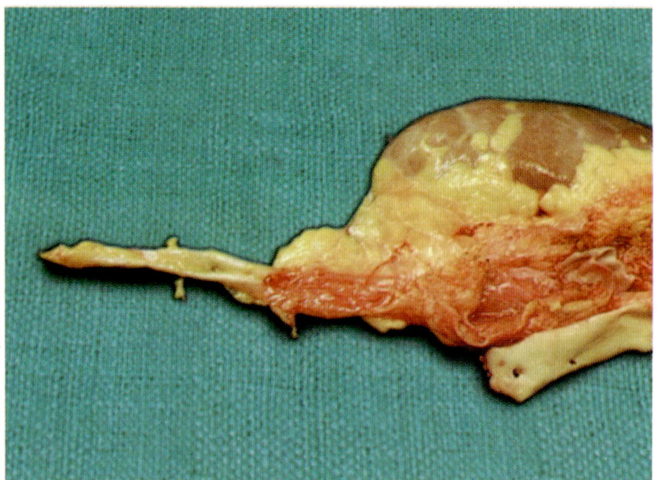

Fig. 3: Less frequent anatomical findings (such as the duplicated ureter illustrated here) should be addressed thoroughly. The blood supply to the ureter (whether single or double) should be preserved in order to avoid preventable post-transplant complications.

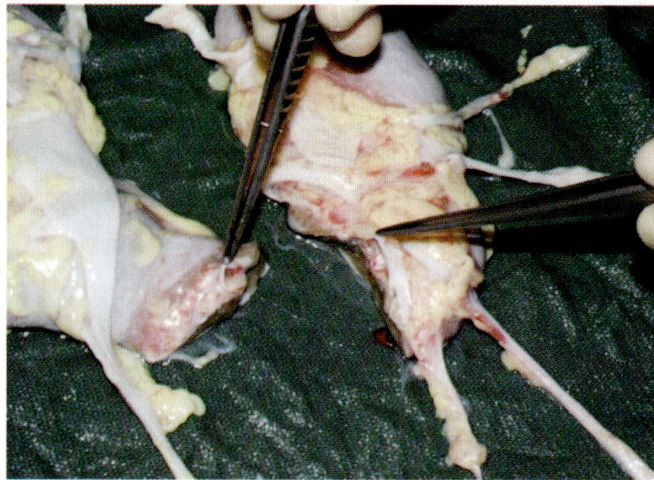

Fig. 4: Ureters in instances of horseshoe kidneys should be evaluated with caution (in addition to the frequent damage that the organ tends to suffer during procurements).

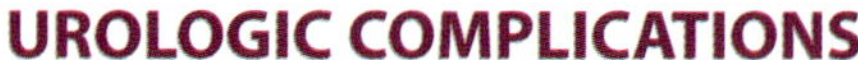

UROLOGIC COMPLICATIONS

- Usually occur within the first 3 months after transplantation
- In most instances, they can be addressed by imaging-guided percutaneous interventions
- Three main categories:
  - Obstructions/strictures (most frequent)
  - Leaks/extravasations
  - Other (least frequent)

URINARY OBSTRUCTION

Origin

- Intrinsic to the ureter
  - Edema (usually in the immediate postoperative period)
  - Ischemia (early in the postoperative period)
  - Fibrosis (delayed)
  - Torsion/redundancy
  - Stones (retained or new stones)
  - Clots (early postoperative or post biopsy)
  - Stent malpositioning
  - Tumors/malignancies
  - Infections
  - Other
- Extrinsic to the ureter
  - Urine leaks
  - Lymphoceles
  - Hematomas
  - Abscesses
  - Compression by the transplant kidney (continuous or intermittent)
  - Compression by the bladder (usually associated with full bladder)
  - Tumors (benign/malignant/urological/nonurological)

Clinical Findings

- Elevated creatinine
- Decreased urinary output
- Pain
- Fevers/chills/urosepsis

Diagnosis

- Imaging studies
  - Ultrasound
  - CT
  - Nuclear medicine
  - MR
- Antegrade ureterography—percutaneous nephrostogram
- Retrograde ureterography—cystoscopy

Treatment

- Percutaneous nephrostomy/stenting
  - Most frequent (and usually most effective) treatment
- Cystoscopy/stenting
  - Operator dependent
  - Outcome associated with anatomical findings such as the site of implantation of the ureter into the bladder

- Percutaneous drainage
  - For extrinsic compression by drainable fluid collections
- Edema
  - Usually resolves with temporary diversion and stenting
- Anastomotic/short strictures:
  - Initial approach with diversion, stenting, and dilatation
  - Reconstruction may be required
  - Outcomes depend on vascular supply of the ureter
- Long strictures (2 cm or longer)
  - Usually require surgical reconstruction
- Stones
  - Require removal
- Clots
  - Usually resolves with temporary diversion and stenting

Anastomosis of native ureter to transplant renal pelvis. In instances where the transplant ureter develops strictures or other types of pathologies that prevent the adequate flow of urine, a reconstruction is necessary. Although reimplantation of the transplant ureter into the bladder is the most frequent procedure, at times this is not possible. In this specific instance (Figs. 5 to 8), mobilization of the bladder was not sufficient to achieve

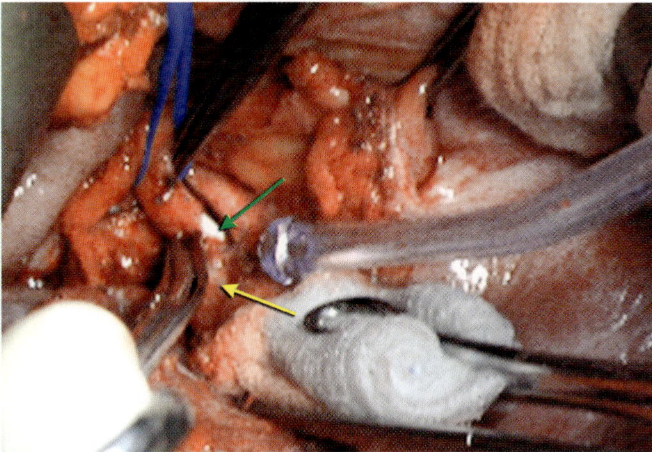

Fig. 5: The strictured ureter was identified and transected at its origin in the renal pelvis. Note the presence of a percutaneously placed ureteral stent (green arrow) within the transplant ureter. The transplant kidney is shown with a yellow arrow.

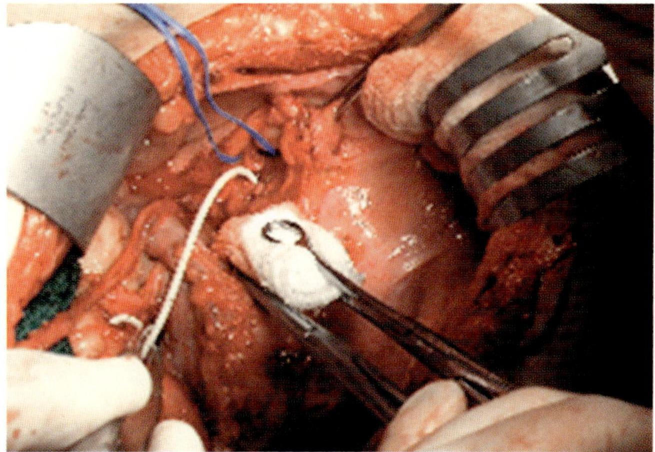

Fig. 6: The transplant ureter is transected and the stent brought out.

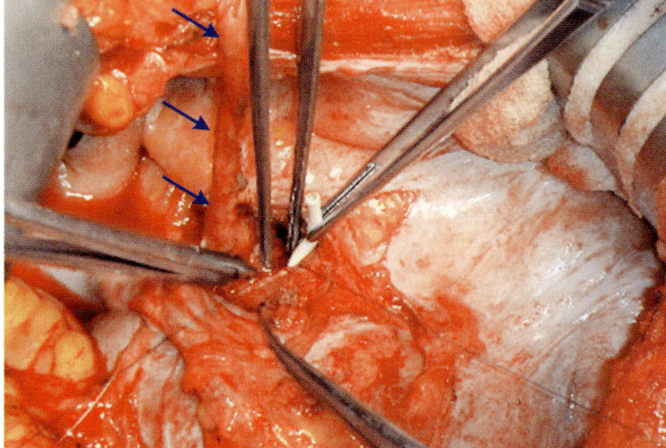

Fig. 7: The ipsilateral native ureter is dissected toward its proximal end, transecting it close to the native kidney. The proximal end (that remains with the native kidney) is tied. Its distal end (arrows) is mobilized, making sure that it is surrounded by connective tissues in order to prevent ischemic changes.

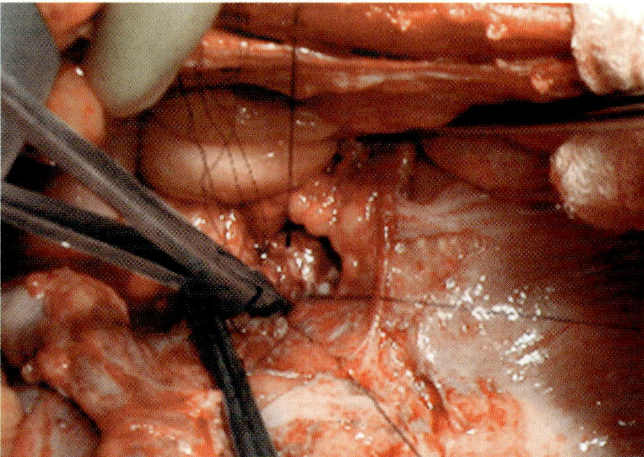

Fig. 8: The native ureter is trimmed to an adequate length and subsequently anastomosed onto the transplant renal pelvis.

a satisfactory anastomosis. The stricture was almost at the renal pelvis, and a decision was made to perform a native ureter to transplant renal pelvis anastomosis.

URINARY LEAKS

Clinical Findings

- Elevated creatinine
- Decreased urinary output
- Pain
- Fevers/chills/urosepsis
- Urine drainage through the wound
- Electrolyte abnormalities
- Usually associated with ureteral ischemia

Diagnosis

- Fluid creatinine much higher than serum creatinine
- Imaging studies
  - Ultrasound
  - CT
  - Nuclear medicine
  - MR
- Aspiration of collection
- Antegrade ureterography—percutaneous nephrostogram
- Retrograde ureterography—cystoscopy

Treatment

Depends on the extent and cause of the leak

Small Leaks

- Initial attempt with placement of urinary catheter and bladder decompression
- Further treatment required if leak does not resolve

Other Leaks

- Percutaneous nephrostomy, stenting, bladder decompression, and percutaneous drainage of the collection
  - Most frequent approach
- Cystoscopy, stenting, bladder decompression, and percutaneous drainage of the collection
  - Operator dependent
- Outcome associated with anatomical findings such as the site of implantation of the ureter into the bladder
- Surgical revision of the anastomosis
  - In instances where the previous treatments failed or the leak is associated with complete disruption of the anastomosis
  - When performing the reconstruction, it is important to make sure that the ureter has an adequate blood supply
  - Surgical possibilities include
    - Reimplantation into the bladder
    - Anastomosis with the ipsilateral native ureter
    - Anastomosis to the contralateral native ureter

PERINEPHRIC FLUID COLLECTIONS

Most kidney transplants have a small perinephric collection in the immediate postoperative period associated with the surgery.

The clinical relevance of perinephric collections is associated with their

- Size
- Etiology
- Physiologic relevance (Fig. 9)

HEMATURIA

Hematuria in transplant patients can have multiple etiologies.

In the immediate postoperative period, almost all recipients have a certain degree of hematuria associated with construction of the ureter to bladder anastomosis.

- In most cases, it is self-limited and resolves spontaneously within days with no treatment
- On occasions clots may form in the bladder and cause urinary outlet obstruction. In such instances, placement of a triple lumen urinary catheter and continuous bladder irrigation are necessary

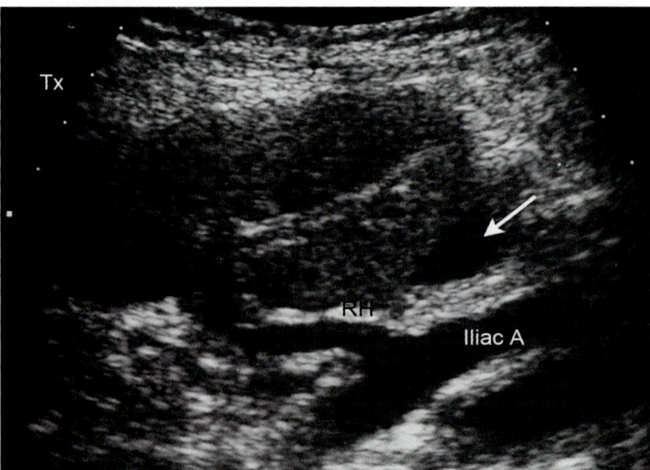

Fig. 9: Ultrasound in the immediate postoperative period showing a small fluid collection (arrow). Such small collections, in the absence of clinical symptoms and no sequential increases in size, can be followed conservatively with serial imaging.

Hematuria after kidney biopsies can result from

- Trauma to the kidney
- Arteriovenous fistulas
- Pseudoaneurysm

Traumatic insertion of urinary catheters can be a cause of hematuria. In such instances, especially in persistent cases, urethral injuries should be considered.

The presence of hematuria not associated with the operative time period should be addressed immediately. A thorough search for infections and tumors (both benign and malignant) of the genitourinary system as well as recurrence of some underlying primary etiologies of renal failure should be instituted.

LYMPHOCELES

Result from lymphatic leaks associated with transection of lymphatics during dissection of the iliac blood vessels and retroperitoneal cavity at the time of transplantation.

Usually Asymptomatic

Tend to Occur Within the First Postoperative Months

Diagnosis by:

- Imaging studies
- Biochemical analysis of the aspirated fluid (electrolytes, BUN and creatinine levels similar to those in blood)
- Exclusion of urinary leaks

Therapeutic interventions should be instituted in instances of

- Clinical manifestations
  - Vascular compression
  - Ureteral compression
  - Pain/discomfort
  - Infections
  - Allograft compromise

Treatments include

- Aspiration (high recurrence rate)
- External drainage (high recurrence rate after removal of the drain)
- Marsupialization
- Sclerosis

RENAL STONES

Renal stones occur very infrequently in transplant allografts (unless they were inadvertently present in the donor and subsequently transplanted onto the recipient)

They usually form in a delayed fashion at least several months post-transplantation

In most cases, recipients have predisposing factors for the formation of stones

Diagnosis is by imaging studies

Treatment

- Asymptomatic stones:
  - Can be followed clinically with serial imaging studies
- Symptomatic stones (associated with infections, obstruction, pain) can be treated with
  - Stents
  - Endourological removal
  - Lithotripsy
  - Surgical removal

FURTHER READING

1. Shapiro R, Simmons R, Starzl T. Renal transplantation. Appleton and Lange. 1997.

CHAPTER 48

Post-Transplant Malignancies

Khalid Al Meshari

Much of our knowledge of malignancy in transplantation comes from large registries such as Israel Penn Transplant Tumor Registry (IPTTR) and Australian New Zealand Dialysis and Transplant Registry (ANZDATR).

Introduction

- Malignancies are common after kidney transplantation
- The distribution of types of cancer post kidney transplantation is different than general population. As compared with cancers in general population, there is up to 100-fold increase of nonmelanoma skin cancer (NMSC), higher incidence of lymphoproliferative disorders, and minimal increase in incidence of common general population cancers (breast, prostate, lung and colon cancers)
- In general, NMSC and oncogenic virus-driven cancers [Epstein–Barr virus (EBV), human papilloma virus (HPV), hepatitis B virus (HBV), hepatitis C virus (HCV), and human herpes virus (HHV-8)] account for 60–70% of post-transplantation malignancy
- Cancer development post kidney transplantation rivals cardiovascular disease as the leading cause of death with a functioning graft
- The rising malignancy rate post kidney transplantation is likely to be due to two major factors:
  - Improved patient and graft survival leading to longer periods of exposure to immunosuppressive agents and therefore longer observation
  - Increase in the mean age of transplant recipients and age alone is known to be a risk factor for malignancy in the general population

Phenotypes

- De novo cancers
- Recurrence of a pretransplant cancer
- Transmission of a cancer from a donor (extremely low incidence)
- Malignancies with increased risk of donor to recipient transmission includes
  - Malignant melanoma
  - Choriocarcinoma
  - Lymphoma
  - Carcinoma of the lung
  - Carcinoma of the breast
  - Carcinoma of the colon
  - Renal cell carcinoma

Risk Factors

- Impaired immune surveillance: the inability of the immune system to eliminate spontaneously occurring cancerous cells
- Immunosuppression:
  - Duration
  - Intensity
  - Type (direct neoplastic action of immunosuppressive drugs)
- Increasing recipient age
- Exposure to environmental carcinogens
- Oncogenic viruses
- Genetic predisposition
- Exposure to UV light:
  - Total sun burden
  - Geographical region
  - Caucasian race

Biology

Post kidney transplantation cancer is much more aggressive in nature and has higher mortality rates as compared with general population.

Immunosuppression: Direct Neoplastic Action

- Antibody induction therapy: Increased risk of post-transplant lymphoproliferative disorder (PTLD) with all lymphocyte depleting preparations (monoclonal and polyclonal)
- Belatacept: An increased risk of PTLD, especially in EBV-negative recipients
- Calcineurin inhibitors (CNI): CSA impairs cellular ability to repair DNA damage, induces TGF-β, and vascular endothelial growth factor (VEGF) that may promote carcinogenesis
- Azathioprine: Associated with increased risk for NMSC. Carcinogenesis is related to damage at DNA level
- Mycophenolate mofetil (MMF): May have protective effect against malignancy
- Sirolimus: It has antineoplastic effects. Direct inhibition of cancer cell replication. Induction of apoptosis. Inhibition of VEGF production and angiogenesis

Oncogenic Viruses (Virally Driven Cancers)

- EBV: PTLD
- HHV8: Kaposi sarcoma
- HBV and HCV: Liver cancer
- HPV: Tongue, mouth, tonsil, anus, vagina and cervical cancer
- Human T-cell lymphotropic virus I and II (HTLV I and II): Leukemia and lymphoma

Post Kidney Transplant Malignancy of Special Consideration (PTLD)

- Second most common malignancy in kidney transplantation and the most common malignancy in pediatric kidney transplantation
- Strongly linked to EBV infection
- It is a spectrum of disease ranging from simple lymphatic hyperplasia to frank lymphoma (Figs. 1 to 5)

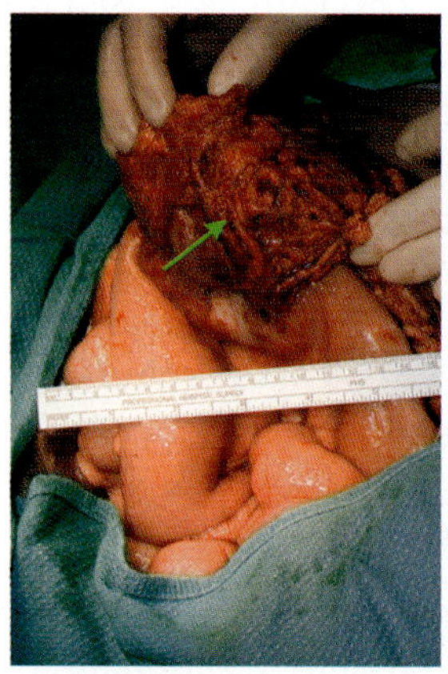

Fig. 1

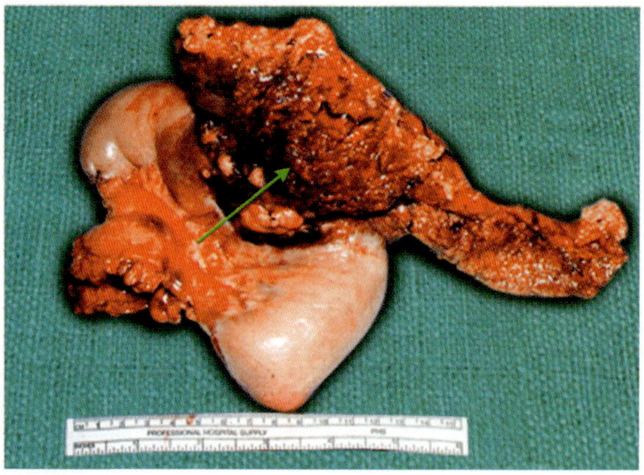

Fig. 2

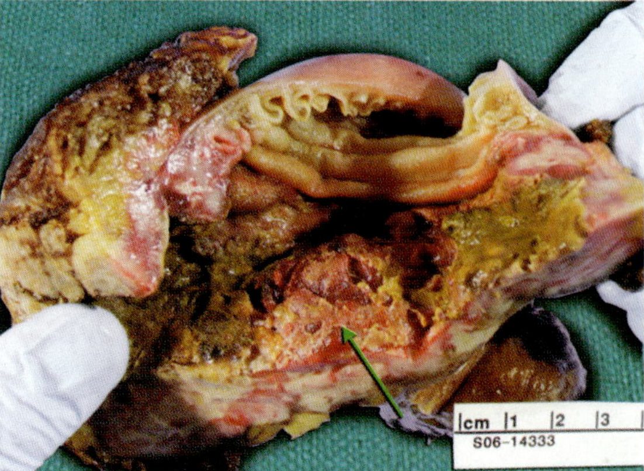

Fig. 3

Figs. 1 to 3: Kidney pancreas recipient who presented with small bowel obstruction. Workup revealed post-transplant lymphoproliferative disorder (PTLD). PTLD encompasses a variety of white blood cell pathologies frequently associated with Epstein–Barr virus (EBV) infection (either reactivation or primary infection). It has been classically attributed to aggressive immunosuppression. Although previously generally classified under the term PTLD, these tumors vary in aggressiveness, prognosis, and treatment. In this specific instance, massive enlargement of the lymphoid tissue (arrows) caused obstruction of the small bowel (requiring resection).

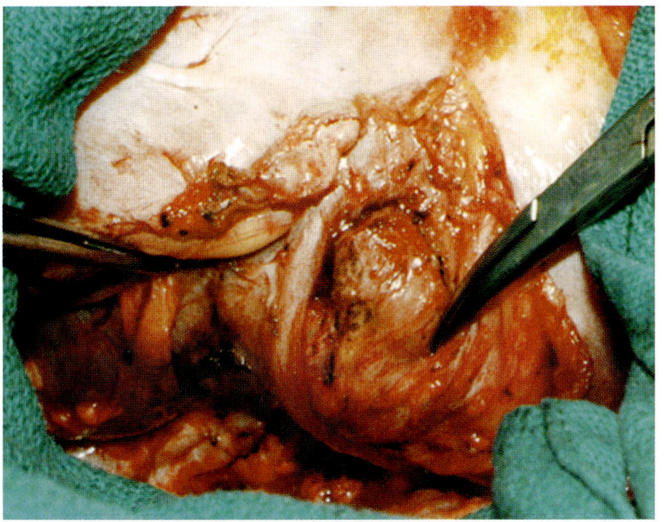

Fig. 4

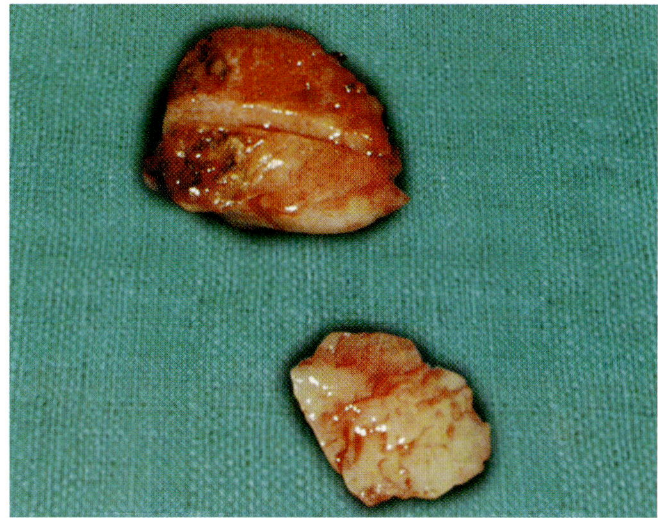

Fig. 5

Figs. 4 and 5: In this other example, a mass in the region of the transplanted kidney was found to be due to post-transplant lymphoproliferative disorder (PTLD). Epstein–Barr virus (EBV) is a DNA virus of the herpes family with a very high incidence in the general population, popularly known as the causative agent of mononucleosis, as well as of non-Hodgkin lymphomas.

- It is a major cause of cancer-related mortality: average mortality rate of 40–60%
- Factors associated with improved survival:
  - Younger age at presentation
  - Solitary site of disease
  - Disease limited to allograft
  - Disease amenable to surgical resection
  - Disease managed and responded to reduction in immunosuppression
- Worst prognostic indicator is the presence of CNS disease
- Management strategies:
  - Reduction in immunosuppression
  - Antiviral therapy (ganciclovir and valganciclovir)
  - Systemic chemotherapy
  - Anti B-cell antibody (anti-CD20 antibody)
  - Surgical incision

Management Guidelines

- General preventive guidelines:
  - Avoid over immunosuppression
  - Skin cancer prevention with sun screen, protective clothing, and avoidance of sun exposure
  - Vaccinations for oncogenic viruses (HBV, HPV)
  - Consider immunosuppressive regimen using MMF and/or sirolimus
  - Appropriate prophylaxis and monitoring for PTLD, particularly EBV-positive donors to EBV-negative recipients
  - Universal CMV prophylaxis
- Pretransplant screening
  - Patients with chronic kidney disease (CKD) have higher risk of cancer compared with the general population
  - Patients with CKD who required immunosuppressive treatment as part of therapy for their underlying kidney disease, or failed prior to kidney transplant, or required other solid organ transplant have additional risk for malignancy
  - Albeit, controversial from cost-effective standpoint, screening for common malignancy in CKD/dialysis patients is recommended. The recommended cancer screening guidelines in the general population are applied to patients with CKD
  - Selective screening for certain types of cancers known to be relatively more common in dialysis patients (e.g., parathyroid cancer, renal and urinary malignancy) is warranted
- Disease-free waiting period for those with cancer

For renal transplant candidates with existing malignancy, recurrent disease may occur earlier and might be more aggressive in phase of immunosuppression. To decrease the chance of recurrence, a disease-free waiting time prior to transplant is recommended as follows:

- 0–2 years:
  - Incidental, localized renal cancer
  - Low-grade bladder cancer
  - Cancers with high cure rates
  - Resected *in situ* carcinoma

- 2 years:
  - Renal cell cancer with 5-year disease-free survival (DFS) of 85–95%
  - Stage I breast cancer
  - Duke A or B1 colon cancer
  - Prostate cancer with 5-year DFS of 85–95%
- 5 years:
  - Large (> 5 cm) renal cell carcinoma
  - Lymphoma
  - Breast cancer > stage I
  - Colon cancer with 5-year DFS of < 80%
  - Prostate cancer with 5-year DFS of < 80%

- Post-transplant malignancy surveillance:
  - PTLD:
    - Antiviral prophylaxis for EBV-negative recipients of EBV-positive kidneys
    - Periodic screening for EBV by PCR for 18 months
    - All patients should have EBV serology checked 6 months after transplantation
  - Cervical cancer (female):
    - Annual pap smear and pelvic examination
    - More frequent examinations if increased risk factors: HPV positive or previous abnormal pap smear
  - Prostate cancer (male):
    - Yearly PSA
    - Men over 50: yearly rectal examination and/or prostate ultrasound
  - Liver cancer:
    - Hepatitis B or C-infected recipients: check alpha-fetoprotein (AFP) yearly, ultrasound of the liver every other year
  - Colorectal cancer:
    - Recipients > 50 years of age: fecal blood test yearly, flexible sigmoidoscopy every 5 years and full colonoscopy every 2 years
  - Skin cancer:
    - Annual self examination and physician examination and biopsy of all suspicious lesions
  - Kaposi sarcoma:
    - Yearly examination of skin, nose, mouth, or throat
    - More frequent examination of recipients of Arab, Jewish, or Mediterranean decent

FURTHER READING

1. Feng S, Buell J, Chari R, et al. Tumors and Transplantation: The 2003 third annual ASTS state-of-the-art winter symposium. AM J Transplant. 2003; 3:1481-87.
2. Gutierrez-Dalmau A, Campistol J. Immunosuppressive therapy and malignancy in organ transplant recipients. Drugs. 2007, 67(8):1167-98.
3. Kasiske B, Kukla A, Thomas D, et al. Lympoproliferative disorders after adult kidney transplant: Epidemiology and comparison of registry report with claims-based diagnoses. Am J Kidney Dis. 2011;58(6):971-80.
4. Malignancy risks after kidney transplantation. Special issue: KDIGO clinical practice guideline for the care of kidney transplant recipients. AM J Transplant. 2009;9 (Suppl 3):S82-S90.
5. Miao Y, Everly J, Gross T, et al. De novo cancers arising in organ transplant recipients are associated with adverse outcomes compared with the general population. Transplantation. 2009;87(9):1347-59.
6. Vajdic C, McDonald S, McCredie M, et al. Cancer incidence before and after kidney transplantation. JAMA 2006;296(23):2823-31.

CHAPTER 49

Vaccinations

Jay Weinstein

INTRODUCTION

Infectious agents are a major cause of morbidity and mortality in end stage renal disease, dialysis, and kidney transplant patients.[1-6] Furthermore, these agents can contribute to rejection of the transplanted organ and to the subsequent development of certain types of cancers.[2,7-9] One way to lessen the risk of infections is by active immunization. Historically, vaccination of adult dialysis and renal transplanted patients has been underutilized.[2,10,11] Such suboptimal vaccination makes immunosuppressed patients unnecessarily vulnerable to preventable infections.

PRINCIPLES

It has been well described that patients with end-stage organ disease respond poorly to active immunizations.[1,10,12] It has also been documented that patients with solid organ transplants receiving immunosuppressive therapy have impaired cellular and humoral immunity also limiting their ability to respond to vaccinations.[8,10,13,14] The first 6 months post-transplant is usually considered the period of the highest risk of rejection and is the point of greatest immunosuppression and the poorest response to vaccination.[1,7,10,13,15] To date there is no controlled trial on the optimum time to vaccinate a kidney transplant patient. However, some general principles exist.

If possible, transplant patients should receive all age-appropriate and risk-specific vaccines recommended by the Advisory Committee on Immunization Practices (ACIP) Centers for Disease Control and Prevention prior to transplantation.[21,27,28] Inactivated vaccines are safe in the post-transplant patient receiving immunosuppressive therapy.[8,20] However, the antibody response may be suboptimal and may rapidly decline.[12] Therefore, whenever possible inactivated vaccines should be given as early as possible in the transplant process for evaluation to ensure the optimal response to vaccination.[8,20] If not possible, most transplant centers wait 3–6 months post-transplant to immunize patient with inactivated vaccines.[8,10,19]

Live vaccines are contraindicated in adult immunosuppressed patients.[8,12,16,17] Titers should be checked once a patient is considered a candidate for transplant surgery. If titers are nonimmune, booster vaccines should be given as early as possible.[8,15,19] Titers can be checked as soon as 1 month after revaccination for successful immunization.[15] Also, be aware that titers have not been well studied in immunosuppressed patients and may not guarantee immunity against the disease. Patients can shed viruses up until 5 weeks postvaccination with live viruses. Therefore, transplant surgery should not be performed 1–2 months after immunization with a live vaccine.[12,15]

However, there are several small studies in the pediatric population that showed live attenuated vaccines, such as MMR and varicella may be given safely to seronegative post-transplant patients.[28] Large studies will be needed to identify the post-transplant population who failed to receive pretransplant vaccines and whether post-transplant patients who remain seronegative may benefit from these live vaccines.[21]

Equally important as the immunization of the transplanted patient is the proper immunization of close household contacts and health-care workers who will care for the immune-suppressed patient.[8,19-22] Updating the vaccination of household contacts and health-care workers will minimize the transplant patients' exposure to infectious viral and bacterial agents. It is safe to immunize close contacts of transplant patients with live viruses except for the typhoid, smallpox, and oral polio vaccines.[19,20]

BACILLUS CALMETTE-GUÉRIN (BCG) VACCINE

- Live vaccine derived from an attenuated bacterium Mycobacterium bovis
- The BCG vaccine is contraindicated in solid organ transplant recipients[6,12,13]
- Still used in many parts of the world with a high incidence of tuberculosis to prevent tuberculosis meningitis in children and military tuberculosis[23]
- Not routinely used in the United States
- Postvaccination BCG tuberculin reactivity has been well described
- Tuberculin reactivity unlikely to persist for > 10 years after vaccination but will be quantitate gold TB test negative

Haemophilus Influenzae Vaccine

- In adult chronic renal disease or kidney transplant recipients, the Haemophilus influenzae type b vaccine is not routinely recommended, but may be given to high-risk individuals who are asplenic or hypogammaglobulemic patients[13,15]
- Although rare in adult transplant patients, infection has a high mortality[15,18]
- Inactivated conjugated vaccine available alone or combined with DTaP or with recombinant hepatitis B[18,24]

HEPATITIS A VACCINE

- ACIP guidelines recommend hepatitis A vaccine (two doses of hepatitis A vaccine 6–12 months apart) for dialysis and kidney transplant patients in the following categories:[14]
  - Chronic liver disease
  - In outbreak of epidemics
  - Traveling into known endemic areas
  - Using intravenous drugs
  - Men who have sex with men
- Dialysis and kidney transplant patients are more at risk of developing severe hepatitis when exposed to hepatitis A[23,23a]
- Most industrialized countries have a low endemic hepatitis A virus transmission[23]
- FDA licensed two inactivated vaccines in the United States. Havrix (GlaxoSmithKline) and Vaqta (Merck)—two doses given 6–12 months apart are recommended[24,25]

HEPATITIS B VACCINE

- ACIP recommends that immunocompromised patients should receive four intramuscular doses of 40 µg Engerix vaccine at 0, 1, 2, and 6 months intervals or three doses of 40 µg Recombivax vaccine intramuscularly at 0, 1, and 6 months intervals[3,24,25]
- The incidence of hepatitis B infection has dramatically declined among dialysis patients since the introduction of the hepatitis B vaccine in 1977[14]
- Hepatitis B may progress more rapidly, more severely, and may reactivate (from latent infection) more frequently in immunocompromised patients[2,4]
- Hepatitis B vaccines available in the United States are recombinant vaccines: Recombivax HB (Merck) and Engerix-B (GlaxoSmithKline)[24,25]
- Monitoring of hepatitis B antibody titers can be useful 1–2 months after the vaccination series. Titers of hepatitis B antibodies < 10 mlU/mL are not protective and require a booster[2,8,14]

Human Papilloma Virus Vaccine

- Human papilloma virus infection is the most common sexually transmitted disease in the United States and is associated with the development of cervical cancer, squamous cell carcinoma of the skin, oropharyngeal cancer, anogenital cancer and respiratory papillomatosis[21,24–26]
- Two vaccines are licensed in the United States: Cervarix, a bivalent inactivated vaccine that protects against type 16 and 18. Gardasil, a quadrivalent which includes 16 and 18, which are the major causes of cervical cancer, and 6 and 11, the most common viruses to cause genital warts
- ACIP recommends all male or female patients ages 11 to 12 years old be vaccinated with three doses: 0, 1–2 months and third dose six months after first. Vaccination is recommended in all women 13 to age 26 years old and men ages 13–21 years old who have not received the vaccine. Males aged 22 through 26 years are also candidates to receive the vaccine.[27,28] Most experts recommend the HPV vaccine in solid organ transplant patients if they meet ACIP criteria prior to surgery[21,26]

Influenza

- Influenza virus is a major cause of pneumonia in dialysis patient and renal transplant patients. Influenza virus is grouped into types A, B, C and is further subdivided by protein on the virus. Influenza A virus has the propensity to rapidly mutate and cause pandemics[7,24,25]

- The FDA licensed four types of influenza vaccines in 2013-2014: the trivalent inactivated vaccine branded as Afluria, Flublok, Flucelvax, and Fluzone. Some brands are thimerosal-free: a high-dose inactivated influenza vaccine Fluarix and FluLaval. A quadrivalent inactivated vaccine has recently been approved by the FDA. Finally, Flumist, a live attenuated virus, is available which may be given nasally to patients aged 2-49 years of age.[24,25,29] A recombinant influenza vaccine is expected to be on the market for patients with egg allergies soon
- ACIP recommends all persons 6 months or older to receive yearly vaccines and specifically the inactivated vaccine in solid organ transplant patients[7,13,14,16,18,27,28,32,33,34]

MEASLES, MUMPS, AND RUBELLA VACCINE

- Contraindicated in adult transplant recipients
- Live-attenuated virus vaccines
- Measles mumps and rubella are rare but potentially serious infectious agents in immunosuppressed patients[26]
- Most adult transplant patients have already been immunized. Patients born prior to 1957 are assumed to be immune[1]
- In the United States, the vaccine is available as M-M-R II (Merck) and ProQuad [measles, mumps, rubella, and varicella (Merck)][24,25]
- Serology for measles, mumps, and rubella should be obtained as soon as the patient is determined to be a transplant candidate. A booster is recommended if titers are found to be nonprotective prior to transplantation[1]

Meningococcal Vaccine

- The conjugated meningococcal vaccine should be considered for adult chronic kidney disease and renal transplant recipients in high-risk groups such as[27,28]
  - Functional asplenia
  - Complement deficiency
  - Traveling to high-risk areas such as sub-Sahara Africa
  - Attending the Hajj in Mecca Saudi Arabia
- A single dose of conjugated vaccine is recommended prior to travel[23]
- Two doses of conjugated vaccine 2 months apart plus a booster every 5 years for asplenic or complement deficient patients[21,28]
- Neisseria meningitidis is an exclusively human pathogen found in the nasopharyngeal mucosa of 10% of the population
- Six subgroups (A, B, C, W135, X, and Y) account for most life-threatening cases (such as meningitis and sepsis)
- Two types of vaccines are licensed in the United States the 4-valent polysaccharide (Menomune by Sanofi) and the 4-valent conjugated vaccine (Menactra by Sanofi) (Menveo Novartis). Both protect against A, C, Y, W-135. Neither contains live bacteria[18,24]
- Advisory committee on immunization practices (ACIP) recommends vaccination of all children and teens 11–18 years of age, as well as all those adults in high-risk groups[28]
- All college aged students should receive the conjugated vaccine[21,28,29]

PNEUMOCOCCAL VACCINE

- Chronic renal failure and kidney transplant patients should be immunized every 3–5 years. ACIP recommends adding the 13-valent conjugated vaccine for wider coverage[5,9,13,14,28]
- Two major types of vaccines are licensed in the United States. An inactivated 23-valent polysaccharide vaccine (Pneumovax by Merck, Pnu-Imune 23 by Wyeth) (not recommended for infants under 2 years of age), a 7-valent (Prevnar by Wyeth) and 13-valent (Prevnar by Wyeth) conjugated vaccines for the pediatric population. The 13-valent conjugated vaccine will replace the 7-valent vaccine[18,24,25]
- The 13-valent conjugated vaccine should be given first followed 8 weeks later by the 23-valent polysaccharide vaccine. Patients immunized with the 23-valent polysaccharide vaccine should receive the 13-valent conjugated vaccine at least 1 year after the 23-valent polysaccharide vaccine
- Monitoring of titers is not necessary[2,3,14,23]
- Studies have shown a higher incidence of invasive pneumococcal disease in solid organ transplant recipients[9,13]
- ACIP recommends that all patients 19–64 years of age with chronic lung, heart, and other chronic medical conditions as well as transplant patients and all those ≥ 65 years old should receive a one time dose of the 23-valent polysaccharide vaccine[27,28]

POLIOVIRUS VACCINE

- Transplant recipients who have never been immunized for polio should receive three doses of the inactivated polio vaccine 4 weeks apart. A one time booster of inactivated polio administered intramuscularly should be given to all transplant patients traveling to high-risk areas of the world. Some experts recommend a booster prior to travel if the vaccine had not been given within 10 years[23]

- ACIP recommends that four doses of the inactivated polio vaccine should be given to all children (including pediatric transplant recipients) at 2, 4, 16–18 months and a booster at 4–6 years of age[27,28]
- Polio has been eradicated from the United States and the Western Hemisphere
- The polio vaccine is available in the United States as an inactivated virus IPOL (Aventus) or as a combination with DTaP and hepatitis B called Pediarix (GlaxoSmith-Kline). Oral polio vaccine is no longer administrated in the United States[18,24]

RABIES VACCINE

- Rabies is a deadly disease caused by a virus spread by the bite or saliva of a rabid bats, raccoons, skunks, foxes ferrets, cats, and dogs
- Almost 100% fatal in unvaccinated cases[6]
- Rabies vaccine is available in two forms: Human diploid cell vaccine (Imovax rabies, Sarnoff) and purified chicken embryo vaccine (RabAvert, Novartis). Both contain inactivated virus and are approved for pre- and postexposure[18,24,25,29]
- Pre-exposure vaccination should be offered to patients in frequent contact with potentially rabid animals as well as to travelers who will spend > 1 month in countries with a high incidence of rabies infection, who will likely come into contact with rabid animals, and who will have limited access to medical treatment[14,28]
- Pre-exposure vaccination consists of three intramuscular doses at 0, 7 and 21–28 days. A booster to maintain immunity is recommended every 2 years for those at continued risk.[24,25,29]
- Chronic renal disease or kidney transplant patients who need pre-exposure prophylaxis for rabies should receive four intramuscularly doses on day 0, 7, 21, and 28[30]
- Postexposure prophylaxis (in patients who were not previously vaccinated) consists of five intramuscular doses over four weeks, with the awareness that the immune response will likely be inadequate. Rabies immune globulin should be administered at the same time[30]
- One or more serum samples should be tested for rabies virus neutralizing antibody by the RFFIT to ensure that an acceptable antibody (titers > 0.5 IU/mL) response has developed after completing the series
- Pre-exposure vaccinated patients should also receive two postexposure doses on day 0 and 3. Some expects will also give rabies immunoglobulin[30]

Rotavirus Vaccine

- A common cause of serious diarrhea in children
- A human bovine reassortant live attenuated rotavirus vaccine, Rotateg, was licensed for use in children between ages of 6-32 weeks[21]
- Contraindication in adult transplant recipients[24,25,29]

SMALLPOX VACCINE

- Contraindicated in transplant and immunosuppressed patients
- Smallpox was eradicated worldwide in 1980
- Although vaccination is no longer recommended, bioterrorism remains a concern
- The smallpox vaccine [smallpox (Vaccinia) Vaccine Acambis Inc.] was a live-attenuated vaccinia (pox type) virus. It is administrated by 15 puncture wounds in the skin with a bifurcated needle dipped into the vaccine. If successful, a blister forms in 3 days[18,24]
- High levels of immunity persisted in immunocompetent patients for 3–5 years. Revaccination was required every 10 years

Tetanus, Diphtheria, Pertussis Vaccines

- Most experts recommend Tdap every 5 years in organ transplant recipients and monitoring diphtheria titers every 2 years[2,3,13]
- Tetanus, diphtheria, and pertussis are found in the environment
- There has recently been a surge in the number of case of whooping cough caused by pertussis
- Studies have shown a rapid decline in tetanus antibodies but especially with antibodies to diphtheria after a booster Td within 6–12 months[2,3,14,15]
- There are several different types of inactivated vaccines: TT—tetanus toxoid for tetanus booster alone, Td is tetanus toxoid with low concentration diphtheria for booster in adults, DT—tetanus toxoid with full concentration diphtheria for use in children, DTaP—tetanus toxoid with full concentration diphtheria and acellular pertussis (limited to children because of reactions in adults), and Tdap—tetanus toxoid with reduced concentration of diphtheria and acellular pertussis (used in adults)[24,25]

VARICELLA VACCINE

- The live-attenuated varicella vaccine is contraindicated in transplant recipients[5,13,24,25]

- Primary varicella infection (although uncommon) can have disastrous consequences in transplant patients, causing disseminated visceral infection, hemorrhagic pneumonia, encephalitis, disseminated intravascular coagulation, and death if untreated
- Serology for varicella zoster should be obtained as soon as a patient is determined to be a candidate for transplant. If serology is non-protective, a booster should be given at least 4 weeks prior to the transplant surgery. Two doses at least 3 months apart should be given in nonimmunized pediatric patients[1,2,21]

VARICELLA ZOSTER VACCINE

- The live-attenuated virus vaccine (Zostavax) is contraindicated in transplant recipients.[5] ACIP recommends the vaccine in patients aged 60 or older
- Reactivation of varicella zoster in immunocompromised patients tends to be benign and usually involves 1–3 dermatomes. However, 20–30% of cases of reactivation of varicella zoster present as cutaneous disseminated disease[2,4]

TRAVEL VACCINES

- Organ transplant recipients who travel abroad should review with their transplant centers all routine immunizations including Tdap, influenza, and pneumococcal and should check measles and varicella titers[23]
- Strong consideration should be given to visiting with a travel medicine "expert" several months prior to embarking[23]
- It is recommended that if possible travel should be limited during the first 3–6 months after transplantation, since this is the period of maximum immunosuppressive therapy[6,23,30]
- Routine prophylaxis with N.N-diethyl-m-toluamide (DEET) repellent and other mosquito avoidance techniques such as netting is recommended in areas where malaria is a concern
- Transplant patients should be advised to avoid risky behavior such as tattoos and sexual contact with non-traveling partners
- Hepatitis B vaccine should be advised for travelers having new sexual partners while traveling, living in endemic areas for prolong periods of time, or likely to need transfusion of blood products
- Polio vaccine should be given as a onetime booster dose in patients who received primary polio immunization and are traveling to sub-Sahara Africa or South America[6,15,24,25,30]
- Hepatitis A vaccine should be given as two doses 6–12 months apart. Titers should be checked for seroconversion. If traveling urgently, intramuscular gamma globulin offers protection for 2–3 months. However, even a single dose of hepatitis A vaccine offers excellent protection (the second dose extends the duration of protection)[6,24,25,30]
- Salmonella typhi vaccination is available in two forms: typhi ImVi (an injectable inactivated vaccine) and Vivotic (an oral live-attenuated vaccine). Transplant patients should only receive the inactivated vaccine. Live vaccines are contraindicated[30]
- Yellow fever vaccine is contraindicated in transplant patients because it is a live-attenuated virus vaccine. Patients should be discouraged form traveling to such areas in South America and sub-Saharan Africa (at least during the peak season). Travel companions of transplant patients may receive the vaccine[23,31]
- Japanese encephalitis vaccine is a killed vaccine given in three doses on day 0, 7, and 30 days. It should be given to patients traveling to endemic areas in Asia. Its effectiveness has not been well studied in solid organ transplant patients. Hypersensitivity reactions occur in 0.6% of recipients. Transplant patients should be observed carefully for signs of graft injury[30]

REFERENCES

1. Chow J, Golan Y. Vaccination of solid-organ transplantation candidate. Clin Infect Dis 2009;49:1550–6.
2. Cohn J, Blumberg EA. Immunization for renal transplant candidates and recipients. Nature Clin Pract Nephrol 2009; 5:46–53.
3. Janus N, Vacher L-V, Karie S, et al. Vaccination and chronic kidney disease. Nephrol Dial Transplant 2008; 23:800–7.
4. Rubin RH. Infectious complications of renal transplantation. Kidney Int 1993;44:221–36.
5. Hasley PB, Arnold RM. Primary care of the transplant patient. Am J Med 2010;123:205–12.
6. Committee to Advise on Tropical Medicine and Travel (CATMAT). An Advisory Committee Statement. The immunocompromised traveller. 2007 Apr 1;33 (ACS-4): 1–10.
7. Frishman J. Infection in solid-organ recipients. NEJM 2007; 357:2601–14.
8. Serrano B, Bayas J-M, Bruni L, et al. Solid organ transplantation and response to vaccination. Vaccine 2007; 25:7331–8.
9. Kumar D, Humar A, Plevneshi A, et al. Invasive pneumococcal disease in solid organ transplant recipients–10 year prospective. Am J Transplant 2007;7:1209–14.

10. Nelsin-Kotton C. Vaccinations in kidney transplant patients: searching for optimal protection. Clin J Am Soc Nephrol 2009; 6:2099–101.
11. Thervet E. Vaccination in solid-organ transplant candidates: time for a benefit/risk assessment. Clin Kid J 2012;5:193–4.
12. Burrough M, Moscona A. Immunization of pediatric solid organ transplant candidates and recipients. Clin Infect Dis 2000;30:857–60.
13. Duchini A, Goss JA, Karpen S, et al. Vaccinations for adult solid-organ transplant recipients: current recommendations and protocols. Clin Micrbiol Rev 2003;16:357–64.
14. Dinitis-Pensey Forrest GN, Cross AS, Hise MK. The use of vaccines in adult patients with renal disease. Am J Kidney Dis 2005;46:997–1011.
15. Sester M, Gartner BC, Girndt M, et al. Vaccination of the solid organ transplant recipient. Transplant Review 2008;22: 274–84.
16. Morine D, Hibberd P. Vaccine recommendations: challenges and controversies vaccines for transplant recipient. Infect Dis Clin N Am 2001;15:273–305.
17. Knoll G. Canadian Society of Transplant and Canadian Nephrology Commentary on the 2009 clinical practices guideline for the care of kidney transplant recipient. Am J Kid Dis 2009;56:219–46.
18. Bllout A, Goffin E, Yombi JC, et al. Vaccination for adult organ transplant recipient: current recommendations. Transplant Proc 2005;37:2826–7.
19. Tamma PD. Vaccine in immunocompromised patient. Pediatr Rev 2010;23:38–40.
20. Danzinger-Isakov L, Kumar D. Guidelines for vaccination of solid organ transplant candidate and recipients. AM J Transplant 2009; (Supp 4):S256–62.
21. Avery RK, Michaels M. Update on immunizations in solid organ transplant recipients: what clinicians need to know. Am J Transplant 2008;8:9–14.
22. Gupta G, Unruh ML, Nolin TD, et al. Primary care of the renal transplant patient. J Gen Intern Med 2010;25:731–40.
23. Kotton CN, Hibbert PL and the AST infectious Disease Community of Practice. Travel medicine and the solid organ transplant recipient. Am J Transplant 2009;9: S273–81.
23a. Boggild AK, Sano M, Humanr A, et al. Travel pattern and risk behavior in solid organ transplant recipients. J Travel Med 2004;11:37–43.
24. Centers for Disease Control and Prevention Vaccines and Immunizations. http://www.cdc.gov/vaccines/
25. National Network for Immunization Information. http://www.immunizationinfo.org/
26. Hibberd PL. Immunization in the solid organ transplant candidate and recipients. Uptodate 2012.
27. Centers for Disease Control and Prevention MMWR Morbidity land Mortality Weekly report Recommendation and Reports /Vol. 60/ No.2 January 28 2011 General Recommendations on Immunization Recommendation of the Advisory Committee on Immunization Practices (ACIP)
28. Centers for Disease Control and Prevention MMWR Morbidity and Mortality Weekly report Recommendation and Reports/Vol. 60/No.7 November 25 2011 Immunization of Healthcare Personnel. Recommendation of the Advisory Committee on Immunization Practices (ACIP)
29. Vaccine information for the public and health professionals from the immunization action coalition. http://www.vaccineinformation.org/
30. Jong EC, Freedman DO. Advising travelers with specific needs 2012 chapter 8 Approach to the Immunocompromised Traveler 2012 CDC Travel YellowBook
31. KDIGO Clinical Practice Guidelines for the Care of Kidney Transplant Recipients. Am Journal of Transplantation 2009;9(Suppl 3):522–51.
32. Avery RK, Ljungman P. Prophylactic measure in the solid-organ recipient before transplantation. Clin Infect Dis 2001; 33:S15–21.
33. Slifkin M, Doron S, Syndman D. Viral prophylaxis in organ transplant patients. Drugs 2004;24:2763–92.
34. Arness T, Pedersen R, Dierkhising R, et al. Varicella zoster virus-associated disease in adult kidney transplant recipients: incidence and risk-factor analysis. Transplant Infect Dis 2008; 10:260–8.
35. Kwak EJ, Julian K, the AST Infectious Disease Community of Practice. Human papillomavirus infection in solid organ transplant recipients. Am J Transplant 9 (Supp 4): S151–60.
36. Stelzmueller I, Wiesmayr S, Swenson BR, et al. Rotavirus enteritis in solid organ transplant recipients: an underestimated problem? Transplant Infect Dis 2007;9:281–5.
37. Azevendo LS, Lasmar EP, David-Neto E. Yellow fever vaccination in organ transplanted patients: is it safe? A multicenter study. Transplant Infect Dis 2012;14:237–41.

CHAPTER 50

Obstetric and Gynecologic Care

Jessica Lee, Andrew W Menzin

OBSTETRIC AND GYNECOLOGIC CARE AFTER TRANSPLANTATION

Pregnancy

- Until recently, delaying pregnancy for up to 24 months after transplantation was recommended
  - Currently pregnancy may be considered after 1 year from transplantation if the following criteria are met:
    - No graft rejection in past year
    - Stable graft function
      - For renal transplants, require serum creatinine < 1.5 mg/dL with minimal proteinuria
    - Low risk of infections such as CMV, toxoplasmosis
    - Not currently taking teratogenic medications
    - Immunosuppressant dosing at stable maintenance levels
- It is important to individualize timing for each patient
  - The better optimized graft function, the greater likelihood of successful maternal, and fetal outcomes
- All pregnancies post-transplant are considered high-risk
  - Need close surveillance by transplant physicians and high-risk perinatologists
  - Goals of pregnancy
    - Maintain maternal health and graft function with stable immunosuppressant dosing
    - Minimize pregnancy complications such as preterm delivery, hypertensive disorders, and fetal growth restriction
- Cesarean deliveries only for obstetric indications
  - Pelvic kidney transplants not indication for cesarean delivery
  - Even with thoracic transplant recipients, cesarean sections would not prevent cardiac overload
  - Concern that cesarean section would increase risk of maternal infection if presence of significant immunosuppression
- Pregnancy complications
  - Hypertension
    - Common in renal and hepatic transplant patients
    - Aggressive management required: Early use of antihypertensive medications when mild hypertension arises
      - Blood pressure should be kept close to normal
      - May lead to fetal growth restriction
    - Preeclampsia
      - Difficult to diagnose due to high incidence of preexisting hypertension and proteinuria
      - Approximately three to four times more common than in general population
        - May lead to higher rates of cesarean delivery
    - HELLP syndrome in hepatic patients may be difficult to diagnose
      - Elevation of liver enzymes may be due to HELLP or due to progression of hepatic disease
  - Preterm delivery (< 37 weeks gestation)
    - Common: Up to 50% of infants are born premature
      - Mean gestational age at delivery in renal transplant patients: 34 weeks
    - As a result, have complications of premature delivery especially those at < 34 weeks gestation
      - Neonatal death
      - Cerebral palsy
      - Blindness, deafness
      - Learning disabilities, low intelligence quotients

- Low birth weight (< 2500 g)
  - Up to 20% of infants
  - May lead to early delivery
  - Increased incidence partially due to increased risk of hypertensive disorders
    - Serial sonograms to monitor fetal growth recommended
- Graft rejections
  - Difficult to detect
  - Must maintain immunosuppression to avoid rejection
  - Acute rejection associated with poorer pregnancy outcomes and recurrent rejection episodes after delivery
  - Lung transplant patients have higher rate of rejection for unknown reasons
- Immunosuppressants
  - Dosing
    - Few studies on optimal immunosuppressants in pregnancy and dosing
    - Need frequent monitoring of serum drug levels
      - Changes in blood volume during pregnancy
      - Persistent vomiting, that is, hyperemesis gravidarum patients
  - Fetal exposure
    - All immunosuppressants cross placenta at varying degrees
    - No evidence of increased incidence of congenital anomalies associated with calcineurin inhibitors, azathioprine, or steroids
      - In US registry data, mycophenolate mofetil shown to have increased miscarriage rate (42%) and structural malformations (27%)
        - Recommended to avoid, starting 6 weeks prior to conception
      - Other immunosuppressants not shown to conclusively increase miscarriage or structural anomaly rates
    - Question of possibility of immunosuppressants increasing risk of autoimmune disease later in life unanswered as of yet
      - Need long-term follow-up of exposed children
    - Breastfeeding
      - Lack of reported adverse effects
      - Current consensus is that benefits of breastfeeding outweigh theoretical risks of immunosuppressant exposure
- Preconception counseling
  - Honest conversations regarding risks need to be discussed prior to conception
    - Parents need to be prepared to potentially care for disabled child
      - Also need to consider who will take care of child
        - In case of parental disability or death due to unexpected illnesses and/or graft dysfunction

Contraception

- Fertility, in those of reproductive age, often returns to normal after transplantation
  - As early as 3 weeks post-transplantation
- Pregnancy soon after transplantation prior to stabilization of graft is not recommended
  - Allow time for resolution of postoperative complications, completion of viral prophylaxis, establishment of immunosuppressive regimen, and stability of the graft
  - American Society of Transplantation recommends counseling on contraception prior to transplantation
- Most effective
  - Intrauterine device (IUD)
    - Three available in United States: Copper containing Paragard, and two levonorgestrel releasing Mirena and Skyla
    - All with similar efficacy and safety
    - Duration of efficacy: Paragard—10 years; Mirena—5 years; Skyla—3 years
      - Prompt return to fertility after removal of IUD
    - Drug interactions
      - Paragard contains copper and therefore no anticipated drug interactions
      - Mirena and Skyla both with low levels of systemic levonorgestrel (20 mcg/day and 14 mcg/day, respectively). Drug interactions are unlikely
    - Decrease in efficacy with immunosuppression?
      - IUDs induce local intrauterine inflammatory reaction
        - Thought to be due to macrophage reaction
      - Majority of immunosuppressants act on T-cells, no effect on macrophages
      - No known evidence of effect of immunosuppressants on copper ions or levonorgestrol
    - Increased risk of infection due to immunosuppression?
      - Lack of studies in transplant population
      - In studies with HIV+ patients, no significant increase in infection rates among HIV+
      - WHO classifies IUD as category 2 contraceptive for HIV+
        - No increased risk
  - Depot medroxyprogesterone acetate (DMPA, Depo-Provera)

        - Intramuscular injection slowly released over 12-week period of time
            - Must return to office every 12 weeks for injection
        - No known drug interactions with common immunosuppressants
            - Hepatic metabolism but not contraindicated in setting of normal liver function following transplant
        - Delayed return to fertility?
            - Ovulation may not return for up to 1 year
            - Average time 6 months
    - Etonogestrel Implant (Nexplanon)
        - Implant in subcutaneous tissue of upper extremity
        - Duration of efficacy: 3 years
        - No known drug interactions with common immunosuppressants
            - Hepatic metabolism but not contraindicated in setting of normal liver function following transplant
- Moderately effective
    - Combined oral contraceptives
        - Contraindicated in following patients
            - Personal history of MI, CVA, or DVT
                - Caution with prolonged immobilization
                    - Increased risk of DVT
                    - Should not be started until postoperative recovery is complete
            - Smokers over the age of 35
            - Migraine headaches with focal aura
            - Uncontrolled hypertension
            - Active liver disease or hepatic adenoma
        - Combined oral contraceptive pills
            - Hepatic metabolism but not contraindicated in setting of normal liver function following transplant
            - Metabolized by cytochrome P450 3A4 system
                - Shared by common immunosuppressants: glucocorticoids, cyclosporine, tacrolimus and sirolimus
                    - Increase bioavailability of these
                    - One study with women on oral contraceptive pills and oral steroids showed no difference in serum levels of drugs and serum cortisol
                    - No clear data on other immunosuppressants
                - Can take oral contraceptives continuously without placebo pills to maintain steady concentrations of immunosuppressants
        - Vaginal ring (NuvaRing)
            - Monthly use
            - Avoid hepatic first-pass metabolism so minimal effect on immunosuppressants metabolized by liver
            - Lack of studies demonstrating efficacy and safety in post-transplant patients
    - Less effective
        - Barrier methods
            - No contraindications for transplant patients regardless of immune status
            - High failure rate
                - Male condoms: 18% in first year with typical use
                - Female condoms: 21%
                - Diaphragms: 16%
            - High noncompliance rates
            - Reasonable for patients with infrequent intercourse or without current sexual partner
    - Emergency contraception
        - Pregnancy can be prevented up to 5 days after episode of unprotected intercourse in up to 85% of pregnancies that would have otherwise occurred
        - No known contraindications to use of emergency contraception
        - Progestin only (Plan B) is preferred

Effects on Menses and Ovarian Function

- Delayed puberty
    - Common
    - 1–2 years later than average
    - Prolonged length of puberty
    - Delayed age of final adult height
- Menstrual irregularities
    - Common prior to transplantations
    - Especially in solid organ transplant patients
    - Range from amenorrhea to menometrorrhagia
    - May have acute vaginal bleeding directly postopertive
    - Typically return of normal menses occurs several months following transplantation
        - Primarily influenced by overall health statues and normal graft function (i.e., normal serum creatinine)
        - With the exception of cases of premature ovarian failure
- Premature ovarian failure
    - Typically occurs after radiation therapy
    - Risk increases with increasing age

- Also can occur with some immunosuppressants (i.e., alkylating agents)
  - GnRH agonists may help prevent premature ovarian failure during alkylating chemotherapy
    - Mechanism not fully elucidated
- Presents with amenorrhea/oligomenorrhea and/or exaggerated menopausal symptoms (hot flashes, sleep disturbances, mood disturbances)
  - Most common presenting symptoms: lack of sexual desire and lack of vaginal lubrication
- Fertility preservation with oocyte fertilization/cryopreservation
- Can alleviate vasomotor symptoms with hormone replacement therapy if eligible
  - Individualize therapy based on immunosuppressants
  - If not a candidate for hormone therapy, can try SSRI/SNRI
  - Alternative interventions may include
    - Meditation/Relaxation
    - Exercise
    - Acupuncture

Cervical Screening

- Vast majority of cervical cancer are caused by high-risk types of human papillomavirus (HPV): 16, 18, 31, 33, or 35
- Incidence in immunocompromised populations increased
  - Seen in renal and bone marrow transplant patients
  - CDC has deemed cervical cancer to be an AIDS-defining condition
- Allogeneic hematopoietic stem cell patients found to have 13-fold increased risk of cervical squamous cell carcinoma
- No clear-cut guidelines set as of yet
- Many propose cervical Pap smears every 6–12 months with reflex HPV testing
  - Colposcopy is needed for further evaluation of abnormal Pap smears
    - Include atypical squamous cells of undetermined significance (ASCUS) with positive high-risk HPV testing, low-grade squamous intraepithelial lesions, high-grade squamous intraepithelial lesions, atypical glandular cells, or cancer
- HPV vaccination shown to reduce incidence of cervical and other genital tract dysplasia in healthy populations
  - Currently recommended for females and males aged 9–26 years
  - Most efficacious when vaccination precedes exposure to HPV infection
  - Unclear of duration of immunity after vaccination in transplant patients
    - Some transplant centers start reimmunization between 6 and 12 months post-transplant
    - National Institute of Health clinical trials regarding vaccine in transplant recipients currently underway

Genital Graft-Versus-Host Disease

- Seen in survivors after allogeneic hematopoietic stem cell transplantation
- Affects vulva and vagina
- Reported in 25–49% of patients
- Symptoms: dryness, burning, pruritus, pain to touch, dyspareunia, amenorrhea, cyclic pain (due to hematocolpos or hematometra), and dysuria
- Signs: erythema, tenderness, erosions, fissures, vaginal synechiae, leukokeratosis, vaginal stenosis, or shortening
- Early recognition integral to successful management
  - Lysis of vaginal synechiae followed by intravaginal or topical estrogen
  - Vaginal dilators for resolution of vaginal stenosis or shortening
  - High-potency topical immunosuppressants such as clobetasol propionate

FURTHER READING

1. Armenti VT, Constantinescu S, Mortiz MJ, et al. Pregnancy after transplantation. Transplant Rev 2008; 22:223–40.
2. Centers for Disease Control and Prevention. HPV vaccine information for clinicians - fact sheet. www.cdc.gov/std/hpv/stdfact-hpv-vaccine-hcp.htm
3. del Mar Colon M, Hibbard JU. Obstetrics considerations in the management of pregnancy in kidney transplant recipients. Adv Chronic Kidney Dis 2007; 14:168–77.
4. Deshpande NA, James NT, Kucirkaa LM, et al. Pregnancy outcomes in kidney transplant recipients: a systematic review and meta-analysis. Am J Transplant 2011; 11:2388–404.
5. Estes CM, Westhoff C. Contraception for the transplant patient. Semin Perinatol 2007; 31:372–7.
6. Kim JM, Song RK, Kim MJ, et al. Hormonal differences between female kidney transplant recipients and health women with the same gynecologic conditions. Transplant Proc 2012; 44:740–3.
7. Lowenstein BR, Vain NW, Perrone SV, et al. Successful pregnancy and vaginal delivery after heart transplantation. Am J Obstet Gynecol 1988; 158:589–90.

8. Malouf MA, Hopkins PM, Singleton L, et al. Sexual health issues after lung transplantation: importance of cervical screening. J Heart Lung Transplant 2003; 23:894–7.
9. Mass K, Quint EH, Punch MR, et al. Gynecological and reproductive function after liver transplantation. Transplantation 1996; 62:476–9.
10. McKay DB, Josephson MA. Pregnancy after kidney transplantation. Clin J Am Soc Nephrology 2008; 3:S117–25.
11. McKay DB, Josephson MA. Pregnancy in recipients of solid organs: Effects on mother and child. N Engl J Med 2006; 254:1281–93.
12. McKay DB, Josephson MA. Reproduction and transplantation: report on the AST Consensus Conference on Reproductive Issues and Transplantation. Am J Transplant 2006; 5:1592–9.
13. Ortiz M, Croxatto H. Copper-T intrauterine device and levonorgestrel intrauterine system: biological bases of their mechanism of action. Contraception 2007; 75:S16–30.
14. Paulen ME, Folger SG, Curtis KM, et al. Contraceptive use among solid organ transplant patients: a systematic review. Contraception 2010; 82:102–12.
15. Pietrzak B, Cyganek A, Jabiry-Zieniewicz K, et al. Function of the ovaries in female kidney transplant recipients. Transplant Proc 2006; 38:180–3.
16. Rodrigues I, Grou F, Joly J. Effectiveness of emergent contraceptive pills between 72 and 120 hours after unprotected sexual intercourse. Am J Obstet Gynecol 2001; 18:531–7.
17. Shanis D, Merideth M, Pulanic TJ, et al. Female long-term survivors after allogeneic hematopoietic stem cell transplantation: evaluation and management. Semin Hematol 2012; 49:83–94.
18. Sucato GS, Murray PJ. Gynecologic health care for the adolescent solid organ transplant recipient. Pediatric Transplant 2005; 9:346–56.
19. Tauchmanova L, Carrano R, Sabbatini M, et al. Hypothalamic-pituitary-gonadal axis function after successful kidney transplantation in men and women. Human Reprod 2004; 19:867–73.
20. Van Diemen-Steenvoorde R, Donckerwolcke RA, Brackel H, et al. Growth and sexual maturation in children after kidney transplantation. J Pediatrics 1987; 110:351–6.
21. World Health Organization. Medical Eligibility Criteria for Contraception–4th edition, Geneva: WHO Press, 2009.
22. Zieman M, Hatcher RA, Cwiak C, et al. Managing contraception. 2010-2012. Georgia: Bridging the Gap Foundation, 2010.

CHAPTER 51

The Role of Quality Management for Monitoring and Improving: A Transplant Program

Yosef D Dlugacz, Andrea Restifo

The basis of any quality management (QM) program is to gather valid and accurate information in order to assess processes and improve outcomes. Because healthcare services, including transplant services, are highly complex and involve many individuals, changing processes and ingrained habits of behavior can be difficult and requires conscious effort. Change often necessitates a cultural change and certainly takes time. There are no quick fixes in QM.

Generally, a robust QM program involves:

- A formalized multidisciplinary QA/PI program
- A formal communication structure
- A consistent peer review process
- Accurate documentation of errors
- Plan for improvement

In order to accomplish the above:

- Clinical and operational indicators need to be developed

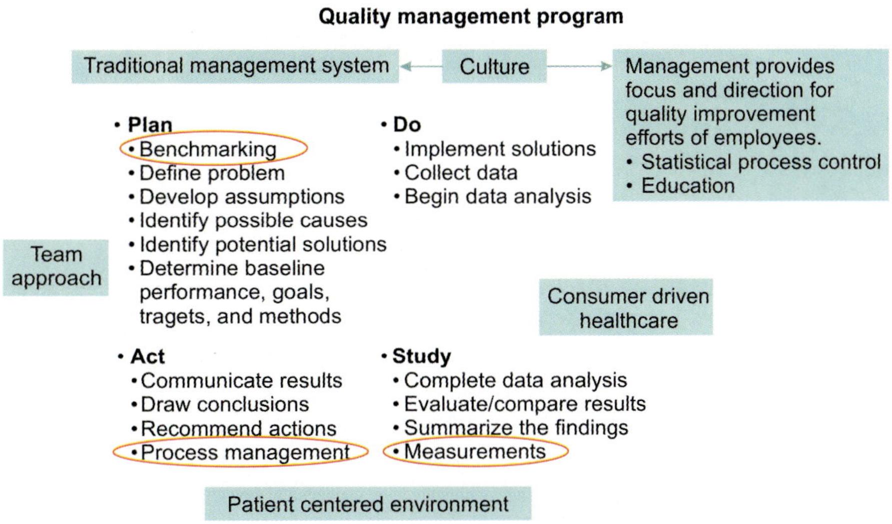

Quality management program

Traditional management system ← Culture → Management provides focus and direction for quality improvement efforts of employees.
- Statistical process control
- Education

Team approach

- **Plan**
  - Benchmarking
  - Define problem
  - Develop assumptions
  - Identify possible causes
  - Identify potential solutions
  - Determine baseline performance, goals, tragets, and methods
- **Do**
  - Implement solutions
  - Collect data
  - Begin data analysis
- **Act**
  - Communicate results
  - Draw conclusions
  - Recommend actions
  - Process management
- **Study**
  - Complete data analysis
  - Evaluate/compare results
  - Summarize the findings
  - Measurements

Consumer driven healthcare

Patient centered environment

- An adverse event reporting process must be established and communicated
- Accountability has to be explicitly articulated
- Process and outcome variables have to be defined
- Indicators for donor and recipient must be developed
- Once defined, indicator must reflect, pre-, acute- and post-transplant process
- Transplant criteria have to be developed
- Analytics have to be developed
- Table of measures, incorporating critical variables, has to be developed

To assess and evaluate a transplant program, data are required about

- Volume of transplants performed over time
- Average LOS
- Patient demographics

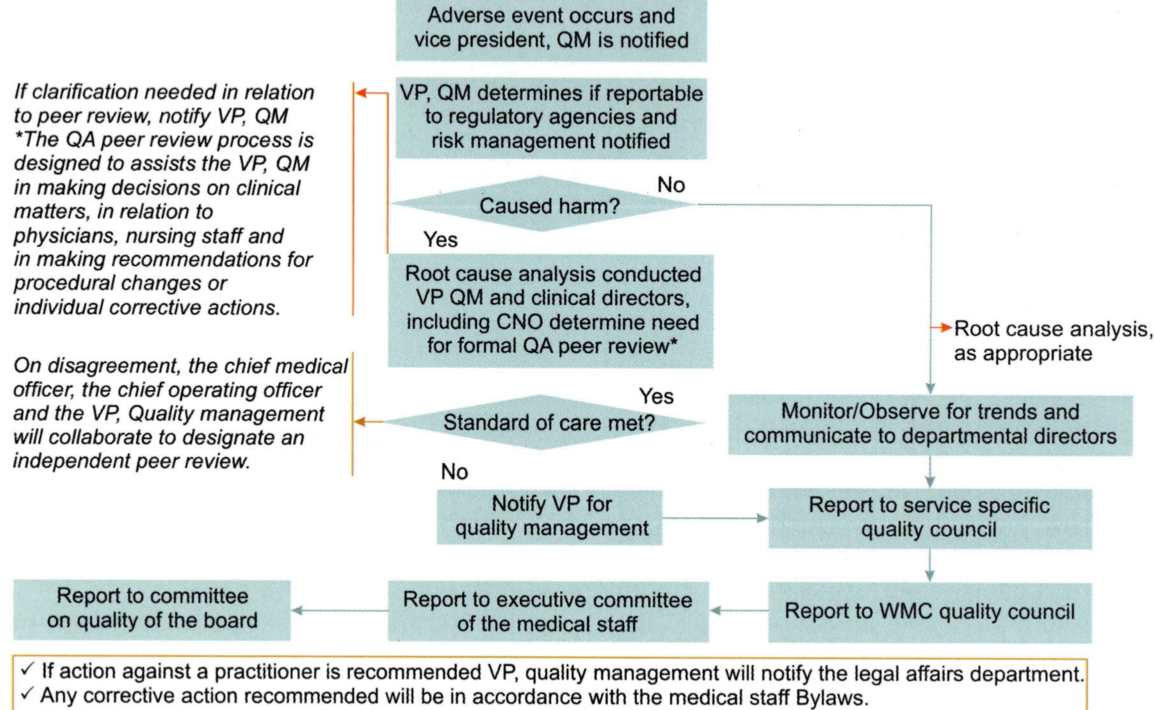

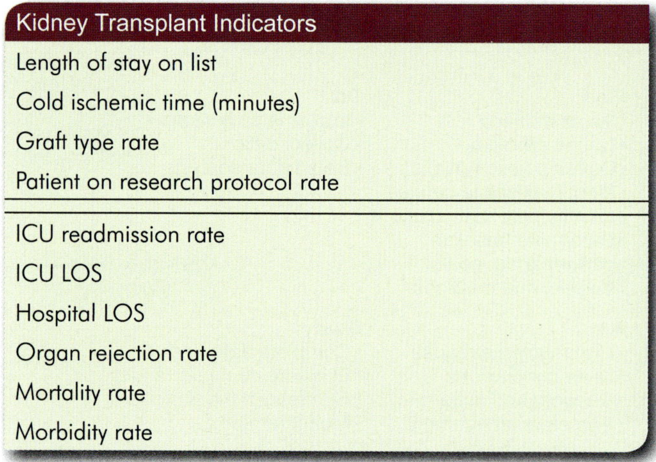

Kidney Transplant Indicators
Length of stay on list
Cold ischemic time (minutes)
Graft type rate
Patient on research protocol rate
ICU readmission rate
ICU LOS
Hospital LOS
Organ rejection rate
Mortality rate
Morbidity rate

Kidney Transplant Indicators

For patients that undergo kidney transplant

	Numerator	*Denominator*
Total # of transplants		
Hospital ALOS	Hospital LOS	Total # of transplants
Readmission to ICU/PACU rate	# of readmissions to ICU/PACU	Total # of transplants
Unplanned returns to the OR rate	# of unplanned returns to the OR	Total # of transplants
Infection rate	# of infections	Total # of transplants
Readmission to hospital rate	# of readmissions to the hospital	Total # of transplants
Survival rate	# of alive patients (disposition <> 20)	Total # of transplants
Rejection rate	# of rejections	Total # of transplants
Kidney graft distribution	ECD, DCD, ECD+DCD, STD	Total # of transplants
Graft function distribution	Immediate, delayed, slow function, no function	Total # of transplants
Graft outcome distribution	Functioning, graft failure, Nephrectomy	
Rejection type distribution	Hyperacute, acute cellular, acute antibody, CAN	
Rejection treatment (Meds) distribution	Steroids, thymoglobulin, OKT3, campath, rituximab (rituxan), plasmapheresis, IVIG, other	
Average cold ischemic time		

For all patients that are referred for a kidney transplant

Avg time from referral to first appointment

Avg time from first appointment to outcome

The indicators can be aggregated monthly, quarterly and/or annually.
Quarterly and/or semi-annual comparisons can be done.

Criteria for Transplant Indicator; Development and Selection

- *Requirement*
  - Multidisciplinary team
  - Clinical relevance
  - Measurable
- *Methods*
  - Brainstorming sessions
  - Evidenced based literature/research
- *Characteristics*
  - Quantifiable (numerators/denominators)
  - High validity and reliability

- Complications (infection, return to the OR)
- Outcomes analysis
- Discharge disposition of patients

To promote change and to transform the culture of a transplant service to achieve improved outcomes, individual physician subjectivity needs to be superseded by objective norms, variables, evidence-based measures, and statistical analysis of aggregated data.

Collaboration is essential for everyone involved in the program, including clinical and administrative leadership and the members of the transplant team. Effective analysis of errors requires a straightforward acknowledgement of the complexity of the process and the likelihood of errors occurring. Unless an appreciation of complexity is accepted, prevention and improvement efforts will remain superficial.

To successfully evaluate transplant services, many factors, services, and people have to coordinate their efforts and issues of prioritization have to be defined.

Assessment has to include evaluation of the elements of structure, process, and outcome.

Gap analysis of program practice and policies with regulatory standards should be conducted.

To implement a QM program, it needs leadership involvement.

Physicians, surgeons, and other disciplines must work together and respect each other's opinions to understand the indicator or the problems they face.

QM should lead to process improvement and outcome.

This type of work must be constantly maintained and cultivated by the director or chairman of the transplant program.

Kidney Transplant: Table of Measures

	Numerator	*Denominator*
Total # of transplants		
Hospital ALOS	Hospital LOS	Total # of transplants
Readmission to ICU rate	# of readmissions to ICU	Total # of transplants
Pre-transplant nutrition consults rate	# of pre-transplant nutrition consults	Total # of transplants
Unplanned returns to the OR (excluding re-transplant) rate	# of unplanned returns to the OR	Total # of transplants
Re-transplant rate	# of re-transplants	Total # of transplants
Adverse drug reaction rate	# of adverse drug reaction	Total # of transplants
Ventilator associated pneumonia index	# of ventilator associated pneumonia	# of ventilator days in ICU
Line related bacteremias index	# of line related bacteremias	# of line days in ICU
Other nosocomial infections rate	# of other nosocomial infections	Total # of transplants
Rejection of organ rate	# of organ rejections	Total # of transplants
Readmission to hospital rate	# of readmissions to the hospital	Total # of transplants
Survival rate	# of alive patients (disposition <> 20)	Total # of transplants
New onset diabetes		

Quality management: Review of adverse events

Adverse event occurs:
Follow "***Quality management adverse patient event reporting***" as per QA/PI plan

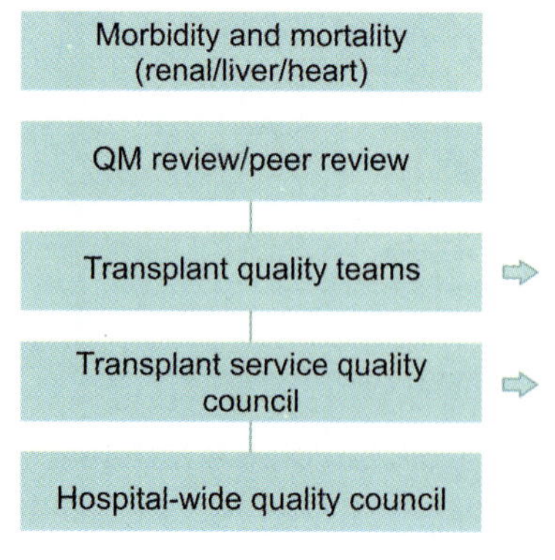

- If a particular case determined not to meet standard of care and requiring further review, the case(s) is transmitted to VP, QM by transplant administrator
  - Multidisciplinary review process
  - RCA conducted
  - May include an external peer review
- Share RCA findings, patterns and trends (lessons larned)
- Share RCA findings, patterns and trends
- Share aggregated data and lessons learned among services
- Surgical services representative communicates data to surgical services quality council

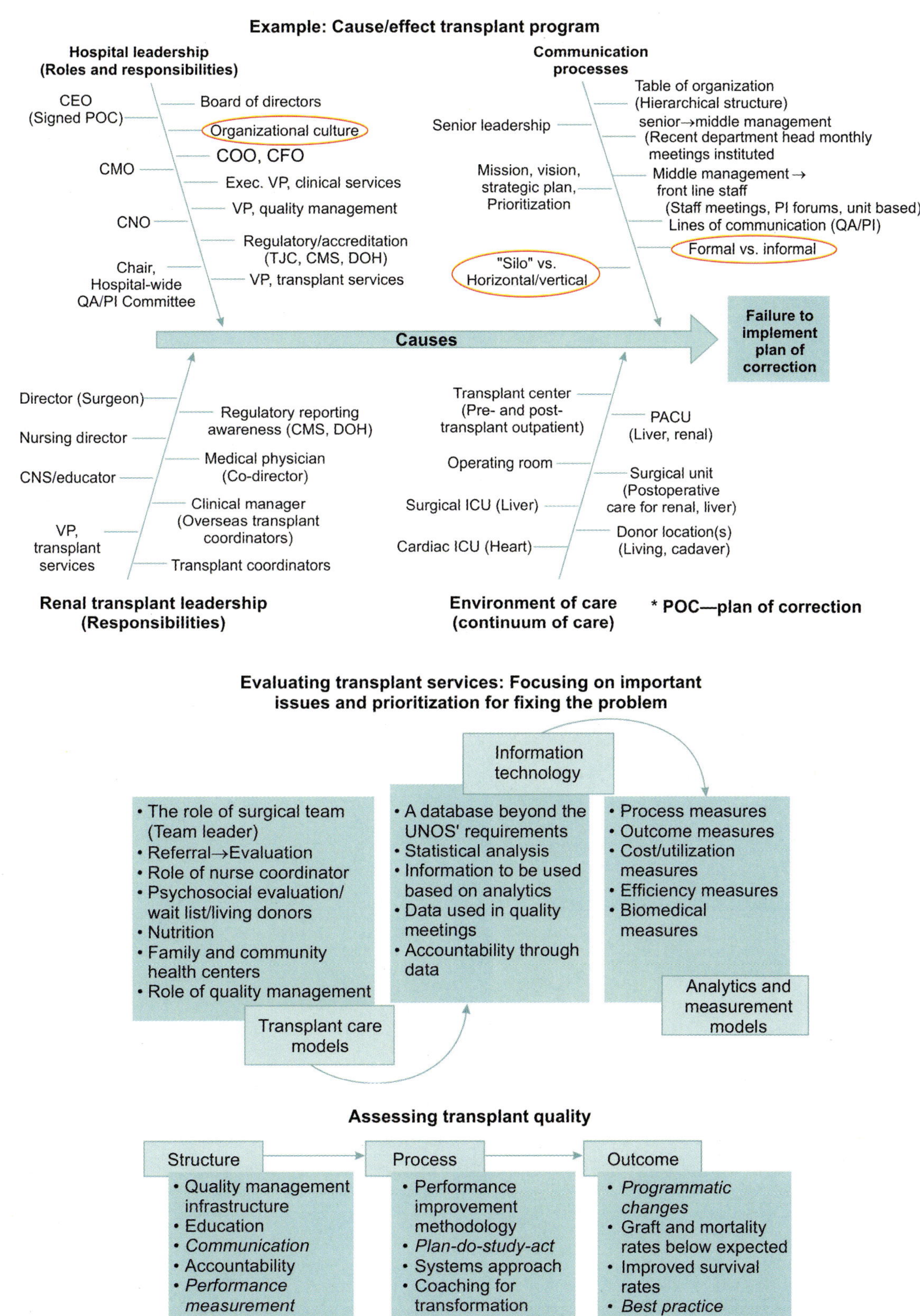
Example: Cause/effect transplant program
Hospital leadership (Roles and responsibilities)
CEO (Signed POC)
Board of directors
Organizational culture
COO, CFO
CMO
Exec. VP, clinical services
VP, quality management
CNO
Regulatory/accreditation (TJC, CMS, DOH)
Chair, Hospital-wide QA/PI Committee
VP, transplant services
Communication processes
Table of organization (Hierarchical structure)
Senior leadership
senior→middle management (Recent department head monthly meetings instituted
Mission, vision, strategic plan, Prioritization
Middle management→ front line staff (Staff meetings, PI forums, unit based)
Lines of communication (QA/PI)
Formal vs. informal
"Silo" vs. Horizontal/vertical
Causes
Failure to implement plan of correction
Director (Surgeon)
Regulatory reporting awareness (CMS, DOH)
Nursing director
Medical physician (Co-director)
CNS/educator
Clinical manager (Overseas transplant coordinators)
VP, transplant services
Transplant coordinators
Transplant center (Pre- and post-transplant outpatient)
PACU (Liver, renal)
Operating room
Surgical unit (Postoperative care for renal, liver)
Surgical ICU (Liver)
Donor location(s) (Living, cadaver)
Cardiac ICU (Heart)
Renal transplant leadership (Responsibilities)
Environment of care (continuum of care)
* POC—plan of correction
Evaluating transplant services: Focusing on important issues and prioritization for fixing the problem
Information technology
• The role of surgical team (Team leader)
• Referral→Evaluation
• Role of nurse coordinator
• Psychosocial evaluation/ wait list/living donors
• Nutrition
• Family and community health centers
• Role of quality management
• A database beyond the UNOS' requirements
• Statistical analysis
• Information to be used based on analytics
• Data used in quality meetings
• Accountability through data
• Process measures
• Outcome measures
• Cost/utilization measures
• Efficiency measures
• Biomedical measures
Analytics and measurement models
Transplant care models
Assessing transplant quality
Structure
• Quality management infrastructure
• Education
• Communication
• Accountability
• Performance measurement
• Continuum of care
• Team approach
Process
• Performance improvement methodology
• Plan-do-study-act
• Systems approach
• Coaching for transformation
• Leveraging EMR–analytics
• Data validation
Outcome
• Programmatic changes
• Graft and mortality rates below expected
• Improved survival rates
• Best practice

CHAPTER 52

Epigenetics in Transplantation

Nirupama Chandel, Ashwani Malhotra, Pravin C Singhal

Epigenetics is spontaneous phenomenon where environment may modify a particular gene expression without any alteration in nucleotide sequence. Since transplanted organ resides in an altered environment, there are multiple scenarios, (1) cells in transplanted organ may react with circulating blood cells and cytokines (2) circulating cells may react in response to cells of transplanted organ, and (3) immunosuppressive drugs, which are administered to the recipient may alter the milieu for the transplanted organ as well as for other host organs (Fig. 1). Although several studies displayed the outcome of these interactions in term of immunity and clinical manifestations, the occurrence of alterations in gene expression—epigenetics—has not been investigated in general, and in kidney transplant recipients in particular.

Epigenetics is the heritability in gene expression patterns molded by mechanisms not involving the general nucleotide sequence change.[1] Organism's phenotype heritable changes can occur during the lifespan due to mechanisms other than changes in nucleotide sequence, which clear the role of environment in the development and evolution. Chromatin, the unit formed by DNA, histone, and associated proteins, may undergo various forms of remodeling, leading to either facilitation or hindrance of transcription (Fig. 2). As chromatin is not bound so loosely that transcription can easily occur; DNA must first be uncoiled from the histones for the transcription factors to be able to bind to their matching sequences.[2] Correspondingly, tighter winding of promoters or enhancers can hide them from transcription factors or polymerases. DNA methylation/demethylation and histone acetylation are all modifiers of epigenetic chromatin modeling.[3] DNA methylation involves the addition of methyl group to C-5 position carbon of cytosine ring catalyzed by DNA methyltransferase enzyme. DNA methylation often associated with the transcriptional silencing of the gene, whereas histone acetylation involves the removal of the positive charge from the histones, thereby decreasing the interaction of the N-terminal of histones with the negatively charged phosphate groups of DNA. As a consequence, the condensed chromatin is transformed into a more relaxed structure that is associated with greater levels of gene transcription. Thus, in general, methylation decreases whereas acetylation is associated with increased transcription (Fig. 2).

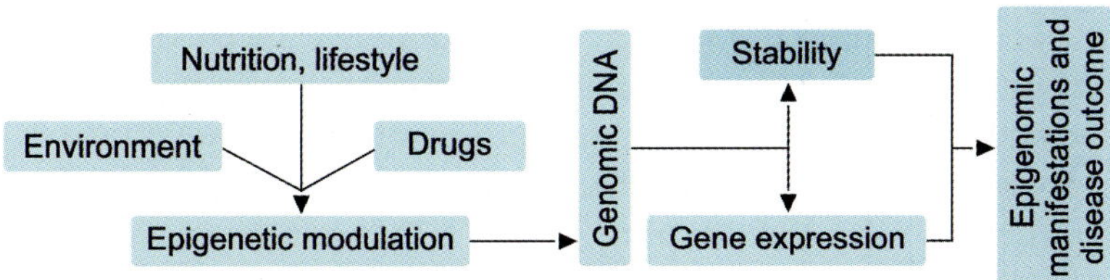

Fig. 1: Schematic diagram of different stimuli, epigenetic mechanisms and gene-activating events leading to epigenomic manifestations.

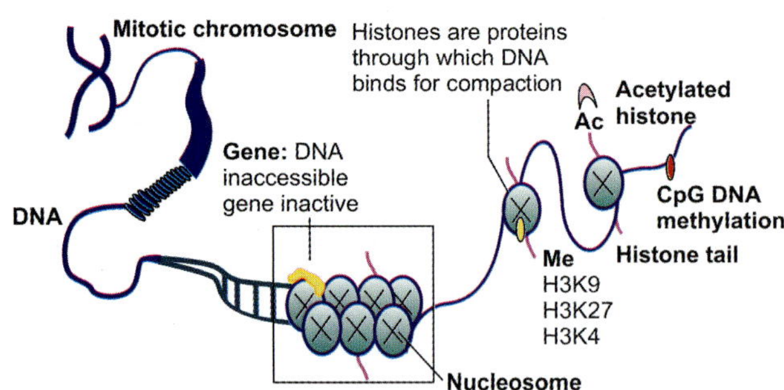

Fig. 2: Mechanisms of inheritable epigenetics. Mammalian gene expression is tightly controlled by genetic as well as epigenetic mechanisms.

EPIGENETICS IN ORGAN TRANSPLANTATION

Organ transplantation is the treatment of choice for patients with end-stage organ failure. Surgical techniques have been refined to such an extent that they no longer decide the fate of a transplanted organ. Issues related to optimal use of immunosuppressive drugs play a major role in determining the long-term outcome of the allograft. In recent studies, occurrence of epigenetic changes and success of transplanted organ has been linked to some extent. It has been shown that epigenetic changes are at least partly involved in transplant outcomes; therefore, it is worth investigating the use of epigenetic markers for prediction of transplant outcome, severity of rejection, T-cell tolerance, and modification of inflammatory response. Studies showed that epigenetic changes during transplantation may contribute to protein dysfunction, thereby influencing transplantation outcome.[4-6] The current immunosuppressive treatment regimen in organ transplant recipients involves a significant reduction in the acute rejection rates; however, allograft nephropathy, a major determinant of long-term graft survival, continues to take its toll.[7,8] The current practice involves starting these agents in a standard prefixed dose, and subsequent titration based on drug-level monitoring. However, patients receiving similar dosing schedules exhibit several fold variation in their drug levels and by the time measurements are made and corrections are initiated, the graft has already been exposed to toxic concentration of the drug. Protocol biopsy studies revealed that grafts exposed chronically to inappropriate concentrations of calcineurine inhibitors universally exhibit variable histological features of toxicity. Environmental toxins have been demonstrated to affect epigenetic transgenerational phenotypes. Anway et al.[9] and Skinner et al.[10] in their studies demonstrated that male infertility resulting from the anti-androgenic fungicide vinclozolin, a potent toxin, was transferred to the next (F1) generation. Additionally, the offspring of rats exposed to vinclozolin had higher rates of immune abnormalities, kidney disease, prostate disease, and breast cancer because of the reprogramming of methylation state of the genome during germ cell development. Since drug toxicity may reprogram the epigenicity status of genes, even the best epigenetic treatment will unlikely to preclude the use of immunosuppressive drugs in their regime. Therefore, it would be advisable to investigate the effect of epigenetic drugs when administered in concert with immunosuppressive drugs. In studies where rats were transplanted with hearts and survival time was observed with/without a histone deacetylases (HDACs) inhibitor and immunosuppressive drugs, the outcome was different. The administration of the HDAC inhibitor prolonged survival time, whereas combined use of both the drugs resulted in the best survival rates. The lack of interstitial infiltration into the graft was seen as a promising effect of the combined treatment.[11,12] In 1993, Schneeberger et al.[13] demonstrated aggravated graft complications such as chronic rejection due to hypoxia-induced factor (HIF)-α hypoxic conditions during ischemia-reperfusion (I/R) injury. Histone modification has been shown to be involved in HIF-α overexpression; the later may activate the MHC chain expression favoring the activation of immune system.[14] One may draw the conclusion that the monitoring of histone modification and HIF-α levels would be therapeutically beneficial.[15] These authors suggested the combination of oxygenation and HDAC inhibitors with continued histone acetylation for the reduction in I/R injury area.

TRANSPLANTATION-INDUCED IMMUNE RESPONSE

The long-term outcome of an otherwise technically perfect graft is largely predicted by the magnitude of immunologically mediated responses against it. HDAC inhibitors can also manipulate the T-cell activation and induction to self-tolerance.[16] Trichostatin A, a potent HDAC inhibitor, has been demonstrated to enhance T-cell expression of Foxp3 (a Treg protein), which leads to immunosuppressive phenotype. However, Foxp3 has been found to be highly susceptible for cytosine phosphate guanosine (CpG) methylation.[17,18] Since T cells play a vital role in graft acceptance or rejection, it would be of great advantage if one would be able to reduce the amount of immunosuppressive drugs depending on host's epigenetic

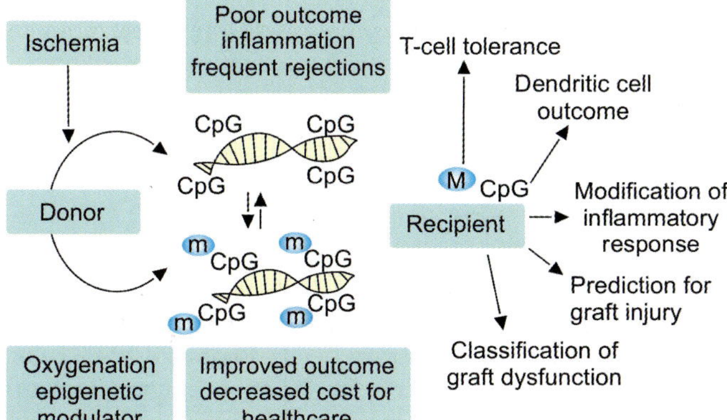

Fig. 3: Impact of epigenetic changes in transplantation outcome.

behavior (Fig. 3). Another important target for the improved graft outcome is complement system. Pratt et al.[5] showed the methylation/demethylation status of C3 complement gene promoter. Parker et al.[4] displayed methylation in regulatory sites of the C3 promoter status through employing pyrosequencing technique in transplanted tissues. In another study, Mehta et al.[1] identified a CALCA promoter hypermethylation as an indicator of post-transplant kidney injury. CALCA gene belongs to calcitonin gene-related peptides that participates in calcium ion (Ca^{2+}) and phosphorus metabolism. It inhibits renal tubular cell reabsorption of Ca^{2+} allowing it to be excreted in the urine. They investigated the methylation of promoter regions in grafted tissues, and found hypermethylation of the CALCA gene promoter in transplant patients with acute tubular necrosis. They observed that the transplant recipients had a higher rate of promoter hypermethylation when compared with healthy controls. Reddy et al.[19] in a follow-up study demonstrated the effect of HDAC inhibitors in graft versus host disease. Suberoylanilide hydroxamic acid (SAHA), an HDAC inhibitor, apart from its anti-tumor activity, reduced secretion of inflammatory cytokines and influenced dendritic cells by enhancing the expression of indoleamine 2, 3-dioxygenase (IDO). IDO is an immunomodulatory enzyme, which is important for the tryptophan catabolism. In human and murine cells, IDO inhibits antigen-specific T-cell proliferation and suppresses T-cell responses in vitro. Its expression is an inducible feature of specific subsets of dendritic cells and also important for T-cell regulatory properties.[20] Treatment with SAHA involves the mechanism of binding of acetylated histone H4 to the IDO promoter that has a potential to attenuate the acute graft versus host disease.[19]

NONSPECIFIC OUTCOME

Nonspecific effects are main concern with epigenetic drugs. For example, azacytidine, a demethylating agent, is going to affect methylation status all over the genome and not only to the specific affected organ. Thus, "It's a mixed blessing," says Rudolf Jaenisch at the Whitehead Institute in Cambridge, Massachusetts. "If you generally inhibit the methyltransferase, then you protect one tissue but you induce cancer in another." Timothy Bestor of Columbia University in New York points out that: "the drugs under development and in trials have genome wide effects, and this lack of specificity and the lack of known targets mean that side effects are likely to be severe." In Bestor's view, "convincing evidence of a beneficial effect of DNA methylation inhibitors in cancer has not appeared despite great effort." He suggested that "the extent of pathogenic gene silencing by DNA methylation may have been greatly overestimated."

In summary, epigenetics is no longer an underestimated issue in transplantation medicine. Further optimization of this issue would not only improve therapeutic approaches but would also decrease the drug load, associated side effects, and cost. Enhanced molecular understanding of epigenetics and its role in the transplant outcome would also open a new window to the diagnostic tools and important biomarkers.

REFERENCES

1. Mehta TK, Hoque MO, Ugarte R, et al. Quantitative detection of promoter hypermethylation as a biomarker of acute kidney injury during transplantation. Transplant Proc 2006;38:3420–6.
2. Mellor J. Dynamic nucleosomes and gene transcription. Trends Genet. 2006;22:320-9.
3. Verga-Weisz PD, Becker PB. Regulation of higher order chromatin structure by nucleosome-remodeling factors. Curr. Opin. Genet. Dev 2006;16:151-6.
4. Parker MD, Chambers PA, Lodge JP, et al. Ischemia-reperfusion injury and its influence on the epigenetic modification of the donor kidney genome. Transplantation 2008;86:1818–23.
5. Pratt JR, Parker MD, Affleck LJ, et al. Ischemic epigenetics and the transplanted kidney. Transplant Proc 2006; 38:3344–6.
6. Schildberg FA, Hagmann CA, Bohnert V, Tolba RH. Improved transplantation outcome by epigenetic changes. Transpl Immunol 2010;23:104–10.
7. de Mattos AM, Olyaei AJ, Bennett WM. Pharmacology of immunosuppressive medications used in renal diseases and transplantation. Am J Kidney Dis 1996;28:631–67.

8. Stoffels B, Tolba RH, Schildberg FA, et al. Komplikationen durch immunsuppressive Therapie nach Lebertransplantation-eine retrospektive 12-Jahres-Analyse des Transplantationszentrums Bonn. Chir Gastroenterol 2008; 24:226–33.
9. Anway MD, Cupp AS, Uzumcu M, et al. Epigenetic transgenerational actions of endocrine disruptors and male fertility. Science 2005;308:1466–1469.
10. Skinner MK, Manikkam M, Guerrero-Bosagna C. Epigenetic transgenerational actions of endocrine disruptors. Reprod Toxicol, in press, 2010.
11. Kinugasa F, Nagatomi I, Nakanishi T, et al. Effect of the immunosuppressant histone deacetylase inhibitor FR276457 in a canine renal transplant model. Transpl Immunol 2009;21:198–202.
12. Kinugasa F, Yamada T, Noto T, et al. Effect of a new immunosuppressant histone deacetylase (HDAC) inhibitor FR276457 in a rat cardiac transplant model. Biol Pharm Bull 2008;31:1723–6.
13. Schneeberger H, Schleibner S, Illner WD, et al. The impact of free radical-mediated reperfusion injury on acute and chronic rejection events following cadaveric renal transplantation. Clin Transpl 1993, 219–32.
14. Wei L, Lu J, Feng L, et al. HIF-1alpha accumulation upregulates MICA and MICB expression on human cardiomyocytes and enhances NK cell cytotoxicity during hypoxia-reoxygenation. Life Sci 2010;87:111–9.
15. Granger A, Abdullah I, Huebner F, et al. Histone deacetylase inhibition reduces myocardial ischemia-reperfusion injury in mice. FASEB J 2008;22:3549–60.
16. Moon C, Kim SH, Park KS, et al. Use of epigenetic modification to induce FOXP3 expression in naive T cells. Transplant Proc 2009;41:1848–54.
17. Floess S, Freyer J, Siewert C, et al. Epigenetic control of the foxp3 locus in regulatory T cells. PLoS Biol 2007;5:e38.
18. Lal G, Zhang N, van der Touw W, et al. Epigenetic regulation of Foxp3 expression in regulatory T cells by DNA methylation. J Immunol 2009;182:259–73.
19. Reddy P, Sun Y, Toubai T, et al. Histone deacetylase inhibition modulates indoleamine 2,3-dioxygenase-dependent DC functions and regulates experimental graft-versus-host disease in mice. J Clin Invest 2008;118:2562–73.
20. Hwang SL, Chung NP, Chan JK, et al. Indoleamine 2, 3-dioxygenase (IDO) is essential for dendritic cell activation and chemotactic responsiveness to chemokines. Cell Res 2005;15: 167–75.

CHAPTER 53

Ischemia Reperfusion

Matthew Giangola, Salil Rajayer, Michael Kuncewitch, Adam Khader, Ping Wang

Renal ischemia/reperfusion injury (renal I/R) involves several complex pathophysiological mechanisms that are incompletely understood. Broadly, cellular injury is in part due to the anoxic cell death incurred during the ischemic period, as well as the buildup of free radicals. However, with the return of blood flow comes an accumulation of inflammatory cells and mediators, reactive oxygen species (ROS), and reactive nitrogen species (RNS). The subsequent biochemical derangements in intracellular homeostasis together work to induce further cell death from inflammation, apoptosis, and necrosis.[1] These events may lead to delayed graft function in the case of transplant recipients or increases in complications, length of hospital stay, and cost of care for those experiencing I/R injury.

Hemodynamics

- The kidneys receive about 1 L/min of blood flow, or roughly 20% of the total cardiac output, equating to about 605 mL/min of renal plasma flow[2]
- The amount that is filtered by the glomeruli is usually 125 mL/min. Hence, the kidney receives a vastly larger supply of blood than that which is needed for metabolism
- Underperfusion of the kidney occurs when the mean arterial pressure is decreased below the kidney's autoregulatory threshold of a systolic pressure of 80 mm Hg

Pathophysiology

- Early phase
  - Decrease in ATP and anerobic metabolism leads to increases in local phospholipases, ROS, free radicals and calcium disregulation, associated with:[3]
    - eNOS/iNOS imbalance
    - Alterations in intracellular pH
    - Increases in ROS and RNS
    - Cellular lipid peroxidation
    - Mitochondrial damage with activation of caspases, leading to apoptosis
  - There is subsequent activation of TLR-2, TLR-4 and PPAR binding, leading to cytokine production
    - Upregulation of inflammatory transcription factors (NF-kB, hypoxia-inducible factor-1, etc.) leads to increases in proinflammatory cytokines (TNF-α, IL-1β, IL-6, etc.)
  - Late phase
    - Increased chemotactic factors (IL-8, platelet-activating factor) and receptors (ICAM, L-selectin) causing adhesion and migration
    - Increased migration of neutrophils and lymphocytes
    - Increased oxidative stress and immunologic damage

Figures 1 to 3 illustrate progression of ischemia reperfusion changes.

Recently, animal experimental models of renal I/R injury have allowed investigators to focus on a number of important basic mechanisms involved in the regulation of renal function, for example, modulation of renal blood flow, medullary oxygenation, and tubuloglomerular feedback.[6]

Future therapeutic considerations and targets renal ischemia reperfusion:

- Antioxidants and antioxidant enzymes
  - Enzymatic antioxidants
  - Nonenzymatic antioxidants
- Hormonal mediators
- Nitric oxide mediators
- Phosphodiesterase inhibitors
- Erythropoietin and its synthetic derivatives
- Mitochondrial fatty acid metabolism[7]
- Stem cell modulation

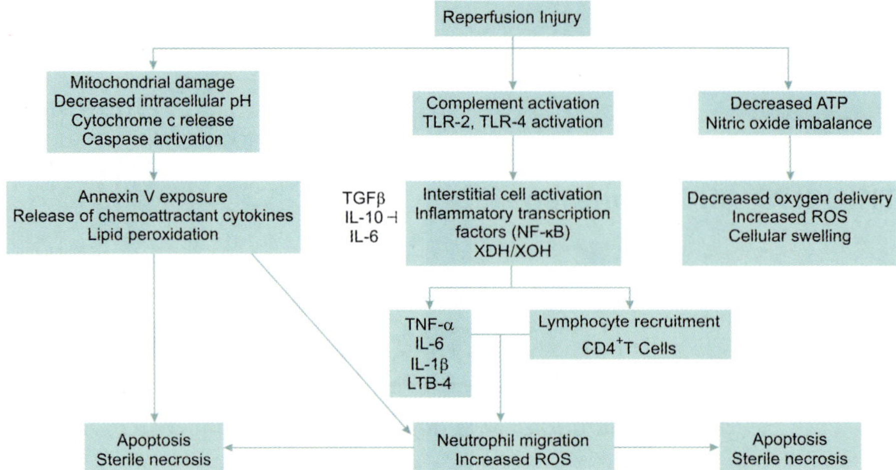

Fig. 1: Progression of reperfusion injury. Initial ischemic insult leads to decreased ATP and cellular damage. Early changes such as mitochondrial damage and caspase activation lead to eventual apoptosis. Activation of complement and toll-like receptors (TLR) engage a pathway that increases inflammation and damage.[4] Ultimately, neutrophil chemotaxis and migration mediate clearance of apoptotic cells.

Histologically, this is manifested by:

- Cellular edema
- Flattening of the epithelial brush border
- Distorted glomeruli and alterations in Bowman's space
- Microhemorrhage and coagulative necrosis
- Tubular casts.[5]

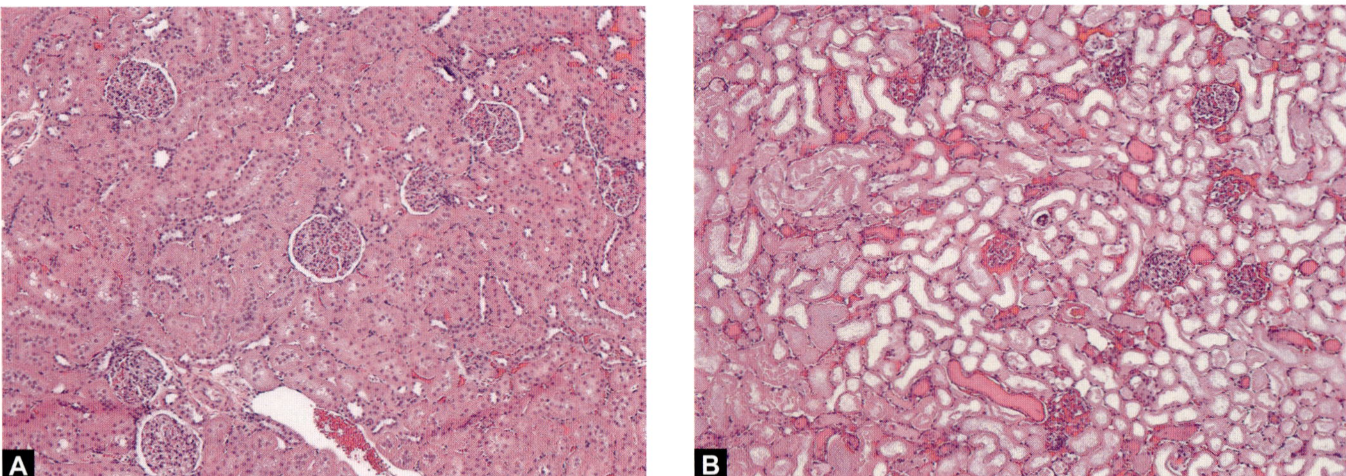

Figs. 2A and B: Renal cortex of normal (A) rat kidney and cortex 24 hours after 90 minutes of complete ischemia followed by reperfusion (B).

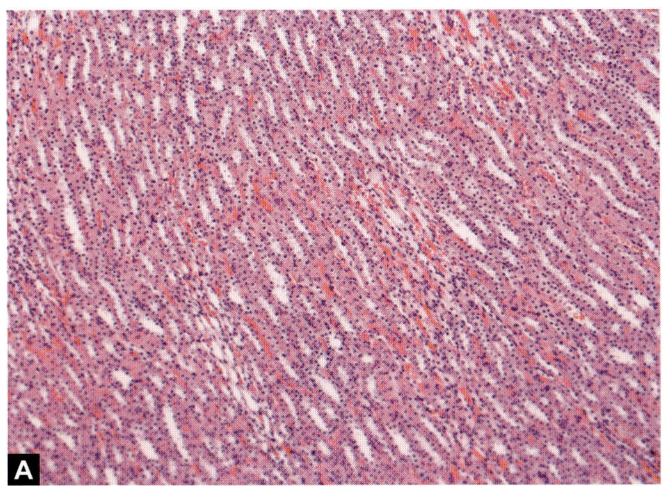

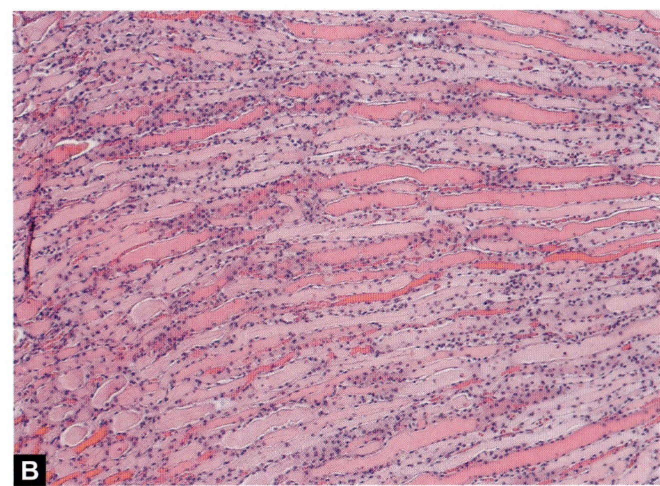

Figs. 3A and B: Renal medulla of normal (A) rat kidney and cortex 24 hours after 90 minutes of complete ischemia followed by reperfusion (B).

REFERENCES

1. Kuncewitch M, Yang WL, Molmenti E, et al. Wnt agonist attenuates liver injury and improves survival after hepatic ischemia/reperfusion. Shock 2013;39:3–10.
2. Eaton DC. Vander's renal physiology. In: Pooler JP (ed.), Renal blood flow and glomerular filtration. 7th edn.
3. Jennette JC. Hepetinstall's pathology of the kidney. 6th edn. 2006.
4. Amura CR, Renner B, Lyubchenko T, et al. Complement activation and toll-like receptor-2 signaling contribute to cytokine production after renal ischemia/reperfusion. Mol Immunol 2012;52:249–57.
5. Bonventre JV, Yang L. Cellular pathophysiology of ischemic acute kidney injury. J Clin Invest 2011;121:4210–21.
6. Chatterjee PK. Novel pharmacological approaches to the treatment of renal ischemia-reperfusion injury: a comprehensive review. Naunyn Schmiedebergs Arch Pharmacol 2007;376:1–43.
7. Idrovo JP, Yang WL, Nicastro J, et al. Stimulation of carnitine palmitoyltransferase 1 improves renal function and attenuates tissue damage after ischemia/reperfusion. J Surg Res 2012; 177:157–64.

CHAPTER 54

Pediatric Kidney Transplantation

Christine Sethna, Nataliya Chorny, Amit Basu, Adam Khader, Jose Prince, Ernesto P Molmenti, Ron Shapiro

Kidney transplantation in the pediatric population is the therapy of choice for children with end-stage renal disease (ESRD). Compared with dialysis, transplantation provides for

- Increased survival (75–87% 5-year survival for dialysis vs. 94–97% for transplant)
- Enhanced quality of life
- Improved physical, cognitive, and psychosocial development

End-Stage Renal Disease

The etiology of ESRD in children is different compared with adults where acquired renal disease predominates.

- In younger children, the leading cause of ESRD is congenital/cystic or hereditary (Table 1)
- In older children and adolescents, glomerular disease and glomerulonephritis (GN) are more prevalent

Contraindications to Kidney Transplantation

- Pre-existing malignancy, especially with metastasis (2 years after cure for most malignancies)
- Autoimmune disease (disease "burnout" for at least 1 year)
- Severe devastating neurological dysfunction
- Active hepatitis B infection

Manifestations of ESRD in Children Include

- Delayed physical growth
- Osteodystrophy
- Delayed puberty
- Diminished neurologic and cognitive function
- Increased somnolence and fatigue
- Hypertension, cardiomegaly and dyslipidemia
- Anemia

Table 1: Causes of pediatric ESRD

FSGS	14.4%
Aplasia/hypoplasia/dysplasia	14.2%
Obstructive uropathy	12.6%
Reflux nephropathy	3.5%
SLE nephritis	3.2%
HUS	3.1%
Chronic GN	3.0%
Polycystic disease	2.9%
Congenital nephrotic syndrome	2.6%
Prune belly	2.0%
Medullary cystic disease	2.0%
Idiopathic crescentic GN	1.8%
Familial nephritis	1.8%
MPGN–type I	1.6%
Unknown	7.5%
Other	23.7%

Epidemiology

- The incidence of ESRD in the United States is 16 per million
- Kidney transplantation is the most common form of therapy for ESRD in children
- The transplant population has grown 19% between 2000 and 2008 with a point prevalence rate of 60.6 per million
- An estimated 800 pediatric kidney transplants are performed each year
- The percentage of living-related donors (LRDs) in pediatrics is greater than in adults. Eighty percent of living donor kidneys come from parents

Pediatric Kidney Transplantation

Allocation of organs for pediatric transplantation is done by United Network for Organ Sharing (UNOS)

- On the UNOS waiting list, pediatric patients are given priority based on age
- The share 35 policy change allocates kidneys from deceased donors (DD) < 35 years to be offered first to pediatric patients < 18 years of age. This resulted in an overall increase in the number of transplants with a reduction in wait time

The vast majority of children with ESRD are candidates for transplantation

- Pre-emptive transplantation accounts for 25% of kidney transplants
- Most centers require the recipient to weigh 8–10 kg prior to transplant (12–24 months)
- Bladder dysfunction should be evaluated prior to transplantation and a multidisciplinary plan instituted. All medical and surgical comorbidities have to be satisfactorily addressed prior to transplantation

Transplant multidisciplinary teams include the following:

- Nephrologist(s)
- Surgeon(s)
- Transplant nurse coordinator(s)
- Social worker(s)
- Psychologist
- Dialysis unit nurses
- Urology service
- Nutritionist
- Pharmacologist(s)
- Infectious disease
- Immunogenetics
- Financial counselor

Surgical Approach

Recipients < 10 kg

- Midline incision
- Intraperitoneal location
- Mobilization of the right colon and distal ileum
- Implantation of the kidney onto the aorta and IVC—as cephalad as possible
- Bilateral native nephrectomies can be performed at the time of transplantation or as a procedure of its own
- Steps to prevent torsion include suturing the kidney (best to leave a bit of perinephric fat attached) to the abdominal wall prior to placing the colon over the kidney and suturing the peritoneum to the abdominal wall

Recipients 10–30 kg

Surgical approach and vessels for implantation determined on an individual basis.

Recipients > 30 kg

- Lower quadrant incision
- Retroperitoneal location
- Implantation of the kidney onto the external iliac vessels
- The anastomoses are usually performed to the common (rather than to external) iliac vessels. This approach allows for the kidney to fit comfortably (and with no compression) within the retroperitoneum

Intraoperative Management

- Optimal hydration should be maintained, especially in small recipients, to ensure adequate renal perfusion
  - An adult kidney may lead to the sudden uptake of approximately 250 mL of blood at the time of reperfusion. Blood transfusions are often needed in small recipients
  - Lack of adequate volume infusion (which sometimes may represent as much as 50% of the total blood volume) can lead to severe hypotension, potential thrombosis of the newly implanted allograft, or delayed graft function
  - Central venous pressure (CVP) of 20 cmH_2O should be maintained during clamp and 12–15 cmH_2O before removal of clamps
  - On release of the aortic and IVC clamps, the ischemic lower extremities and new kidney are reperfused, which may cause hypothermia and acidosis
  - Replacing urine volume with IV fluids
  - Frequently monitoring serum electrolytes and correcting any abnormalities
- Prior to reperfusion, IV furosemide (1 mg/kg) and 20% mannitol (0.5–1.0 g/kg) are administered
- Dopamine can be added to achieve adequate blood pressure (MAP 65–70 mm Hg)
- Acidosis should be monitored and treated
- Special anesthesia considerations:
  - Operating room temperature set at 32°C
  - All prep solutions and fluids are warmed
  - Hypothermia aggressively corrected with warm saline abdominal lavage
  - CVP, arterial pressure, cardiac activity, oxygen saturation, ABG, electrolytes, and hemoglobin are monitored
- Externally warming the kidney after unclamping

- Avoidance of nitrous oxide anesthesia to prevent intestine distension
- The infant's abdomen must accommodate a new, large organ, which in addition to receiving a large percentage of the cardiac output, may impede respiration and decrease venous return

Postoperative Period—Initial 24–48 hours

- Urinary volume is replaced milliliter for milliliter using 1% dextrose ¼ normal saline with sodium bicarbonate
- Replacement of insensible losses
- Hypertension is common, but antihypertensive medications are used sparingly to avoid decreased renal perfusion
- Electrolytes abnormalities can occur and should be carefully monitored and corrected
- Keep small child intubated in early postoperative phase if there are signs of pulmonary edema
- Continuous EKG monitoring, pulse oximeter, CVP monitoring, CXR, daily weight, I/O
- Perioperative IV antibiotics for 24 hrs
- BUN, creatinine, Ca, phos, Mg, lytes, CBC, ABG, coagulation studies, UA
- Gastritis prophylaxis
- Renal US Doppler immediately postoperative
- Glycemic control
- Wound and catheter care
- Urologic care—keep Foley catheter in bladder for 5 days
- Infection surveillance and prevention
- Additional diuretics (furosemide 1–2 mg/kg/dose, 20% mannitol 0.3–0.5 g/kg/dose), sodium bicarbonate (1 mEq/kg), and fluids (normal saline 10 mL/kg bolus) should be administered as needed
- As kidney function improves, urine replacement is switched to daily fluid intake of 150–200% maintenance fluids

Discharge Planning

- Focus on parent, caretaker, and patient education
- Medication boxes and notebook/checkbox systems
- Outpatient schedules for laboratory assessment and clinic visits

Outpatient Management

- Evaluate by laboratory tests or clinic visits daily during the first few weeks after transplant
- GFR estimates once creatinine reaches nadir
- Hypertension—avoid ACEI for 3 months
- Worsening hypertension—Doppler studies of the renal artery
- Post-transplant bone disease—vitamin D supplements if indicated by high PTH
- Hyperlipidemia
- Dental examination 6 monthly
- Ophthalmology yearly
- Gynecological follow-up yearly, if age >18 years, sexually active or has irregular bleeding
- Non adherence—psychosocial dynamics, body image and transplant meds
- Immunizations—withheld until 1-year post tx; resume as per AAP recommendations
- Nutrition—tube feeds versus oral feeds; high phosphorus diet; diet low in saturated fats
- Aerobic and weight-bearing exercise
- Growth and development—< 1 year old have acceleration of growth following transplant
  Adolescents have deceleration of growth following transplant
- Quality of life—importance of returning to school

Immunosuppression Protocols

- Induction:
  - Thymoglobulin/alemtuzumab/basiliximab/daclizumab
  - Corticosteroids
  - Induction with a biological agent is used in approximately 60% of recipients (NAPRTCS)
  - Anti CD25 monoclonal antibodies when added to standard therapy decreased the incidence of acute rejection episodes and steroid-resistant rejection episodes
  - Thymoglobulin has been found to be safe and effective in preventing acute rejection episodes in the short term
- Maintenance:
  - Calcineurin Inhibitor: Tacrolimus/cyclosporine
  - Antiproliferative: Mycophenolate mofetil (MMF)/azathioprine. Two-third of the recipients get MMF; 10–15% get sirolimus and 2% get azathioprine
  - Corticosteroids. 85% of recipients get steroids. Retarded skeletal growth, hypertension, obesity, diabetes mellitus, hyperlipidemia, osteoporosis, and aseptic necrosis of bone are important side effects of steroids. Increasing tendency to use lower daily maintenance doses or alternate day dosing of steroids
  - Complete steroid avoidance can be achieved using tacrolimus in combination with MMF and an extended course of Dacluzimab (Stanford)
  - Steroid avoidance has also been achieved using alemtuzumab preconditioning and Tacrolimus/MMF maintenance immunosuppression (Pittsburgh)

- Overall acute rejection rates at 6 months were lower; 1-year graft survival rates were higher; and mean total steroid dose was higher from transplant to 6 months in patients treated with tacrolimus than those treated with cyclosporine
- DD kidney transplant patients have an acute rejection rate of 18% when taking MMF compared with 60% when taking azathioprine
- More frequent dosing of sirolimus is appropriate in children as the mean drug half-life is 12 hours as compared with a half-life of 96 hours in adults
- Eighty percent of recipients were receiving a three-drug regimen at 6 months post-transplant [North American Pediatric Renal Trials and Collaborative Studies (NAPRTCS), 2003]

- Because of adverse side effects of steroids, steroid-free and early steroid withdrawal protocols have been used in children with success as stated above, but long-term outcome data is awaited
- Regimens are usually center specific; individualization is needed to address specific situations
  - Induction with antilymphocytic agents allows delayed introduction of CNI in patients with delayed graft function
  - Induction with antilymphocytic agents provides intensified immunosuppression in highly sensitized recipients
  - In a child with a prior h/o malignancy, a two-drug regimen or even monotherapy is used
  - Child with a prior h/o malignancy, antilymphocytic agents are avoided
  - Child with prior malignancy, living donor preferred to get best HLA matches
- Other post-transplant medications:
  - Bactrim
  - Valganciclovir
  - Nystatin
  - Aspirin
  - Antihypertensives
  - Lipid lowering agents

Outcomes

- Patient survival after transplantation is superior than achieved by dialysis
- 1-year patient survival: LRD 98%, DD 97%
- 5-year patient survival: LRD 95%, DD 92%
- Causes of patient death are infection (31%), cardiopulmonary disease (16%), and malignancy (11%)
- 45% of patients who die have a functioning graft at time of death
- 1-year graft survival: LRD 96%, DD 94%
- 5-year graft survival: LRD 86%, DD 78%
- Causes of graft failure: Chronic renal allograft dysfunction (33%)
  - Acute rejection (15%)
  - Vascular thrombosis (11%)
  - Disease recurrence (7%)
  - Nonadherence (4.5%)
  - Primary nonfunction (2%)
  - Infection (2%)
  - Malignancy (1%)
  - Death due to other causes (9%)
- Risk factors for graft failure:
  - Donor source (LRD better than DD)
  - Recipient age (children < 2 years lower survival)
  - Donor age
  - Recipient age (children < 2 years lower survival)
  - Ethnicity (African American with poorer outcome)
  - HLA matching
  - Delayed graft function

Complications

Early Complications

- Vascular complications are inversely proportional to recipient size
- Vascular thromboses represent a technical cause of allograft loss
- Torsion of allograft pedicle and graft infarction can occur
- Other vascular complications (such as renal artery stenosis) are also encountered
- Urinary obstruction and urinary leaks
- Wound infections
- Accelerated acute and acute rejection
- Delayed graft function—ATN
- Postoperative bleeding and hematoma formation
- Lymphocele

Late Complications

- Bacterial infection
- UTI
- Pneumonia
  - Wound infection
- Viral infection
  - EBV
  - CMV
  - BKV
  - VZV
- Fungal infection

- Post-transplant lymphoproliferative disease (EBV related)
- Other malignancies
- Diabetes mellitus—medication related
- Cardiovascular disease. Children and adolescents with ESRD have a > 10-fold risk of cardiovascular death as young adults
- Recurrence of the primary disease in transplant—FSGS, CNF, HUS, primary oxalosis, MPGN
- Chronic transplant nephropathy
- Medication—nonadherence in the adolescent
- Tacrolimus nephrotoxicity
- Erythrocytosis (occasionally seen)
- Neurologic and psychiatric complications

FURTHER READING

1. Ellis D, Gilboa N, Bellinger M, Shapiro R. Renal transplantation in infants and children. In: Renal Transplantation by Ron Shapiro, Richard Simmons, Thomas E. Starzl (eds.), Appleton and Lange: Stamford, CT 1997.
2. McDonald RA. Post-transplant management. In: Tejani AH, Fine RN, Harmon WE (eds), Pediatric solid organ transplantation. Wiley, Hoboken, NJ 2000.
3. NAPRTCS 2011 Annual report—patients on dialysis https://web.emmes.com/study/ped/annlrept/annualrept2011.pdf
4. Sampaio M, Poomipanit N, Kuo HT, et al. Induction therapy in pediatric kidney transplant recipients discharged with a triple drug immunosuppressive regimen. Pediatr Transplant 2010; 14:770–8.
5. Sarwal M, Rianthavorn P, Ettenger RB. Kidney transplantation in children. In: Morris PJ, Knechtle SJ (eds), Kidney transplantation: principles and practice. 6th edn. Saunders, Philadelphia 2008.
6. So SKS. Pediatric kidney transplantation. In: Flye MW (ed), Atlas of organ transplantation. Saunders, Philadelphia 1995.
7. US Renal Data System, USRDS 2012 Annual Data Report: Atlas of End-Stage Renal Disease in the United States, National Institutes of Health, National Institute of Diabetes and Digestive and Kidney Diseases, Bethesda, MD 2011.
8. Vassilios PE, Najarian JS. Surgical technique and management. In: Tejani AH, Fine RN, Harmon WE (eds), Pediatric solid organ transplantation. Wiley, Hoboken, NJ 2000.
9. Vukevic Z, Ellis D, Bellinger M, et al. Donor evaluation, surgical technique and postoperative management. In: Fine RN, Webber SA, Olthoff KM, Kelly DA, Harmon WE (eds), Pediatric solid organ transplantation. 2nd edn. Wiley, Hoboken, NJ 2007.

CHAPTER 55

Renal Transplant Pathology

Megan L Troxell, John C Papadimitriou, Cinthia B Drachenberg

NORMAL KIDNEY (FIGS. 1 TO 6)

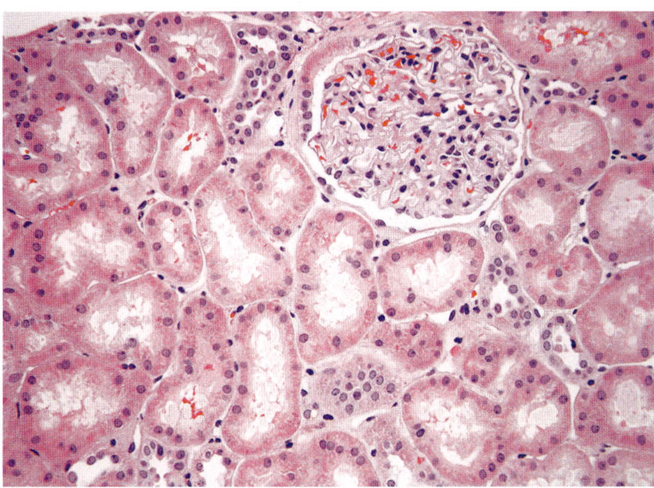

Fig. 1: Normal renal cortex. The normal renal cortex is composed of closely spaced proximal and fewer distal tubules, with interspersed glomeruli. This hematoxylin and eosin (H&E) stain demonstrates the abundant pink granular cytoplasm of proximal tubules, while the few distal tubules are lined by flatter, relatively paler epithelial cells (just below glomerulus at 5 o'clock, and upper center). The tubules are back to back, without intervening fibrous tissue or inflammatory cell infiltrates. A normocellular glomerulus is shown.

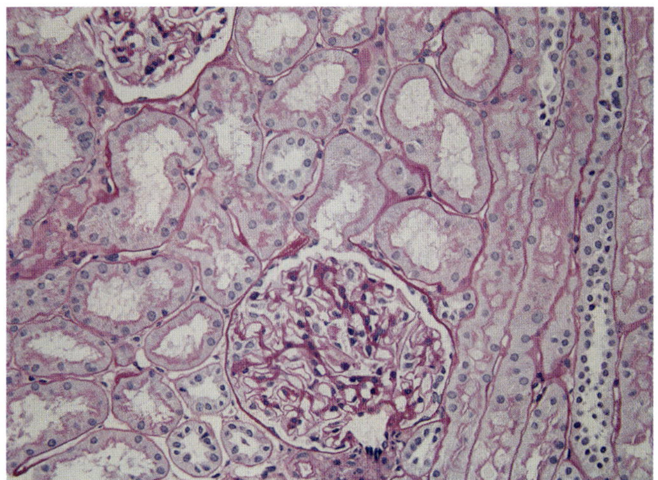

Fig. 2: Normal renal cortex. The periodic acid Schiff (PAS) is helpful in delineating tubular and glomerular basement membranes. The proximal tubules have a luminal brush border that stains weakly magenta with PAS. Distal tubules lack this brush border and have a smaller diameter; a long vertical distal tubule can be seen at far right. Again, the tubules are very closely spaced. The urinary pole of this normal glomerulus is also shown, where Bowman's space is contiguous with the proximal tubular lumen (12 o'clock). PAS staining is quite useful in demonstrating certain pathologic features such as hyaline changes and lymphocytes permeating in tubules, which will be illustrated below.

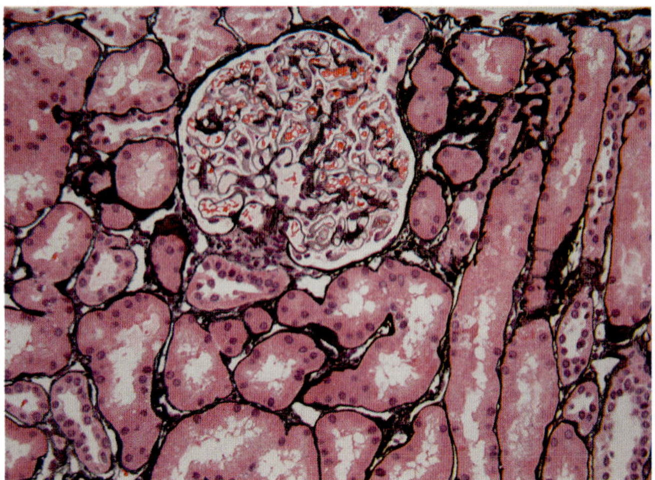

Fig. 3: Normal renal cortex. Silver stains, such as the Jones silver stain shown here, also stain basement membranes and are especially useful in evaluating glomerular pathology. In this normal glomerulus, the urinary pole is seen (at 2 o'clock), as is the juxtaglomerular apparatus with the macula densa (at 6–7 o'clock). The macula densa is the specialized portion of the distal tubule that provides tubular glomerular feedback within individual nephrons.

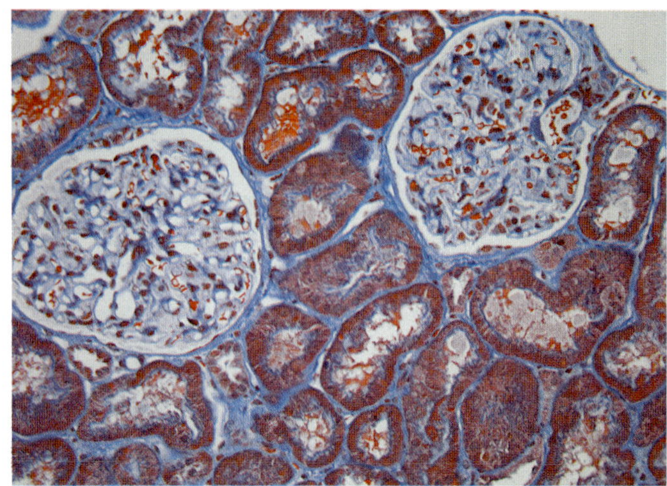

Fig. 4: Normal renal cortex. Trichrome stains are especially important in determining the extent of interstitial fibrosis in a renal allograft. Collagen is stained blue in this Masson's trichrome, or may be stained green in other trichrome preparations. A normal kidney should have minimal fibrous tissue between tubules in the cortex, as is shown here. Adequacy criteria for the renal allograft biopsy include two cores of renal cortex (as rejection may be patchy), sampling at least 10 glomeruli, although more is generally preferred. C4d staining may be performed on sections of cortex and medulla; some pathologies involve the medulla first/preferentially (polyoma virus infection, acute interstitial nephritis), yet an adequate sample of cortex is essential for assessment of rejection.

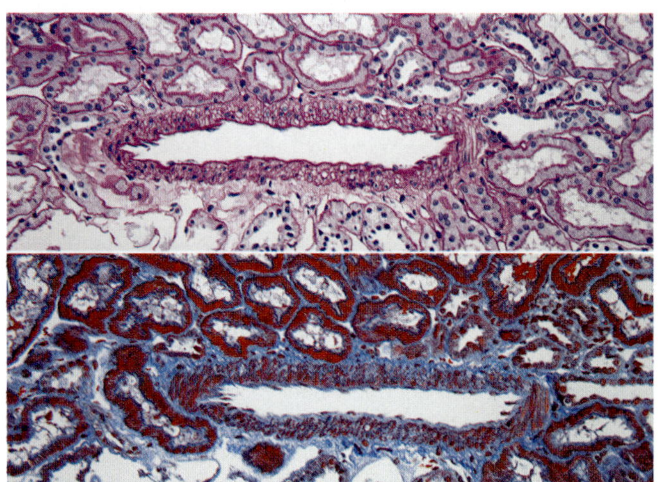

Fig. 5: Normal artery. Normal arteries are composed of three layers, the outmost adventitia, which is often imperceptible in small arteries, the medial smooth muscle layer, and the innermost intimal layer. In medium and large arteries, the internal elastic lamina separates the media and intima. The normal intima should be composed of a single cell layer of flat endothelium with no, or only minimal, fibrous tissue. The top panel is a periodic acid Schiff (PAS) stain, which highlights the cell membranes of the myocytes in the media; the bottom panel shows the same artery with trichrome stain. Note that there is minimal blue staining fibrous tissue in the intima.

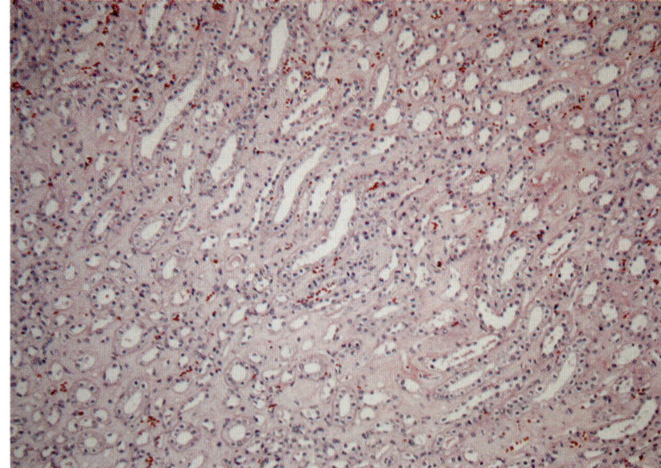

Fig. 6: Normal renal medulla. This low-power image shows a transition between outer medulla—upper right, and deep medulla—lower left. Deep/inner medulla contains only thin limbs of Henle, collecting ducts and vasa recta, while the outer medulla contains thick limbs as well. The medulla lacks inflammatory cells, but tubules are normally separated by fibrous tissue. Hematoxylin and eosin (H&E) stain.

ALLOGRAFT REJECTION

The individual histopathologic features of rejection will be illustrated according to the 1997–2008 Banff criteria (Table 1).[1-5] Then examples of different Banff classes of rejection will be provided. However, not all centers apply the Banff criteria strictly; the comparative clinical trials in transplantation (CCTT) classification system is one such alternative schema, and is summarized in Tables 2A and B.[6-8]

Table 1: *Diagnostic categories for renal allograft biopsies:* Banff 2007 update[1-5]

1. *Normal*
2. *Antibody mediated changes*

Acute/Active ABMR; all 3 features must be present for diagnosis

i. Histologic evidence of acute tissue injury, including one or more of the following:
- Microvascular inflammation (g > 0 and/or ptc > 0)
- Intimal or transmural arteritis (v > 0)
- Acute thrombotic microangiopathy, in the absence of any other cause
- Acute tubular injury, in the absence of any other apparent cause

ii. Evidence of current/recent antibody interaction with vascular endothelium, *including at least one of the following*:
- Linear C4d staining in peritubular capillaries (C4d2 or C4d3 by IF on frozen sections, or C4d > 0 by IHC on paraffin sections)
- At least moderate microvascular inflammation ([g + ptc] ≥ 2)
- Increased expression of gene transcripts in the biopsy tissue indicative of endothelial injury by validated method

iii. Serologic evidence of donor-specific antibodies (HLA or other antigens)
- [Biopsies showing 2 of the 3 features are designated as "suspicious" for ABMR]

Chronic, Active ABMR; all three features must be present for diagnosis

i. Morphologic evidence of chronic tissue injury, including one or more of the following:
- Transplant glomerulopathy (cg > 0), if no evidence of chronic TMA
- Severe peritubular capillary basement membrane multilayering (requires EM, defined as ≥ 7 layers in 1 cortical ptc, and ≥ 5 in 2 additional)
- Arterial intimal fibrosis of new onset, excluding other causes
- Increased expression of gene transcripts in the biopsy tissue indicative of endothelial injury by validated method

ii. Evidence of current/recurrent antibody interaction with vascular endothelium, including *at least one of the following*:
- Linear C4d staining in peritubular capillaries (C4d2 or C4d3 by IF on frozen sections, or C4d > 0 by IHC on paraffin sections)
- At least moderate microvascular inflammation ([g + ptc] ≥ 2)
- Increased expression of gene transcripts in the biopsy tissue indicative of endothelial injury, if thoroughly validated

iii. Serologic evidence of donor-specific antibodies (HLA or other antigens)

C4d staining without evidence of rejection; all 3 features must be present for diagnosis

i. Linear C4d staining in peritubular capillaries (C4d2 or C4d3 by IF on frozen sections, or C4d > 0 by IHC on paraffin sections)

ii. No glomerulitis, no peritubular capillaritis, no intimal arteritis, no chronic glomerulopathy or ptc lamination, no TMA, no acute tubular injury (in the absence of other apparent causes) [g = 0, ptc = 0, cg = 0 (by LM and by EM if available), v = 0]

iii. No acute cell-mediated rejection (Banff 97 type 1A or greater) or borderline changes

3. *Borderline changes*: 'suspicious' for acute T-cell mediated rejection (may coincide with categories 2, 5, 6)
   - Focal tubulitis (t-t3) with minor interstitial infiltration (i0, i1) or
   - Focal interstitial infiltration (i2, i3) with mild (t1) tubulitis, see below
4. *T-cell mediated rejection* (may coincide with categories 2, 5, 6)
   - *Type IA*: Significant interstitial infiltration (> 25% of parenchyma affected, i2 or i3) and foci of moderate tubulitis (t2)
   - *Type IB*: Significant interstitial infiltration (> 25% of parenchyma affected, i2 or i3) and foci of severe tubulitis (t3)
   - *Type IIA*: Mild-to-moderate intimal arteritis (v1)
   - *Type IIB*: Severe intimal arteritis comprising > 25% of the luminal area (v2)
   - *Type III*: 'transmural' arteritis and/or arterial fibrinoid change and necrosis of medial smooth muscle cells with accompanying lymphocytic inflammation (v3)

Contd...

Contd...

Chronic active T-cell-mediated rejection
'Chronic allograft arteriopathy' (arterial intimal fibrosis with mononuclear cell infiltration in fibrosis, formation of neo-intima)
5. *Interstitial fibrosis and tubular atrophy*, no evidence of any specific etiology (may include nonspecific vascular and glomerular sclerosis, but severity graded by tubulointerstitial features)
I. Mild interstitial fibrosis and tubular atrophy (< 25% of cortical area)
II. Moderate interstitial fibrosis and tubular atrophy (26–50% of cortical area)
III. Severe interstitial fibrosis and tubular atrophy (> 50% of cortical area)
6. *Other*: Changes not considered to be due to rejection—acute and/or chronic; may include isolated glomerulitis (g), chronic glomerular (cg), or chronic vascular (cv) lesions and coincide with categories 2–5 above.

Table 2A: CCTT criteria for diagnosis of acute cellular rejection[6]

Type I: At least 5% of the cortex must have interstitial mononuclear infiltration with at least 2 of the following 3 features:
Edema
Tubular degeneration/injury
Activated lymphocytes
In addition, tubulitis must be present, with at least 3 tubules affected in 10 serial high-power fields (40x) from the areas with the most infiltrate.
Type II: Arterial or arteriolar mononuclear cell endothelial inflammation (endothelialitis or endarteritis) is present (with or without features of type I).
A threshold of at least one cell under the endothelium is required
A lymphocyte adherent to the luminal surface of an endothelial cell is not sufficient.
Type III: Arterial or arteriolar fibrinoid necrosis or transmural inflammation is present and may or may not be accompanied by thrombosis, parenchymal necrosis/recent infarction, or hemorrhage.

Table 2B: Comparison of Banff and CCTT classification schemes for cellular rejection[1,6,7]

Category	Banff	CCTT
Tubulointerstitial	Borderline	Type I
	Type I	Type I
Vascular	Type II	Type II
Fibrinoid necrosis	Type III	Type III

Acute Cellular Tubulointerstitial Lesions (Figs. 7 to 16)

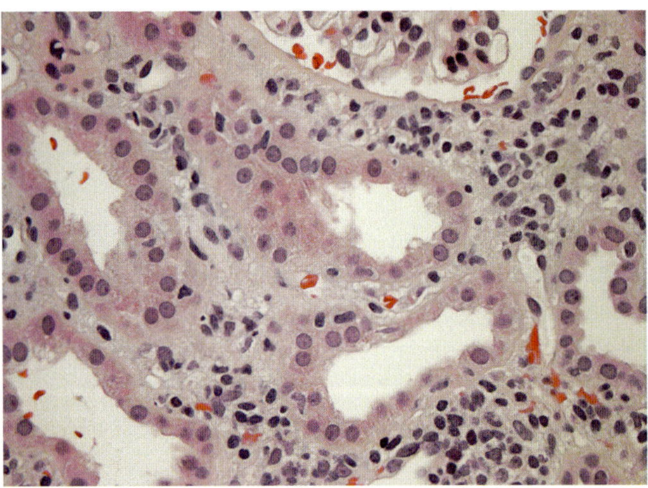

Fig. 7: Interstitial inflammation and tubulitis. This hematoxylin and eosin (H&E) stain shows both mononuclear interstitial inflammation and tubulitis. Tubulitis is defined as the inflammatory cells crossing the tubular basement membrane, admixed with tubular epithelial cells. Mononuclear cells include T-cell lymphocytes, B-cell lymphocytes, monocytes and plasma cells, but not eosinophils or neutrophils. The inflammatory cells have dark blue, irregular nuclei, while the tubular epithelial nuclei are generally larger, rounder, paler pink-purple, with nucleoli. On H&E stain, it may be difficult to discern interstitial from tubular inflammation, as tubular basement membranes are not readily apparent. Periodic acid Schiff (PAS) stains are quite helpful for this (Figs. 8 to 11). Tubules are also separated by inflammation and edema in this image. Based on the finding of one to four mononuclear cells per tubular cross section, this field is scored as t1 per Banff classification (Table 3).

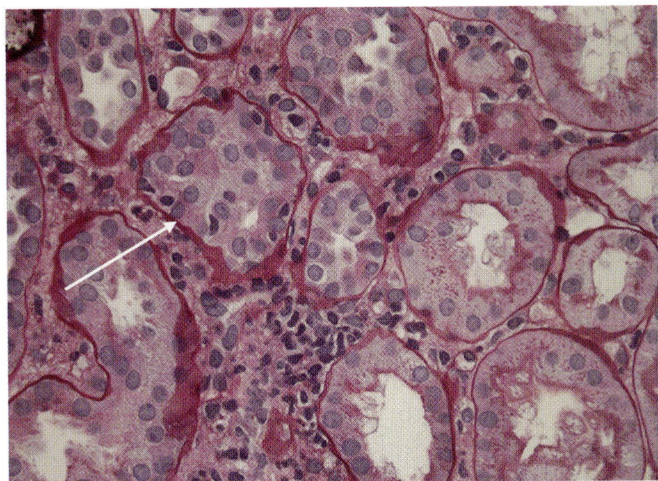

Fig. 8: Interstitial inflammation and tubulitis. This periodic acid Schiff (PAS) stain is from the same biopsy as Figure 7. The outlines of the tubular basement membrane are clearly seen on PAS-stained sections. One tubule (arrow) contains seven lymphocytes, and could be classified as Banff t2 (see Table 3). It is important to note that assessment of acute rejection in a renal allograft is currently based on inflammation in nonatrophic areas of cortex; overall inflammation may also be reported. Tubules with moderate-to-severe atrophy should not be assessed. Tubular atrophy is illustrated in Figures 100 to 104.

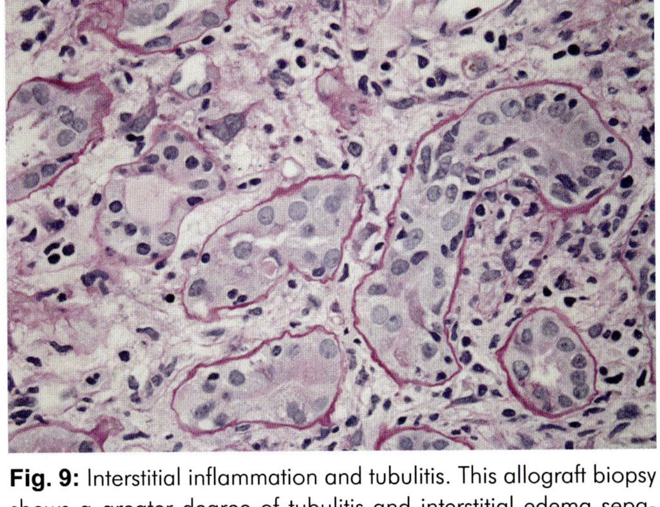

Fig. 9: Interstitial inflammation and tubulitis. This allograft biopsy shows a greater degree of tubulitis and interstitial edema separating the tubules. Although there are >10 mononuclear cells within the elongated tubule to the right of the field, this tubule is cut in longitudinal rather than cross section, and is thus best classified as t2 (Table 3). A periodic acid Schiff (PAS) stain nicely contrasts the irregular darker blue nuclei of inflammatory cells, with the rounder pale nuclei of tubular epithelial cells.

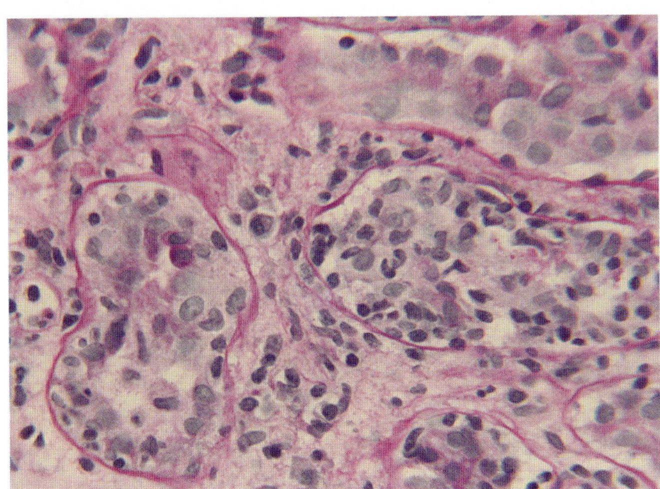

Fig. 10: Interstitial inflammation and tubulitis. There are innumerable mononuclear cells in the tubule to the right of the field, qualifying as a Banff t3 lesion (> 10 cells/cross section, see Table 3), periodic acid Schiff (PAS) stain.

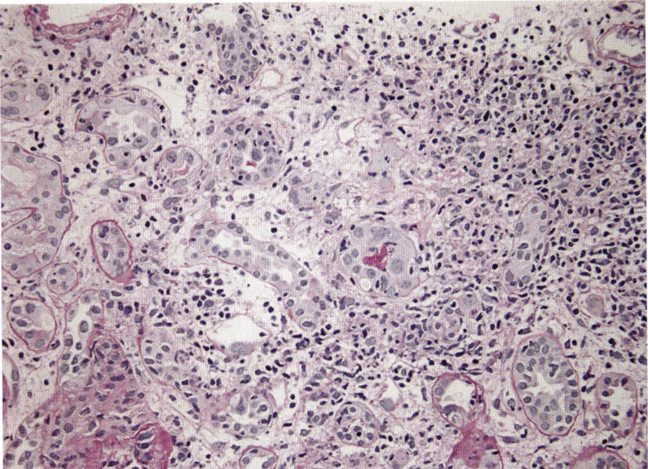

Fig. 11: Interstitial inflammation, edema and tubulitis. A lower power view of a periodic acid Schiff (PAS) stain shows tubulitis and brisk inflammation between tubules (interstitial inflammation). Again, this should be scored in nonatrophic areas of renal cortex. The overall percentage of inflamed parenchyma in the biopsy determines the "i" score (see Table 3).

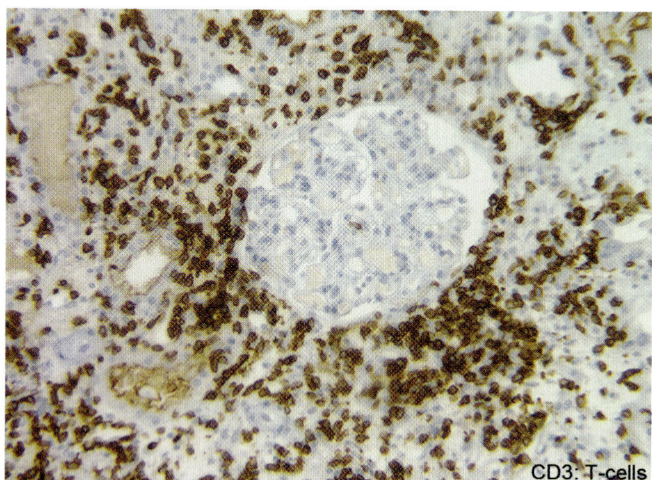

Fig. 12: Interstitial inflammation and tubulitis, T-cell stain. This CD3 immunohistochemical (IHC) stain highlights T-cell lymphocytes, seen in abundance in tubules and the interstitium. The brown reaction product indicates positive T-cell lymphocyte membrane staining, against the blue hematoxylin counter stain. A glomerulus is in the center, almost completely devoid of inflammation.

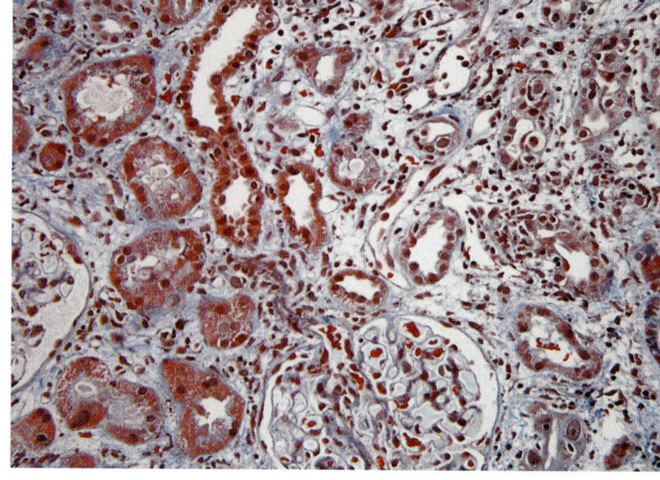

Fig. 13: Interstitial inflammation, edema, and tubulitis, trichrome stain. Interstitial inflammation and edema are seen on trichrome stain. In the right portion of the field, tubules are separated by pale blue, fine reticular staining, indicative of edema. This pattern contrasts with the denser blue pattern of interstitial fibrosis (see Fig. 101). Tubulitis is present in several tubules in the upper right; however, mononuclear cells may be difficult to identify on trichrome stains.

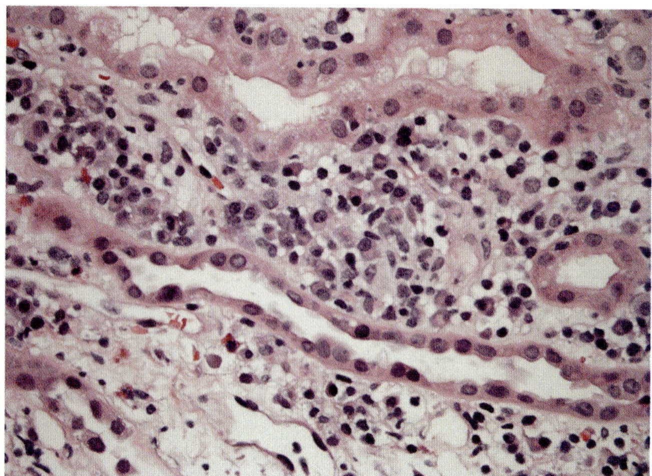

Fig. 14: Interstitial inflammation, plasmacytic. In some allografts, the inflammatory cell infiltrate is particularly rich in plasma cells, as shown here. The plasma cells in the interstitium have eccentric purple cytoplasm, with a pale pink paranuclear area ("hof") and a so-called "clock-face" nuclear chromatin pattern. Mononuclear cell tubulitis is also seen in the longitudinally sectioned tubule above. Plasma cell rich infiltrates have been associated with worse graft outcome and if severe should also prompt consideration of post-transplant lymphoproliferative disorder (see Fig. 142).[9] Hematoxylin and eosin (H&E) stain.

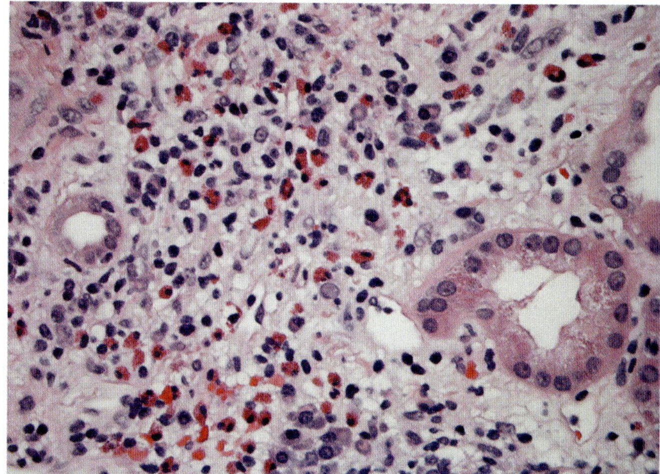

Fig. 15: Interstitial inflammation, eosinophilic. The inflammatory infiltrate in this rejection is particularly rich in eosinophils. While admixed eosinophils are certainly a characteristic of acute cellular rejection, the differential diagnosis of an eosinophil-rich infiltrate also includes acute interstitial nephritis, which could be due to drugs or other agents, as in native kidneys. Eosinophils are seen best on Hematoxylin and eosin (H&E) stain, as shown here, and may be relatively inapparent on periodic acid Schiff (PAS), silver and trichrome staining.

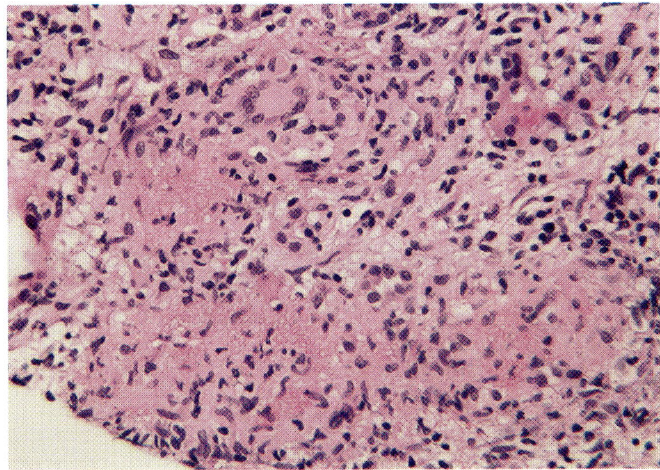

Fig. 16: Interstitial inflammation, granulomatous. This allograft biopsy shows granulomatous inflammation, in a biopsy with acute cellular rejection. Importantly, granulomas on biopsy should prompt consideration of infectious etiologies (bacterial, mycobacterial, fungal, viral) in the immunocompromised host. Other causes of granulomatous inflammation in native and allograft kidneys include sarcoid, lymphoma (PTLD), ANCA-associated vasculitis, and other autoimmune conditions, as well as crystal or paraprotein nephropathy, and tubular rupture (hematoxylin and eosin, H&E stain shown).[10]

Acute Cellular Vascular Lesions (Figs. 17 to 23)

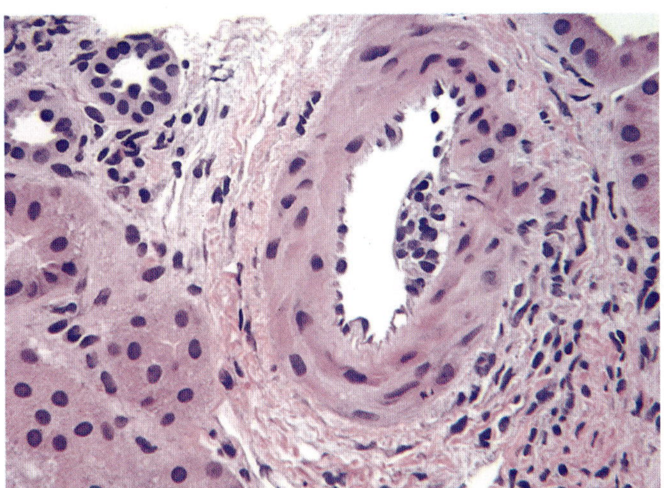

Fig. 17: Intimal arteritis (endothelialitis). Endothelialitis is defined as mononuclear inflammation beneath the endothelium, often associated with reactive endothelial cells and intimal edema. The Banff "v" criteria are based on the degree of luminal narrowing due to intimal arteritis in the most severely affected artery (Table 3). As this focus shows < 25%, luminal narrowing, it is classified as Banff v1 (hematoxylin and eosin, H&E stain).

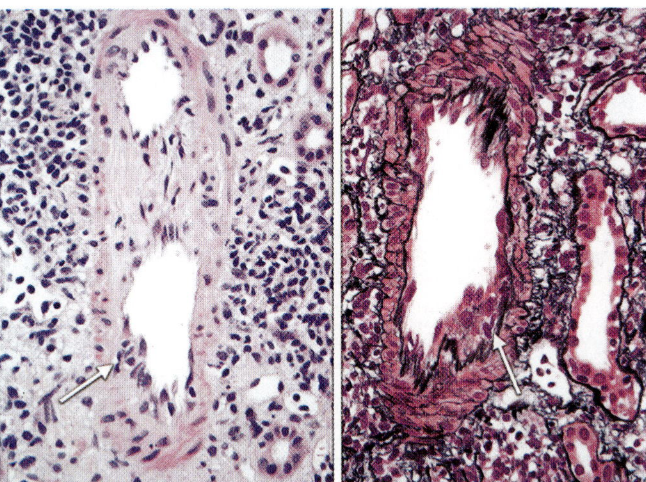

Fig. 18: Intimal arteritis, early. This intimal arteritis is shown on hematoxylin and eosin (H&E) (left) and silver stain (right). White arrows in each panel indicate the few subintimal lymphocytes admixed with reactive endothelial cells. There are cells within a dilated peritubular capillary (capillaritis) and tubulitis to the right of the arrow in the right panel.

Table 3: Banff component scores for tubulitis, interstitial inflammation and vasculitis[1–5]

Quantitative criteria for tubulitis (t)
t0-No mononuclear cells in tubules
t1-One to 4 cells/tubular cross sections (or 10 tubular cells)
t2-Five to 10 cells/tubular cross sections (or 10 tubular cells)
t3-Greater than 10 cells/tubular cross section, or the presence of at least 2 areas of tubular basement membrane destruction accompanied by i2/i3 inflammation and t2 tubulitis elsewhere in the biopsy
Quantitative criteria for mononuclear cell interstitial inflammation (i)
i0-No or trivial interstitial inflammation (<10% of unscarred parenchyma)
i1-10–25% of parenchyma inflamed
i2-26–50% of parenchyma inflamed
i3-greater than 50% parenchyma inflamed
Quantitative criteria for intimal arteritis (v)
v0-No arteritis
v1-Mild-to-moderate intimal arteritis in at least 1 arterial cross section
v2-Severe intimal arteritis with at least 25% luminal area lost in at least 1 arterial cross section
v3-Transmural arteritis +/– arterial fibrinoid change and medial smooth muscle necrosis with lymphocytic infiltrative in vessel
Quantitative criteria for early allograft glomerulitis score (g)
g0-No glomerulitis
g1-Glomerulitis in <25% of glomeruli
g2-Segmental or global glomerulitis in 25–75% of glomeruli
g3-Glomerulitis (mostly global) in >75% of glomeruli
Minimal criteria for glomerulitis is newly defined as complete or partial occlusion of >1 glomerular capillary by leukocyte infiltration and endothelial cell enlargement[5]
Quantitative criteria for vascular fibrous intimal thickening (cv)
cv0-No chronic vascular changes
cv1-Vascular narrowing of up to 25% luminal area by fibrointimal thickening of arteries +/– breach of internal elastic lamina or presence of foam cells or occasional mononuclear cells (in the most affected vessel)
cv2-Increased severity of changes described above with 26-50% narrowing of vascular luminal area .
cv3-Severe vascular changes with >50% narrowing of vascular luminal area
Quantitative criteria for interstitial fibrosis (ci)
ci0-Interstitial fibrosis in up to 5% of cortical area
ci1-Mild-interstitial fibrosis in 6–25% of cortical area
ci2-Moderate-interstitial fibrosis in 26–50% of cortical area
ci3-Severe-interstitial fibrosis in >50% of cortical area
Quantitative criteria for tubular atrophy (ct)
ct0-No tubular atrophy
ct1-Tubular atrophy in up to 25% of the area of cortical tubules
ct2-Tubular atrophy involving 26–50% of the area of cortical tubules
ct3-Tubular atrophy in > 50% of the area of cortical tubules
Quantitative criteria for allograft glomerulopathy (cg)
cg0-No glomerulopathy-double contours in < 10% of peripheral capillary loops in most severely affected glomerulus
cg1-Double contours affecting up to 25% of peripheral capillary loops in the most affected of nonsclerotic glomeruli
cg2-Double contours affecting 26–50% of peripheral capillary loops in the most affected of nonsclerotic glomeruli
cg3-Double contours affecting more than 50% of peripheral capillary loops in the most affected of nonsclerotic glomeruli
cg scoring for electron microscopic analysis has been proposed[5]

Contd...

Contd...

Quantitative criteria for mesangial matrix increase (mm)
mm0-No mesangial matrix increase
mm1-Up to 25% of nonsclerotic glomeruli affected (at least moderate matrix increase)
mm2-26–50% of nonsclerotic glomeruli affected (at least moderate matrix increase)
mm3- > 50% of nonsclerotic glomeruli affected (at least moderate matrix increase)
Quantitative criteria for arteriolar hyaline thickening (ah)
ah0-No PAS-positive hyaline thickening
ah1-Mild-to-moderate PAS positive hyaline thickening in at least one arteriole
ah2-Moderate-to-severe PAS positive hyaline thickening more than one arteriole
ah3-Severe PAS-positive hyaline thickening in many arterioles
Alternative quantitative scoring for hyaline arteriolar thickening (aah)[3]
aah0-No typical lesions of CNI arteriolopathy
aah1-Replacement of degenerated smooth muscle cells by hyaline deposits present in only one arteriole, no circumferential involvement
aah2-Replacement of degenerated smooth muscle cells by hyaline deposits present in more than one arteriole, but no circumferential involvement
aah3-Replacement of degenerated smooth muscle cells by hyaline deposits with circumferential involvement, independent of the number of arterioles involved
Quantitative criteria for peritubular capillaritis[3]
ptc0-No significant cortical ptc, or < 10% of PTCs with inflammation
ptc1- ≥10% of cortical peritubular capillaries with capillaritis with max 3–4 luminal inflammatory cells
ptc2- ≥10% of cortical peritubular capillaries with capillaritis with max 5–10 luminal inflammatory cells
ptc3- ≥10% of cortical peritubular capillaries with capillaritis with max > 10 luminal inflammatory cells

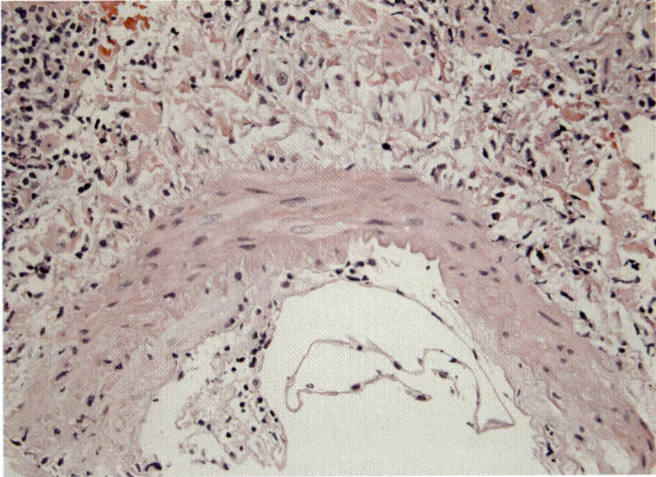

Fig. 19: Intimal arteritis (endothelialitis). A partial cross section of a larger artery shows numerous lymphocytes associated with the endothelial layer that is detaching from the artery wall. This is also a Banff v1 lesion. However, inflammatory cells simply marginating along a vessel wall would not warrant a diagnosis of rejection. Hematoxylin and eosin (H&E) stain.

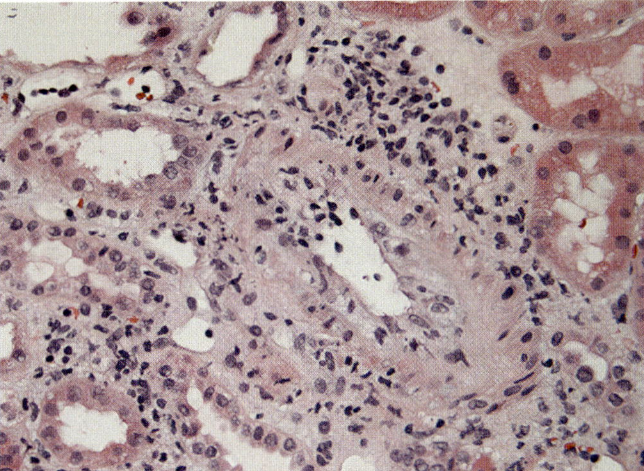

Fig. 20: Intimal arteritis (endothelialitis). The small artery in the center contains numerous mononuclear cells enmeshed in the intimal layer (top left of vessel). The remainder of the vessel demonstrates an edematous, hypercellular reactive intima with foam cells, and would qualify as a Banff v2 lesion based on loss of > 25% luminal area. Peritubular capillaritis is also seen in the far upper left of image (see section "Antibody-mediated rejection" below). Hematoxylin and eosin (H&E) stain.

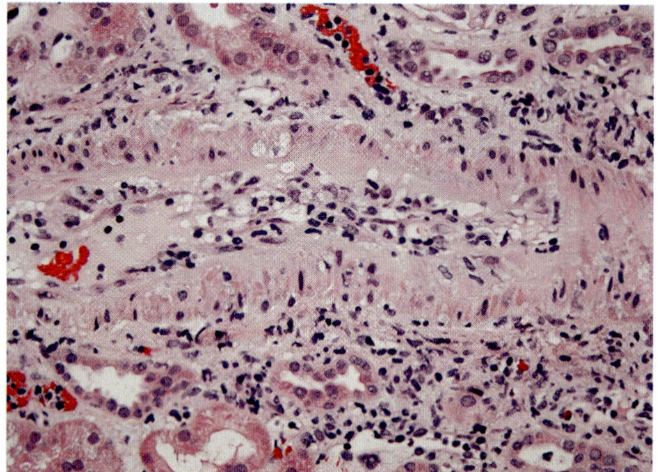

Fig. 21: Intimal arteritis, severe. An even more severe example of intimal arteritis, with numerous mononuclear cells, endothelial cells, and myofibroblasts resulting in marked narrowing of the arterial lumen, v2 lesion. Hematoxylin and eosin (H&E) stain.

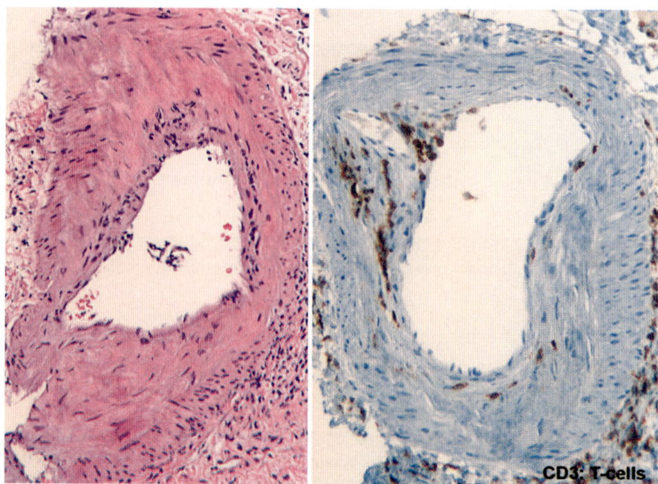

Fig. 22: Intimal arteritis (endothelialitis), T-cell stain. This composite image shows an Hematoxylin and eosin (H&E)-stained section (left) of an artery with endothelialitis. A CD3 T-cell stain is shown in the right panel on a deeper section of the same artery. In this example, there is also paucicellular fibrous tissue in the intima (see section "Chronic Allograft Damage").

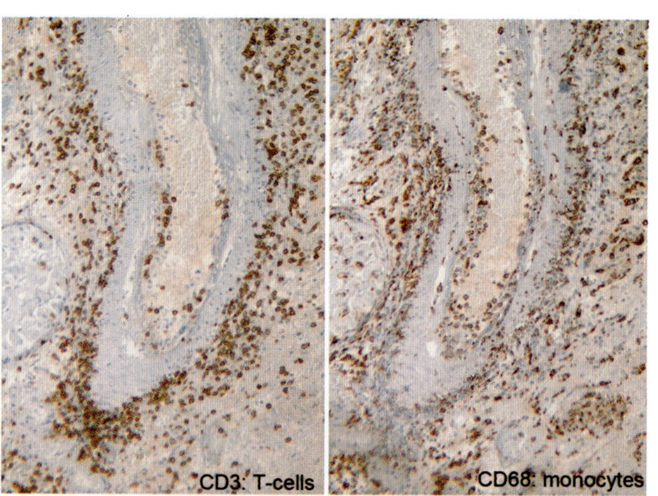

Fig. 23: Intimal arteritis (endothelialitis), T-cell and monocyte markers. A CD3 stain for T-cell lymphocytes is shown in the left panel and highlights the T-cell component of the vascular inflammation in this v1 lesion. In the right panel, a CD68 stain shows a greater number of monocytes associated with the endothelium and in the vascular lumen. Many T-cells and monocytes are also seen in the interstitium surrounding the artery.

Vascular Lesions in Banff Type III Rejection (Figs. 24 to 27)

Fibrin and fibrinoid necrosis and/or transmural inflammation of arteries characterizes severe rejection. It is not entirely clear whether this is a manifestation of acute cellular, acute antibody-mediated rejection, or both. Fibrin is not readily apparent on periodic acid Schiff (PAS) stains, as it is pale with a smudged texture. Fibrin is bright pink on hematoxylin and eosin (H&E) stains, most silver stain counterstains and is readily apparent on trichrome stains, as bright red.

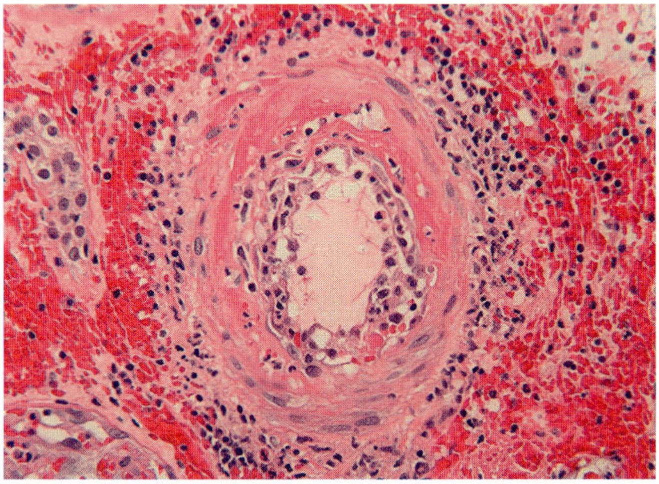

Fig. 24: Arterial fibrinoid necrosis. A small artery contains numerous intimal mononuclear cells (endothelialitis, Banff v2). However, the bright pink fibrinoid/necrotic material in the intima and partially replacing the arterial media characterizes a Banff v3 lesion. Hematoxylin and eosin (H&E) stain.

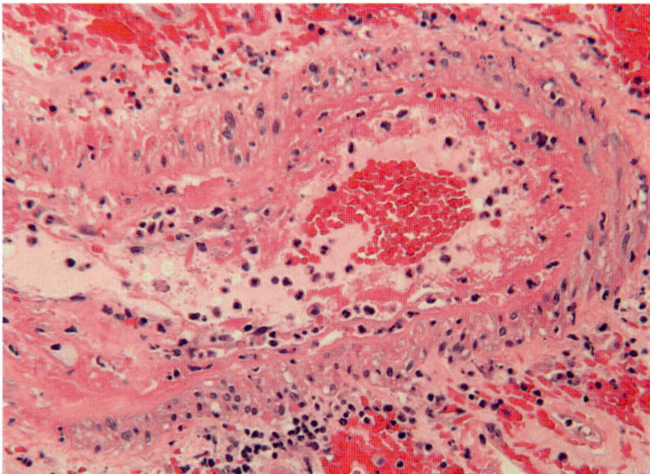

Fig. 25: Arterial fibrinoid necrosis. A longitudinal section of an artery shows mononuclear and neutrophilic inflammation, with some apoptotic debris in the media (upper portion). Importantly, there is also abundant brightly eosinophilic material with a fibrillary texture, characteristic of fibrin, Banff v3 lesion. Hematoxylin and eosin (H&E) stain.

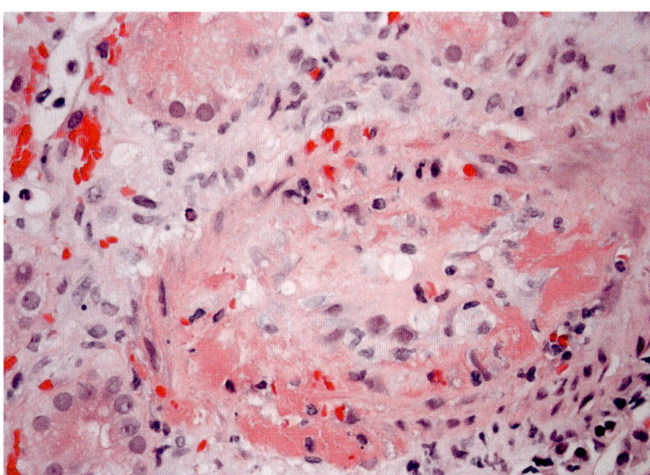

Fig. 26: Arterial fibrinoid necrosis. This small caliber artery demonstrates several foci of fibrinoid necrosis, along with sparse inflammation in the intima and media, Banff v3. Hematoxylin and eosin (H&E) stain.

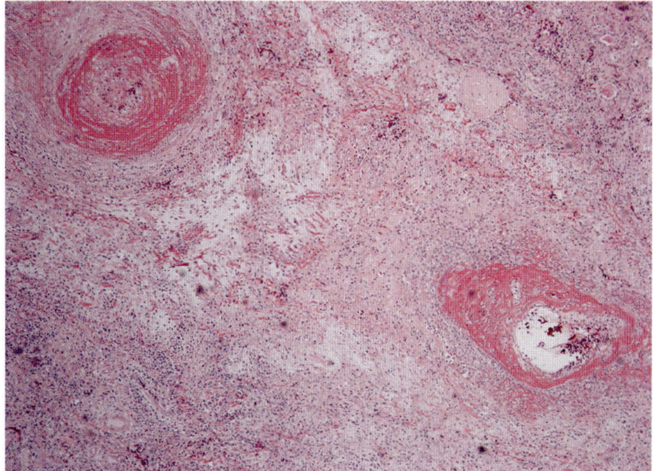

Fig. 27: Arterial fibrinoid necrosis, allograft nephrectomy. This allograft nephrectomy specimen had severe acute rejection, with concentric fibrinoid necrosis of large arteries, as seen in the lower right and upper left of the field. The intervening renal parenchyma has essentially been destroyed, and there is a brisk inflammatory infiltrate.

Acute Antibody-Mediated Rejection (Figs. 28 to 41)

Definitive diagnosis of antibody-mediated rejection requires clinicopathologic correlation. As listed in Table 1, evidence of antibody-endothelial interaction (esp. C4d staining), histologic evidence of antibody-associated graft injury, and demonstration of circulating donor-specific antibodies are required for diagnosis.

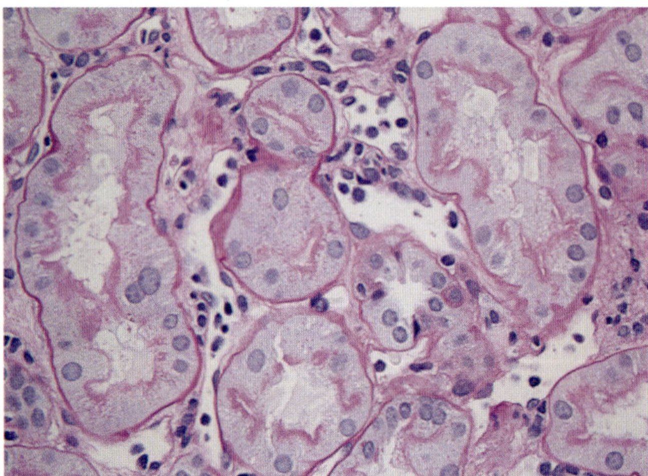

Fig. 28: Peritubular capillaritis. Peritubular capillaries are universally present in renal parenchyma between tubules, but are usually inconspicuous. This periodic acid Schiff (PAS)-stained section shows dilated peritubular capillaries containing mononuclear inflammatory cells (compare with Fig. 2). Peritubular capillaritis is a histologic hallmark of antibody-mediated rejection, though it is seen rarely other conditions, such as severe acute tubular necrosis.

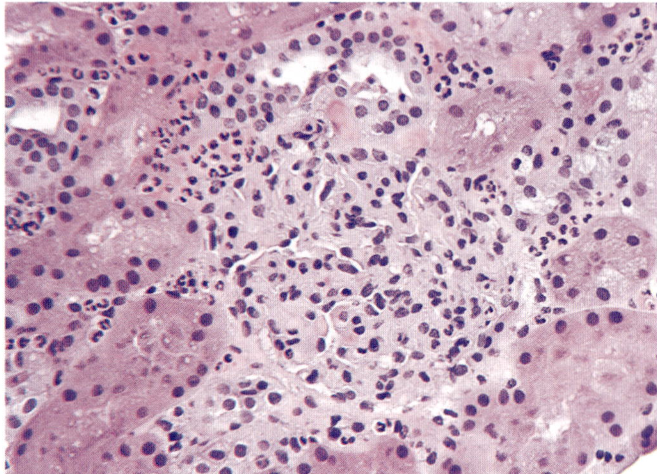

Fig. 29: Peritubular capillaritis. On lower power, neutrophils are extremely abundant within peritubular capillaries, and the central glomerulus is also hypercellular. Often peritubular capillaritis is considerably more subtle than shown here. The Banff 2007 update proposed a threshold and scoring scheme for peritubular capillaritis (ptc, Table 3).[3] This would represent a ptc3 lesion by virtue of >10 cells per peritubular capillary lumen. Hematoxylin and eosin (H&E) stain.

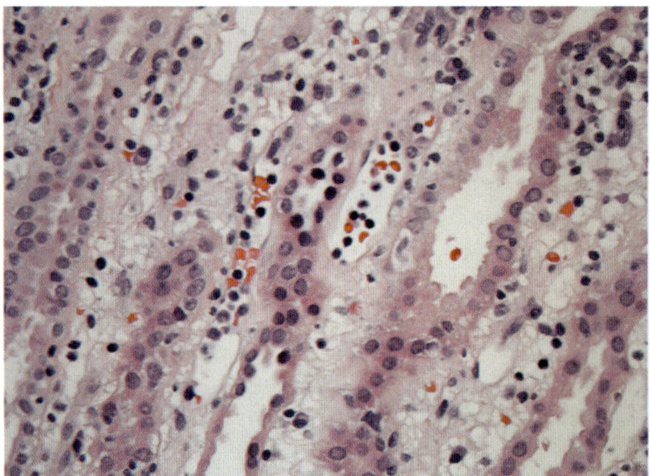

Fig. 30: Peritubular capillaritis. Here, peritubular capillaries contain mostly mononuclear cells. This field also shows tubular injury in that tubular epithelial cells are flattened and beginning to slough into the lumen. There is interstitial inflammation, including plasma cells. The rare tubulitis is suggestive of combined acute antibody-mediated and cellular rejection, a very common occurrence. Hematoxylin and eosin (H&E) stain.

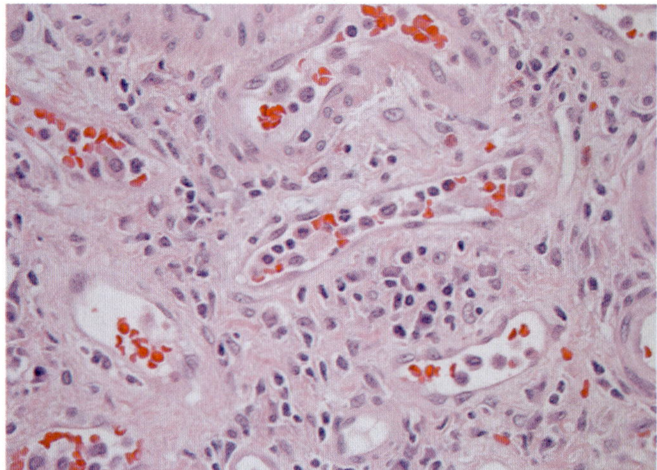

Fig. 31: Peritubular capillaritis. Capillaries are filled with mixed inflammatory cells, including neutrophils and mononuclear cells with pink cytoplasm—these are monocytes. No tubules are seen in this image. Hematoxylin and eosin (H&E) stain.

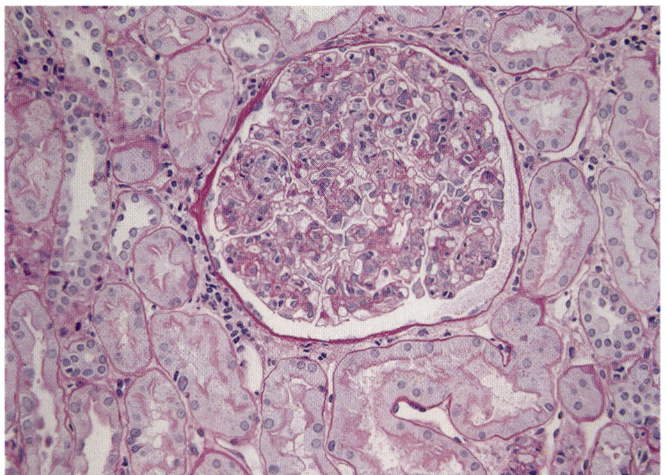

Fig. 32: Glomerulitis. Although the red and white blood cells must constantly pass through glomeruli, few cells are seen within glomerular capillaries in sections of normal kidney or normal allograft. Accumulation of leukocytes within capillary lumina is termed glomerular capillaritis, or glomerulitis, as shown here. The glomerular capillaries contain inflammatory cells, compared with normal glomeruli in Figures 1 to 3. Some of the surrounding peritubular capillaries are prominent, but do not contain cells. Glomerulitis is again a hallmark of antibody-mediated rejection, but is not entirely specific, as it may also rarely be associated with glomerulonephritides, etc. The Banff 1997 publication glomerulitis scoring criteria are listed in Table 3 (g scores).[1] Periodic acid Schiff (PAS) stain.

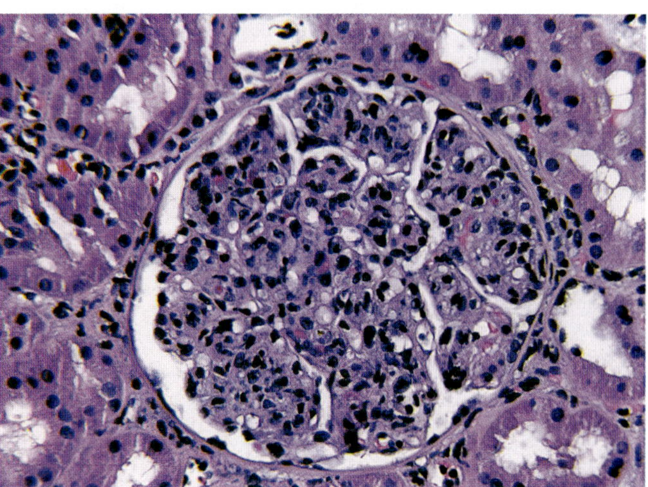

Fig. 33: Glomerulitis. This glomerulus is markedly hypercellular. There is a brisk infiltrate of inflammatory cells. The architectural changes including accentuated lobularity, lytic changes of the mesangium, and capillary wall alterations are also suggestive of a component of chronic injury (chronic allograft glomerulopathy, discussed in Figures 55, 115 to 118). Hematoxylin and eosin (H&E) stain.

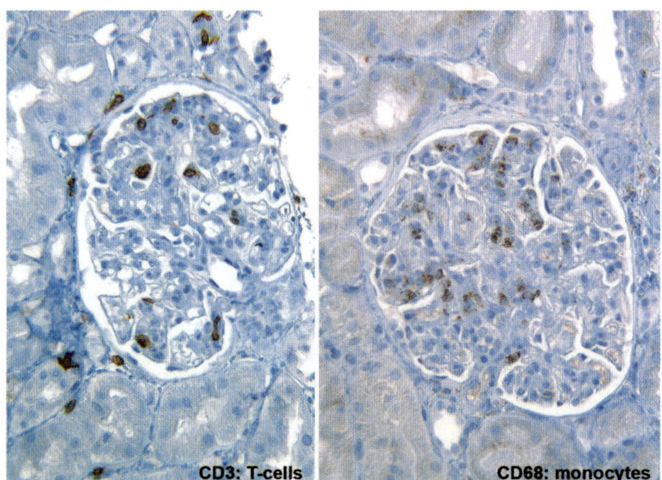

Fig. 34: Glomerulitis, T-cell and monocyte markers. In antibody-mediated rejection, many of the cells infiltrating the glomeruli are monocytes.[11] The left panel shows glomerulitis as stained by the T-cell marker CD3, with a paucity of positive cells. The right panel shows a glomerulus stained with the monocyte marker CD68; granular cytoplasmic staining highlights many monocytes in glomerular capillaries. The brown reaction product indicates positive staining, against the blue hematoxylin counter stain.

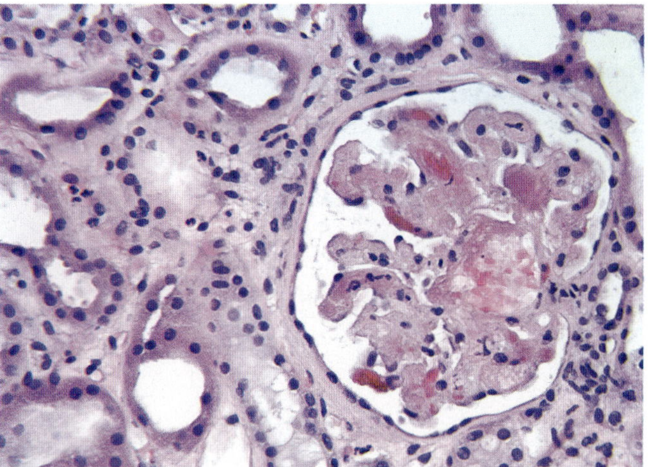

Fig. 35: Glomerular fibrinoid necrosis. Fibrin in glomeruli is also a feature of antibody-mediated rejection, as illustrated here. Other examples of fibrin thrombi (calcineurin inhibitor toxicity, recurrent disease, etc.) are discussed in section "Thrombotic Microangiopathy". Hematoxylin and eosin (H&E) stain.

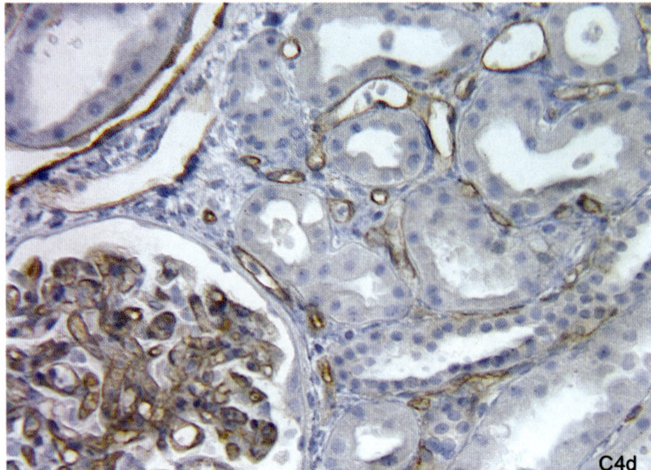

Fig. 36: C4d staining, immunohistochemistry. The complement cascade is activated at sites of antibody-mediated injury, yet most of the complement split-products are rapidly removed. However, an antibody to the "d" fragment of C4 (C4d, also similar with C3, split-product C3d) binds covalently to endothelial surfaces and can be detected by immunostaining. IHC detection of C4d staining is shown on the case with fibrin thrombi (see Fig. 35 above). The brown reaction product is positive against a blue (hematoxylin) counterstain. In this context, the C4d-positivity provides support for an antibody-mediated mechanism. However, there are rare instances in which C4d deposition is seen without morphological evidence of active rejection, for instance, in grafts that are ABO-incompatible.[3] The significance of this finding remains an area of active research, and careful clinicopathologic correlation is needed in this situation.

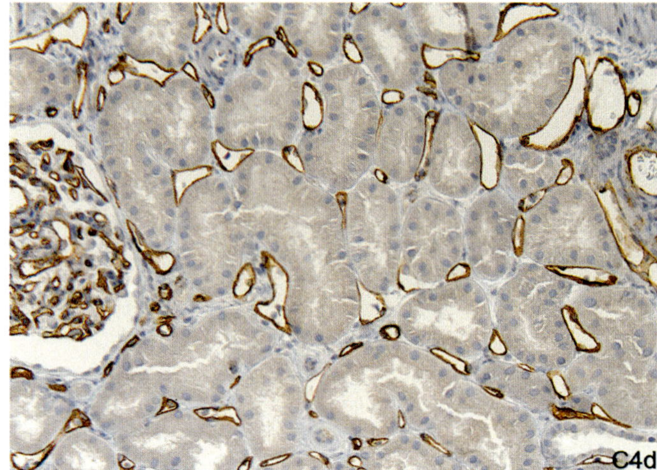

Fig. 37: C4d staining, immunohistochemistry. The peritubular and glomerular capillaries stain strongly for C4d. With the IHC technique on formalin-fixed paraffin embedded (FFPE) tissue sections, normal glomeruli should show no C4d staining. Linear glomerular staining, as shown here, might be associated with antibody-mediated glomerular endothelial injury. Antibody deposits in glomerulonephritis also show C4d staining in a different pattern, for instance, in recurrent membranous glomerulonephritis (see Fig. 134)

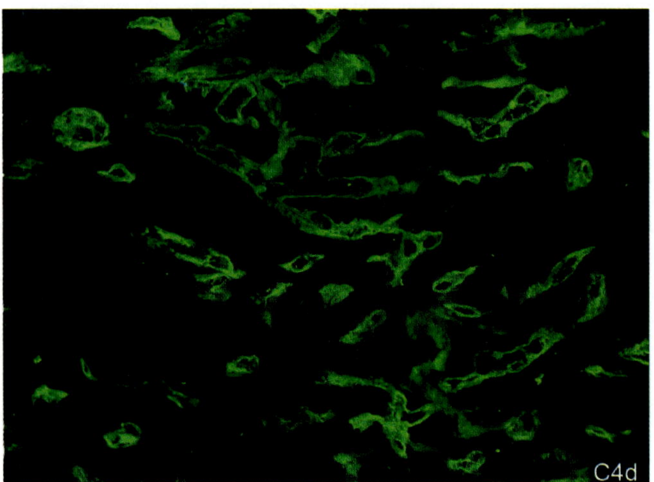

Fig. 38: C4d staining, immunofluorescence (IF). C4d antibody staining of frozen tissue with the IF method highlights peritubular capillaries strongly and diffusely (here, FITC conjugated antibodies are green in darkfield fluorescence microscope). There are proposed criteria for scoring and interpretation of C4d staining (Table 4),[3] which differ somewhat between the IHC–FFPE method (considered somewhat less sensitive), and the IF method on frozen sections of fresh tissue (considered more sensitive). Nevertheless, many labs perform successful C4d staining and interpretation of FFPE sections, which do not require a separate fresh tissue specimen.

Table 4: C4d scoring in peritubular capillaries[3]

Score	Biopsy area positive (%)	Interpretation: IF	Interpretation: IHC
C4d0 negative:	0%	Negative	Negative
C4d1 minimal:	1<10%	Negative	Unknown
C4d2 focal:	10–50%	Unknown	Positive?
C4d3 diffuse:	>50%	Positive	Positive

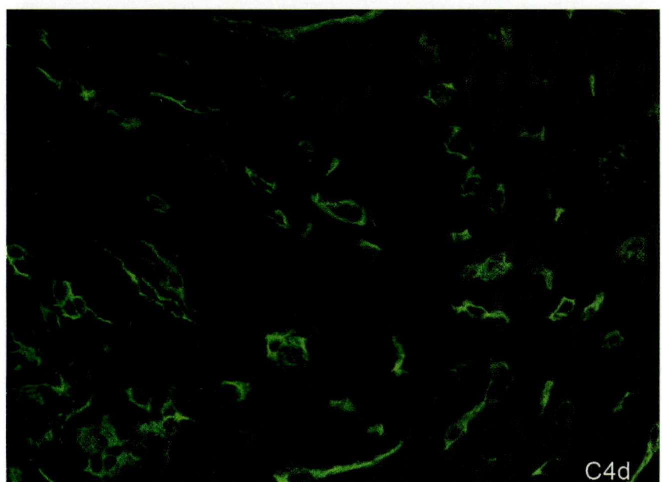

Fig. 39: C4d staining, immunofluorescence. The C4d staining is slightly less intense than Figure 38 above, but is still diffusely positive. Guidelines recommend that the minimal specimen size for C4d interpretation is at least 5 high-power microscopic fields of cortex and/or medulla without scarring or infarction.[3]

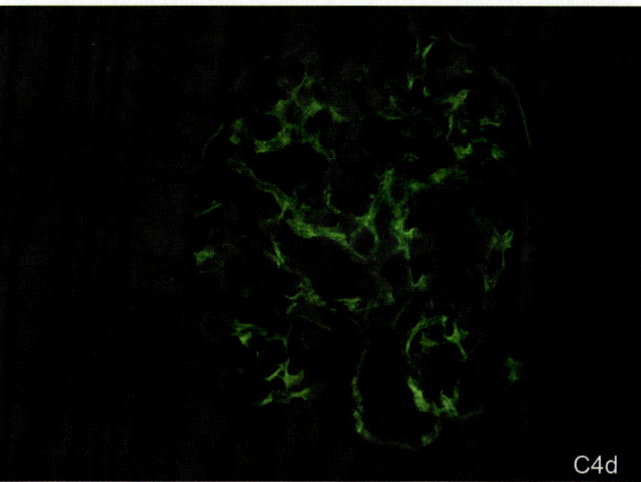

Fig. 40: C4d staining, immunofluorescence, normal glomerulus. With this method on frozen sections, normal glomeruli shows a mild degree of C4d staining, mostly mesangial. This can serve as a helpful internal control. However, other patterns of glomerular C4d staining may suggest additional pathology (antibody-mediated glomerular endothelial injury, glomerulonephritis, *see* Fig. 37).

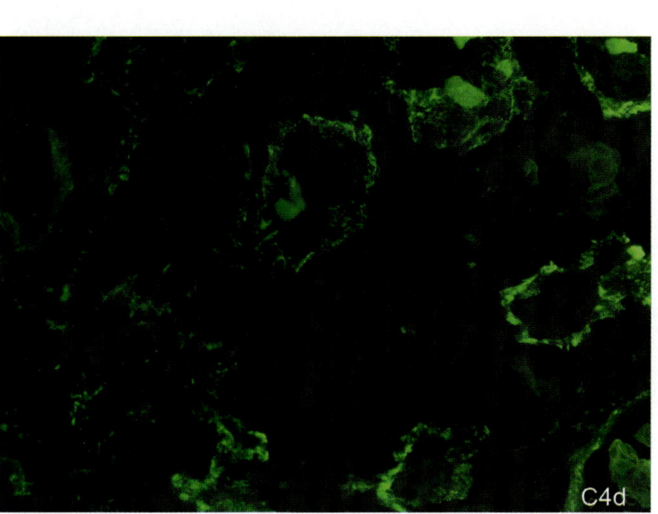

Fig. 41: C4d staining, immunofluorescence, tubular staining. C4d reactivity within tubular basement membranes, shown here, may sometimes be difficult to distinguish from peritubular capillary staining by IF. Correlation with corresponding hematoxylin and eosin (H&E)-stained sections may be helpful. Tubular basement membrane C4d staining occurs preferentially in atrophic tubules, or in cases of polyoma virus infection.

Examples of Acute Cellular and/or Acute Antibody-Mediated Rejection with Banff Grading (Figs. 42 to 47)

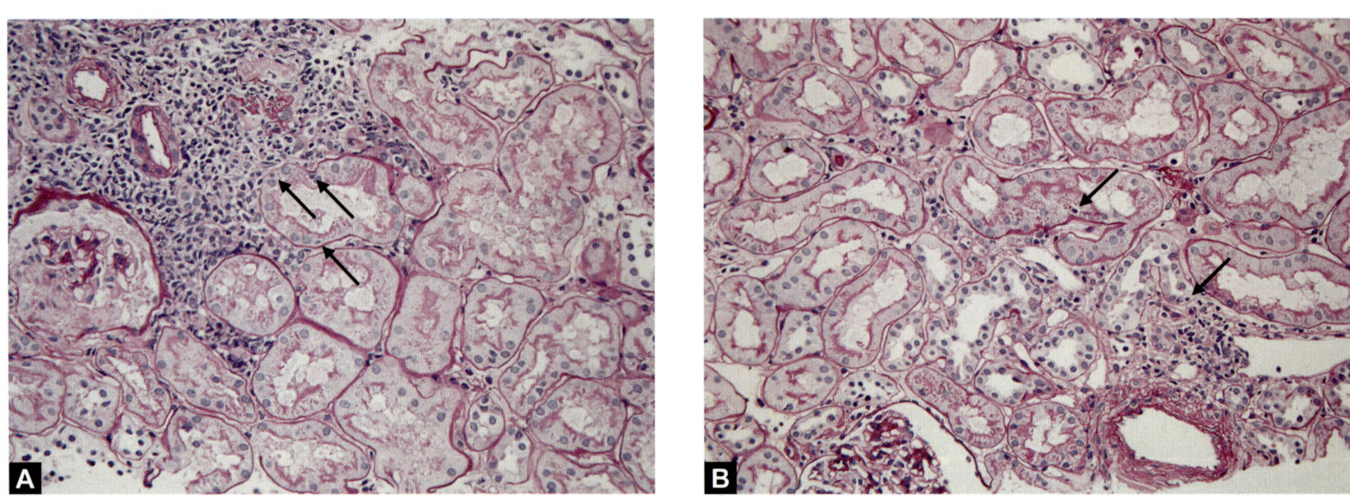

Figs. 42A and B: Banff Borderline. Panel A shows a focus of interstitial inflammation in the upper left, with rare lymphocytes in the adjacent tubule (arrows, t1). Panel B also shows a rare tubulitis (arrows) in an area of scant interstitial inflammation. Based on <10% interstitial inflammation in this biopsy specimen, and scant tubulitis (i0, t1), this biopsy specimen is classified as Borderline.

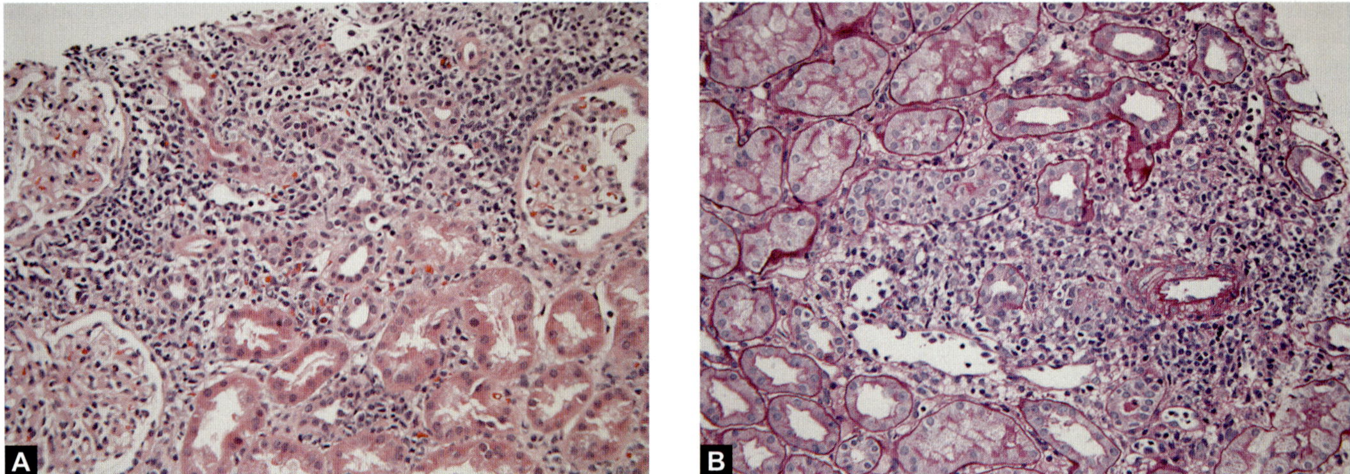

Figs. 43A and B: Banff IA acute rejection. The hematoxylin and eosin (H&E) image in panel A demonstrates a brisk mononuclear cell infiltrate in the interstitium and tubules (especially upper left-center). The periodic acid Schiff (PAS) image in B shows another focus of inflammation and tubulitis (center). Based on inflammation in > 25% of the biopsy specimen (i2) and moderate tubulitis (t2), this biopsy meets criteria for Banff IA acute rejection.

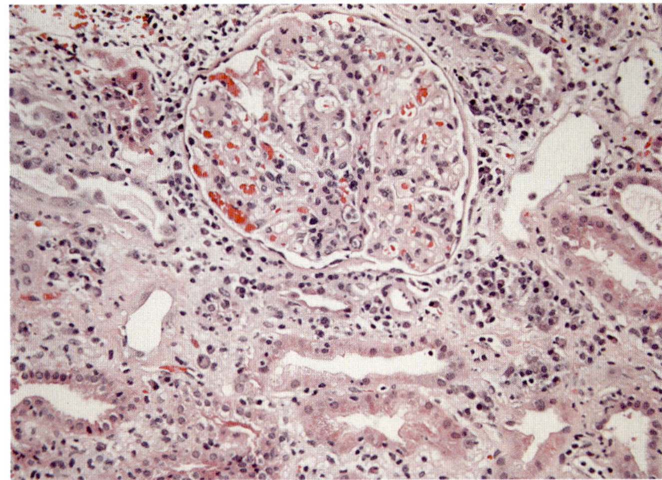

Fig. 44: Banff type IB acute rejection. This image shows a brisk interstitial inflammatory cell infiltrate with a prominent plasma cell component; review of the entire specimen showed >50% inflamed parenchyma (i3). In addition, there is readily apparent tubulitis even on this hematoxylin and eosin (H&E) stain (t3). There was no endothelialitis (v0). These features are diagnostic of acute cellular rejection, Banff type IB. Further, the illustrated glomerulus is abnormal in that there are numerous mononuclear cells in capillary loops (glomerulitis, g2 based on involvement on 25–75% of glomeruli). Glomerulitis is generally regarded as a feature of antibody-mediated rejection; together with positive peritubular capillary C4d (not shown) and unknown donor-specific antibody status, this is "suspicious" for antibody-mediated rejection. Diagnosis summary: Banff type IB, suspicious for antibody-mediated rejection.

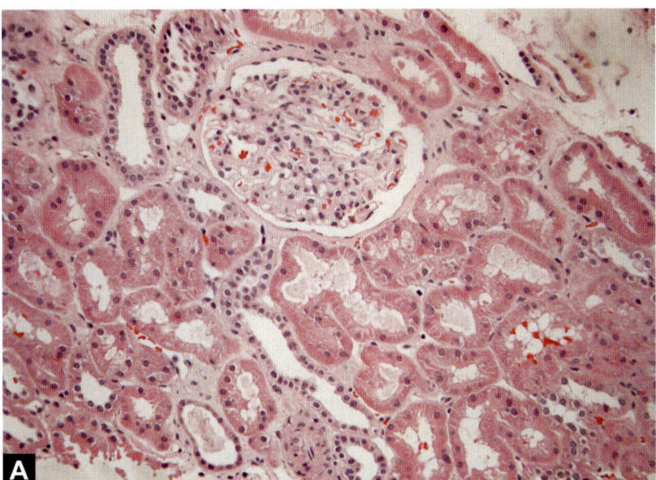

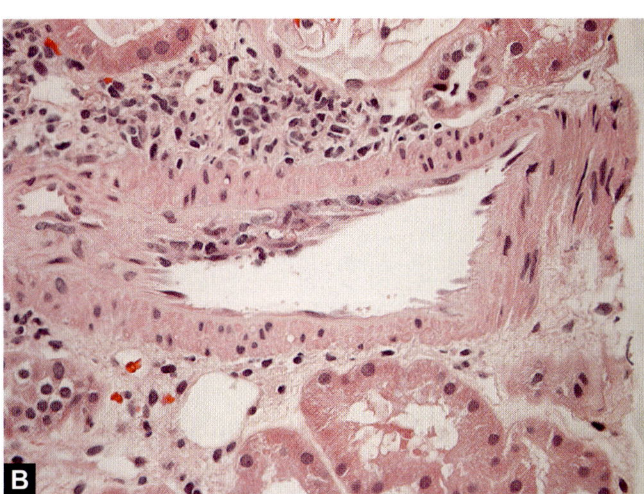

Figs. 45A and B: Banff type IIA acute rejection. On a 1-year surveillance biopsy, interstitial inflammation and tubulitis were essentially absent, panel A (i0, t0). However, shown in panel B is a single artery with endothelialitis (v1). This mandates a diagnosis of acute cellular rejection, Banff type IIA. Hematoxylin and eosin (H&E) stains.

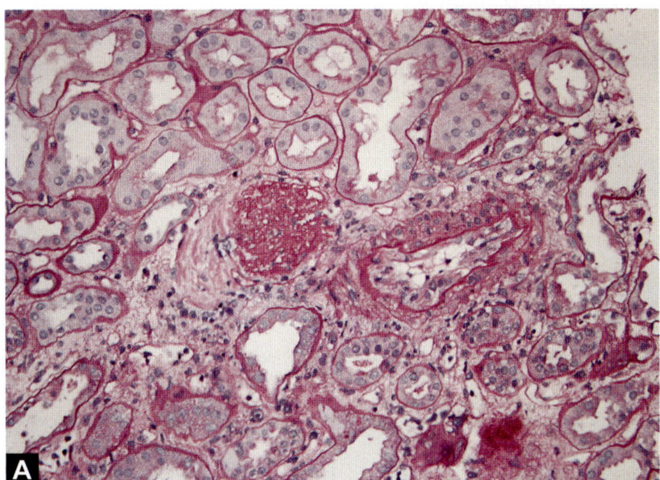

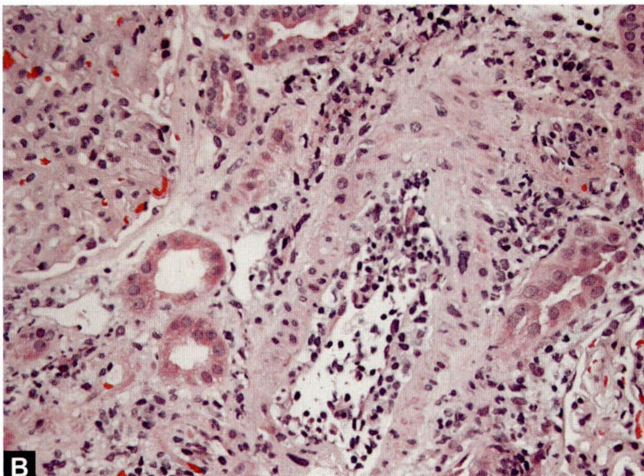

Figs. 46A and B: Banff type IIB acute rejection. Panel A shows a globally sclerotic glomerulus at center. Just to the right there is an artery with mild endothelialitis (v1). Below the artery is a small focus of tubulitis (t1). However, in panel B, there is severe intimal arteritis, with >25% narrowing of the lumen (v2), mandating a diagnosis of Banff type IIB acute rejection.

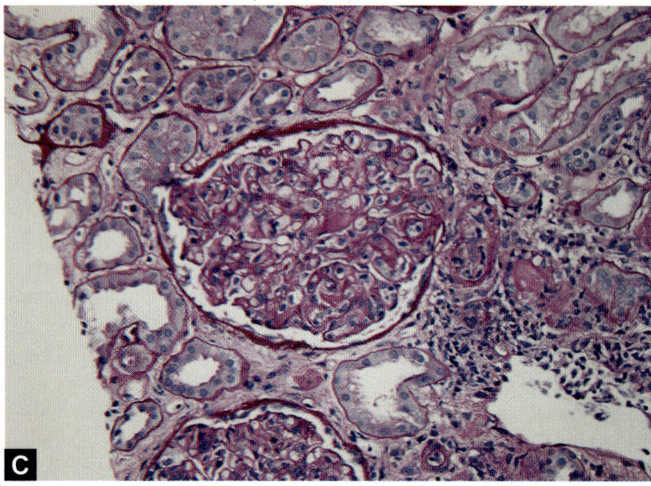

Fig. 46C: In addition, panel C (periodic acid Schiff, PAS stain) shows mild glomerulitis, along with endothelialitis of the afferent arteriole, and inflammation of the vein at lower right (venulitis).

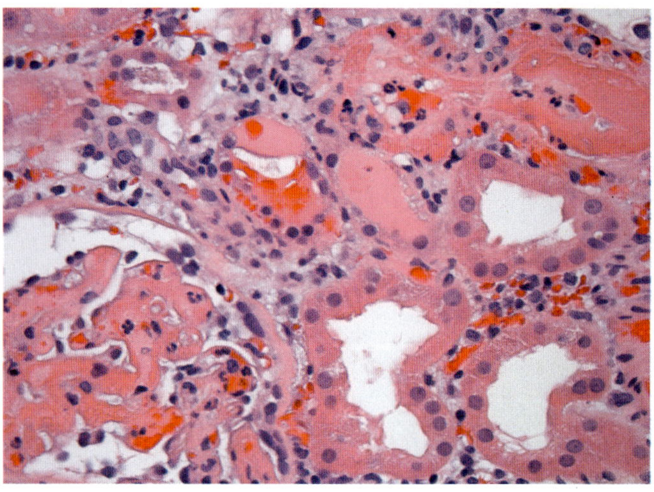

Fig. 47: Banff type III acute rejection. This allograft biopsy had scattered interstitial inflammation with injured tubules, but negligible tubulitis (i1, t0). However, there was prominent fibrinoid necrosis of arteries and arterioles (upper right, v3). In addition, many glomeruli contained fibrin thrombi (lower left). These features are indicative of Banff type III rejection, likely with a component of antibody-mediated rejection in light of the fibrin thrombi, and in correlation with positive C4d and donor-specific antibody results (not shown). Hematoxylin and eosin (H&E) stain.

Chronic Allograft Rejection (Figs. 48 to 55)

Chronic allograft rejection is associated with many histopathologic changes the kidney (Table 5). These include interstitial fibrosis, tubular atrophy, vascular changes, glomerulosclerosis, and glomerulopathy. However, many of these histologic changes are not specific for rejection, and can result from other causes of kidney injury such as drug toxicity, infection, arteriosclerosis, hypertension, and obstruction. Allograft vasculopathy/arteriopathy, glomerulopathy and mesangial matrix increase, as well as peritubular capillary multilayering are associated with chronic rejection and will be illustrated here, as well as in section "Glomerular Processes". Other changes are addressed in section "Chronic Allograft Damage".

Table 5: Histopathologic changes that may be seen in calcineurin-inhibitor toxicity, many non-specific

Morphology	Figure numbers
Isometric vacuolization of tubules (acute)	78–80
Arteriolar medial smooth muscle swelling/ vacuolization	111
Arteriolar medial hyalinosis	107–111
"Striped" atrophy	105
Juxtaglomerular apparatus hyperplasia	111
Calcification	75–76
Thrombotic microangiopathy/fibrin thrombi	56–63
Focal segmental glomerulosclerosis (FSGS)	122–124

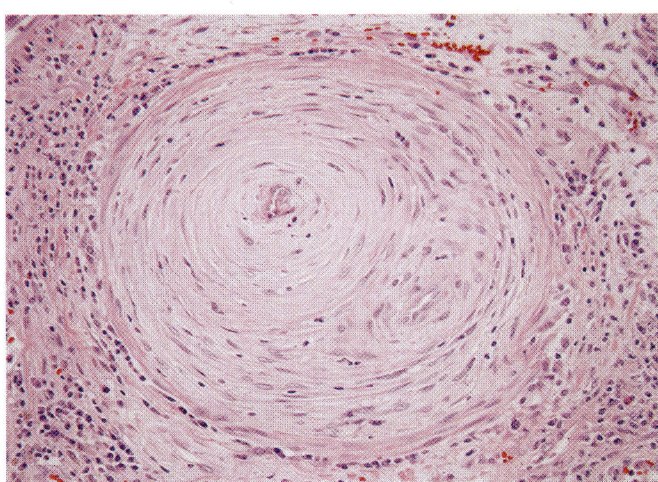

Fig. 48: Allograft vasculopathy/arteriopathy. This artery is nearly occluded by a concentric and relatively cellular pattern of myofibroblastic-like cells and pale, loose matrix. There are rare inflammatory cells entrapped within, but endothelialitis is not evident. Elastin stains would not highlight these intimal changes (not shown), and these features are characteristic of severe allograft vasculopathy, which can be graded by the Banff schema, here cv3 as there is > 50% luminal narrowing (cv, Table 3).[1]

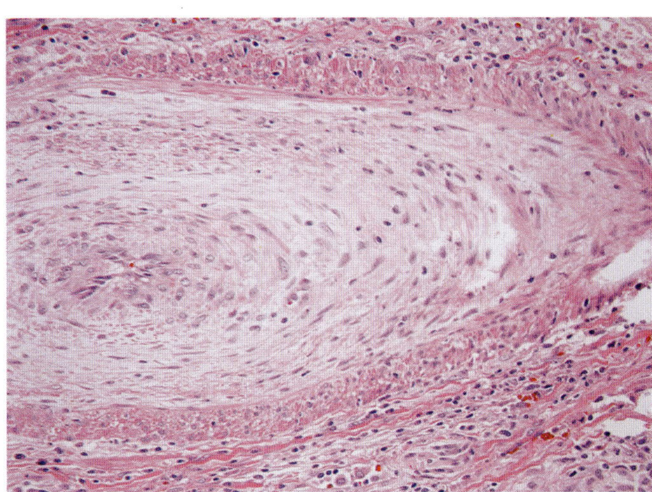

Fig. 49: Allograft vasculopathy/arteriopathy. A longitudinal section of an artery with marked concentric and cellular fibrointimal thickening. Hematoxylin and eosin (H&E) stain.

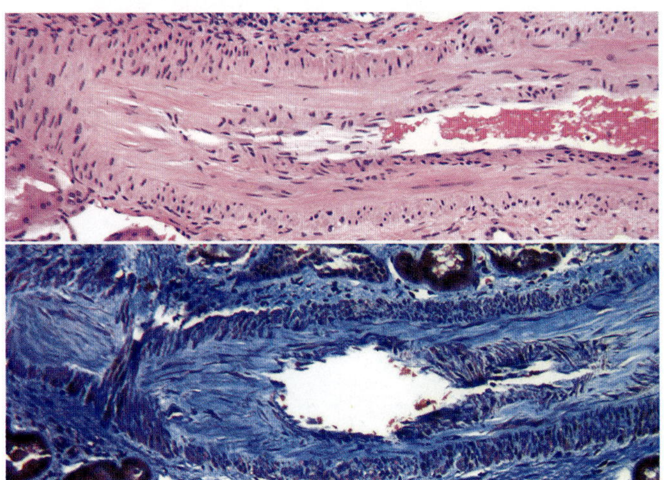

Fig. 50: Allograft vasculopathy/arteriopathy. This artery demonstrates a well-developed neointima, characterized by an intimal layer of smooth muscle cells. This is nicely apparent on the trichrome stain (lower panel) in which the smooth muscle cell cytoplasm stains red. There is an intervening layer of dense fibrosis between this and the media. Top: Hematoxylin and eosin (H&E) stain; bottom: trichrome stain.

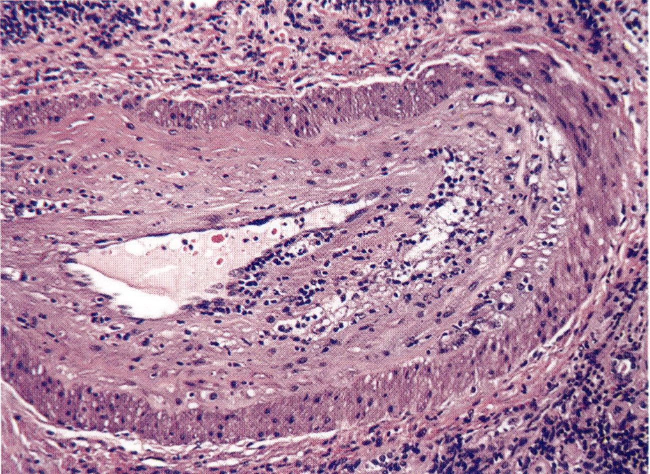

Fig. 51: Chronic active allograft vasculopathy/arteriopathy. Intimal foam cells, as seen here at right, are also characteristic of allograft vasculopathy. In addition, there is an active endothelialitis, with numerous inflammatory cells underlying the endothelium, as well as involving the fibrointimal layer (Banff v2, type 2A acute rejection and cv3). Taken together, these features are diagnostic of chronic active allograft arteriopathy. Hematoxylin and eosin (H&E) stain.

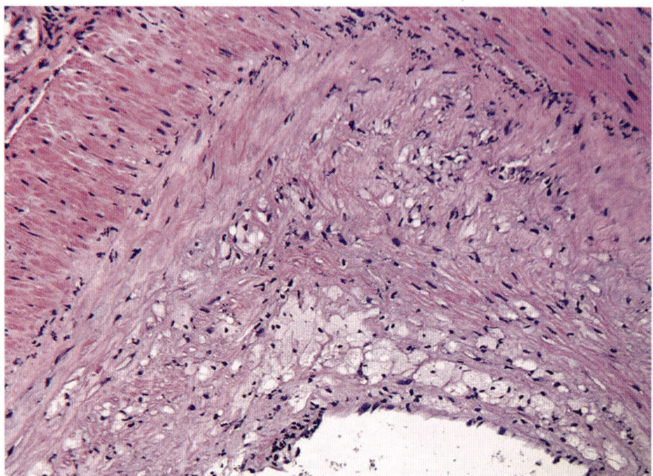

Fig. 52: Chronic active allograft vasculopathy/arteriopathy. A large (arcuate) caliber artery with a very thick fibrointimal proliferation also contains foam cells. Active inflammation is seen scattered throughout the fibrointimal tissue, and underlying the endothelium, again diagnostic of chronic active allograft arteriopathy. Hematoxylin and eosin (H&E) stain.

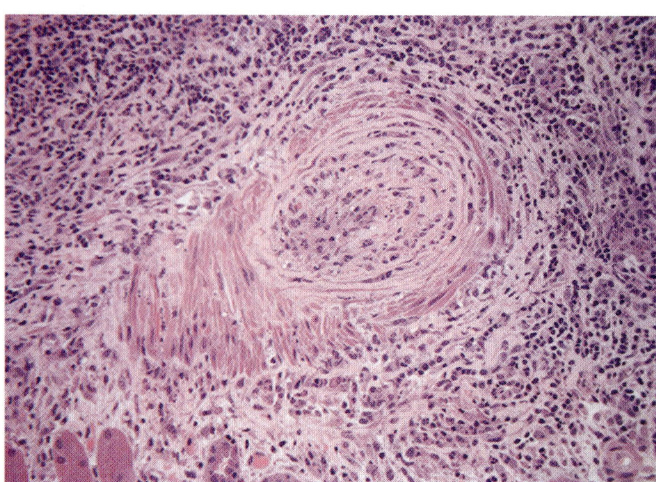

Fig. 53: Chronic active allograft vasculopathy/arteriopathy. This artery is occluded by concentric intimal fibrosis, myofibroblasts, and a dense inflammatory cell infiltrate. There is also a dense interstitial inflammatory cell infiltrate and tubulitis seen focally at bottom center. Hematoxylin and eosin (H&E) stain.

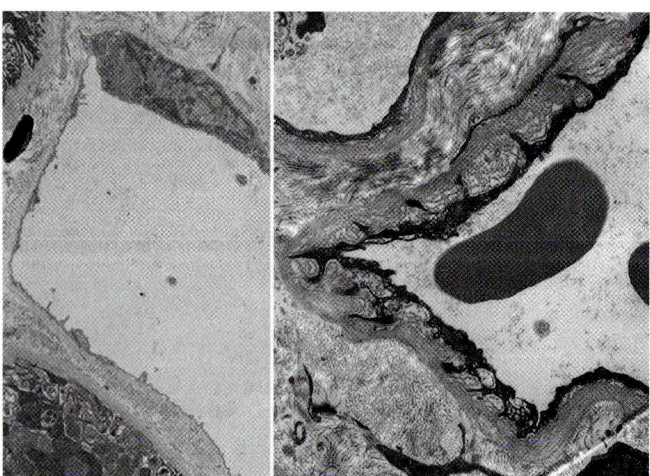

Fig. 54: Peritubular capillary multilayering, electron microscopy. The electron micrograph at left shows a normal peritubular capillary, characterized by a single layer of endothelium and endothelial basal lamina. The image at right shows a slightly higher power of a peritubular capillary with prominent basement membrane multilayering, an indication of chronic allograft damage attributed to antibody-mediated rejection. This electron microscopic feature can be used to assess antibody-mediated rejection in situations where C4d immunostaining might not be informative (ABO-incompatible, C5 inhibitor treatment, etc.)

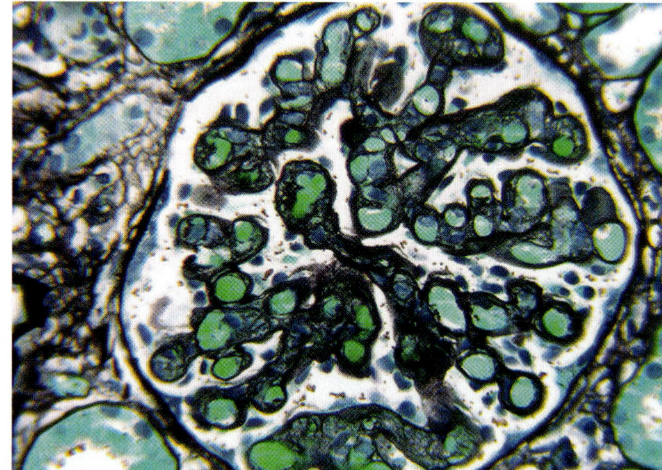

Fig. 55: Transplant glomerulopathy. This glomerulus shows duplication of glomerular basement membranes in a case of antibody-mediated rejection. This is an example of transplant glomerulopathy, although basement membrane double contours may also be seen in thrombotic microangiopathy (TMA) associated with other causes, or membranoproliferative glomerulonephritis (MPGN). The Banff schema classifies allograft glomerulopathy based on the percentage of capillary loops involved in the most affected glomeruli (see Table 3). Transplant/allograft glomerulopathy is discussed in more detail section "Glomerular Processes". This is a silver stain with a green counterstain.[1]

THROMBOTIC MICROANGIOPATHY (FIGS. 56 TO 63)

Thrombotic microangiopathic (TMA) changes are relatively rare in renal allografts and prompt a differential diagnosis including entities unique to the allograft such as antibody-mediated rejection and calcineurin inhibitor toxicity. Even less frequently, TMA in allografts may be due to entities such as recurrent or de novo hemolytic uremia syndrome (HUS), thrombotic thrombocytopenic purpura (TTP), malignant hypertension, scleroderma, radiation damage, and viral infection. Other histopathologic findings in the allograft biopsy, along with clinical correlation, generally narrow the diagnosis.

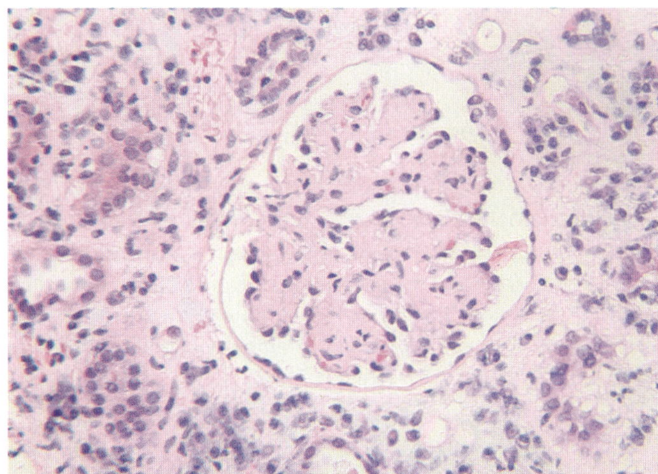

Fig. 56: Thrombotic microangiopathy (TMA), glomerulus. This glomerulus appears nearly "bloodless" with capillary loops occluded by swollen endothelial cytoplasm and rare red blood cell fragments. In addition, it is shrunken and does not fill Bowman's space, likely due to microangiopathic changes in the afferent arteriole, not shown in this image. Hematoxylin and eosin (H&E) stain.

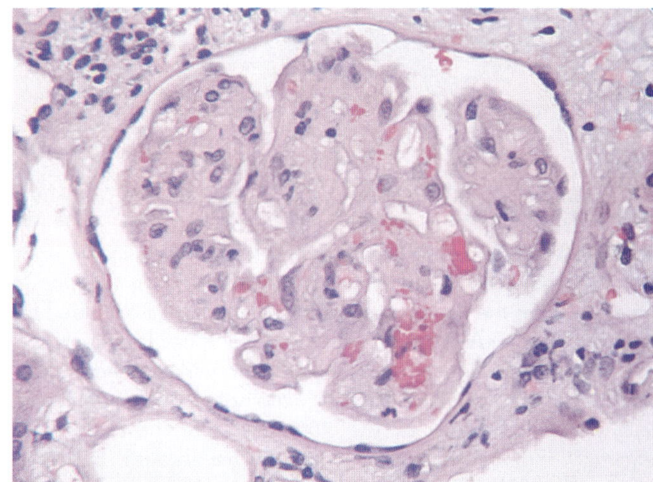

Fig. 57: Thrombotic microangiopathy (TMA), glomerulus. Red blood cell fragments are more apparent in this glomerulus with TMA. No fibrin thrombi are present. Hematoxylin and eosin (H&E) stain.

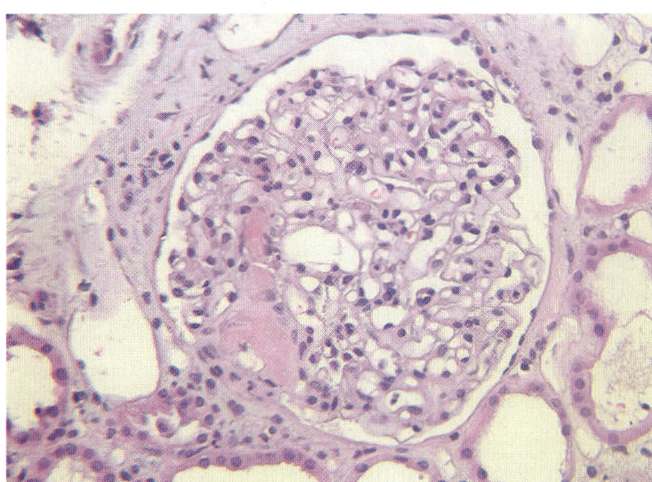

Fig. 58: Fibrin thrombi, glomerulus. Prominent but segmental bright pink fibrin thrombi are seen in the glomerulus at 7–9 o'clock.

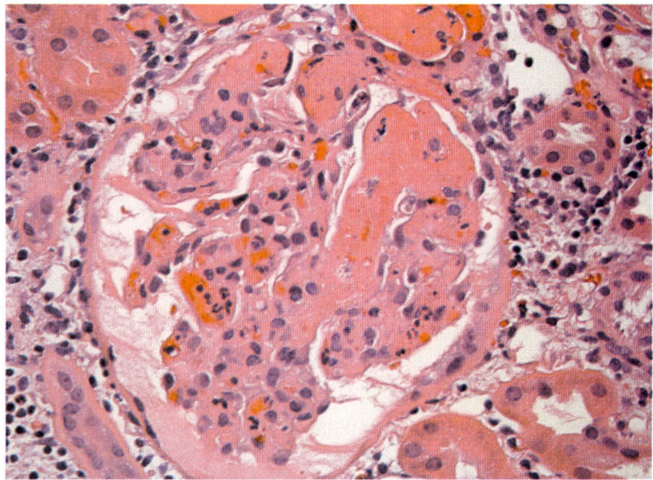

Fig. 59: Fibrin thrombi, glomerulus. Large fibrin thrombi fill the upper portion of this glomerulus. Numerous leukocytes and erythrocytes also occupy the glomerulus. Ischemic retraction of the glomerular tuft is suggestive of arterial or arteriolar lesions. There is also a brisk interstitial inflammatory cell infiltrate with edema. This patient presented with malignant hypertension shortly after transplant. Other pathologic and laboratory indication of antibody-mediated rejection were absent, yet clinical suspicion remains high. Hematoxylin and eosin (H&E) stain.

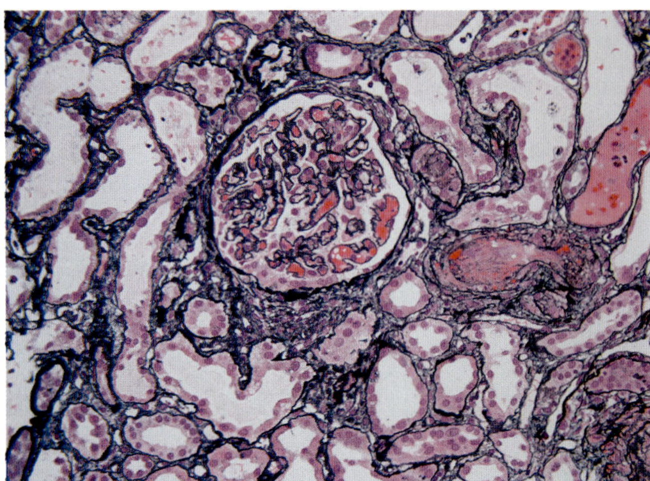

Fig. 60: Thrombotic microangiopathy. The arteriole in the right of this silver-stained image shows small amounts of pink fibrinous material within the lumen and media. The lumen is occluded by fibrin and reactive/edematous cells. Red blood cell fragments are also present. Consequently, the tubules show marked ischemic and reactive changes including ectasia, vacuolization and sloughing of cells, and enlarged nuclei. The glomerulus also shows ischemic retraction and wrinkling of the basement membranes, but there is no endothelial cell swelling or fibrin thrombi in this glomerulus.

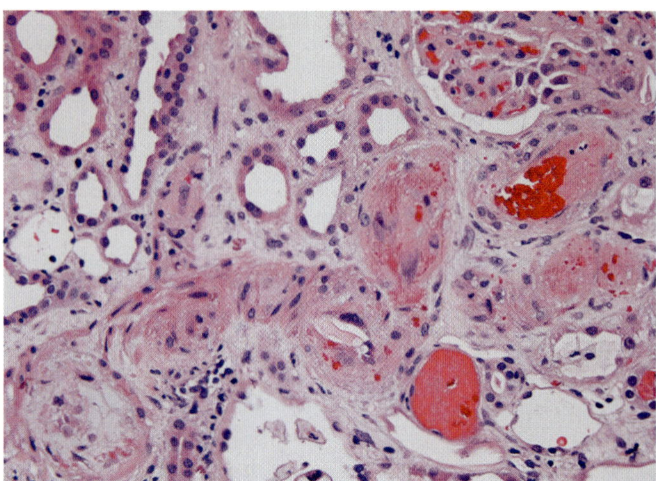

Fig. 61: Thrombotic microangiopathy. A high power view of small tortuous arterioles from the same case as Figure 60 demonstrates occlusion (left), with numerous red blood cell fragments as well as fibrin thrombi (center and right). Hematoxylin and eosin (H&E) stain.

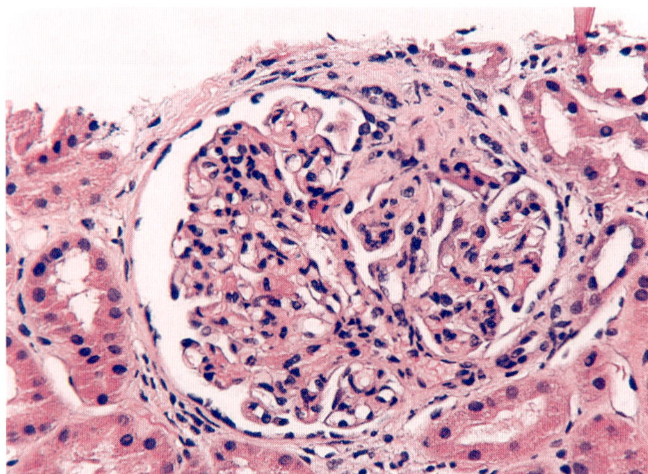

Fig. 62: Thrombotic microangiopathy (TMA), healing. Some residual acute capillary hypercellularity and occlusion remains in this image of healing TMA. There is large area of scarring and adhesion of the glomerular tuft to Bowman's capsule apparent in the upper right of the glomerulus (at 2 o'clock). Hematoxylin and eosin (H&E) stain.

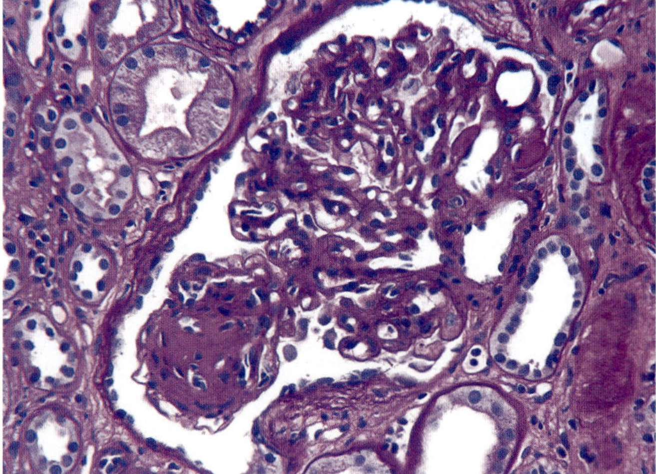

Fig. 63: Thrombotic microangiopathy (TMA), healing. This glomerulus demonstrates nodular mesangial sclerosis (lower left) along with two instances of hyaline accumulation (upper right), following an episode of TMA. These histologic features are shared with diabetic glomerulopathy; thus careful correlation with clinical history and prior pathology is essential. Periodic acid Schiff (PAS) stain.

ACUTE TUBULAR DAMAGE AND SEQUELAE OF DELAYED GRAFT FUNCTION (FIGS. 64 TO 80)

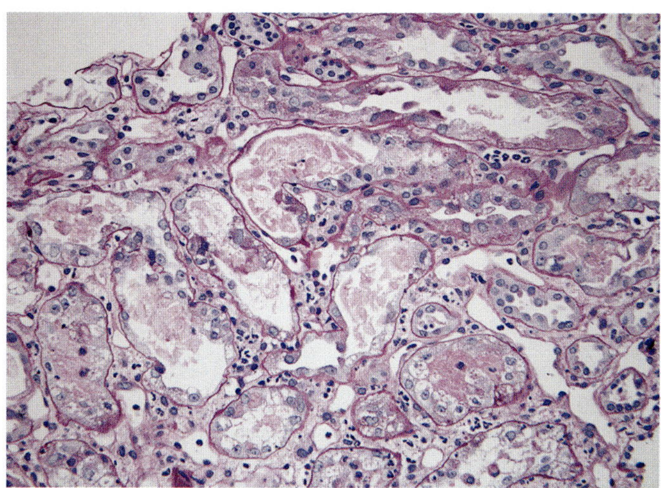

Fig. 64: Acute tubular necrosis/injury (ATN). This is a florid example of ATN. There are many tubular epithelial cells that have detached from the tubular basement membrane, resulting in cell debris and granular cast material filling some tubular lumina. Remaining tubular epithelial cells have vacuolated cytoplasm, and are flattened out. Tubular nuclei are large and reactive appearing. Remarkably, there is a brisk neutrophilic infiltrate within peritubular capillaries. In this case, peritubular capillaritis is in response to the severe ATN, rather than representing antibody-mediated rejection. Periodic acid Schiff (PAS) stain.

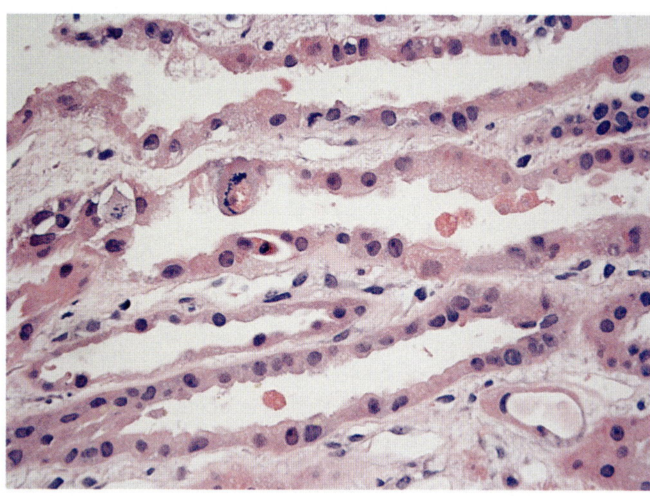

Fig. 65: Acute tubular necrosis/injury (ATN).This high power hematoxylin and eosin (H&E) image shows many injured tubules with atypical mitotic figures, and several epithelial cell remnants in the tubular lumina.

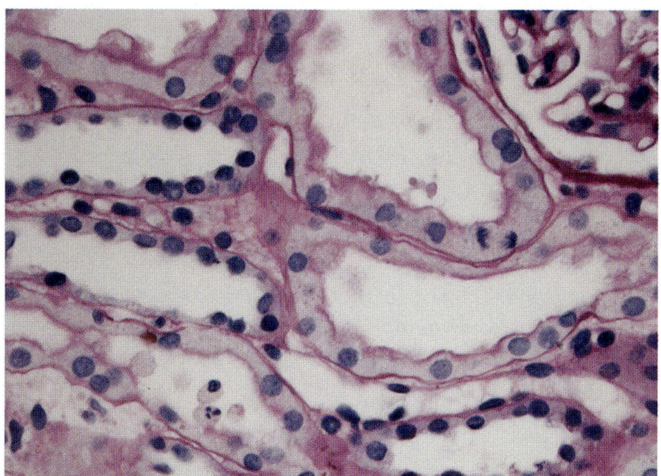

Fig. 66: Acute tubular necrosis/injury (ATN). A tubular mitotic figure is seen on this high power image of a periodic acid Schiff (PAS) stain, in a case with less floridly abnormal tubular epithelial cells. Cell debris is seen in the tubule at lower left.

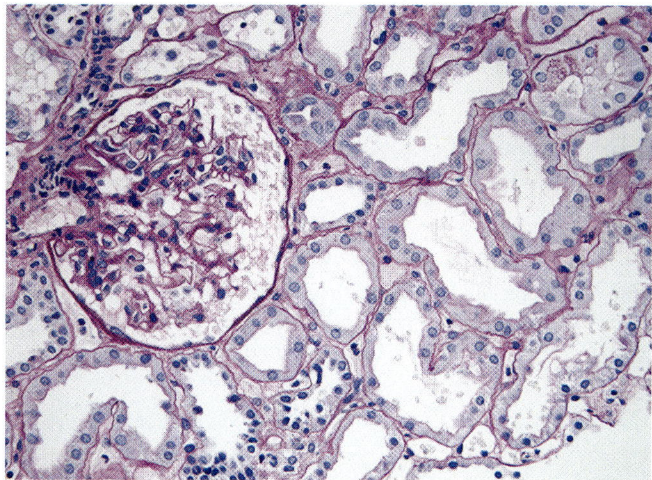

Fig. 67: Acute tubular necrosis/injury (ATN). This ATN case shows relatively mild histological changes, characterized by flat tubular epithelial cells without the characteristic normal light magenta brush border. Few cells are sloughing into the tubular lumen (upper left). The glomerulus also appears to be ischemic, affected by the same process impacting the tubules. Periodic acid Schiff (PAS) stain.

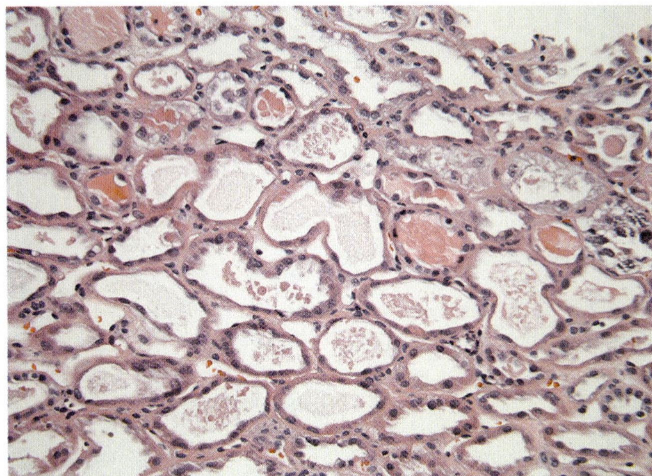

Fig. 68: Delayed graft function/chronic acute tubular necrosis (ATN). Tubules are injured and ectatic, with many pink granular and protein casts. The extensive calcification, seen as the purple staining material in the upper tubules, are indicative of a more chronic process, as may been seen in delayed graft function. Hematoxylin and eosin (H&E) stain.

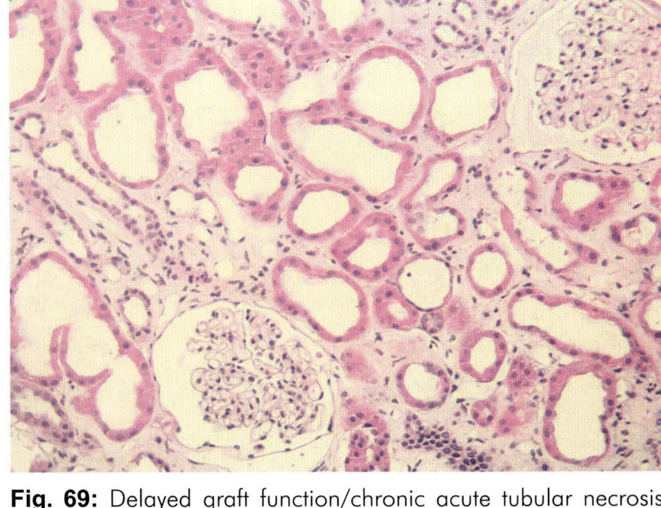

Fig. 69: Delayed graft function/chronic acute tubular necrosis (ATN). Histologic changes associated with delayed graft function include ectatic proximal tubules. Interstitial fibrosis, causing separation of the tubules, is indicative of chronicity. Hematoxylin and eosin (H&E) stain.

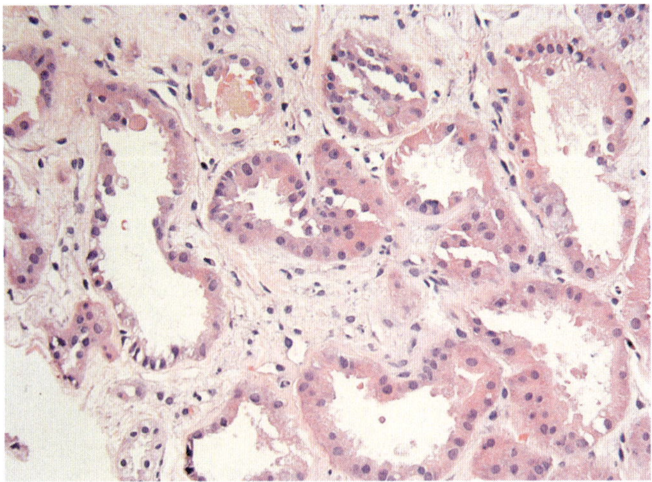

Fig. 70: Acute tubular necrosis/injury (ATN). Acute and chronic ATN with granular casts, epithelial cell sloughing and vacuolization, as well as interstitial fibrosis. Hematoxylin and eosin (H&E) stain.

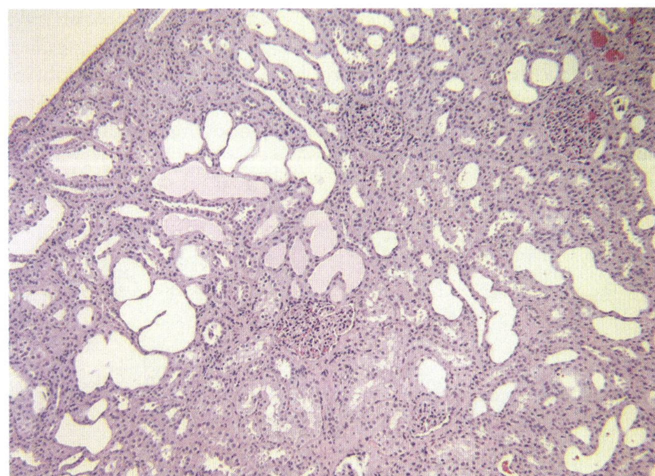

Fig. 71: Urinary outflow obstruction. On low power, tubules are markedly dilated; there are also scattered inflammatory cell infiltrates between tubules. Hematoxylin and eosin (H&E) stain.

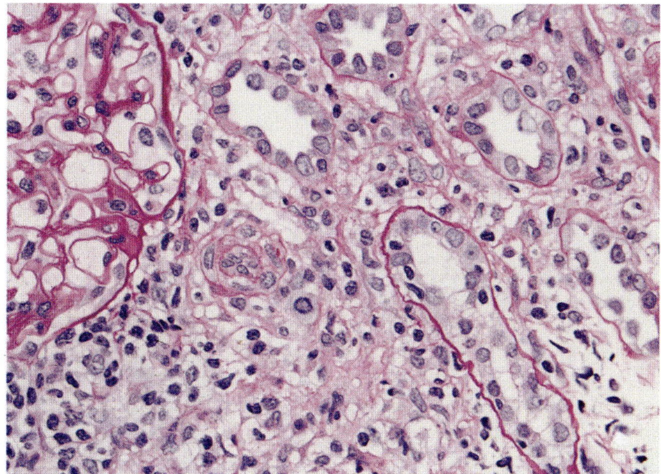

Fig. 72: Ureteral obstruction. There are focal areas of mononuclear cell tubulitis, in early atrophic tubules, and interstitial inflammation. This field would mimic acute cellular rejection; however, other histopathologic features of obstruction were seen, as illustrated in Figures 73 and 74. Periodic acid Schiff (PAS) stain.

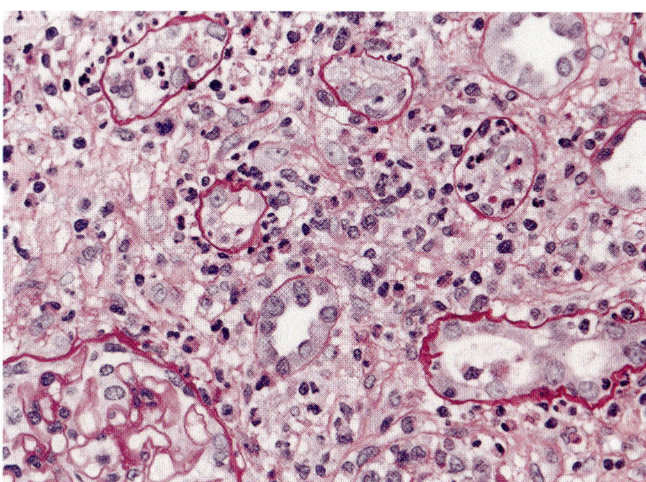

Fig. 73: Ureteral obstruction. Neutrophils are seen within tubules and in the interstitium. This pattern of inflammation raises consideration for various infections including pyelonephritis, as well as reflux and obstruction. This is a periodic acid Schiff (PAS) stain from the same case as Figure 72.

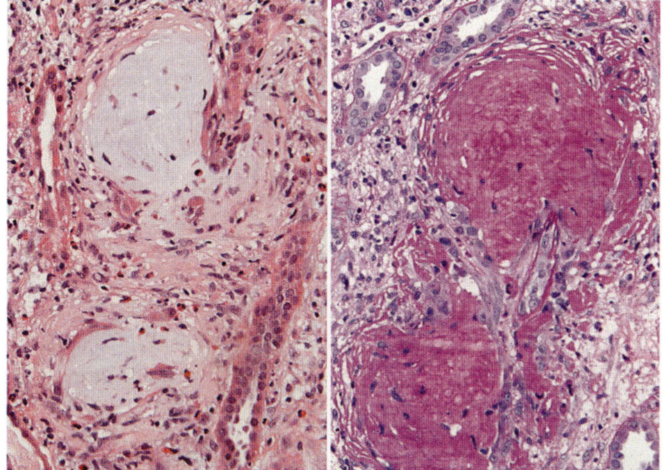

Fig. 74: Tamm–Horsfall protein aggregates in obstruction. Large aggregates of Tamm–Horsfall protein are seen extruded from the tubules in the interstitium, another feature of obstruction. On hematoxylin and eosin (H&E) stain, Tamm–Horsfall protein is pale (left), while it is brightly magenta on periodic acid Schiff (PAS) stain (right). Tamm–Horsfall protein casts have similar staining qualities, yet are generally much more subtle.

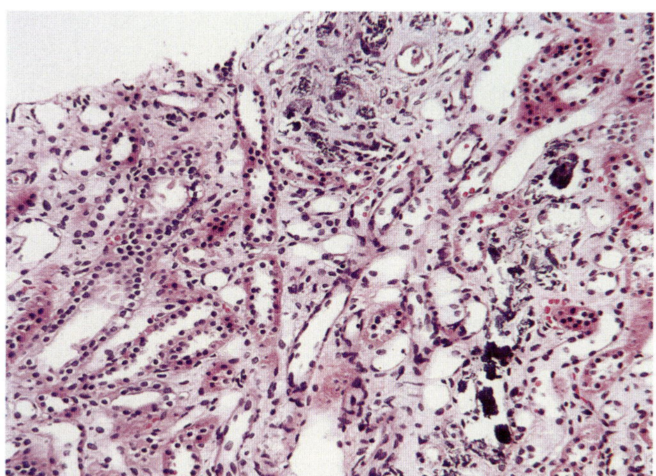

Fig. 75: Nephrocalcinosis. Numerous dark purple calcifications are seen on this hematoxylin and eosin (H&E) stain, usually calcium phosphate. Tubular calcifications are commonly seen in the context of prolonged tubular injury or stasis, but have other causes, as shown below.

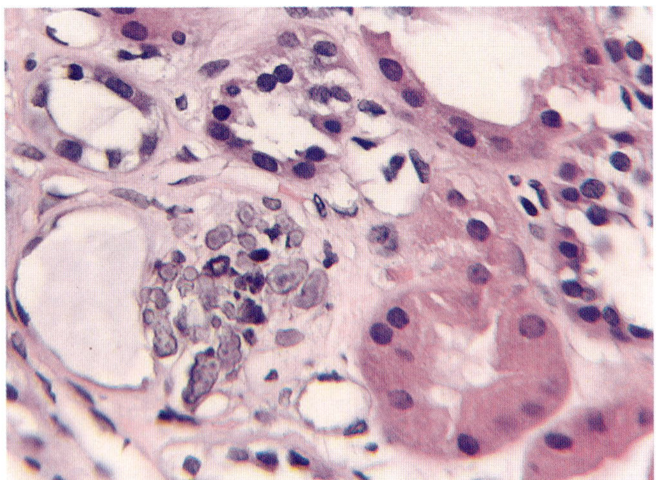

Fig. 76: Nephrocalcinosis. High power image of calcifications, in this case attributed to calcineurin inhibitor toxicity.

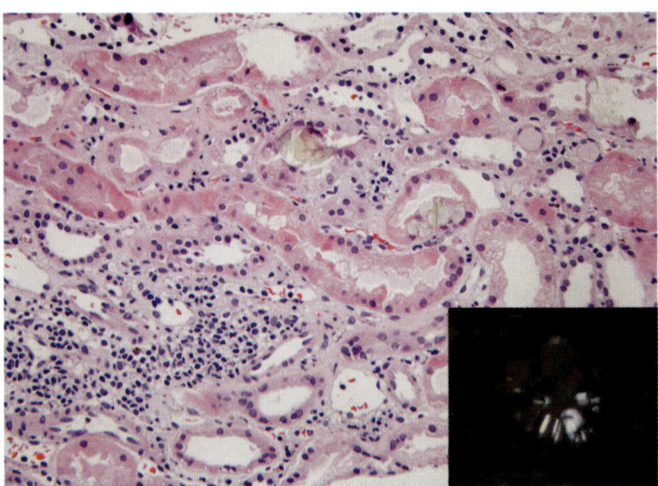

Fig. 77: Oxalate nephropathy. Numerous translucent fan-shaped calcium oxalate crystals are present in tubules (upper central & right); they are brightly birefringent in polarized light (inset). There is acute tubular injury, focal interstitial inflammation (left) without tubulitis, and interstitial fibrosis. Oxalate is excreted by allografts early post-transplantation; however, oxalate crystals are injurious to renal tubules and when seen on biopsy, should prompt further clinical investigation.

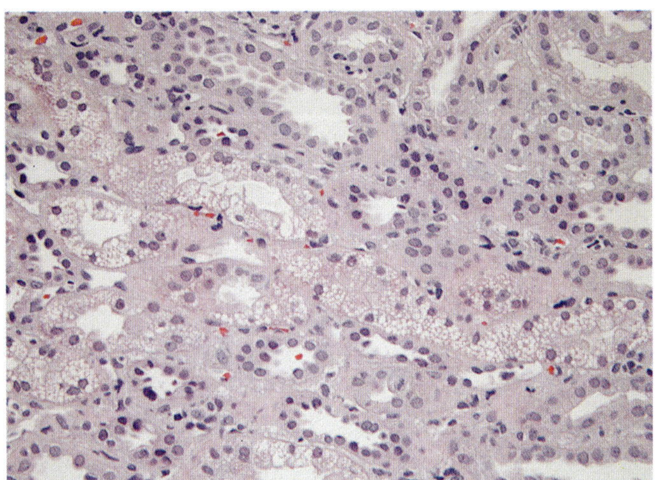

Fig. 78: Isometric vacuolization of tubules. Isometric vacuolization describes small clear vacuoles of uniform size within tubular epithelial cells. Focal isometric vacuolization is associated with calcineurin inhibitor toxicity, but it is not specific. More diffuse vacuolization of tubules is seen with contrast agents used for imaging studies, osmotic agents (some of which may be components of therapeutic agents including IVIg), etc. Hematoxylin and eosin (H&E) stain.

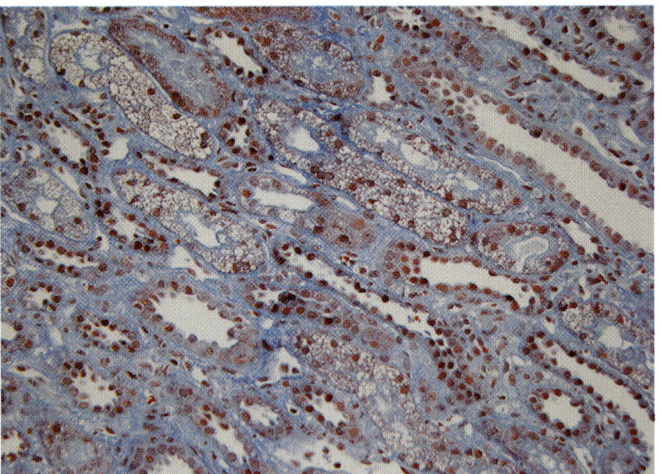

Fig. 79: Isometric vacuolization of tubules. Trichrome stain.

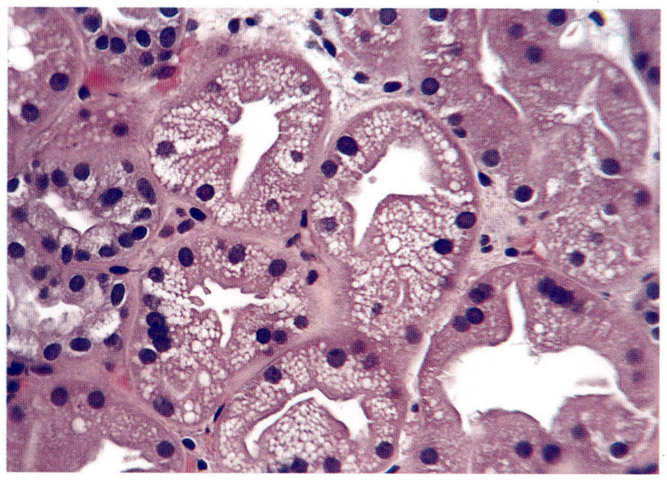

Fig. 80: Isometric vacuolization of tubules. High power, hematoxylin and eosin (H&E) stain.

ALLOGRAFT INFECTIONS (FIGS. 81 TO 99)

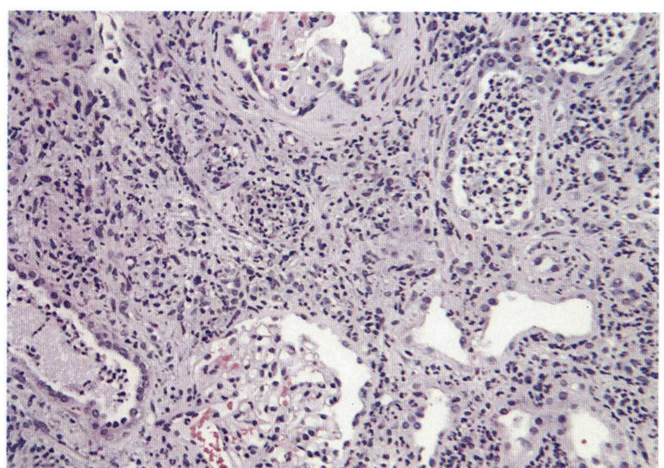

Fig. 81: Pyelonephritis. This is an example of pyelonephritis with a brisk interstitial and intratubular neutrophilic infiltrate, including microabscess formation. Hematoxylin and eosin (H&E) stain.

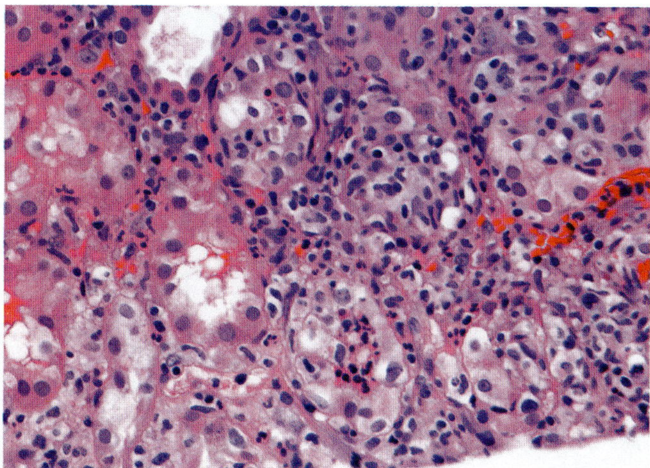

Fig. 82: Pyelonephritis. Higher power image of neutrophilic infiltrates. Hematoxylin and eosin (H&E) stain.

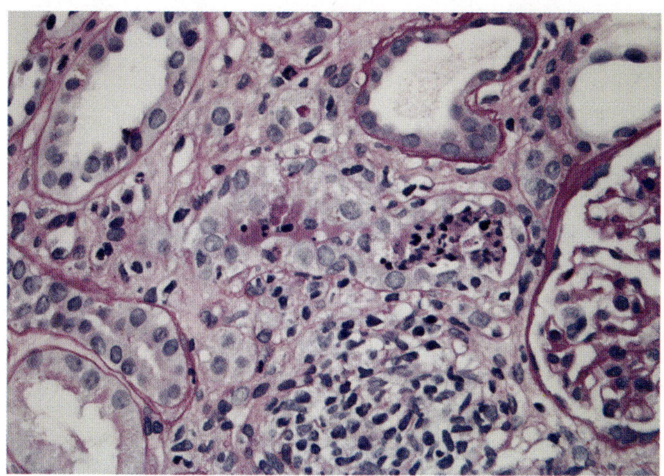

Fig. 83: White blood cell cast. A white blood cell cast is shown in the tubule at center, composed of neutrophils and neutrophilic debris. Lymphocytic interstitial inflammation is seen below. The differential diagnosis includes pyelonephritis, other infections, as well as reflux. Periodic acid Schiff (PAS) stain.

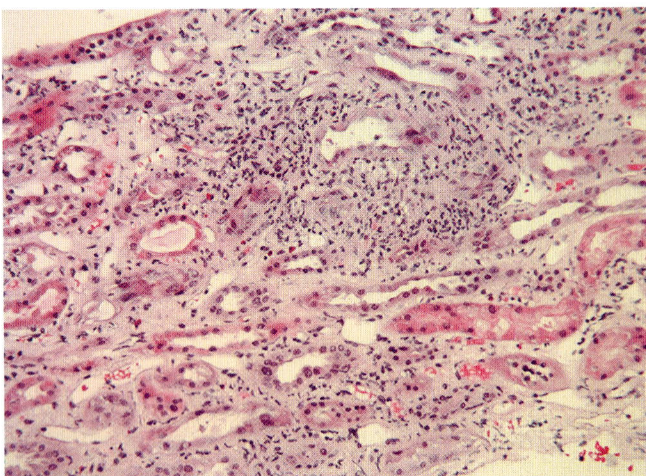

Fig. 84: Polyoma virus nephropathy. Infection by polyoma virus, usually BK polyoma virus, is an important cause of graft dysfunction. At low power, the interstitial inflammation and tubulitis may mimic acute rejection. However, careful examination reveals viral cytopathic change in the form of nuclear viral inclusions, illustrated in subsequent Figures 84 to 93. A high index of suspicion is needed for diagnosis of polyoma virus in allograft biopsies, and can be confirmed by immunostaining. Hematoxylin and eosin (H&E) stain is shown here.

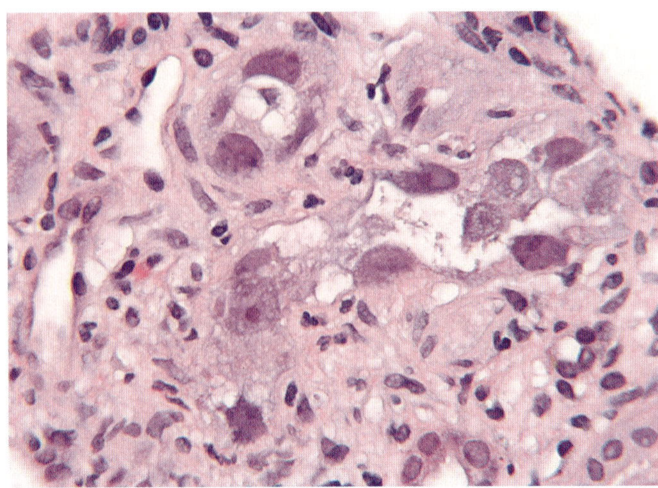

Fig. 85: Polyoma virus nephropathy. High-power view of smudgy nuclei/viral inclusions in polyoma viral nephropathy. Hematoxylin and eosin (H&E) stain.

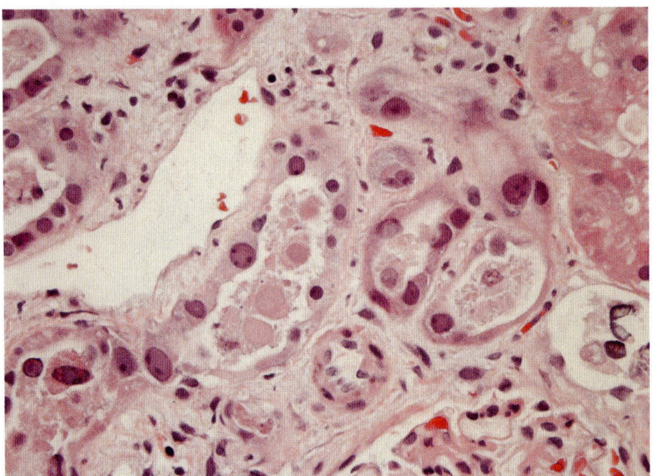

Fig. 86: Polyoma virus nephropathy. All of the larger, paler nuclei contain virus, although the inclusions are not well demarcated. In addition, virally infected non-viable cells are seen as the light pink material sloughed into the lumen of the central tubule. This is a case of JC viral infection, with histologic features indistinguishable from BK. Hematoxylin and eosin (H&E) stain.

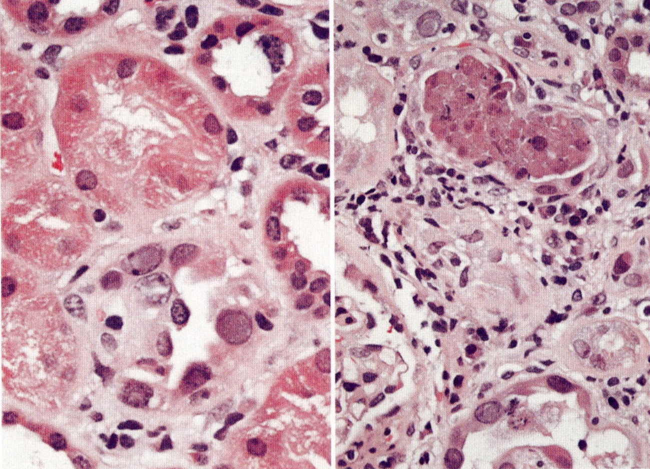

Fig. 87: Polyoma virus nephropathy. Left: Compare the virally infected nuclei, with punched out nuclear pale inclusions in the bottom tubular cross section, to the uninfected proximal tubular cell nuclei in the upper tubule. Right: Numerous viral inclusions are present, along with a cast at top, composed of dead virally infected cells, and an interstitial inflammatory cell infiltrate.

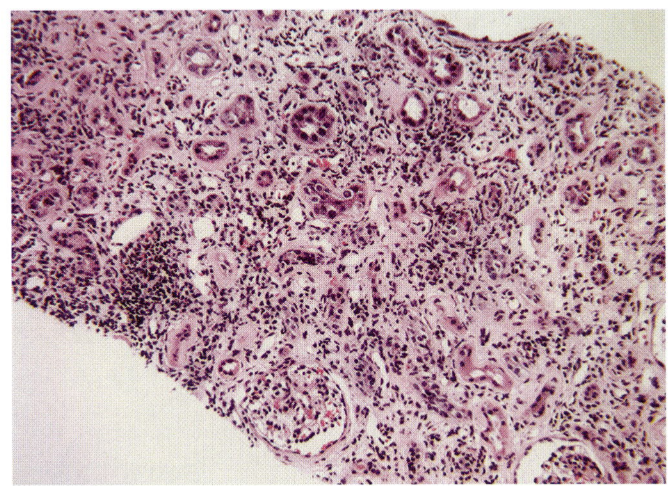

Fig. 88: Polyoma virus nephropathy. Advanced polyoma virus nephropathy with extensive tubular atrophy, interstitial fibrosis, along with ongoing inflammation and viral inclusions. Various grading systems for polyoma viral nephropathy have been proposed, all of which incorporate extensive interstitial fibrosis (irreversible) as a predictor of poor clinical outcome.[12]

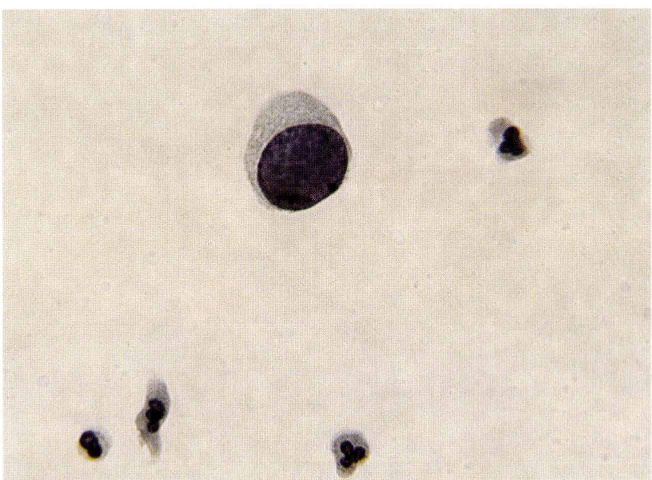

Fig. 89: Polyoma virus nephropathy, decoy cell. Polyoma virus infected cells shed into the urine can be seen as "decoy" cells. On urine cytology, these may mimic a neoplastic process due to their marked nuclear atypia and high nuclear:cytoplasmic ratio. The nuclei are large and glassy, as shown here on this Papanicolaou stain. A few acute inflammatory cells (neutrophils) are also seen.

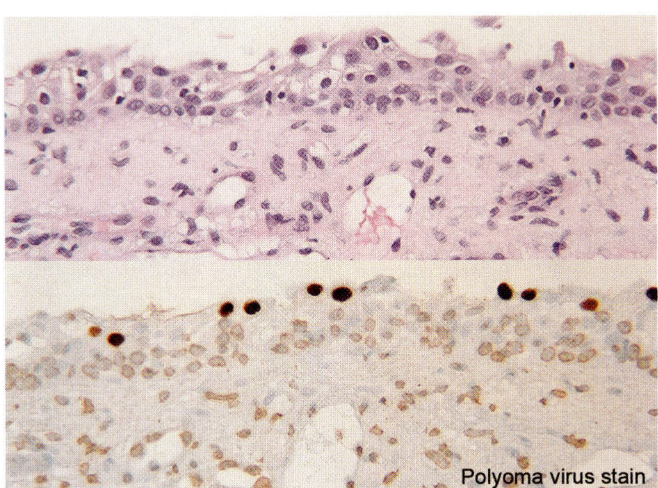

Fig. 90: Polyoma virus in urothelium. The upper hematoxylin and eosin (H&E) stain shows rare superficial urothelial cells with mildly atypical nuclei. The polyoma virus immunostain in the lower panel highlights several positive nuclei from the same case. Brown stain is positive against the blue counterstained background.

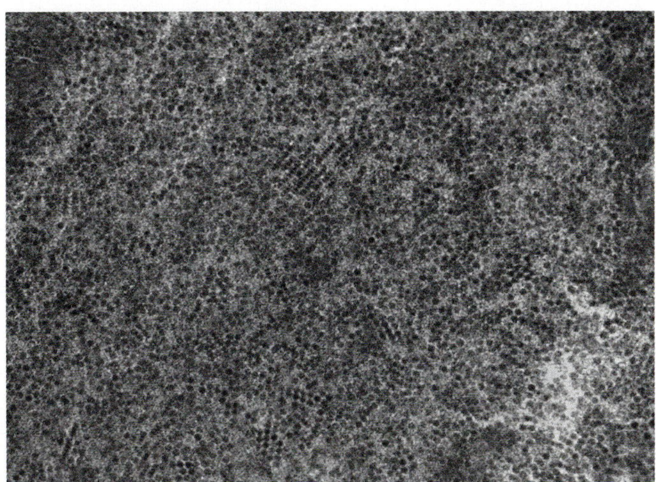

Fig. 91: Polyoma virus nephropathy, electron microscopy. Viral particles (30-50 nm) aligned in a characteristic lattice can be seen in polyoma virus infected nuclei by electron microscopy. Image courtesy of Mike Rudine and Robert Kayton, Oregon Health and Science University.

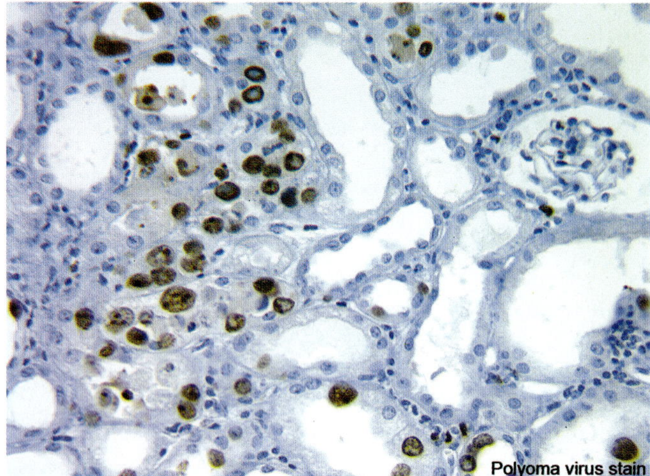

Fig. 92: Polyoma virus nephropathy, immunostain. Immunostaining for polyoma virus highlights virally infected nuclei and is important in confirming the specific diagnosis. Many laboratories utilize antibodies to SV40 (simian virus) polyoma virus that cross react with both BK and JC polyomavirus. Brown stain is positive against the blue counterstained background.

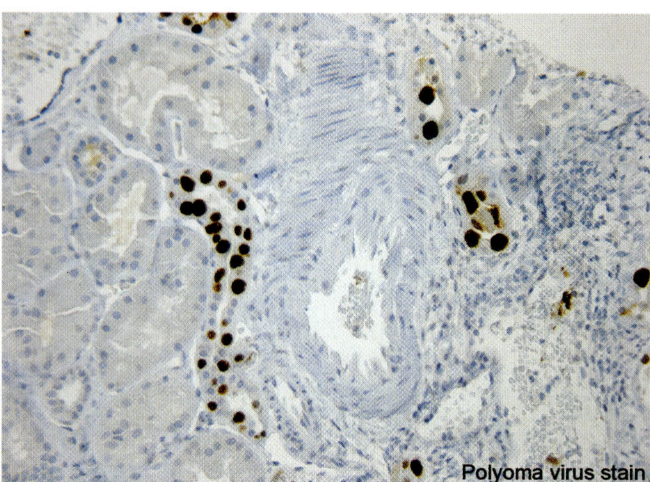

Fig. 93: Polyoma virus nephropathy, immunostain. This polyoma virus immunostain highlights JC virus in the nuclei of renal tubular epithelial cells, same case as Figure 86. Brown stain is positive against the blue counterstained background.

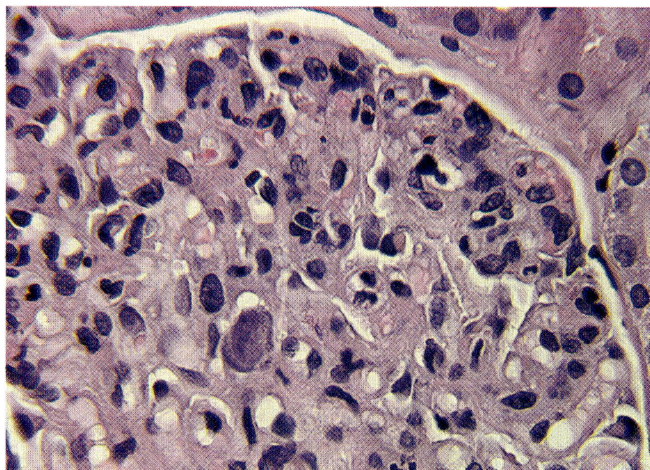

Fig. 94: Cytomegalovirus (CMV) nephropathy. CMV virus preferentially infects endothelial cells. In this example, CMV virus is seen in glomerular endothelium. There is a large light purple "smudged" nuclear inclusion, along with surrounding cytoplasmic granules, in the center of the image. Otherwise, the glomerulus is hypercellular. Hematoxylin and eosin (H&E) stain.

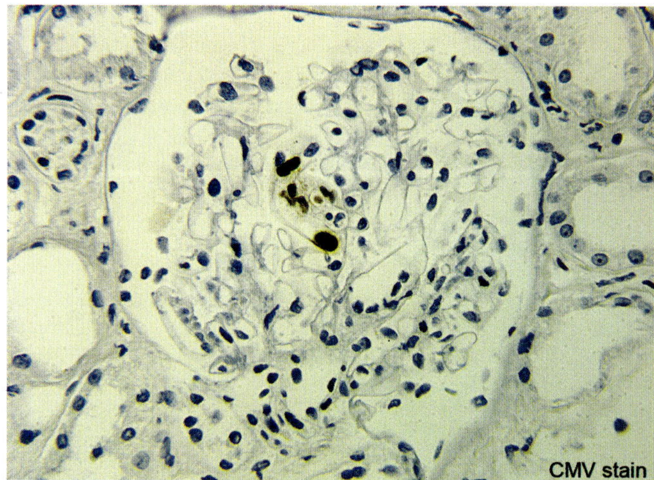

Fig. 95: Cytomegalovirus (CMV) nephropathy. CMV virus can also be demonstrated by a specific immunostain, as shown in this glomerulus at lower power. Brown stain is positive against the blue counterstained background.

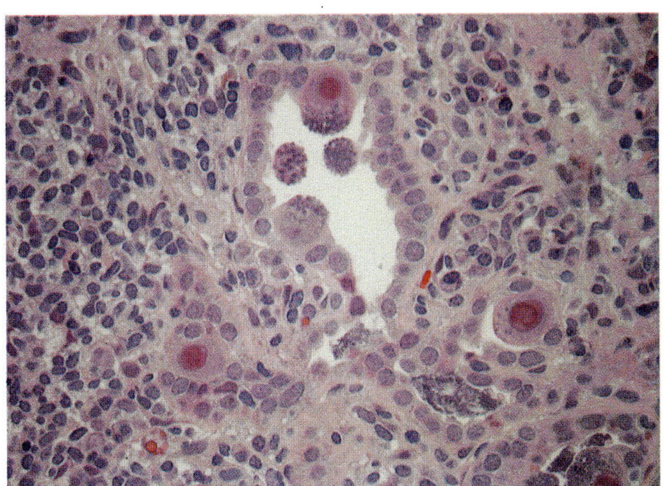

Fig. 96: Cytomegalovirus (CMV) nephropathy. In this case, CMV virus is seen in renal tubular epithelial cells. The bright red nuclear and purple granular cytoplasmic inclusions are readily apparent. In this case, CMV virus was also confirmed by immunostaining (not shown).

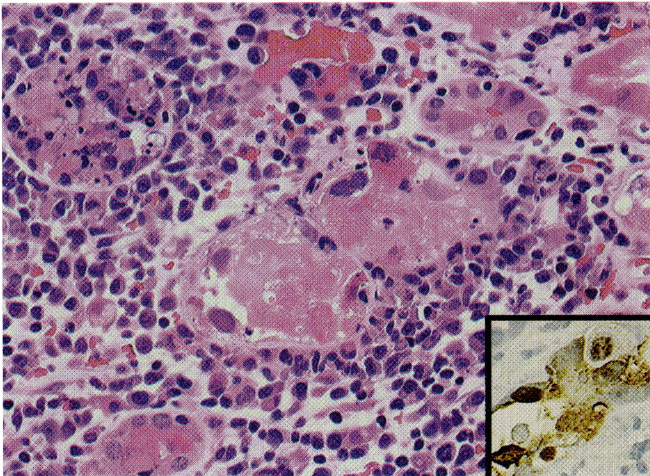

Fig. 97: Adenovirus. The tubules in center contain several viral inclusions on hematoxylin and eosin (H&E) stain. There is tubular injury with cellular and viral debris, and a brisk mononuclear cell infiltrate.[13] An adenovirus IHC stain is shown in the inset (IHC: brown positive against a blue counterstain). Images courtesy of Dr. Erika R. Bracamonte, University of Arizona Medical Center.

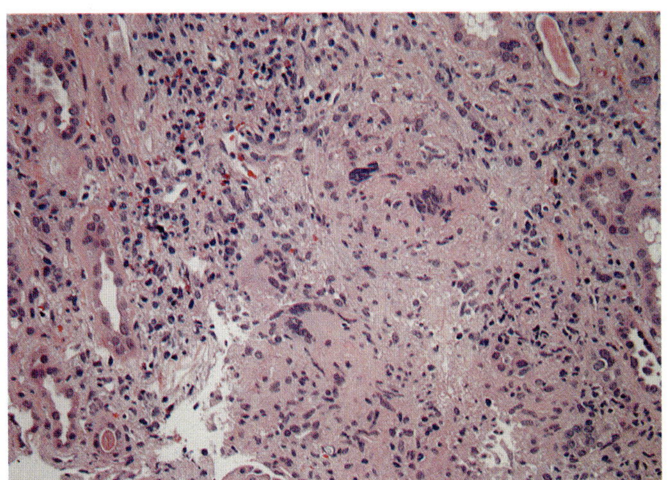

Fig. 98: Granulomatous interstitial nephritis, fungal infection. Granulomatous inflammation is seen with prominent multinucleated giant cells, center. Lymphocytic and eosinophilic inflammation is seen at left. Fungal, mycobacterial, viral and other infections must be ruled out when granulomas are seen in renal allograft biopsy; however, granulomatous inflammation may also been seen in other settings including rejections (see Fig. 16).[10,2] Hematoxylin and eosin (H&E) stain.

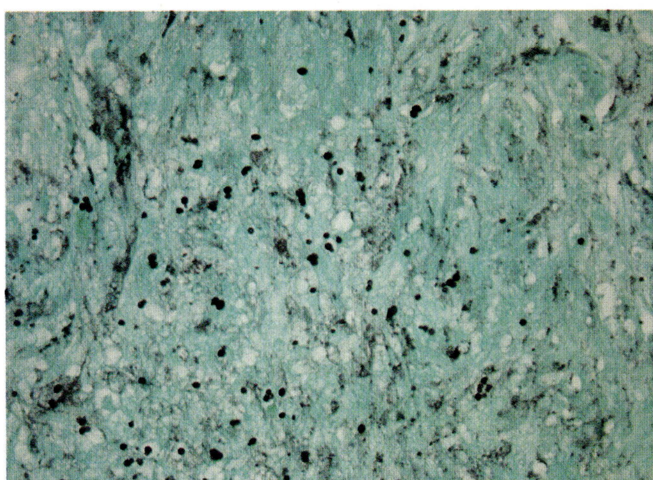

Fig. 99: Granulomatous interstitial nephritis, fungal infection. A Grocott Methenamine silver (GMS) stain highlight small yeast forms in the granulomas seen in Figure 98; histoplasma antigen was detected in urine.

CHRONIC ALLOGRAFT DAMAGE (FIGS. 100 TO 114)

Allograft injury from a variety of insults can result in permanent damage, and it may be difficult to determine

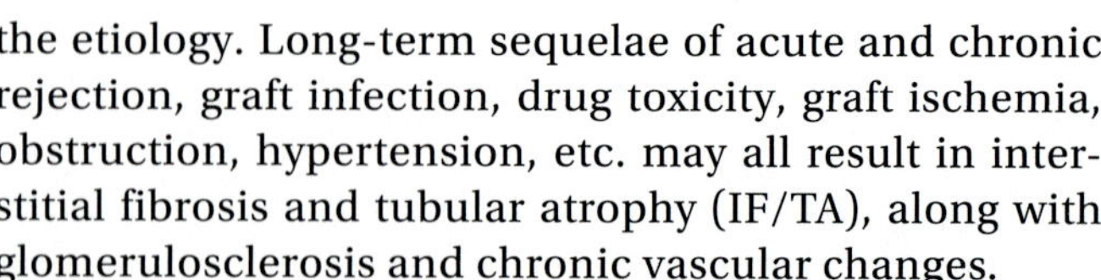

the etiology. Long-term sequelae of acute and chronic rejection, graft infection, drug toxicity, graft ischemia, obstruction, hypertension, etc. may all result in interstitial fibrosis and tubular atrophy (IF/TA), along with glomerulosclerosis and chronic vascular changes.

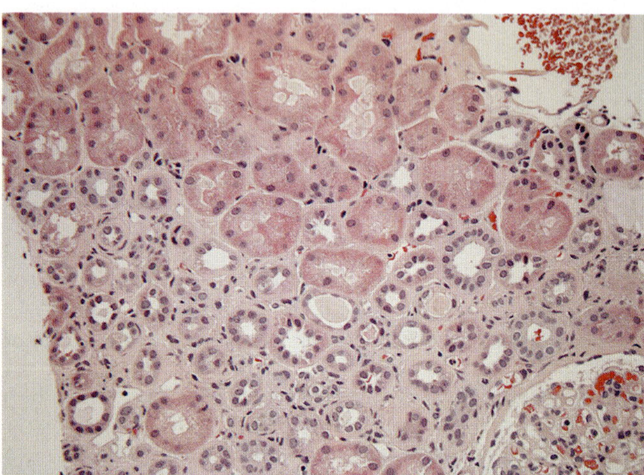

Fig. 100: Tubular atrophy and interstitial fibrosis. On hematoxylin and eosin (H&E) stain, normal cortical tubules are back-to-back with minimal intervening fibrous tissue, as in the upper portion of this H&E image. Tubular atrophy is seen as tubules with smaller cross section, as at bottom. Tubules are also more widely spaced due to interstitial fibrosis.

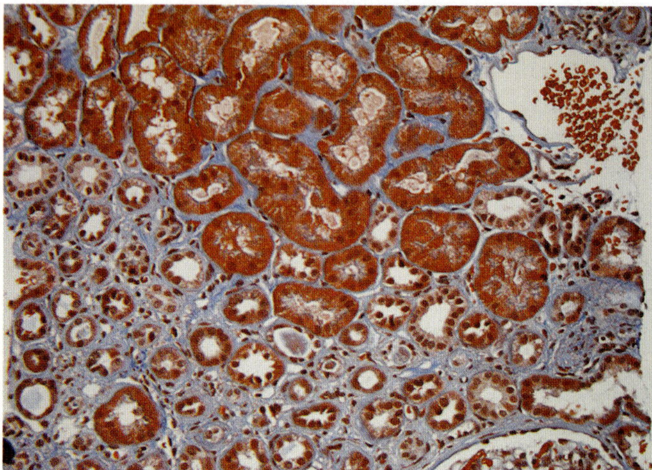

Fig. 101: Tubular atrophy and interstitial fibrosis. A trichrome stain of the same field as Figure 100 highlights the interstitial fibrosis in blue.

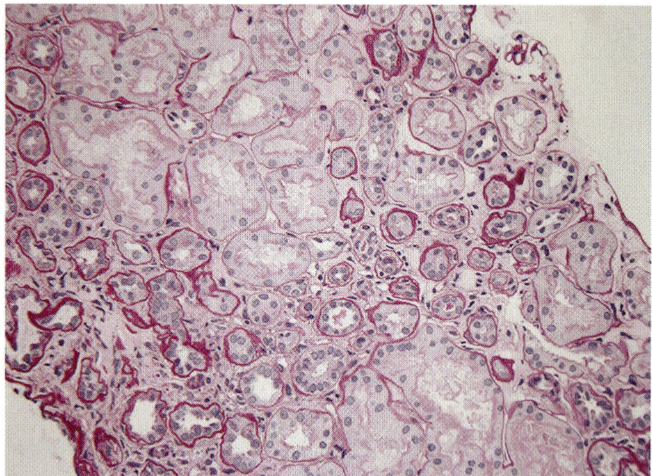

Fig. 102: Tubular atrophy and interstitial fibrosis. On periodic acid Schiff (PAS) stain, atrophic tubules have thick, wrinkled basement membranes, which stain dark magenta. The increased fibrous tissue between tubules also stands out as pale pink.

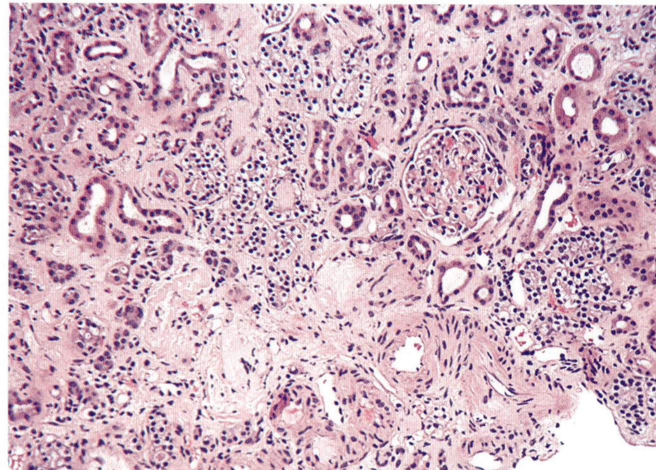

Fig. 103: Diffuse tubular atrophy and interstitial fibrosis. Hematoxylin and eosin (H&E) stain.

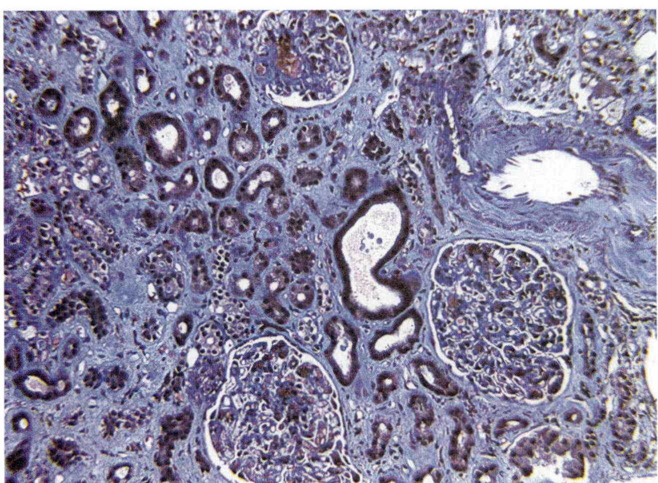

Fig. 104: Diffuse tubular atrophy and interstitial fibrosis. The trichrome stain on the same biopsy specimen as Figure103 highlights extensive fibrosis between tubules (blue). Further, there is fibrous intimal hyperplasia of the artery in the upper right.

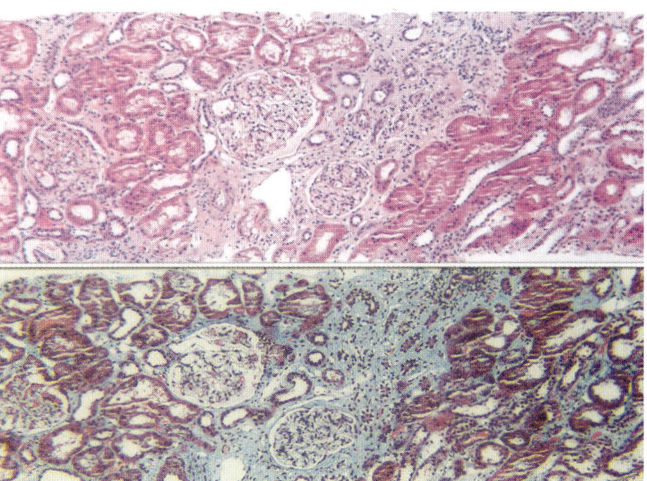

Fig. 105: Striped atrophy. This image shows so-called "striped" atrophy, where a zone of atrophic cortex alternates with zones of nearly normal cortex. The atrophic tubules are shrunken, and widely separated by fibrous tissue, blue on the lower trichrome stain. This finding has been associated with calcineurin inhibitor toxicity, but is not specific, as it can be seen in chronic graft injury from other causes.

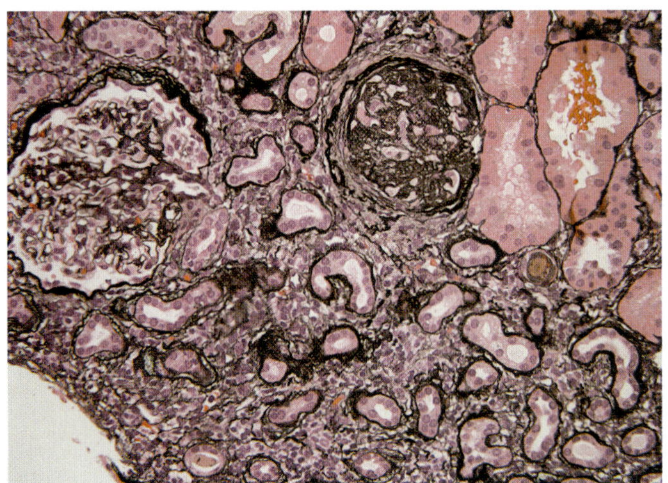

Fig. 106: Global glomerulosclerosis interstitial fibrosis and tubular atrophy. Jones silver stain shows a globally sclerotic glomerulus at center. The tubules to the upper right are healthy, whereas the bottom part of the field shows tubular atrophy with interstitial fibrosis and a mononuclear cell infiltrate. The glomerulus at left is slightly ischemic, but otherwise normal.

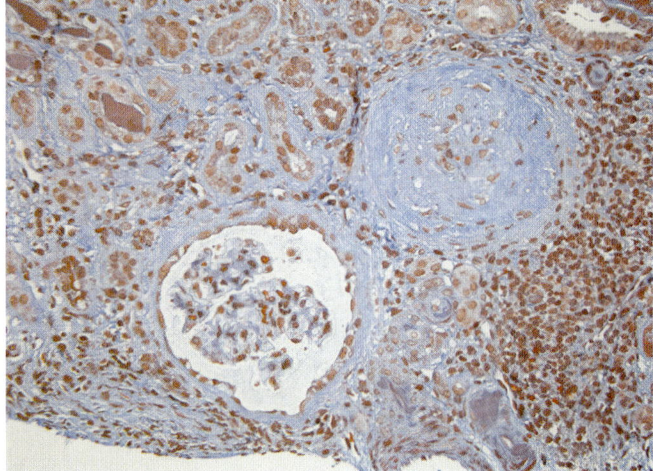

Fig. 107: Global glomerulosclerosis, interstitial fibrosis and tubular atrophy. The globally sclerotic glomerulus on this trichrome stain appears as a dense blue ball. The glomerulus below and to the left is shrunken and ischemic, and does not fill Bowman's space. There is diffuse interstitial fibrosis and tubular atrophy in the remainder of the field. The small arteries/arterioles at lower right contain reddish hyaline material, seen better in Figure 108.

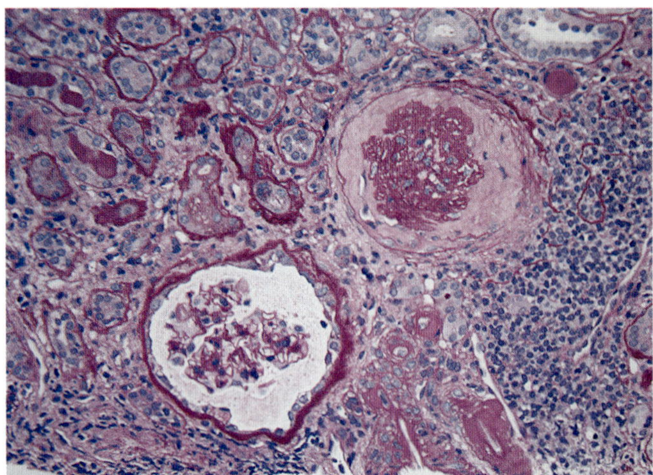

Fig. 108: Global glomerulosclerosis interstitial fibrosis and tubular atrophy with inflammation. Periodic acid Schiff (PAS) stain on the same field as Figure 107 shows global glomerulosclerosis. In addition, hyaline change in the small vessels at bottom right is readily apparent as bright magenta. Atrophic tubules stand out with thick wavy basement membranes. Mononuclear cells infiltrate the interstitium, as well as atrophic tubules (tubulitis). Tubulitis in zones of atrophic tubules is not currently considered an indication of active cellular rejection, however, scoring of total graft inflammation may have significance and is under investigation.[4]

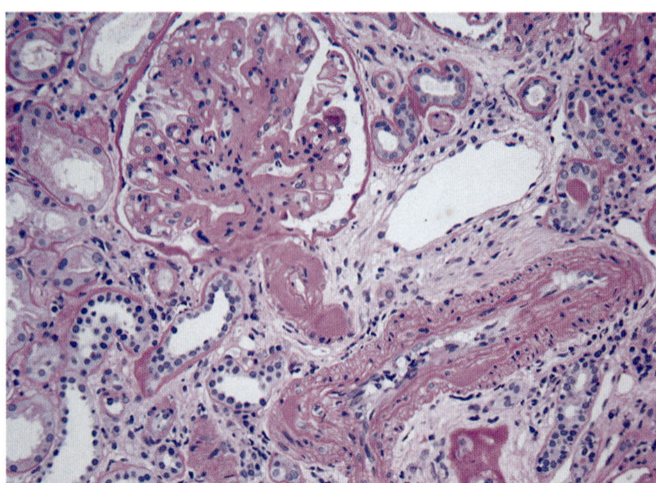

Fig. 109: Massive arteriolar hyaline. The arteriole associated with the glomerulus is extensively involved by hyaline, as is the small artery at lower right. The artery contains intimal inflammatory cells in addition (endothelialitis) and is thus diagnostic of Banff type II rejection. The glomerulus shows mesangial sclerosis, as well as capillary wall reduplication, likely due to chronic rejection (allograft glomerulopathy). While hyaline in the media of arterioles is associated with calcineurin inhibitor toxicity, arteriolar hyaline is also commonly seen in diabetic nephropathy, hypertension, etc., although the hyaline is said to be more intimal in these situations. Periodic acid Schiff (PAS) stain.

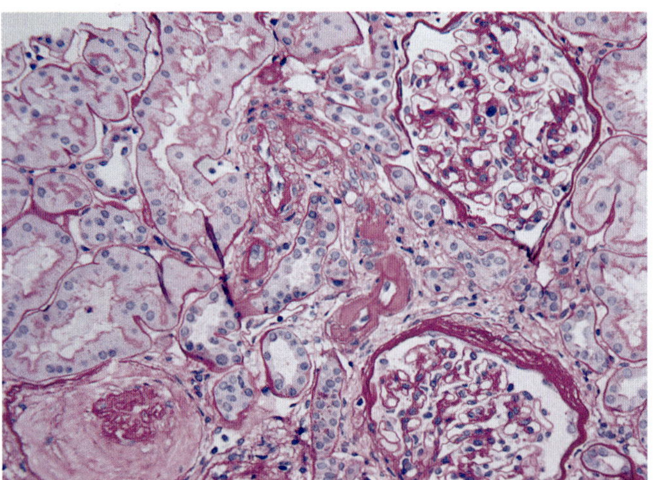

Fig. 110: Arteriolar hyalinosis. Several arterioles in the center contain circumferential hyaline. The glomerulus at lower right shows ischemic change in that the glomerulus is shrunken and there is periglomerular fibrosis. The glomerulus at lower left is globally sclerotic. Two different hyalinosis grading schemes have been proposed by Banff (Table 3).[1] Periodic acid Schiff (PAS) stain.

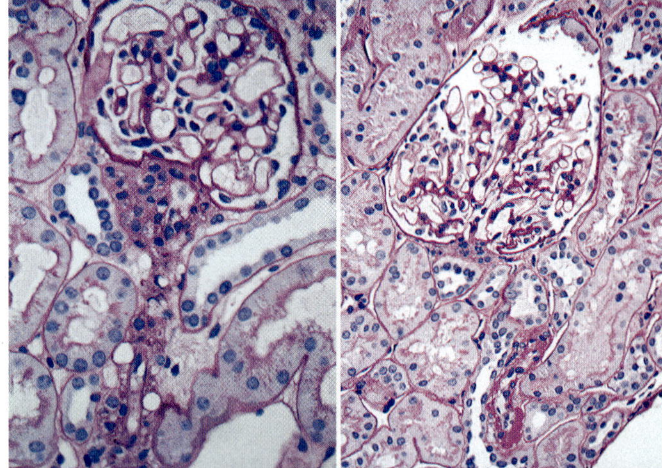

Fig. 111: Arteriolar medial vacuolization and hyaline. Vacuolization and injury of arteriolar myocytes is thought to be an early effect of calcineurin inhibitors, leading to arteriolar medial hyalinosis. The left panel shows large clear vacuoles in the arteriole leading to the glomerulus. Also, the juxtaglomerular apparatus is quite large (immediately below the glomerulus at 6–7 o'clock). At lower power, the right panel shows another glomerulus and arteriole from the same case, with arteriolar hyalinosis. Periodic acid Schiff (PAS) stain.

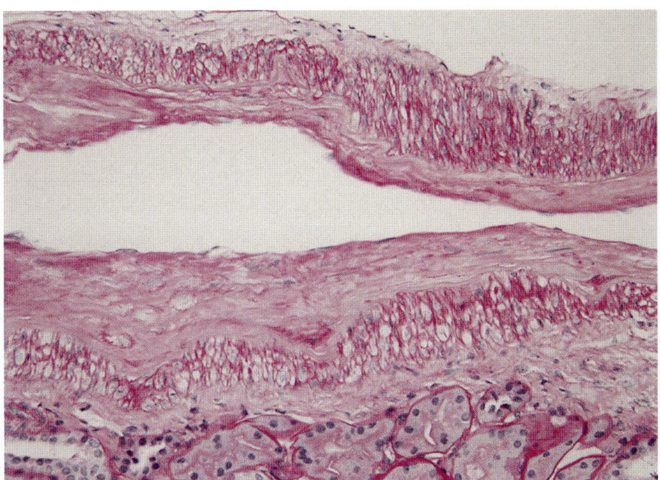

Fig. 112: Arterial fibrous intimal hyperplasia. A longitudinal section of an artery shows demarcation between the medial smooth muscle of the artery and the paucicellular pale fibrous tissue that narrows the lumen. Since the intimal hyperplasia is eccentric and paucicellular, it is less likely to be related to chronic rejection. Examples of chronic vascular lesions characteristic of rejection are presented in section "Allograft Rejection". Periodic acid Schiff (PAS) stain.

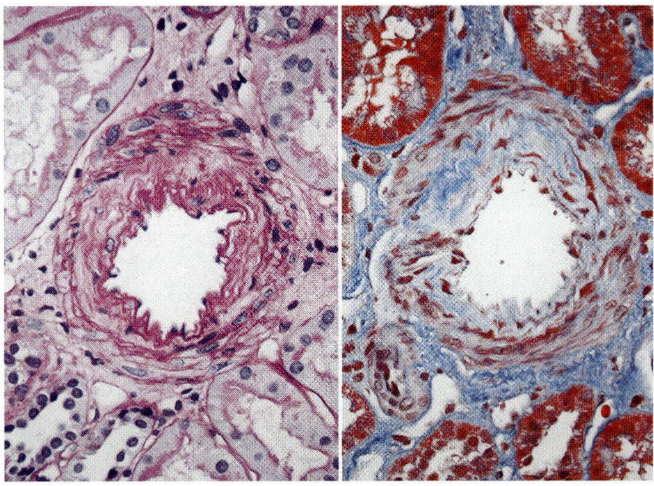

Fig. 113: Donor vascular disease. This fibrous intimal hyperplasia is a result of donor vascular disease (arteriosclerosis). Left: Periodic acid Schiff (PAS) stain, right: trichrome stain.

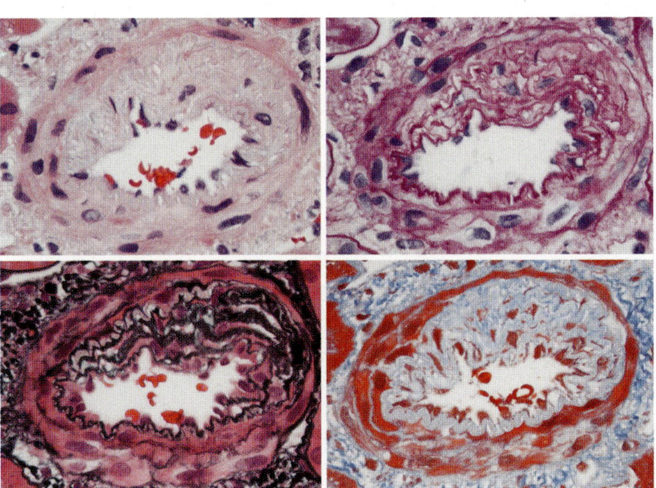

Fig. 114: Eccentric intimal fibrosis. Abundant elastic fibers in the intimal proliferation are generally seen in arteriosclerosis and not in vascular changes due to chronic rejection. These are pale on hematoxylin and eosin (H&E) (upper left), and stain black on silver, elastic, EVG or VVG stains (lower left). Periodic acid Schiff (PAS) stain (upper right) and trichrome (lower right) also highlight the intimal multilamellation.

GLOMERULAR PROCESSES (FIGS. 115 TO 134)

Glomeruli in allografts may be affected by immune-mediated processes, or by recurrent or de novo glomerular disease.[1,14,15]

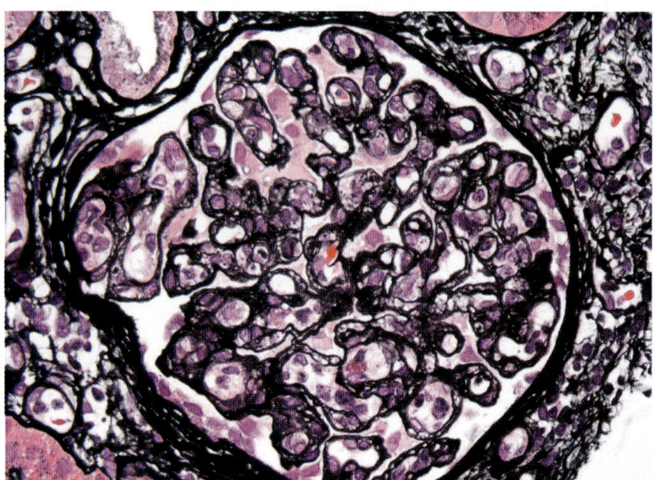

Fig. 115: Transplant glomerulopathy. Chronic antibody or cell-mediated rejection may cause glomerular injury. Most typically, glomerular endothelial injury causes new basement membrane formation, resulting in so-called "duplication" of glomerular basement membranes, imparting a "double-contour" or "tram-track" appearance on silver-stains, as is shown here. Although this appearance is characteristic of allograft glomerulopathy, it is also seen in membranoproliferative glomerulonephritis (MPGN) and chronic thrombotic microangiopathy. MPGN may be distinguished by immunofluorescence, as it is immune-complex mediated.

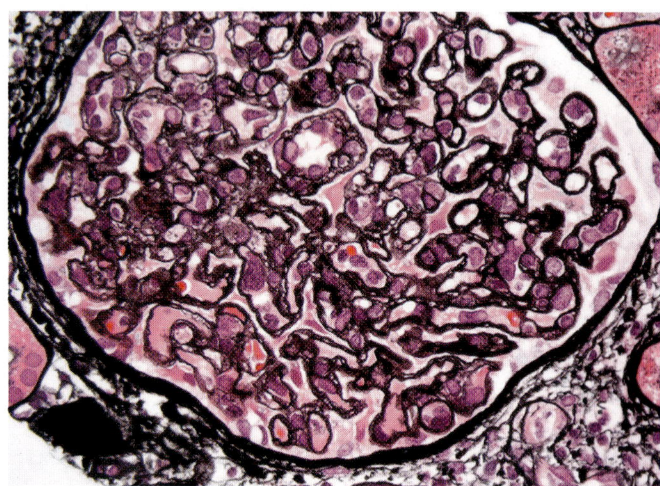

Fig. 116: Transplant glomerulopathy. This silver stain shows multilayer glomerular basement membranes, some with cell nuclei in between layers. Additional examples are in section "Allograft Rejection", chronic rejection.

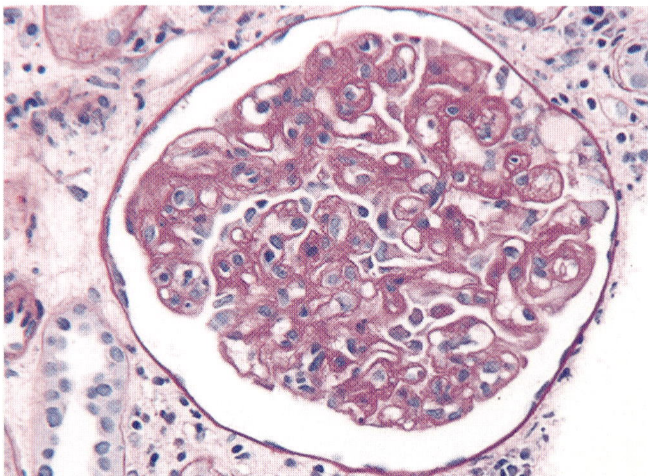

Fig. 117: Transplant glomerulopathy. On periodic acid Schiff (PAS) stain, thick, multilayered capillary loops are apparent. There is also increased mesangial matrix, another feature of allograft glomerulopathy.

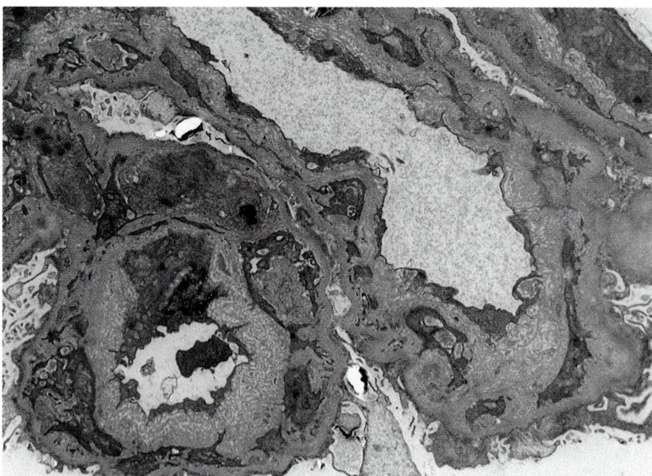

Fig. 118: Transplant glomerulopathy, electron microscopy. Two glomerular capillary loops are shown. Each has an outer layer of (original) glomerular basement membrane, and then cell cytoplasm, and multiple layers of loose new basement membrane lined by injured, non-fenestrated endothelial cells.

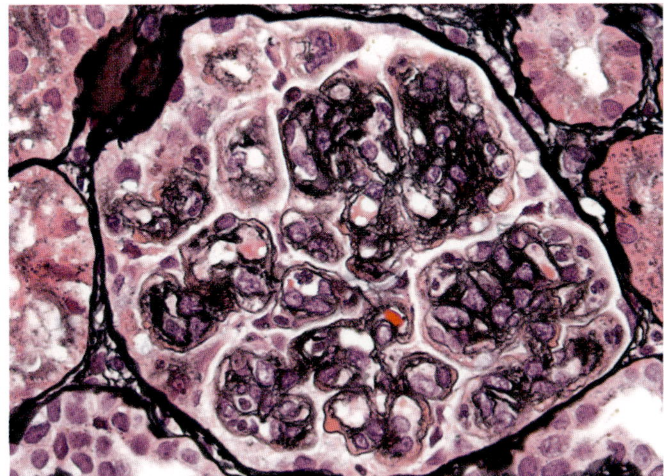

Fig. 119: Membranoproliferative glomerulonephritis (MPGN). This allograft biopsy showed glomeruli with prominent glomerular basement membrane duplication. However, this is an example of recurrent MPGN. The pink material between basement membrane layers represents mostly immune deposits, and was strongly positive on immunofluorescence studies.

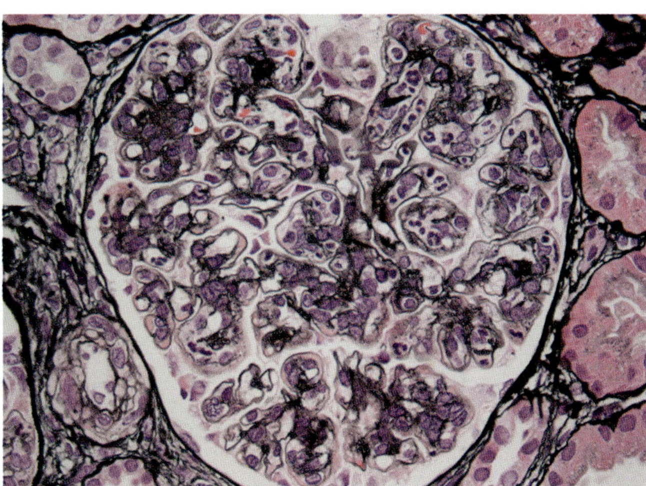

Fig. 120: Membranoproliferative glomerulonephritis (MPGN). This glomerulus has focal "tram-track" basement membranes, but also prominent neutrophilic infiltrates in capillary loops. Besides MPGN, neutrophilic exudates can be seen in lupus, postinfectious glomerulonephritis and antibody-mediated rejection (capillaritis).

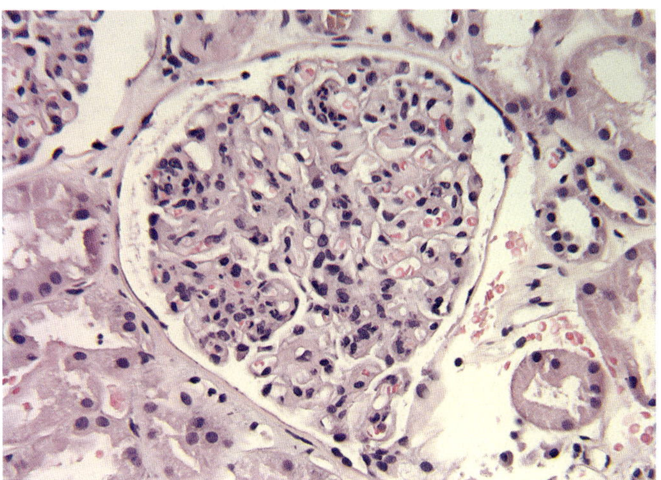

Fig. 121: Postinfectious glomerulonephritis. This glomerulus contains numerous neutrophils, along with segmental endocapillary proliferation (7–10 o'clock).

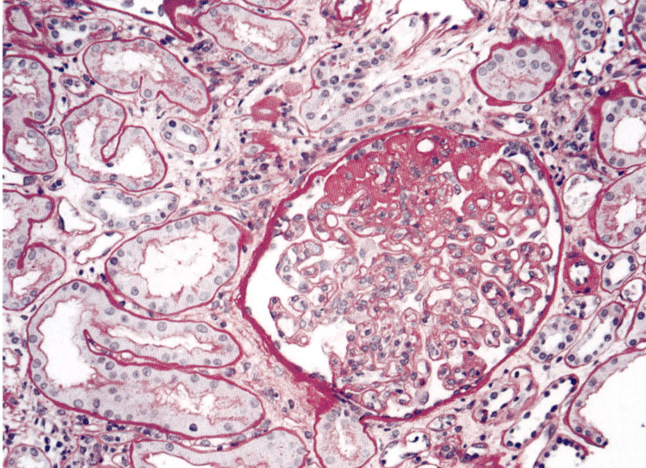

Fig. 122: Transplant glomerulopathy and focal segmental glomerulosclerosis (FSGS). This periodic acid Schiff (PAS) stain demonstrates double-contoured glomerular basement membranes. In addition, there is a large zone of segmental sclerosis, characterized by consolidated bright magenta basement membrane and hyaline (10–12 o'clock). Given the evidence of chronic glomerular damage (glomerulopathy), the FSGS is likely associated with hyperfiltration as an end-result of (mal) adaptive response after graft injury damages a significant fraction of the allograft nephrons.

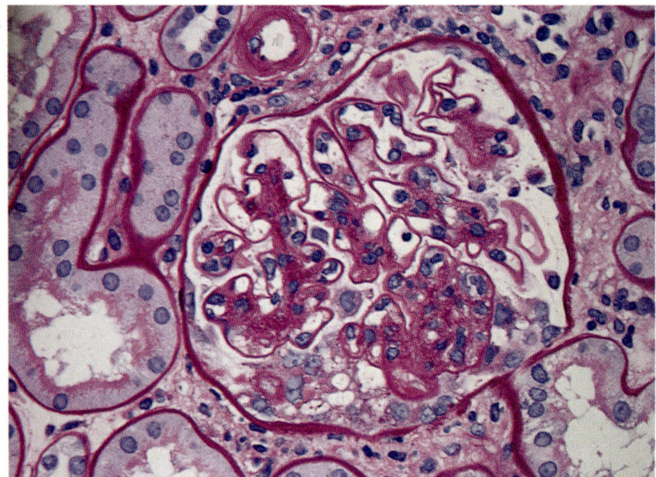

Fig. 123: Focal segmental glomerulosclerosis (FSGS). This FSGS was seen in the setting of diabetes and hyperfiltration, a (mal) adaptive response. FSGS associated with calcineurin inhibitor toxicity might also be considered here, given the arteriolar hyaline seen in upper middle. Periodic acid Schiff (PAS) stain.

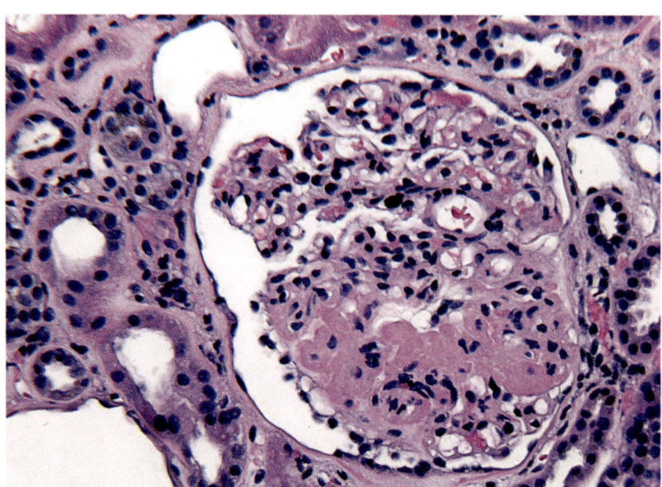

Fig. 124: Focal segmental glomerulosclerosis (FSGS). A segmental scar with hyalinosis in the bottom portion of the glomerulus. Hematoxylin and eosin (H&E) stain.

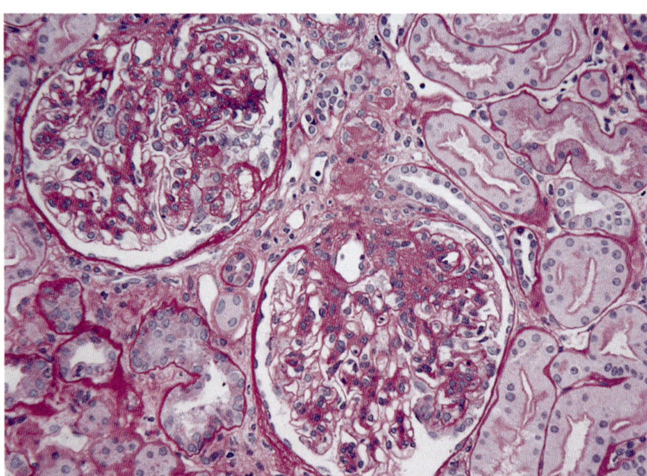

Fig. 125: Focal segmental glomerulosclerosis (FSGS), recurrent. Two glomeruli with lesions of FSGS are seen (both at 4–5 o'clock); these are characterized by prominent, reactive podocytes and less apparent glomerular scarring at this stage. The upper left glomerular tuft has an adhesion to Bowman's capsule. The lower right glomerular arteriole also contains hyaline (arteriole is in center, toward the top of the field). Periodic acid Schiff (PAS) stain.

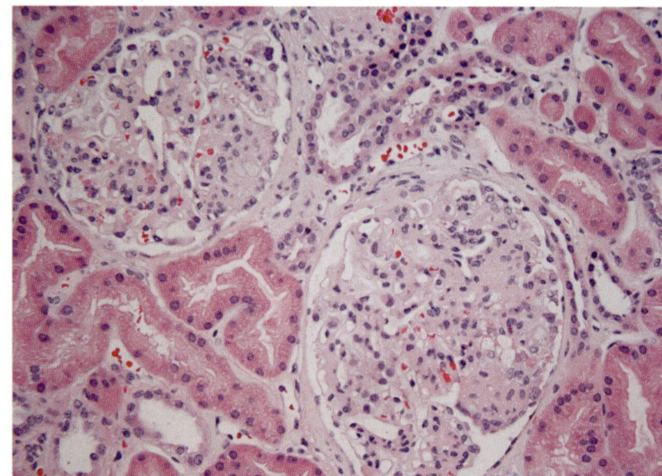

Fig. 126: Focal segmental glomerulosclerosis (FSGS), recurrent. The same two glomeruli as Figure 125. Segmental sclerosis may not be as obvious on hematoxylin and eosin (H&E) stain. Here, the upper left glomerulus contains endocapillary foam cells, consistent with the cellular variant of FSGS.

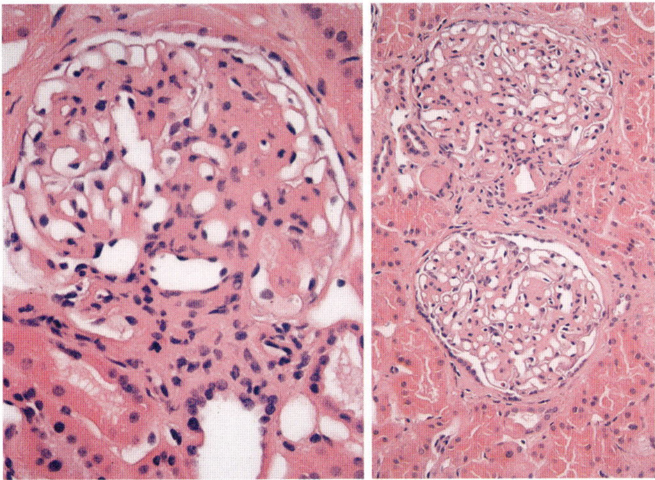

Fig. 127: Diabetic nephropathy, donor-derived. This donor kidney biopsy had evidence of diabetic nephropathy. The glomerulus on the left has mesangial widening by pink basement membrane material, although they do not appear nodular. The glomeruli on the right have diffuse but mild mesangial expansion. There is also arteriolar hyalinosis, as seen at the top glomerular arteriole, and also to the left of that glomerulus (7 o'clock).

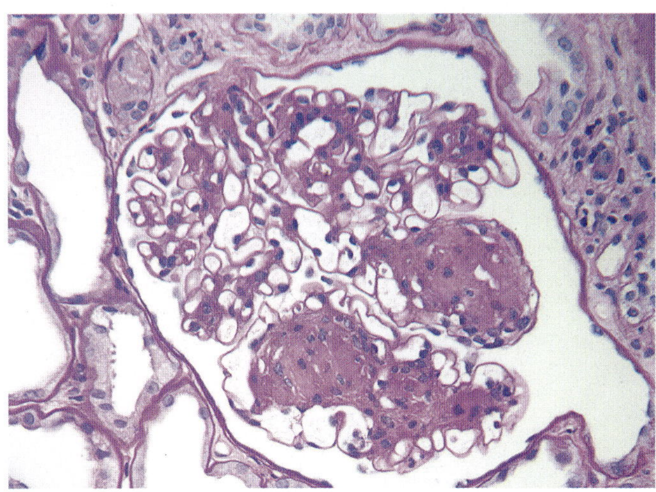

Fig. 128: Diabetic nephropathy. Several eccentric Kimmelstiel-Wilson nodules are shown. Periodic acid Schiff (PAS) stain.

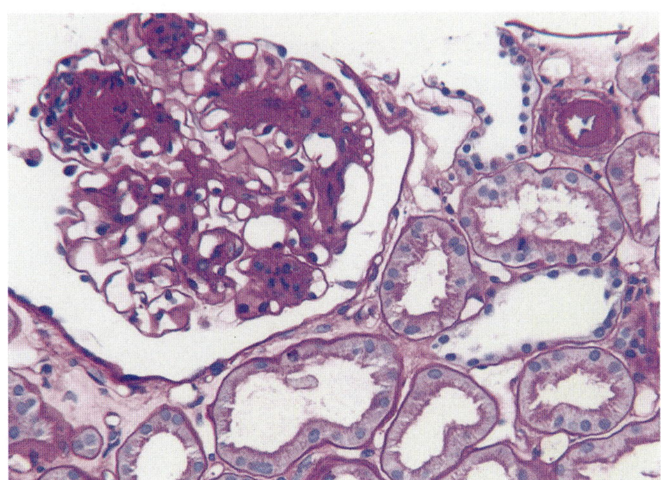

Fig. 129: Diabetic nephropathy. Prominent mesangial nodules are seen in most segments of the glomerulus; arteriolar hyaline is seen at right.

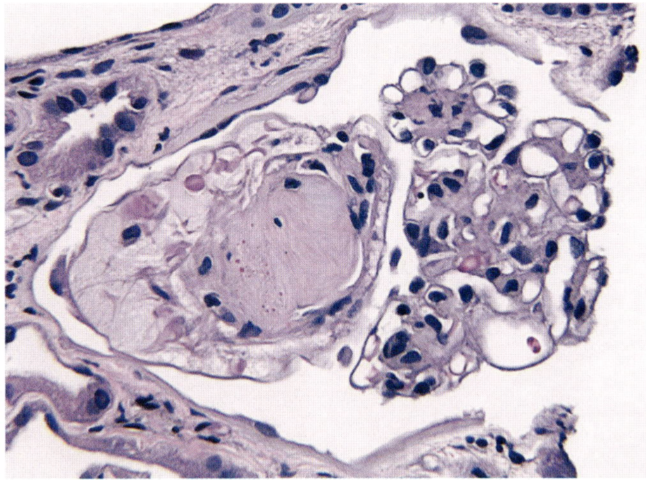

Fig. 130: Diabetic nephropathy. A large microaneurysm is seen surrounding the Kimmelstiel-Wilson nodule in the left side of the glomerulus.

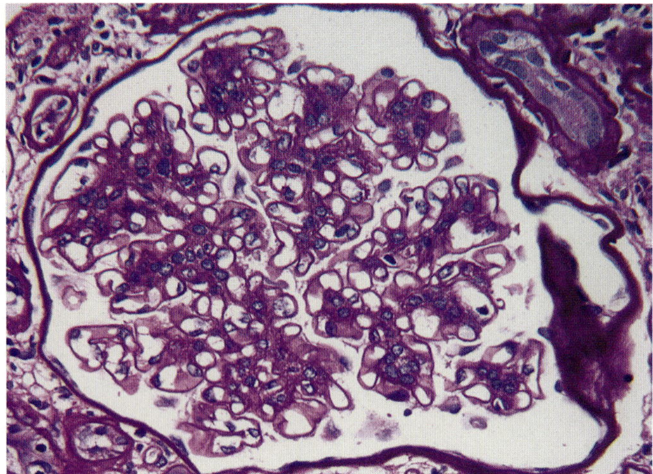

Fig. 131: Mesangioproliferative glomerulonephritis. This glomerulus has increased mesangial matrix, bright magenta on this periodic acid Schiff (PAS) stain, and also has increased mesangial cellularity. This particular example of mesangioproliferative glomerulonephritis is Hepatitis C related, but could also represent recurrent IgA nephritis, diabetic nephropathy, etc.

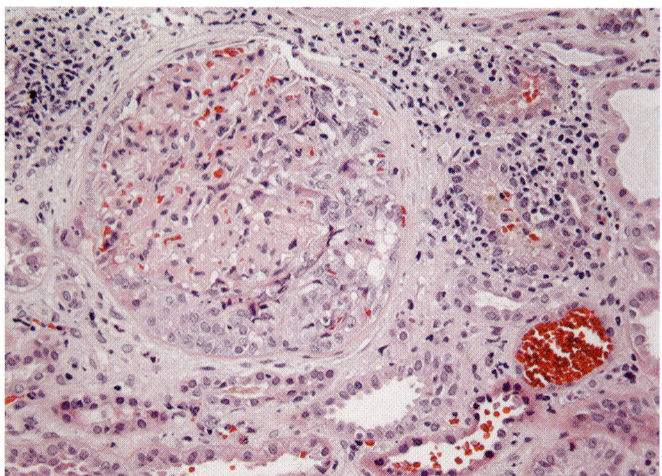

Fig. 132: Recurrent crescentic glomerulonephritis. Recurrence of crescentic glomerulonephritis in an allograft is quite rare, but is very important to recognize. The larger cells at the circumference of the glomerulus (1–7 o'clock) are a crescent compressing the glomerular tuft, and may be more readily apparent on periodic acid Schiff (PAS) and silver stains. The red blood cells and hemosiderin in tubules are also an indication of glomerular bleeding. Hematoxylin and eosin (H&E) stain.

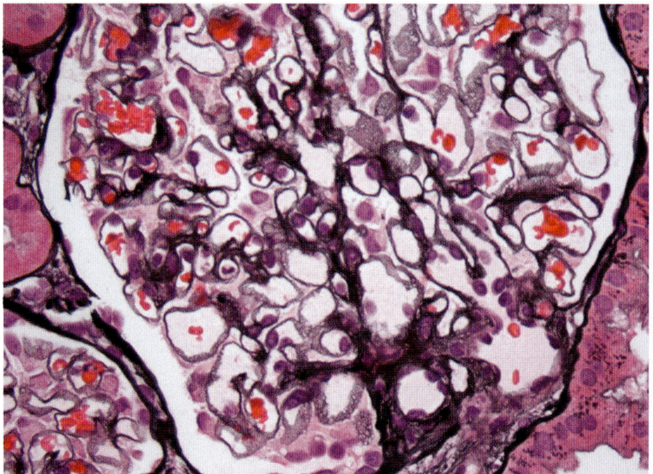

Fig. 133: Recurrent membranous glomerulonephritis. The glomerular basement membranes appear irregular, seemingly containing "bubbles" on silver stain. These are immune complex deposits within the glomerular basement membrane, which do not take up silver stain and thus appear pale. There has been considerable glomerular basement membrane remodeling around the deposits; a more typical appearance of membranous glomerulopathy is simply "spikes" on the outer aspect of the basement membrane.

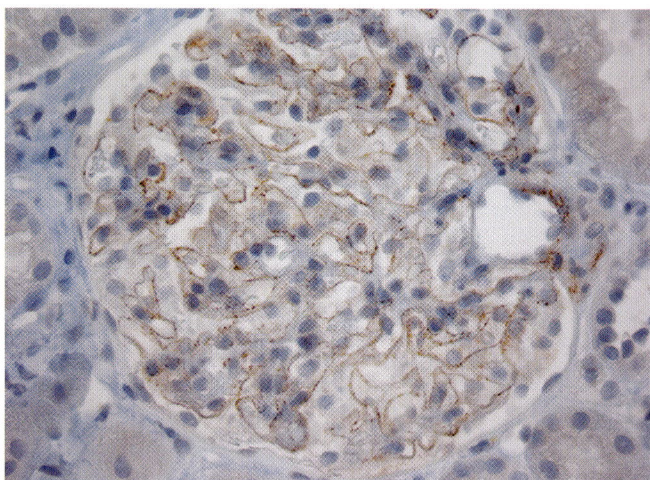

Fig. 134: Recurrent membranous glomerulonephritis, C4d stain. Sparse membranous deposits along capillary loops are highlighted in brown on this C4d immunostain. Aberrant C4d staining in glomeruli on immunohistochemical or immunofluorescence studies can be a clue to immune-complex mediated glomerular disease in the allograft, and prompt further investigation.

OTHER PATHOLOGIC FINDINGS IN RENAL ALLOGRAFTS (FIGS. 135 TO 144)

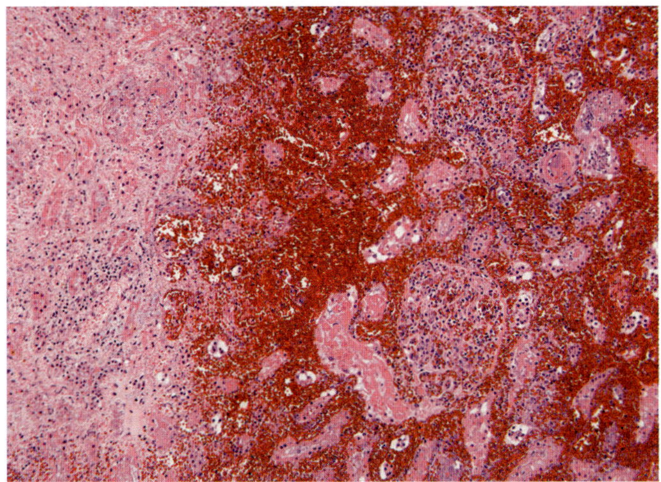

Fig. 135: Hemorrhagic infarct in allograft nephrectomy. The renal parenchyma is extensively hemorrhagic; there are numerous infiltrating inflammatory cells. The renal parenchymal tissue is non-viable.

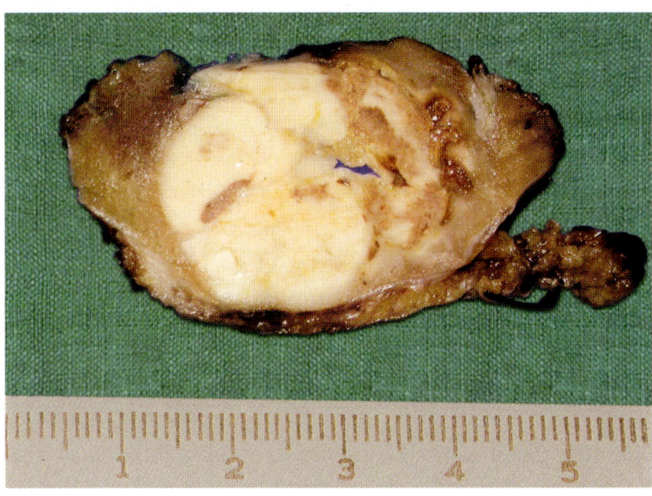

Fig. 136: Renal allograft carcinoma, resected by partial nephrectomy. Gross photo of the sectioned specimen, tumor is white-tan.

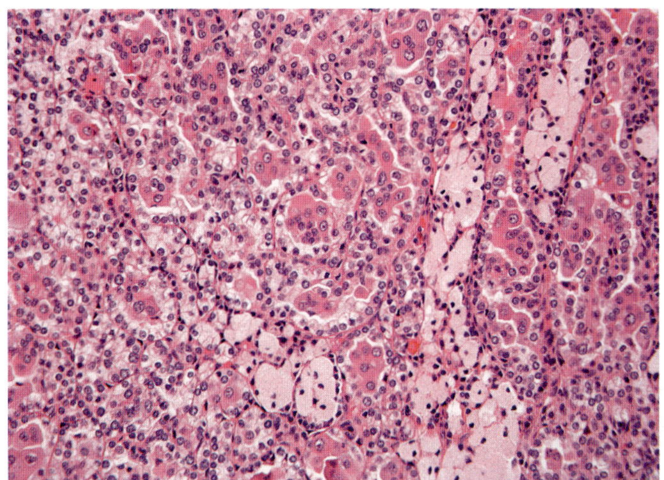

Fig. 137: Renal allograft carcinoma. Microscopic image of the tumor shown in Figure 136 shows that the tumor is composed of small clear and granular cells with intervening foamy histiocytes, most consistent with a variant of papillary renal cell carcinoma. Hematoxylin and eosin (H&E) stain.

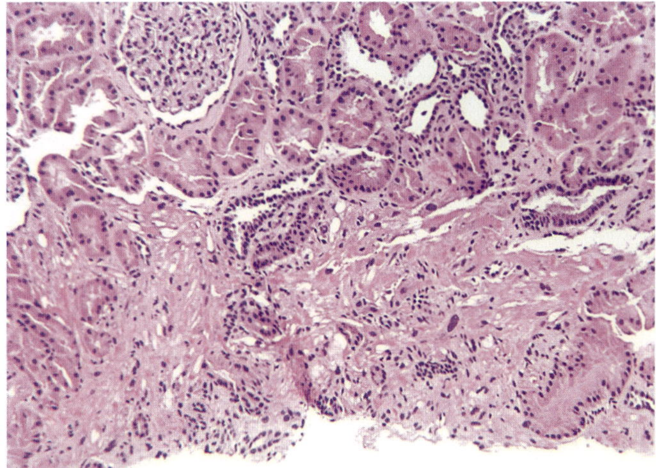

Fig. 138: Renal allograft angiomyolipoma, needle biopsy. The area devoid of tubules along the bottom of needle biopsy core is occupied by atypical spindle cells and vessels; a fatty or lipomatous component is not prominent in this case. Angiomyolipomas usually have benign behavior and rarely may cause problems due to hemorrhage. They are common in tuberous sclerosis patients, but are certainly seen in other settings as well.

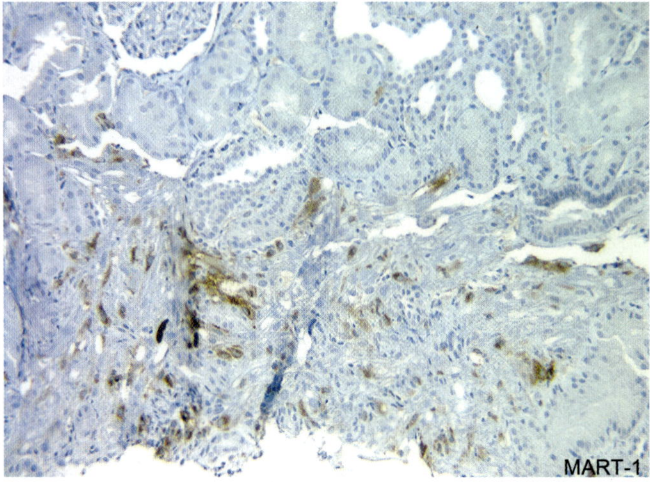

Fig. 139: Renal allograft angiomyolipoma, MART-1 stain. The diagnosis of angiomyolipoma can be confirmed by immunostaining. This family of tumors (PEComas) should be positive for MART-1/ Melan-A and HMB-45, although the staining is often patchy, as seen here (positive brown staining against blue counterstain).

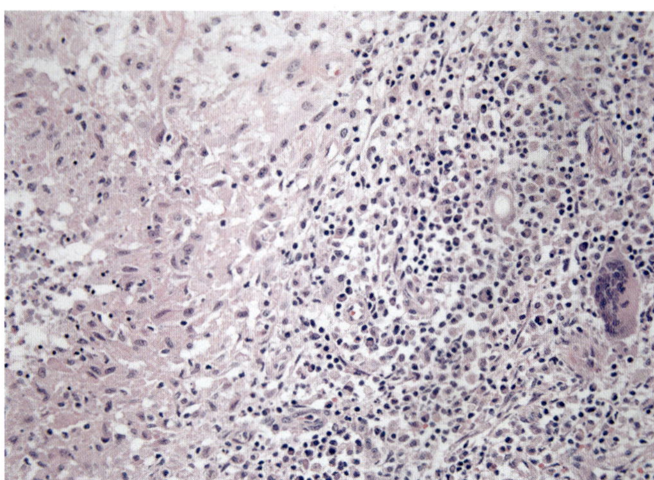

Fig. 140: Xanthogranulomatous pyelonephritis. Xanthogranulomatous pyelonephritis is an inflammatory mass-lesion; in this example, pink histiocytes are seen in the left part of the field, with mononuclear inflammatory cells and one multinucleated giant cell at right. Histiocytes may contain remarkable amounts of lipid, such that they may grossly or microscopically mimic renal cell carcinoma (not shown). Xanthogranulomatous pyelonephritis is most often associated with urinary obstruction (especially stones), and urine cultures can be positive for a variety of bacterial organisms.

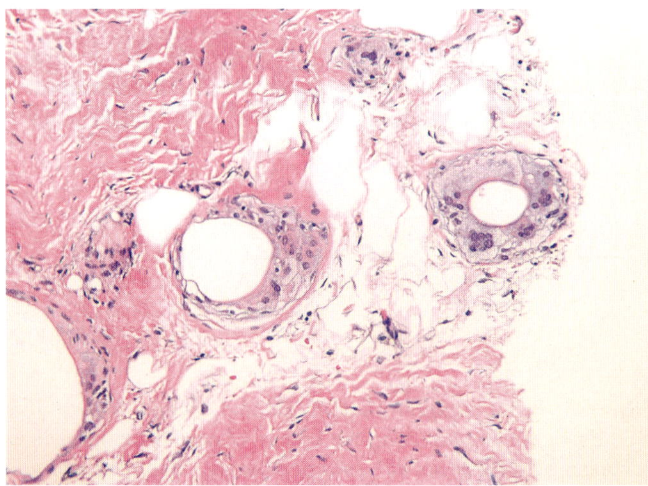

Fig. 141: Foreign body giant cells in renal allograft capsule. These multinucleated giant cells are seen in the fibrous capsule surrounding the renal allograft, a reaction at the surgical site. They may be seen on renal allograft biopsy if the needle throw passes through the fibrous capsule. This foreign body type of giant cell reaction is not associated with infection.

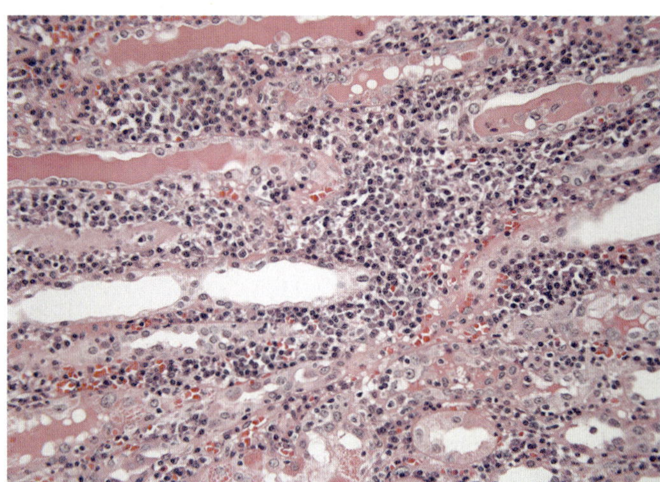

Fig. 142: Post-transplant lymphoproliferative disorder (PTLD). This allograft nephrectomy contains a very dense, predominantly plasmacytic inflammatory infiltrate. While plasma cell rich infiltrates may be seen in rejection, this degree of plasmacytic inflammation should raise suspicion of PTLD. These plasma cells were demonstrated to be kappa-monoclonal (not shown), essentially diagnostic of plasmacytoma-like PTLD. PTLD often occurs in the transplanted organ, but may occur elsewhere in the recipient. The current classification of PTLD is shown in Table 6.[16]

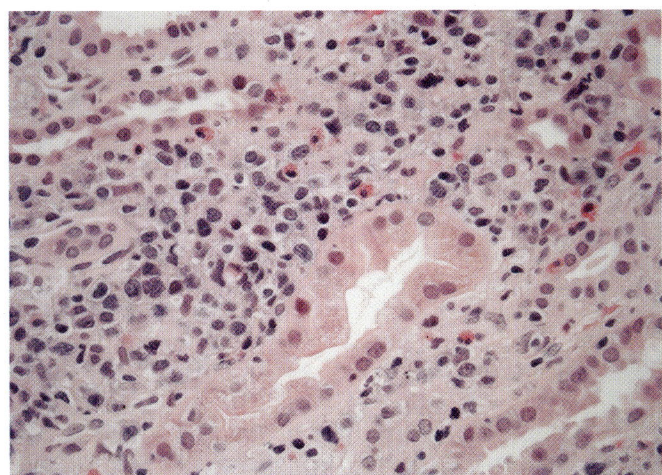

Fig. 143: Post-transplant lymphoproliferative disorder (PTLD). A lymphocytic and eosinophilic infiltrate with some large atypical lymphoid cell nuclei was seen focally in this allograft biopsy. Elsewhere, there was tubulitis and micro-infarcts, raising a large differential, including rejection, drug hypersensitivity reaction, rejection, and vasculitis. In this case Epstein–Barr virus (EBV) staining, shown in Figure 144, was very helpful in coming to the diagnosis of PTLD, polymorphic type.

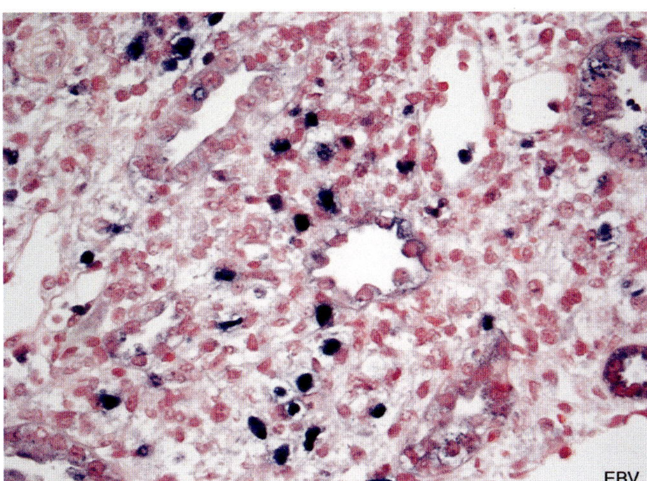

Fig. 144: Post-transplant lymphoproliferative disorder (PTLD), Epstein–Barr virus (EBV) in situ hybridization. The EBV early RNA (EBER) is highlighted in blue against a red counterstain. Approximately 80% of PTLDs are EBV positive.

Table 6: Classification of post-transplant lymphoproliferative disorder (PTLD)[16]

Early PTLD
Plasmacytic hyperplasia
Infectious mononucleosis-like
Polymorphic PTLD
Monomorphic PTLD
Subclassify further as per lymphoma
Classical Hodgkin PTLD

REFERENCES

1. Racusen LC, Solez K, Colvin RB, et al. The Banff 97 working classification of renal allograft pathology. Kidney Int 1999; 55:713–22.
2. Racusen LC, Colvin RB, Solez K, et al. Antibody-mediated rejection criteria—an addition to the Banff '97 classification of renal allograft rejection. Am J Transplant 2003; 3:708–14.
3. Solez K, Colvin RB, Racusen LC, et al. Banff 07 classification of renal allograft pathology: updates and future directions. Am J Transplant 2008; 8:753–60.
4. Sis B, Mengel M, Haas M, et al. Banff '09 meeting report: antibody mediated graft deterioration and implementation of Banff working groups. Am J Transplant 2010; 10:464–71.
5. Haas M, Sis B, Racusen LC, et al. Banff 13 meeting report. Am J Transplant 2014:14(2): 272-83.
6. Colvin RB, Cohen AH, Saiontz C, et al. Evaluation of pathologic criteria for acute renal allograft rejection: reproducibility, sensitivity and clinical correlation. J Am Soc Nephrol 1997;8:1930–41.
7. Colvin RB. Renal transplant pathology. In: Jennette JC, Olson JL, Schwartz MM, Silva FG (eds), Heptinstall's pathology of the kidney. 5th edn. Philadelphia: Lippencott-Raven, 1998:1409–540.
8. Nickeleit V. The pathology of kidney transplantation. In: Ruiz P (ed), Transplantation pathology. Cambridge: Cambridge University Press, 2009:45–110.
9. Charney DA, Nadasdy T, Lo AW. Plasma cell-rich acute renal allograft rejection. Transplantation 1999;68:791–97.
10. Meehan SM, Josephson MA, Haas M. Granulomatous tubulointerstitial nephritis in the renal allograft. Am J Kid Disease 2000;36:E27.
11. Magil AB, Tinckam K. Monocytes and peritubular capillary C4d deposition in acute renal allograft rejection. Kidney Int 2003;63:1888–93.
12. Masutani K, Shapiro R, Basu A et al. The Banff 2009 working proposal for polyomavirus nephropathy: a critical evaluation of its utility as a determinant of clinical outcome. Am J Transplant 2012;12:907–19.
13. Storsley L, Gibson IW. Adenovirus interstitial nephritis and rejection in an allograft. J Am Soc Nephrol 2011; 22:1423–27.
14. Choy BY, Chan TM, Lai KN. Recurrent glomerulonephritis after kidney transplantation. Am J Transplant 2006; 6:2535–42.
15. Ivanyi, B. A primer on recurrent and de novo glomerulonephritis in renal allografts. Nat Clin Pract Nephrol 2008; 4:446–57.
16. Tsao L, Hsi ED. The clinicopathologic spectrum of post-transplantation lymphoproliferative disorders. Arch Pathol Lab Med 2007;131:1209–18.

CHAPTER 56

Candidate Imaging

Mariano Volpacchio, Catherine D'Agostino, Christopher Palestro, et al.

THROMBOSIS OF THE ABDOMINAL AORTA (FIGS. 1 TO 6)

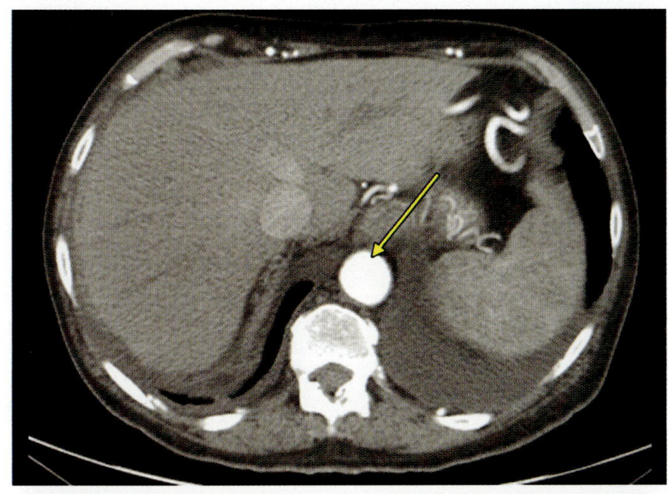

Fig. 1: A patent enhancing upper abdominal aorta (yellow arrow).

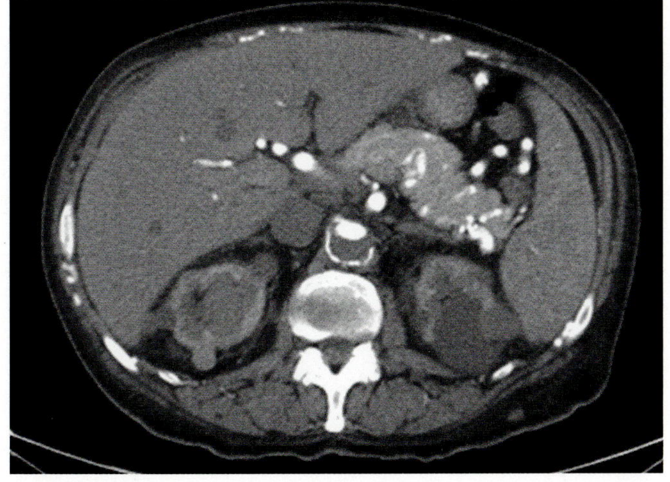

Fig. 2

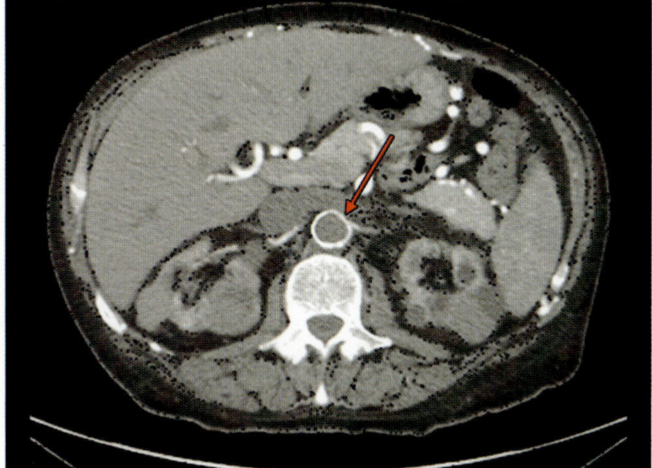

Fig. 3

Figs. 2 and 3: Thrombosis of the mid-portion of the aorta (red arrow).

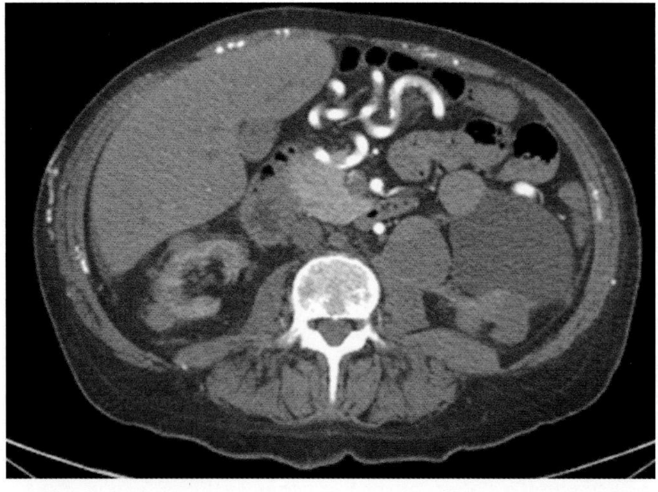

Fig. 4: The distal aorta and external iliac arteries are not patent.

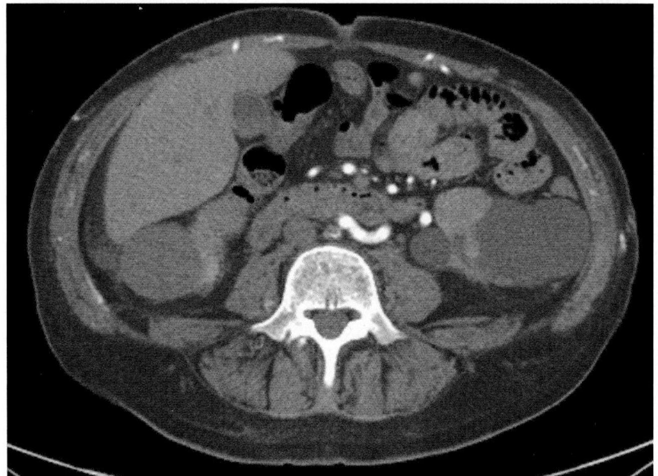

Fig. 5

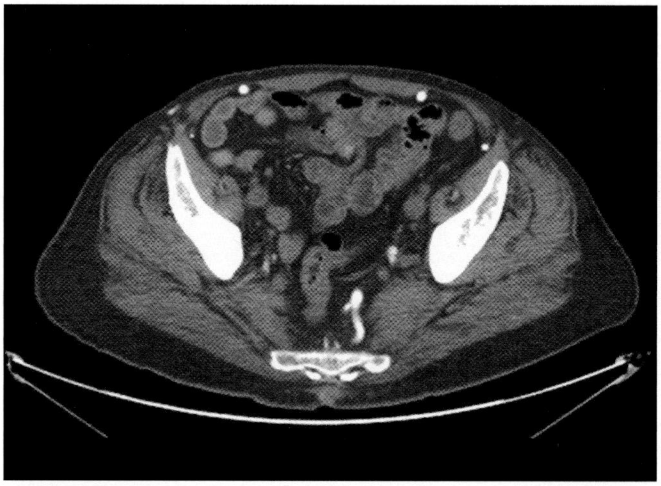

Fig. 6

Figs. 1 to 6: Sequential CT images obtained during pre-transplant evaluation. The distal aorta and external iliac arteries are not patent (Figs. 4 to 6). The prominent inferior epigastric arteries as well as the multiple collaterals throughout the body reflect collateralization of flow. Notice the multiple acquired cysts in both native kidneys, some of them hyperattenuating due to hemorrhagic changes (of concern for malignancies).

RENAL PATHOLOGIES (FIGS. 7 TO 10)

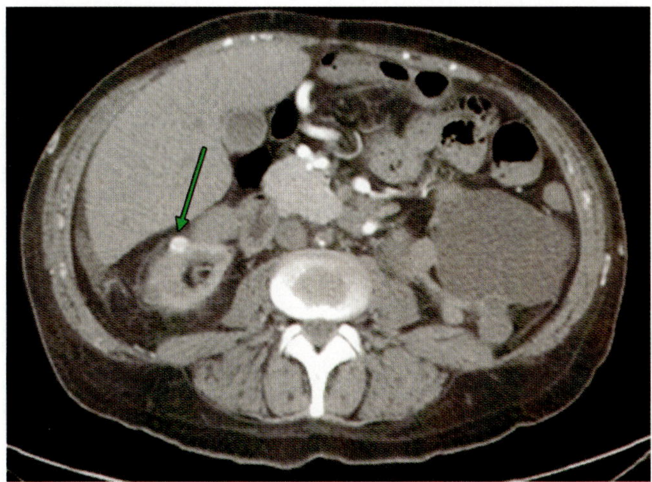

Fig. 7: Pretransplant evaluation CT image that shows a hyperattenuating lesion that could, on an unenhanced scan, represent either a hyperdense cyst (Bosniak 2) or a solid mass. This lesion exhibited a brisk enhancement suggesting a small renal cell carcinoma as was subsequently proven by microscopic tissue examination in the right kidney. All suspicious lesions should be thoroughly evaluated to exclude malignancies.

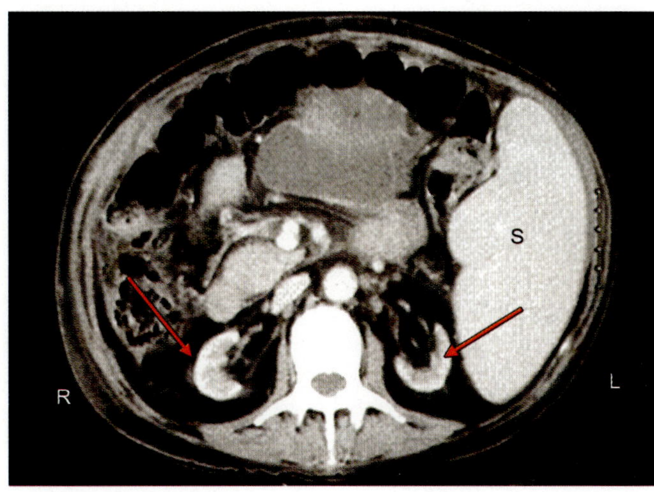

Fig. 8: Pretransplant evaluation CT showing atrophic native kidneys (red arrows). Note the splenomegaly (S).

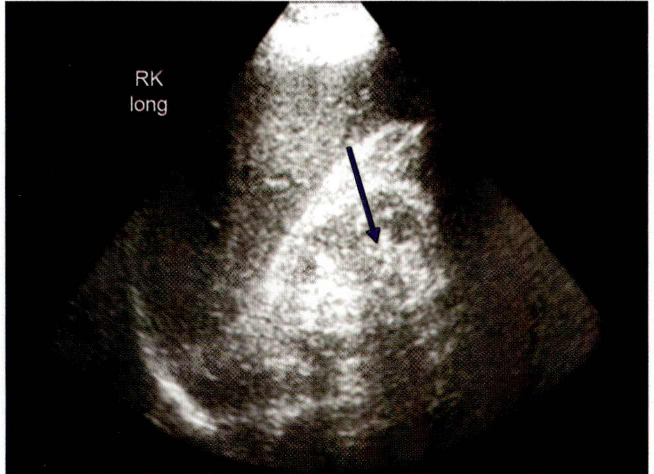

Fig. 9: Longitudinal US showing a small, echogenic right native kidney with a calculus (blue arrow) projecting an acoustic shadow.

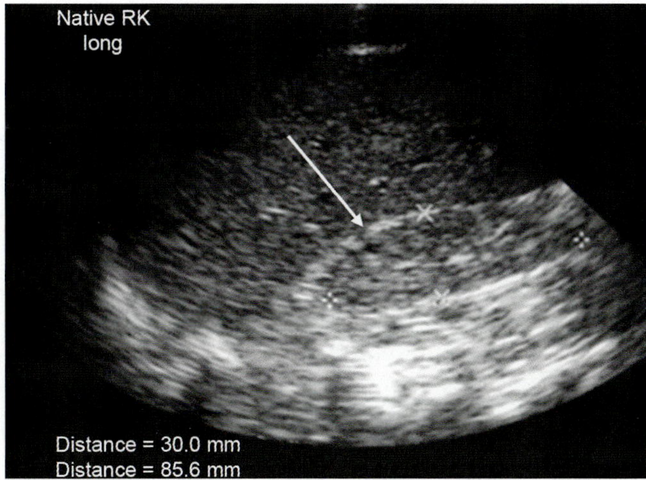

Fig. 10: Longitudinal US of a small native kidney (white arrow) showing loss of corticomedullary differentiation, typical of end-stage kidney disease (small native kidney encircled by asterisks).

RENAL CELL CARCINOMA OF THE NATIVE KIDNEYS (FIGS. 11 AND 12)

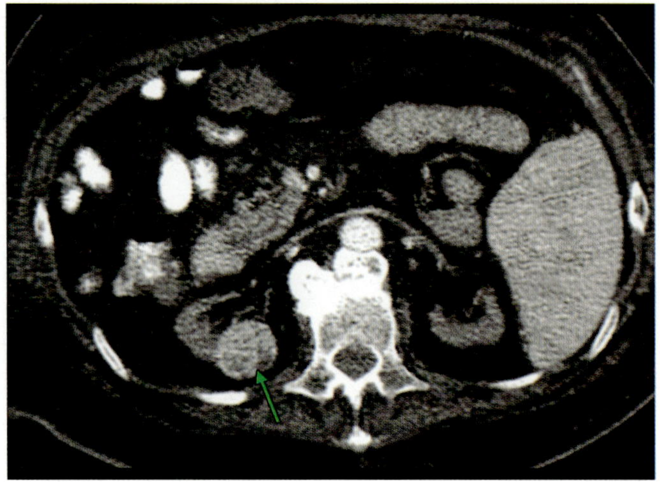

Fig. 11: Axial contrast-enhanced CT image showing a rounded, heterogeneously enhancing mass (green arrow) emerging from the posterior aspect of the atrophic right native kidney. This is a typical appearance of a renal cell carcinoma. Patients on long-term dialysis treatment are more susceptible to the development of diverse lesions, among which are carcinomas. These cancers are usually smaller and less aggressive than those affecting the rest of the population and, not uncommonly, multiple.

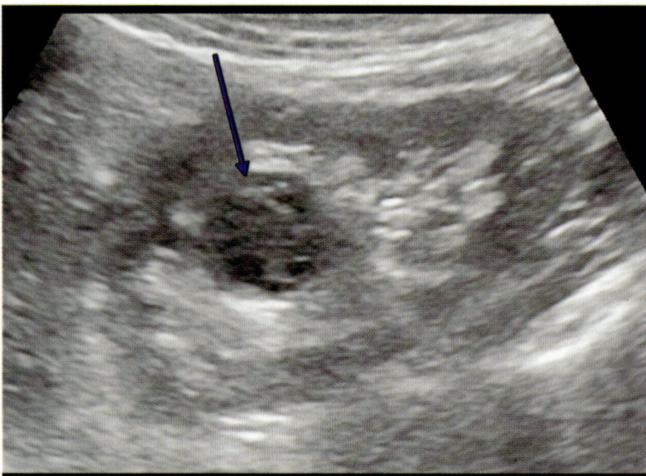

Fig. 12: Longitudinal ultrasound of the left native kidney showing a rounded, hypoechoic, heterogenous mass (blue arrow) corresponding to a renal cell carcinoma.

GALLBLADDER PATHOLOGIES (FIGS. 13 TO 15)

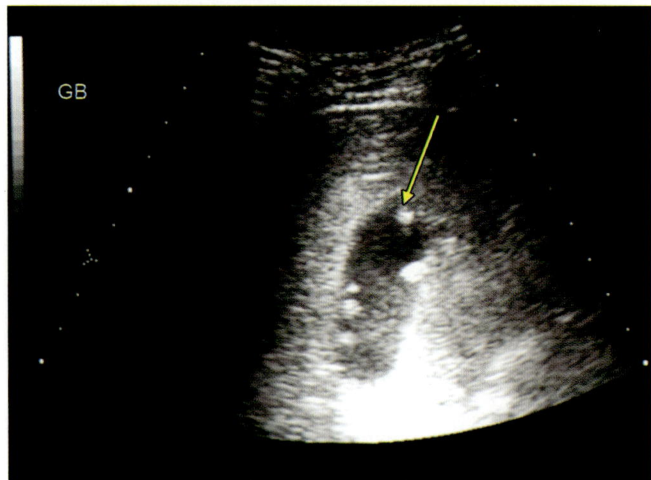

Fig. 13

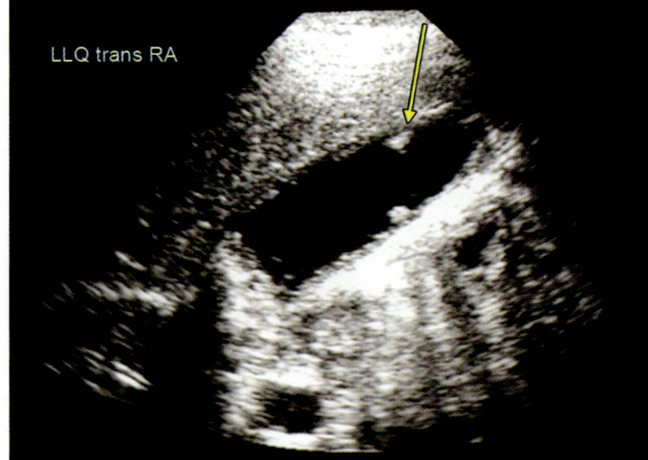

Fig. 14

Figs. 13 and 14: Pretransplant ultrasound images showing small polyps (yellow arrows) emerging from the gallbladder wall.

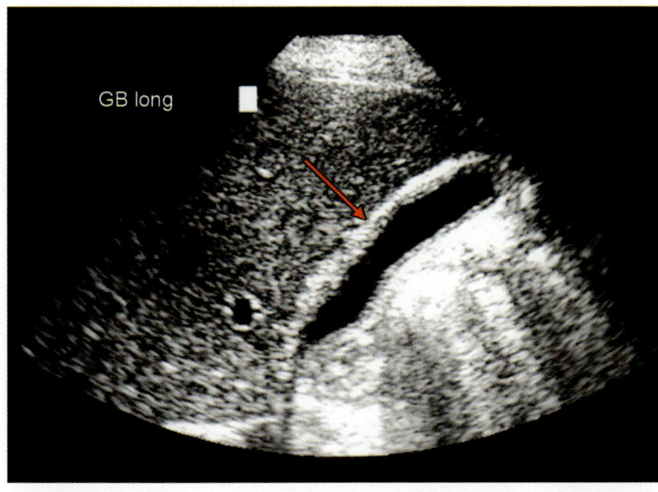

Fig. 15: Pretransplant ultrasound evaluation shows a thickened gallbladder wall (red arrow). Although this is a nonspecific finding, clinical correlation is crucial in order to exclude cholecystitis.

VENOUS THROMBOSES (FIGS. 16 TO 19)

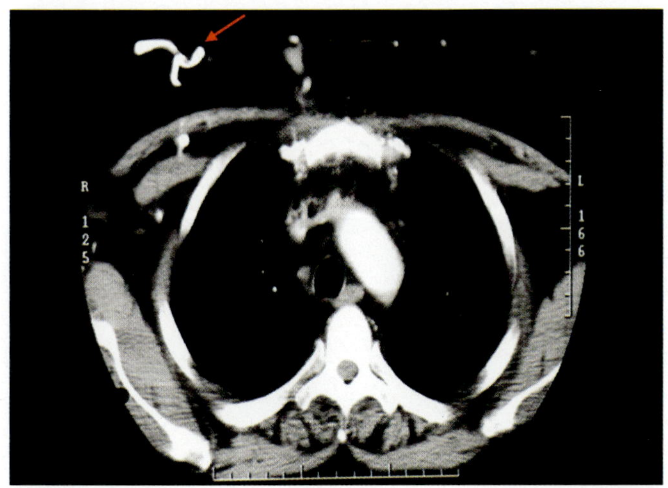

Fig. 16

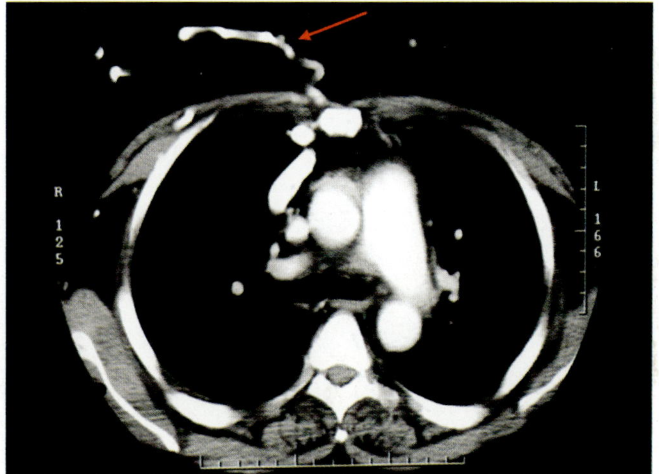

Fig. 17

Figs. 16 and 17: Pretransplant evaluation CT reveals a filiform nonenhancing left brachiocephalic vein as well as multiple prominent collateral vessels (red arrows) in the chest wall.

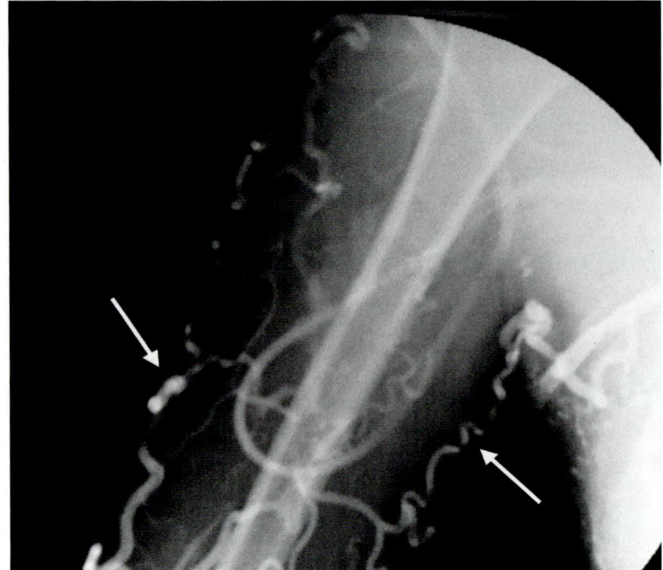

Fig. 18: A venography study failed to opacify the brachiocephalic vein (consistent with the diagnosis of thrombosis). Again, multiple subcutaneous collateral vessels (white arrows) can be seen.

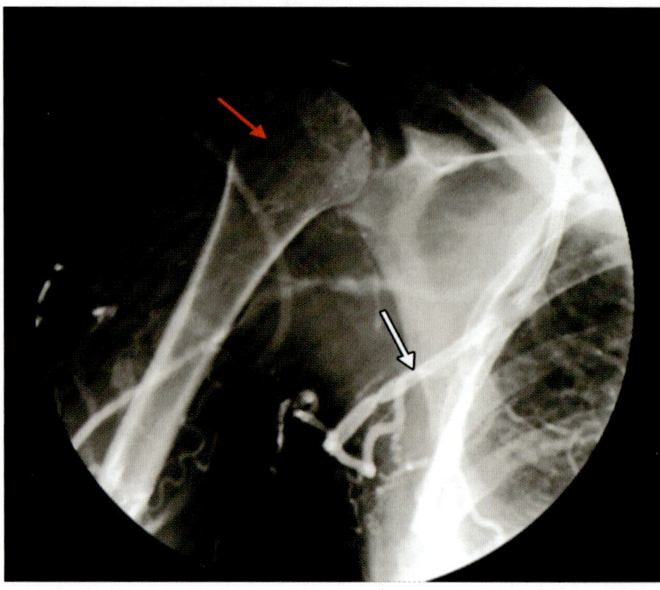

Fig. 19: Thrombosis of the subclavian vein with chest wall collaterals (white arrow). Osteoporosis can also be noted (red arrow).

VARIOUS FINDINGS (FIGS. 20 AND 21)

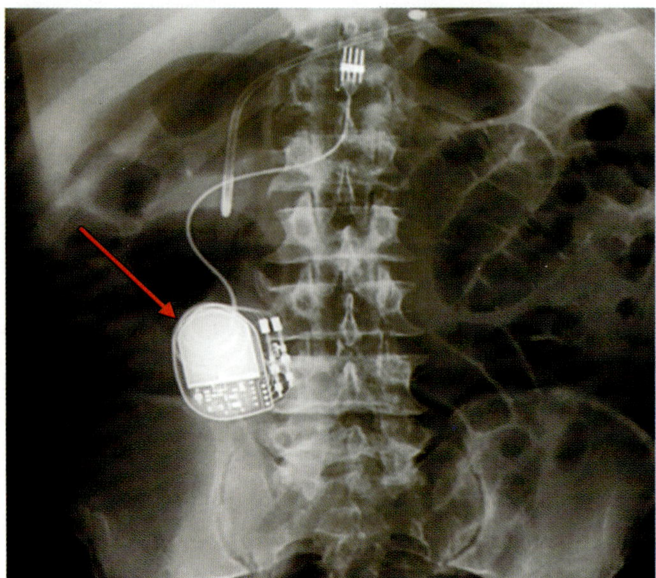

Fig. 20: Electrical stimulator seen on a plain film of the abdomen (red arrow).

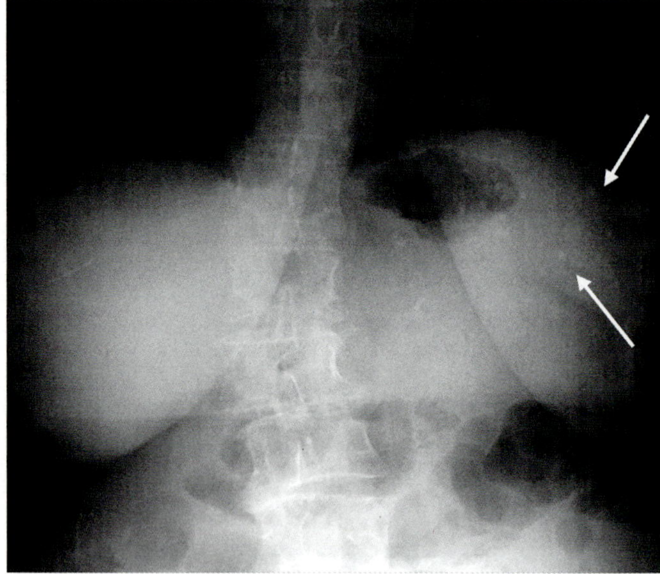

Fig. 21: Calcified splenic granulomata (white arrows) on a plain film of the abdomen.

ATRIAL THROMBUS (FIGS. 22 TO 27)

Transplant candidate with end-stage renal disease secondary to lupus who was found to have right atrial mass during routine cardiac evaluation not present in a previous echocardiogram obtained 3 months earlier prior to placement of a dialysis catheter.

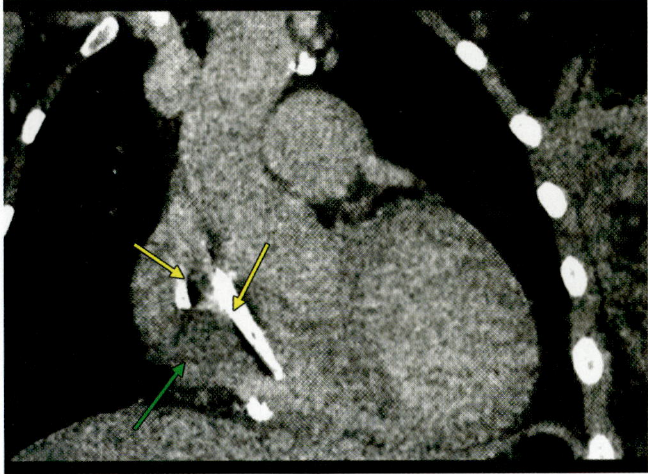

Fig. 22

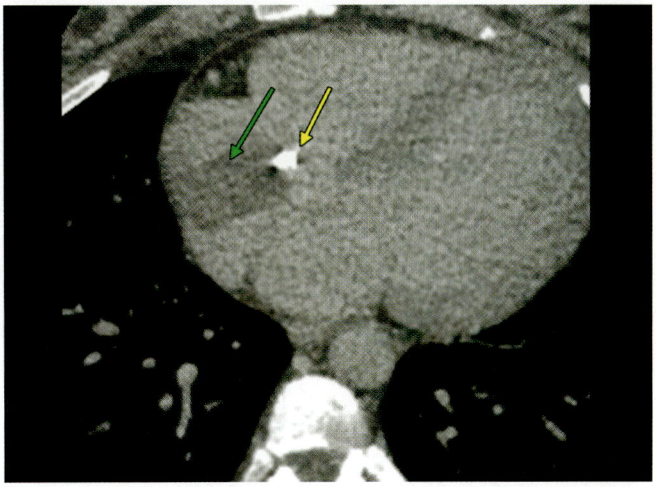

Fig. 23

Figs. 22 and 23: CT images confirmed the presence of a mass (green arrows) believed to be a thrombus adjacent to the dialysis catheter (yellow arrows) in the right atrium. The mass was found to be anchored to the atrial wall, with no attachment to the dialysis catheter and no associated tricuspid regurgitation on transesophageal echocardiogram.

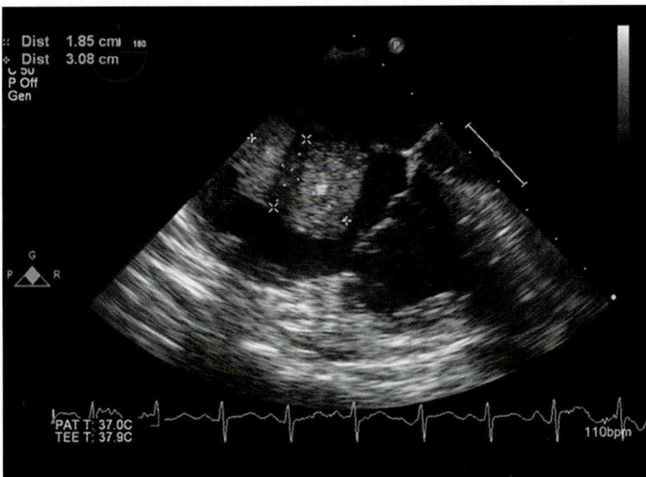

Fig. 24: Transesophageal echo (TEE): Mid-esophageal four-chamber view showing a 1.85 cm × 3.08 cm mass in the right atrium.

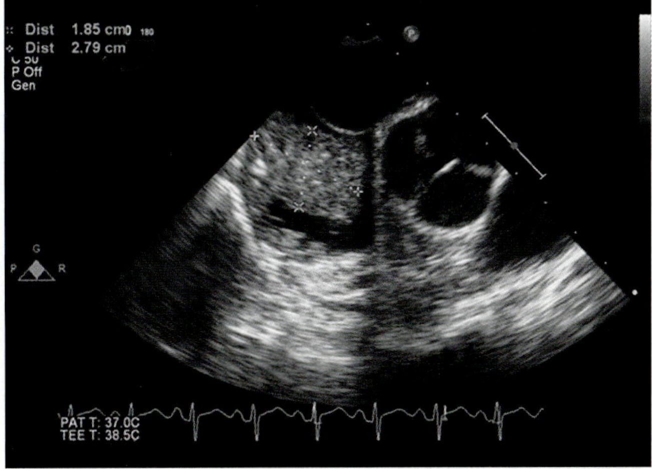

Fig. 25: Transesophageal echo (TEE): Mid-esophageal short-axis view at the level of aortic valve showing a 1.85 cm × 2.79 cm mass (encircled by asterisks) attached to the right atrial free wall and sparing the interatrial septum.

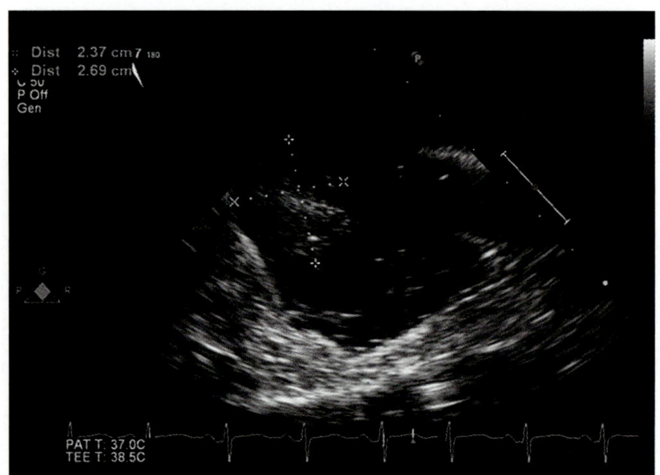

Fig. 26: Transesophageal echo (TEE): Bicaval view displaying a 2.37 cm × 2.69 cm mass attached to the right atrial free wall and sparing the inter-atrial septum. A catheter is seen in the superior vena cava (SVC), the tip of which ends in the right atrium and does not appear to be associated with the mass.

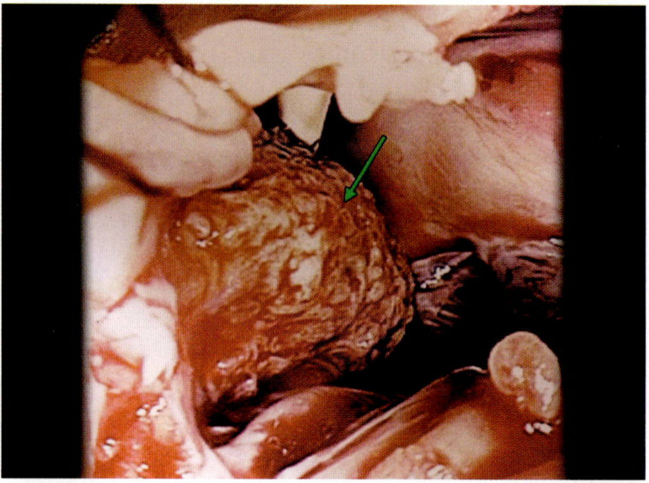

Fig. 27: Attempts to lyse it with TPA in the setting of anticoagulation failed. The size of the mass (almost the entire right atrial cavity) in association with the presence of bacteremia prompted the decision to proceed with surgical resection. This figure shows an intraoperative view of the mass (green arrow), determined to be a thrombus by pathological examination.

CHAPTER 57

Donor Evaluation

Mariano Volpacchio, Catherine D'Agostino, Christopher Palestro, et al.

RETROAORTIC LEFT RENAL VEIN (FIGS. 1 TO 8)

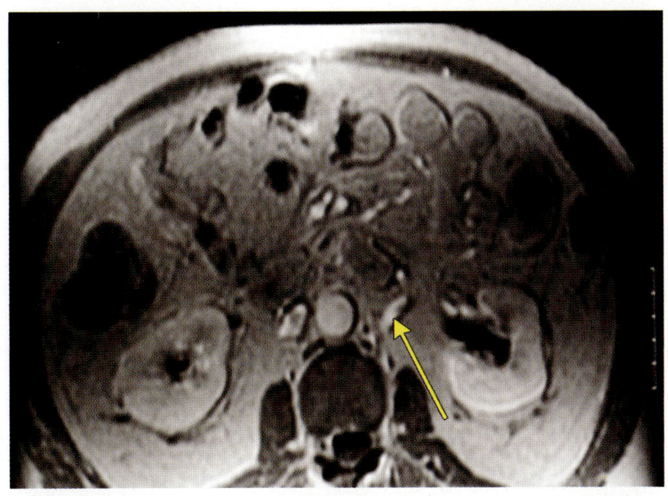

Fig. 1

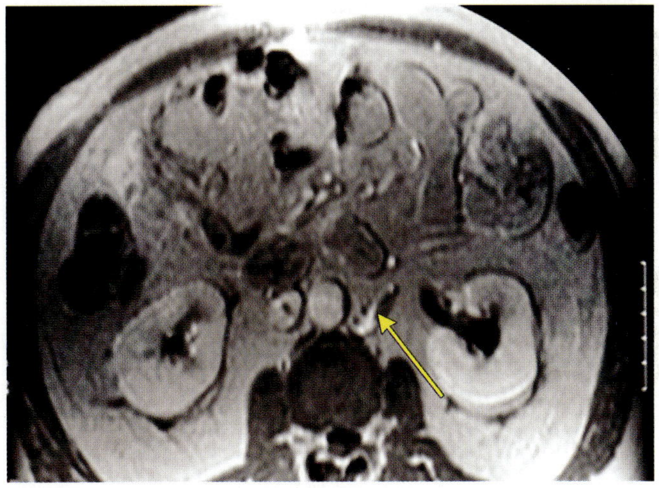

Fig. 2

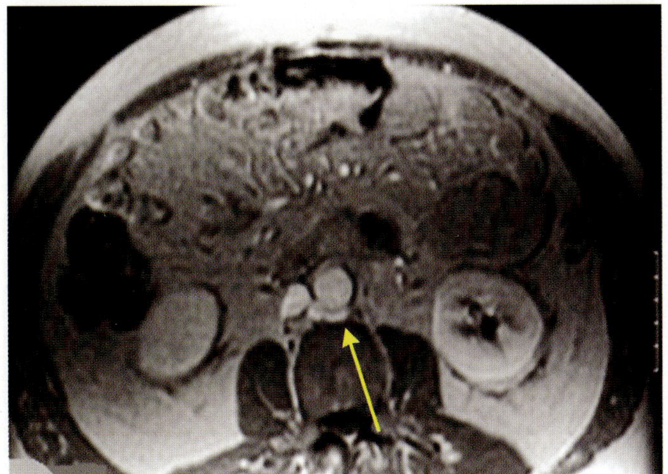

Fig. 3

Figs. 1 to 3: MRI images.

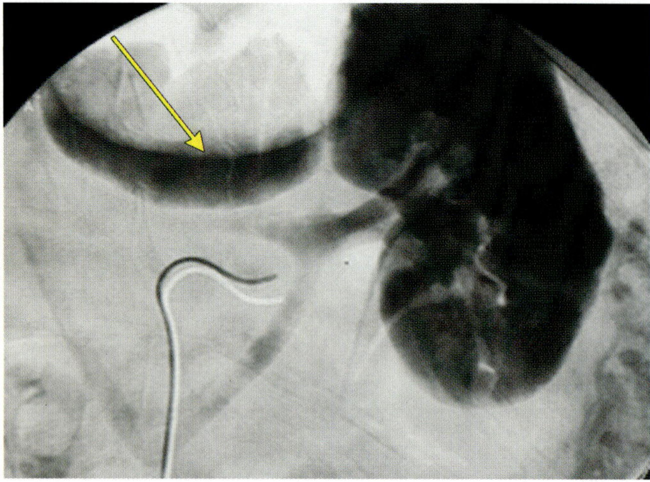

Fig. 4: Venous phase renal angiogram.

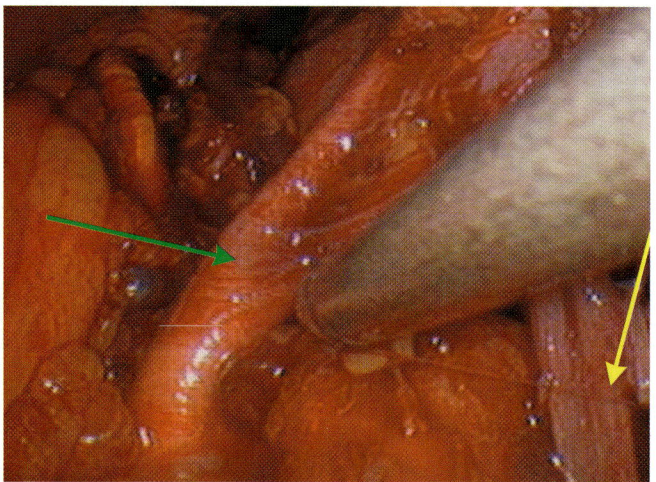

Fig. 5

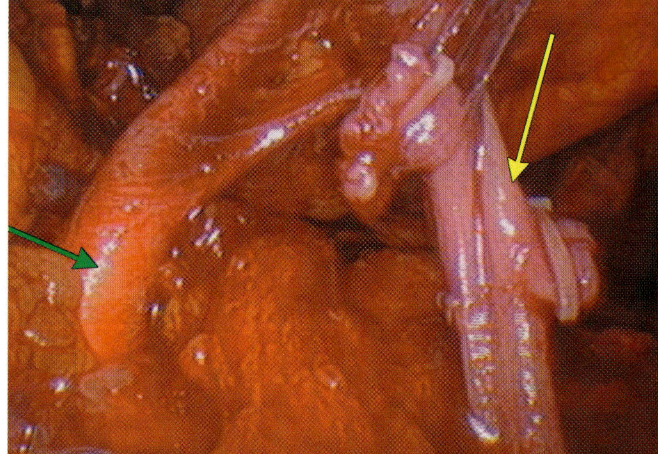

Fig. 6

Figs. 1 to 6: Evaluation of a live donor with a retroaortic left renal vein. (Fig. 4) Figures 5 and 6 depict intraoperative views. The retroaortic left renal vein is shown with yellow arrows. Green arrows point to the left renal artery.

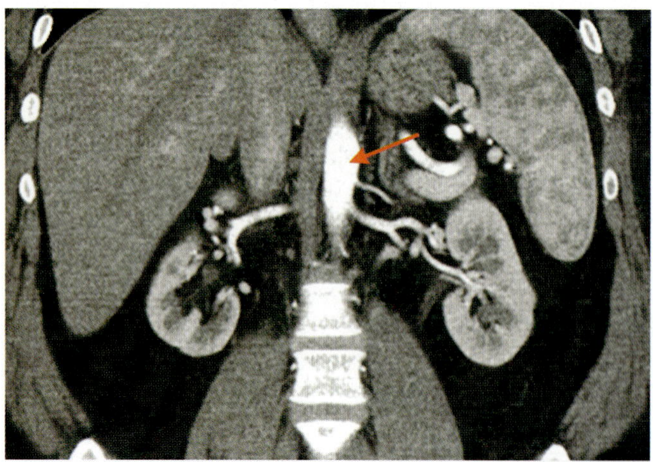

Fig. 7

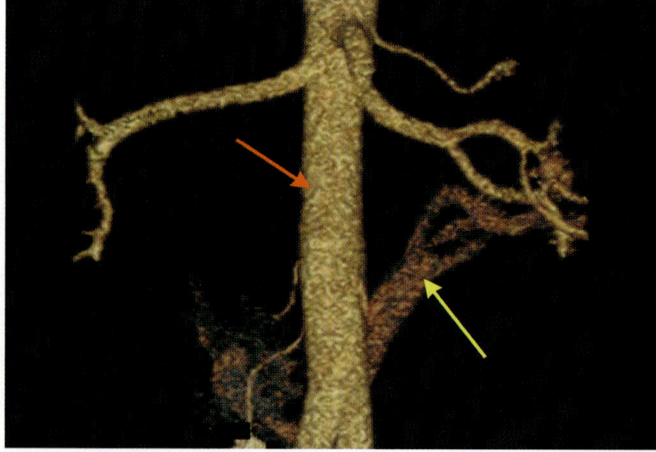

Fig. 8

Figs. 7 and 8: Additional images depicting a retroaortic left renal vein (yellow arrow) and the aorta (red arrows).

CIRCUMAORTIC LEFT RENAL VEIN (FIGS. 9 TO 12)

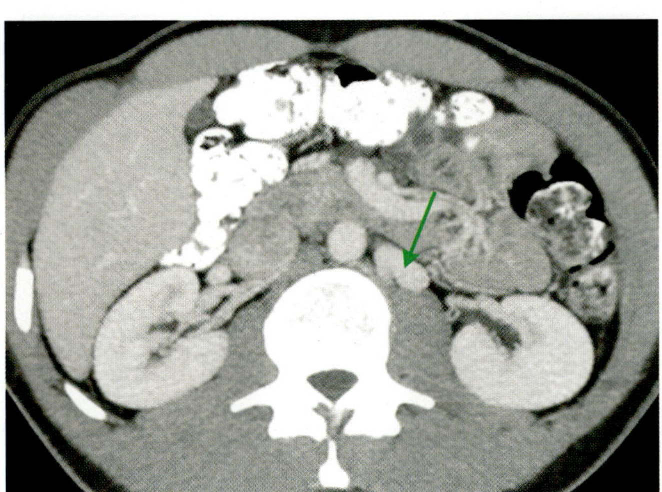

Fig. 9

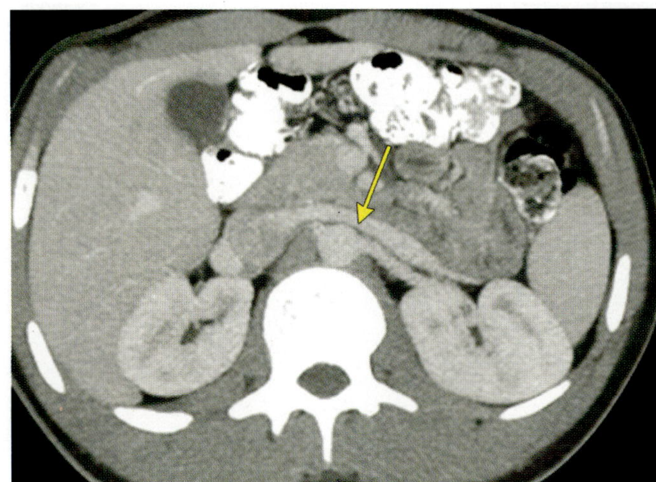

Fig. 10

Figs. 9 and 10: A common trunk is shown with a green arrow. The anterior branch is shown with a yellow arrow.

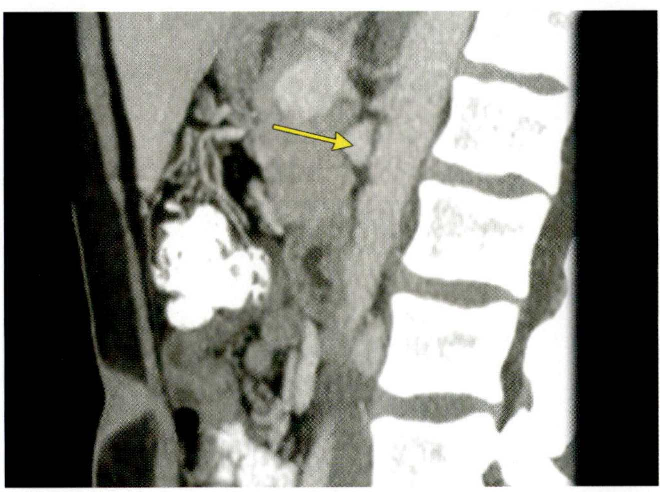

Fig. 11

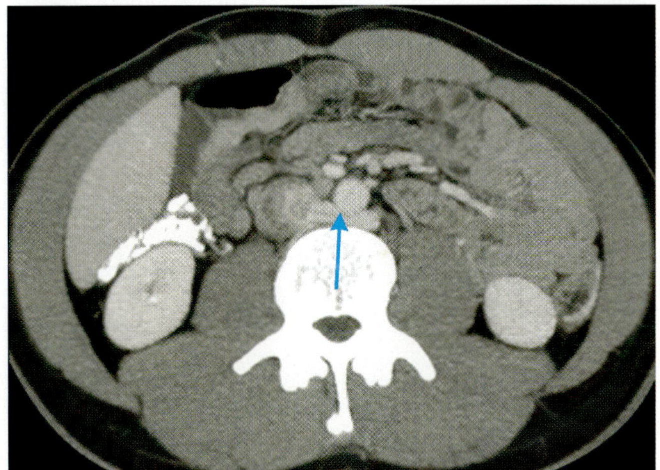

Fig. 12

Figs. 9 to 12: Axial and sagittal CT images showing a circumaortic left renal vein. (Fig. 9) A common trunk is shown with a green arrow; (Figs. 10 and 11) The anterior branch (yellow arrows) can be seen passing through the aortomesenteric angle; (Fig. 12) The posterior branch (blue arrow) drains into inferior vena cava.

DOUBLE RENAL VEIN (FIGS. 13 TO 15)

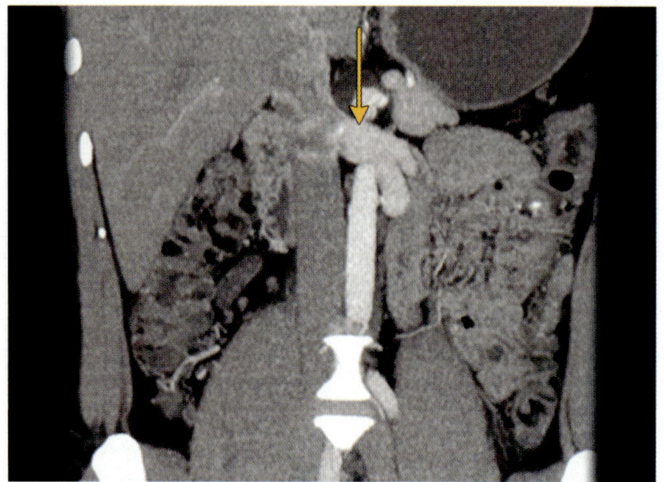

Fig. 13

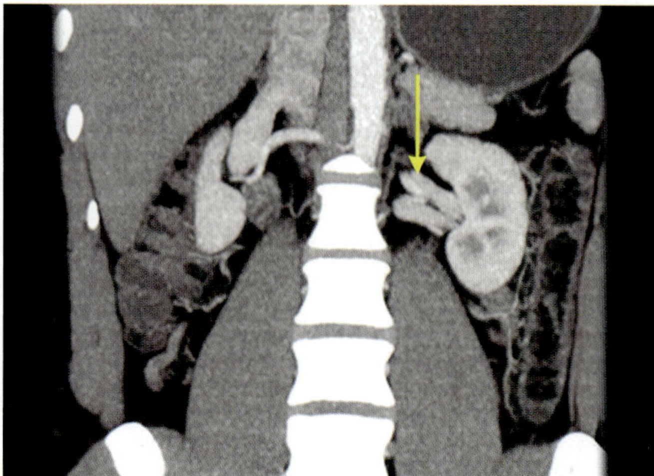

Fig. 14

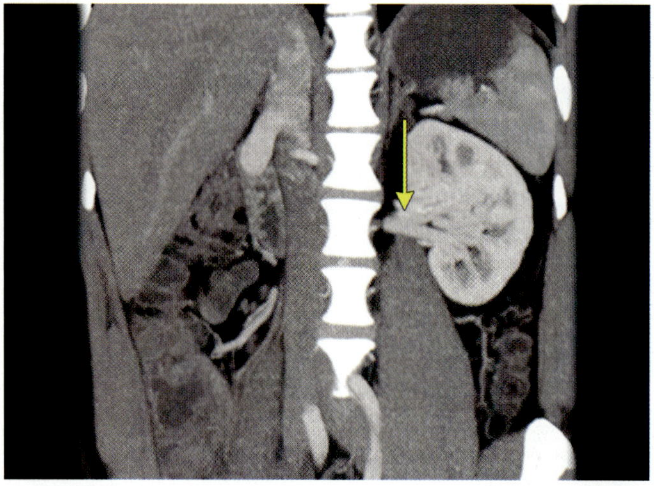

Fig. 15

Figs. 13 to 15: Consecutive coronal CT images showing a duplicated left renal vein (yellow arrows) draining as a common single trunk into the inferior vena cava (orange arrow).

ECTOPIC KIDNEY (FIGS. 16 AND 17)

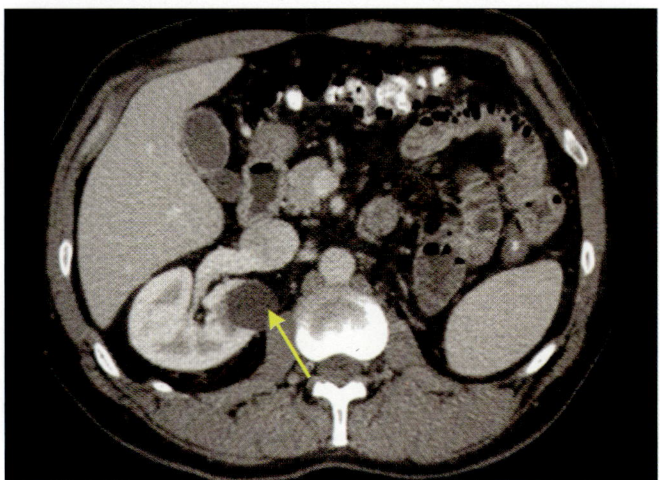

Fig. 16

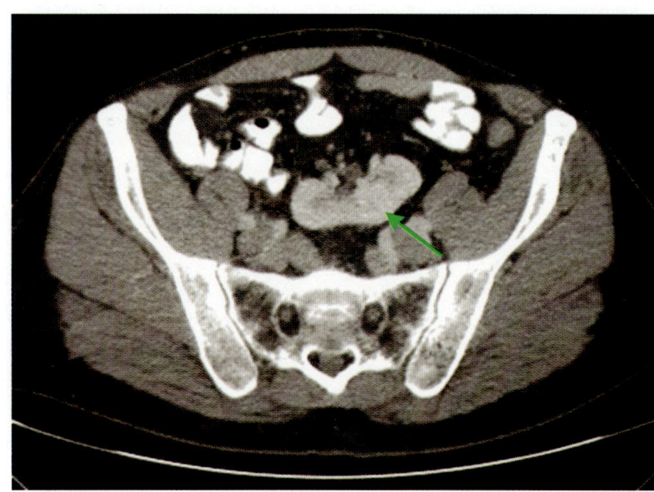

Fig. 17

Figs. 16 and 17: (Fig. 16) Axial CT image showing an empty left renal fossa; (Fig. 17) A more caudal view shows a malrotated left kidney (green arrow) in the pelvis. Notice also the simple cortical cyst in the right kidney (yellow arrow, Fig. 16).

HORSESHOE KIDNEY (FIGS. 18 AND 19)

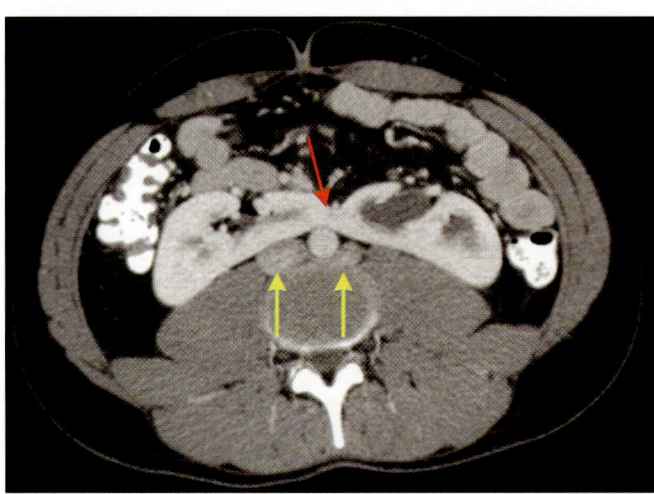

Fig. 18

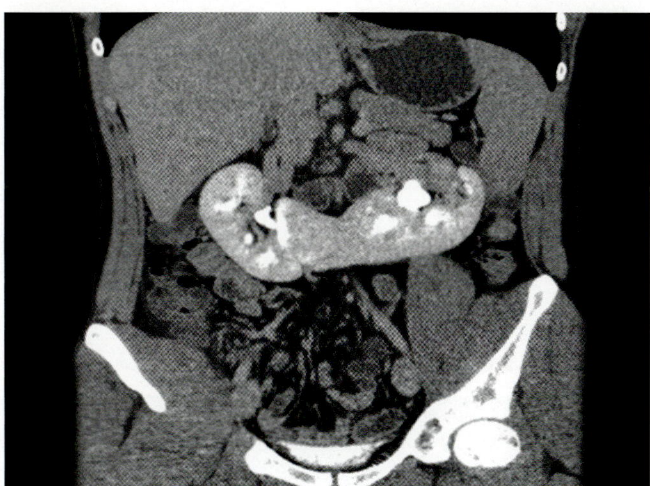

Fig. 19

Figs. 18 and 19: (Fig. 18) Axial corticomedullary phase CT image showing a horseshoe kidney fused ventral to the great vessels (red arrow). Notice also the duplicated IVC (yellow arrows); (Fig. 19) A coronal excretory phase image shows normal contrast material opacification of the collecting system which is located superficially and oriented ventrally.

RENAL AGENESIS (FIGS. 20 TO 22)

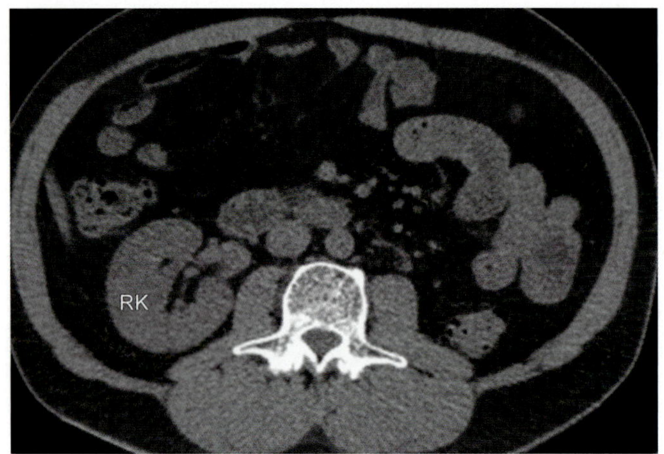

Fig. 20

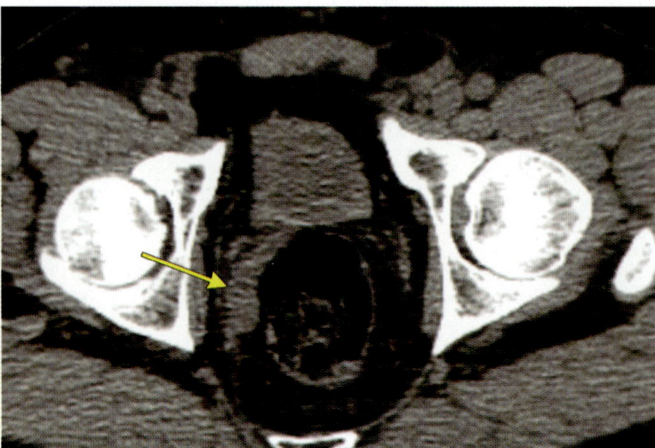

Fig. 21

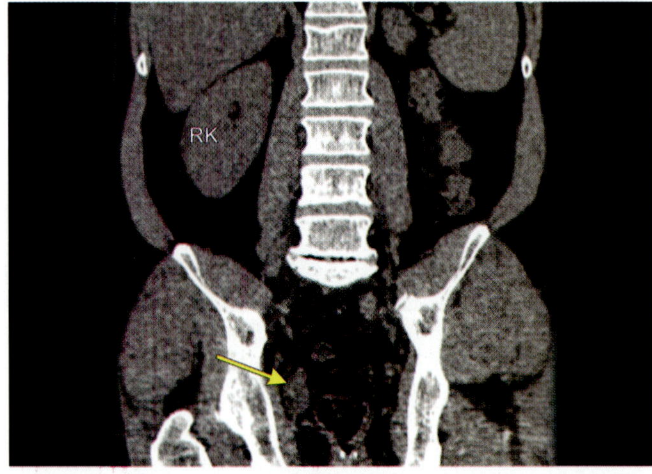

Fig. 22

Figs. 20 to 22: Unenhanced axial CT images showing absence of the left kidney in renal fossa as well as in the pelvis. The ipsilateral (left) seminal vesicle is also absent, confirming renal agenesis rather than atrophy (arrows point at the right seminal vesicle) RK: Right kidney.

SMALL LEFT KIDNEY (FIGS. 23 AND 24)

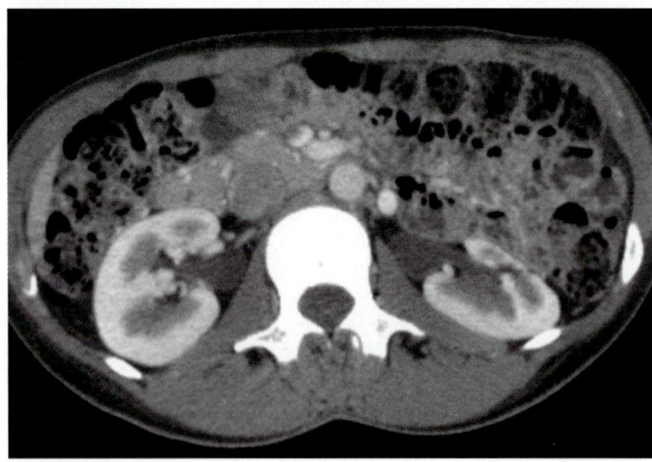

Fig. 23

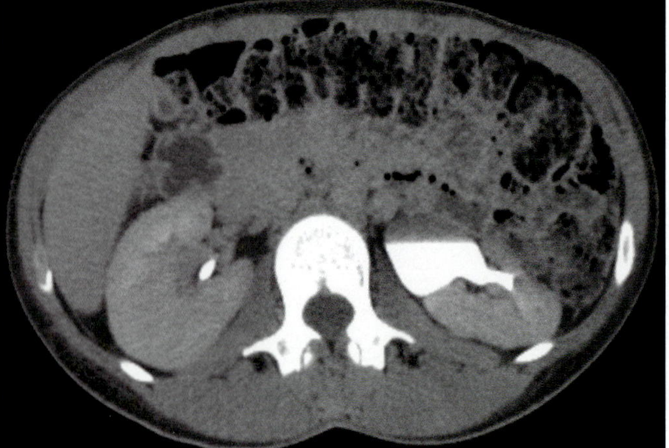

Fig. 24

Figs. 23 and 24: Corticomedullary and excretory phase axial CT images showing a decreased in size left kidney with parenchymal thinning, likely the sequela of previous inflammatory or vascular insults.

CHAPTER 58

Collections

Mariano Volpacchio, Catherine D'Agostino, Christopher Palestro, et al.

PERINEPHRIC COLLECTIONS

- It is not infrequent for kidney transplants to have one or more small perinephric collections in the immediate postoperative period
- Most such collections are small and represent expected sequel of the surgical procedure (i.e. serous or hemorrhagic)
- The clinical relevance of perinephric collections is associated with their:
  - Size
  - Location
  - Etiology
  - Growth
  - Physiologic relevance
- Collections associated with kidney transplantation include but are not limited to:
  - Seromas
  - Hematomas
  - Urinomas
  - Lymphoceles
  - Abscesses
- Because some collections may potentially enlarge and result in functional impairment of the graft, baseline examinations should document their size, location, and extension as a reference for future comparisons
- Although ultrasound (US) is very sensitive in the detection of fluid collections, the sonographic appearance of the collections is nonspecific
- A combination of imaging modalities, chronology relative to the surgery, clinical findings, and laboratory information may assist in suggesting a possible etiology
- Imaging studies, particularly ultrasound, may guide diagnostic and therapeutic drainage procedures

SEROMAS

- The presence of small pockets of serous fluid collections after the transplant surgery is almost an expected finding
- They are usually small, crescent-shaped, well-defined collections of anechoic fluid with no mass effect
- They usually reabsorb progressively
- Seromas are characterized by water attenuation on computed CT and water signal intensity on MRI (Fig. 1)

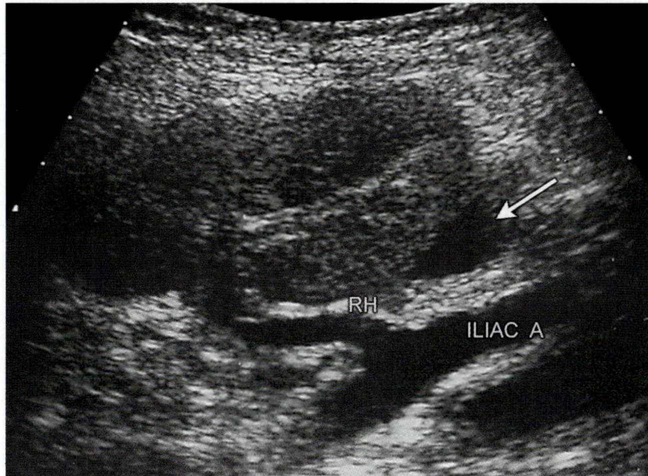

Fig. 1: Ultrasound in the immediate postoperative period showing a collection (arrow) surrounding the posterior aspect of the lower pole of the graft. Such small collections, in the absence of clinical symptoms and no sequential increases in size, can be followed conservatively with serial imaging.

HEMATOMAS

- Blood collections are common postoperatively, but may also result from biopsies, trauma, or spontaneous bleeds
- Hematomas may be subcapsular or extracapsular within the extraperitoneal space
- In the peritoneal space, blood tends to accumulate following the classic patterns of fluid migration within the peritoneal cavity
- Hematomas may also be intraparenchymal and potentially be confused with other masses
- The imaging appearance of hematomas is variable and depends on their stage of evolution
  - In the acute phase hematomas are echogenic on ultrasound
  - In later phases, they tend to be hypoechoic, heterogenous and often septated with progressive decrease in size
  - Their main feature on CT imaging is hyper attenuation, although with time the attenuation decreases and mixed-density collections with occasional fluid-fluid levels may be seen ("hematocrit effect")
  - Although on MRI hematomas can have a variable appearance based on their stage of iron oxidation, they typically show hyperintensity on both T1 and T2 (methemoglobin)

Intraparenchymal Hematoma (Figs. 2 and 3)

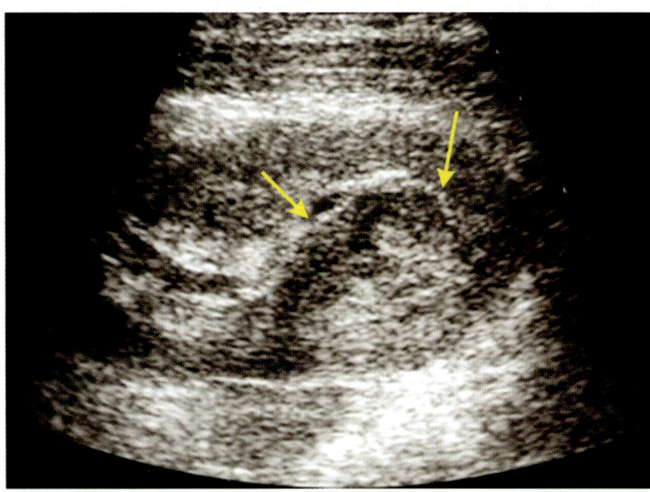

Fig. 2

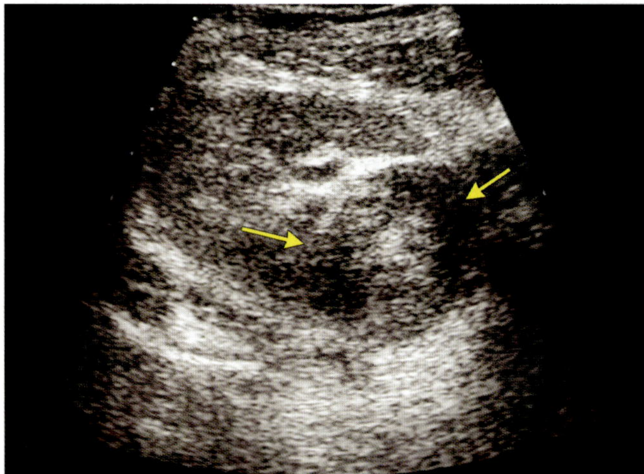

Fig. 3

Figs. 2 and 3: Longitudinal and transverse sonograms show an ovoid mass (arrows) with a central echogenic component and an outer hypoechoic rim located in the posterior region of the graft indenting on the sinus. Although this finding initially raised concerns about the possibility of a mass, the allograft had shown no abnormalities in an ultrasound performed on the previous day. Subsequent exams demonstrated spontaneous resolution of this hematoma in a transplant patient admitted because of low platelet counts and mild pain over the allograft.

Subcapsular Hematomas (Figs. 4 to 7)

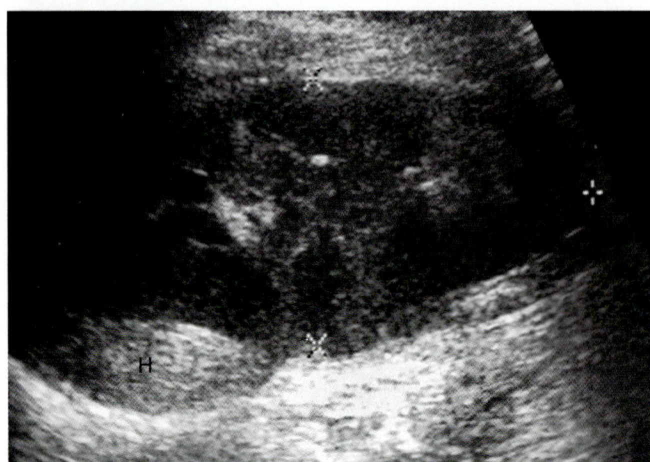

Fig. 4: Sagittal sonogram shows a lenticular-shaped echogenic hematoma (H) indenting on the posterior aspect of the upper pole of the graft (delineated by cursors).

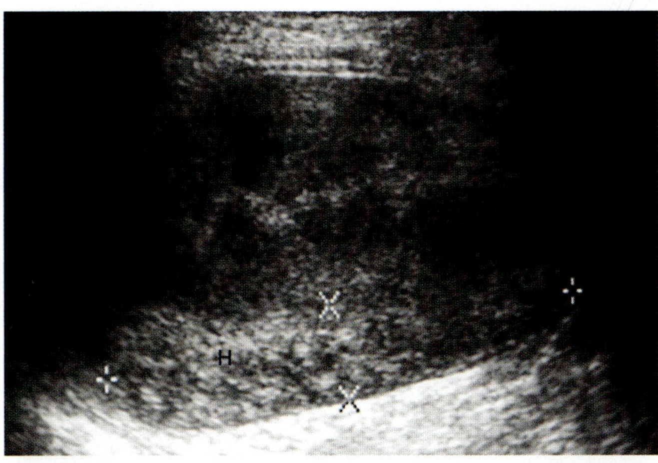

Fig. 5

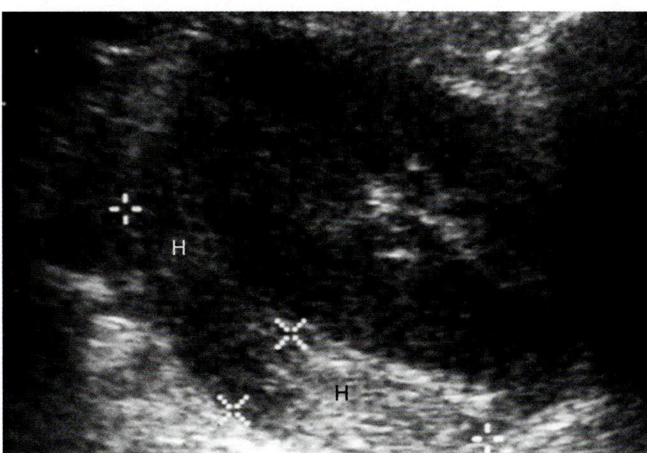

Fig. 6

Figs. 5 and 6: Sagittal and transverse sonograms of a transplant kidney show an elongated hematoma (H and cursors) along the posterior aspect of the graft. Notice the lesser echogenicity by comparison with the preceding case. US is a simple noninvasive modality that allows for a clear depiction of hematomas, their functional implications, and follow-up.

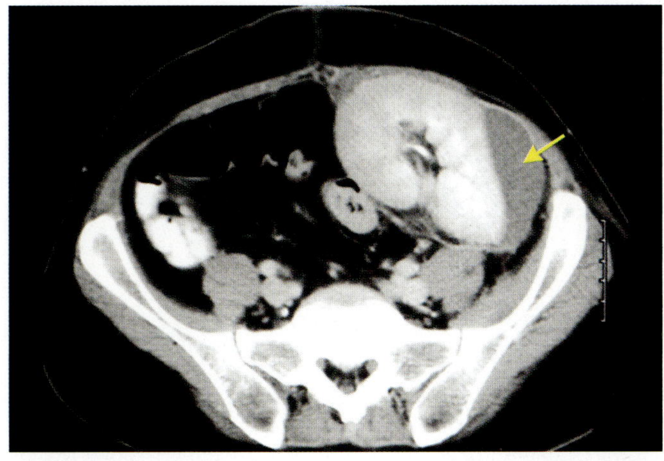

Fig. 7: Axial contrast-enhanced CT shows a semilunar subcapsular fluid collection (arrow) that compresses the allograft contour. This proved to be a subcapsular hematoma. The low attenuation suggests a subacute or chronic stage.

Enlarging Hemorrhagic Collection (Figs. 8 and 9)

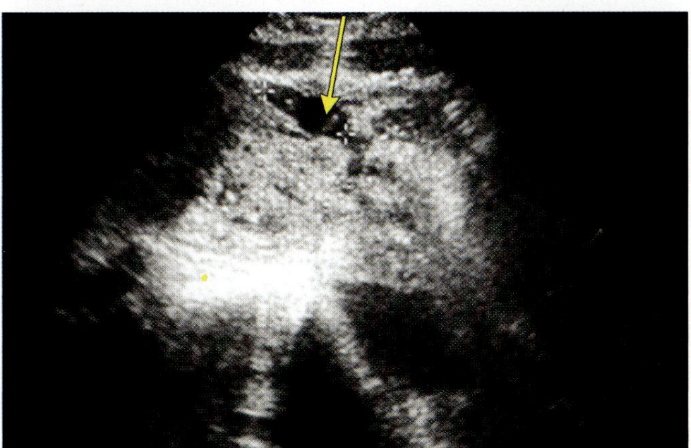

Fig. 8: An initial ultrasound study shows a laminar anechoic fluid pocket (yellow arrow and cursors).

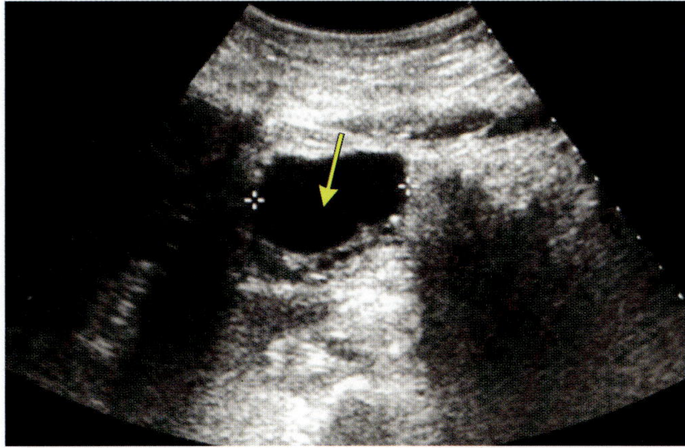

Fig. 9: Follow-up evaluation shows a significant enlargement (yellow arrow and cursors)—prompting aspiration and subsequently exploration. The collection was associated with hemorrhage from the donor ureter.

Perinephric Hematomas (Figs. 10 to 19)

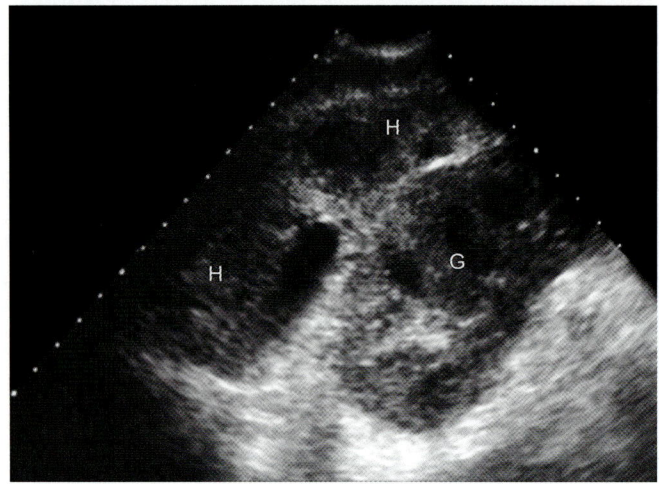

Fig. 10

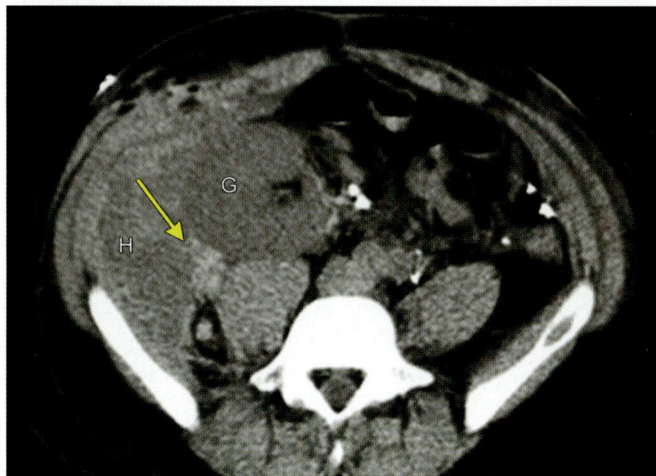

Fig. 11

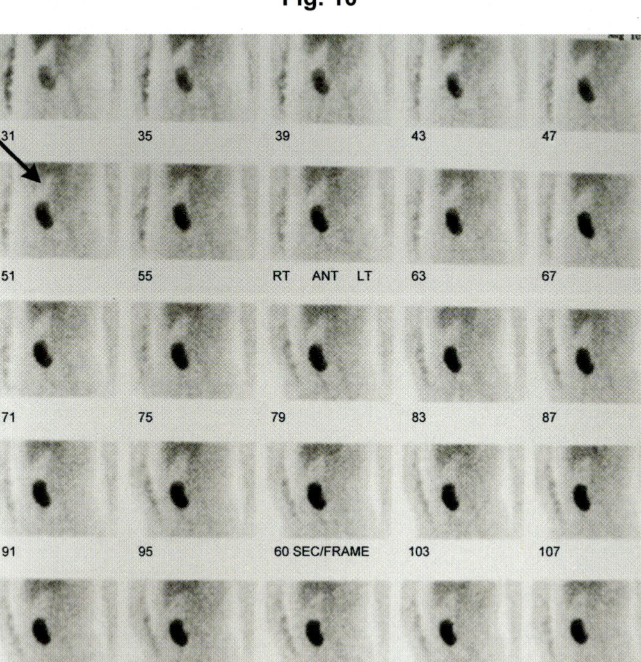

Fig. 12

Figs. 10 to 12: US and CT scan of a perinephric hematoma. (Fig. 10) Sagittal sonogram shows an echogenic hematoma (H) with scattered anechoic foci; (Fig. 11) Axial CT shows typical hyper attenuating areas (yellow arrow) within the large hematoma (H) reflecting the retracting clot. The right lower quadrant allograft (G) is displaced medially. Often these hematomas are a result of biopsies performed on hemorrhagic prone patients. The high attenuation within the hematoma is very suggestive of an evolving clot. The radionuclide image (Fig. 12) shows absence of activity (black arrow) above the allograft, corresponding to the hematoma.

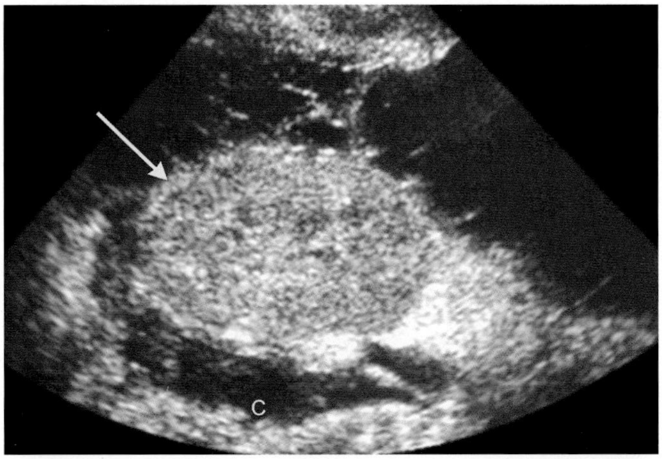

Fig. 13

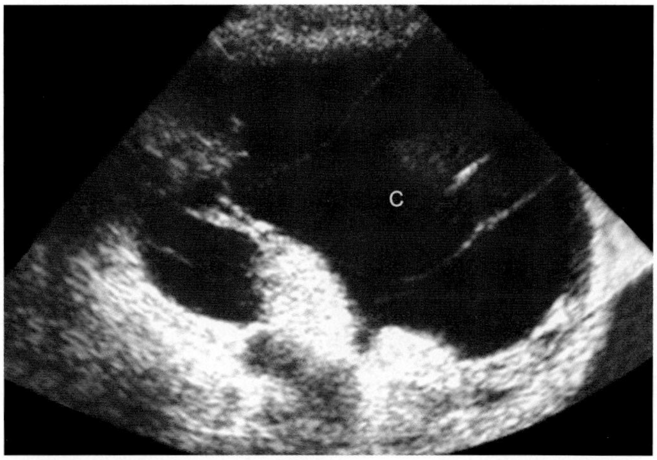

Fig. 14

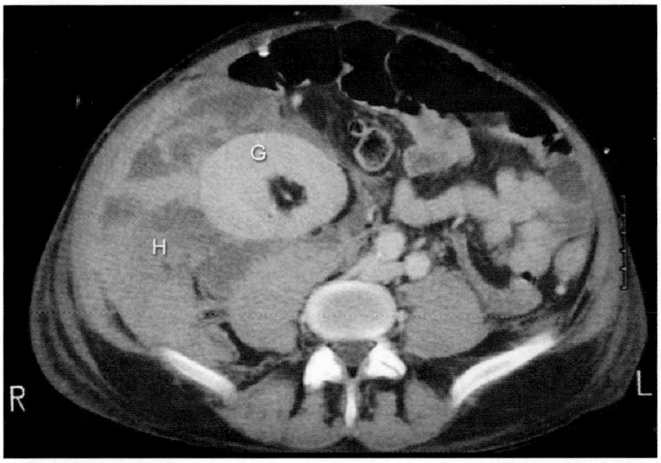

Fig. 15

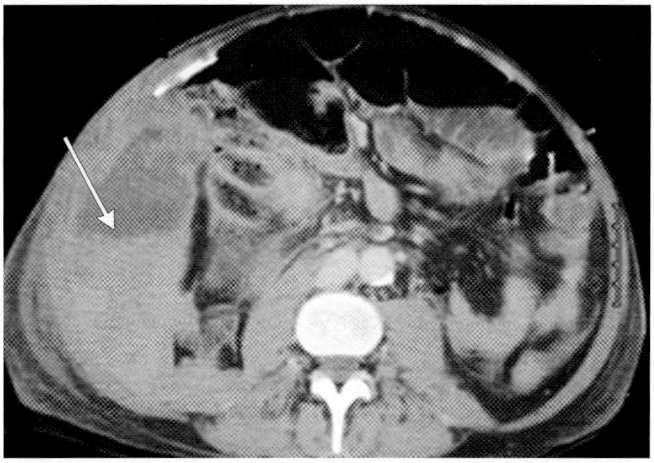

Fig. 16

Figs. 13 to 16: (Figs. 13 and 14) Sagittal ultrasound depicts renal allograft (arrows) with increased echogenicity and decreased cortico-medullary differentiation surrounded by a complex multiseptated collection (C). Doppler evaluation (not shown) revealed an abrupt change of velocity of the renal vein, likely the result of extrinsic compression by the hematoma; (Figs. 15 and 16) Corresponding axial CT images show the typical appearance of extraperitoneal bleeding manifesting as a voluminous mixed-density collection (H) surrounding the graft (G).The high attenuation suggests a hematoma as the etiology of the collection. Note the hematocrit effect (arrow).

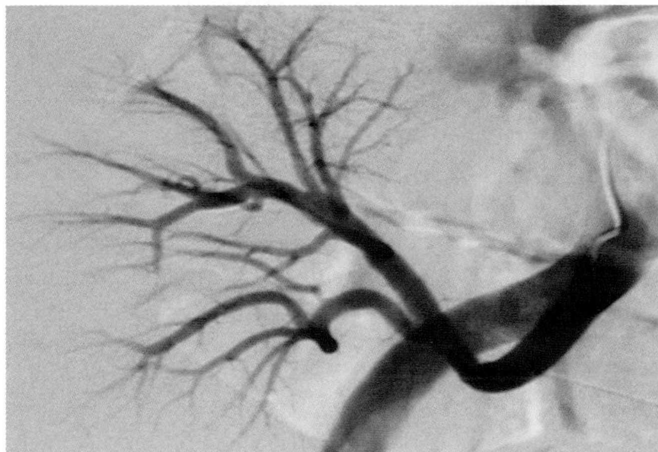

Fig. 17: An angiogram was performed to exclude vascular compromise and bleeding from the graft.

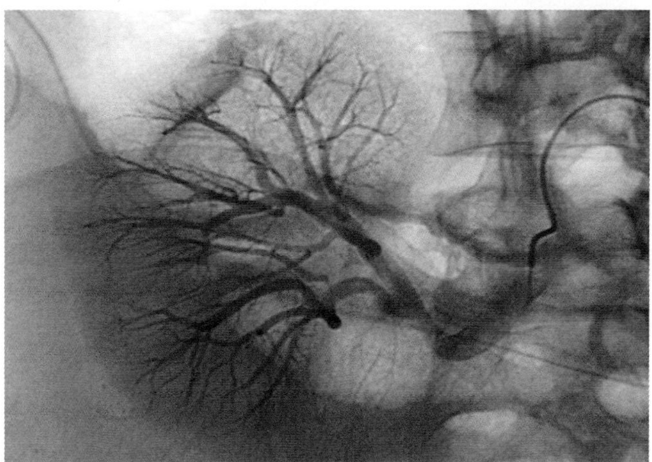

Fig. 18: Arterial and capillary phases depict normal findings and no cause for the bleeding.

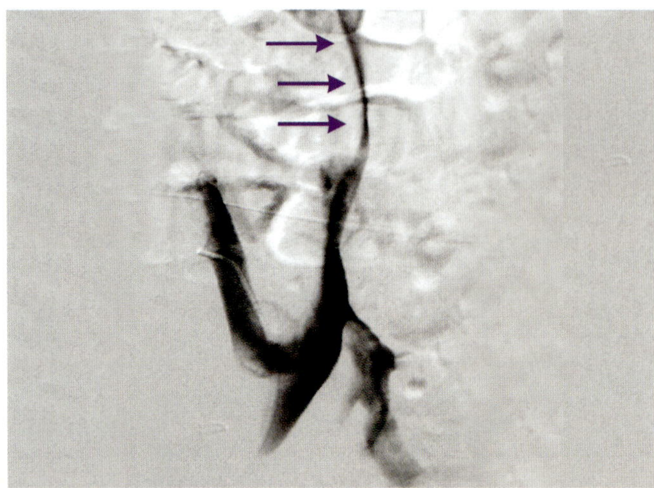

Fig. 19: The venous phase shows compression of the inferior vena cava (arrows) and diminished intrarenal venous flow (consistent with the Doppler findings).

Post-Biopsy Perinephric Hematoma (Figs. 20 to 23)

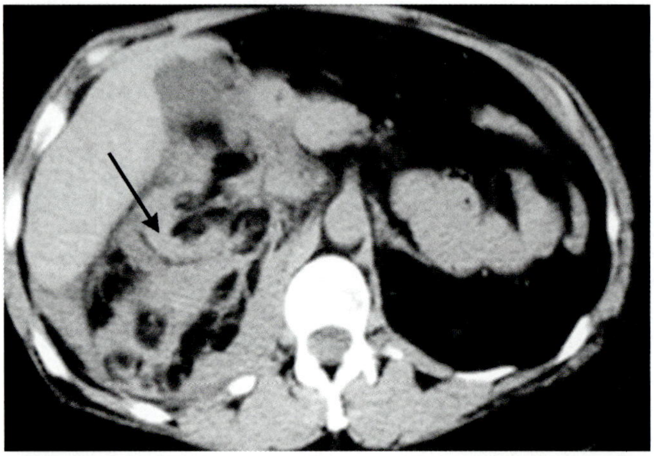

Fig. 20

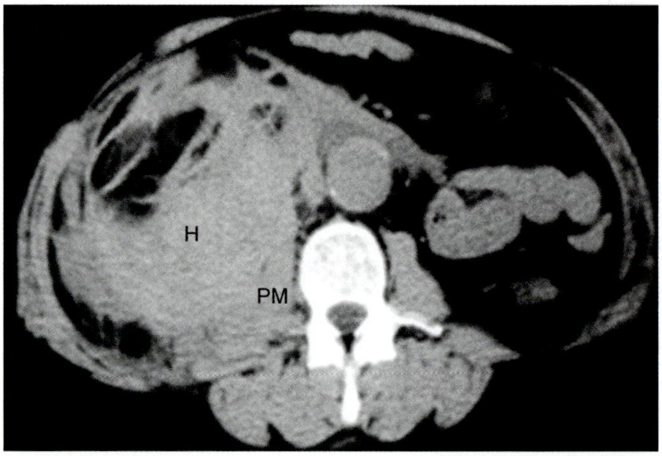

Fig. 21

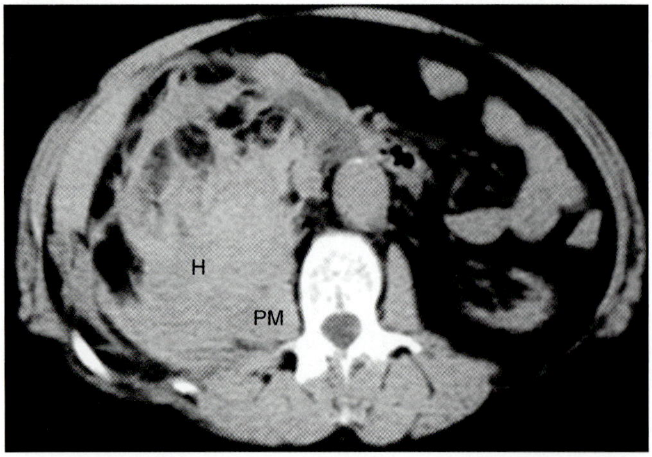

Fig. 22

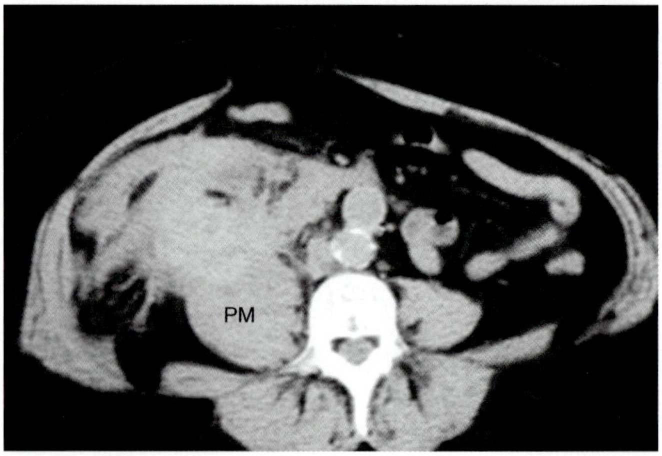

Fig. 23

Figs. 20 to 23: Serial axial CT images show a hyperdense hematoma (H) dissecting along extraperitoneal fat planes, abutting the psoas muscle (PM), and reaching the perirenal fat surrounding the atrophic native kidney (arrow).

Intraperitoneal Hematoma (Fig. 24)

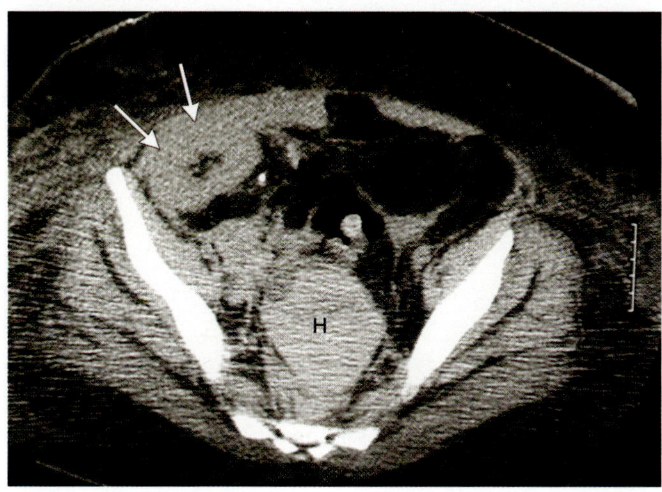

Fig. 24: Axial CT image shows a hyperdense collection of blood (H) located in the cul-de-sac (the most dependent portion of the peritoneal cavity). The fluid distribution within the peritoneal cavity differs relative to that in the extraperitoneal space. A right lower quadrant kidney allograft (arrows) is noted.

Hematomas Post Allograft Nephrectomy (Figs. 25 to 30)

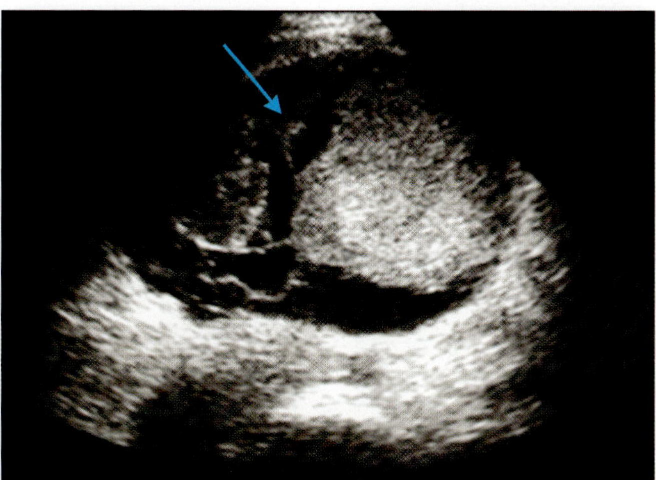

Fig. 25: Ultrasound transverse images show a complex heterogeneous collection (blue arrow) in the nephrectomy bed.

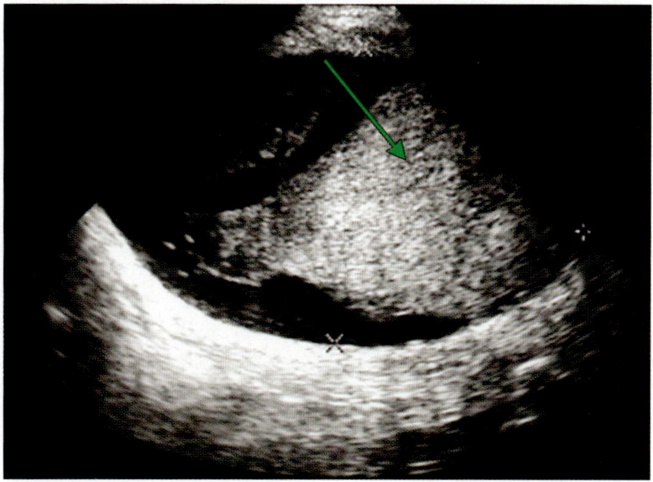

Fig. 26: The central echogenic area (green arrow) with no vascularity on color Doppler imaging represents a blood clot.

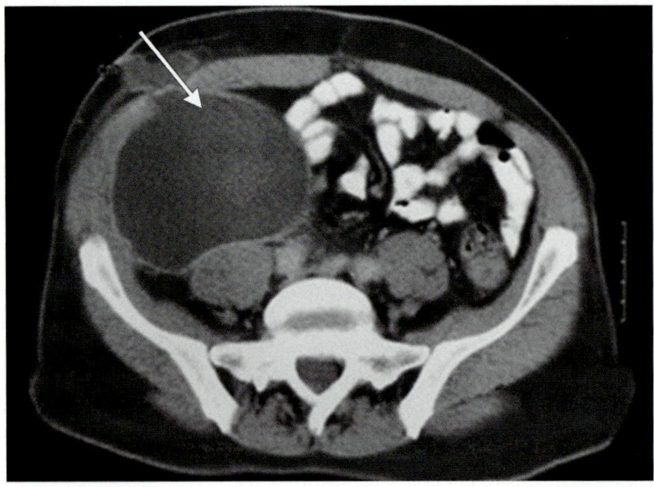

Fig. 27

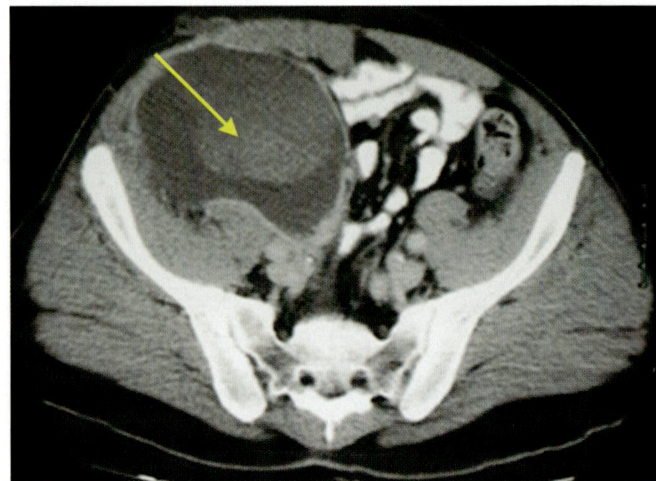

Fig. 28

Figs. 27 and 28: Axial CT images show a large rounded water-attenuation encapsulated collection (white arrow) in the graft nephrectomy bed. Notice the central relative hyperdense region (yellow arrow) that raised concerns for a vascular lesion (such as a pseudoaneurysm) but proved to be a hematoma. While CT provided a valuable correlation to the sonographic findings, Doppler evaluation allowed for the exclusion of a vascular lesion. The outer region reflects the serous component of the hematoma.

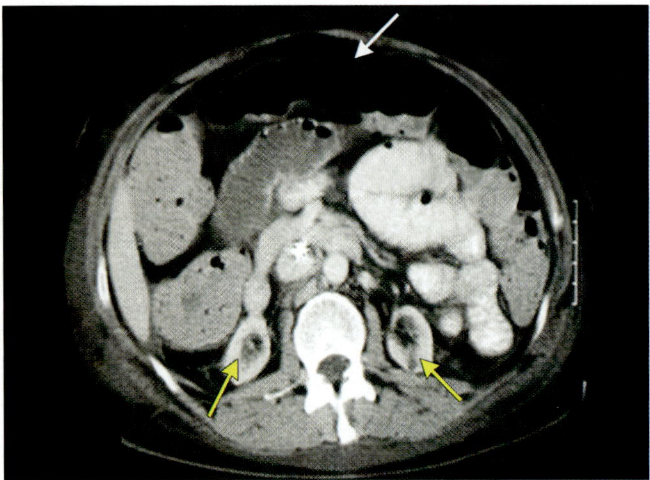

Fig. 29: CT imaging after graft nephrectomy showing atrophic native kidneys (yellow arrows) and a reflex ileus (white arrow).

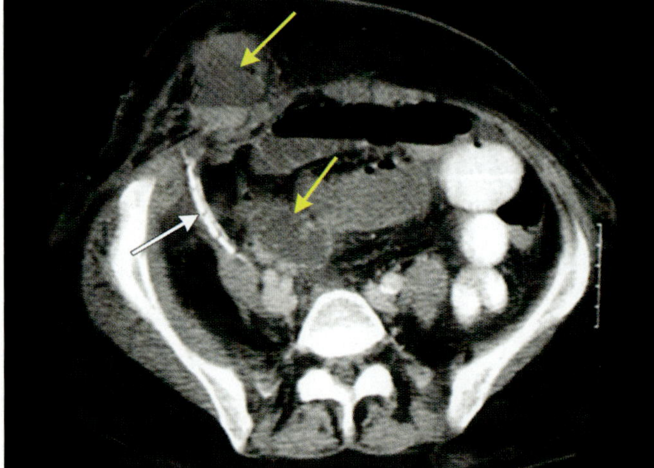

Fig. 30: CT after graft nephrectomy showing two collections consistent with hematomas (yellow arrows) with a drain (white arrow) within the right lower quadrant. Notice the fluid-fluid level in the wall hematoma (hematocrit effect).

Abdominal Wall Hematomas (Figs. 31 to 34)

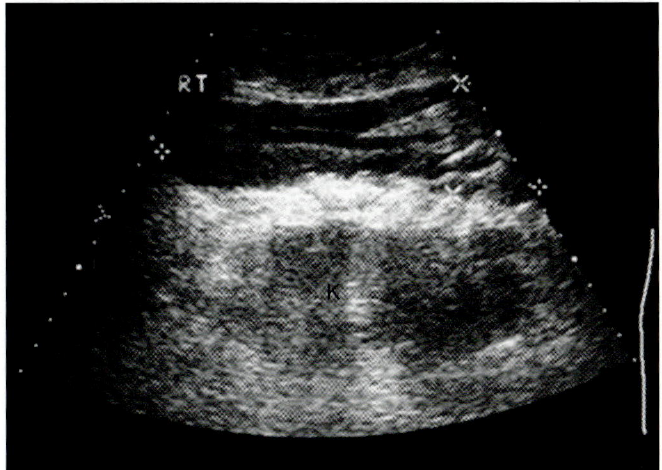

Fig. 31: Transverse sonogram shows a heterogeneous hematoma (delineated by cursors) located superficial to the kidney allograft (K).

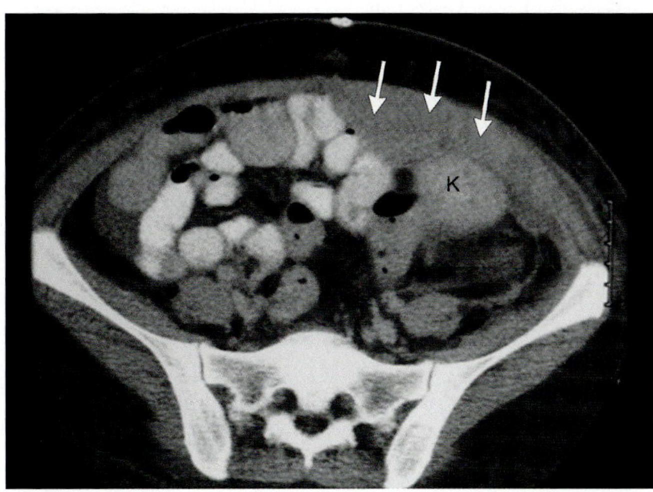

Fig. 32: Axial CT image shows enlargement of the rectus abdominis muscle due to the presence of a heterogeneous, mostly hyperdense hematoma (arrows). Allograft (K).

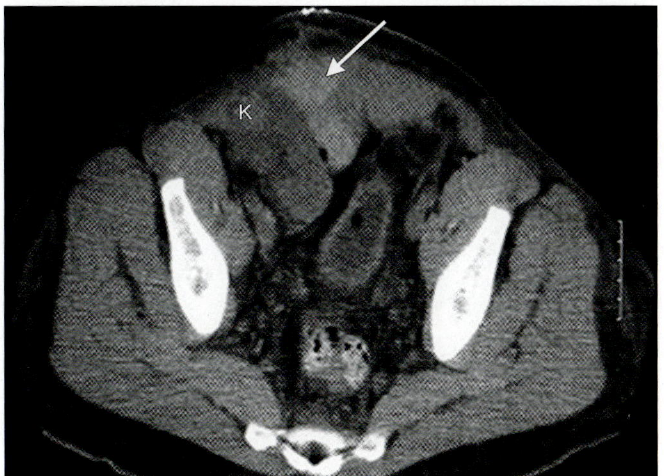

Fig. 33

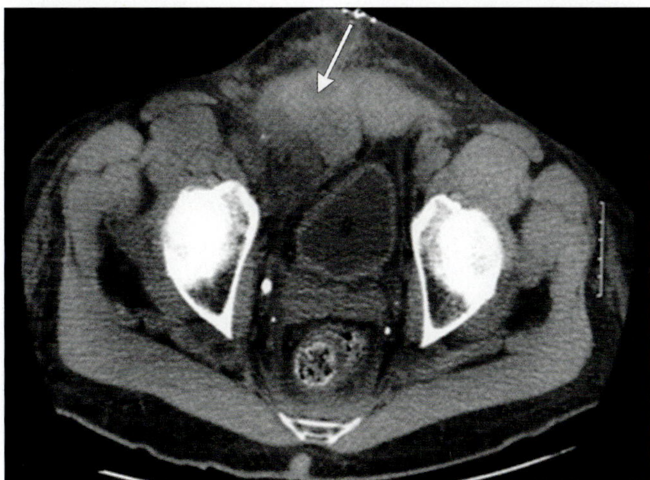

Fig. 34

Figs. 33 and 34: Consecutive axial CT images show a rectus sheath hematoma (arrows) causing muscle enlargement and indenting on the allograft (K).

URINOMAS (FIGS. 35 TO 40)

- Urinomas (urine collections) are a result of urinary leaks from the collecting system and/or bladder
- Most commonly seen at the distal ureter (ureter-bladder anastomosis), but also may occur at any portion of the excretory tract including the calyceal system (although this location is unusual and secondary to segmental infarction)
- Urinary leaks are usually due to ischemic damage
- Urinomas:
  - Are an early complication after surgery
  - Tend to grow relatively rapidly
  - Are usually rounded or lobulated in appearance
  - Are localized between the graft and the bladder, usually near the mid-ureter
  - Appearance in various imaging modalities reflect its fluid:
    - Anechoic on US
    - Water density and signal intensity on CT and MRI respectively
  - Although the aforementioned imaging findings are nonspecific, specificity may be achieved by means of
    - aspiration of the fluid (that has a creatinine value greater than that in blood)
    - antegrade pyelogram
    - nuclear medicine study
      - gradual radioisotope concentration is seen within a collection that initially manifested as a cold defect
      - obtaining delayed scans is indispensable as accumulation of the radiopharmaceutical may take some time
    - contrast material-enhanced CT obtained in the excretory phase may also reveal opacified urine extravasating into the urinoma
    - retrograde pyelogram

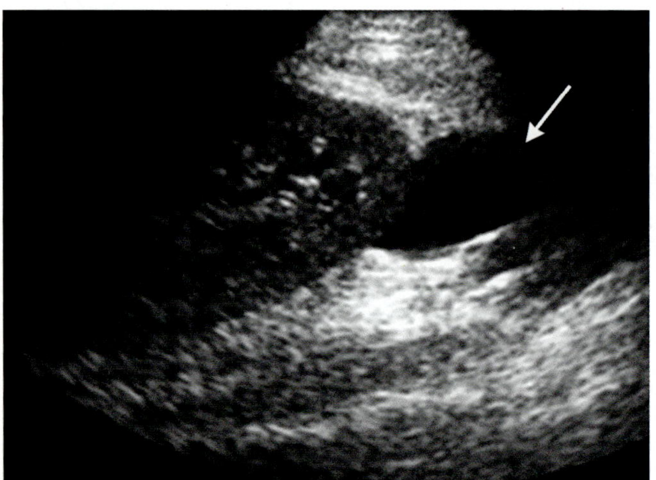

Fig. 35

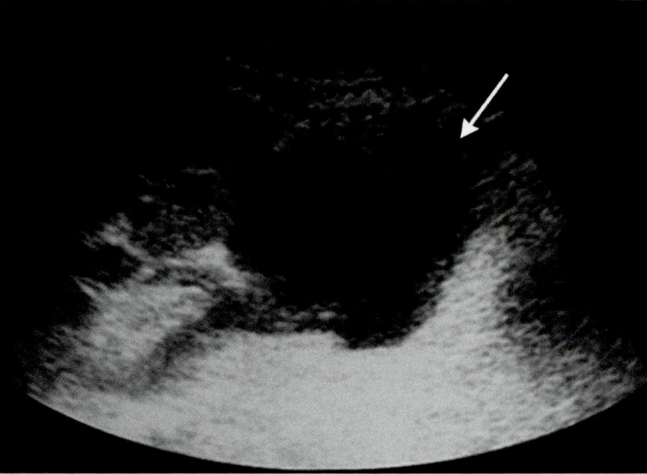

Fig. 36

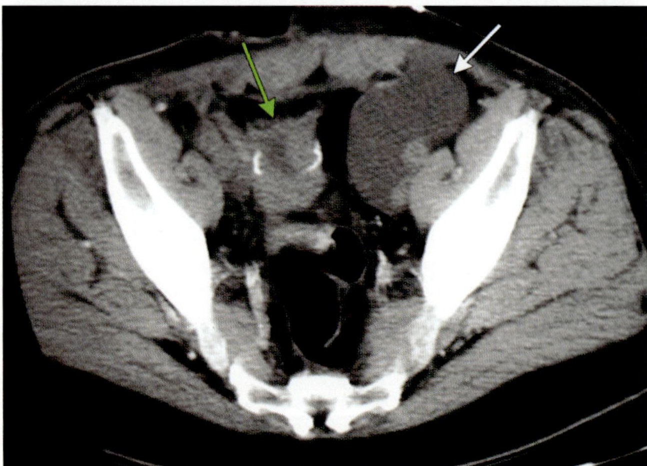

Fig. 37

Figs. 35 to 37: Multiple views of a well-demarcated perinephric transplant fluid collection adjacent to the lower pole of the graft (white arrows) that turned out to be a urinoma. A prospective diagnosis of urinoma based solely on these images is not possible due to the nonspecific appearance of the fluid collection. Note the pancreas transplant at the right lower quadrant (green arrow).

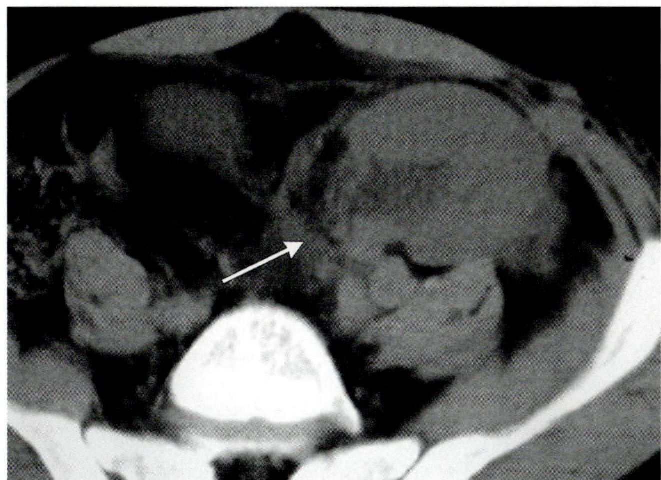

Fig. 38: Axial CT image of the left lower quadrant showing an irregularly shaped fluid collection (arrow) dissecting along fat planes medial to the allograft.

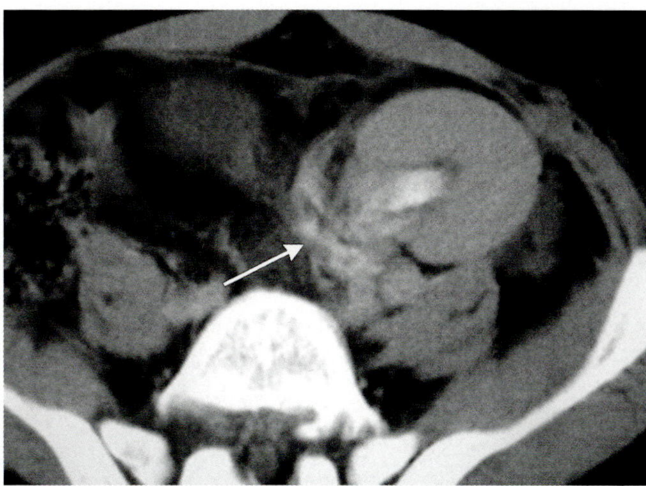

Fig. 39: Excretory phase CT image after contrast material administration. There is progressive enhancement of the collection confirming extravasation of urine (arrow). The irregular infiltration of fat is typical of the extraperitoneal location of the fluid.

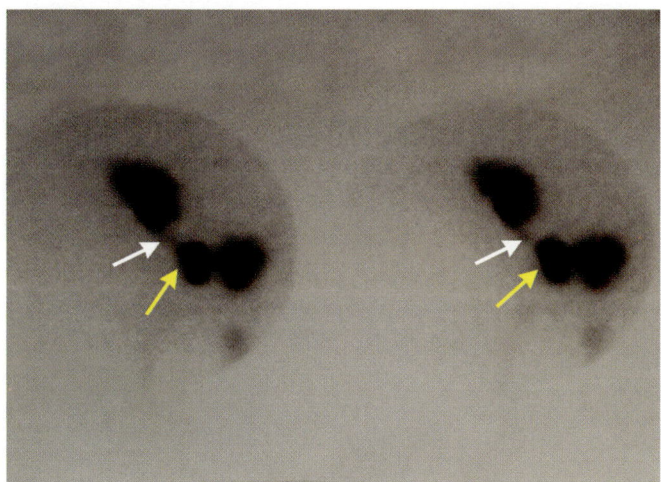

Fig. 40: The nuclear medicine renal scan demonstrates passage of radiotracer from the distal ureter (white arrows) into a bilobed collection, the urinoma, (yellow arrows) adjacent to the bladder.

LYMPHOCELES (FIGS. 41 TO 53)

- Lymphoceles are collections of lymphatic fluid that form in most cases secondary to the disruption of lymphatic channels sustained during the dissection of the iliac vessels at the time of implantation
- They may develop at any time but are usually seen between the 4th and 8th weeks after transplantation
- They are probably the most common peritransplant collections
- Most of them are small and inconsequential but some may become large and cause compression of the graft or the collecting system with ensuing hydronephrosis
- Sonographically lymphoceles are anechoic, round or lobulated, often septated fluid collections, most commonly located between the lower pole of the graft and the bladder
- On CT and MRI they manifest as typical fluid collections with nonspecific characteristics
- Although they have a tendency to recurrence, most do not require aspiration

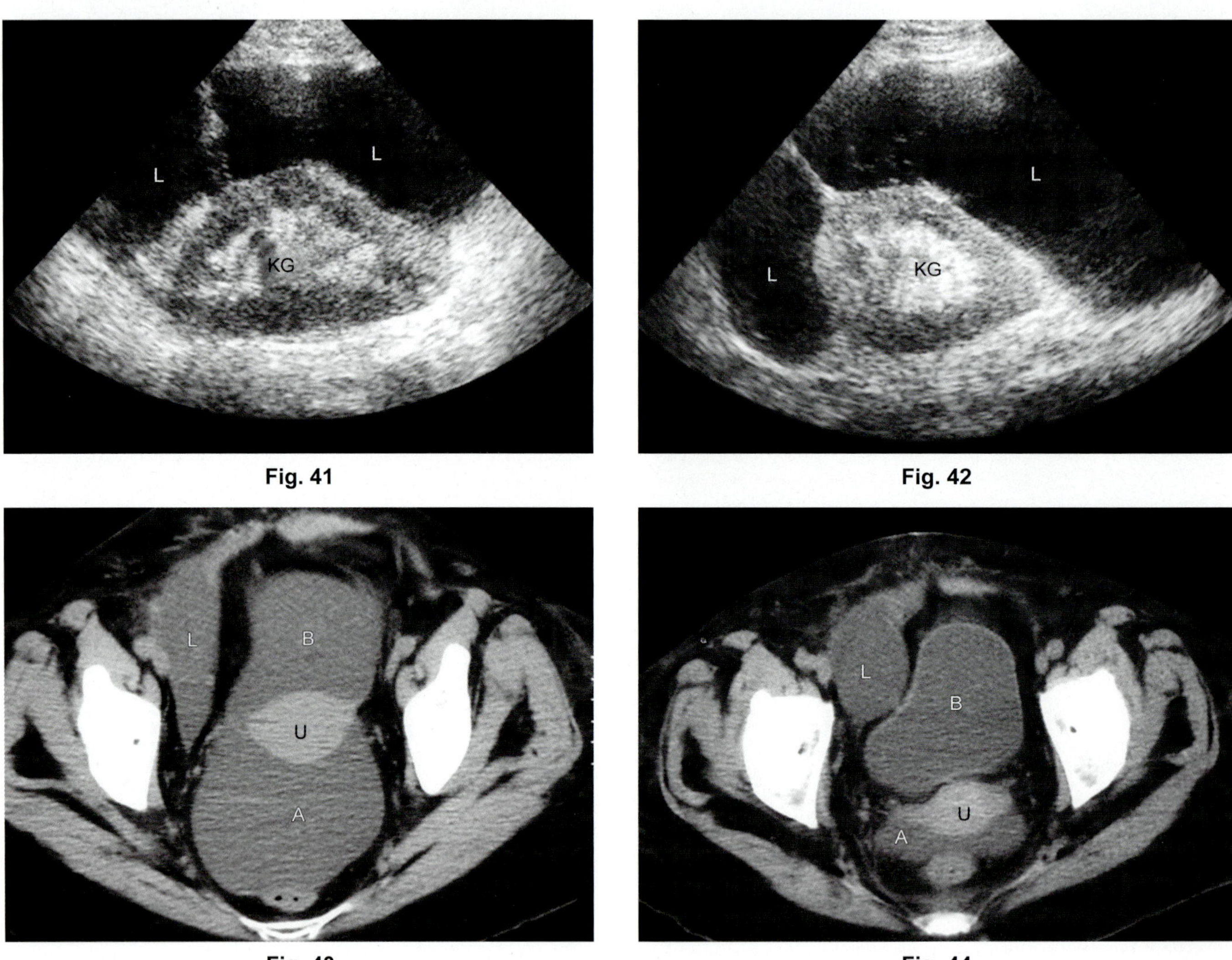

Fig. 41 Fig. 42

Fig. 43 Fig. 44

Figs. 41 to 44: (Figs. 41 and 42) Ultrasound images show a complex heterogeneous fluid collection (L) surrounding the allograft (KG); (Figs. 43 and 44) The corresponding CT images of the same case show a well-demarcated homogeneous fluid collection (L) in the right lower quadrant adjacent to and indenting on the bladder (B). Ascites (A) is seen in the pouch of Douglas. Lymphoceles are homogeneous on CT but usually show septa on US imaging. (U) Uterus.

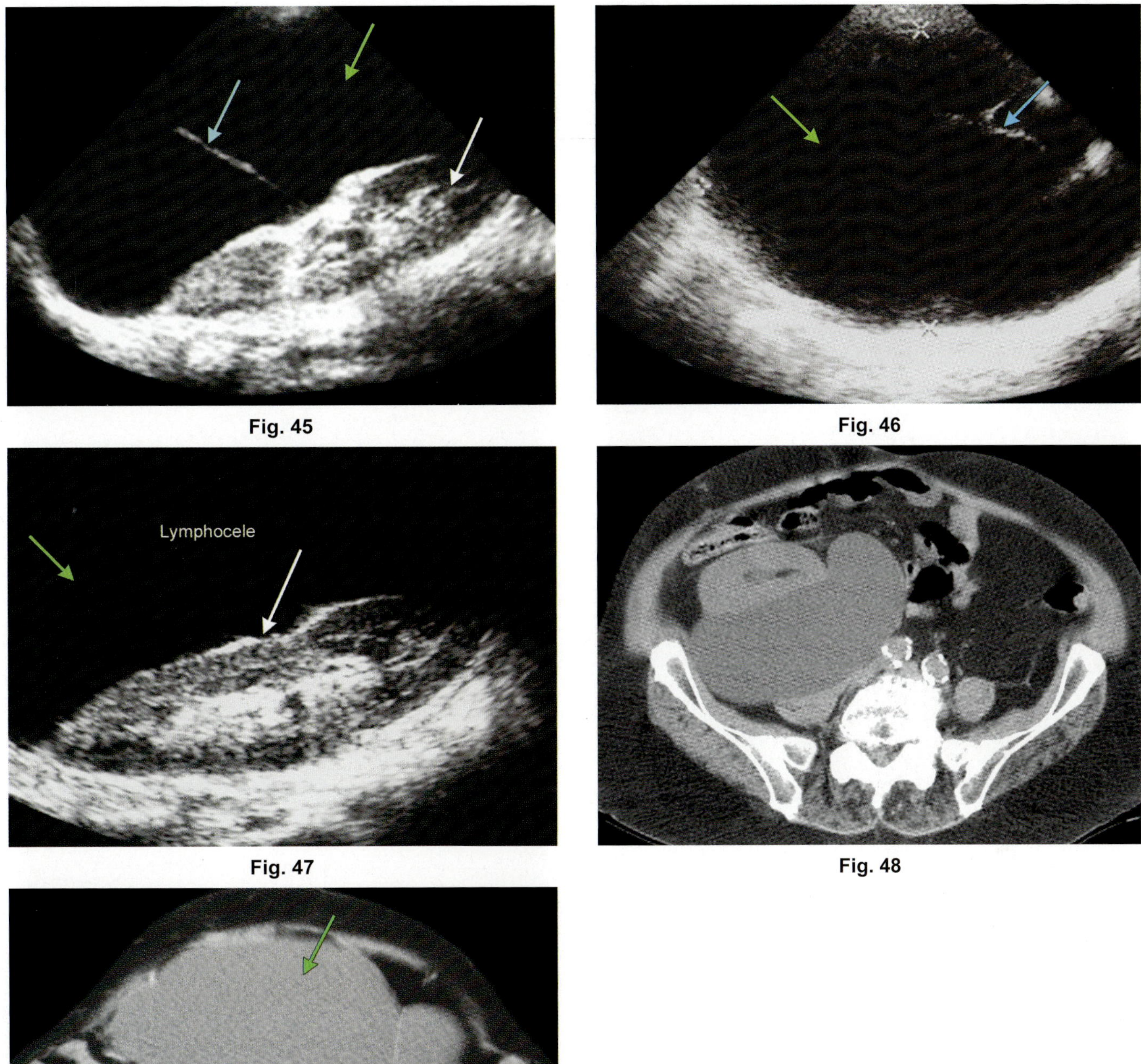

Fig. 45

Fig. 46

Fig. 47

Fig. 48

Fig. 49

Figs. 45 to 49: (Figs. 45 to 47) Ultrasound and (Figs. 48 and 49) CT images of lymphoceles (green arrows) compressing the allografts (white arrows). In the presence of physiologic alterations (such as vascular or ureteral compression) lymphoceles should be drained. Collections of this magnitude may be associated with elevated resistive indices on Doppler US. The multiloculated appearance (blue arrows) is a typical sonographic finding of lymphoceles.

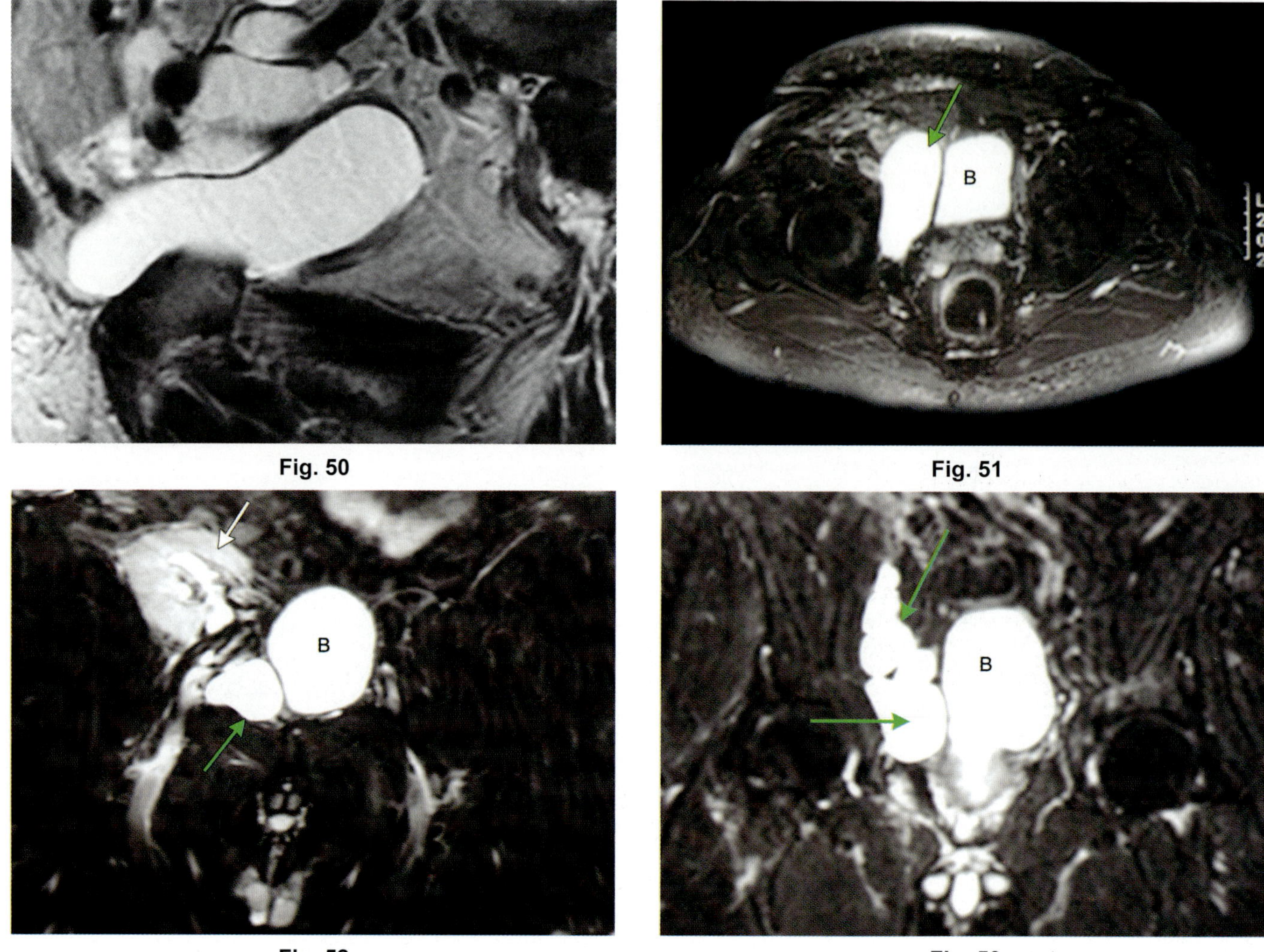

Fig. 50

Fig. 51

Fig. 52

Fig. 53

Figs. 50 to 53: MRI images of a lymphocele. (Fig. 50) T2-weighted sagittal; (Fig. 51) T2-weighted fat saturated axial and (Figs. 52 and 53) coronal images illustrate a right-sided hyperintense multiloculated collection compatible with a lymphocele (green arrows) indenting on the bladder contour (B). Note the normal appearing right lower quadrant kidney graft (white arrow).

Lymphoceles and Hydronephrosis (Figs. 54 to 57)

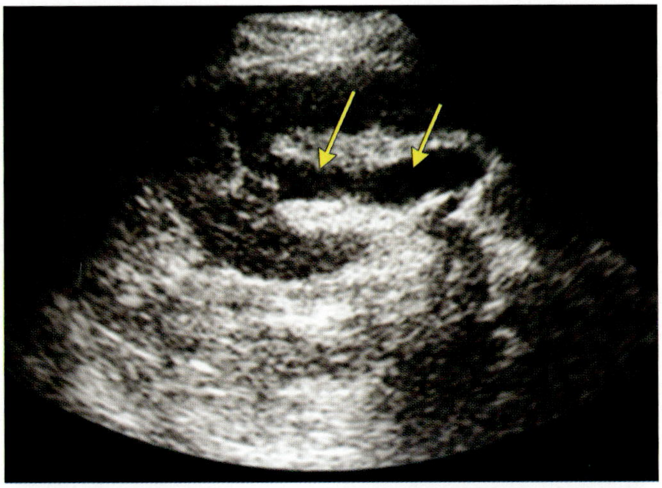

Fig. 54

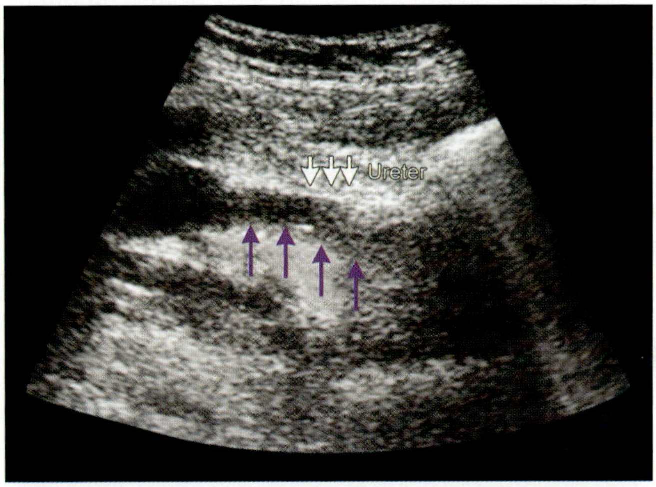

Fig. 55

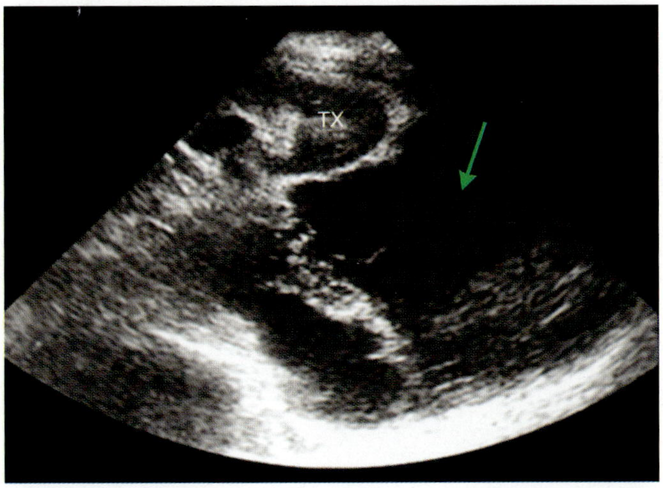

Fig. 56

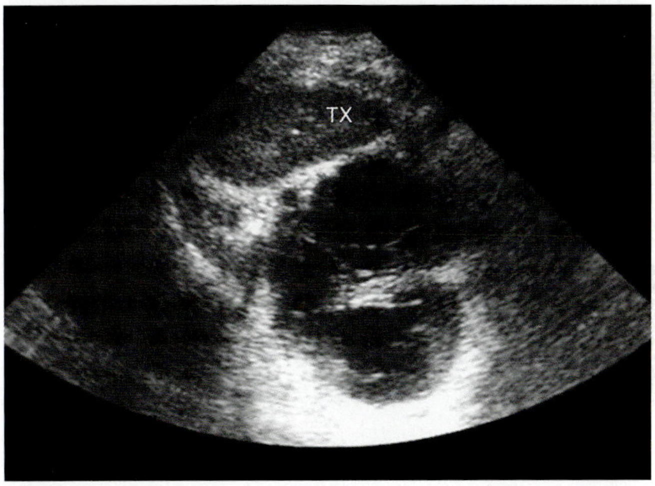

Fig. 57

Figs. 54 to 57: (Fig. 54) Sequential ultrasound images show hydronephrosis (yellow arrows) and (Fig. 55) ureteral dilatation (purple and white arrows) (Figs. 56 and 57) These figures show a complex multiseptated fluid collection (green arrow) adjacent to the hydronephrotic graft (TX). The presence of septa is typical of lymphoceles although not specific. As illustrated in this case, lymphoceles may exert a mass effect and result in graft dysfunction.

ABSCESSES (FIGS. 58 TO 68)

- Purulent collections may be seen at any time after transplantation, but most commonly occur in the early postoperative period
- Although clinical and laboratory findings may suggest their infectious nature, abscesses may also have a silent or atypical presentation
- Since transplant patients are more susceptible to infections than non-immunosuppressed individuals, imaging is crucial in the evaluation as well as in the diagnostic and/or therapeutic drainage of collections
- Imaging is also important to exclude other causes of infections
- Abscesses manifest as fluid-containing lesions or collections within or outside of the allograft
- Ultrasound usually reveals low-level echoes within the abscesses
- Abscesses may even be solid-appearing
- Abscesses are often well-defined with a ring-enhancing capsule on CT or MRI
- The presence of gas is less frequent but adds specificity to the diagnosis

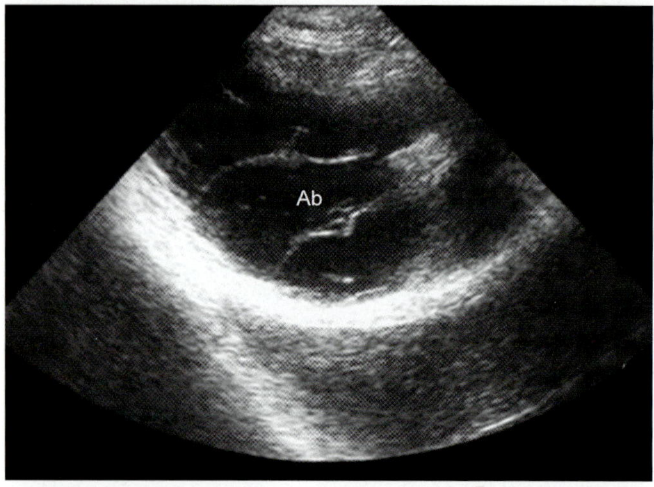

Fig. 58: Transverse ultrasound image showing a multilocular fluid collection consistent with an abscess (Ab) in a patient with fever and an elevated white blood cell count.

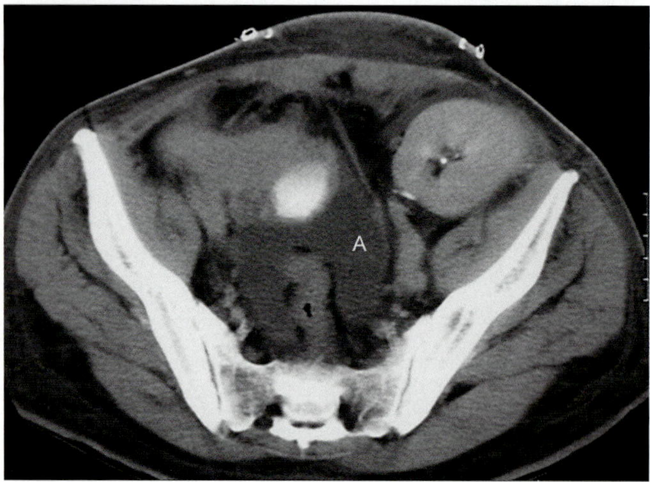

Fig. 59

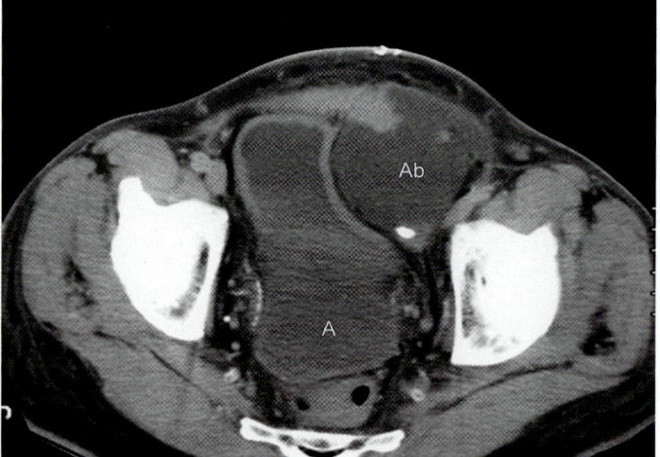

Fig. 60

Figs. 59 and 60: Axial CT images show an encapsulated fluid collection surrounding the allograft and compressing the bladder. Notice also the presence of ascites (A).

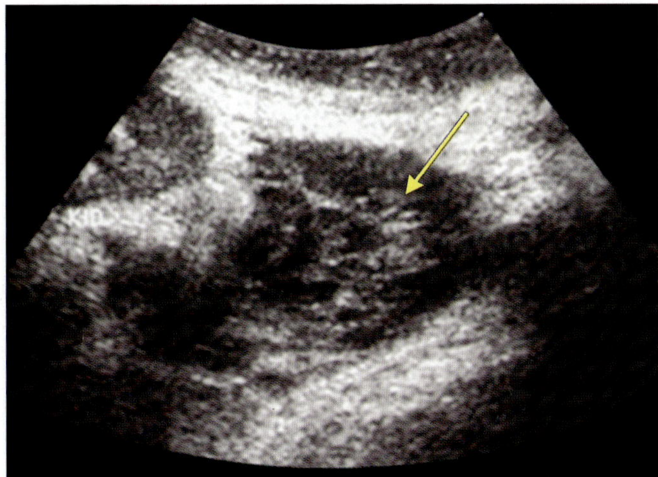

Fig. 61: US of a complex perinephric collection with multiple irregular echoes (yellow arrow) between the allograft and the bladder. Purulent material was aspirated.

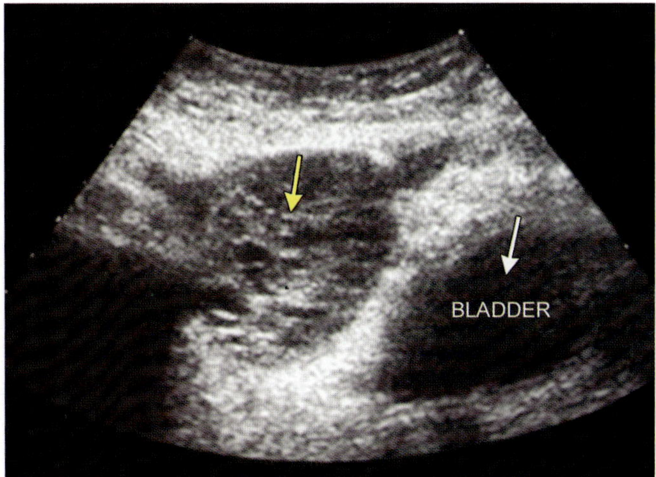

Fig. 62: Perinephric collections (yellow arrow) should not be confused with urine within the urinary bladder (white arrow).

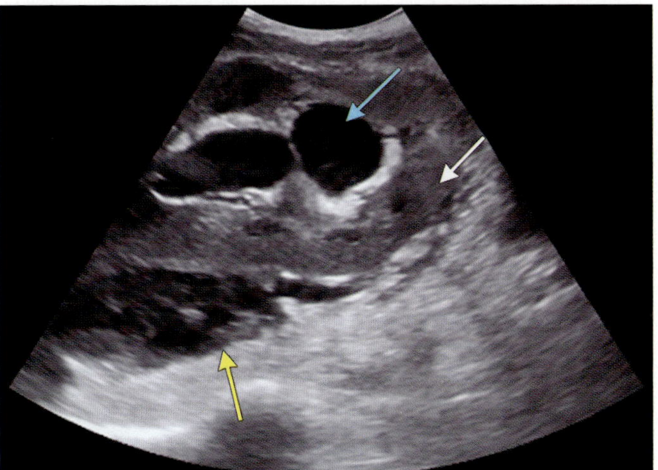

Fig. 63

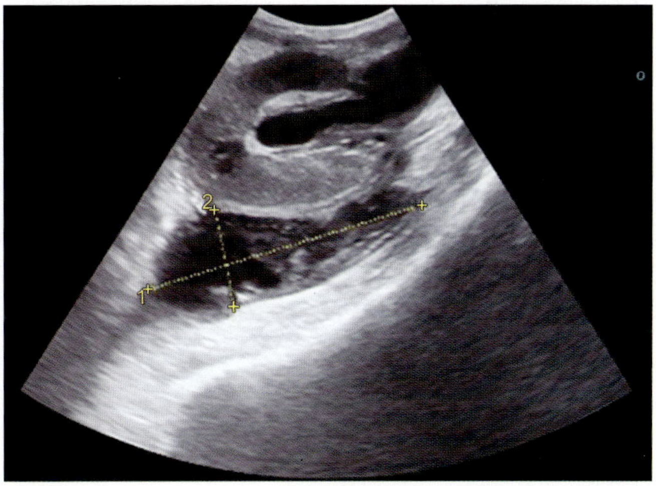

Fig. 64

Figs. 63 and 64: Sagittal views of a transplanted kidney (white arrow) with a perinephric collection (subsequently identified as an abscess) shown by a yellow arrow in Figure 63 and by markers in Figure 64. Note as well the presence of hydronephrosis (blue arrow).

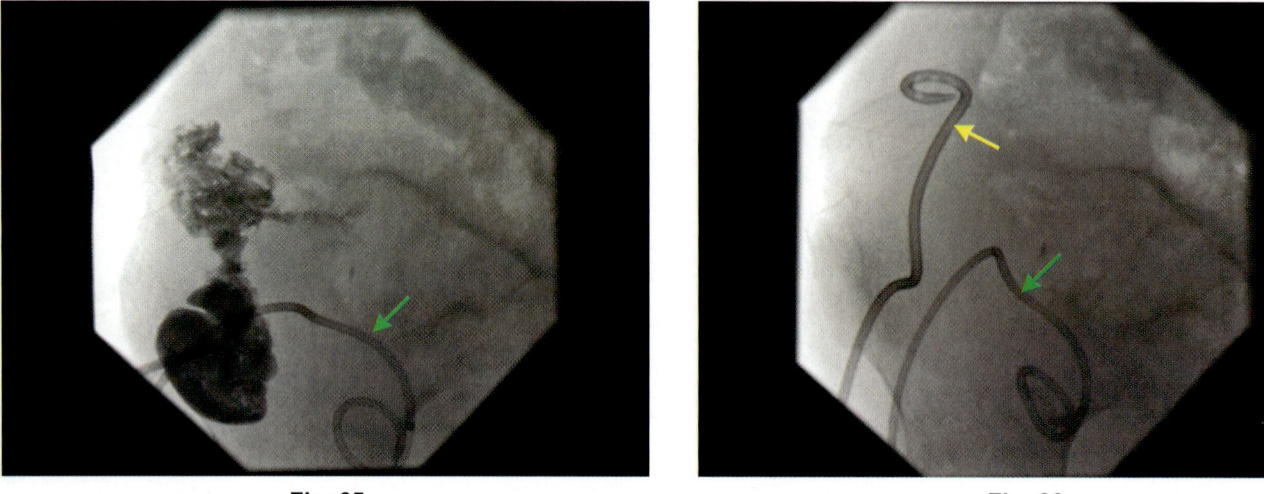

Fig. 65 Fig. 66

Figs. 65 and 66: (Fig. 65) The abscess was identified and drained (Fig. 66) percutaneously (yellow arrow). The green arrow shows a nephrostomy tube placed to decompress the hydronephrosis.

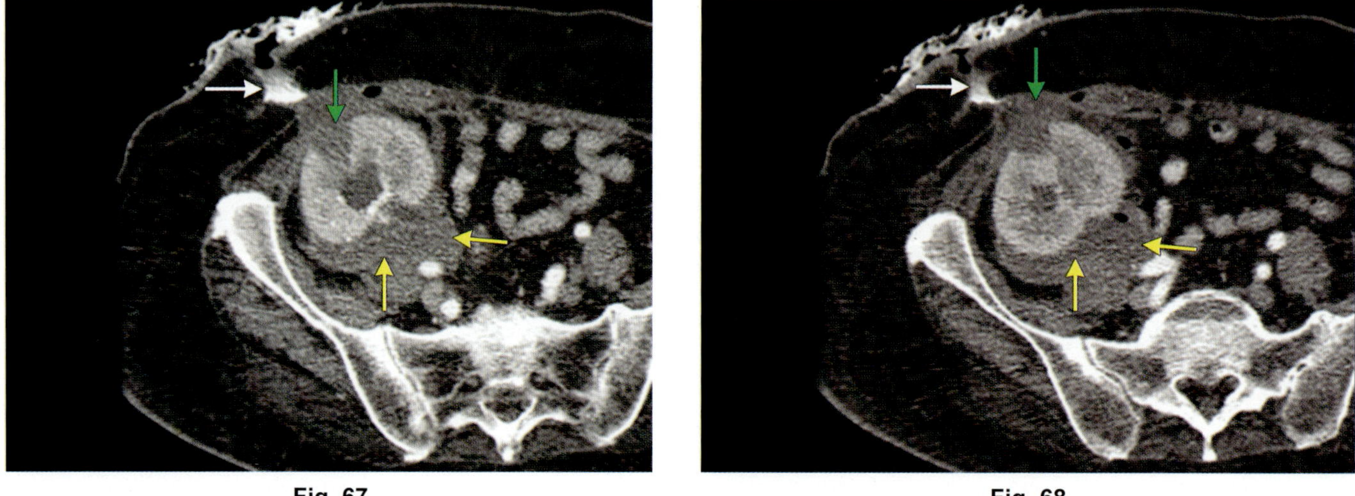

Fig. 67 Fig. 68

Figs. 67 and 68: Axial CT images show a perinephric fluid collection (yellow arrows) with gas bubbles located posterior to the allograft. This proved to be an abscess on aspiration. A second smaller collection can be seen deep to the abdominal wall (green arrows). Notice contrast leaking through a defect in the wall consistent with a urinary fistula (white arrows).

MISCELLANEOUS COLLECTIONS (FIGS. 69 TO 76)

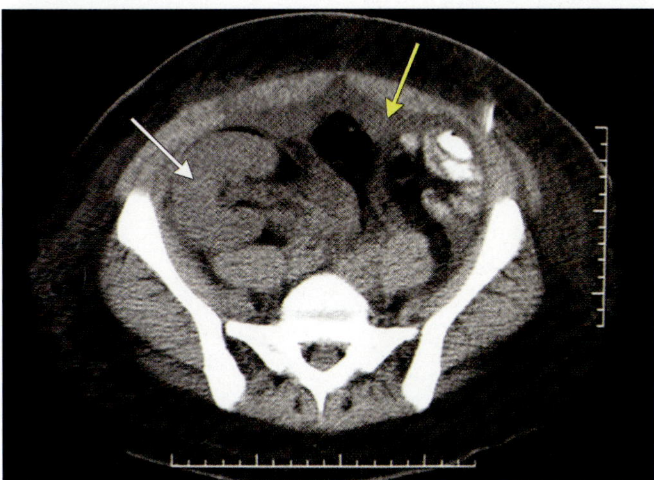

Fig. 69: Intraperitoneal fluid. CT axial image illustrating the presence of intra-peritoneal fluid (yellow arrow). Note the extra-peritoneal location of the allograft (white arrow), the lack of any prominent amount of extraperitoneal fluid, and the clear outline of the intraperitoneal ascitis.

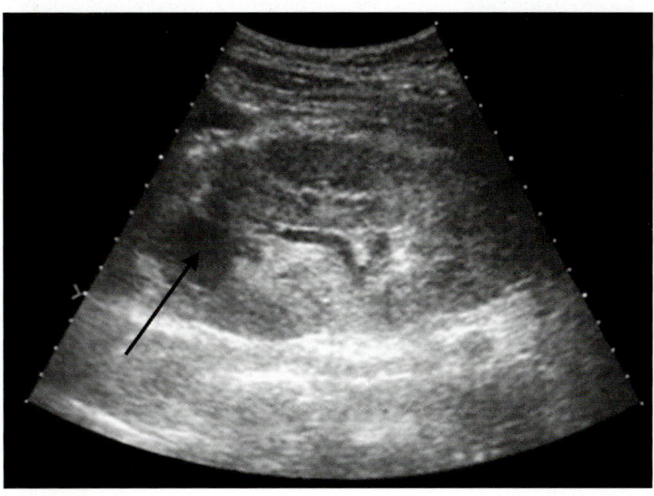

Fig. 70: Renal cyst. Longitudinal ultrasound shows a rounded fluid-containing structure (arrow) consistent with a simple cyst in the allograft.

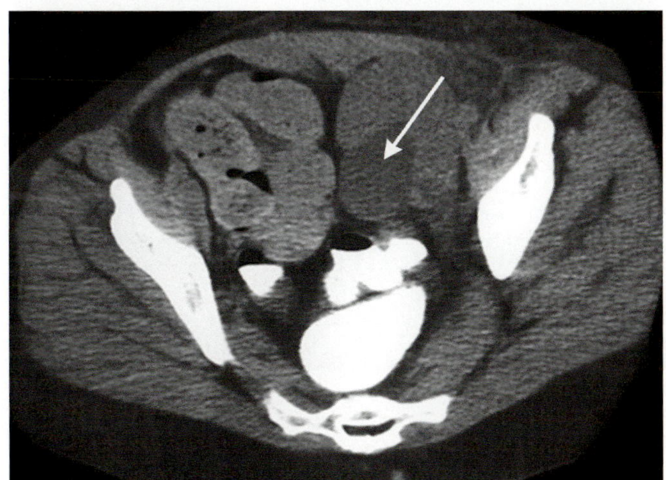

Fig. 71: Hydronephrosis. Cysts and fluid collections should not be confused with hydronephrosis of the allograft, as shown in this image (arrow) where the dilated renal pelvis is indicated by an arrow.

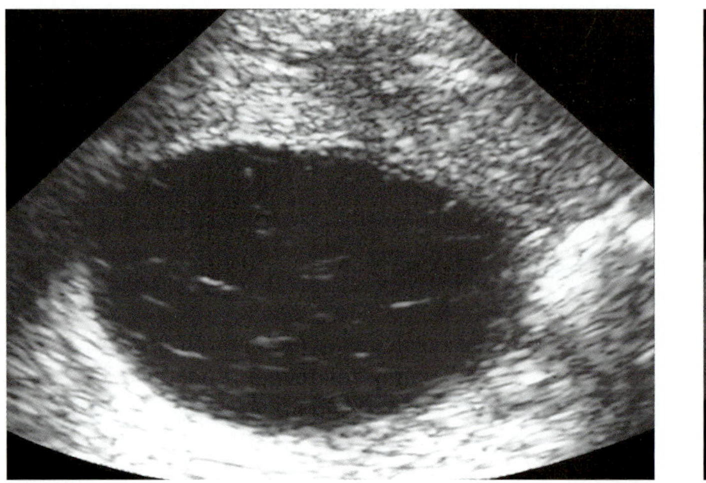

Fig. 72

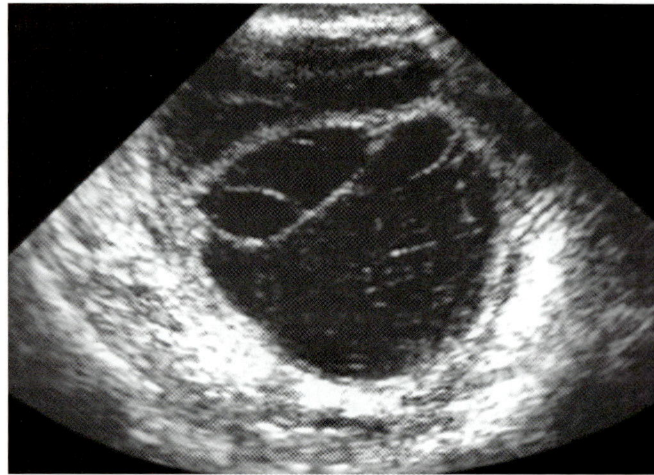

Fig. 73

Figs. 72 and 73: Hemorrhagic ovarian cyst. Young female transplant recipient with right lower quadrant pain, fever, and leukocytosis. US evaluation demonstrates a complex, septated cystic mass with low-level echoes consistent with a hemorrhagic ovarian cyst.

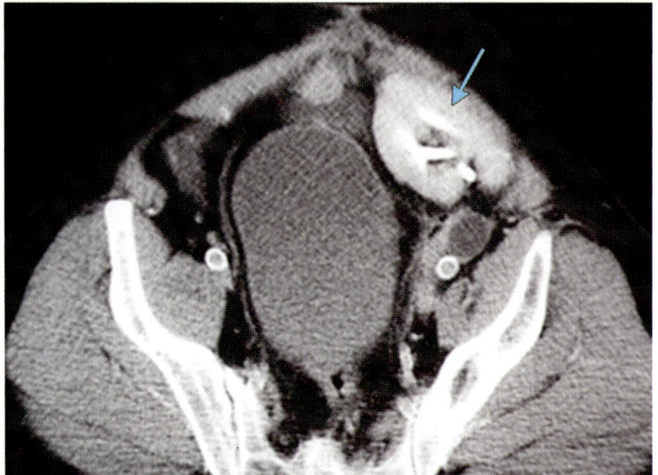

Fig. 74

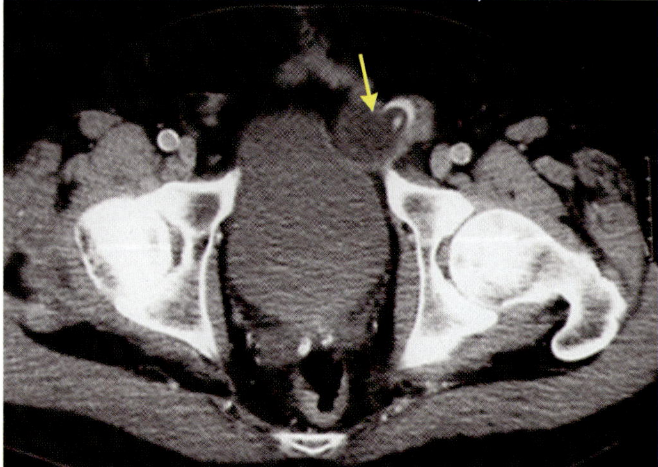

Fig. 75

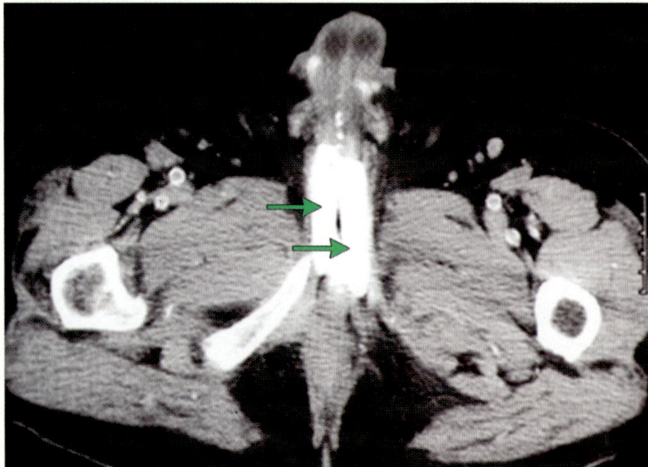

Fig. 76

Figs. 74 to 76: Sequential axial CT images in a patient with a left lower quadrant renal transplant (blue arrow) showing a rounded fluid-filled structure (yellow arrow) indenting the anterolateral bladder wall. Although this could be misleading to the diagnosis of a collection, careful scrutiny of consecutive images shows it represents the insufflation device of a penile prosthesis (green arrows). Notice the extensive vascular calcifications in this diabetic patient who had undergone a simultaneous pancreas kidney transplantation.

CHAPTER 59

Parenchymal Imaging

Mariano Volpacchio, Catherine D'Agostino, Christopher Palestro, et al.

NORMAL STUDY (FIGS. 1 AND 2)

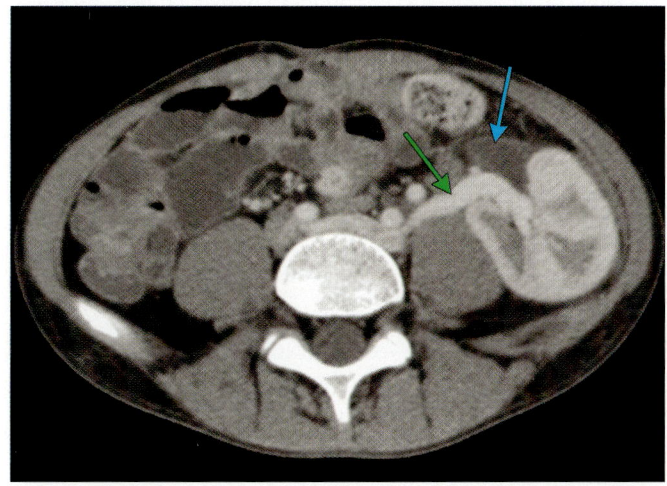

Fig. 1

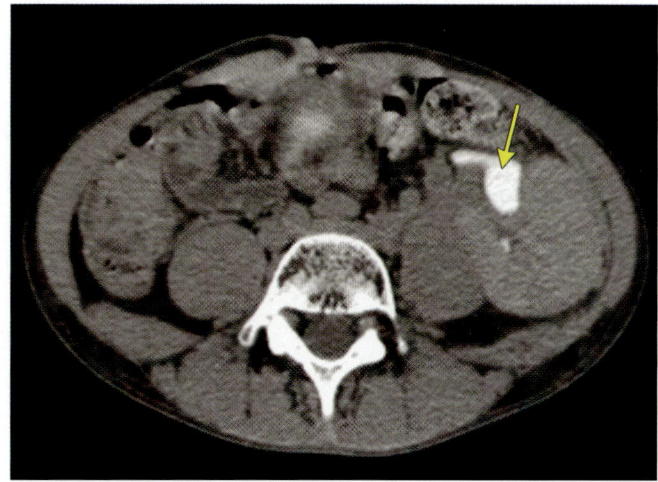

Fig. 2

Figs. 1 and 2: CT of a normal transplant kidney in the left lower quadrant. (Fig. 1) On the corticomedullary phase the extrarenal pelvis (blue arrow) could be potentially misinterpreted as a cystic lesion or a perirenal fluid collection. (Fig. 2) The excretory phase shows filling with excreted opacified urine (yellow arrow) confirming a normal finding. Notice normal donor renal vein joining to the recipient left external iliac vein (green arrow).

ALLOGRAFT CYST (FIGS. 3 AND 4)

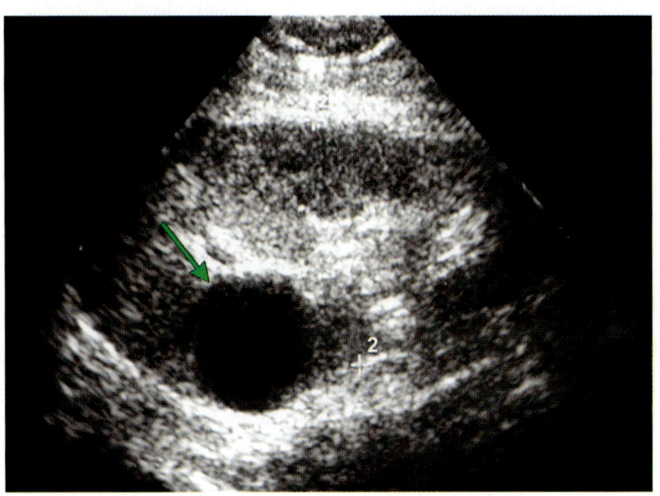

Fig. 3

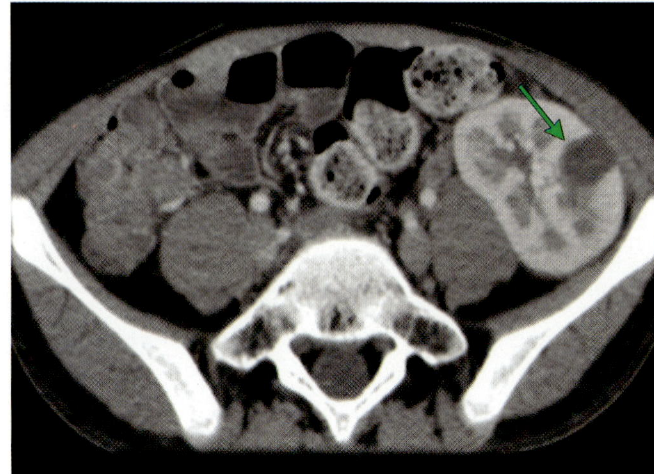

Fig. 4

Figs. 3 and 4: Renal allograft cysts (green arrows). Transplanted kidneys may contain cysts. It is important to determine prior to transplantation that such cysts have no current or potential malignancy. When in doubt, an MRI of the kidneys or a biopsy should always be obtained. These findings have to be thoroughly discussed with the potential recipient prior to implantation.

ACUTE TUBULAR NECROSIS (FIGS. 5 TO 11)

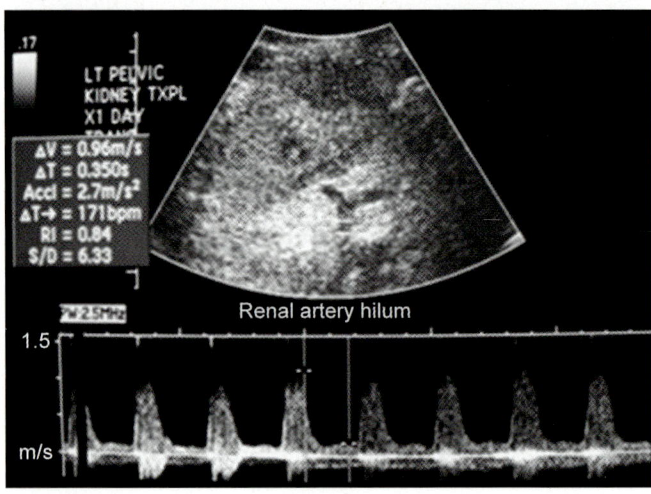

Fig. 5

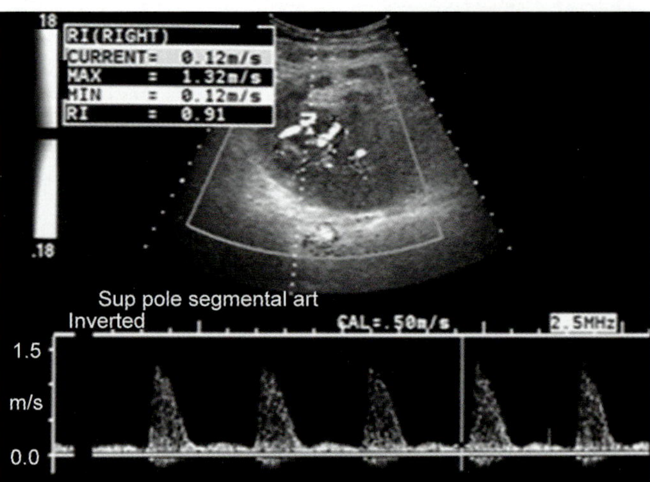

Fig. 6

Figs. 5 and 6: Serial images illustrating increasing resistive index (RI) on consecutive days—diagnosis of acute tubular necrosis (ATN) confirmed by biopsy.

$$RI = \frac{\text{peak systolic velocity (PSV)} - \text{end diastolic velocity (EDV)}}{\text{peak systolic velocity (PSV)}}$$

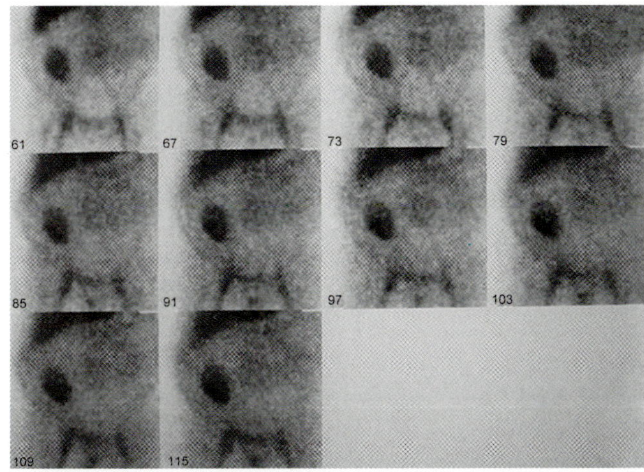

Fig. 7: Images from a ^{99m}Tc-MAG3 renal scan allograft with acute tubular necrosis (ATN). There is renal cortical uptake of tracer but no excretion.

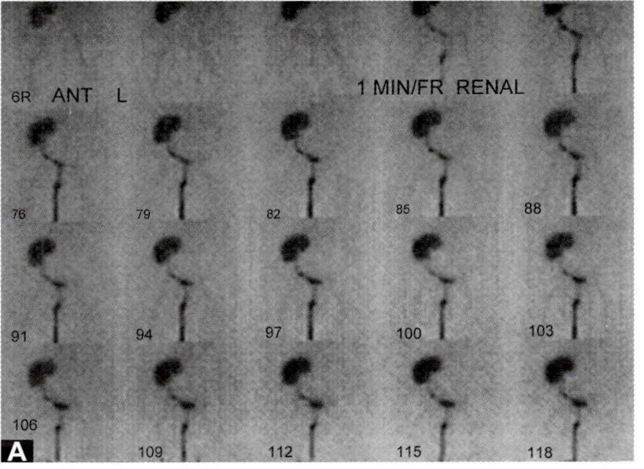

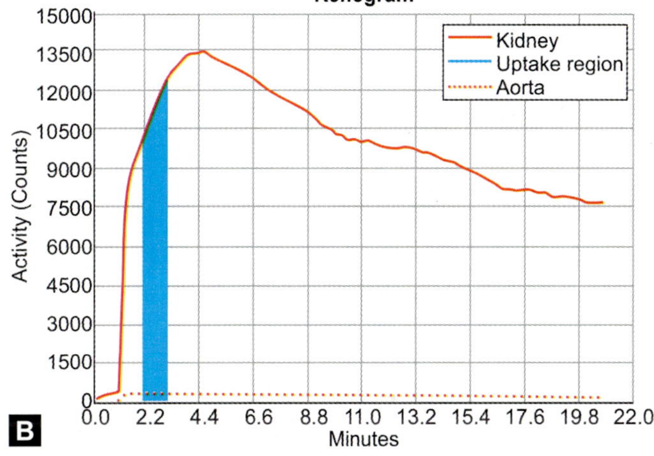

Figs. 8A and B: In this case of mild ATN, there is some radiotracer draining via an open urinary catheter.

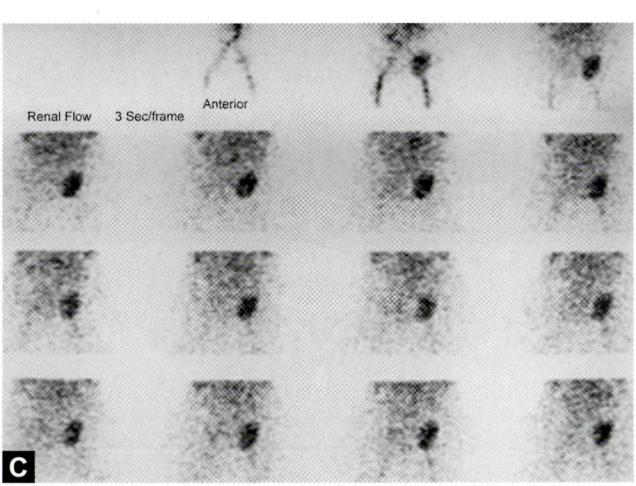

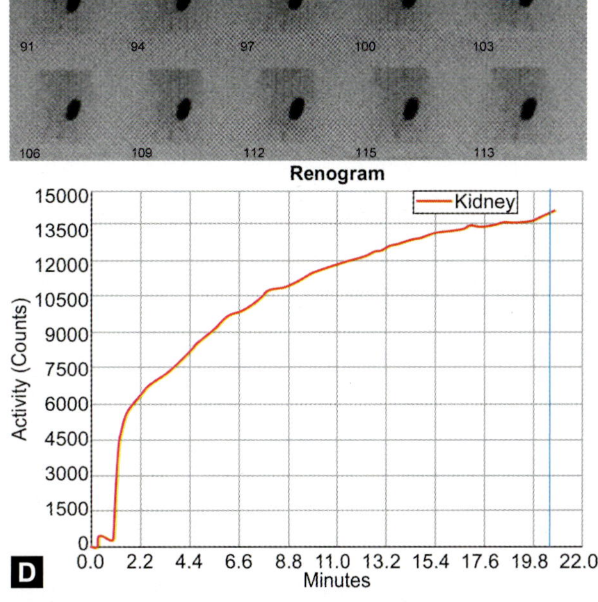

Figs. 8C and D: There is normal flow to the transplant, with continually increasing cortical activity over time. This is the classical presentation of ATN on a ^{99m}Tc-MAG3 renal scan.

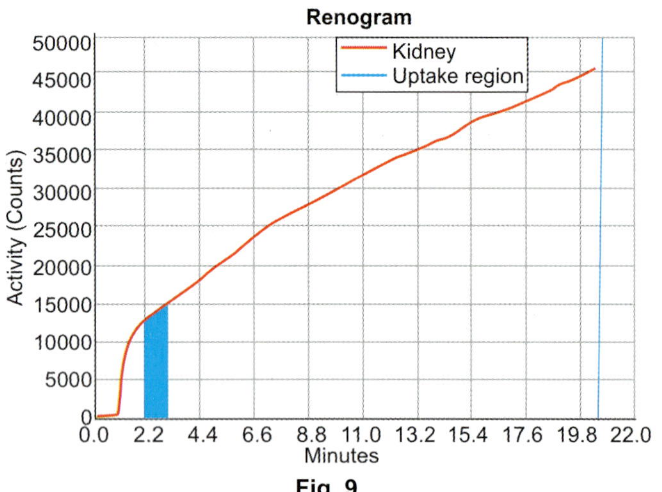

Fig. 9

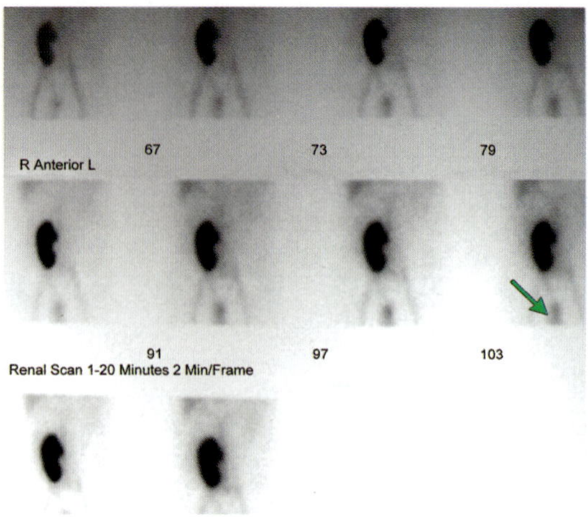

Fig. 10

Figs. 9 and 10: Both the renogram and the images from the ^{99m}Tc-MAG3 renal scan demonstrate continually increasing cortical activity over time. There is minimal drainage from the collecting system with only faint bladder activity identified (green arrow).

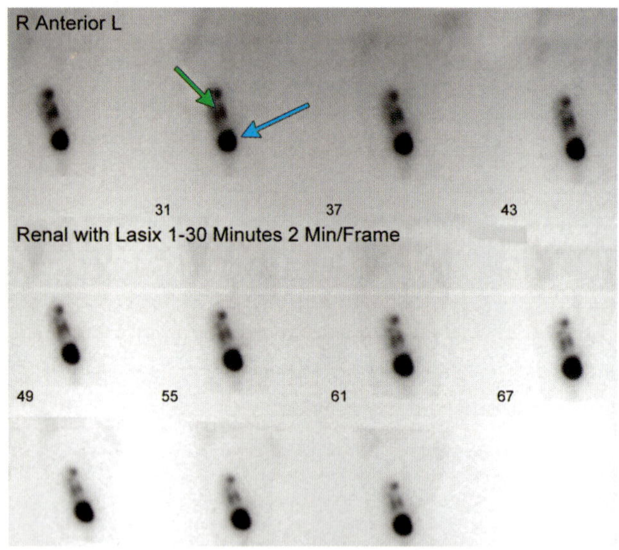

Fig. 11: A follow-up study after resolution of ATN shows normal cortical transit of activity with prompt visualization of the collecting system (green arrow) and urinary bladder (blue arrow).

ACUTE CELLULAR REJECTION (FIGS. 12 TO 22)

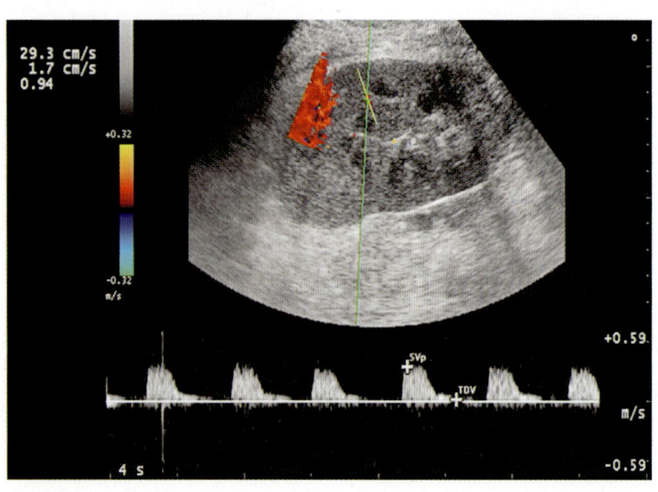

Fig. 12: Transplant recipient who presented with pain over the allograft and decreased urine output—resistive index of 0.94. Although abnormal, it is a nonspecific finding. Notice the enlarged, rounded graft in this patient with acute rejection (diagnosed by biopsy).

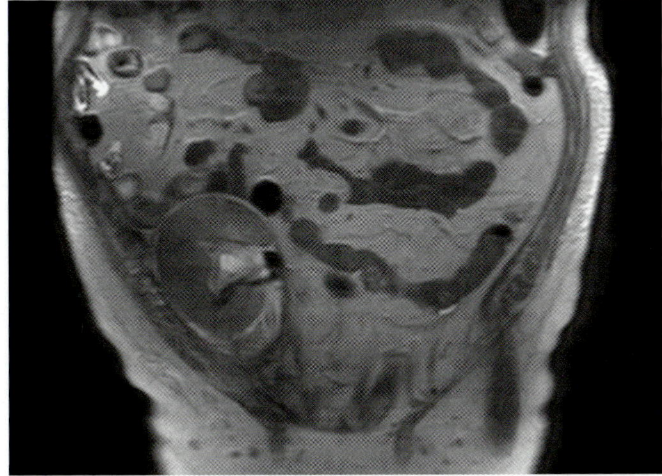

Fig. 13: T2-weighted coronal MRI showing a rounded right lower quadrant renal allograft with loss of normal corticomedullary differentiation. Notice the edematous sinus and perirenal fat in contrast with the remaining intraperitoneal and extraperitoneal fat. Although morphologic and vascular changes found in acute rejection are nonspecific, their presence may be a clue for more specific testing (such as a biopsy in this case of rejection).

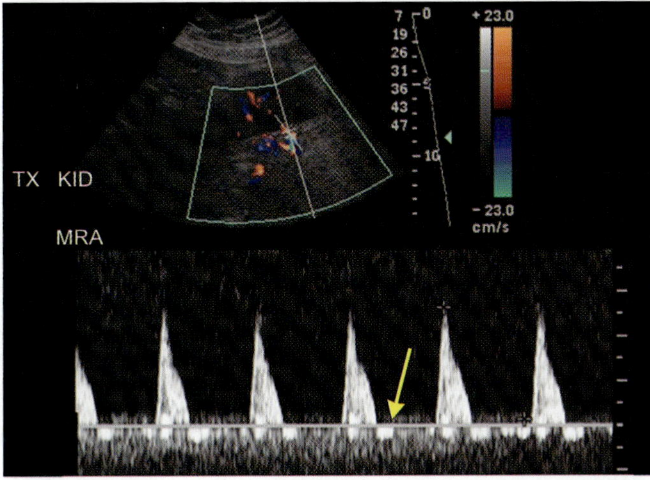

Fig. 14

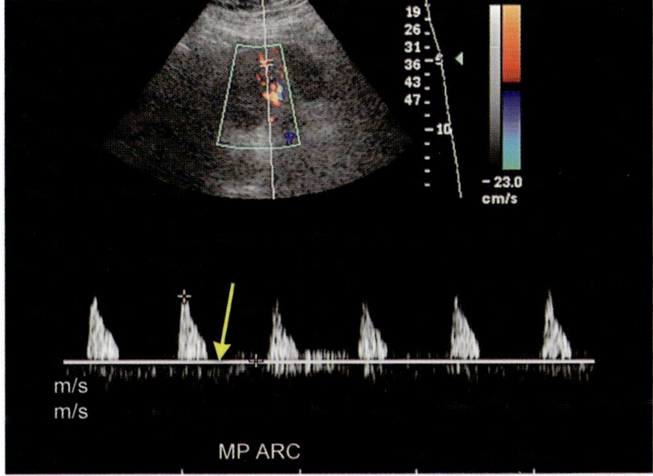

Fig. 15

Figs. 14 and 15: Absent or reversed diastolic flow (yellow arrows) on pulsed Doppler ultrasound examination. Biopsy showed acute cellular rejection. Follow-up examination after treatment revealed normal waveforms.

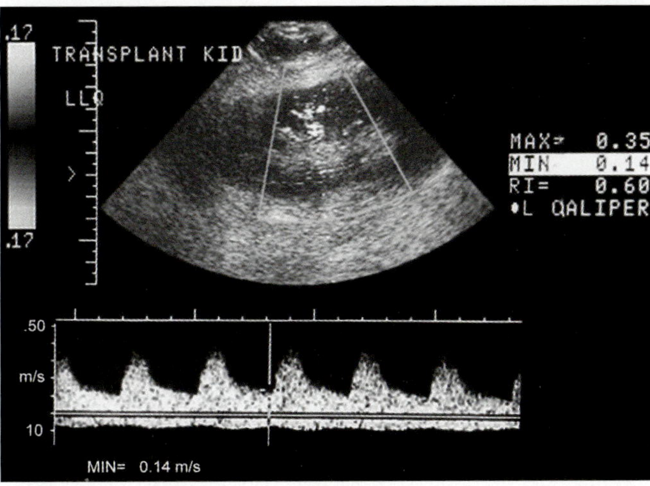

Fig. 16

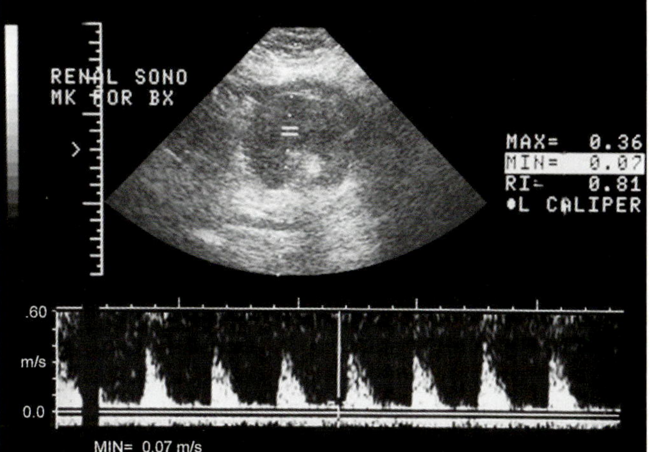

Fig. 17

Figs. 16 and 17: Duplex Doppler US imaging of the same patient showing increasing resistive index over a period of 16 days associated with the onset of rejection (biopsy proven).

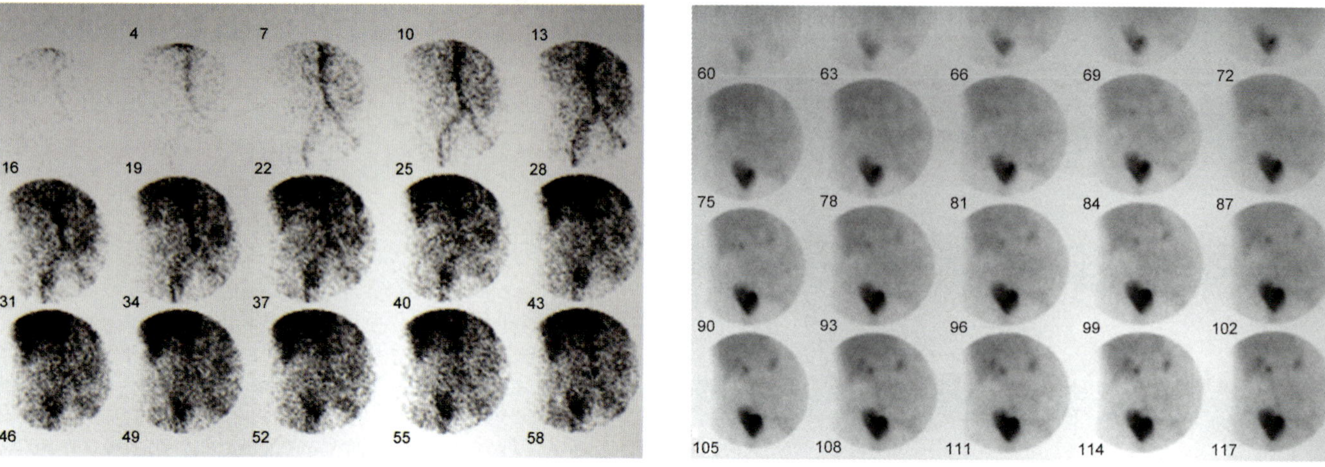

Fig. 18

Fig. 19

Figs. 18 and 19: (Fig. 18) Nuclear medicine image showing decreased perfusion of the allograft in a patient with acute cellular rejection (ACR); (Fig. 19) On the functional images there is delayed uptake and markedly delayed cortical transit with minimal excretion. The scan appearance of ACR can be similar to that of ATN, except that in ACR both flow and function are compromised, while in ATN function is compromised, but flow usually is preserved.

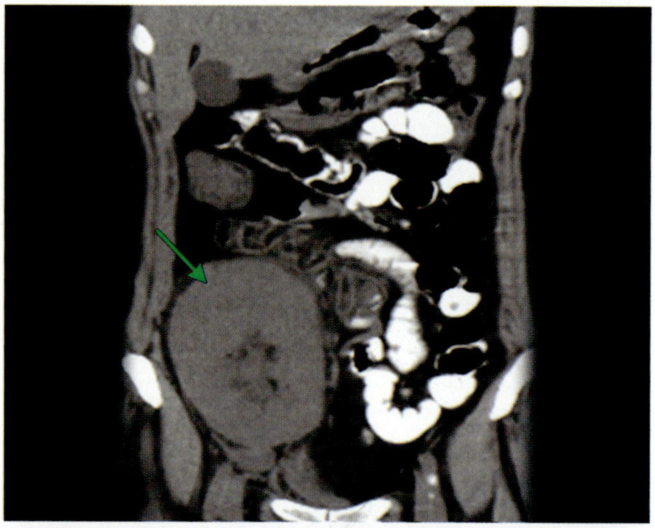

Fig. 20

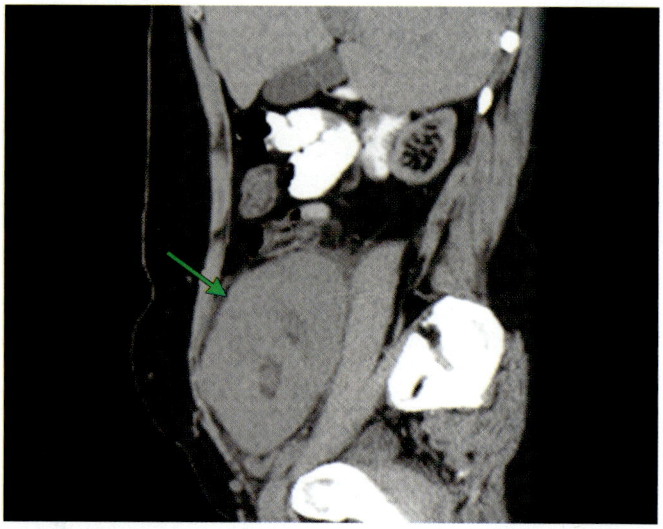

Fig. 21

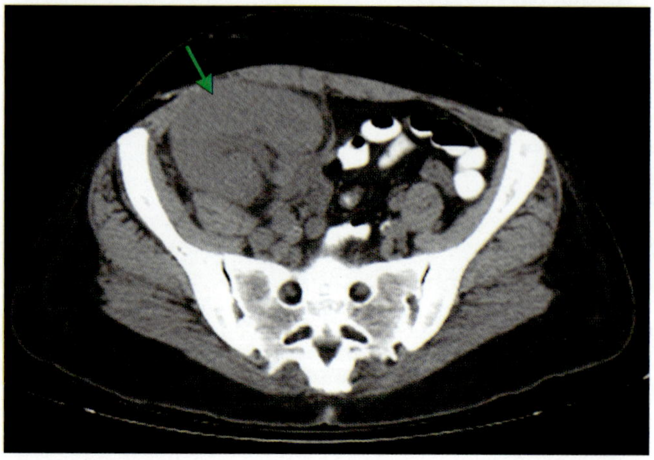

Fig. 22

Figs. 20 to 22: CT Images of a transplant kidney (green arrows), severely enlarged due to acute rejection after discontinuation of immunosuppression. Notice also the subtle increased density of perirenal fat due to edematous changes.

HEMATOMA RESEMBLING RENAL MASS (FIGS. 23 AND 24)

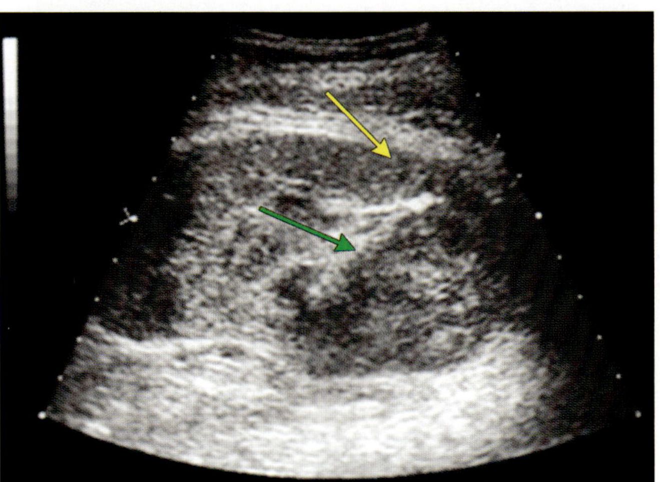

Fig. 23

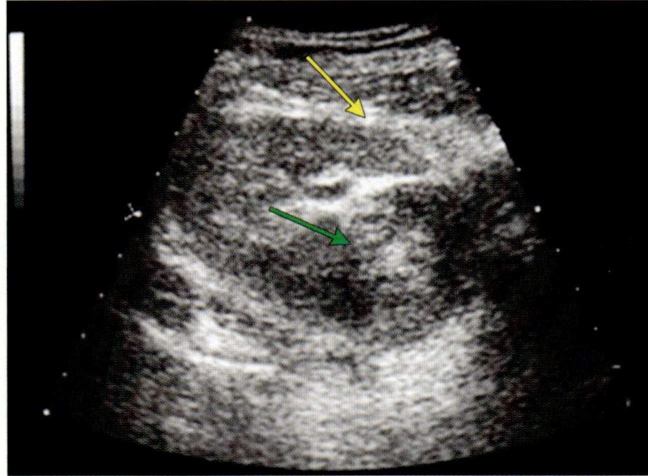

Fig. 24

Figs. 23 and 24: Renal transplant hematoma. One day prior to the ultrasound examination, patient underwent a biopsy of the kidney transplant without apparent complications except for minor pain over the allograft. Follow-up sonography revealed a hematoma (solid mass-green arrows) in the lower pole of the transplant kidney (yellow arrows) mimicking a neoplasm (ultrasound study of the transplant kidney at the time of the biopsy was normal).

CALCIFIED FAILED ALLOGRAFTS (FIGS. 25 AND 26)

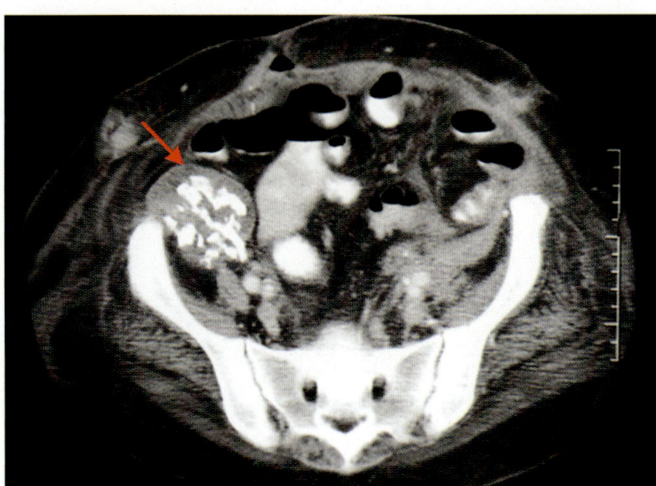

Fig. 25: Axial CT image showing coarse calcifications in a right lower quadrant graft (red arrow), that is also decreased in size. Patient subsequently underwent a retransplant on the left side (that had to be removed emergently as a result of a ruptured pseudoaneurysm).

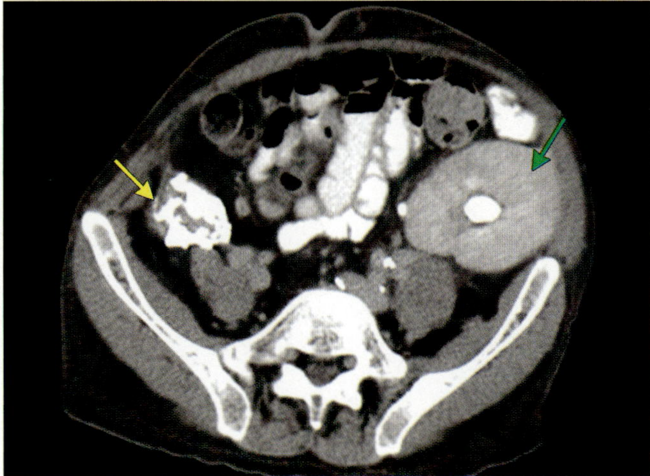

Fig. 26: Contrast-enhanced axial CT image showing a barely recognizable small, grossly calcified right lower quadrant transplant kidney (yellow arrow). A mildly enlarged left lower quadrant transplant kidney (green arrow) reveals a slightly heterogeneous nephrogram as well as perirenal edema consistent with pyelonephritis.

CHAPTER 60

Urologic Imaging

Mariano Volpacchio, Catherine D'Agostino, Christopher Palestro, et al.

NORMAL URINARY IMAGING (FIGS. 1 AND 2)

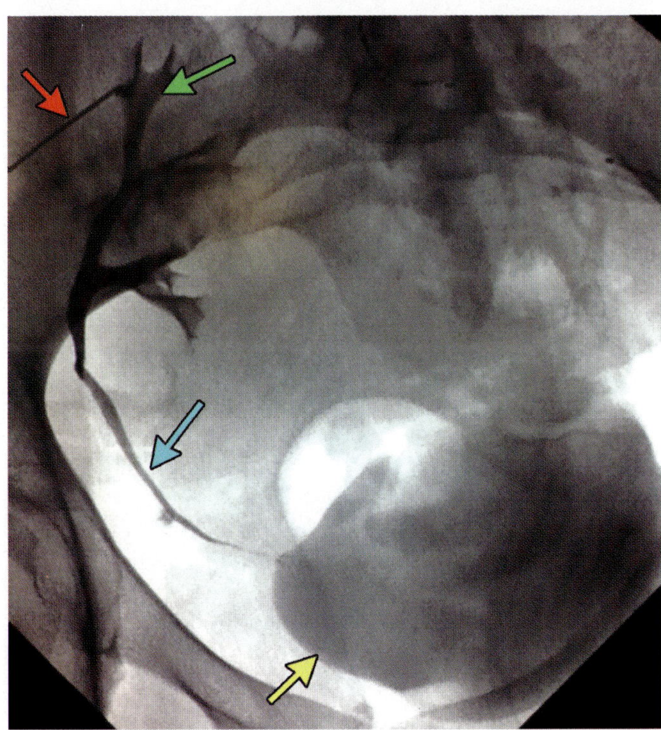

Fig. 1: Normal transplant percutaneous nephrostogram. Note the percutaneous needle (red arrow) used for injection of contrast into the collecting system (green arrow) of the transplant kidney. The ureter (blue arrow) and bladder (yellow arrow) can be identified.

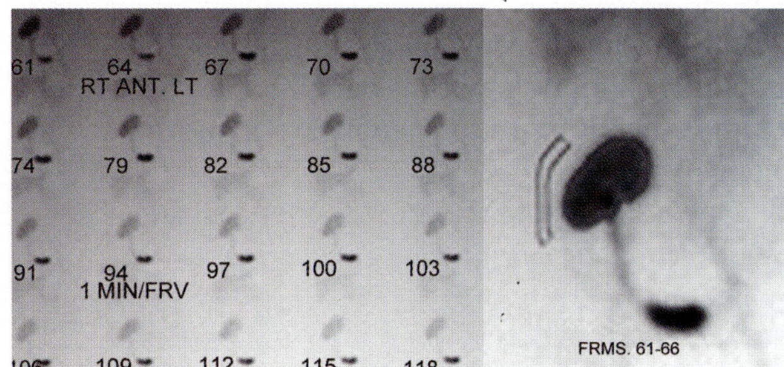

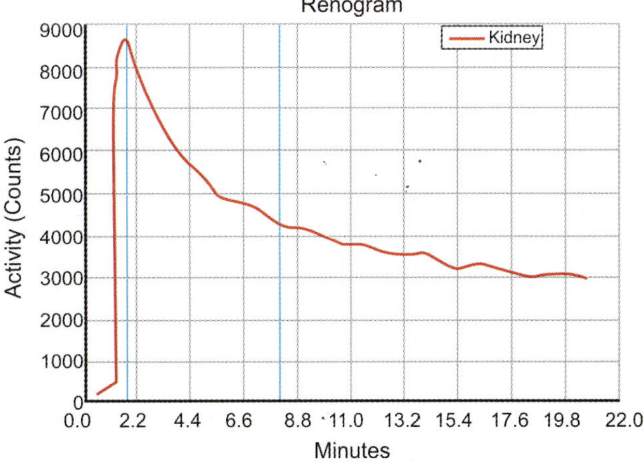

Fig. 2: Normal ^{99m}Tc-MAG3 renal scan. There is normal parenchymal uptake, cortical transit, and excretion of tracer. The renogram curve is typical of normal function.

URINARY OBSTRUCTION (FIGS. 3 TO 24)

- Most obstructions occur at the ureterovesical junction or in the distal transplant ureter
- In the immediate postoperative period, obstructions are usually associated with:
  - Technical factors:
    - Tight anastomosis
    - Torsion/twisting of the ureter
  - Edema
  - Blood clots

- In a more delayed fashion, contributing factors include:
  - Fibrosis
  - Ischemia
  - Rejection
  - Infections
  - Mass effect
  - Adhesions
  - Calculi
- Ultrasound images (usually the initial modality of choice) should be interpreted with caution
  - Dilatation of the collecting system may be absent in:
    - early stages
    - instances of parenchymal fibrosis
  - Most transplant kidneys have a prominent renal pelvis
  - Dilatation of the transplant ureter and collecting system may be due to reflux from a full bladder
  - Dilatation may persist from previous instances of treated obstruction
- Nuclear scintigrams may show clearance of the radiotracer.
- Antegrade pyelograms not only can diagnose obstructions, but also show the site and type of stenosis and may be used as a guide to percutaneous treatment

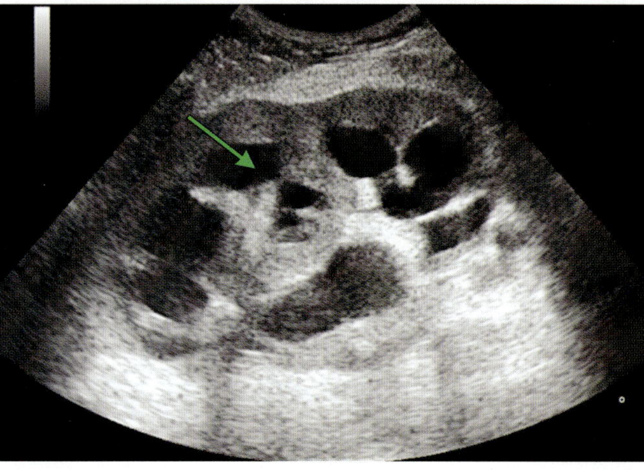

Fig. 3

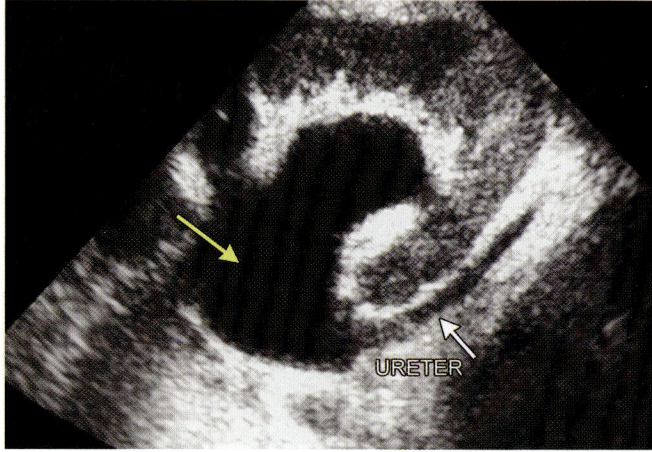

Fig. 4

Figs. 3 and 4: Hydronephrosis. These two ultrasound images show marked dilatation of the collecting system (green arrow), renal pelvis (yellow arrow) and ureter (white arrow). When obtaining such studies, the bladder should be empty in order to avoid an inaccurate reading associated with urinary reflux.

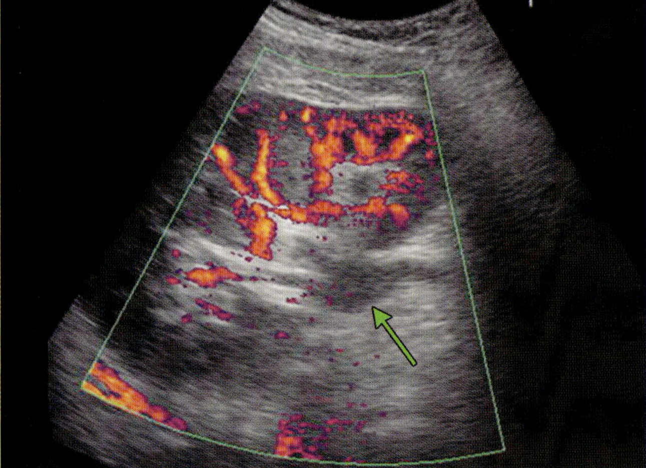

Fig. 5: As shown in the image above, the presence of an extrarenal pelvis (green arrow) is a frequent finding in transplantation and should not be confused with hydronephrosis.

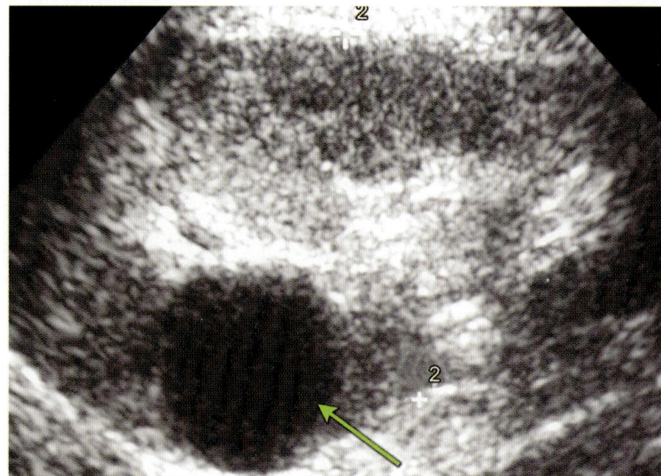

Fig. 6: Renal cysts (green arrow) in the allograft are sometimes also encountered and are part of the differential diagnosis.

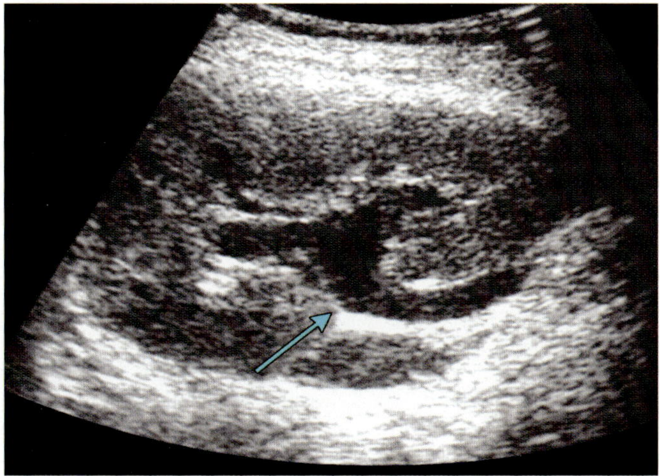

Fig. 7

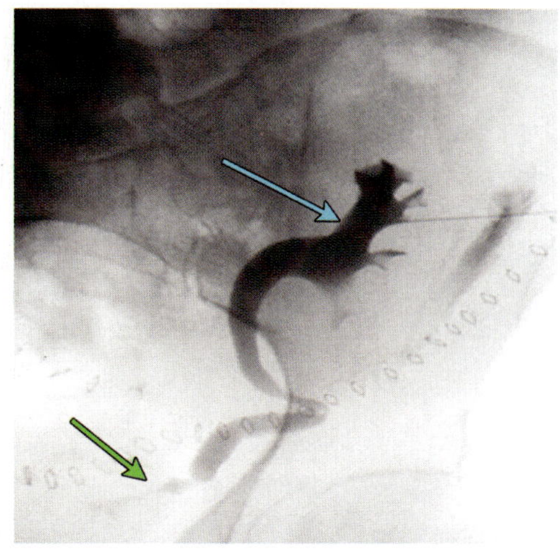

Fig. 8

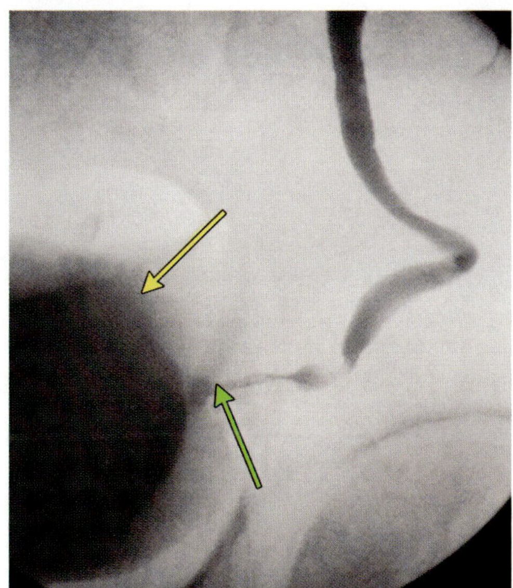

Fig. 9

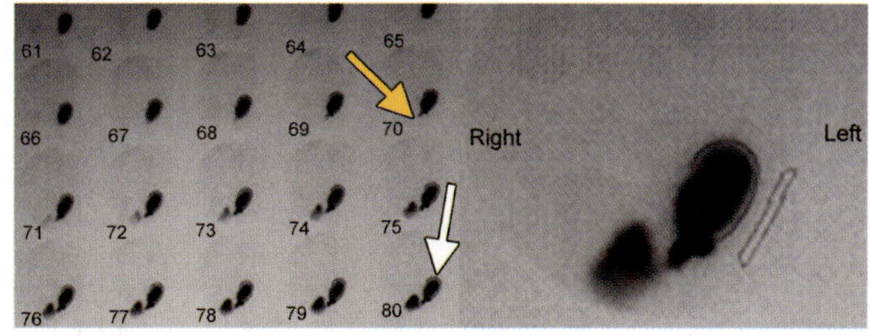

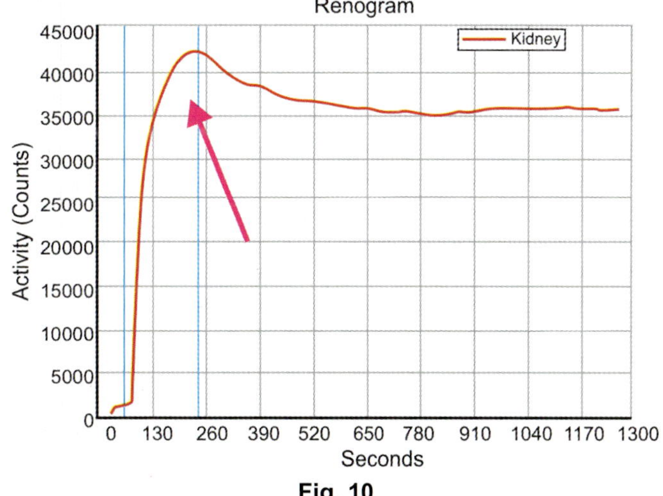

Fig. 10

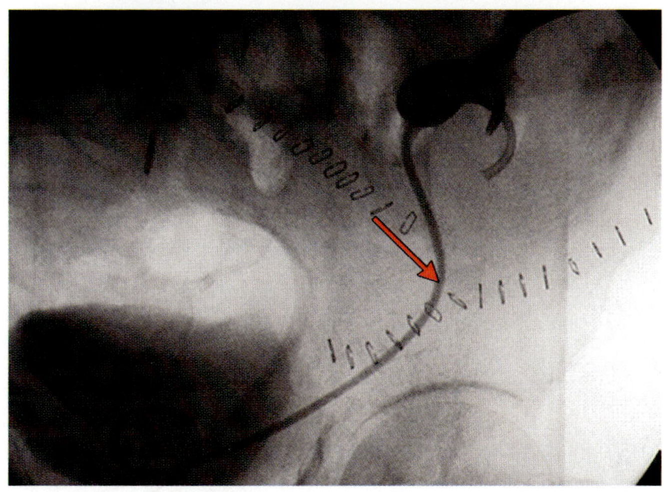

Fig. 11A

Figs. 7 to 11A: (Fig. 7) Patient who presented with hydronephrosis (blue arrows) on US and percutaneous (Fig. 8) nephrostomy studies; (Figs. 8 and 9). Focal strictures (green arrows) were observed at the ureterovesical junction, with some passage of contrast into the bladder (Fig. 9, yellow arrow); (Fig. 10) A ^{99m}Tc-MAG3 renal scan showed preserved flow (pink arrow) to the transplant kidney, with minimal drainage from the collecting system (orange arrow). Note the persistent collecting system activity in the images (white arrow) even at the end of the study; (Fig. 11A) A stent (red arrow) was placed.

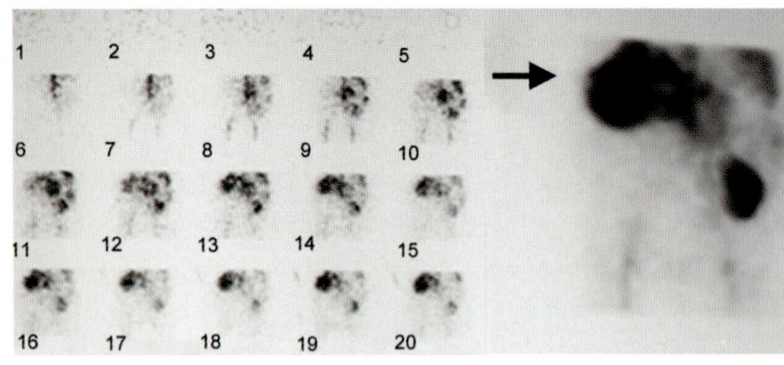

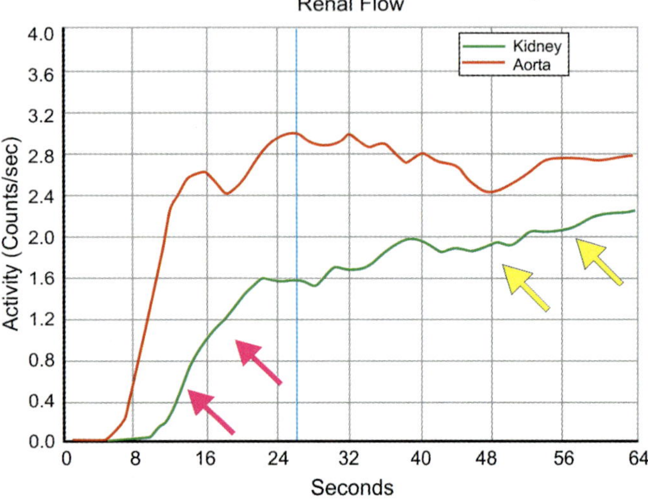

Fig. 11B: ^{99m}Tc-MAG3 renal scan in a case of urinary obstruction demonstrates delayed and diminished perfusion (pink arrows) to the transplant as well as continually increasing cortical activity (yellow arrows). Hepatic activity (black arrow) is clearly seen. The liver is the secondary route of excretion for MAG3.

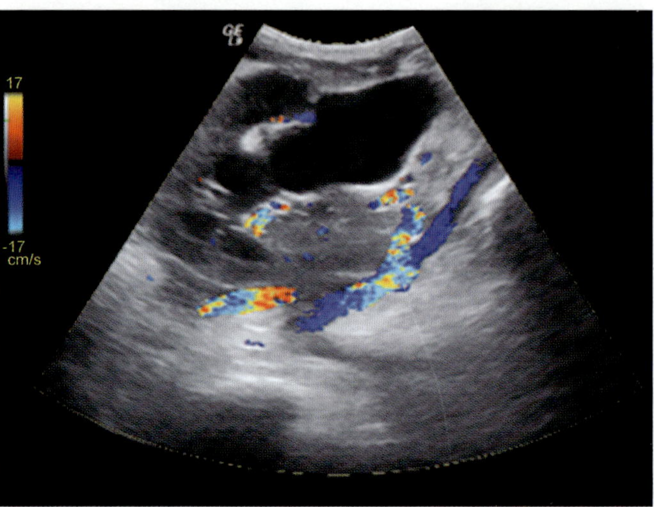

Fig. 12: Hydronephrosis. In this specific instance, the hydronephrosis developed approximately one month after transplantation with a deceased donor graft. Note the iliac vein visualized in blue on color Doppler.

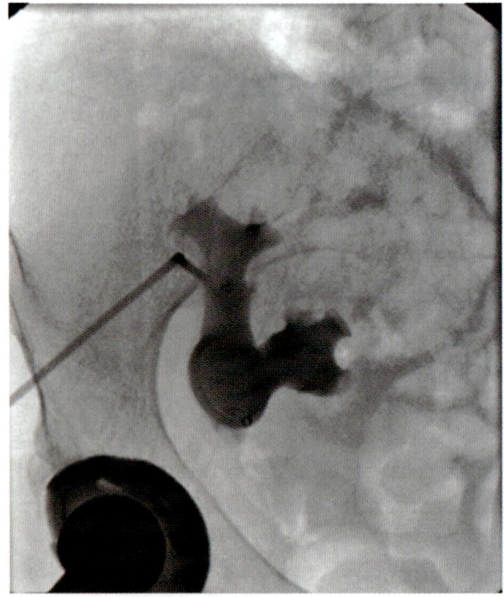

Fig. 13

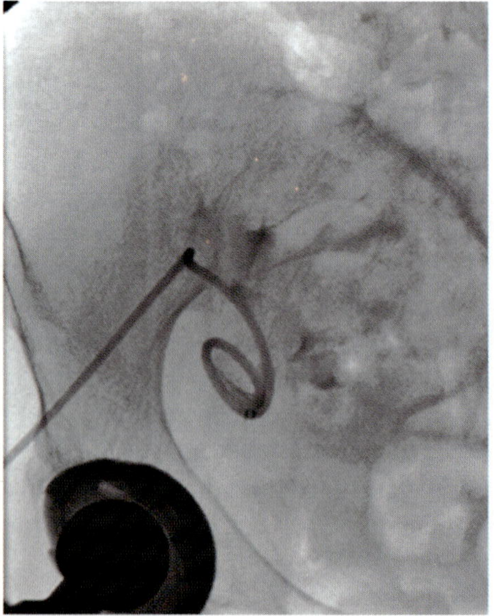

Fig. 14

Figs. 13 and 14: Initial treatment was with percutaneous nephrostomy (Figs. 13 and 14) and subsequent surgical repair. Delayed ureteral strictures in the setting of adequate renal function (and no evidence of obstruction in the initial postoperative period) are frequently due to poor irrigation of the distal donor ureter.

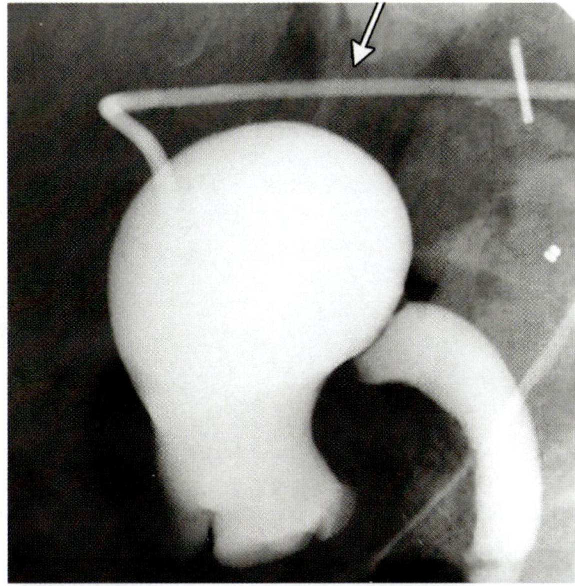

Fig. 15

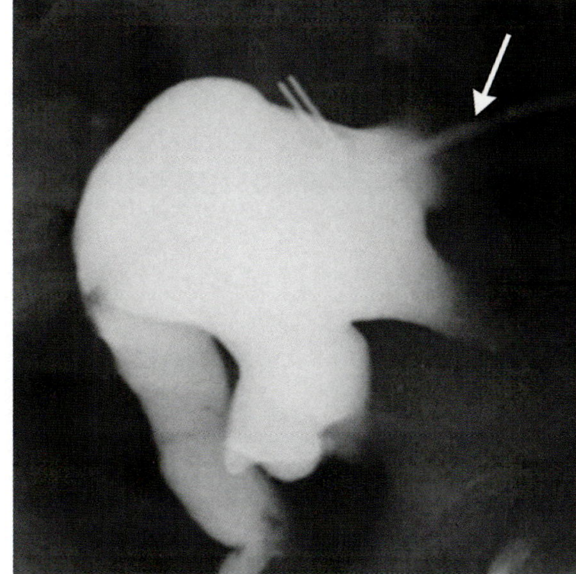

Fig. 16

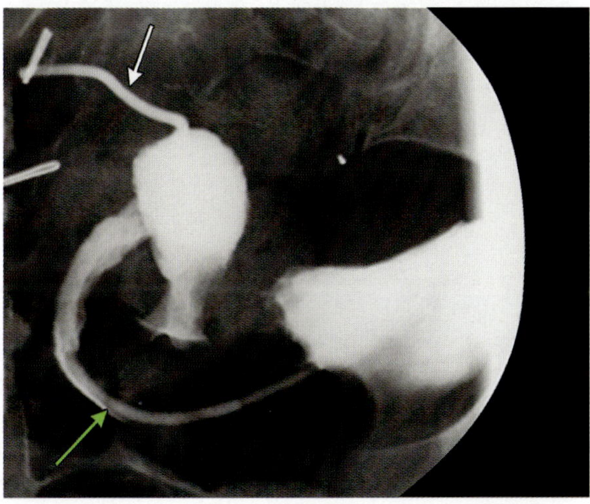

Fig. 17

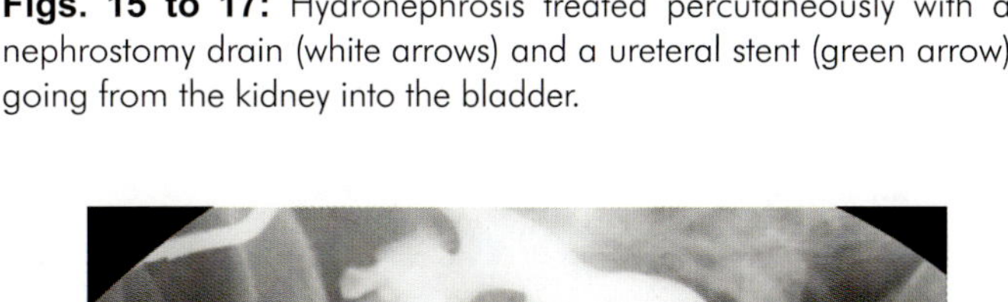

Figs. 15 to 17: Hydronephrosis treated percutaneously with a nephrostomy drain (white arrows) and a ureteral stent (green arrow) going from the kidney into the bladder.

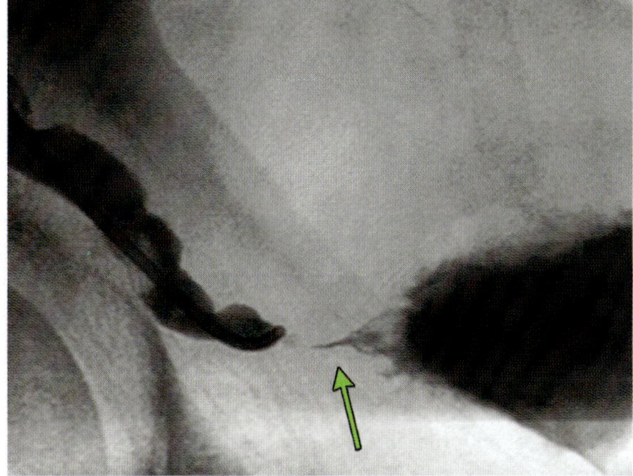

Fig. 18: Stricture at the ureter-to-bladder anastomosis (green arrow).

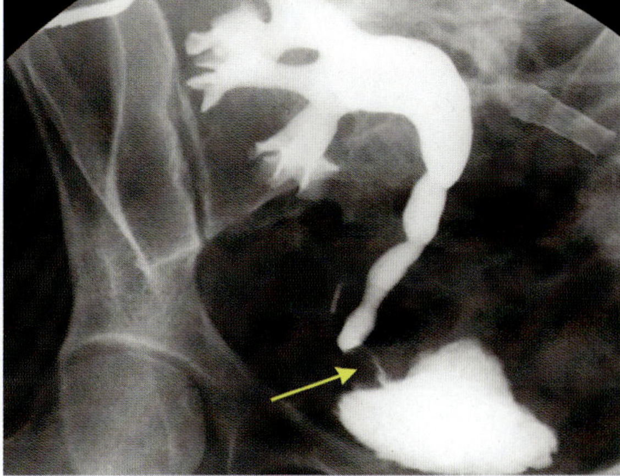

Fig. 19: Stricture (yellow arrow) associated with torsion of the ureter at the time of implantation.

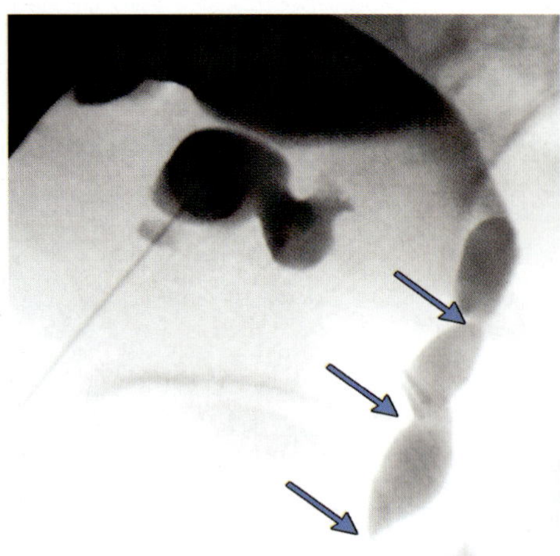

Fig. 20: Ureteral obstruction associated with repeated torsion of the ureter. Note the corkscrew appearance (blue arrows).

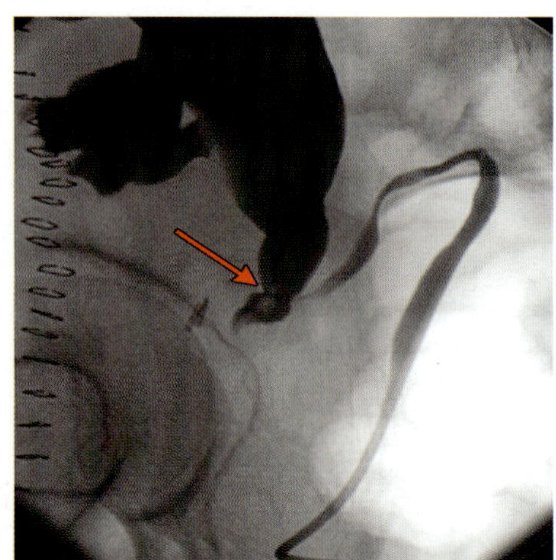

Fig. 21: Obstruction associated with a clot (filling defect, red arrow) in the lumen of the ureter after a ureter-to-ureter anastomosis.

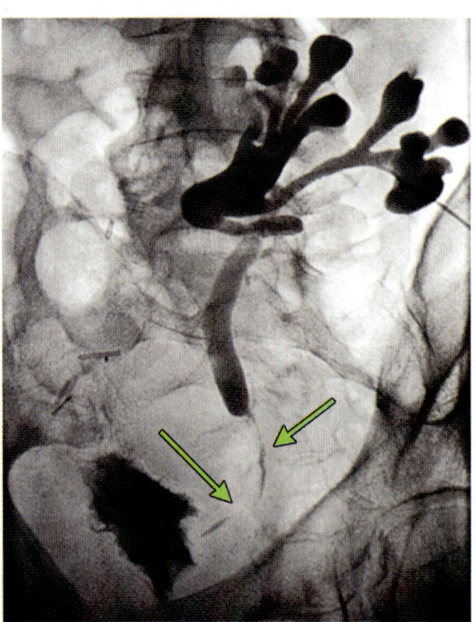

Fig. 22

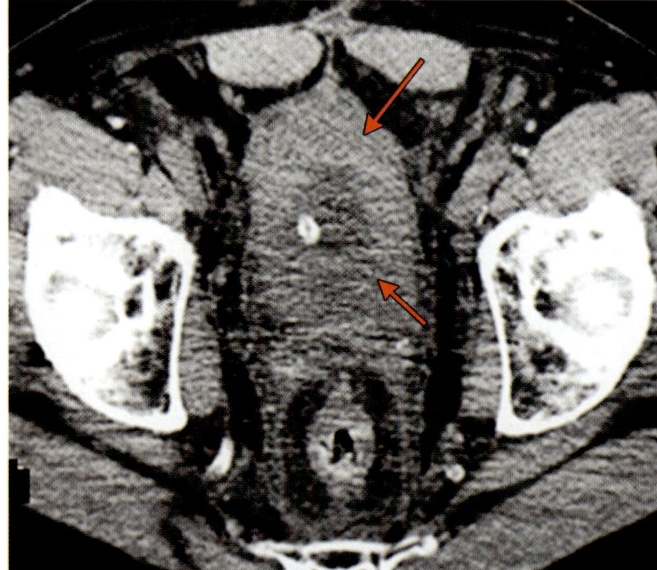

Fig. 23

Figs. 22 and 23: Ureteral obstruction (green arrows) secondary to bladder wall thickening (red arrows) in a bladder-drained pancreas/ kidney transplant. Exocrine pancreatic secretions resulted in marked irritation and thickening of the bladder wall.

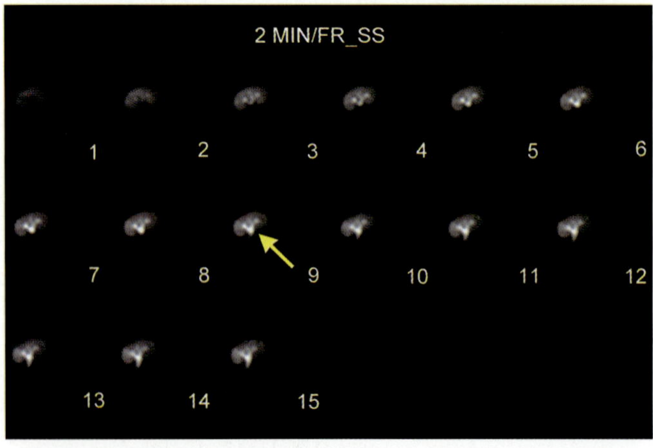

Fig. 24: ^{99m}Tc-MAG3 renal scan performed in a case of ureteral obstruction associated with edema at the ureter to bladder anastomosis. The patient developed increasing creatinine and decreased urine output 48 hours after transplantation in an otherwise uncomplicated case. On the renal scan, the collecting system and proximal ureter (yellow arrow) are clearly visualized, but there is no passage of activity into the urinary bladder. Treatment was with a percutaneous nephrostomy tube and ureteral stent. They were subsequently removed with complete recovery, and no need for further interventions.

URINARY LEAKS (FIGS. 25 TO 36)

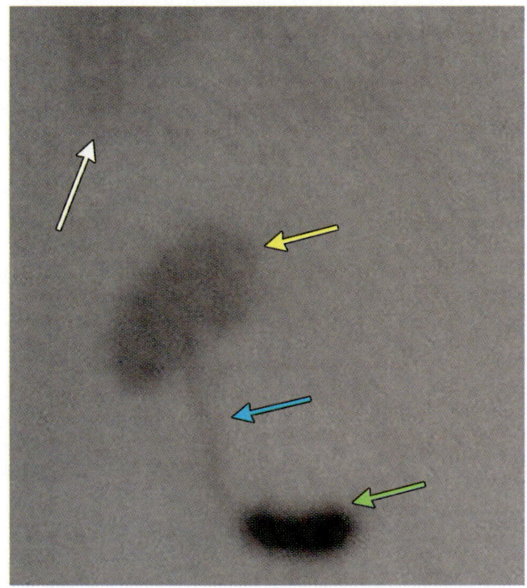

Fig. 25: Image from a normal ^{99m}Tc-MAG3 renal scan showing accumulation of tracer in the cortex of the transplant (yellow arrow), ureter (blue arrow), and bladder (green arrow). Faint hepatic activity (white arrow), which is normal also can be appreciated.

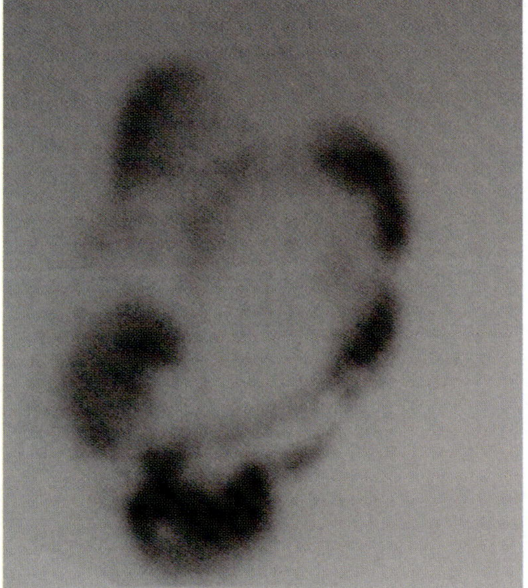

Fig. 26

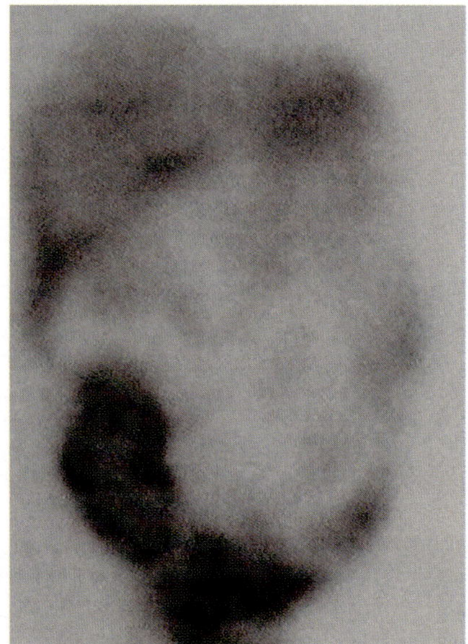

Fig. 27

Figs. 26 and 27: These two images demonstrate urinary extravasation. The radionuclide can be seen throughout the peritoneal cavity around, not within, the liver and bowel.

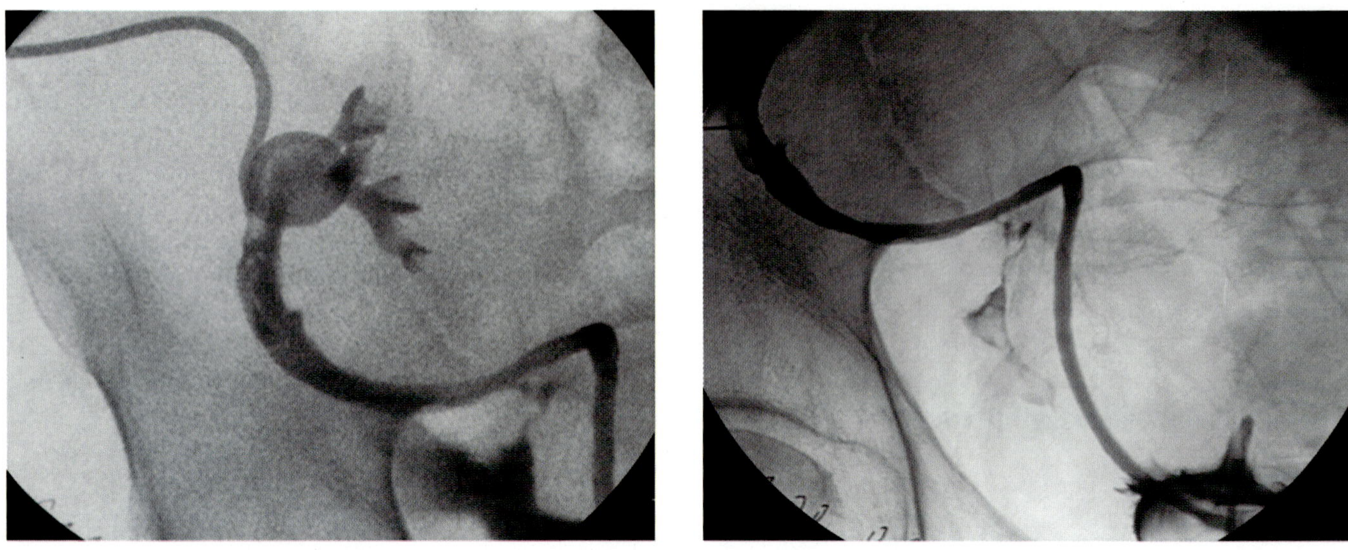

Fig. 28 Fig. 29

Figs. 28 and 29: Small urinary leak treated with percutaneous drainage and with placement of a ureteral stent.

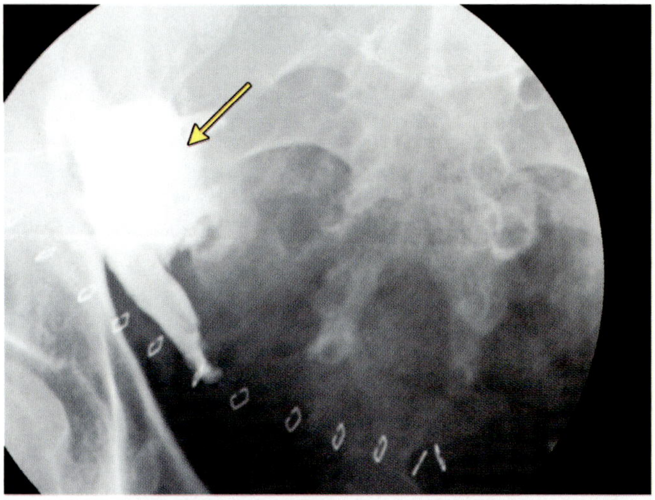

Fig. 30 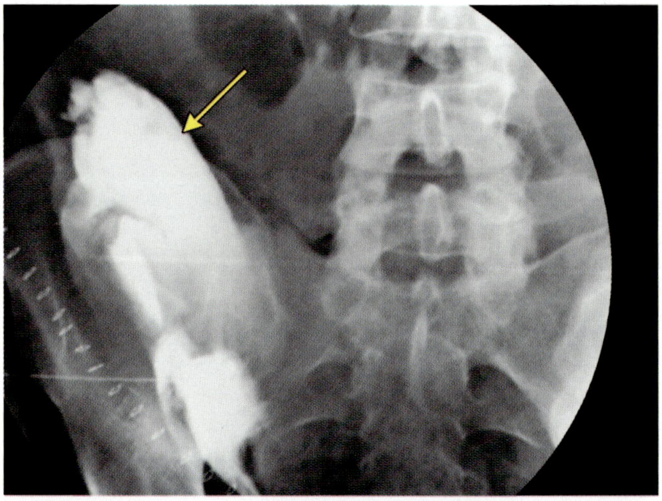 Fig. 31

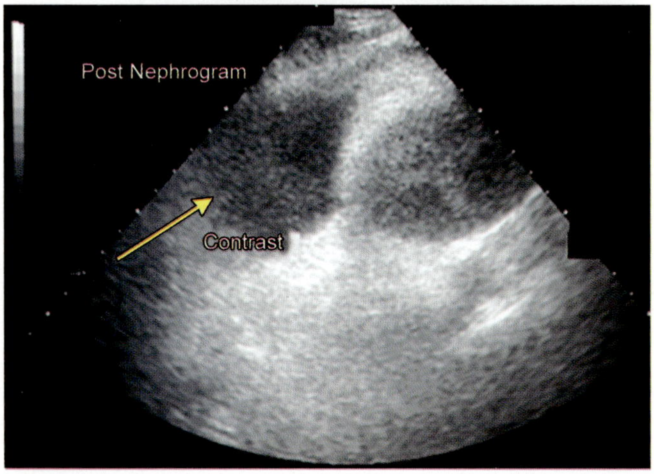

Fig. 32 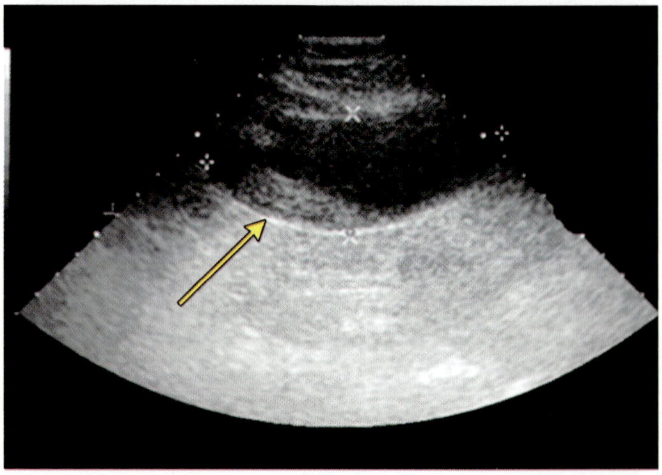 Fig. 33

Figs. 30 to 33: Massive proximal urinary leak (yellow arrows) in a transplant kidney associated with ureteral necrosis.

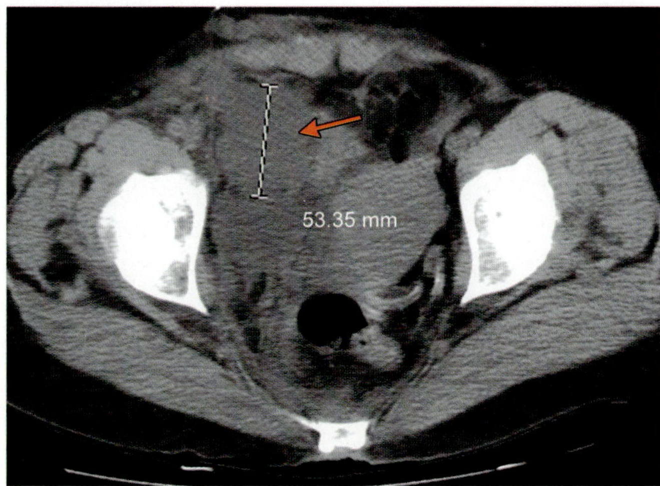

Fig. 34: CT scan showing a fluid collection suspicious for a urinoma (red arrow). A diagnostic aspirate helps to determine the nature of collections. An aspirate creatinine value similar to that in urine confirms the diagnosis of urinoma. An aspirate creatinine value similar to that in blood/serum excludes it.

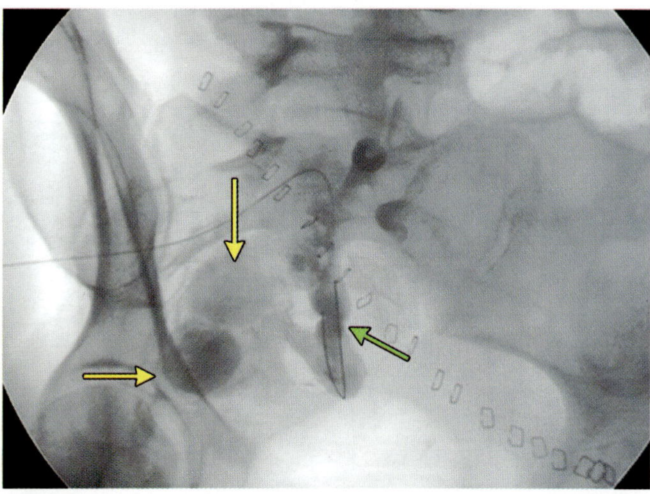

Fig. 35: An antegrade nephrostomy study shows the transplant ureter (green arrow) and a urinary leak associated with a bilobed collection (yellow arrows).

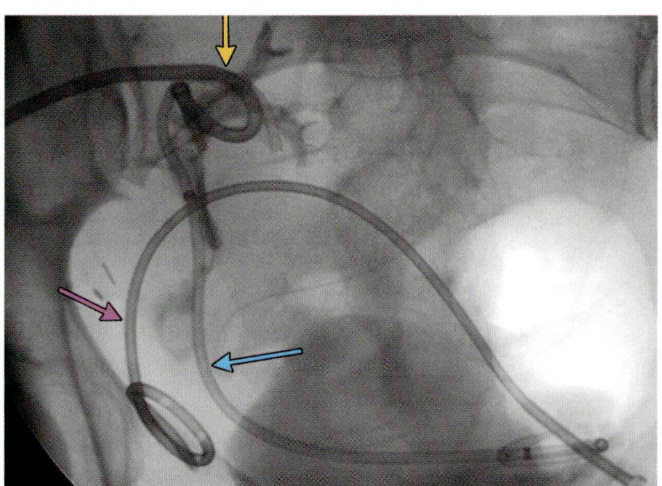

Fig. 36: Treatment included a percutaneous nephrostomy tube (orange arrow), a ureteral stent (blue arrow), and percutaneous drainage (pink arrow) of the collection.

URINARY LEAK AND OBSTRUCTION IN A TRANSPLANT KIDNEY WITH A DOUBLE URETER (FIGS. 37A TO 38)

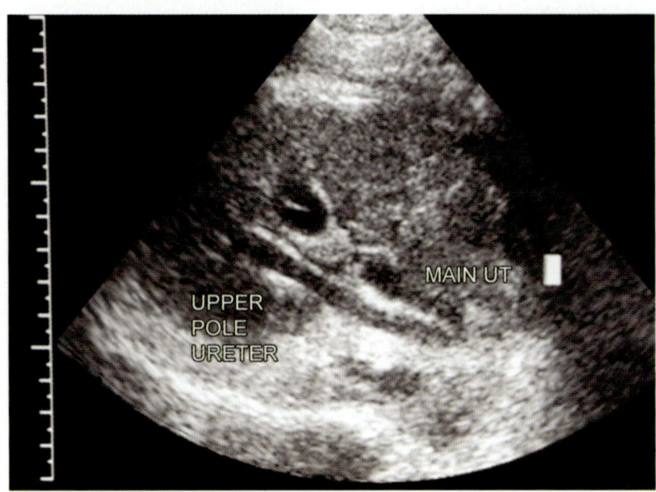

Fig. 37A: Transplanted kidney with double ureter. Ultrasound image showing two ureters: a main ureter (labeled "main UT" in the image) and another ureter from the upper pole (labeled "upper pole ureter").

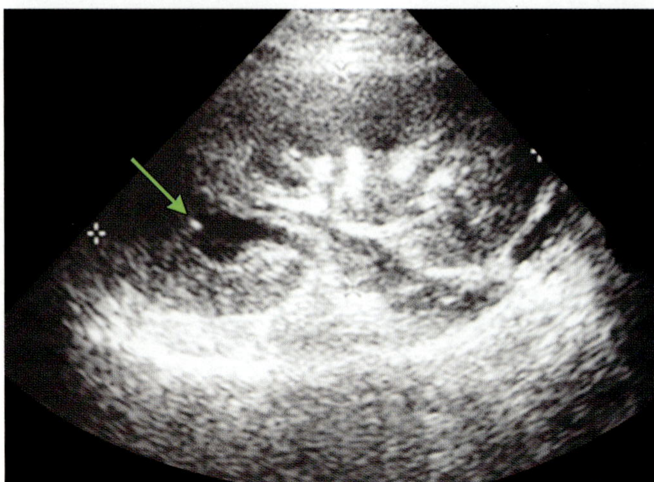

Fig. 37B: Further US imaging shows a prominent upper pole calyx (green arrow).

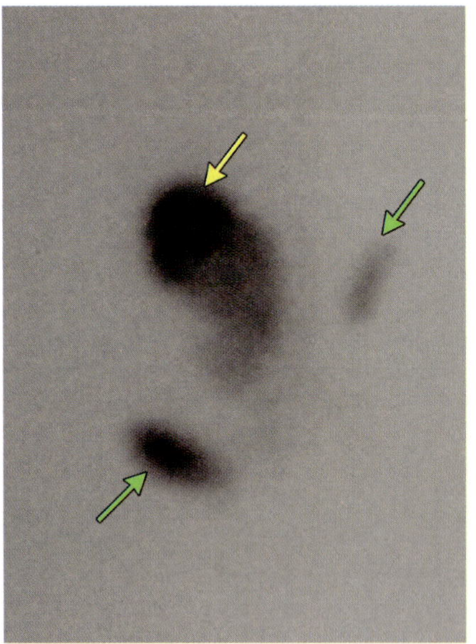

Fig. 38: On the renal scan the upper pole of the kidney shows intense radionuclide accumulation (yellow arrow) in the obstructed upper pole collecting system. Free tracer (green arrows) representing a urinary leak also is seen.

URETER-TO-URETER ANASTOMOSIS—IPSILATERAL (FIGS. 39 TO 42)

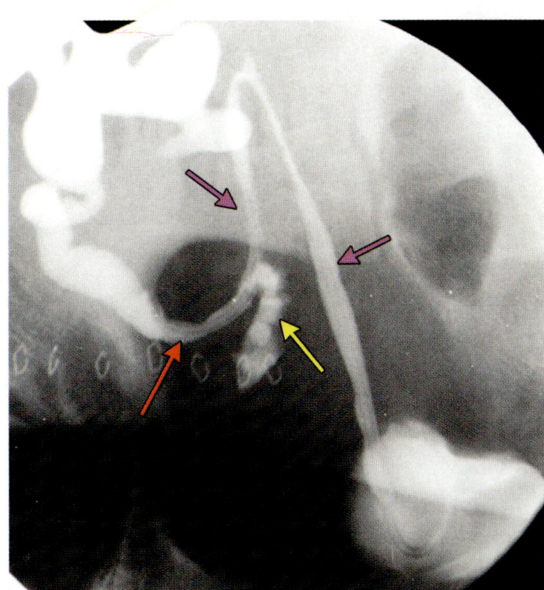

Fig. 39: Anastomosis between transplant ureter (red arrow) and ipsilateral native ureter (pink arrows). The yellow arrow shows a urinary leak at the anastomosis.

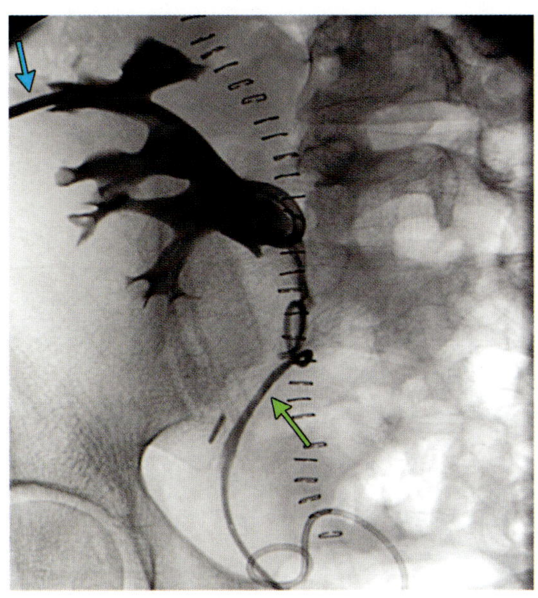

Fig. 40: Transplant to ipsilateral native ureter anastomosis with a ureteral stent (green arrow) in place. Note also the presence of a percutaneous nephrotsomy drain (blue arrow).

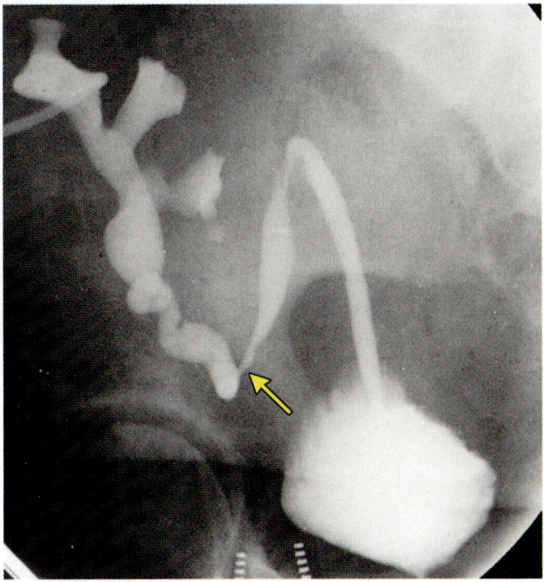

Fig. 41

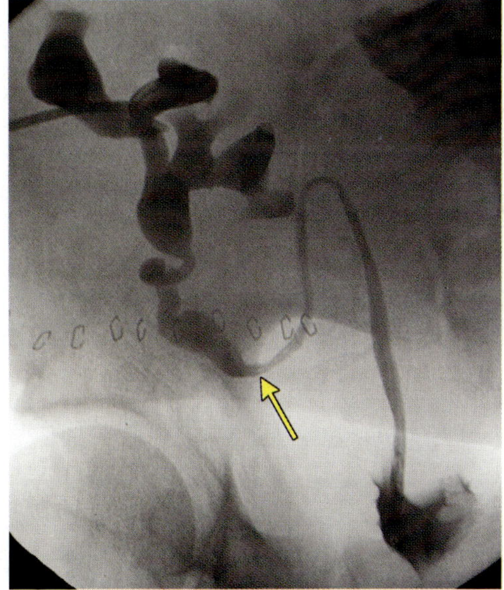

Fig. 42

Figs. 41 and 42: Two examples of transplant to ipsilateral native ureteral anastomoses. The arrows (yellow) point to the site of the anastomoses, that show varying degrees of stenoses.

URETER-TO-URETER ANASTOMOSIS—CONTRALATERAL (FIG. 43)

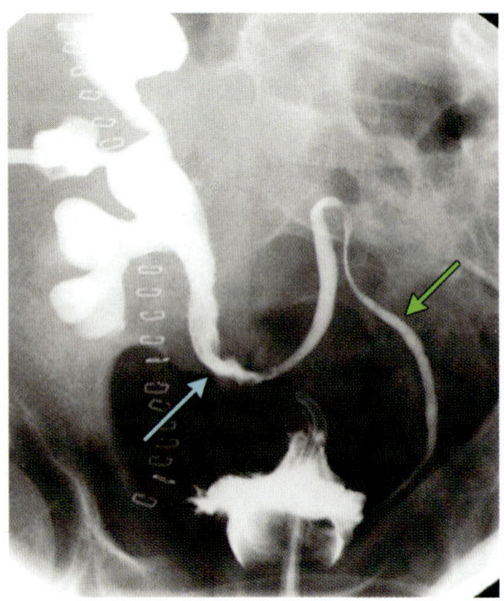

Fig. 43: Anastomosis between the transplant ureter (blue arrow) and the native contralateral (green arrow) ureter.

HEMATURIA (FIGS. 44 TO 46)

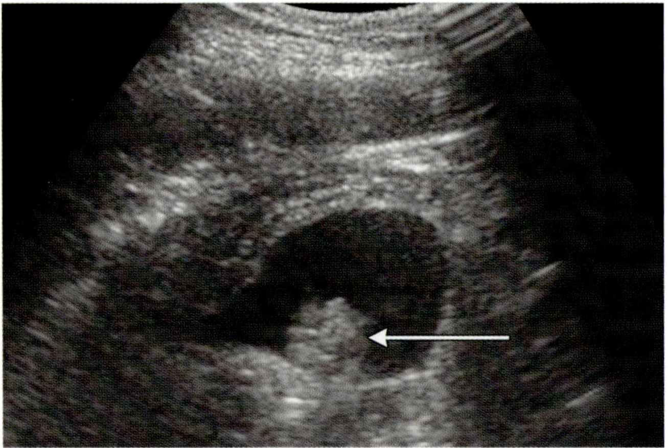

Fig. 44 **Fig. 45**

Figs. 44 and 45: Ultrasound images of intravesical blood clots (white arrows) in the immediate postoperative period. Demonstration of movement with changes in position suggests that the intravesical image is a clot rather than a tumor.

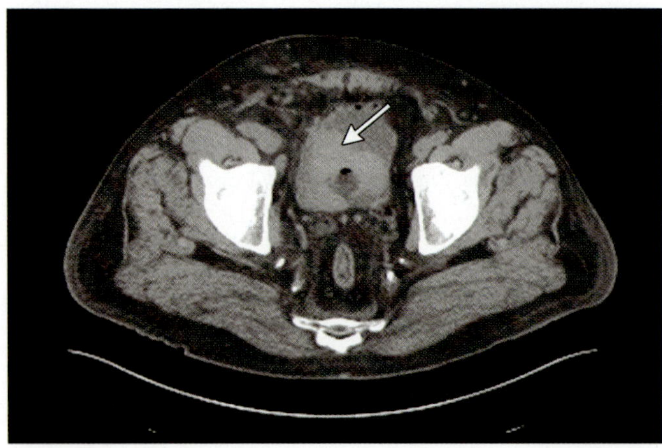

Fig. 46: CT scan showing a urinary catheter surrounded by an intravesical blood clot (arrow). Notice the high attenuation of the clot.

UROTHELIAL THICKENING (FIGS. 47 TO 49)

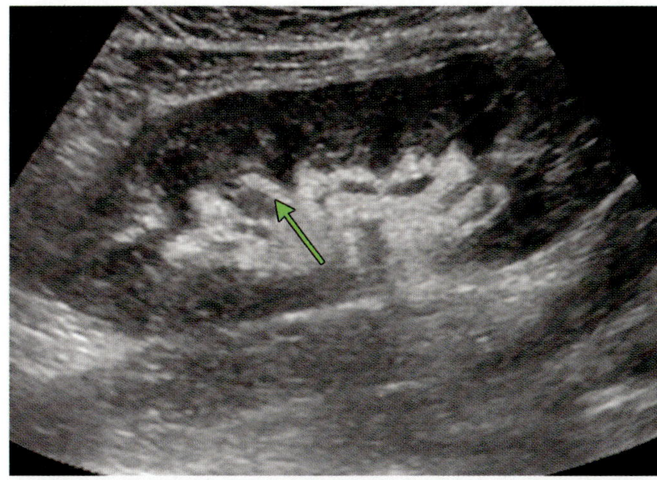

Fig. 47

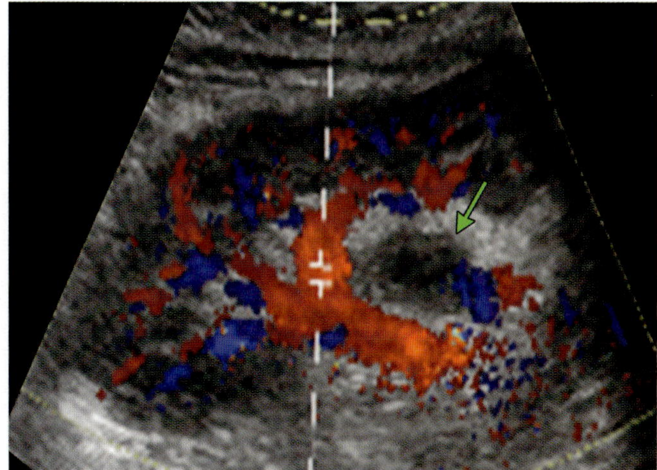

Fig. 48

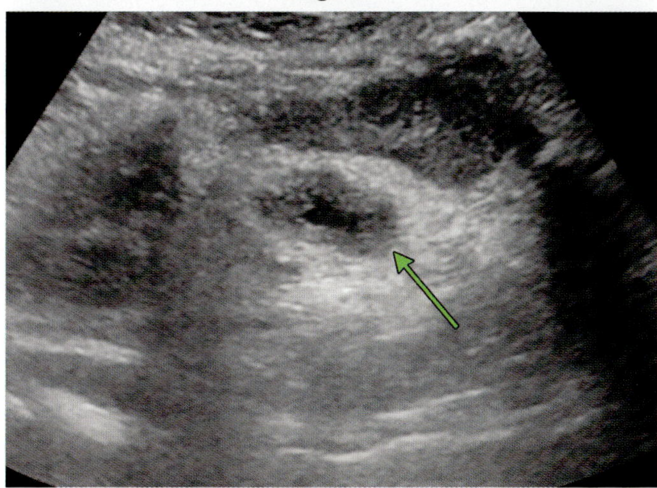

Fig. 49

Figs. 47 to 49: The presence of prominent and thickened urothelium (green arrows) in transplant patients is a nonspecific finding that should be evaluated in order to exclude malignancies, infections, and other pathologies.

COMMUNICATION BETWEEN THE URINARY SYSTEM AND THE ILIAC VEIN (FIG. 50)

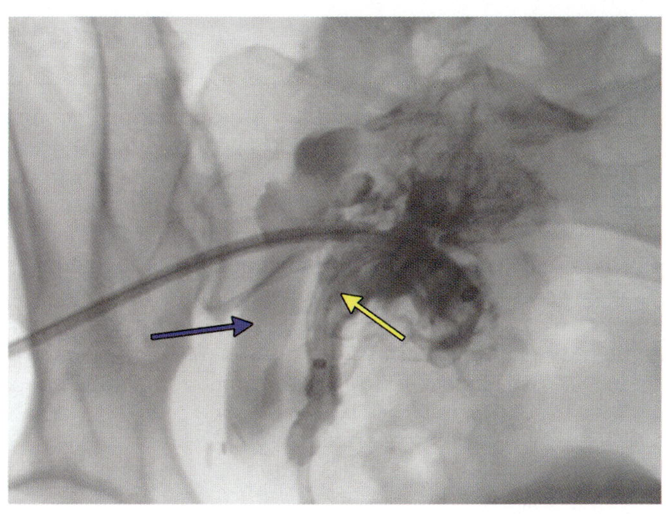

Fig. 50: Study showing injection of contrast into the urinary collecting system (yellow arrow), that also flows into the recipient external iliac vein (blue arrow) confirming the presence of an anomalous communication between these structures.

GAS IN COLLECTING SYSTEM (FIGS. 51 TO 53)

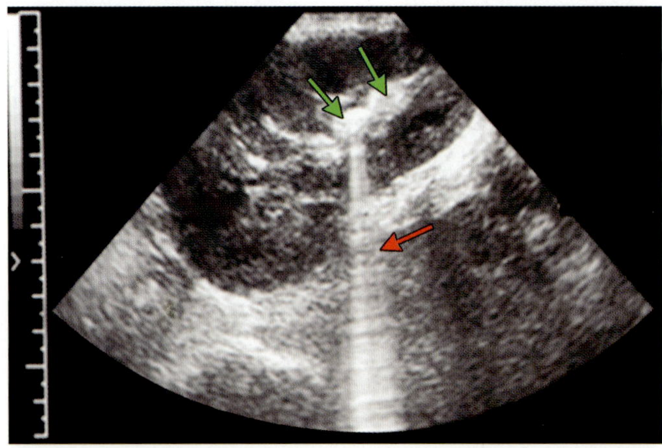

Fig. 51: Ultrasound image showing air (green arrows) in the calyces of a normal functioning kidney 8 hours post-transplantation. There are echogenic foci in the calyces of the mid and lower poles with associated ring-down artifact (red arrow). If the echogenic foci were stones, posterior acoustical shadowing would be seen. As opposed to patients with a long standing renal transplant, the presence of air in the immediate postoperative period may not represent a pathologic finding. In the absence of symptoms, there patients can be followed clinically and with serial images.

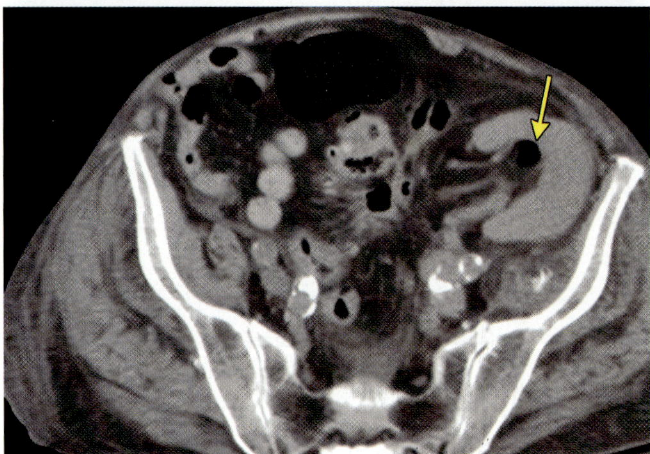

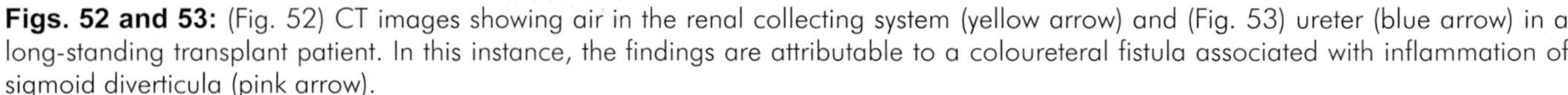

Fig. 52 **Fig. 53**

Figs. 52 and 53: (Fig. 52) CT images showing air in the renal collecting system (yellow arrow) and (Fig. 53) ureter (blue arrow) in a long-standing transplant patient. In this instance, the findings are attributable to a coloureteral fistula associated with inflammation of sigmoid diverticula (pink arrow).

URINARY CALCULI (FIG. 54)

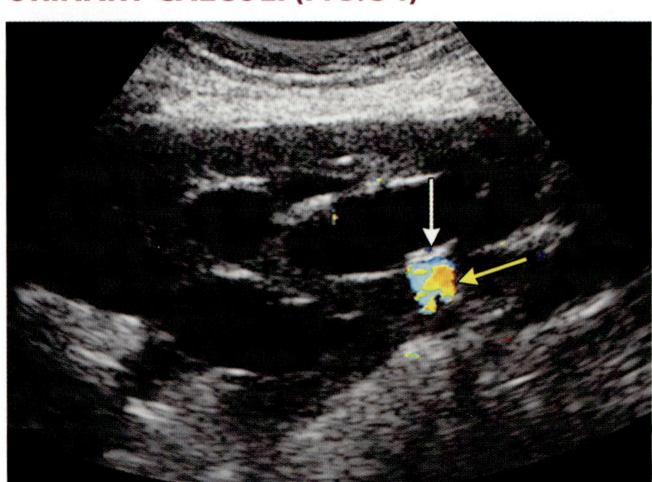

Fig. 54: Longitudinal ultrasound image showing pyelocalycial dilatation and a calculus (white arrow) associated with typical twinkling artifact (yellow arrow). Renal transplant patients have an increased incidence of urinary lithiasis and usually do not experience colicky pain (the ureter is denervate). The twinkling artifact is a useful ancillary finding to recognize calculi. Notice the absence of reverberation artifact (as opposed to the echogenic foci associated with gas in the collecting sysem).

CHAPTER 61

Vascular Imaging

Mariano Volpacchio, Catherine D'Agostino, Christopher Palestro, et al.

- Ultrasound evaluation is a fundamental part of the vascular study of the transplant kidney
- This is especially true with the use of Doppler capabilities
  - Color Doppler allows depiction of the vessels and their anastomoses
  - Duplex Doppler allows for
    - Hemodynamic evaluation through spectral analysis
    - Assessment of multiple vascular functional parameters
    - Noninvasive screening and detection of multiple potential abnormalities that may be ultimately be confirmed with CT angiography, MR angiography, or classic angiography (still the golden standard)
- Although the resistive index (RI) was initially regarded as a specific parameter of graft rejection, subsequent studies and experience proved it could not fulfill its original promise. It is probably associated with both resistance and compliance
- Mean normal RI is 0.6 and a value > 0.8 is considered abnormal
- RI is currently considered a nonspecific marker of graft dysfunction
  - It is usually elevated (> 0.8) in acute rejection, acute tubular necrosis, calcineurin inhibitor toxicity, and renal vein thrombosis
  - It is usually decreased in instances of renal artery stenoses, arteriovenous (AV) communications

$$RI = \frac{\text{peak systolic velocity (PSV)} - \text{end diastolic velocity (EDV)}}{\text{peak systolic velocity (PSV)}}$$

- We routinely obtain a duplex Doppler ultrasound study in the immediate postoperative period upon arrival of the recipient to the postanesthesia care unit
- Such evaluation provides very useful information of the status of the kidney immediately after surgery, and serves as a baseline for future imaging studies
- Duplex Doppler ultrasonography should be the first imaging study (unless otherwise determined by the treating physician) in the evaluation of abnormal renal function

NORMAL STUDIES (FIGS. 1 TO 6)

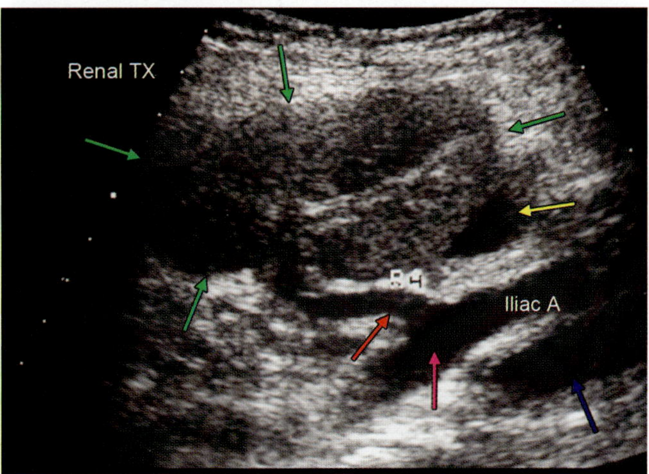

Fig. 1: Normal gray scale US study: Note the renal artery (RA, red arrow) anastomosed in an end-to-side fashion onto the external iliac artery (iliac A, pink arrow). The external iliac vein (blue arrow) lies below the iliac artery. A small postoperative fluid collection can also be seen (yellow arrow). The green arrows outline the transplant kidney.

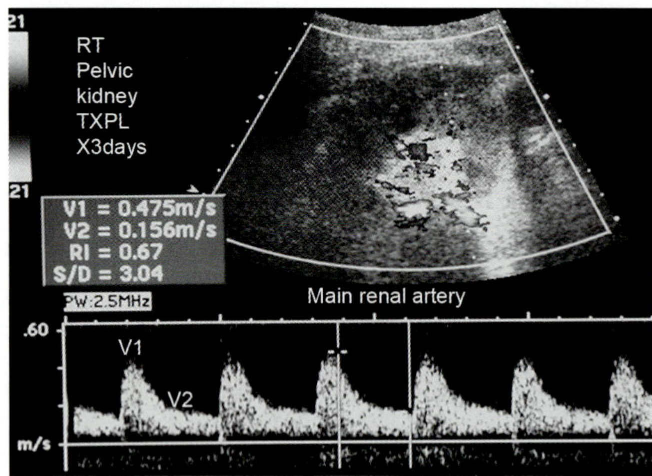

Fig. 2: Normal duplex Doppler ultrasound study. The normal spectral waveform consists of a brisk systolic upstroke (V1) and high diastolic flow (V2). The resistive index (RI) of 0.67 is within normal limits.

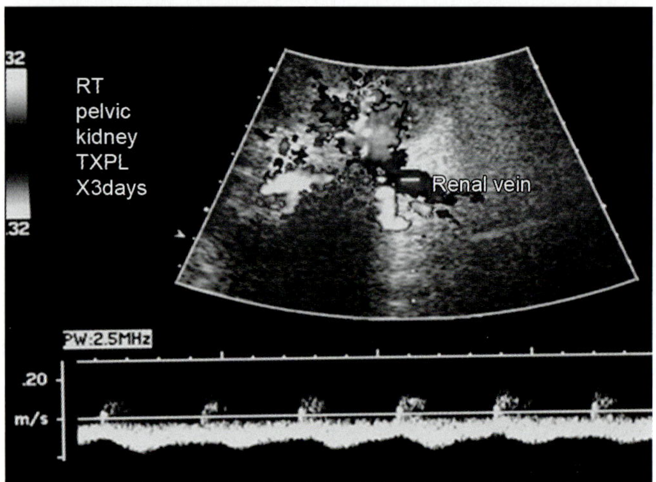

Fig. 3

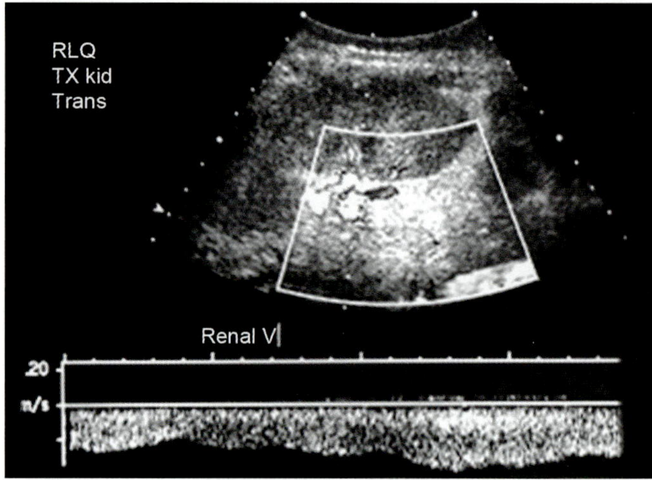

Fig. 4

Figs. 3 and 4: Normal duplex Doppler ultrasound studies of transplant renal veins. Note the venous waveform with mild undulation reflecting normal right atrial pressure changes and mild phasicity reflecting normal respiration.

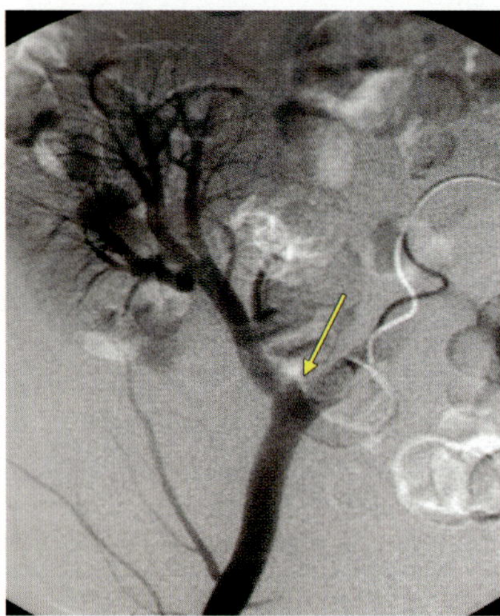

Fig. 5: Normal transplant angiogram: End-to-side anastomosis (yellow arrow) of donor renal artery to recipient *external* iliac artery.

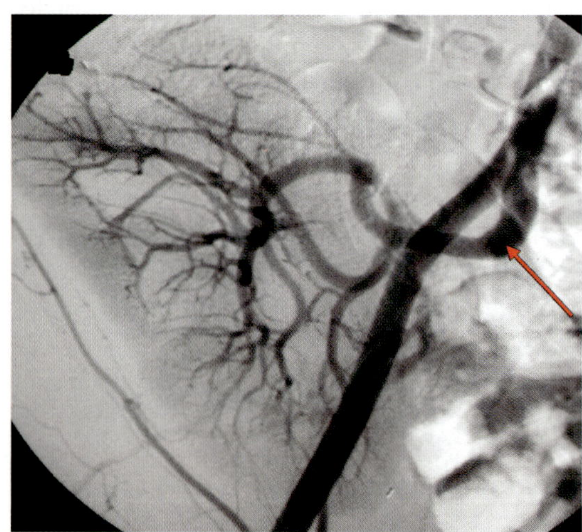

Fig. 6: Normal transplant angiogram: End-to-end anastomosis (red arrow) of donor renal artery to recipient *internal* iliac artery.

ELEVATED RI (FIG. 7)

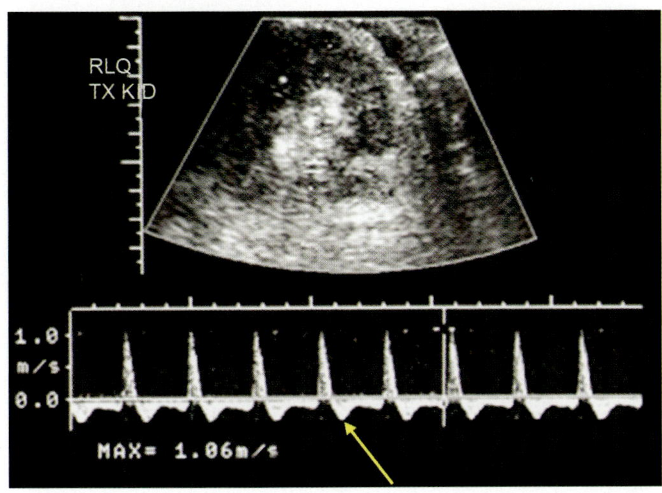

Fig. 7: Elevated resistive index (RI) with reverse of diastolic flow (yellow arrow). A RI of 0.8 or greater is usually considered abnormal. This is a nonspecific finding that could indicate rejection, acute tubular necrosis, cyclosporine toxicity, or renal vein thrombosis.

IMPROVING RI (FIGS. 8 AND 9)

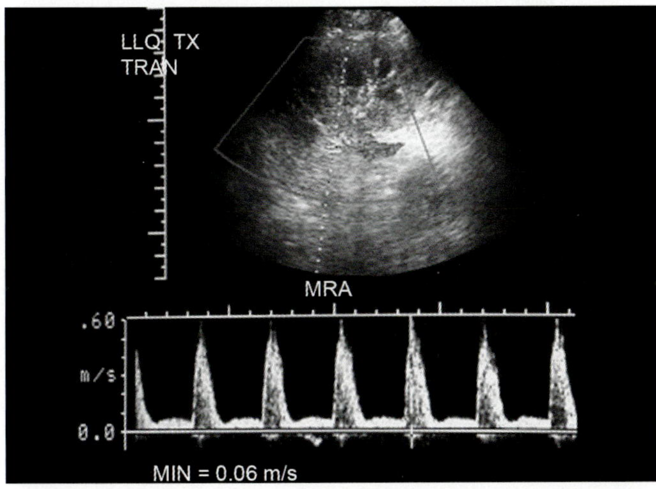

Fig. 8: An elevated resistive index (RI) within the transplant kidney may be secondary to acute tubular necrosis.

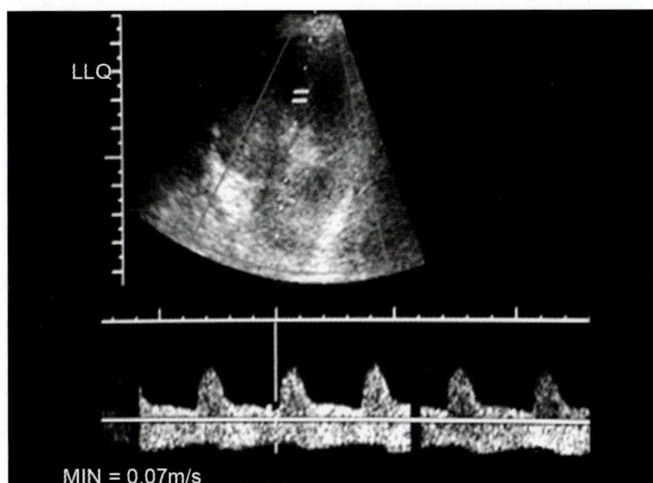

Fig. 9: Improved resistive index (RI) in the same patient associated with improved renal function. Note the increase in diastolic flow.

RENAL ARTERY STENOSIS (FIGS. 10 TO 22)

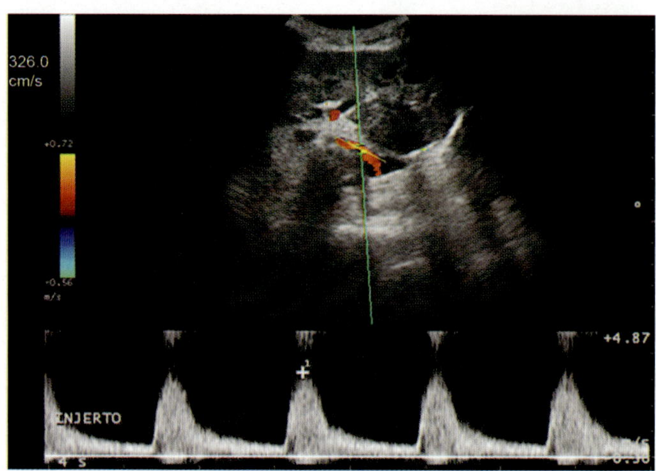

Fig. 10

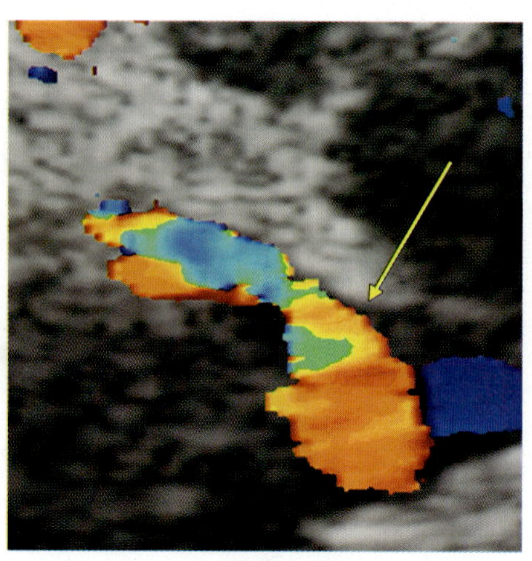

Fig. 11

Figs. 10 and 11: A systolic flow jet was observed in the region of the transplant renal artery to recipient iliac artery anastomosis, with peak systolic velocities > 326 cm/s (normal 180–210 cm/s). Note the aliasing (yellow arrow), an artifact occurring when the velocity in the vessel is too high for the Doppler frequency.

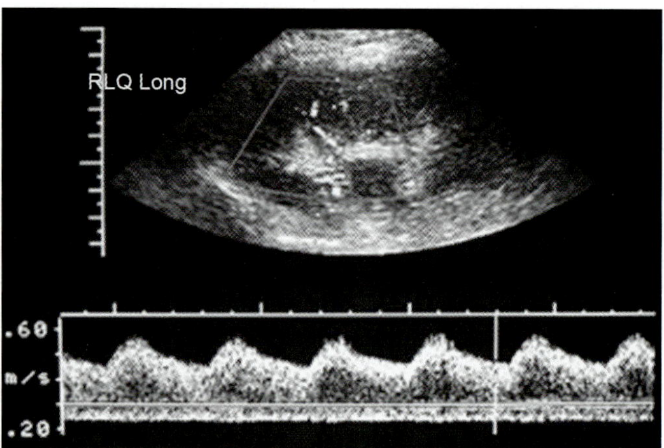

Fig. 12: Evaluation of intrarenal arteries. Tardus–parvus waveform (prolonged systolic rise) and low resistive index (RI) (under 0.5): Indicative of renal artery stenosis.

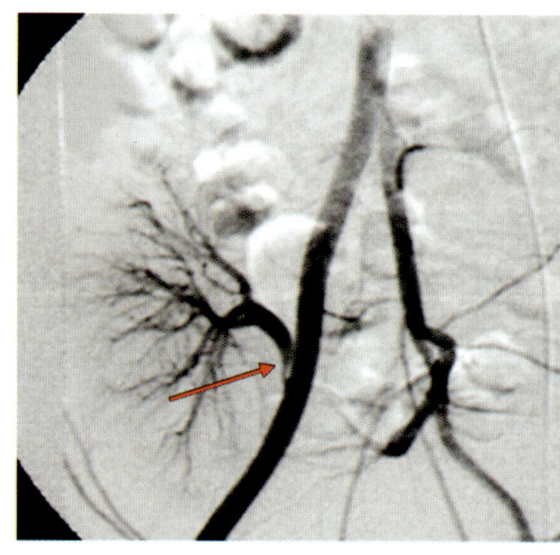

Fig. 13: An angiogram revealed a 75% stenosis (red arrow).

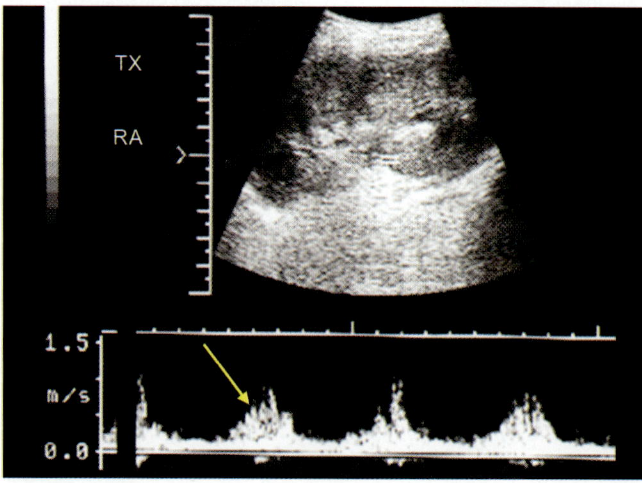

Fig. 14: Abnormal Tardus–parvus arterial waveform in the renal hilum 1 year after transplantation. The slow systolic upstroke (yellow arrow) is highly suggestive of a stenosis proximal to the site being evaluated.

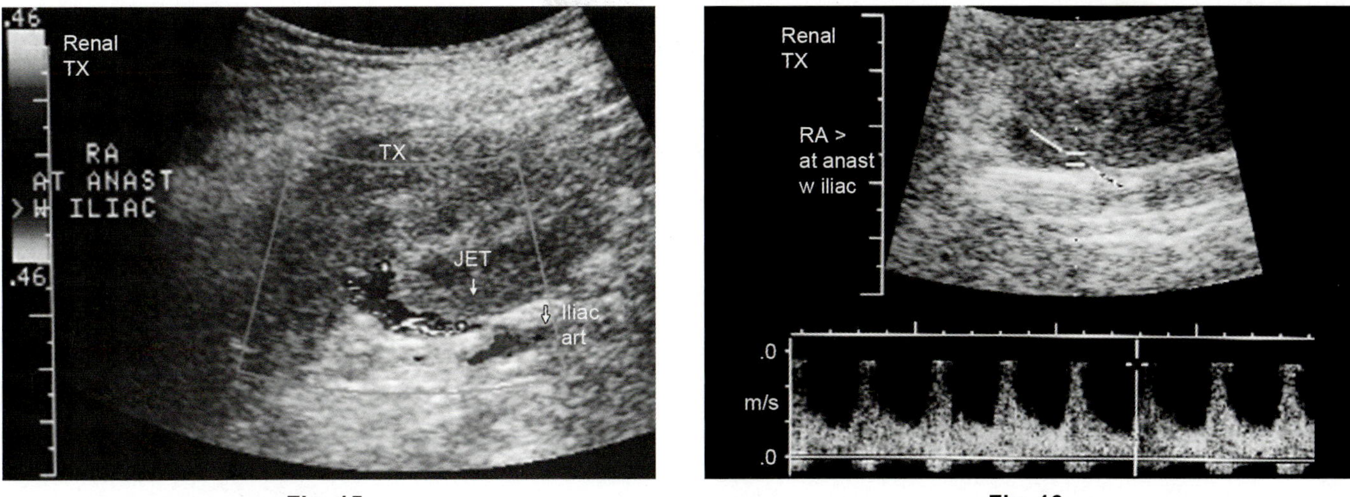

Fig. 15

Fig. 16

Figs. 15 and 16: A systolic flow jet was found in the region of the renal to iliac artery anastomosis (Fig. 15), with peak systolic velocities > 500 cm/s (Fig. 16).

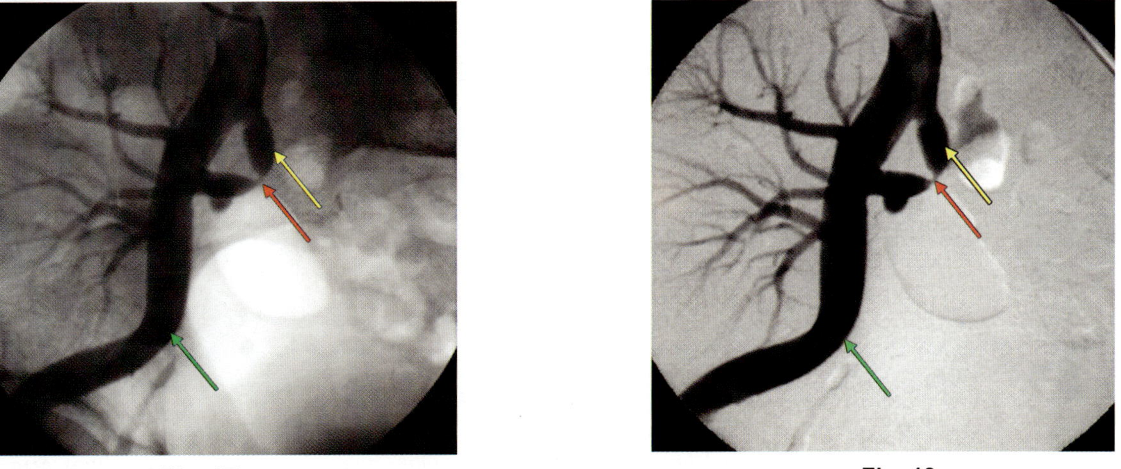

Fig. 17

Fig. 18

Figs. 17 and 18: Renal artery stenosis (red arrows). In this instance, the transplant renal artery had been anastomosed in an end-to-end fashion onto the recipient internal iliac artery (yellow arrows). Note as well the external iliac artery (green arrows). This type of anastomosis carries a greater risk (threefold) of subsequent stenosis by comparison with end-to-side anastomosis.

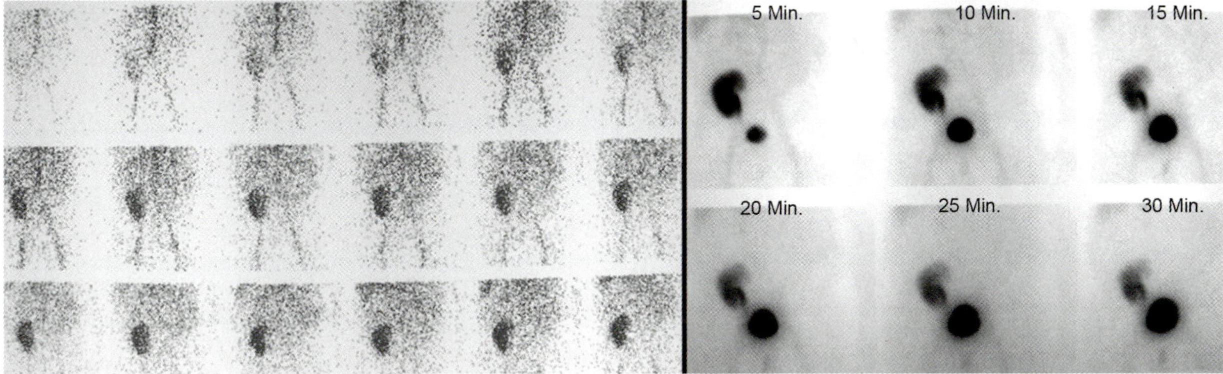

Fig. 19: Flow (left) and functional (right) images from a baseline nuclear medicine scan performed on a patient with renal artery stenosis of the transplanted kidney. Both flow and function are normal.

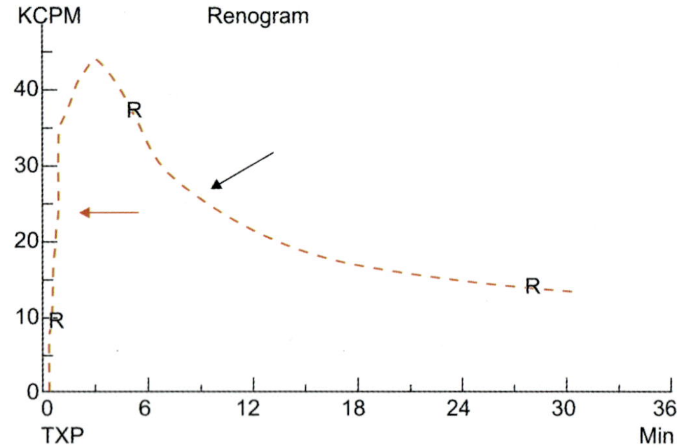

Fig. 20: Renogram from the patient's baseline study confirms normal flow (red arrow) and cortical transit (black arrow).

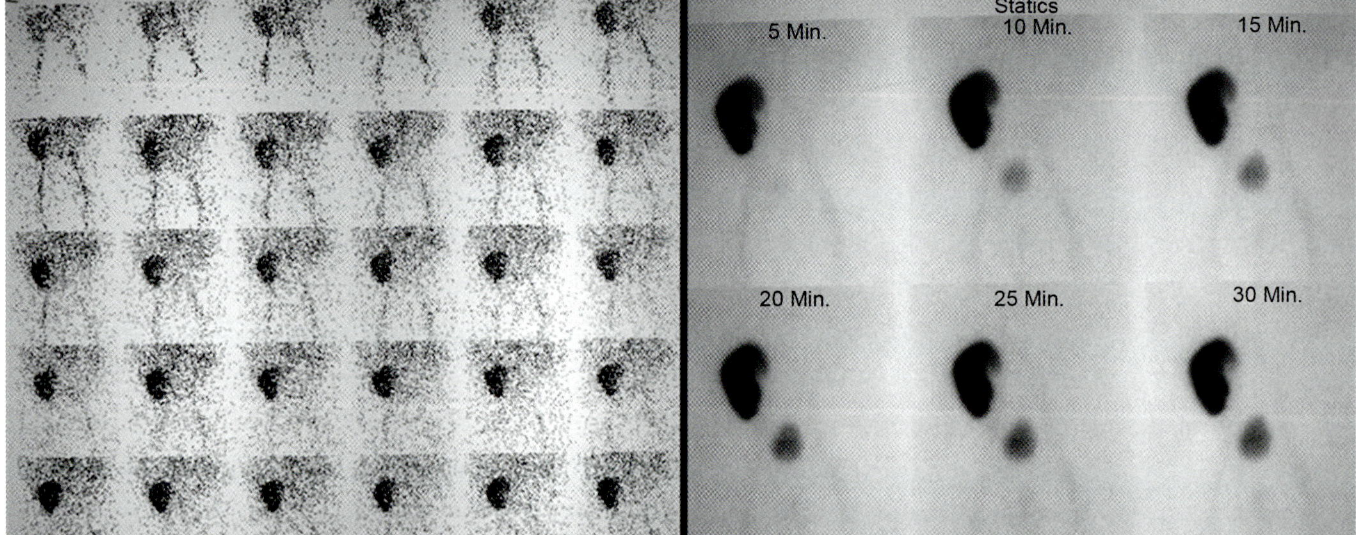

Fig. 21: Flow (left) and functional (right) images from the angiotensin-converting enzyme (ACE) inhibitor nuclear medicine scan performed on the same patient. The flow phase is normal and unchanged from the baseline study. On the functional images, there is markedly delayed cortical transit with considerable residual cortical activity at the end of the study. Normal flow with deterioration of function is the hallmark of hemodynamically significant renal artery stenosis on ACE inhibitor renography (compare with baseline study in Fig. 19).

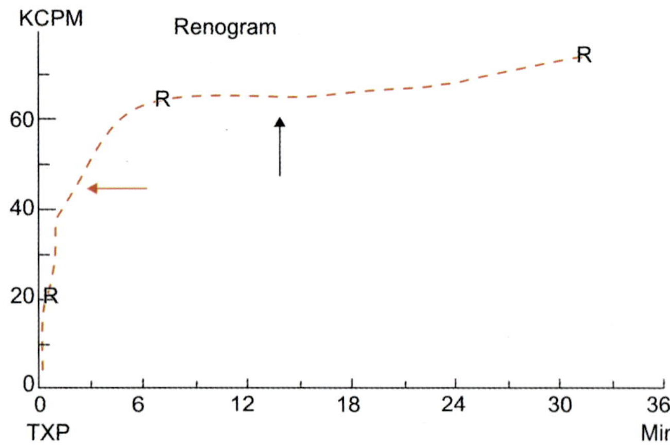

Fig. 22: Renogram from the patient's angiotensin-converting enzyme (ACE) inhibitor study indicates normal flow to the kidney (red arrow). In contrast to the baseline study, however, cortical activity (black arrow) continues to increase over the duration of the test (compare with Fig. 20).

RENAL ARTERY THROMBOSIS (FIGS. 23 TO 26)

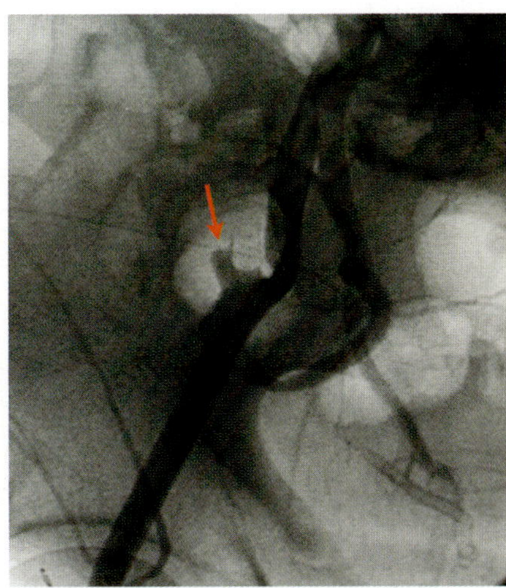

Fig. 23: Angiogram of a renal artery thrombosis. Only the origin (red arrow) of the transplant renal artery is opacified on this angiogram. Notice the abrupt amputation of the graft artery consistent with complete occlusion secondary to thrombosis.

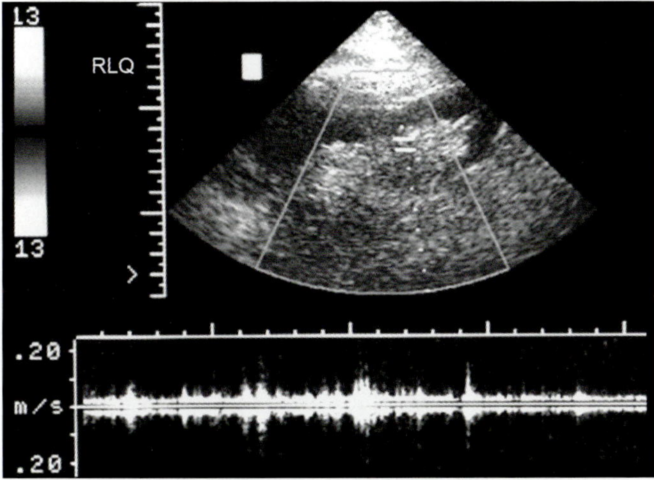

Fig. 24: Renal artery thrombosis: no arterial waveform. Background noise is noted.

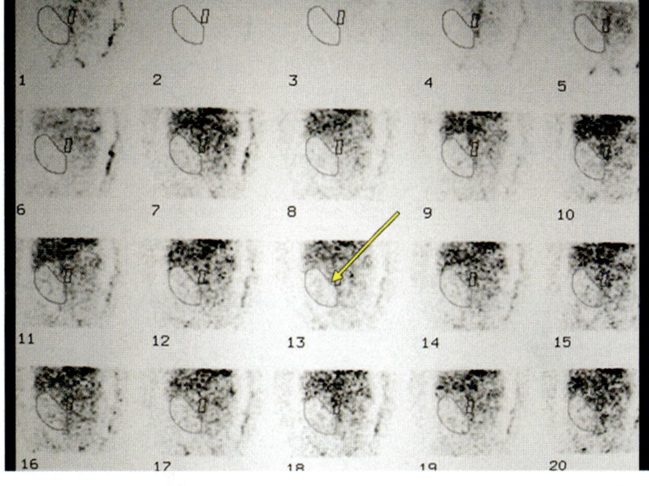

Fig. 25: The flow phase of the nuclear medicine renal scan fails to demonstrate perfusion of the renal allograft (yellow arrow) following renal artery thrombosis.

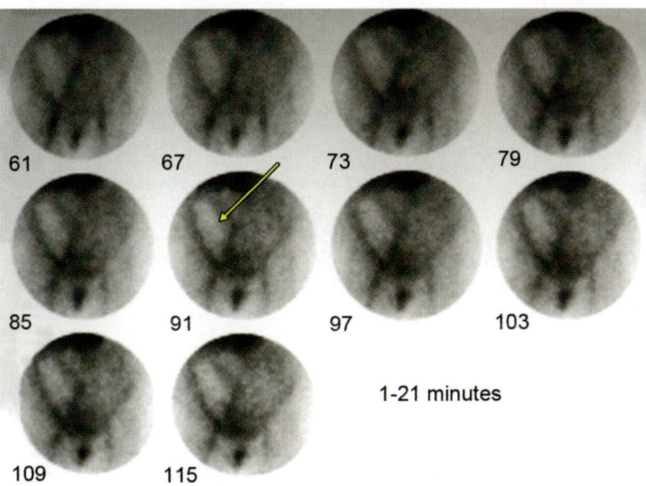

Fig. 26: The appearance of the thrombosed graft on the functional phase of the study is similar to that on the flow phase. There is a photopenic defect (yellow arrow) corresponding to the transplant in the right iliac fossa.

THROMBOSIS OF TRANSPLANT RENAL ARTERY AND EXTERNAL ILIAC ARTERY (FIGS. 27 TO 30)

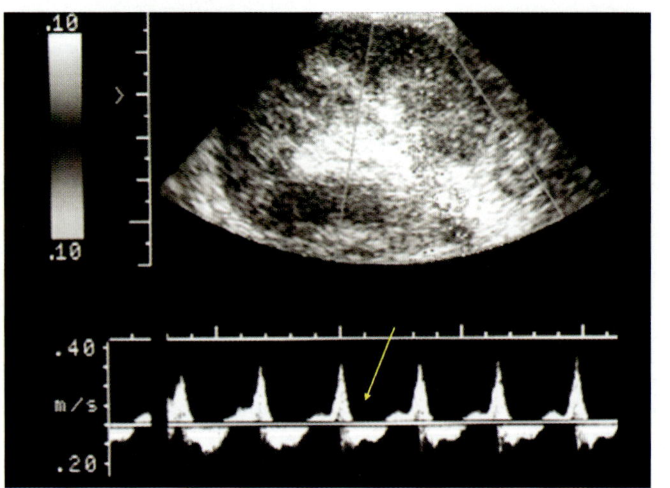

Fig. 27

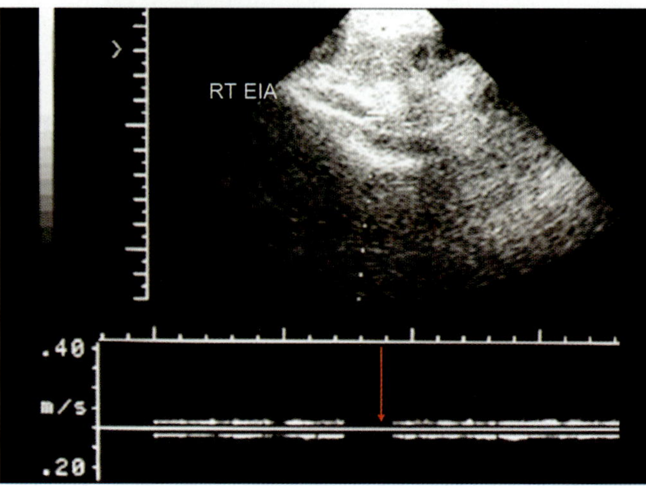

Fig. 28

Figs. 27 and 28: Transplant recipient with history of left to right femorofemoral bypass and retrograde flow supplying the right external iliac and transplant renal arteries. Patient presented with pain over the allograft and deteriorating renal function. Doppler study shows a waveform (Fig. 27, yellow arrow) from a vessel with "systolic and diastolic" components. Although initially it was thought to be an abnormal arterial waveform with diastolic reversal, subsequent evaluation revealed that the waveform originated from the transplant renal vein. The waveform was similar in appearance to that of the inferior vena cava (IVC). Such venous waveforms can be very pulsatile in individuals with chronic heart failure (CHF), especially in the setting of tricuspid regurgitation. No renal artery was found, and no flow could be observed in the right common iliac artery (Fig. 28, red arrow), just background noise.

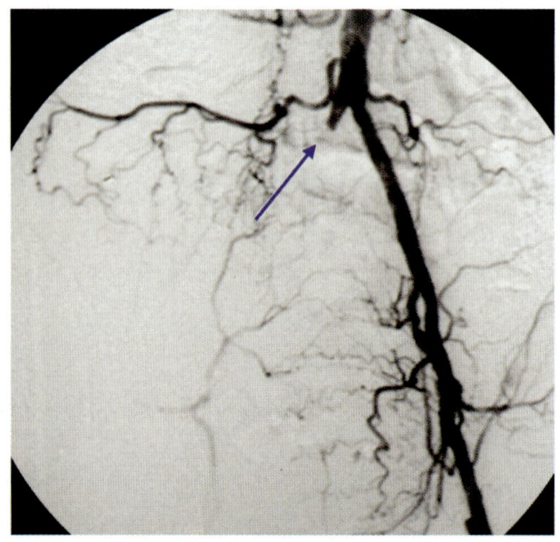

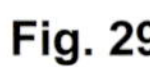

Fig. 29

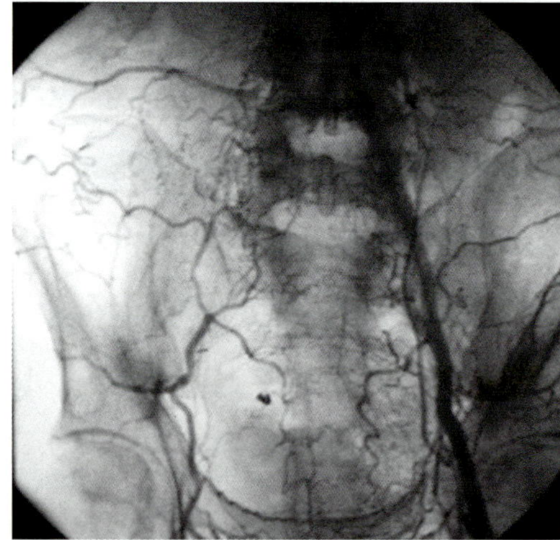

Fig. 30

Figs. 29 and 30: Angiograms shows occlusion of the right common iliac artery (Fig. 29, blue arrow) and of the femorofemoral bypass. There is left to right collateral circulation from the lower lumbar and pelvic arteries.

SEGMENTAL RENAL INFARCTION (FIGS. 31 TO 35)

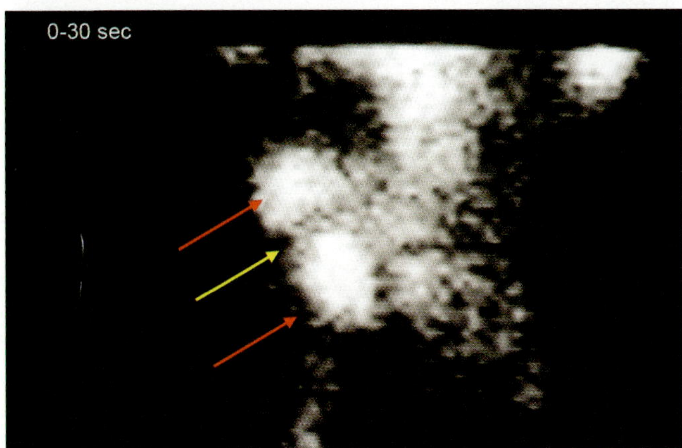

Fig. 31: Group added image from the flow phase of a nuclear medicine scan of renal transplant allograft with three renal arteries. The arteries to the upper and lower poles were patent at the time of transplantation, and the nuclear medicine renal scan demonstrates normal perfusion to the upper and lower halves of the kidney (red arrows). The artery supplying the mid part of the kidney was considerably smaller than the other two arteries and had been injured prior to transplantation. Note the lack of activity in the mid pole of the kidney (yellow arrow), indicating an absence of blood flow to this region.

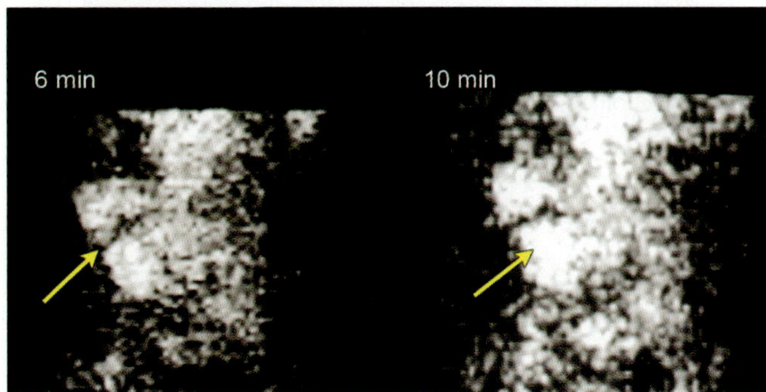

Fig. 32: The appearance of the transplant on the functional phase of the study is similar to that on the flow phase (Fig. 31). There is absent cortical accumulation in the mid part of the kidney (arrows), corresponding to the area supplied by the thrombosed artery.

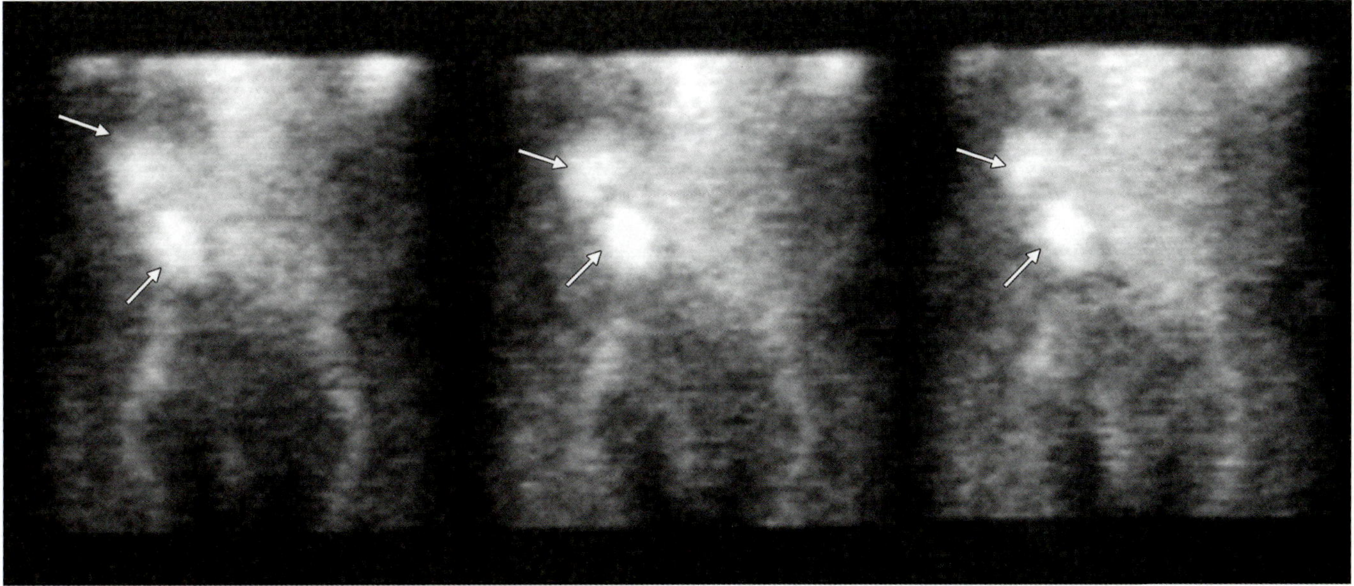

Fig. 33: The arteries to the upper and lower poles of the transplant were patent at the time of surgery, and the renal scan demonstrates good cortical uptake in these regions (white arrows).

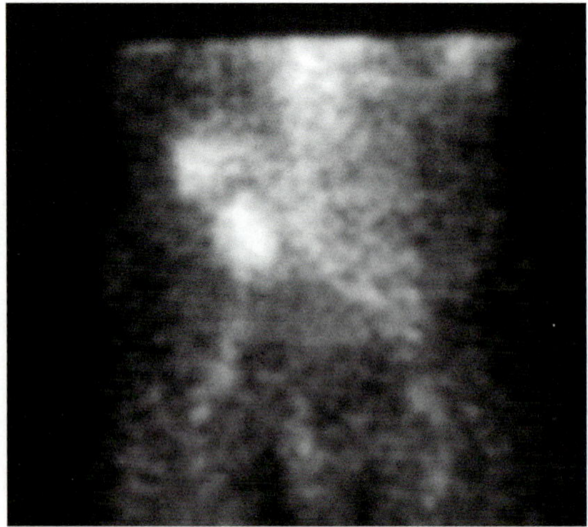

Fig. 34: As this case illustrates, nuclear medicine imaging is a simple noninvasive method for assessing renal vascular patency and function.

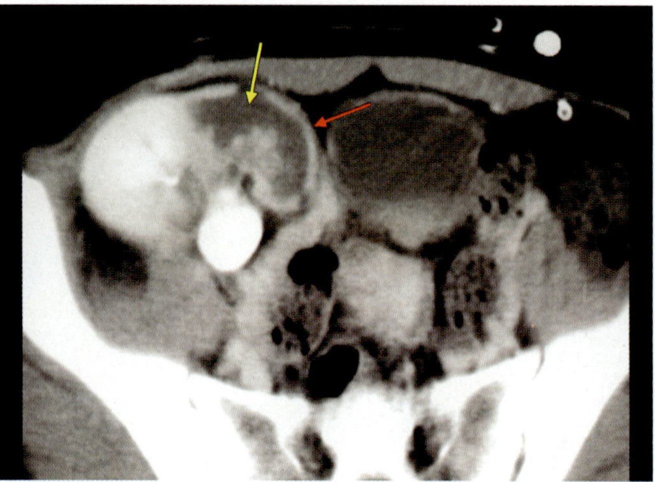

Fig. 35: Contrast-enhanced CT showing a hypoattenuating area in a right lower quadrant (RLQ) graft consistent with a segmental infarction (yellow arrow). Note the well-demarcated borders indicating territorial distribution. The rim sign (red arrow) indicates the viability of peripheral tissue perfused by capsular arteries.

AV FISTULAS (FIGS. 36 TO 44)

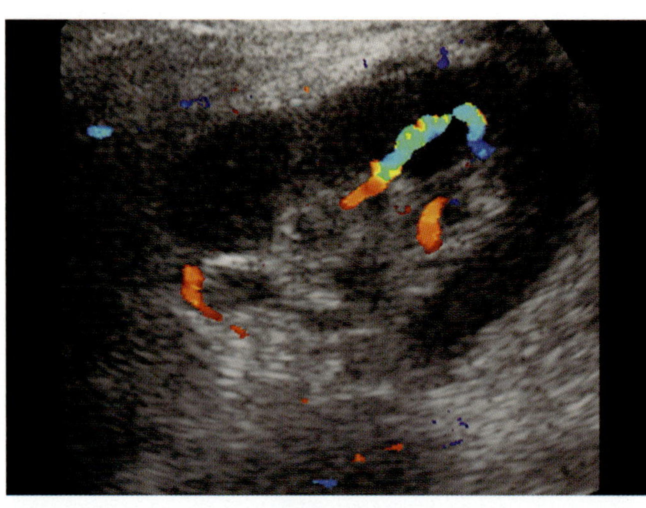

Fig. 36

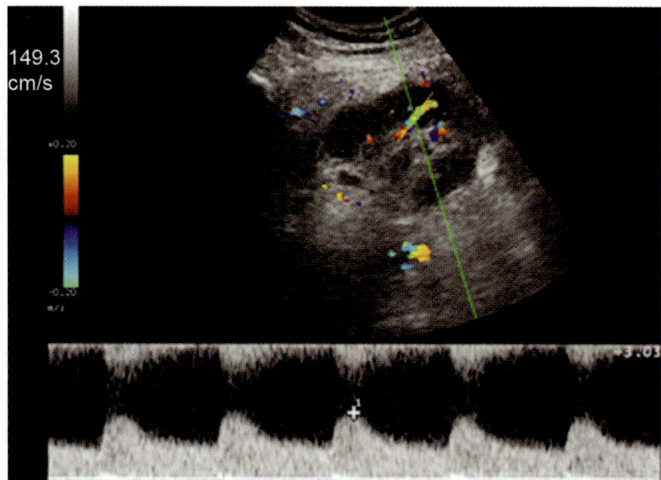

Fig. 37

Figs. 36 and 37: Intrarrenal arteriovenous (AV) fistula. Color (Fig. 36) and duplex Doppler (Fig. 37) images show a dilated feeding artery and a draining vein with turbulent, high-velocity flow (149 cm/s) at the interlobar artery level.

Intrarenal AV fistulas are usually the result of a simultaneous laceration during biopsy procedures of an artery and a vein that result in a fistulous communication between both vessels. Color Doppler shows a focal flurry of disorganized color flow presumably due to vibration of surrounding tissues. The feeding artery and draining vein may be visualized with proper gain and parameter settings. Although the artery shows high-velocity and low-resistance waveforms on spectral analysis, the vein shows pulsatile arterialized flow.

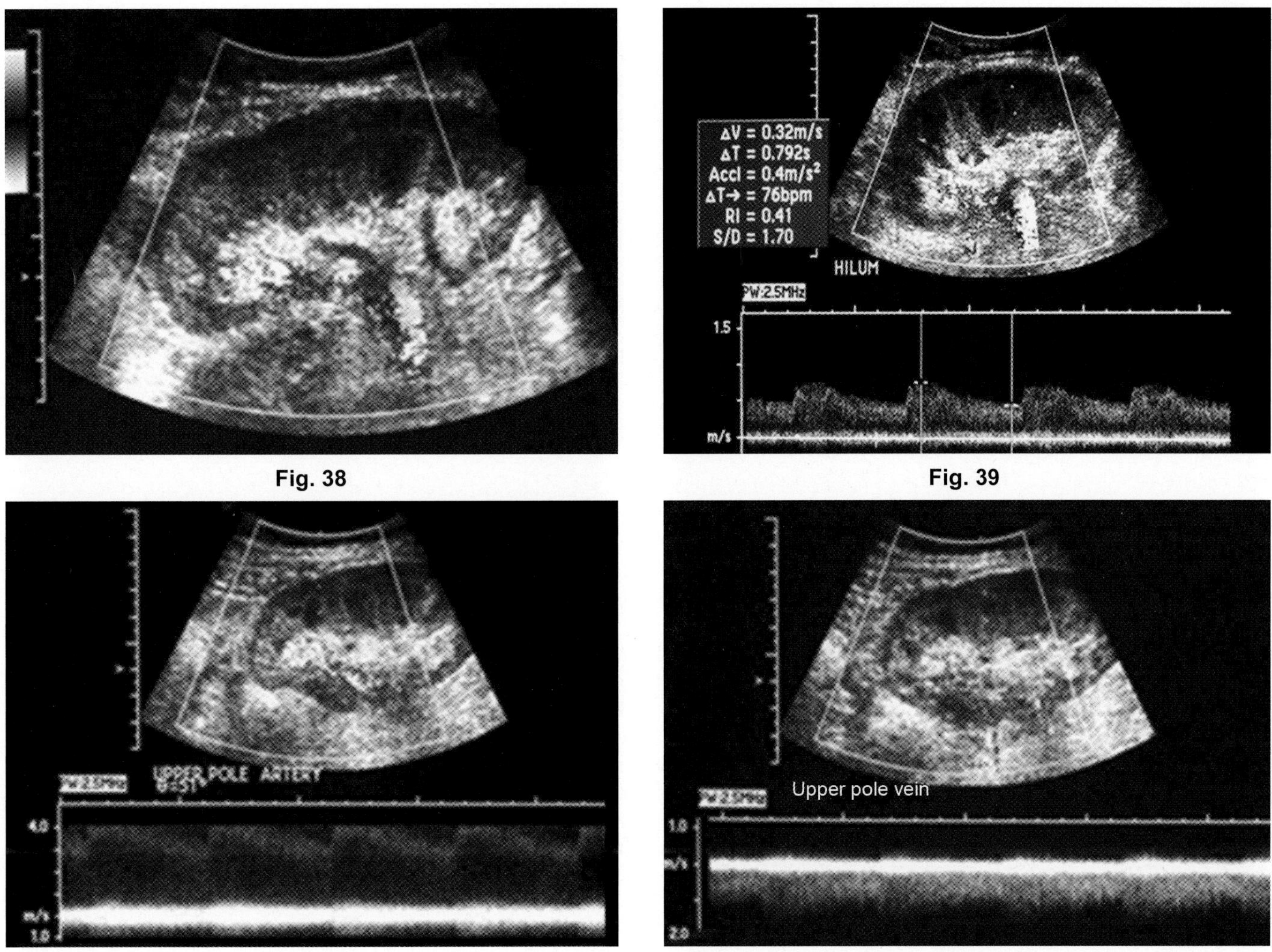

Fig. 38

Fig. 39

Fig. 40

Fig. 41

Figs. 38 to 41: Patient was referred based on "bruit" on physical exam 3 years after kidney transplantation. Doppler study (Fig. 38) showed a "bruit" of tissue vibration indicative of elevated velocity. The transplant renal artery (Fig. 39) was found to have high-velocity flow with peak systolic velocity > 600 cm/s and a low resistance [resistive index (RI) is 0.41] with prominent diastolic flow secondary to lack of resistance from the transplant vein due to the arteriovenous (AV) fistula. Figures 40 (mislabeled as artery) and 41 show pulsatile flow in draining vein.

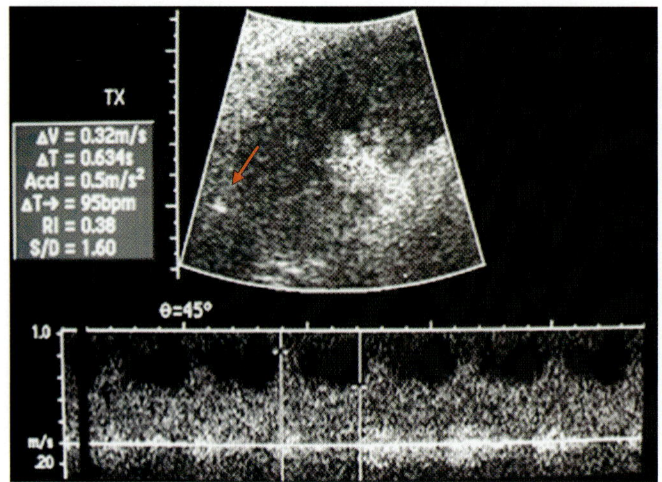

Fig. 42

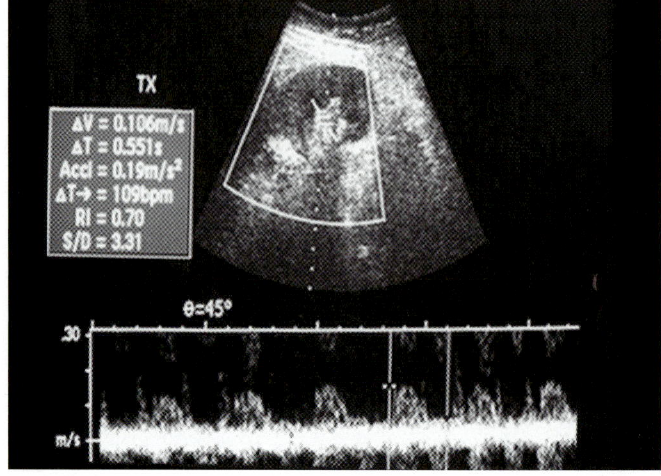

Fig. 43

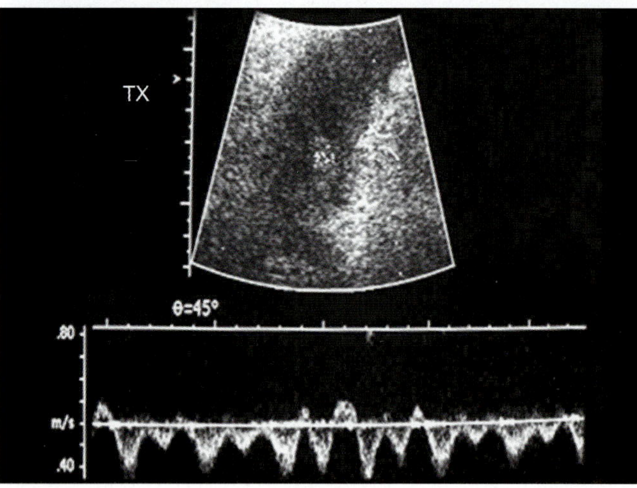

Fig. 44

Figs. 42 to 44: Arteriovenous (AV) fistula after transplant biopsy. A small echogenic area in the upper pole (Fig. 42, red arrow) shows turbulent, high-velocity flow on pulsed Doppler interrogation at the site of the fistula. There is low resistance secondary to the low resistance of the draining vein. The draining vein shows turbulent flow with arterialization of the venous signal (Figs. 43 and 44). This is usually not of clinical concern unless considerable vascular shunting exists, causing ischemia in the transplant kidney. Large AV fistulas can be coiled and occluded. Small AV fistulas often resolve spontaneously.

PSEUDOANEURYSMS (FIGS. 45 AND 46)

Although pseudoaneurysms also usually result from biopsy injuries, the laceration only involves the arterial wall (as opposed to AV fistula in which it involves both artery and vein).

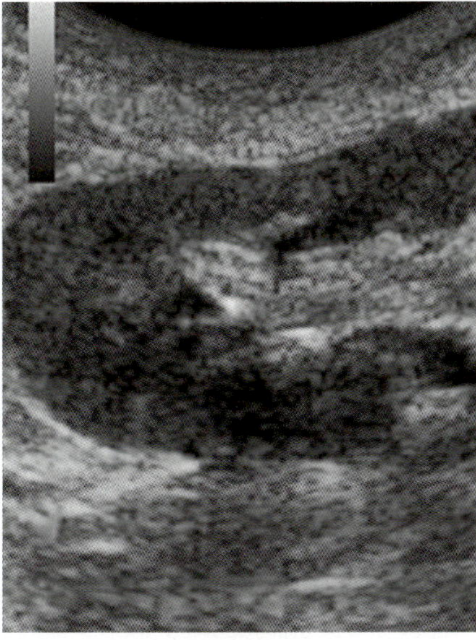

Fig. 45

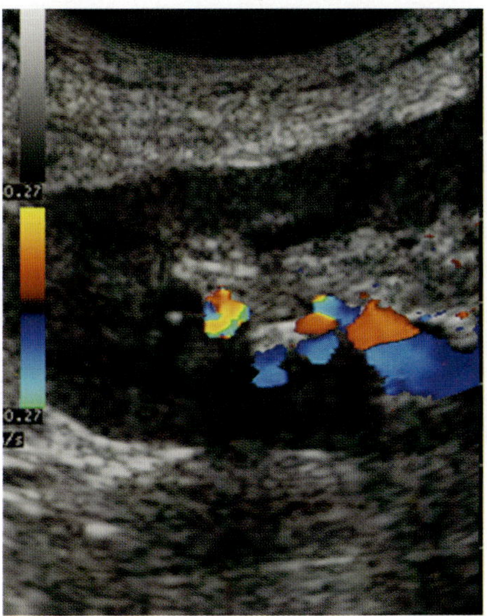

Fig. 46

Figs. 45 and 46: Gray scale ultrasound (Fig. 45) shows a rounded cystic area that on color Doppler evaluation (Fig. 46) demonstrates flow, usually disorganized, often with focal aliasing. A "ying-yang sign" can be seen with color Doppler imaging. A to-and-fro spectral Doppler waveform (not shown here) representing alternating forward and reverse flow can be seen in the pseudoaneurysm neck if the neck is visualized.

RENAL VEIN STENOSIS (FIGS. 47 AND 48)

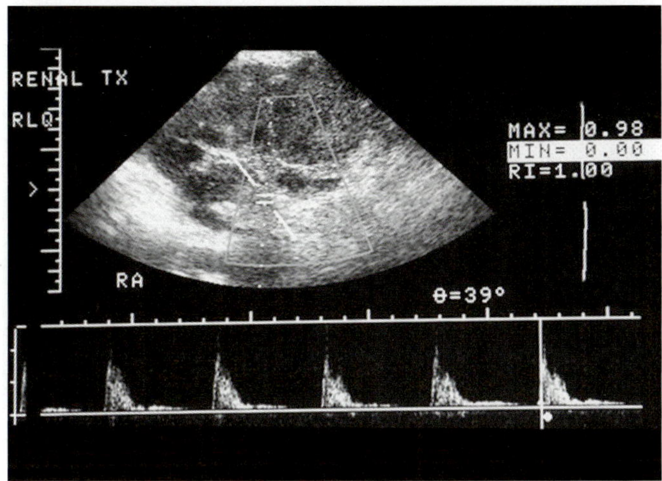

Fig. 47

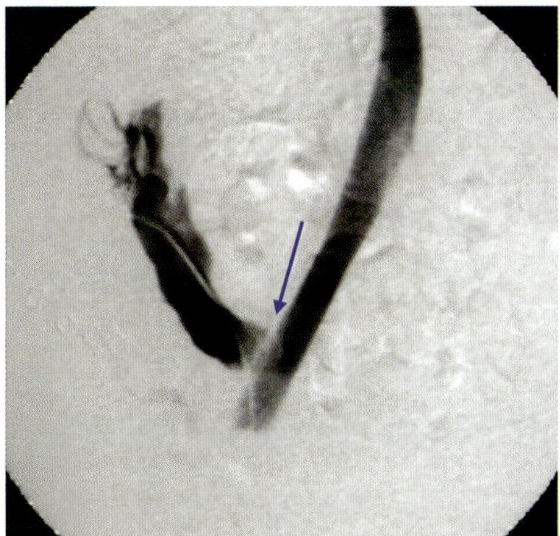

Fig. 48

Figs. 47 and 48: Duplex Doppler ultrasound demonstrates a high resistance arterial waveform with an elevated resistive index (RI) (Fig.47). The renal vein was enlarged with associated distention of the intrarenal veins. These findings prompted a search for a downstream venous obstruction. A stenosis of the renal vein–iliac vein anastomosis was identified on ultrasound and at venography (Fig. 48, blue arrow).

RENAL VEIN TORSION (FIGS. 49 AND 50)

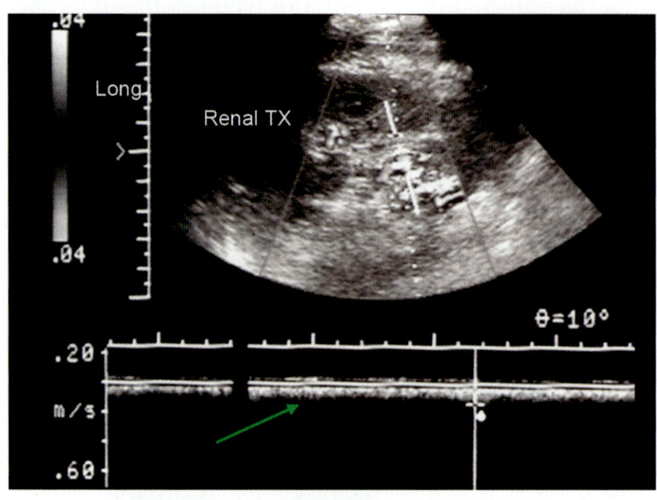

Fig. 49

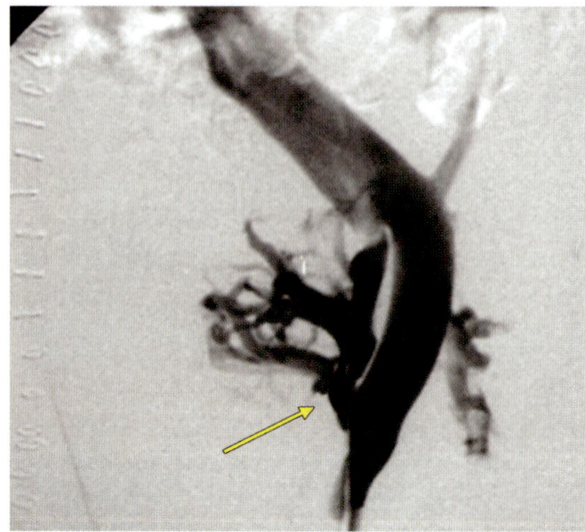

Fig. 50

Figs. 49 and 50: Abnormal ultrasound of a transplant kidney. Pulsed Doppler of renal vein shows low-velocity and monophasic waveform lacking phasicity (Fig. 49, green arrow) indicating a downstream venous obstruction. Angiogram showed a renal vein stricture (Fig. 50, yellow arrow). Patient was taken to the operating room where a kink of the renal vein was identified. The renal allograft was repositioned so to allow the vein and artery to lie in a nontwisted comfortable position. No vascular reconstruction was required.

ABRUPT CHANGE IN RENAL VEIN FLOW VELOCITY ASSOCIATED WITH AN EXPANDING HEMATOMA (FIGS. 51 TO 56)

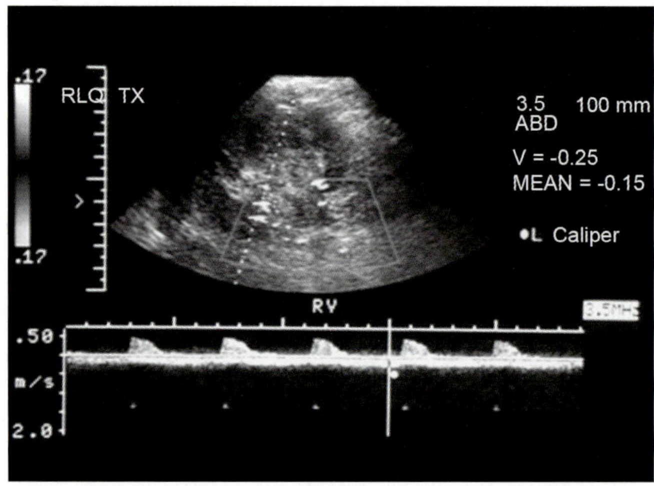

Fig. 51

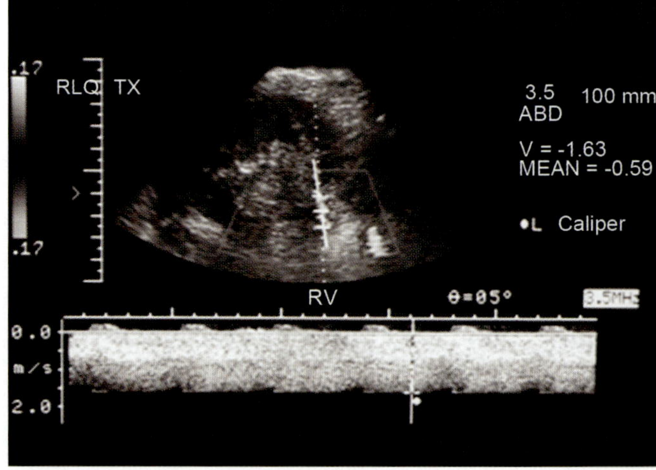

Fig. 52

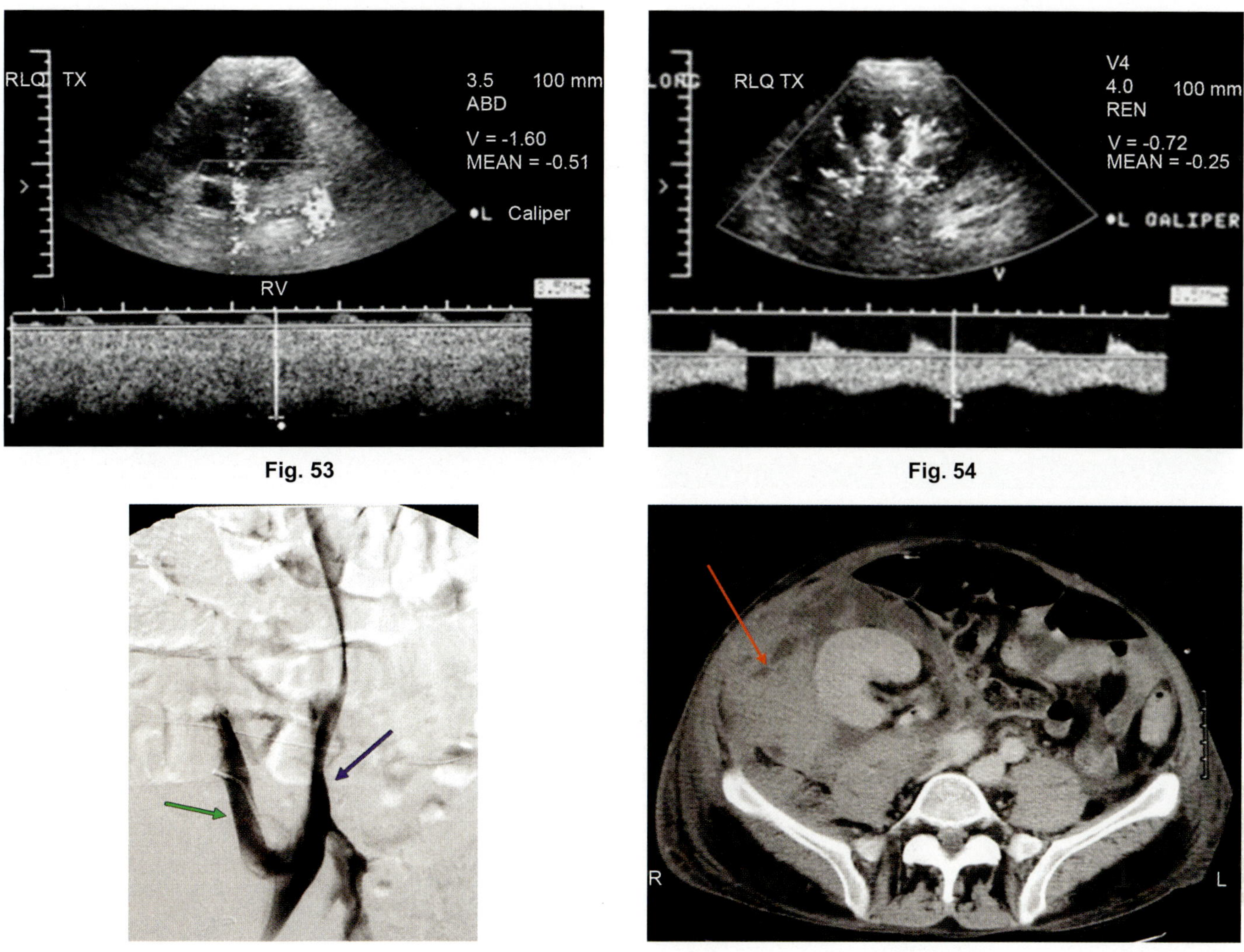

Fig. 53

Fig. 54

Fig. 55

Fig. 56

Figs. 51 to 56: Figs. 51 to 53 show an initial normal spectral waveform of the renal vein on sonography at 09:15 AM. Fig. 54 depicts an abrupt change in venous velocity after a transplant biopsy at 17:00 PM. A venogram shows external compression by a hematoma on the recipient common iliac vein (Fig. 55, blue arrow). Note the transplant renal vein (green arrow). The postbiopsy hematoma seen on CT examination (Fig. 56, red arrow).

RENAL VEIN THROMBOSIS (FIGS. 57 TO 67)

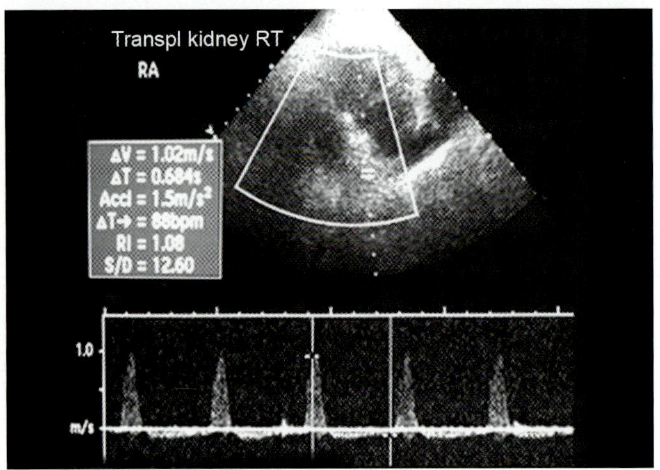

Fig. 57: Renal vein thrombosis with high-resistant arterial waveform secondary to venous outflow obstruction/edema. RI = 1.08.

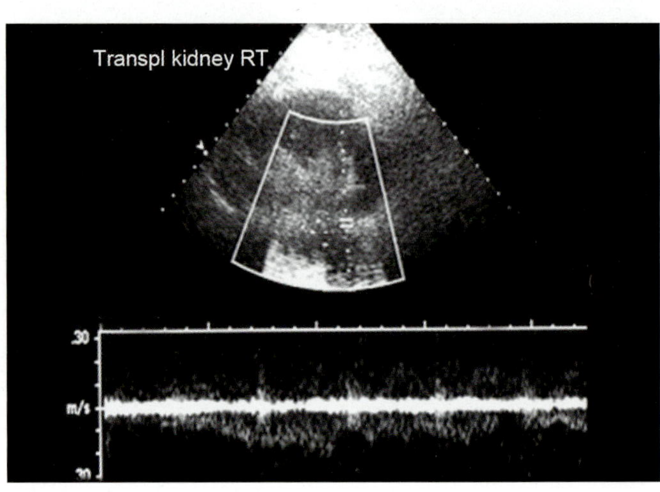

Fig. 58: Renal vein thrombosis with only background noise on Doppler evaluation.

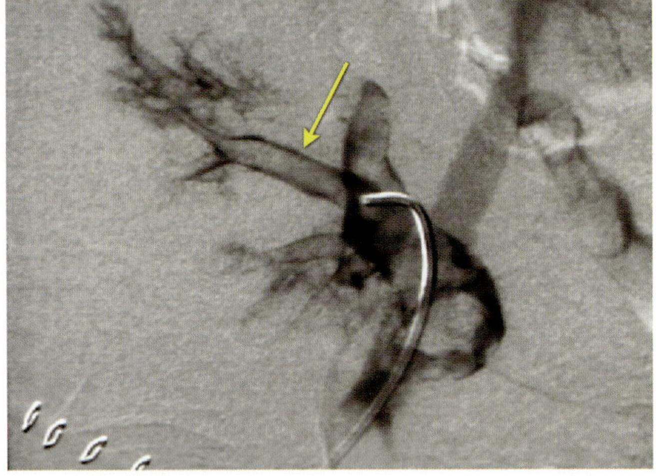

Fig. 59: Renal vein thrombosis (yellow arrow) on venography.

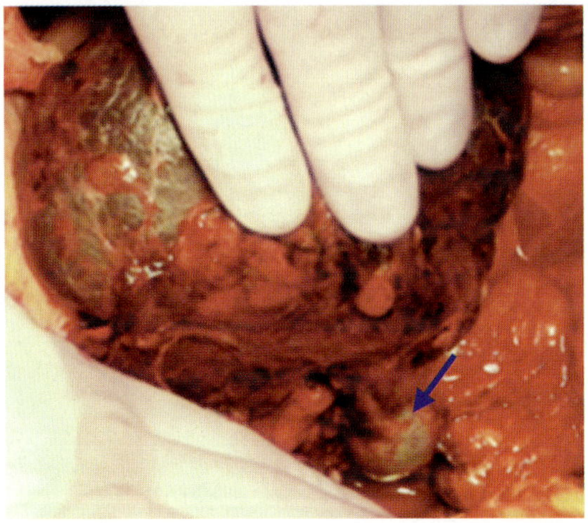

Fig. 60

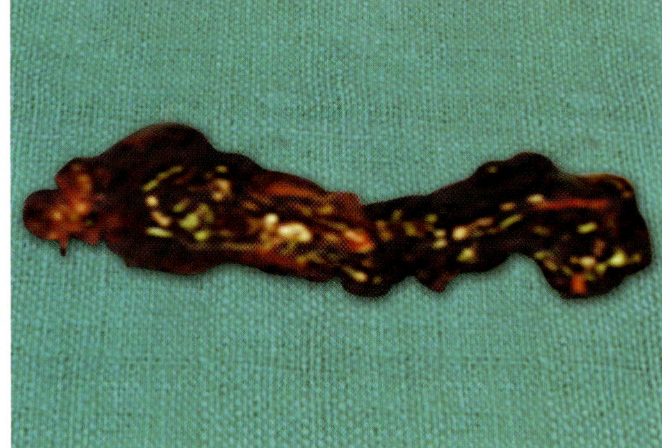

Fig. 61

Figs. 60 and 61: Intraoperative picture of a thrombosed renal vein (Fig. 60, blue arrow). Figure 61 shows the removed thrombus. There is also thrombosis of the allograft.

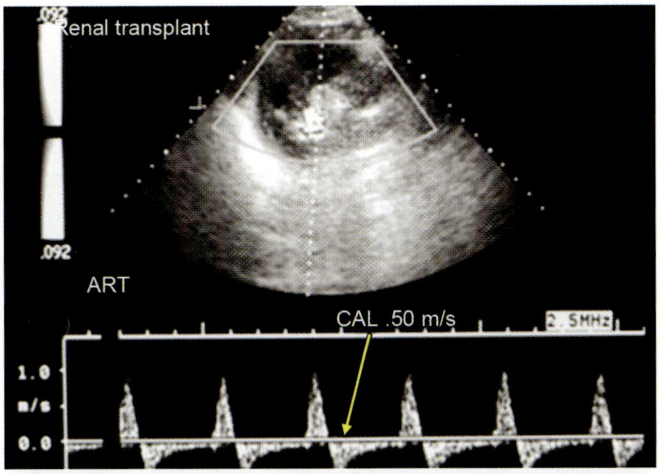

Fig. 62

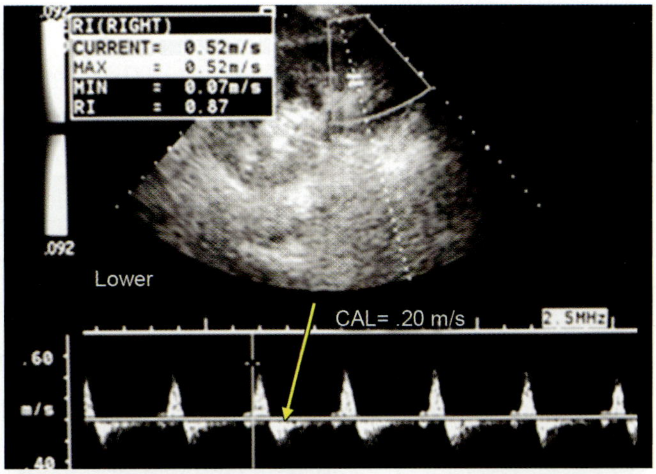

Fig. 63

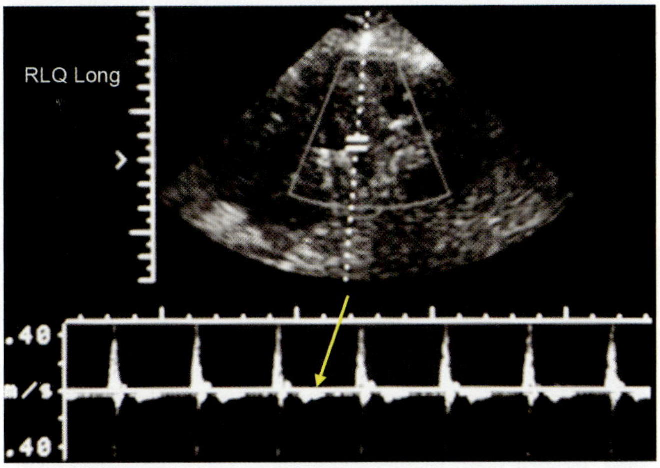

Fig. 64

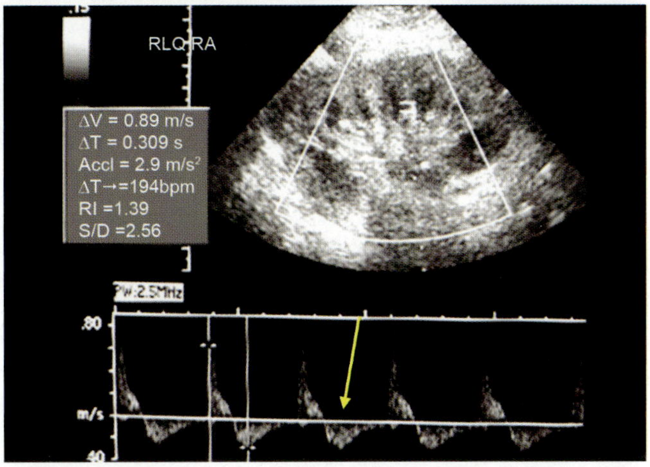

Fig. 65

Figs. 62 to 65: Various examples of duplex Doppler US studies in cases of renal vein thrombosis. Note the abnormal arterial waveforms with high resistance and reversal of flow in diastole (yellow arrows) in the setting of nonvisualization of the renal vein.

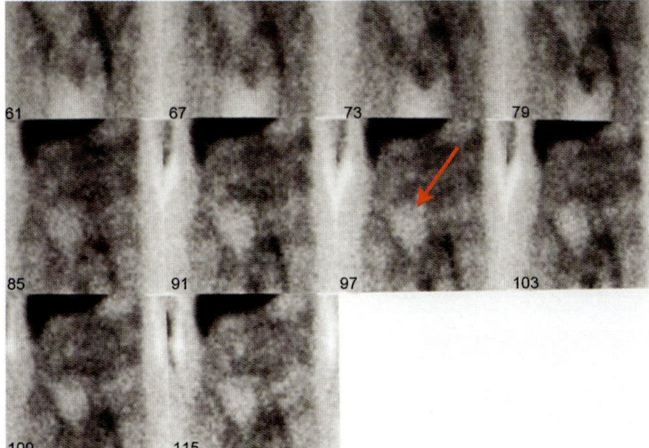

Fig. 66: Late renal vein thrombosis. On the perfusion phase of the renal scan there is no evidence of flow to renal transplant (red arrow) in the right iliac fossa.

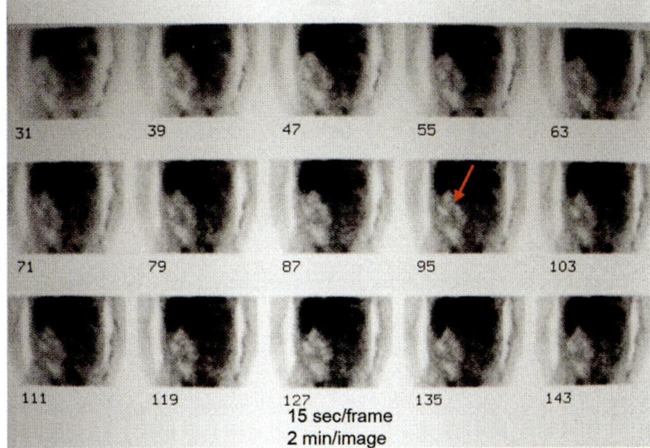

Fig. 67: On the functional phase of the study the kidney appears as a photopenic area (red arrow) with no evidence of cortical uptake of tracer, indicating a complete lack of function. The appearance of the late phase of renal vein thrombosis on the nuclear medicine renal scan is indistinguishable from that of renal artery thrombosis (compare with Fig. 25).

ILIAC VEIN THROMBOSIS

Early Detection and Successful Thrombectomy of an Iliac Vein Thrombosis Presenting with Allograft Dysfunction (Figs. 68 to 71)

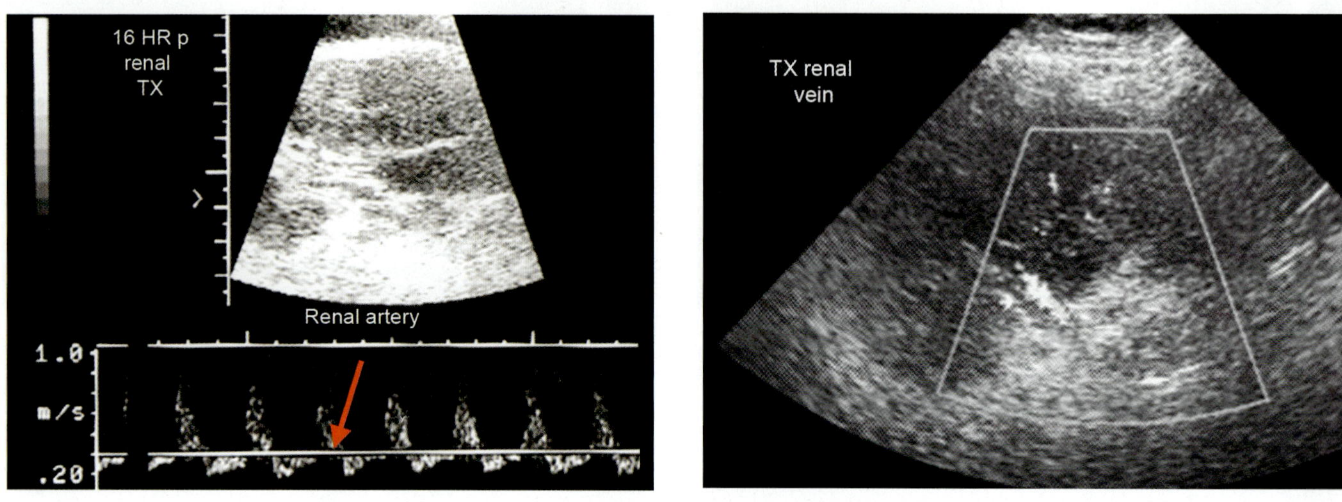

Fig. 68 Fig. 69

Figs. 68 and 69: Kidney transplant recipient with adequate urine output for the first several postoperative hours followed by a marked elevation of creatinine and BUN in association with oliguria unresponsive to intravenous fluids. An emergency duplex Doppler sonography performed 16 hours postoperatively revealed an arterial waveform with a dramatic diastolic reversal of flow (Fig. 68, red arrow). The transplant renal vein was difficult to appreciate (Fig. 69), with vascular flow seen on Doppler only. There was very low PRF (pulse repetition frequency) and an increase in Doppler gain (very slow flow). Differential diagnosis: venous obstruction versus hyperacute rejection.

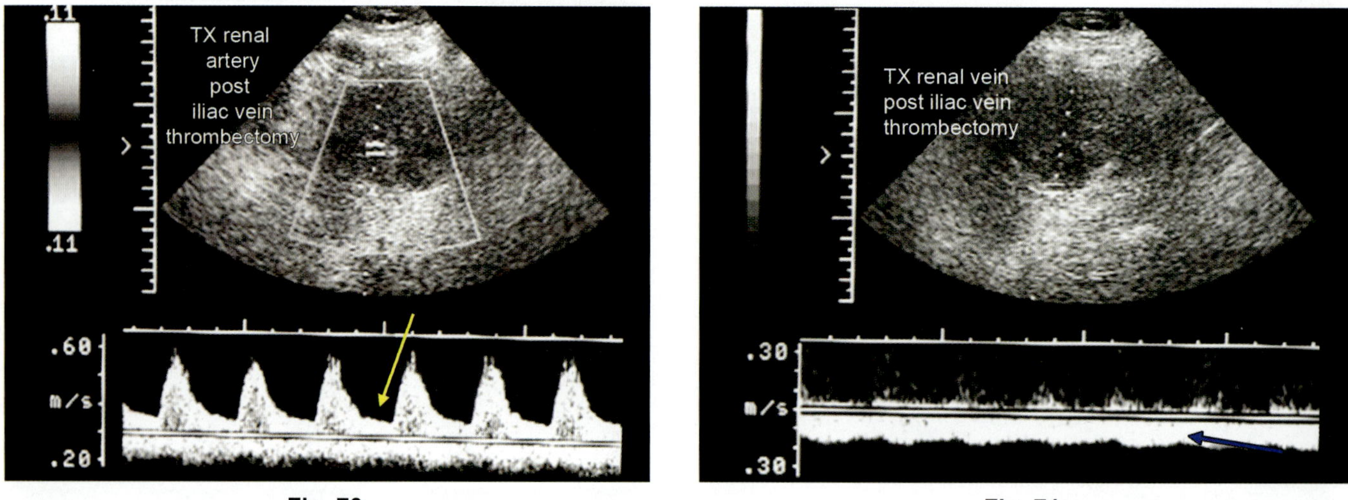

Fig. 70 Fig. 71

Figs. 70 and 71: The patient was explored. A thrombus in the distal external iliac vein was found and removed. The enlarged, edematous transplant kidney improved after the thrombectomy. No gross predisposing factors for the thrombus were identified. A repeat renal artery Doppler showed flow throughout diastole (Fig. 70, yellow arrow) and a normal venous waveform (Fig. 71, blue arrows).

ILIAC ARTERY ANEURYSM (FIG. 72)

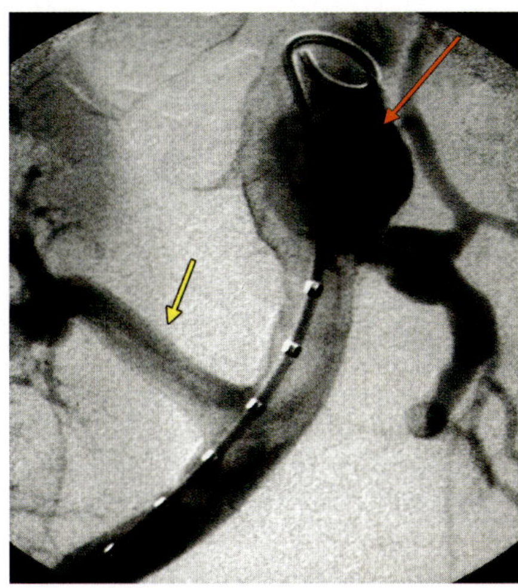

Fig. 72: An angiogram shows a common iliac artery aneurysm (red arrow). Notice the patent transplant renal artery (yellow arrow).

ATRIAL FIBRILLATION (FIGS. 73 AND 74)

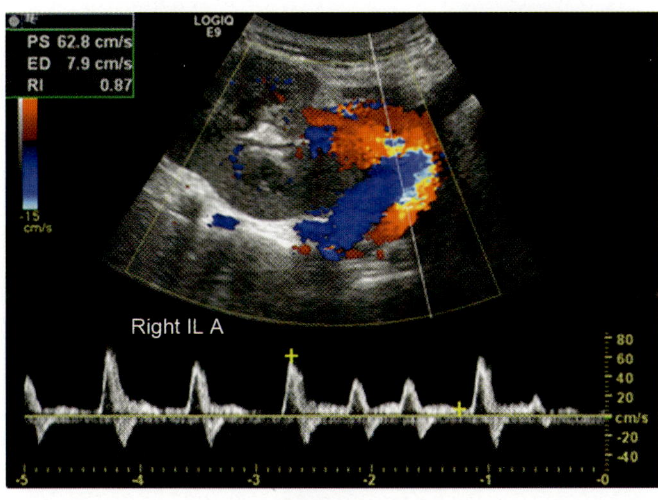

Fig. 73

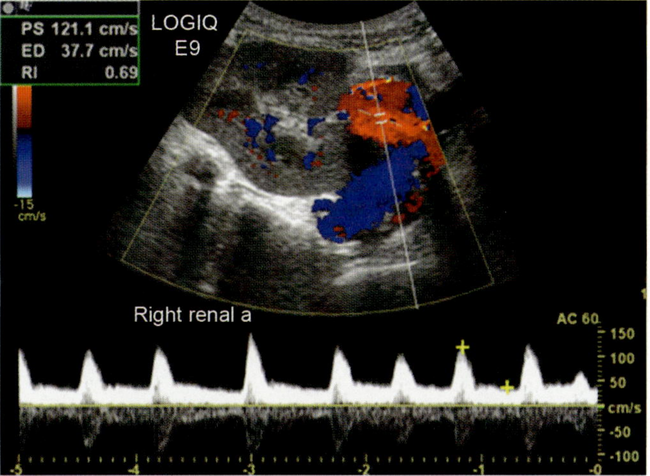

Fig. 74

Figs. 73 and 74: Note the lack of normal regular sinus rhythm of the pulsed Doppler waveforms within the native iliac artery (Fig. 73) and transplant renal artery (Fig. 74).

ACCIDENTAL TRANSECTION OF A SEGMENTAL BRANCH OF THE RENAL ARTERY DURING PROCUREMENT (FIGS. 75 TO 81)

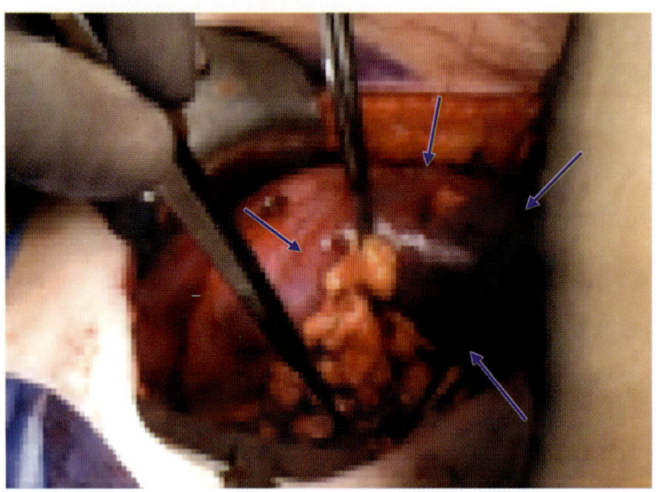

Fig. 75: Live donor kidney transplant in which the branch of the anterior division of the renal artery supplying the anterior middle and lower segments of the kidney was accidentally transected during procurement. Aware of the injury at the time of procurement, it was noted that the involved area had decreased perfusion with preservation fluid. A decision was made to implant the kidney and to evaluate the involved area after reperfusion in the recipient. It was noted that the lower half of the anterior aspect of the allograft remained poorly perfused (blue arrows) and had very diminished Doppler signals.

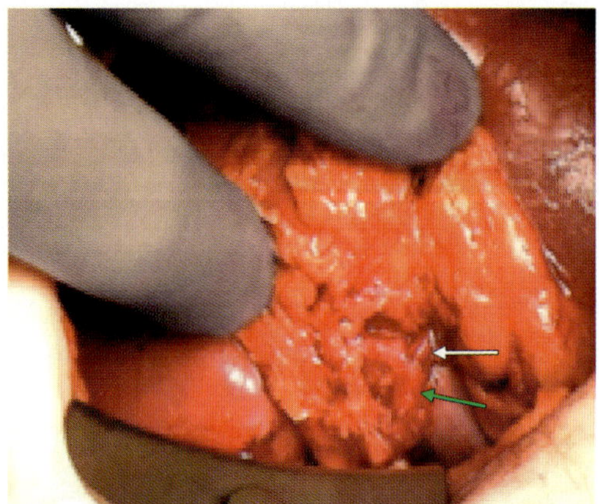

Fig. 76: The transected artery was identified, dissected, and reanastomosed (white arrow) to the anterior division of the renal artery (green arrow).

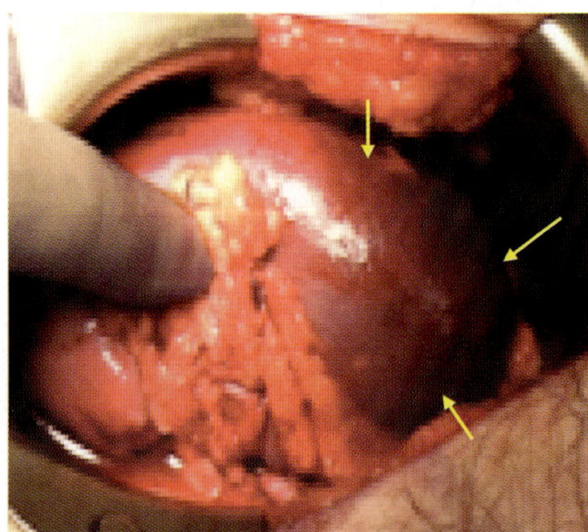

Fig. 77: There was a marked improvement in perfusion (yellow arrows) after this maneuver. Doppler evaluation of the reconstructed artery as well as of its associated parenchyma was found to be adequate.

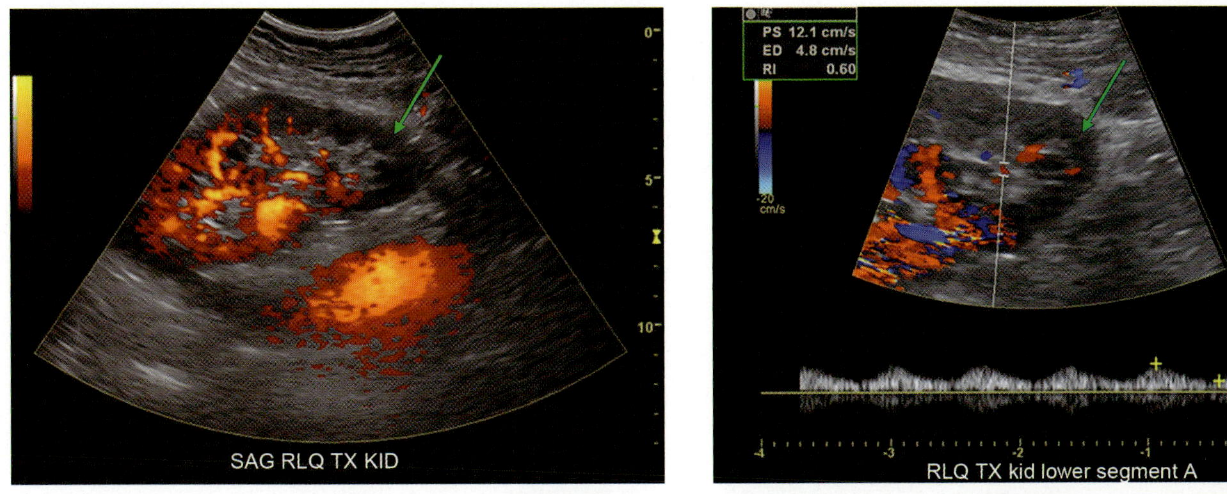

Fig. 78

Fig. 79

Figs. 78 and 79: Color and spectral Doppler images in the immediate postoperative period depict decreased perfusion in the transplant kidney lower pole (green arrows) in association with parvus–tardus waveforms. Since the allograft was producing urine, it was decided to observe and repeat the imaging study.

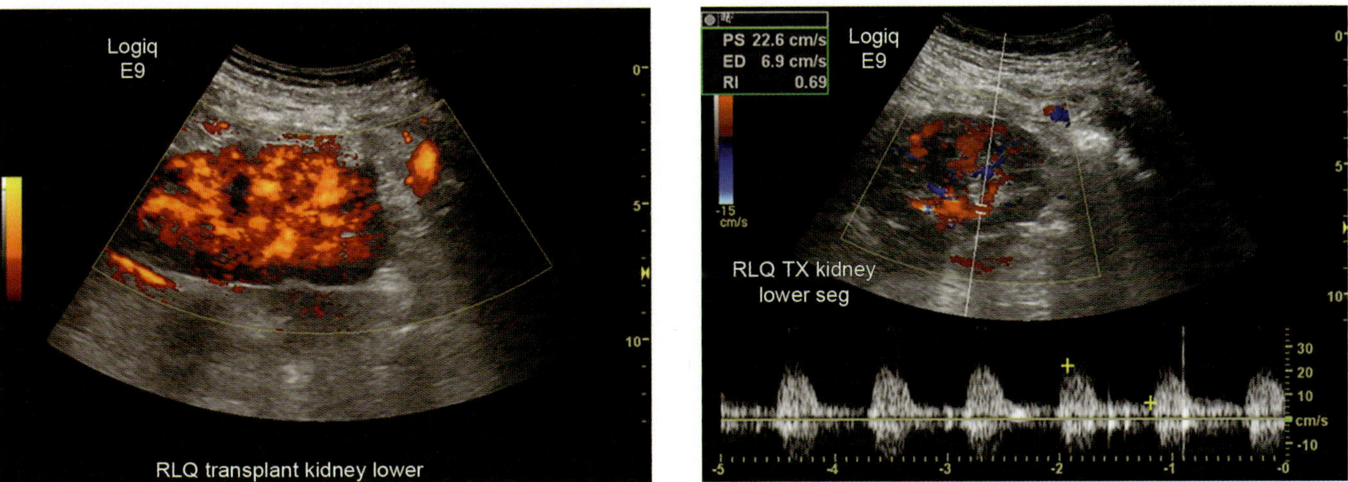

Fig. 80

Fig. 81

Figs. 80 and 81: Imaging 12 hours later demonstrates homogeneous vascularity throughout the entire organ, with normal-appearing waveforms in the lower pole.

HEMI-INFARCTION OF TRANSPLANT KIDNEY (FIGS. 82 AND 83)

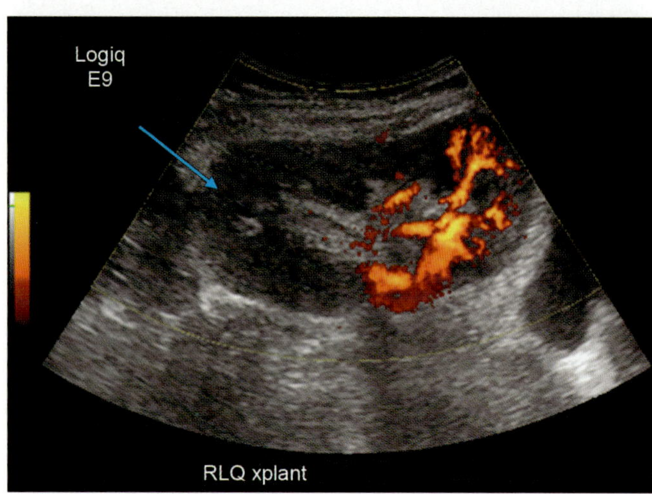

Fig. 82: Recipient 10 years after renal transplantation with a recent history of a single high-velocity reading in the renal artery at the hilum, normal parenchymal resistive indices, and no parvus–tardus waveforms, who presented with an elevated creatinine. Duplex Doppler evaluation of the kidney transplant showed an avascular upper segment (blue arrow).

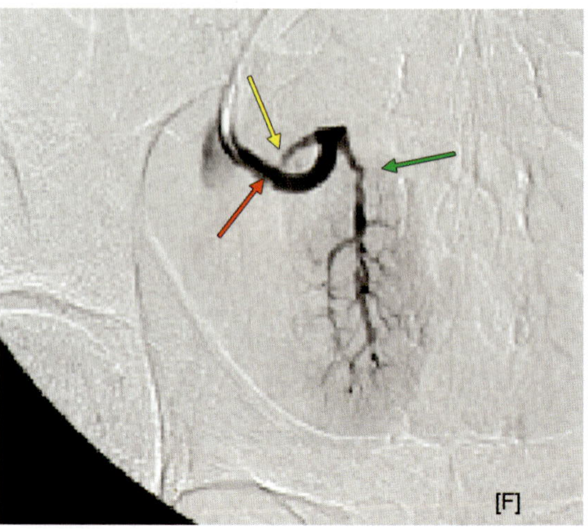

Fig. 83: Contrast examination showed a patent renal artery (red arrow) with occlusion of its branch to the lateral–superior half of the kidney (yellow arrow). The artery supplying the medial–inferior half of the kidney, although patent, showed a beaded wavy appearance (green arrow) suggestive of vasculitis.

CHAPTER 62

Infections and Malignancies

Mariano Volpacchio, Catherine D'Agostino, Christopher Palestro, et al.

INFECTIONS

- Transplant patients (mostly due to their immunosuppression) are susceptible to a wide spectrum of both local and systemic infectious complications
- In the first postoperative month, like in the non-immunosuppressed postoperative population, there is a predominance of nosocomial infections
- Opportunistic infections usually occur during the second to the sixth months after transplantation, when immunosuppression levels are high
- Although imaging findings may at times be suggestive of certain diagnoses, there is considerable overlap and biopsies are necessary until proven otherwise

LUNG INFECTIONS

Aspergillus (Figs. 1 and 2)

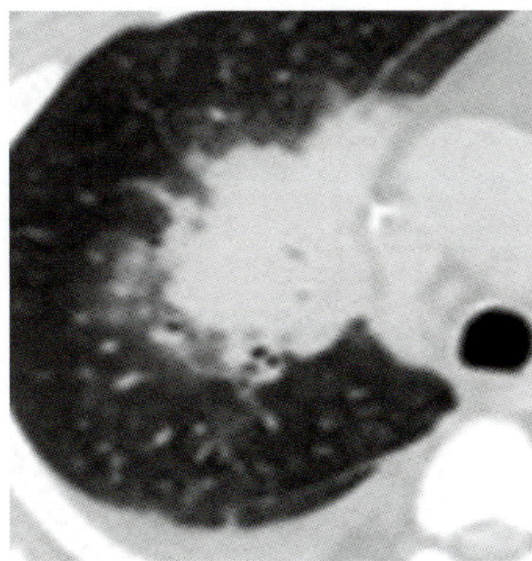

Fig. 1: Angioinvasive aspergillosis. Forty-nine-year-old male who presented 97 days after transplantation with fevers. Coned-down view of right lung shows a rounded paramediastinal mass surrounded by a haze of ground glass (so-called "halo sign") representing perilesional hemorrhage.

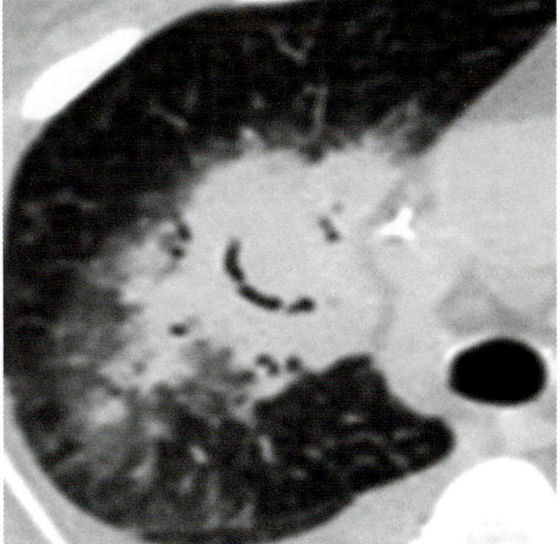

Fig. 2: Subsequent scan after clinical improvement shows incipient cavitation with a classic "crescent sign". This is the typical appearance of an angioinvasive mycotic (particularly aspergillus) infection.

Cryptococcus (Fig. 3)

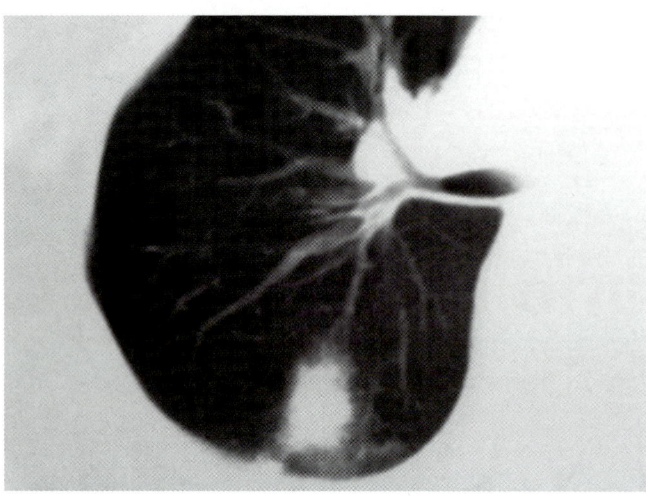

Fig. 3: Forty-eight-year-old female 91-day post-transplantation. Coned-down axial view of right lung shows a soft-tissue opacity surrounded by a thin ground glass halo. Blood and BAL cultures were positive for *Cryptococcus neoformans*.

Ground Glass Opacities [Cytomegalovirus (CMV) and Pneumocystis] (Figs. 4 and 5)

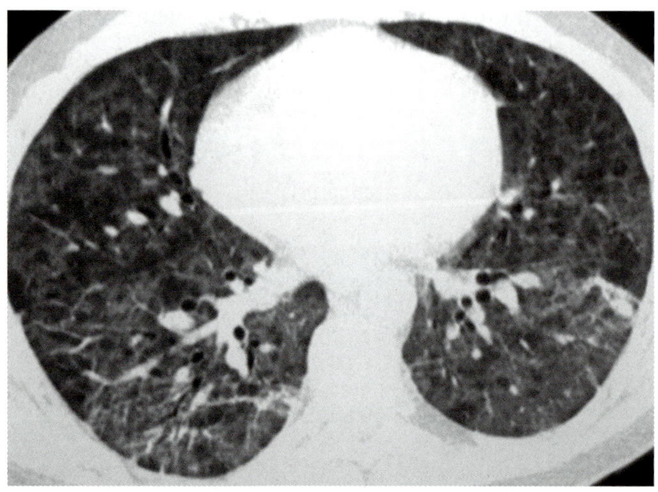

Fig. 4

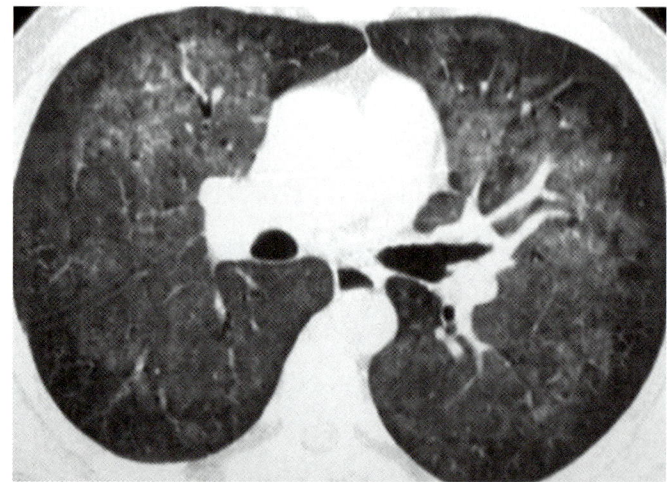

Fig. 5

Figs. 4 and 5: Two examples of diffuse ground glass pulmonary opacities. Both cases were in immunosuppressed transplant patients with complaints of fevers and cough. The ground glass opacities in Figure 4, patchy and geographic in distribution, proved to be CMV. The ground glass opacities in Figure 5, diffuse and with preservation of the mantle, are suggestive (although not diagnostic) of Pneumocystis Jirovecii (as was subsequently proved in this case).

Tuberculosis (TB) (Figs. 6 and 7)

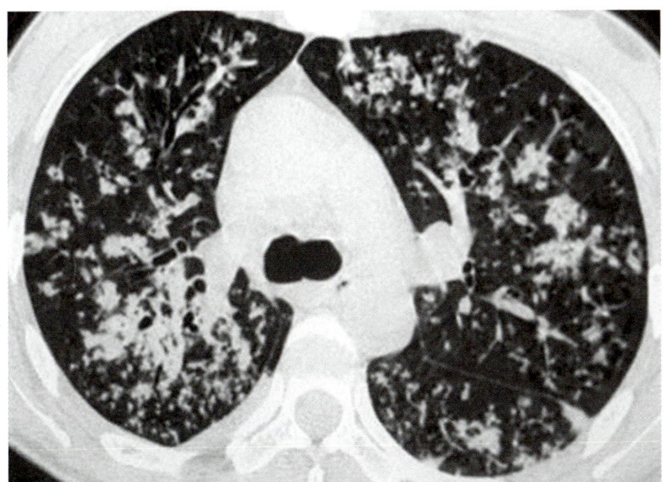

Fig. 6: Tubular branching opacities featuring a tree-in-bud appearance. This pattern is quite typical of endobronchial disseminated TB.

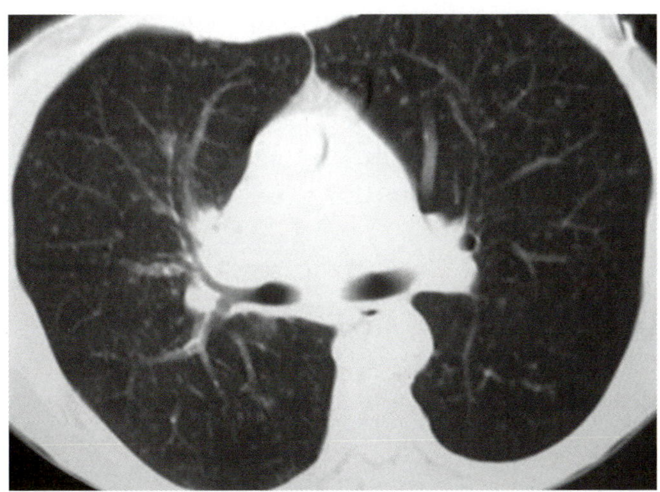

Fig. 7: Miliary pattern of hematogenous TB dissemination seen as very small nodules (so the name of miliary or resembling millet seeds) throughout both lungs.

Histoplasmosis (Fig. 8)

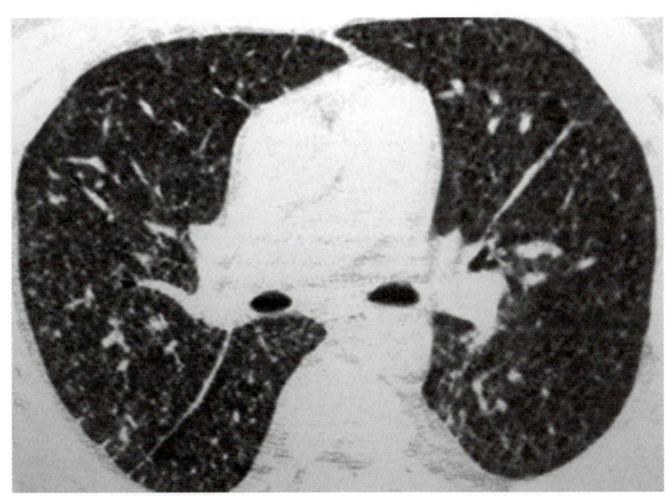

Fig. 8: Axial CT image shows a myriad of tiny nodules randomly distributed in both lungs in a renal transplant patient that proved to be disseminated (miliary) histoplasmosis.

INFECTIOUS LYMPHADENOPATHY

Tuberculosis (Figs. 9 and 10)

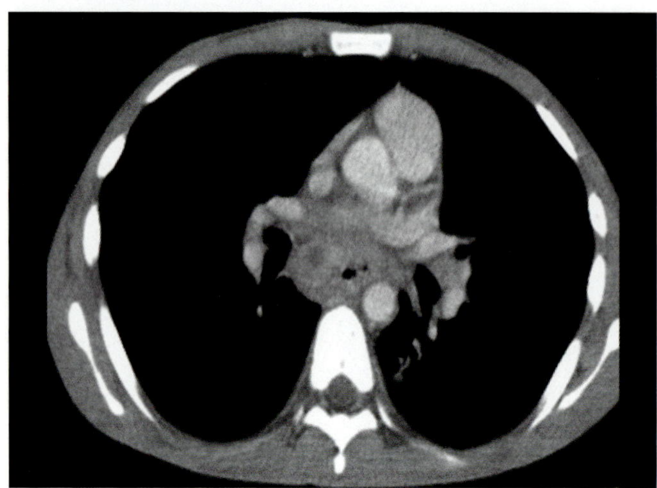

Fig. 9: Thirty-one-year-old transplant patient. Contrast-enhanced axial CT shows a bulky conglomerate of lymph nodes in the posterior mediastinum. Notice the central hypodense areas representing caseous necrosis, a typical finding of TB in immunosuppressed patients.

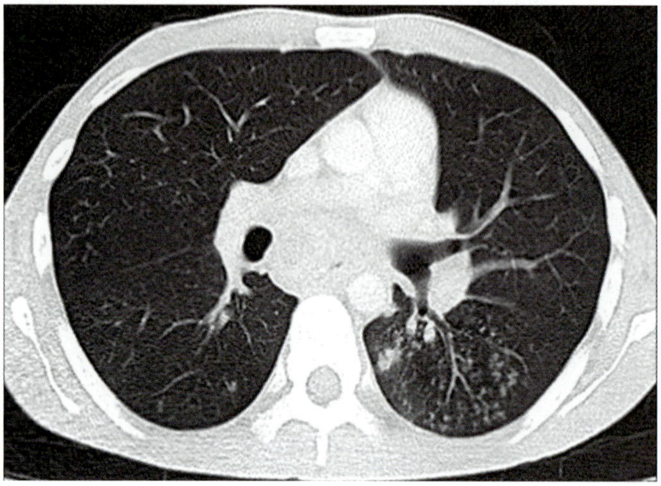

Fig. 10: Lung window corresponding image that shows centrilobular opacities in the posterior right inferior lobe with a "tree-in-bud" pattern. This tree-in-bud-pattern is quite typical of TB although is not specific since it can also be present in other infectious processes.

INTESTINAL INFECTIONS

Pseudomembranous Colitis (Fig. 11)

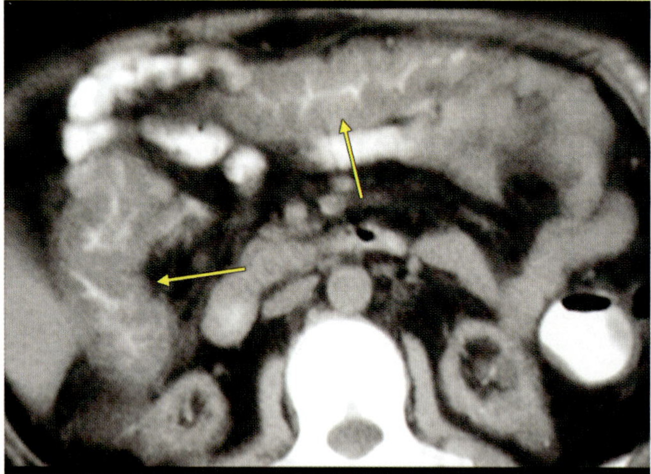

Fig. 11: Abdominal pain, diarrhea, and fever in a transplant patient. An unenhanced axial CT image shows diffuse mural thickening of the colon (arrows). Notice the "accordion" appearance of the transverse and ascending colon, a hallmark of pseudomembranous colitis. The atrophic native kidneys are also seen.

Cytomegalovirus (CMV) (Fig. 12)

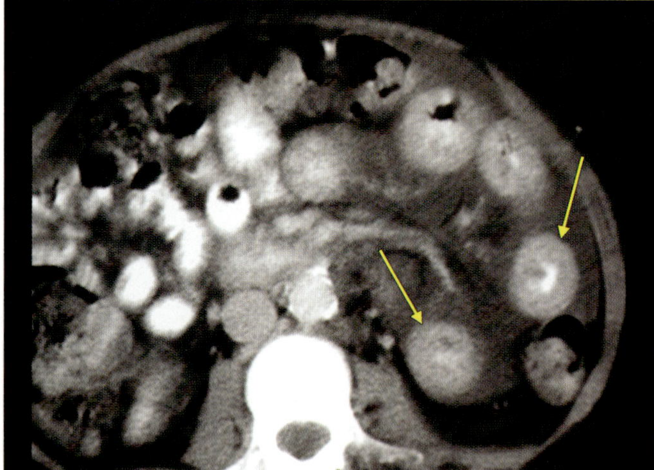

Fig. 12: Concentric mural thickening of the jejunum (arrows) in a transplant with CMV enteritis.

TB (Fig. 13)

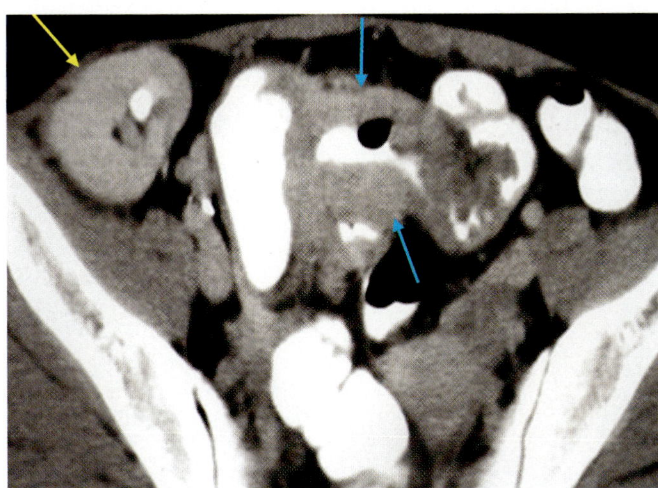

Fig. 13: Abdominal pain with bloody stool in a patient with a transplant kidney (yellow arrow) in the RLQ. This axial CT image shows marked thickening of the distal ileum (blue arrows) with ulcerations in a case of ileocecal Tuberculosis.

PYELONEPHRITIS (FIGS. 14 AND 15)

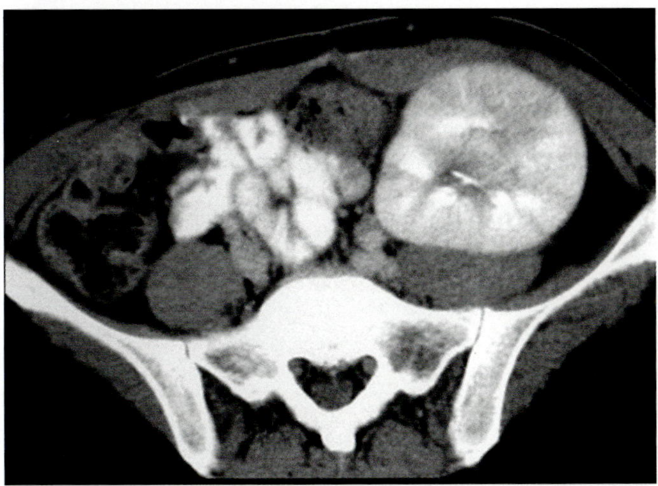

Fig. 14: Axial contrast-enhanced CT image that shows a striated nephrogram consistent with pyelonephritis in a LLQ kidney graft.

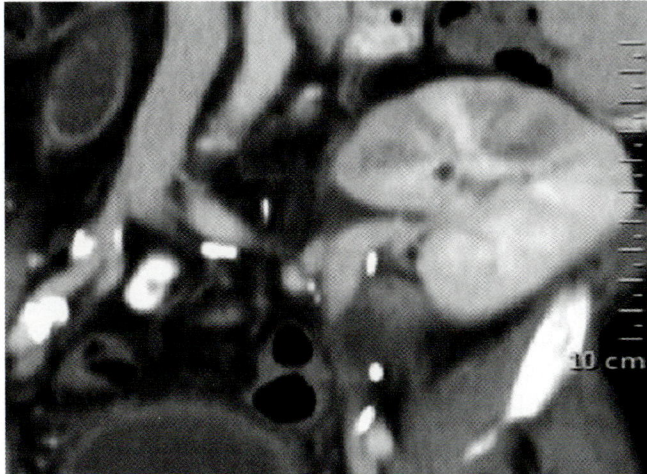

Fig. 15: Coronal reformatted contrast-enhanced CT image that shows a heterogeneous nephrogram with patchy lobular areas of hypoattenuation compatible with pyelonephritis.

SINUS INFECTIONS

Aspergillus (Fig. 16)

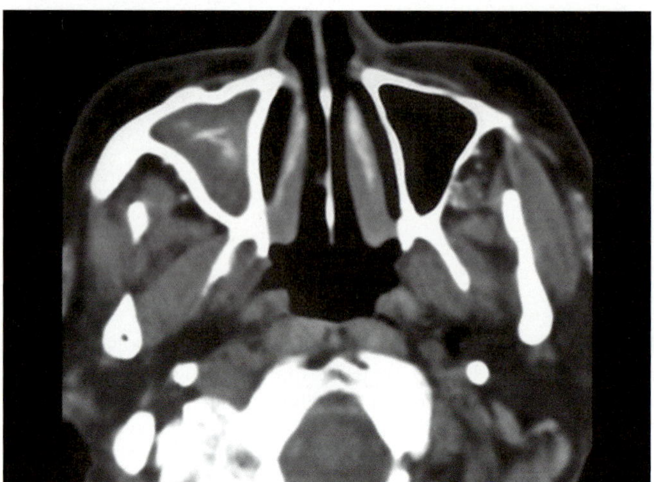

Fig. 16: Imaging protocols in immunosuppressed patients often include evaluation of sinunasal structures. In this transplant febrile patient, the CT image shows a mass with a central hyperdensity occupying the right maxillary antrum. This appearance is often seen in mycotic infections, particularly aspergillus sinusitis as in this instance.

MALIGNANCIES

- Chronic immunosuppression is associated with an increased risk of a wide spectrum of neoplasia
- Post-transplant lymphoproliferative disorders are frequent, affect multiple organs and systems, and present in a variety of ways
- Imaging assessment is crucial in the diagnosis and follow-up of these neoplasias

CNS INFECTIONS

Chagas Disease (Fig. 17)

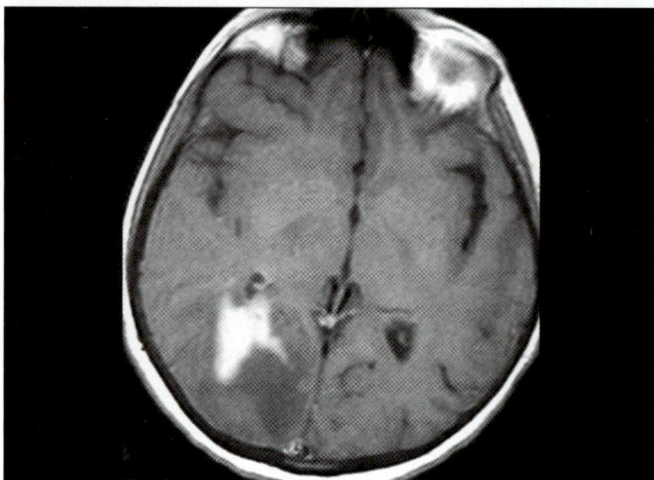

Fig. 17: T1-weighted contrast-enhanced MRI image shows an enhancing solid lesion with adjacent edema in the right occipital lobe. This is a nonspecific finding and a lymphoma could have a similar appearance. This is proved to be Chagas disease in a transplant patient originally from South America.

CNS LYMPHOMA (FIGS. 18 TO 20)

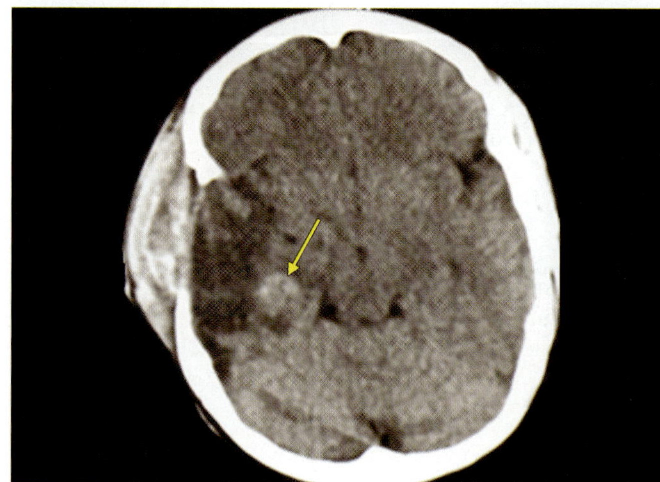

Fig. 18: Rounded heterogeneous hyperdense lesion (arrow) with surrounding vasogenic edema in the temporal lobe. The sequela of a recent craniectomy performed for biopsy purposes can also be observed.

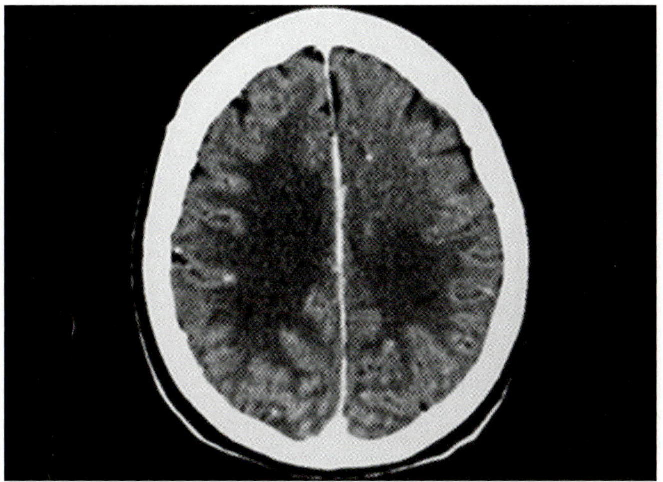

Fig. 19: Diffuse hypodensity in both centrum semiovale.

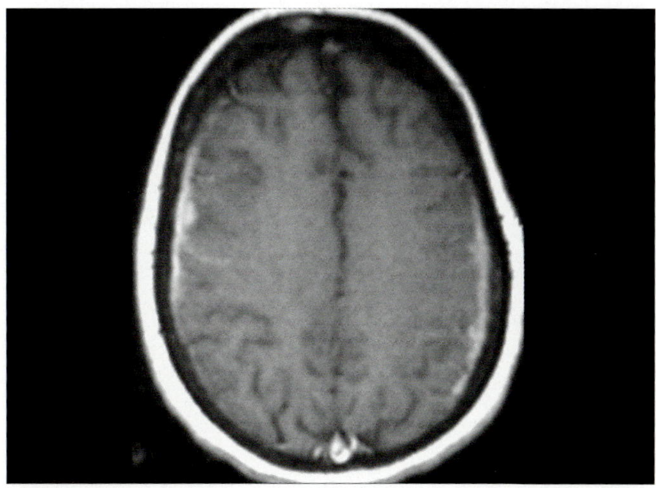

Fig. 20: T1-weighted contrast-enhanced axial MRI showing diffuse dural thickening with increased enhancement. This is an example of lymphomatous meningeal involvement.

POST-TRANSPLANT LYMPHOPROLIFERATIVE DISEASE (PTLD) (FIGS. 21 TO 39)

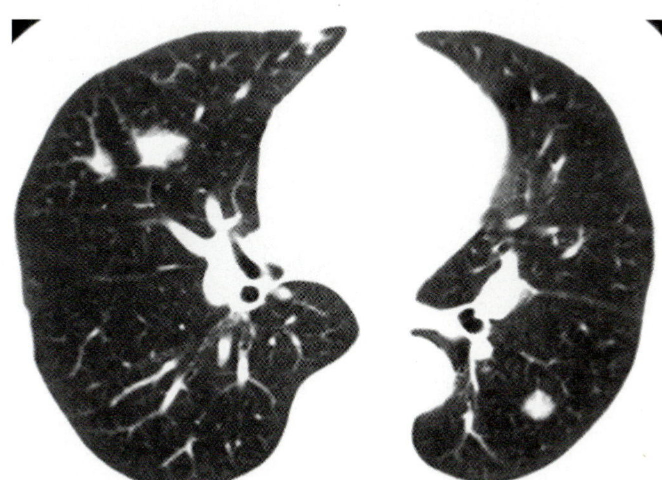

Fig. 21: Axial CT image showing bilateral lung nodules. Unfortunately, this is a nonspecific finding and a tissue sampling (by thoracoscopic or open lung surgery) is mandatory.

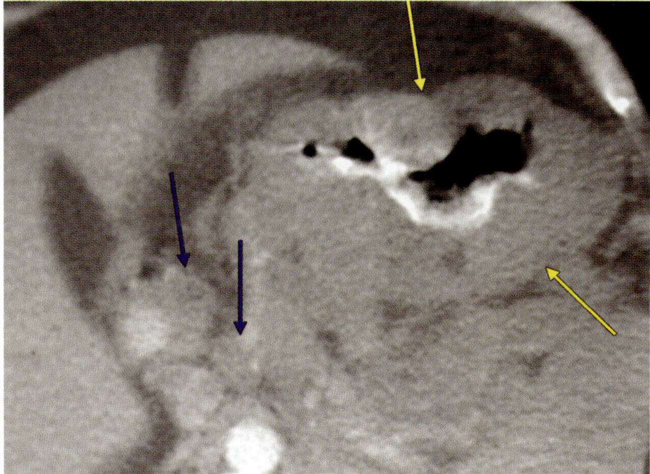

Fig. 22: Contrast-enhanced axial CT image showing marked diffuse gastric wall thickening (yellow arrows) with prominent adjacent lymphadenopathies (blue arrows). Lymphoproliferative processes usually have a predilection for extranodal sites in immunosuppressed patients such as the one depicted here.

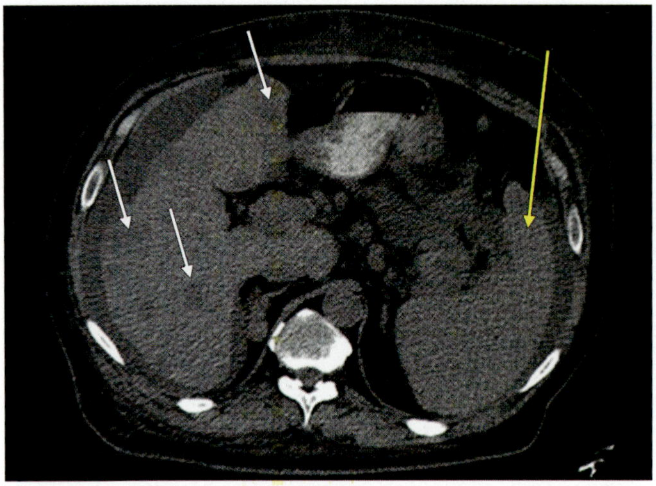

Fig. 23

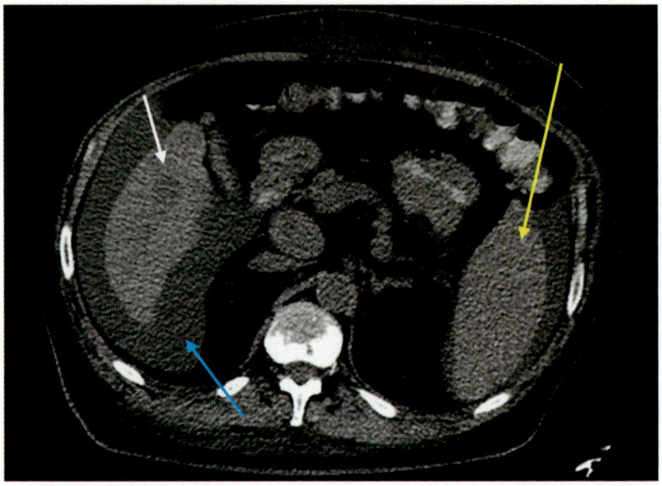

Fig. 24

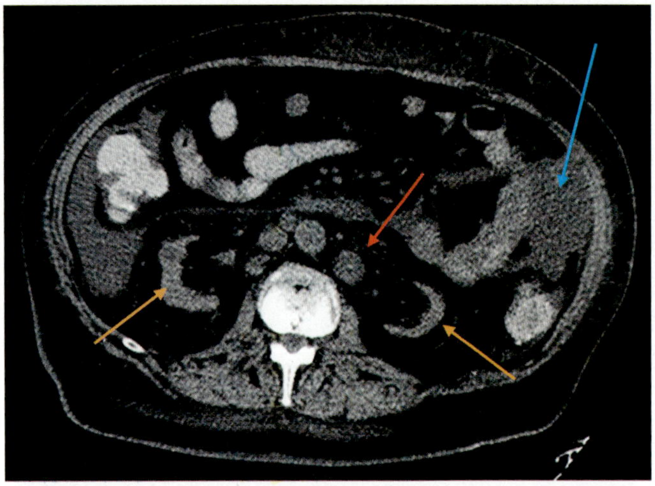

Fig. 25

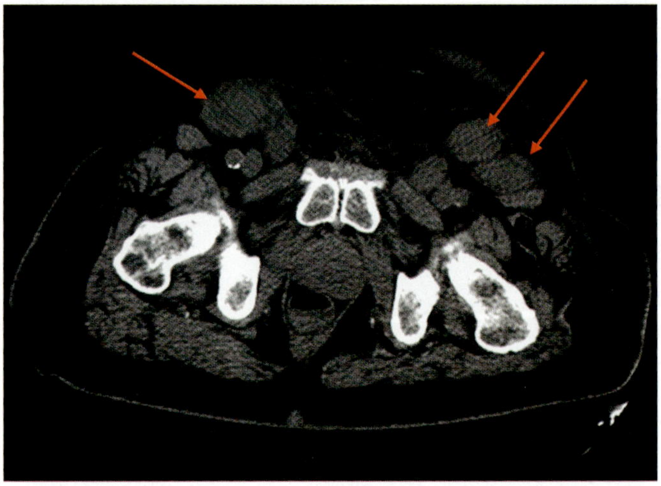

Fig. 26

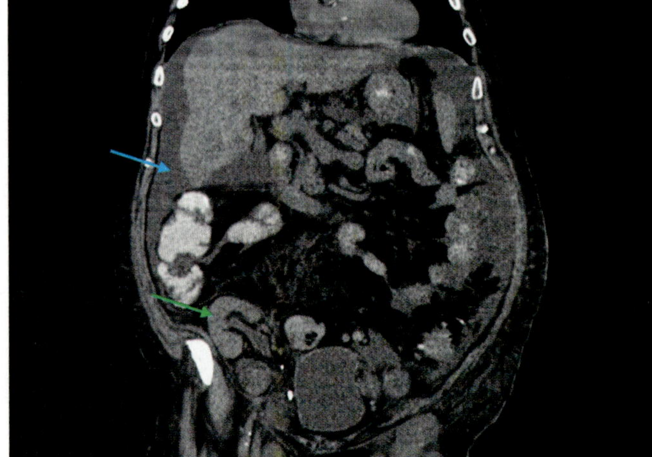

Fig. 27

Figs. 23 to 27: Unenhanced CT images in axial and coronal planes showing multiple low-attenuation liver lesions (white arrows), splenomegaly (yellows arrows), and retroperitoneal and bilateral inguinal lymphadenopathy (red arrows). Ascites is also seen (blue arrows). Note the atrophic native kidneys (orange arrows) and the normal-appearing RLQ kidney graft (green arrow).

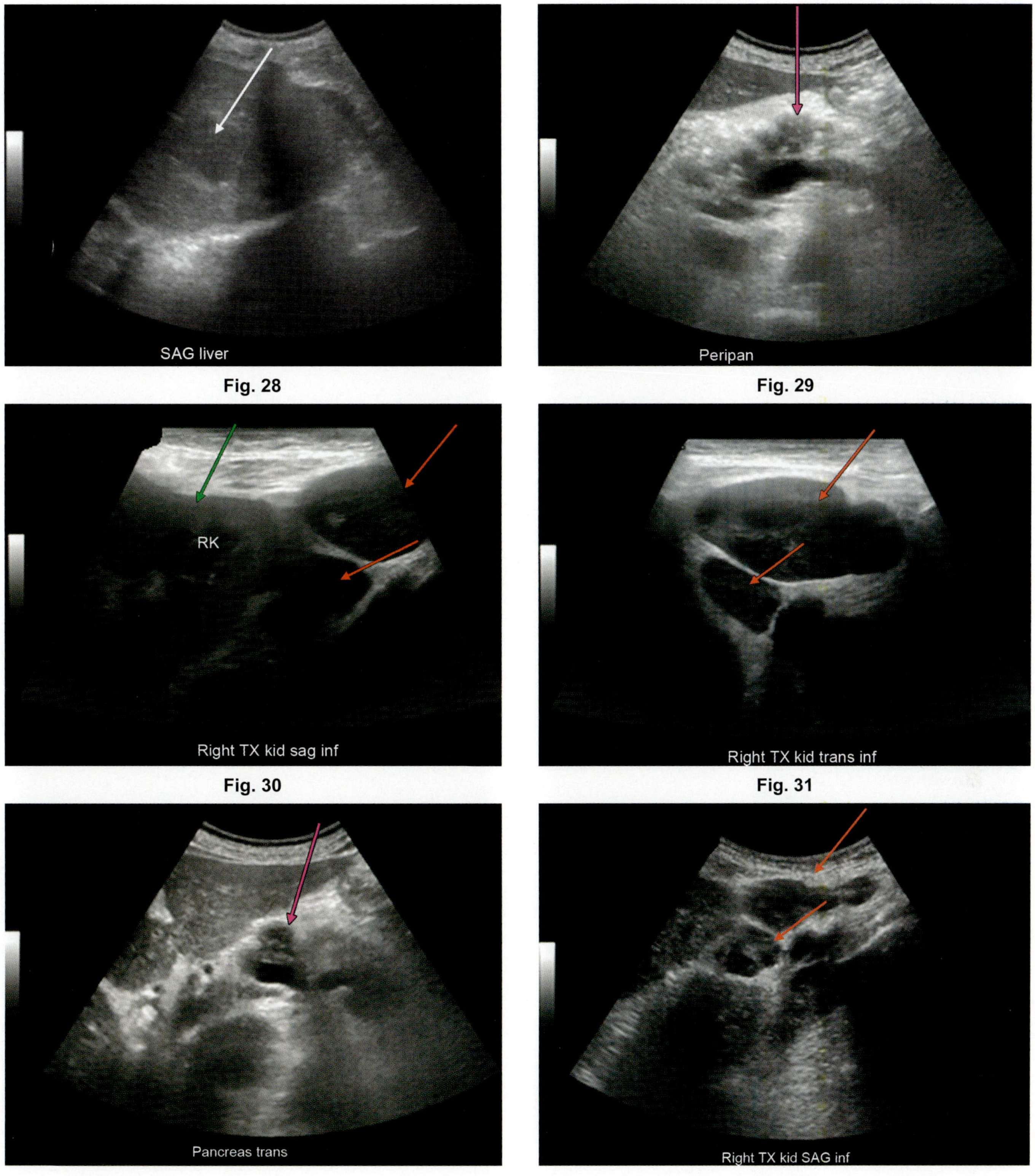

Fig. 28

Fig. 29

Fig. 30

Fig. 31

Fig. 32

Fig. 33

Figs. 28 to 33: Ultrasound images of the abdomen and pelvis reveal liver masses (white arrow), peripancreatic (pink arrows), right iliac, and inguinal lymphadenopathy (red arrows). The transplant kidney is shown with a green arrow.

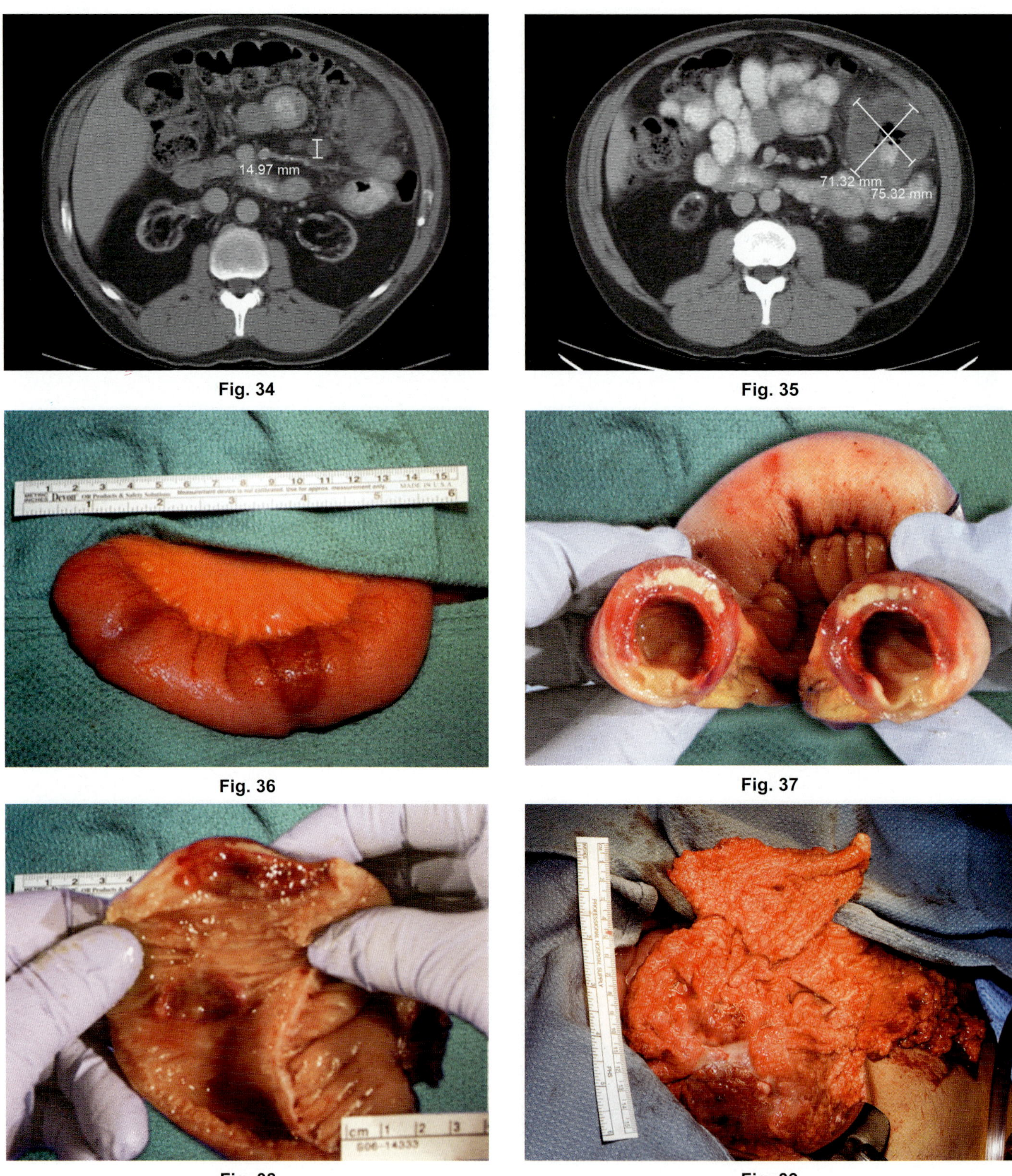

Fig. 34

Fig. 35

Fig. 36

Fig. 37

Fig. 38

Fig. 39

Figs. 34 to 39: CT images (Figs. 34 and 35) and operative specimens (Figs. 36 to 39) in a case of PTLD with gastrointestinal tract involvement. Notice marked circumferential wall thickening shown on CT and its pathologic correlate.

KAPOSI SARCOMA (FIGS. 40 AND 41)

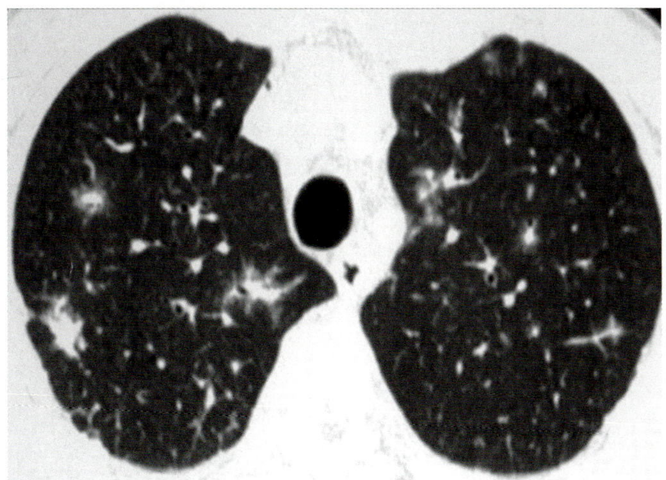

Fig. 40: Axial CT image showing multiple, scattered, irregularly shaped lung nodules. Some of them are surrounded by a subtle halo of ground glass density. This presentation in not uncommon in pulmonary involvement with Kaposi sarcoma.

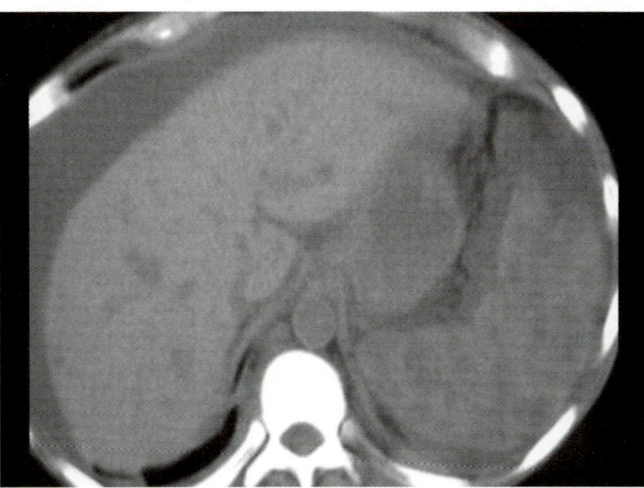

Fig. 41: Axial CT image showing multiple hypoattenuating foci in the spleen. This finding prompted multiple differential diagnoses among which lymphoma and infections were emphasized. However, this proved to be splenic involvement with Kaposi sarcoma.

CHAPTER 63

Various Findings

Mariano Volpacchio, Catherine D'Agostino, Christopher Palestro, et al.

SUPERIOR VENA CAVA (SVC) STENOSIS (FIGS. 1 AND 2)

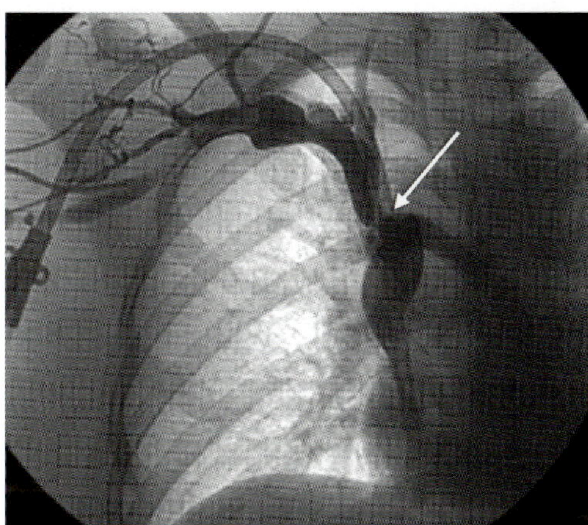
Fig. 1

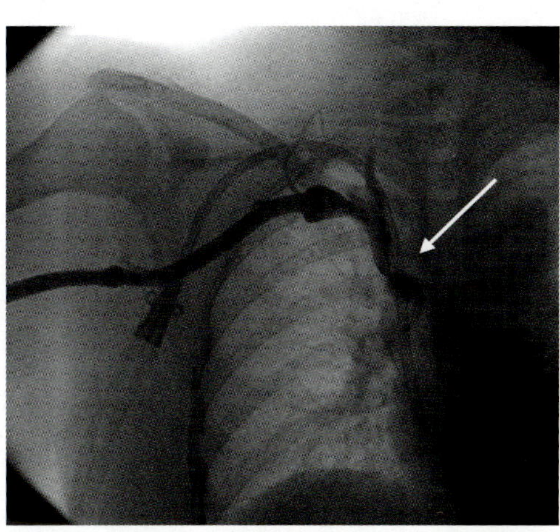
Fig. 2

Figs. 1 and 2: Recipient with no clinical symptoms prior to transplantation who developed edema of the head, neck, and upper torso intraoperatively. A diagnosis of SVC stenosis (white arrows) was made, likely secondary to the previous insertion of multiple dialysis catheters. Given the severity of the clinically findings that did not resolve postoperatively, a surgical repair was required.

FRACTURE (FIGS. 3 AND 4)

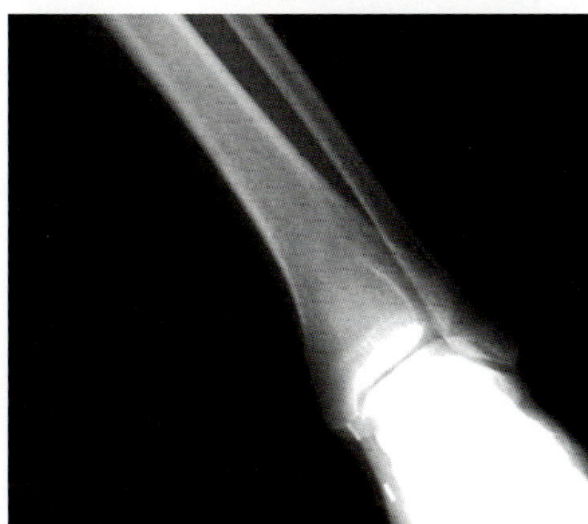
Fig. 3

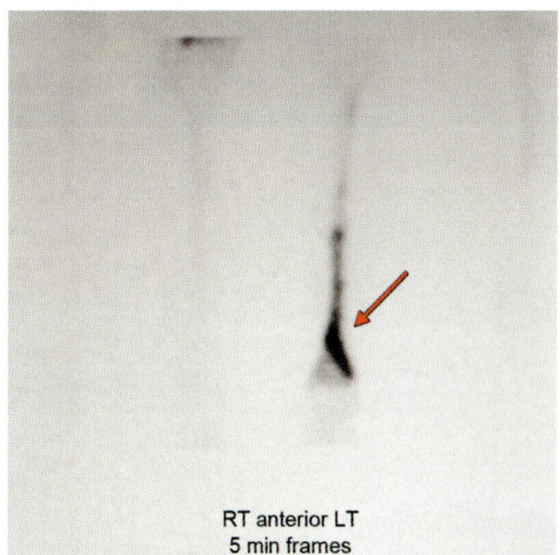

Fig. 4

Figs. 3 and 4: X-ray (Fig. 3) fails to demonstrate an oblique stress fracture of the left tibia. Nuclear medicine bone scan (Fig. 4) shows increased uptake (red arrow) compatible with a fracture. As this case illustrates, whenever pathology is suspected and the initial imaging study is negative, additional imaging studies should be obtained.

OSTEOPENIA (FIG. 5)

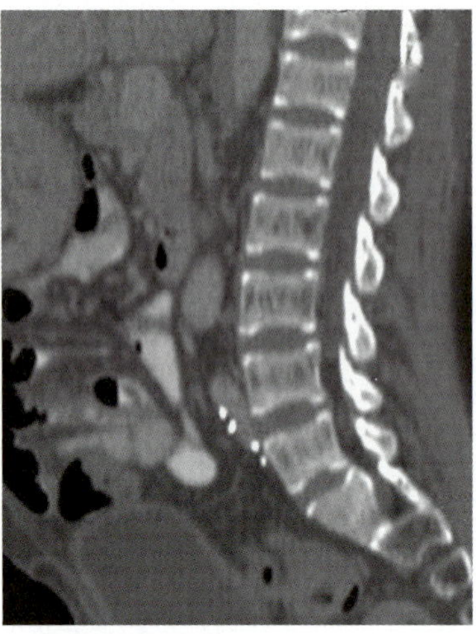

Fig. 5: Sagittal CT scan in a 30-year-old male kidney transplant recipient showing decreased bone density in the lumbar spine, especially in the midportion of the vertebral bodies, in a "rugger jersey" appearance of secondary hyperparathyroidism. Osteopenia is a common finding and is mainly related to chronic steroid use.

POSTOPERATIVE RESIDUAL INTRA-ABDOMINAL GAS (FIG. 6)

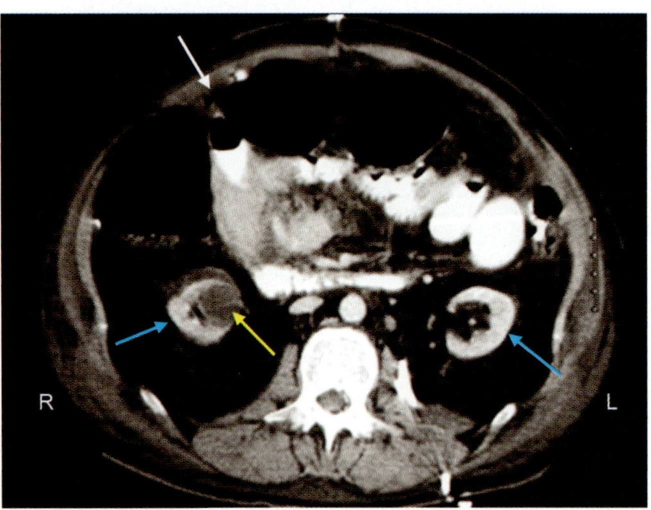

Fig. 6: A small amount of postoperative gas (white arrow) can be seen. Note also the atrophic native kidneys (blue arrows) and a right renal cyst (yellow arrow).

EPIDURAL LIPOMATOSIS (FIG. 7)

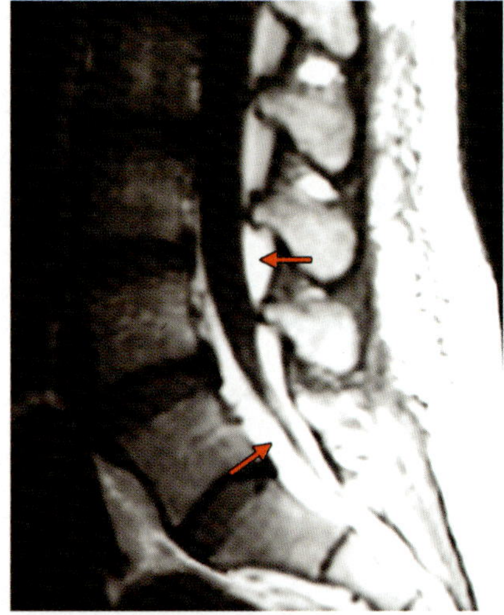

Fig. 7: Sagittal T1-weighted MR image showing epidural lipomatosis (red arrows). Fat has high signal intensity on T1-weighing. Epidural lipomatosis can sometimes be a symptomatic finding associated with the steroid therapy given to transplant patients.

GONADAL PATHOLOGIES (FIGS. 8 TO 10)

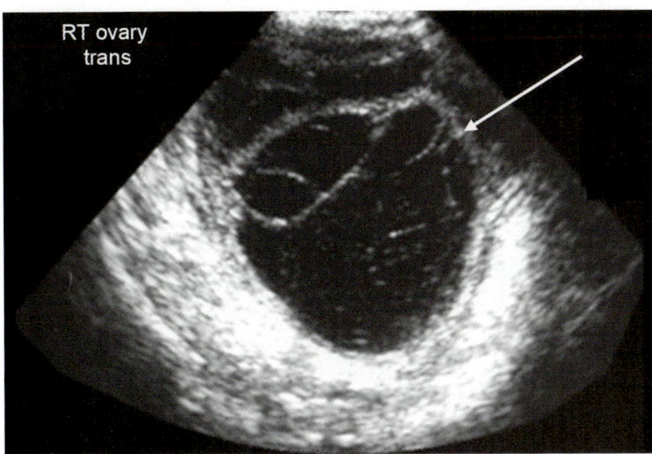

Fig. 8

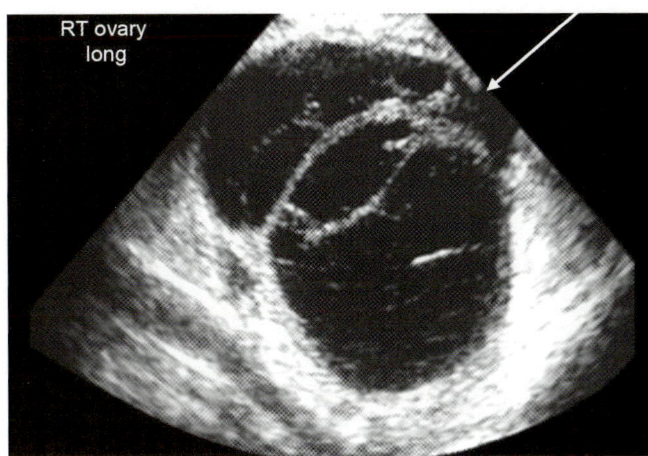

Fig. 9

Figs. 8 and 9: Transvaginal ultrasound images showing a hemorrhagic right ovarian cyst with septations and fine echoes (white arrows).

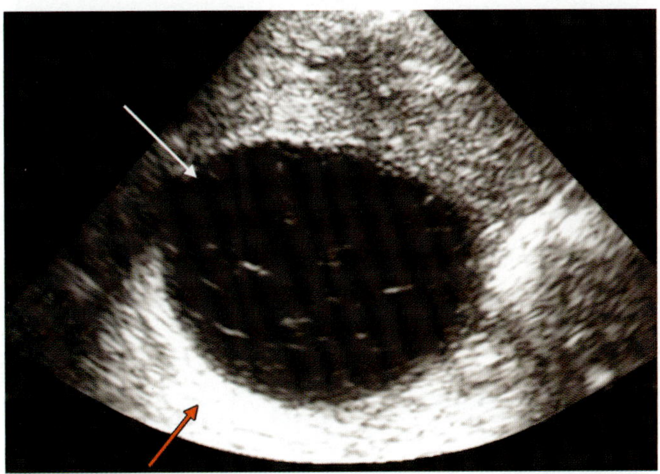

Fig. 10: Ultrasound reveals a mildly complex left ovarian cyst containing a few fine echoes (white arrow). Note the acoustical enhancement (red arrow) posterior to the anechoic cyst.

GASTROINTESTINAL PATHOLOGIES (FIGS. 11 AND 12)

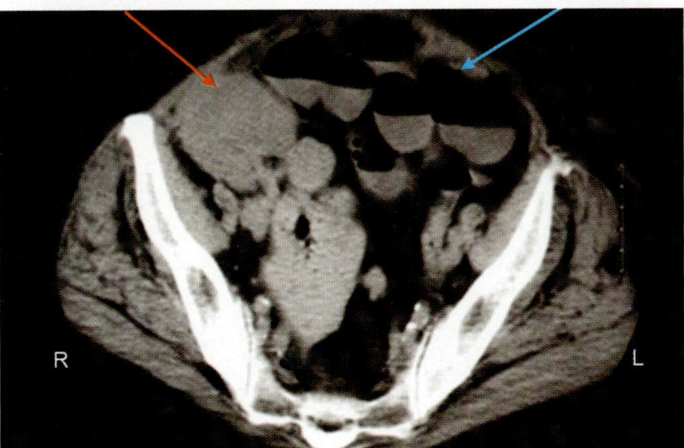

Fig. 11: Small bowel obstruction. Dilated small bowel loops (blue arrow) containing air/fluid levels in a transplant recipient who underwent a hysterectomy 4 months prior to the current presentation. The transplant kidney is shown with a red arrow.

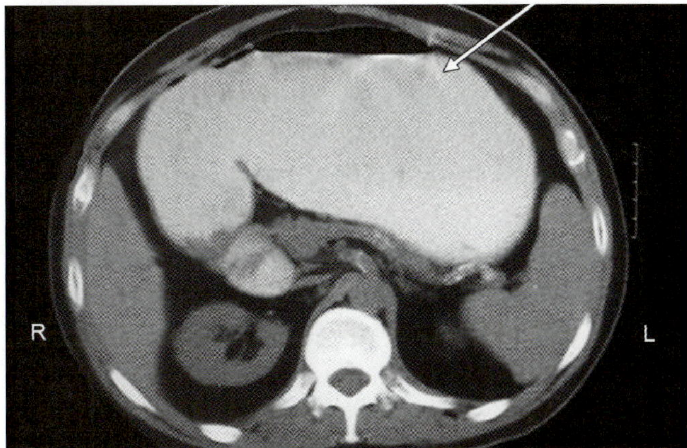

Fig. 12: Dilated stomach (gastroparesis) as seen on a CT examination in a diabetic patient.

APPENDICITIS (FIGS. 13 TO 18)

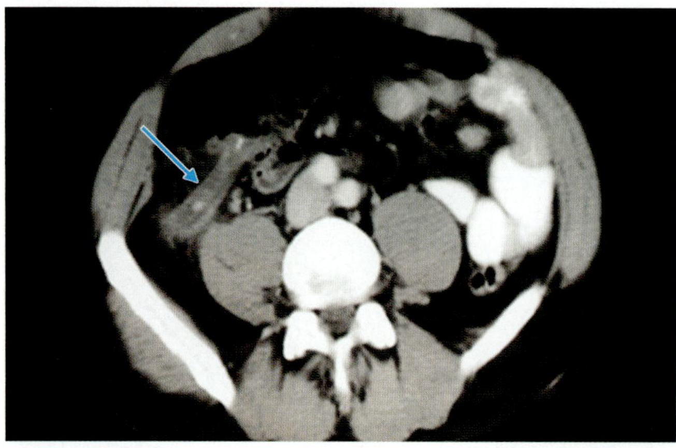

Fig. 13

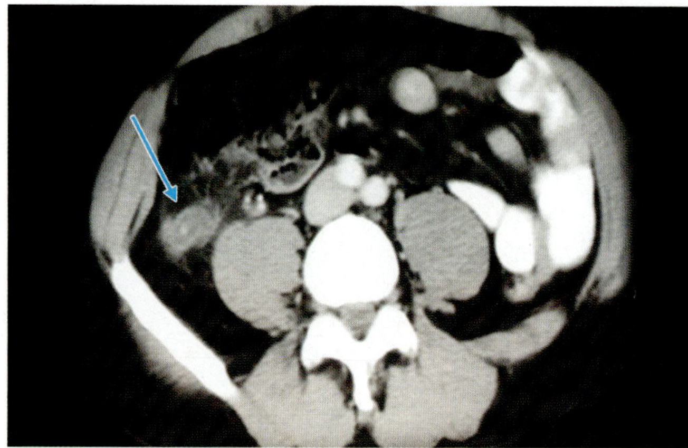

Fig. 14

Figs. 13 and 14: In instances of right lower quadrant pain, the differential diagnosis should include, in addition to pathologies associated with the allograft, all other possible pathologies encountered in the general nontransplant population, such as appendicitis (blue arrows).

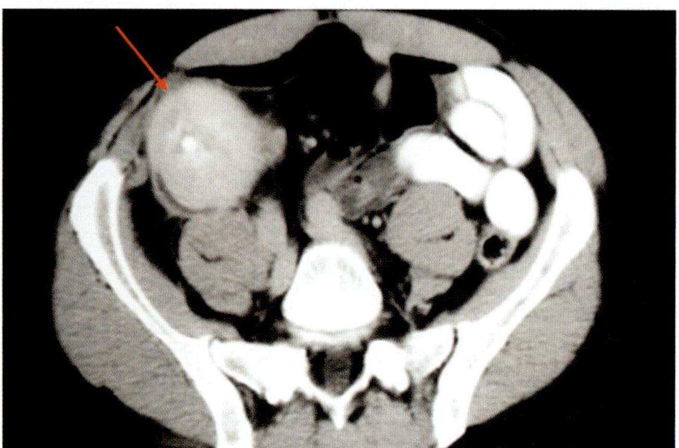

Fig. 15

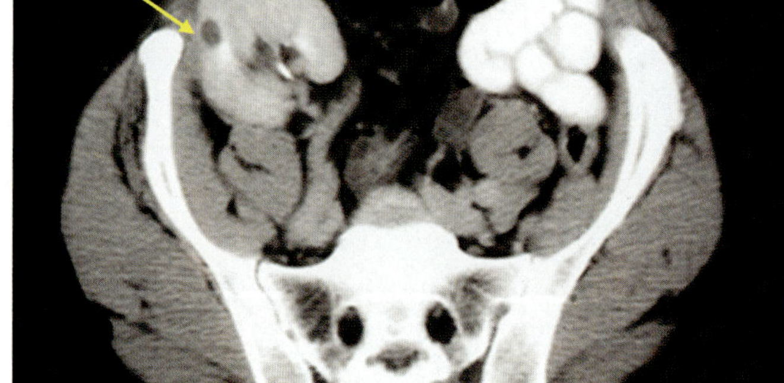

Fig. 16

Figs. 15 and 16: Consecutive axial images show a dilated, fluid-filled appendix with adjacent inflammatory fat stranding. A right iliac fossa transplant kidney (red arrows) with a small renal cyst (yellow arrow) can be seen just below the abnormal appendix.

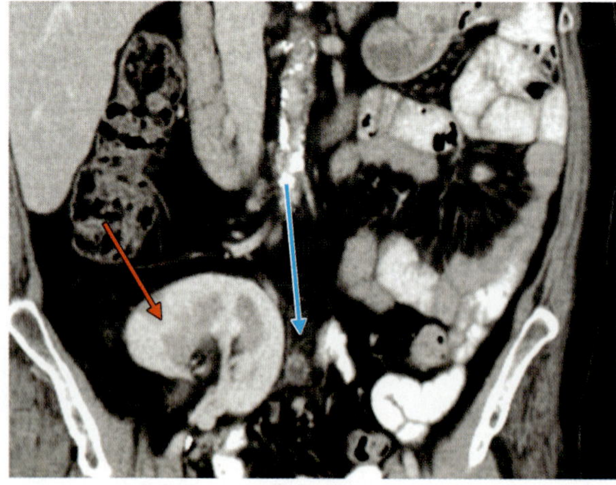

Fig. 17

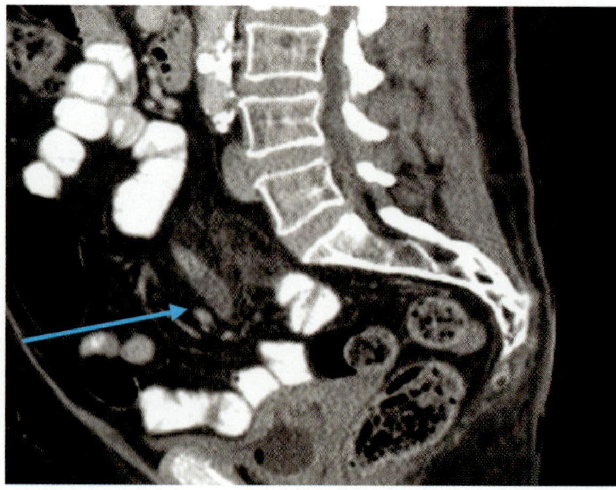

Fig. 18

Figs. 17 and 18: Coronal (Fig. 17) and sagittal (Fig. 18) CT images demonstrate a distended, fluid-filled appendix (blue arrows) with inflammatory changes adjacent to a RLQ transplant kidney (red arrow).

POSTERIOR REVERSIBLE ENCEPHALOPATHY SYNDROME (PRES) (FIGS. 19 AND 20)

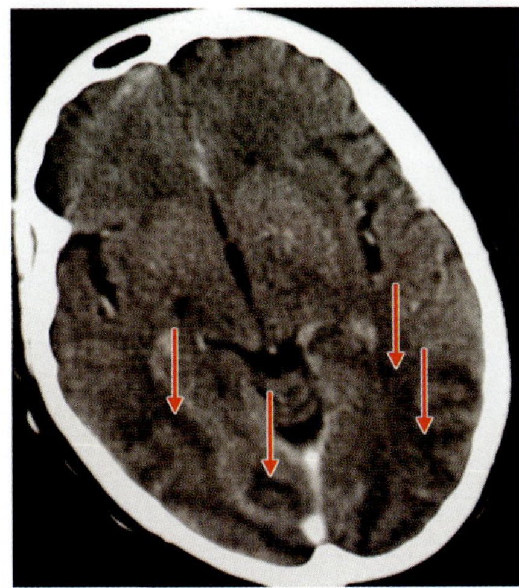

Fig. 19

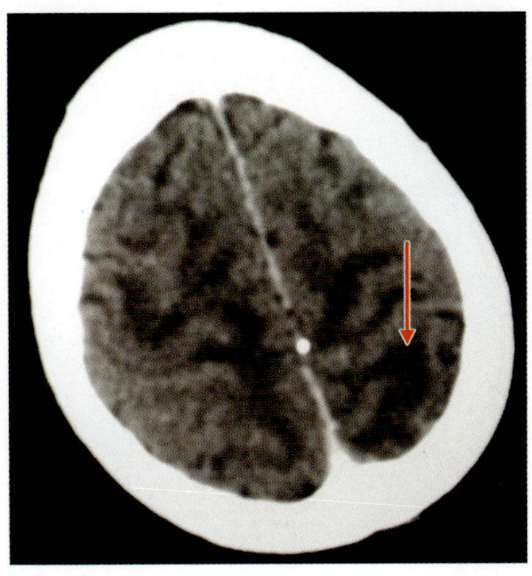

Fig. 20

Figs. 19 and 20: A 62-year-old female kidney transplant recipient who presented with altered mental status, visual disturbance and seizures. Contrast-enhanced axial CT images show bilateral hypoattenuation of subcortical white matter in the occipital and parietal lobes consistent with vasogenic edema in a pattern typical of PRES associated with calcineurin inhibitor toxicity.

CNS PATHOLOGIES (FIGS. 21 AND 22)

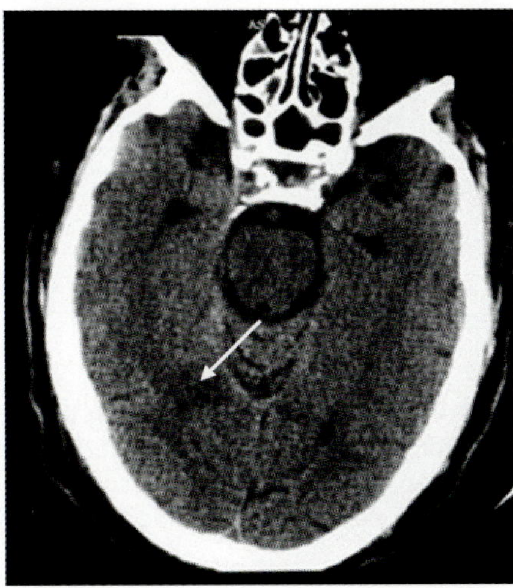

Fig. 21: Axial CT image showing a hypodense nonterritorial infarct (white arrow).

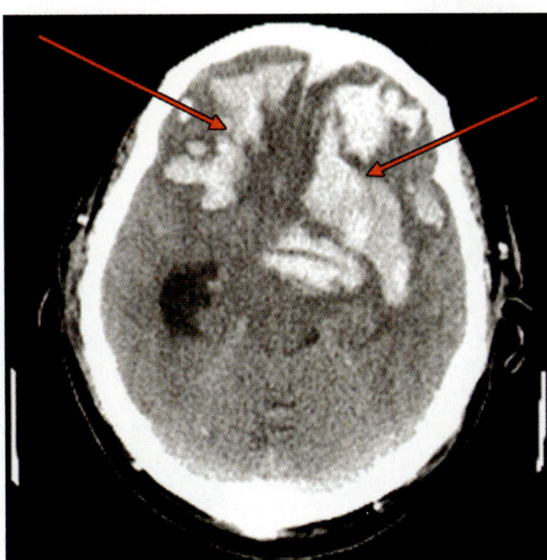

Fig. 22: Extensive bilateral high attenuation intracranial hemorrhage (red arrows) on CT examination.

CARDIOPULMONARY PATHOLOGIES (FIGS. 23 AND 24)

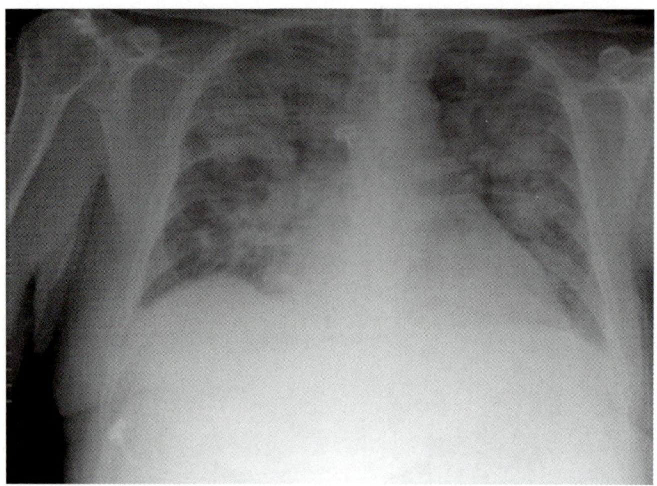

Fig. 23: Plain chest radiograph: pulmonary edema (lung opacities) and vasculitis in a patient with a diagnosis of recurrent IgA nephropathy and a failing allograft. Both findings improved with steroids and plasmapheresis.

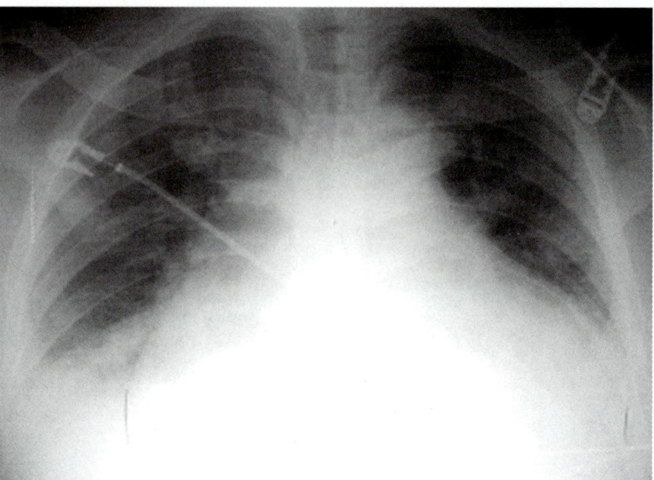

Fig. 24: Plain chest radiograph (acute finding): large, globular cardiac silhouette. Findings are consistent with cardiac tamponade. Echocardiography revealed a large pericardial effusion.

DRUG TOXICITY (FIG. 25)

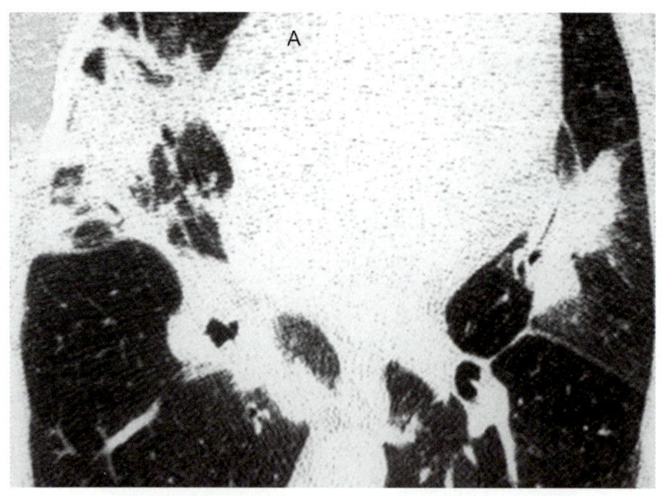

Fig. 25: Coned-down axial CT image showing bilateral consolidations in a transplant patient with low-grade fever, cough and dyspnea. This pattern is compatible with cryptogenic organizing pneumonia that in this patient was secondary to sirolimus toxicity.

LIVER LESIONS (FIGS. 26 AND 27)

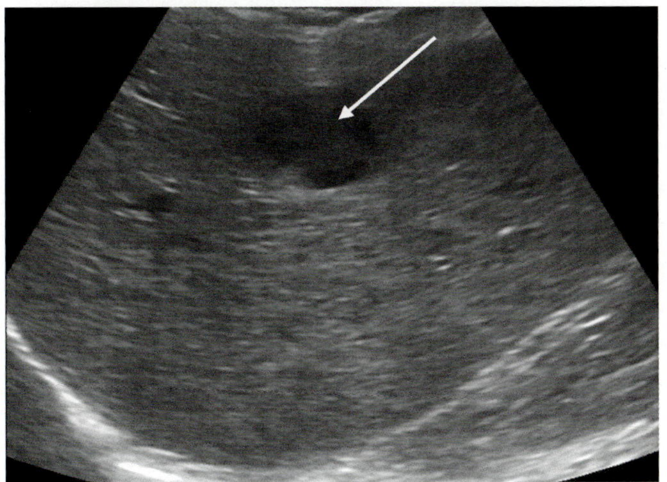

Fig. 26

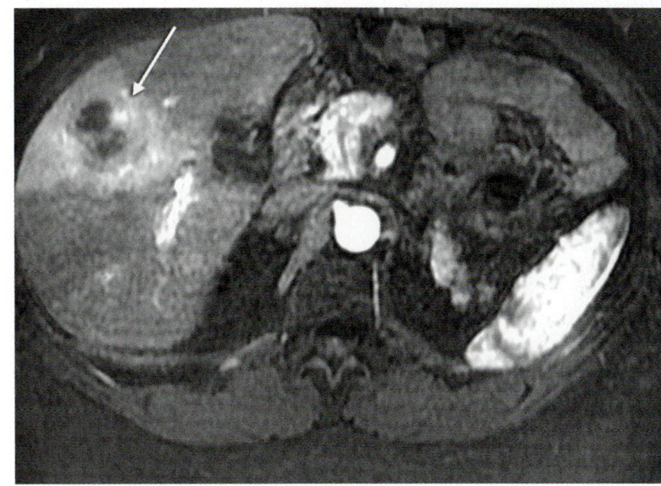

Fig. 27

Figs. 26 and 27: Hypoechoic liver lesion noted on ultrasound (Fig. 26, white arrow) 6 months after transplantation. MRI showed it as a peripherally enhancing lesion (Fig. 27, white arrow). Biopsy showed large B-cell lymphoma.

ABDOMINAL WALL PATHOLOGIES (FIGS. 28 TO 31)

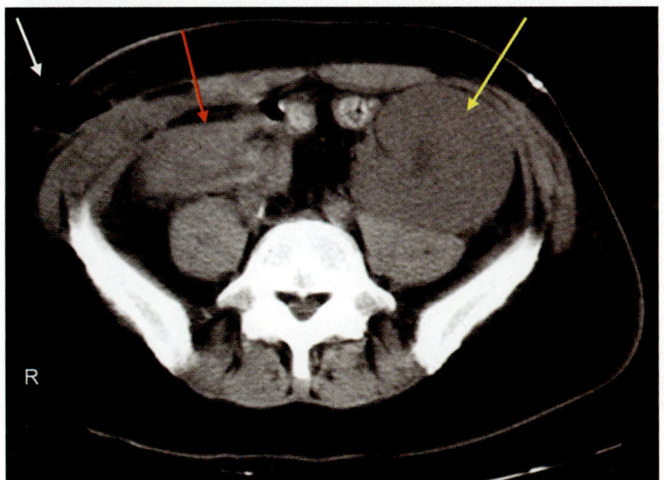

Fig. 28: Abdominal wall defect/open wound (white arrow) in a patient status post simultaneous pancreas (red arrow)/kidney (yellow arrow) transplantation.

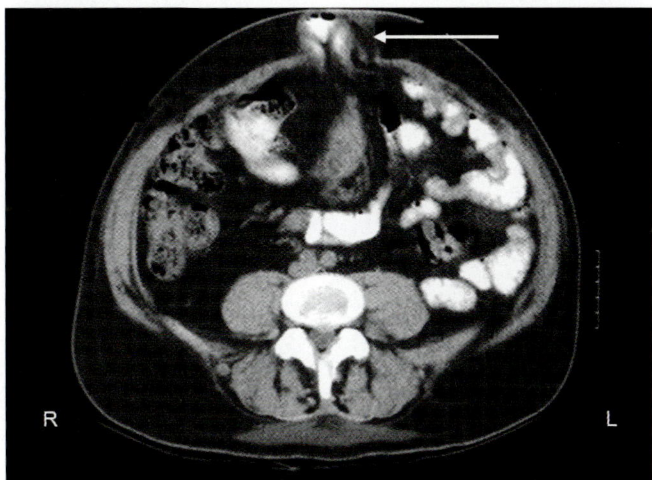

Fig. 29: Axial CT image showing a midline hernia (white arrow) in a recipient status post simultaneous pancreas/kidney transplantation.

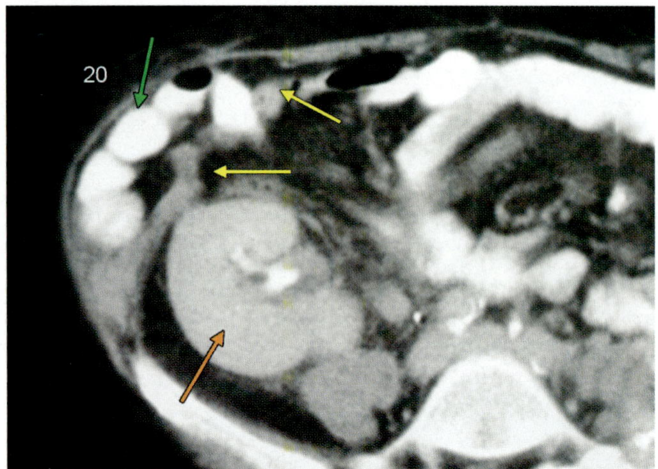

Fig. 30: Axial contrast-enhanced CT image showing a normal-appearing transplant kidney (orange arrow) in the RLQ and an incisional hernia through a partial wall defect (yellow arrows). An opacified ileal loop (green arrow) enters into the defect and is contained by a thinned external oblique muscle.

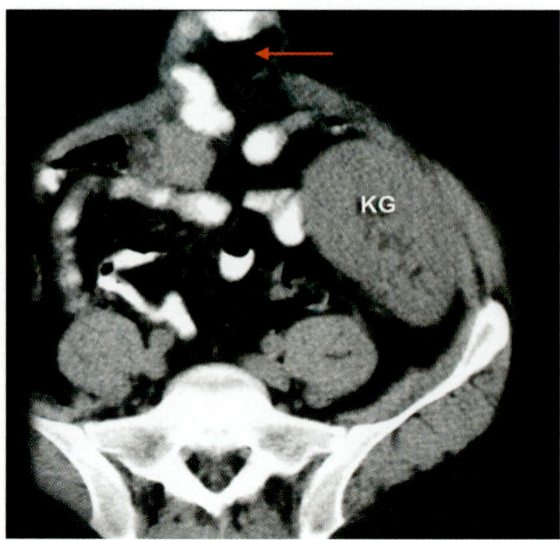

Fig. 31: Axial unenhanced CT image showing a bowel loop (arrow) entering a broad incisional hernia in a patient with rectus muscle diastasis. KG: kidney graft.

INTESTINAL OBSTRUCTION SECONDARY TO ABDOMINAL WALL HERNIA (FIGS. 32 TO 34)

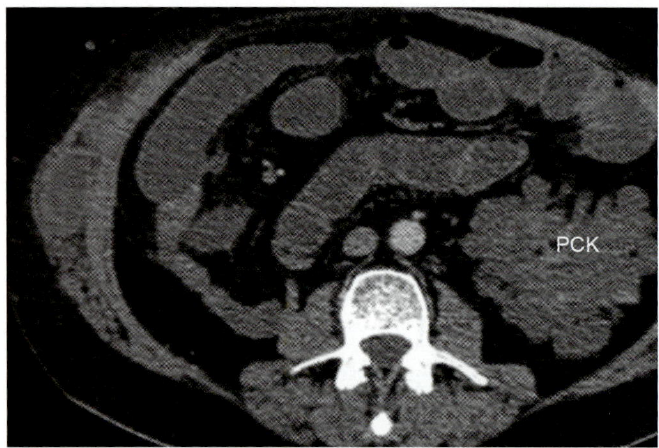

Fig. 32

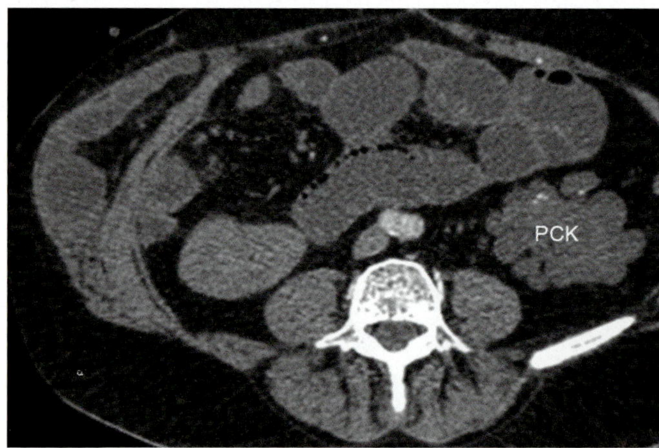

Fig. 33

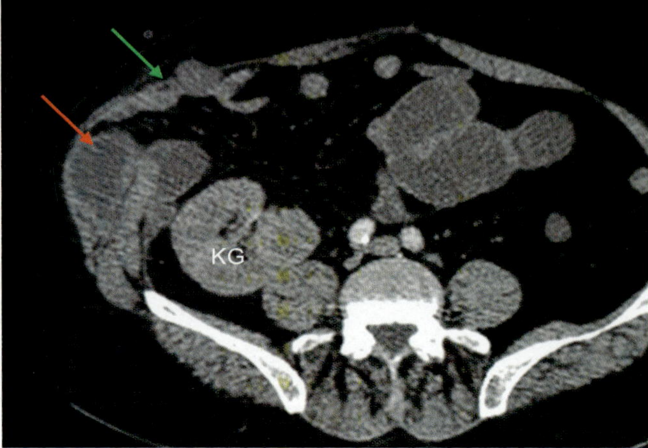

Fig. 34

Figs. 32 to 34: Sequential unenhanced axial CT images showing dilated loops of small bowel consistent with a diagnosis of intestinal obstruction. Notice the dilated afferent loop (red arrow) entering and the collapsed efferent loop (green arrow) leaving the incisional RLQ hernia (Fig. 34). The native left polycystic kidney (PCK) is seen as well as a normal-appearing graft (KG) in the RLQ.

CHAPTER 64

Dermatologic Manifestations of Kidney Disease

Julia R Nunley

INTRODUCTION

Dermatologic conditions are common in the renal transplant recipient and range from skin signs of systemic diseases that cause chronic kidney disease to findings that are unique to the uremic condition to cutaneous malignancies and infections associated with transplantation (Table 1). This chapter demonstrates a wide variety of these cutaneous changes; it also includes some of the adverse cutaneous drug reactions that may be seen in this group of patients.

Table 1: Dermatologic conditions seen in diseases causing chronic kidney disease

Metabolic disorders
Diabetes mellitus
Acanthosis nigricans
Eruptive xanthomas
Necrobiosis lipoidica
Diabetic dermopathy
Amyloidosis
Macroglossia
Purpura
Atherosclerosis/cholesterol emboli
Blue toes
Cutaneous necrosis
Petechiae
Splinter hemorrhage

Contd...

Contd...

Connective tissue diseases
Progressive systemic sclerosis
Calcinosis cutis
Cutaneous sclerosis
Distal digital infarct
Nail fold capillaries
Sclerodactyly
Telangiectasia
Vitiligo-like depigmentation
Polyarteritis nodosa
Palpable purpura
Nodules
Ulcers
Systemic lupus erythematosus
Chronic cutaneous lupus (discoid lupus)
Livedo reticularis
Nonbullous neutrophilic dermatosis
Palpable purpura
Purpura
Subacute cutaneous lupus
Wegener's granulomatosis
Palpable purpura
Petechiae
Saddle nose deformity

Contd...

Contd...

Hepatitis viruses
Hepatitis C
Lichen planus
Porphyria cutanea tarda
Hypertrichosis
Milia
Photosensitivity
Sclerodermatous changes
Vesicles/bullae
Hypertrichosis (on temples)
Necrolytic acral erythema
Mixed cryoglobulinemia
Digital infarct
Livedo reticularis
Palpable purpura
Hepatitis B
Polyarteritis nodosa
Genetic disorders
Fabry disease
Angiokeratomas of lower abdomen
Tuberous sclerosis
Ash leaf macule
Facial angiofibromas
Periungual fibromas
Shagreen patch
Nail patella syndrome
Dermatologic conditions associated with the uremic condition
Alopecia
Arterial steal syndrome
Calcinosis cutis
Calciphylaxis
Kyrle's (acquired perforating dermatosis)
Nephrogenic systemic fibrosis
Porphyria cutanea tarda
Pruritus-related skin changes

Contd...

Pseudoporphyria cutanea tarda
Uremic frost
Xerosis
Dermatologic conditions associated with renal transplantation
Medication related
Cushingoid changes
Gingival hyperplasia
Disorders of the pilosebaceous unit: acne, folliculitis, hypertrichosis, keratosis pilaris, and sebaceous gland hyperplasia
Immunosuppression related
Infections
Bacterial
Fungal
Mycobacterial
Parasitic
Viral
Malignancies
Actinic keratosis (precancerous)
Basal cell carcinoma
Kaposi sarcoma
Melanoma
Merkel cell carcinoma
Squamous cell carcinoma
Nail changes seen in kidney diseases
Beau lines
Half and half nails (Lindsey nails)
Nail fold capillary abnormalities
Drug reactions
Acute generalized exanthematous pustulosis (AGEP)
Exanthem
Fixed drug reaction
Leukocytoclastic vasculitis
Lichenoid drug reaction
Erythema multiforme
Stevens Johnson
Toxic epidermal necrolysis

Contd...

Dermatologic Conditions Seen in Diseases Causing Chronic Kidney Disease

Metabolic Disorders

Acanthosis nigricans (Figs. 1 and 2): The hyperpigmented, velvety hyperkeratosis of acanthosis nigricans is most commonly found around the neck, although any flexural area may be involved. More advanced cases are frequently studded with skin tags as well. When classic areas such as these are affected, acanthosis nigricans is a reliable marker for insulin resistance; however, skin findings may precede the development of diabetes mellitus by many years. There is no effective topical or systemic treatment of acanthosis nigricans; keratolytic agents and bleaching agents have no effect. However, if the patient can lose the excess weight before the development of diabetes mellitus, the skin changes will resolve. When atypical sites are affected—such the lips and tongue—an internal malignancy, most commonly gastric cancer, must be sought.

Necrobiosis lipoidica (Figs. 3 and 4): Seen in Figure 3 is a classic lesion of necrobiosis lipoidica (NLD) with a shiny, yellowish, atrophic epidermis allowing visibility of the dermal blood vessels deeper in the dermis. The shins are

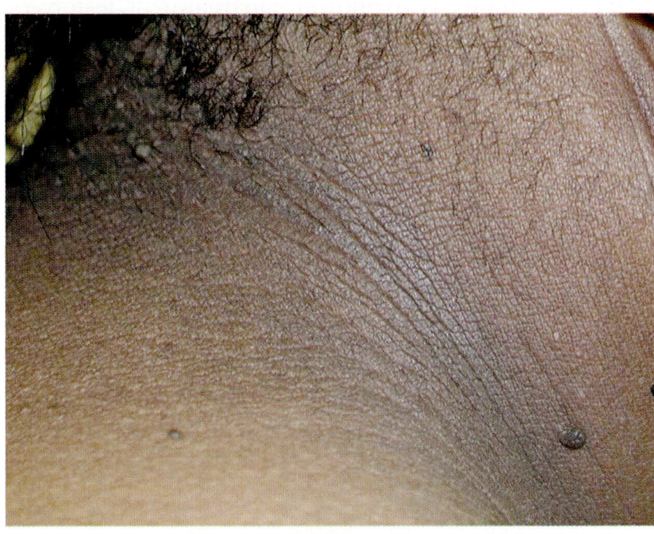

Fig. 1

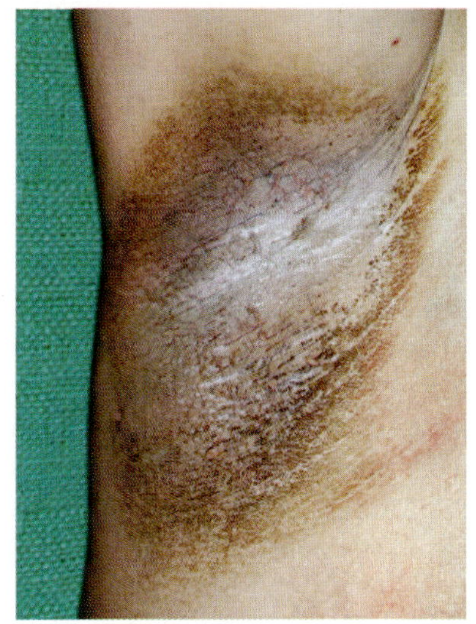

Fig. 2

Figs. 1 and 2: Acanthosis nigricans.

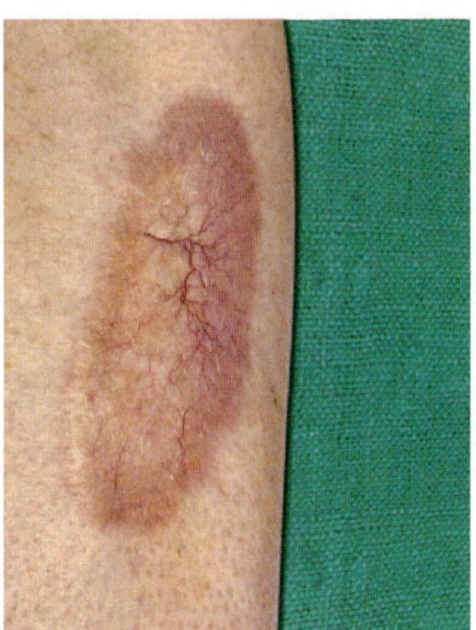

Fig. 3

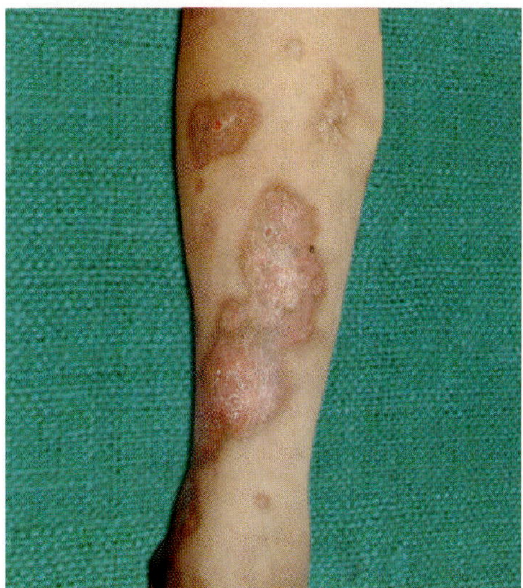

Fig. 4

Figs. 3 and 4: Necrobiosis lipoidica.

most commonly affected, although lesions may be found on the hands, forearms, trunk, and less commonly on the breast, penis, or in surgical sites. Over 95% of patients who develop necrobiosis are diabetic; however, only 0.2% of diabetics are affected. Diabetic control and systemic diabetic complications are unrelated to the development, progression, or severity of NLD.

Lesions of NLD are of cosmetic concern, especially when extensive as seen in Figure 4; however, they are typically asymptomatic. Intralesional steroids are often used to abort the enlargement of the plaques, but there is no effective treatment to eradicate or prevent lesions; their pathogenesis remains unknown. Rarely, lesions will ulcerate; ulcerative NLD is difficult to treat and usually requires topical or systemic immunosuppression.

Eruptive xanthomas (Fig. 5): Seen here are the small, reddish-yellow papules typical for eruptive xanthomas. As a group, xanthomas are characterized by the accumulation of lipid-laden histiocytes and commonly develop in association with a dyslipidemia; the cutaneous presentation and localization often belie the type of dyslipidemia. Tendon xanthomas and palmar xanthomata are associated with hypercholesterolemia as seen in type II and type III hyperlipidemias; xanthelasma (seen in the medial canthi of the eyes) may or not be associated with lipid abnormalities. Eruptive xanthomas, seen here, occur in crops most commonly on the buttocks and extensor surfaces of the extremities and flexural creases. They occur in the setting of hypertriglyceridemia from either a genetic abnormality (type I and V hyperlipidemias) or an underlying systemic disease, most commonly diabetes mellitus; other associated conditions include hypothyroidism and nephrotic syndrome. Insulin is necessary for lipoprotein lipase to properly clear triglycerides. In its absence, marked hypertriglyceridemia may develop. Abdominal pain associated with hepatosplenomegaly, intestinal ischemia, or pancreatitis may occur. Treatment of the diabetic with eruptive xanthomas involves insulin administration as well as dietary alterations. With appropriate treatment, lesions of eruptive xanthoma will spontaneously resolve.

Diabetic dermopathy (Fig. 6): Otherwise known as "brown spots of diabetes," diabetic dermopathy is more subtle than other cutaneous manifestations of diabetes mellitus but is probably the most relevant. Thought to be related to diabetes-related vascular changes, it is seen more commonly in patients with long-standing, poorly controlled diabetes mellitus and is associated with diabetic neuropathy and other vascular complications. Lesions consist of round to oval pink to reddish brown, slightly scaly, atrophic patches most commonly on the shins. Somewhere between 30% and 50% of diabetic patients develop diabetic dermopathy.

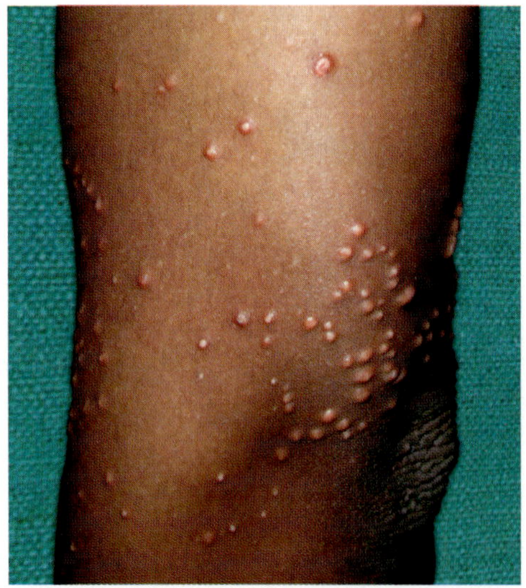

Fig. 5: Eruptive xanthomas.

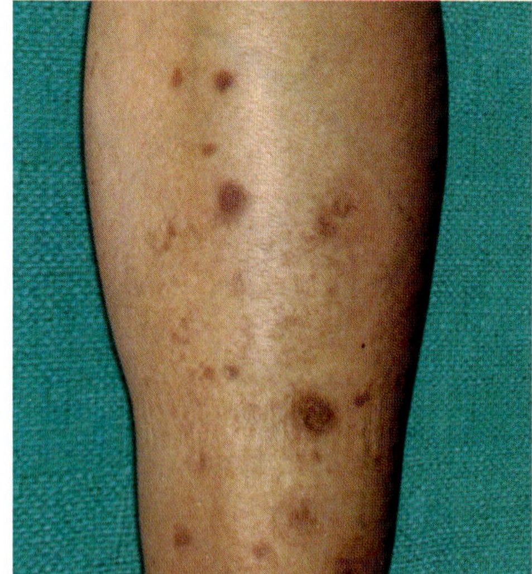

Fig. 6: Diabetic dermopathy.

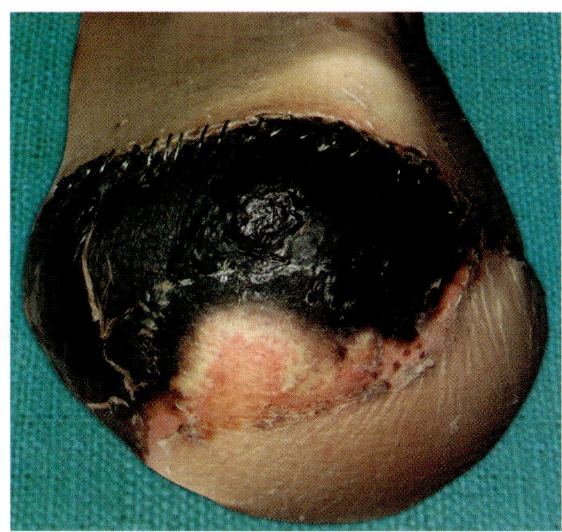

Fig. 7

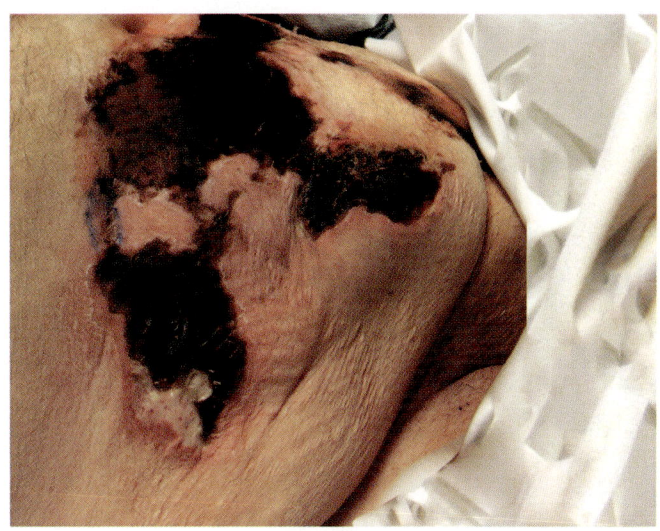

Fig. 8

Figs. 7 and 8: Cholesterol emboli.

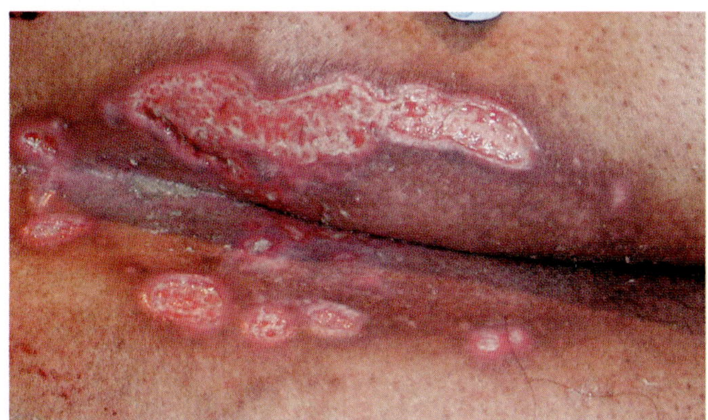

Fig. 9: Aortic occlusion.

Cholesterol emboli (Figs. 7 and 8): Cholesterol emboli are seen in the setting of significant atherosclerotic disease. Patients may present with cutaneous stigmata of the embolic phenomenon as well as acute renal failure, or rapidly worsening renal failure, and eosinophilia. Cutaneous changes include livedo reticularis, splinter hemorrhages, and blue toes. Seen here are two unusual examples of extensive skin necrosis resulting from cholesterol emboli. The lesions on the abdomen have the classic morphology of stellate or retiform purpura with escar. This starburst appearance of purpura (stellate purpura) with or without skin necrosis is pathognomonic for a vascular occlusive process. When present, stellate purpura requires a skin biopsy and work up to determine the cause of vascular occlusion—things to consider include cholesterol or mycotic emboli, vasculitis, calciphylaxis, hypercoagulable syndromes, and vasculoinvasive infections such as mucor or fusarium.

Aortic occlusion (Fig. 9): A biopsy of these ulcers revealed extensive cutaneous arterial thrombosis. Evaluation revealed aortic occlusion due to extensive atherosclerosis. Physical examination suggested a vascular problem as she had bilateral pulseless lower extremities.

Connective Tissue Diseases

Progressive systemic sclerosis (scleroderma) (Figs. 10 to 12)

Sclerodactyly (Fig. 10): Sclerodactyly, seen here with the sausage-like digit changes and loss of skin folds over the joints, is a classic finding of scleroderma otherwise known as progressive systemic sclerosis (PSS). The vitiligo-like changes also evident in this picture are not uncommon in PSS, but are under recognized. PSS comes in a limited and diffuse form, defined mostly by skin involvement. Skin involvement of the acral areas, including distal extremities and face, is seen in both forms; marked truncal involvement is only seen in diffuse PSS. Either may have systemic involvement, but when rapidly progressive, diffuse PSS has a worse prognosis, often associated with the development of malignant hypertension and rapidly progressive renal failure.

Calcinosis cutis (Fig. 11): Calcinosis cutis is not uncommon in PSS. When present in limited PSS, it may be part of the CREST syndrome (calcinosis cutis, Raynaud phenomenon, esophageal dysmotility, sclerodactyly, and telangiectasia). Unfortunately it is very difficult to treat. Surgical excision often results in recurrence.

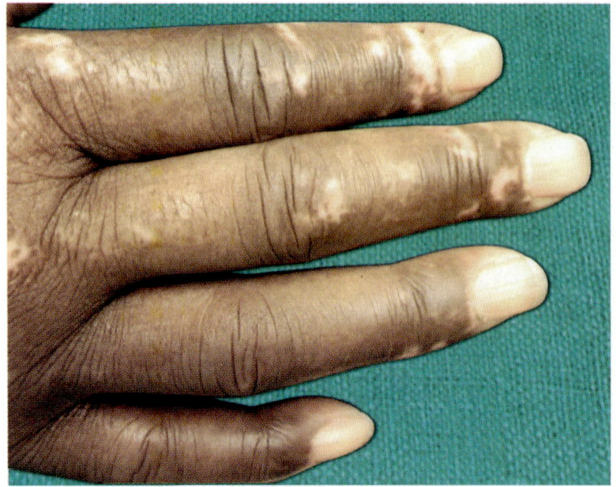

Fig. 10

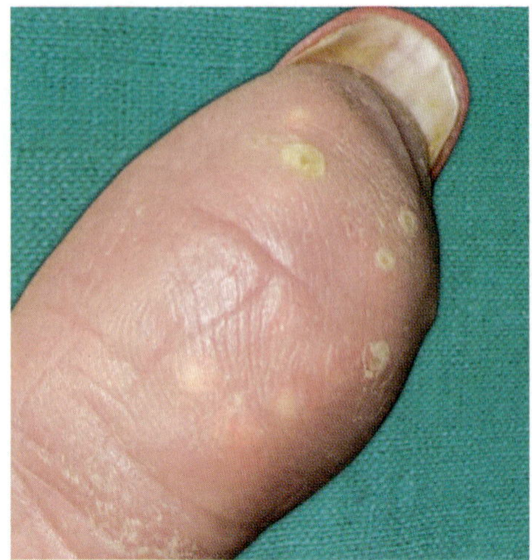

Fig. 11

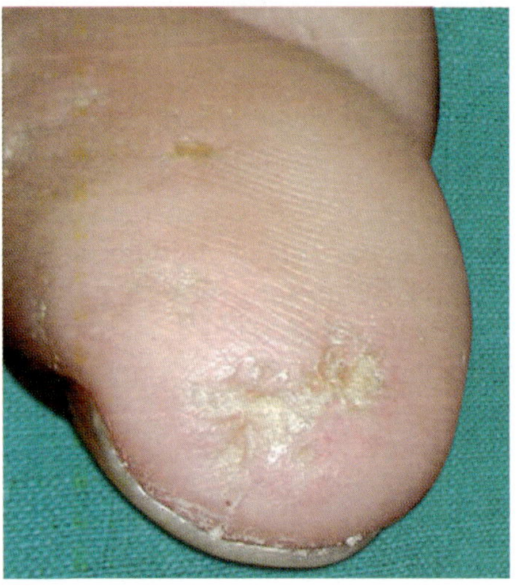

Fig. 12

Figs. 10 to 12: Progressive systemic sclerosis (scleroderma).

Raynaud phenomenon (Fig. 12): Raynaud phenomenon can be seen idiopathically or in association with a connective tissue disease, most commonly PSS. It manifests as a stress or cold-induced transient vasospastic disorder. Severe cases can result in digital pulp infarct (as seen here), distal digital necrosis, and gangrene.

Systemic Lupus Erythematosus (Figs. 13 to 25)

Butterfly rash (Fig. 13): Probably one of the most familiar skin findings associated with systemic lupus erythematosus is the malar "butterfly" rash; however, it is not the most common. At times it is confused with rosacea, a common cutaneous disorder. This confusion is expected since both conditions are photoactivated disorders. When present, the malar rash is a marker of acute lupus and patients should be evaluated for systemic organ involvement.

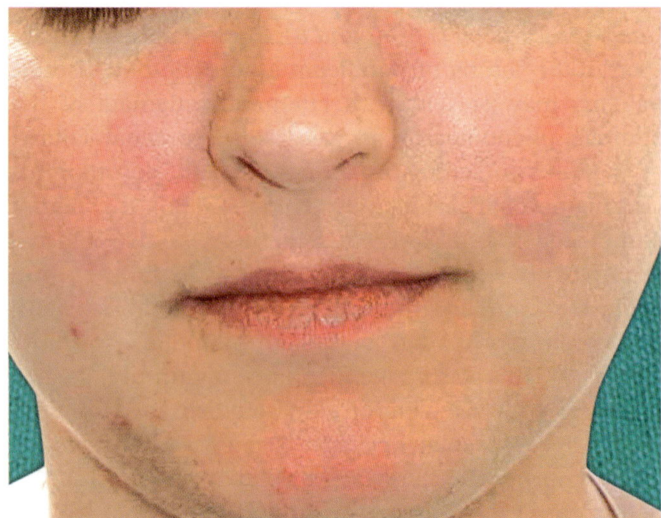

Fig. 13: Butterfly rash.

Chronic cutaneous lupus (Figs. 14 and 15): Chronic cutaneous lupus, AKA discoid lupus erythematosus (DLE) is the most common skin disorder in the spectrum of lupus disorders, but it is uncommonly associated with systemic lupus erythematosus (SLE). Somewhere between 2% and 10% of patients with DLE have or develop SLE. However, DLE can be a devastating disease in its own right with its chronic relentless course resulting in scarring, dyspigmentation, and alopecia. Figure 14 demonstrates a less serious lesion in which repigmentation has occurred, evident by the macules of pigment developing within the area of depigmentation. DLE can be distinguished from vitiligo by the presence of a hyperpigmented border. Figure 15 shows a more advanced process resulting in a permanent scarring alopecia and depigmentation. DLE is a photoactivated process and patients must be routinely advised to utilize sun-protection measures. There is also a small risk of malignant degradation, which would be amplified with extensive sun exposure.

Chronic cutaneous lupus (Figs. 16 and 17): The erythema in these two Figures of DLE demonstrates active inflammation; burnt-out lesions will be white. Involvement of the conchal bowl is pathognomonic for DLE. The crusted lesions are worrisome; they may represent the presence of vasculitis and, thus, the possibility of SLE. They may also represent malignant degradation to squamous cell carcinoma. Treatment of active DLE lesions includes the use of topical or intralesional steroids, oral antimalarial agents, and systemic immune suppression. Systemic steroids are not effective in most cases of cutaneous lupus.

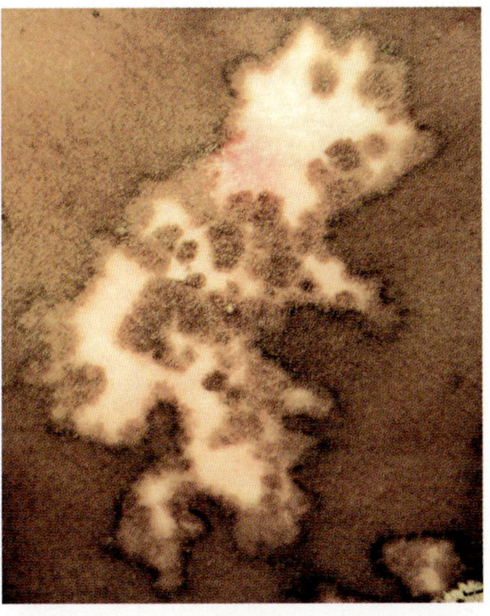

Fig. 14

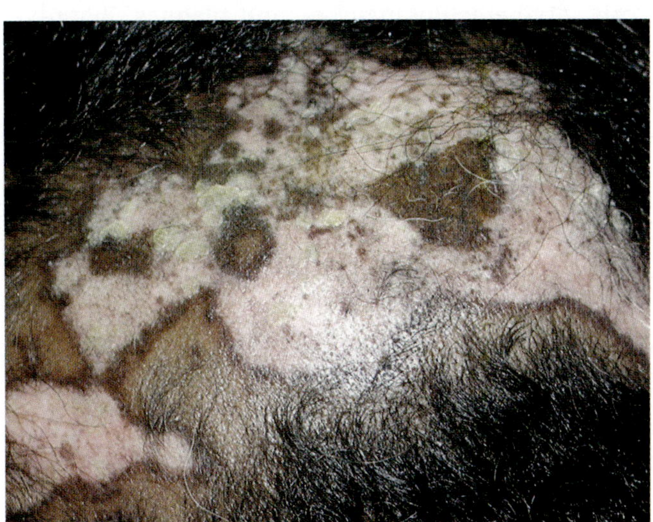

Fig. 15

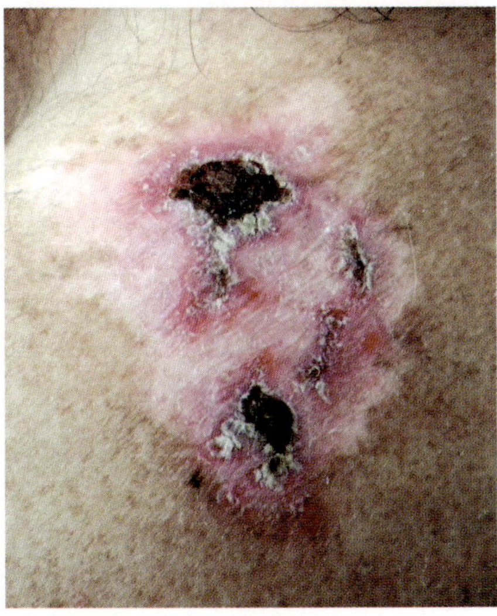

Fig. 16

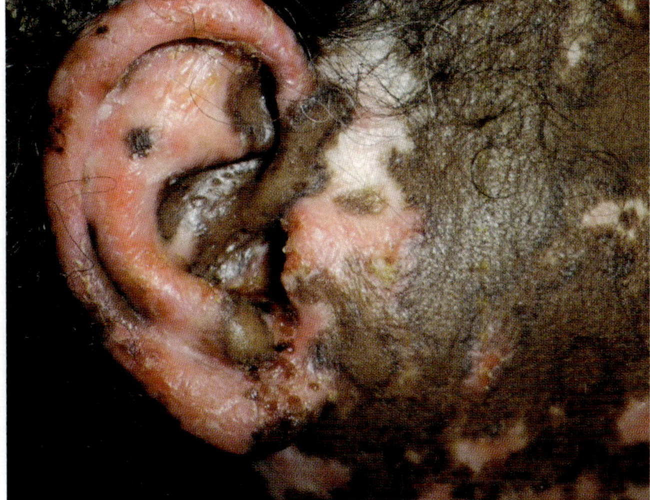

Fig. 17

Figs. 14 to 17: Chronic cutaneous lupus.

Subacute cutaneous lupus erythematosus (SCLE) (Figs. 18 and 19): SCLE is also a photosensitive disorder, but unlike DLE it does not result in scarring, although pigmentary alteration is common. It may be seen in SLE or Sjogren syndrome, or as a drug-induced phenomenon. It has been estimated that approximately 50% of patients with SCLE have SLE and up to 10–20% of cases are drug related; although a multitude of drugs have been implicated, the most common are antihypertensive agents. All races can be affected with various forms of cutaneous lupus; however, SCLE is more common in Caucasian patients and DLE is more common in African-Americans. The Figures here represent the two morphologic patterns of SCLE. Figure 18 demonstrates the psoriasiform type with scaly, erythematous patches, and plaques. Figure 19 is the annular form, with round to oval, mildly scaly, erythematous patches, and plaques.

Lupus panniculitis (Fig. 20): Lupus panniculitis, AKA lupus profundus, is another chronic condition in the spectrum of lupus and affects the subcutis. Between 10% and 50% of patients have or will develop SLE; but only 2–5% of SLE patients develop lupus panniculitis. Up to 70% of lesions have overlying DLE changes, but it is not uniformly present. Examination of an active lesion will reveal tender, deep nodules, or indurated plaques. The differential diagnosis includes calciphylaxis and other causes of panniculitis such as pancreatic panniculitis, polyarteritis nodosa, and α-1-antitrypsin disease. Active disease typically responds to antimalarial agents and other medications commonly used for lupus; the morbidity is associated with atrophic scaring and tissue loss.

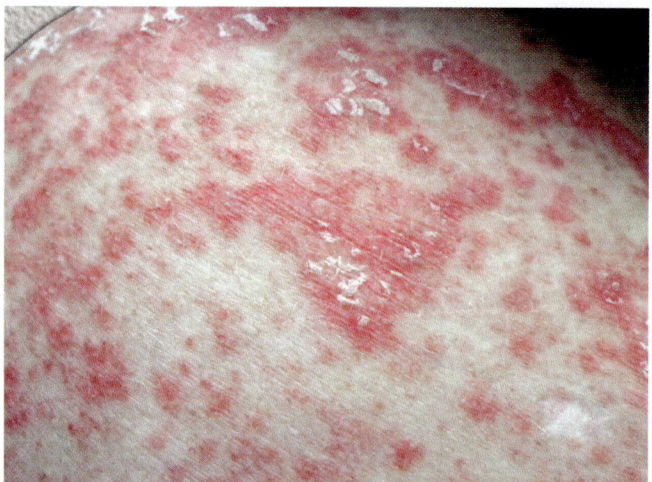

Fig. 18

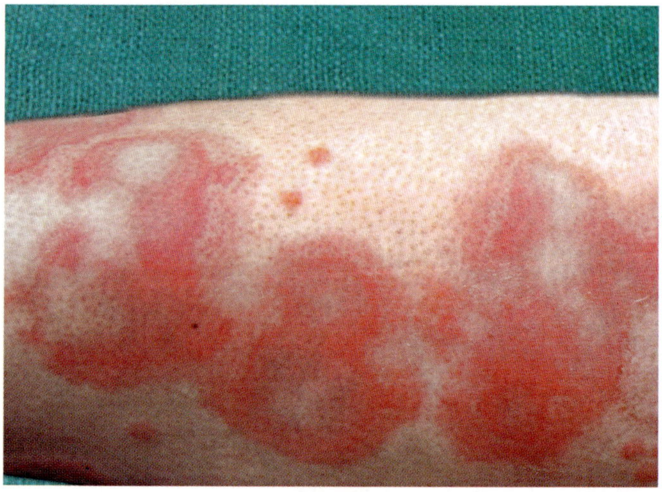

Fig. 19

Figs. 18 and 19: Subacute cutaneous lupus erythematosus.

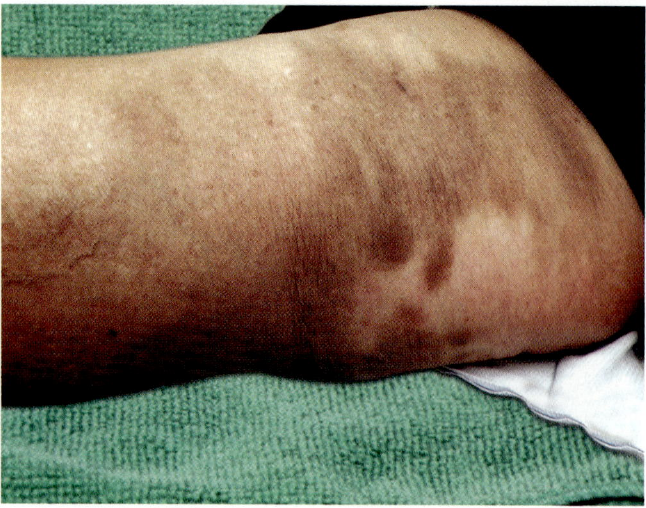

Fig. 20: Lupus panniculitis.

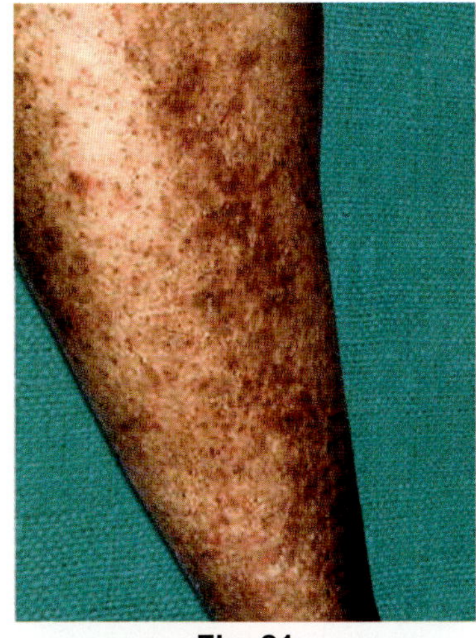

Fig. 21

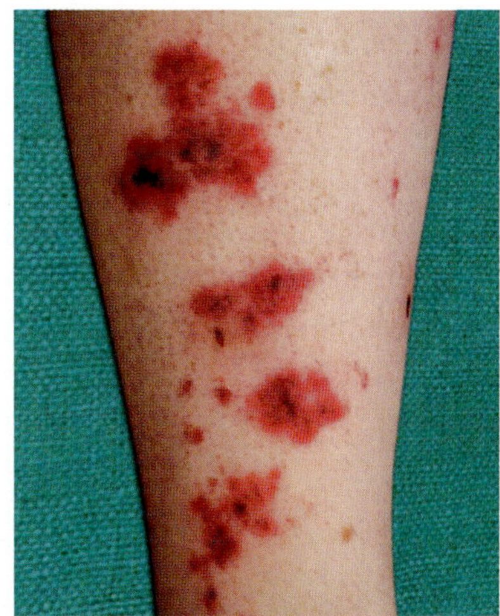

Fig. 22

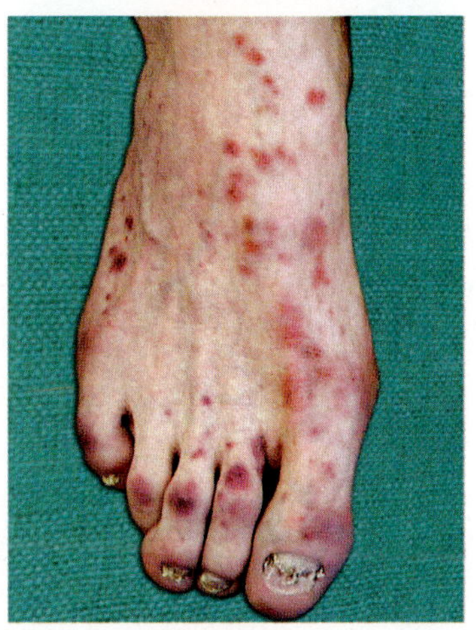

Fig. 23

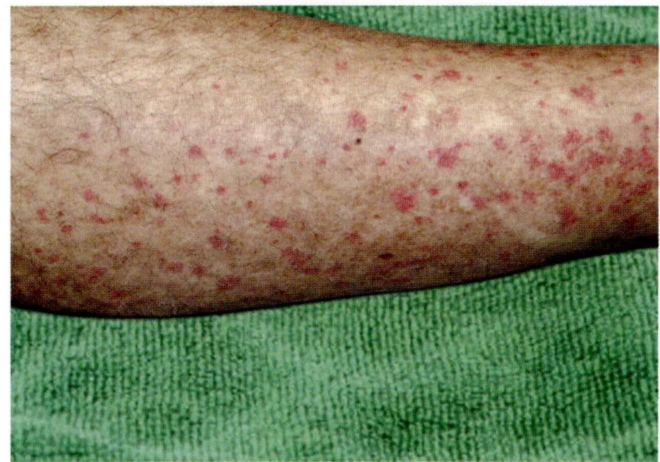

Fig. 24

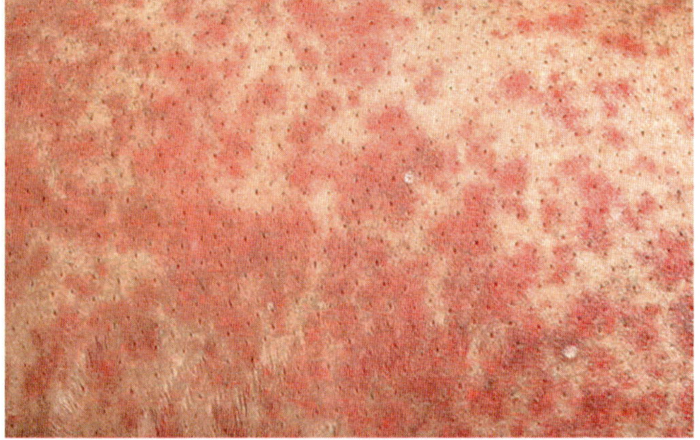

Fig. 25

Figs. 21 to 25: Leukocytoclastic vasculitis.

Leukocytoclastic vasculitis (LCV) (Figs. 21 to 25): LCV is a small vessel vasculitis with a wide variety of causes, although up to 50% of cases are idiopathic. The process may be acute or chronic, systemic, or skin-limited. The most commonly affected organ systems include the skin, joints, gastrointestinal system, and kidneys. The pathogenesis varies with etiology and includes immune complex formation, ANCA-associated processes, and hypersensitivity reactions. Systemic conditions associated with LCV include connective tissue diseases, infections, malignancies, paraproteinemias, and food or drug-induced reactions. The most common connective tissue diseases causing LCV are SLE, rheumatoid arthritis, and Sjogren syndrome. Seen in each Figure is the classic palpable purpura associated with LCV. One cannot determine the cause from visual inspection. Diagnosis depends on histologic findings, including immunofluorescence, along with serologic and systemic evaluation. Figure 21 is due to mixed cryoglobulinemia from chronic hepatitis C; Figure 22 is drug-induced from propylthiouracil; Figures 23 and 14 are idiopathic; and Figure 25 is from a case of chronic Henoch-Schonlein purpura.

Hepatitis Viruses

Hepatitis viruses can account for renal disease and several skin disorders.

Lichen planus (LP) (Figs. 26 to 29): LP is a chronic, often remitting, reactive lymphocytic disorder. Most cases are idiopathic; however, there may be an association between LP and hepatitis C. Lesions are described by the 4 Ps—pruritic, purple, polygonal, papules and are classically found on the volar aspects of the wrists, though any mucocutaneous surface may be affected. Typical lesions are seen in Figures 26 and 27; Figure 28 demonstrates a more hyperpigmented version; Figures 28 and 29 shows an ulcerative lesion with the classic white lacy pattern of Wickham striae on the oral mucosa.

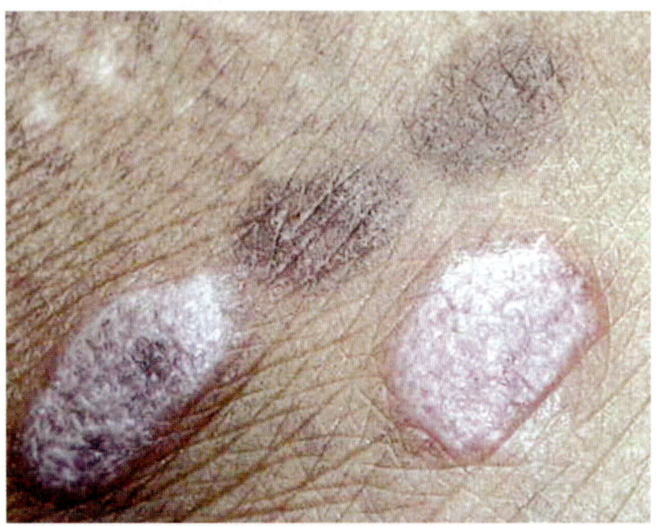

Fig. 26

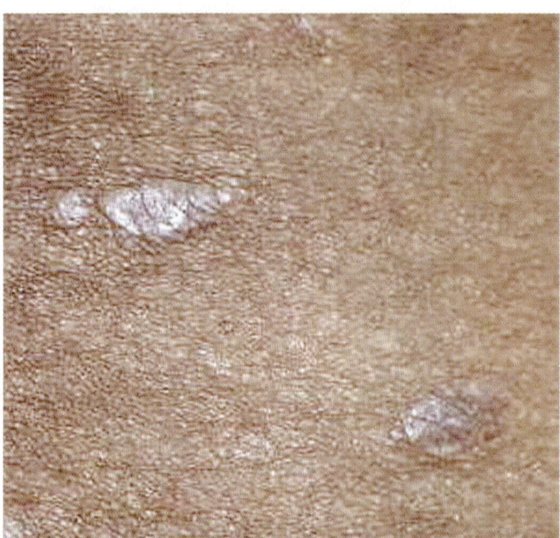

Fig. 27

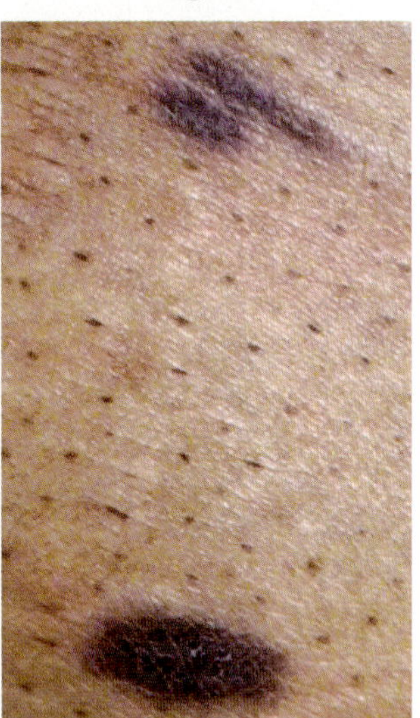

Fig. 28

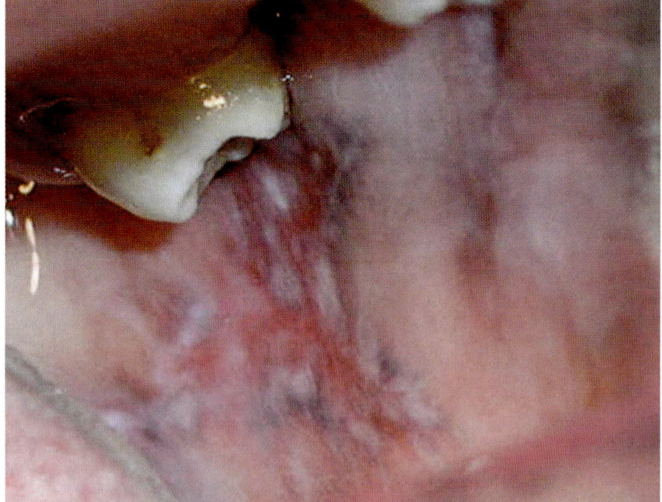

Fig. 29

Figs. 26 to 29: Lichen planus.

Porphyria cutanea tarda (PCT) (Figs. 30 to 33): PCT is a disorder of heme biosynthesis that can be genetic, or acquired. The acquired form is much more common and is due to a hepatic deficiency of the enzyme uroporphyrinogen decarboxylase. Multiple factors contribute to the development of PCT in susceptible individuals; the more common of these factors include chronic hepatitis C (HCV), hemochromatosis; alcoholism, lupus, and multiple medications including estrogens. Elevated serum porphyrins result in a phototoxic reaction when the individual is exposed to ultraviolet light in the Soret band (410 nm). The cutaneous findings include blisters, skin fragility, a peculiar hypertrichosis between the eyebrows and temple, and a late finding of cutaneous sclerosis similar to scleroderma. Figures 30 and 31 demonstrate the typical erosions on the dorsal hands. Patients often don't recognize the preceding blister since the fragile blister easily ruptures; however, at times large bullae may be seen. Any area that is sun exposed may develop blisters. Figure 32 shows how the scalp can be affected. Disruption of the sweat glands and resultant healing after blistering cause the tiny white papules of milia seen in Figure 33. The initial course of treatment is sun avoidance and phlebotomy. Most patients have marked iron overload with ferritin levels into the thousands. The condition may also respond to eliminating triggers and treating the underlying HCV.

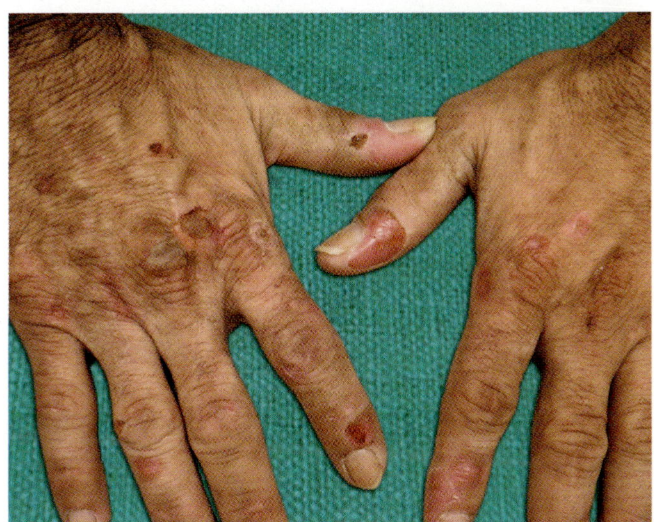

Fig. 30

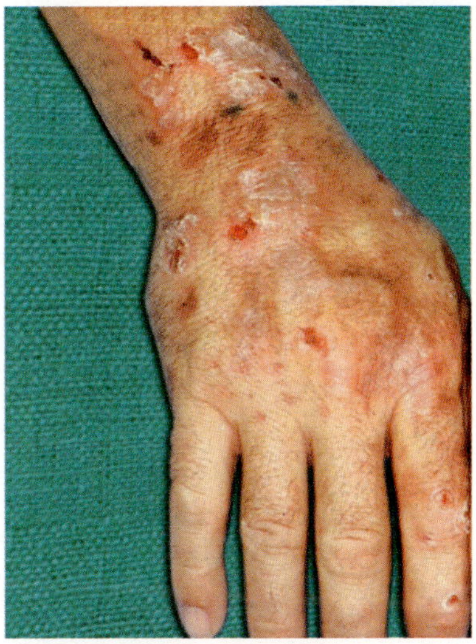

Fig. 31

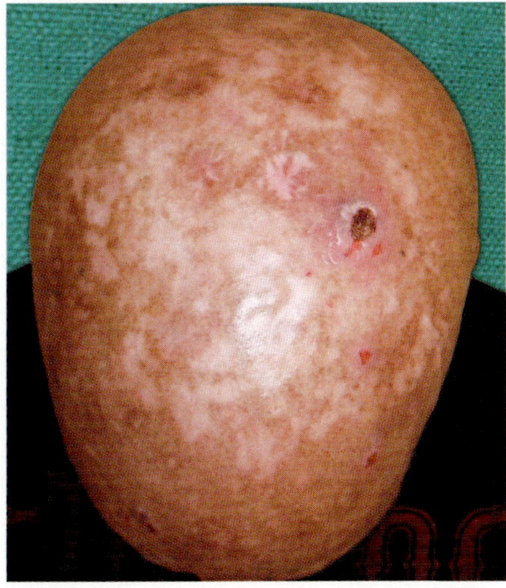

Fig. 32

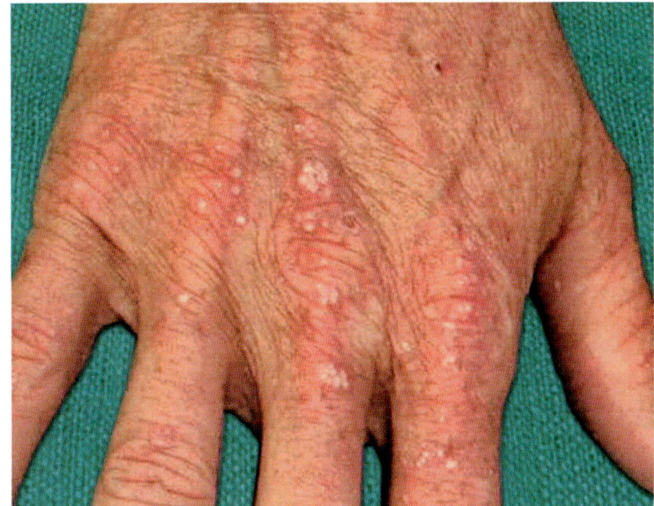

Fig. 33

Figs. 30 to 33: Porphyria cutanea tarda.

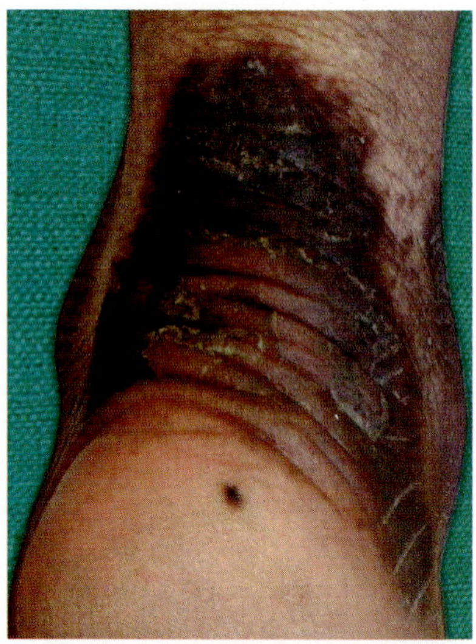

Fig. 34

Fig. 35

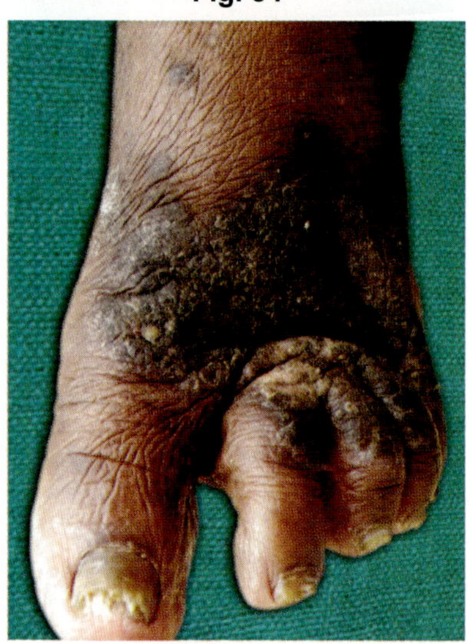

Fig. 36

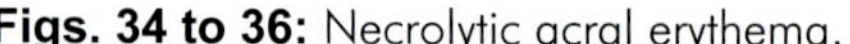

Figs. 34 to 36: Necrolytic acral erythema.

Necrolytic acral erythema (NAE) (Figs. 34 to 36): NAE is a rare condition most commonly seen in patients with HCV; only a few cases have been reported without HCV. It mimics other necrolytic dermatoses such as that associated with glucagonoma. Skin findings consist of dusky to erythematous to hyperpigmented scaly plaques. The distribution is limited to acral sites; dorsal feet are uniformly affected. Some lesions are asymptomatic; others have a burning sensation; when associated with significant pruritus lesions may be mistaken for lichen planus. The pathogenesis of NAE is poorly understood; theoretical causes include metabolic aberrations including liver dysfunction, hypoalbuminemia, diabetes mellitus, and zinc deficiency.

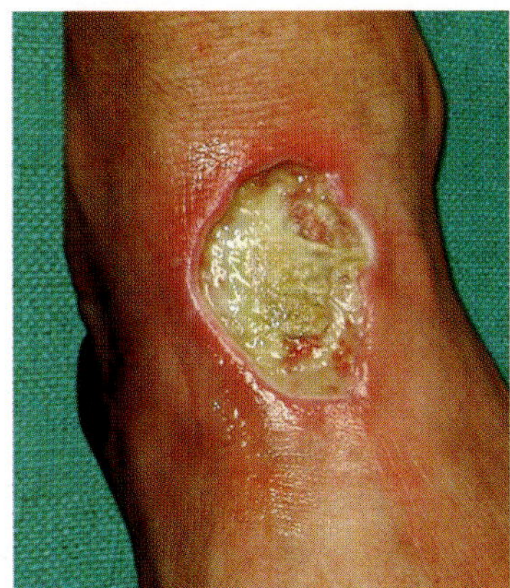

Fig. 37

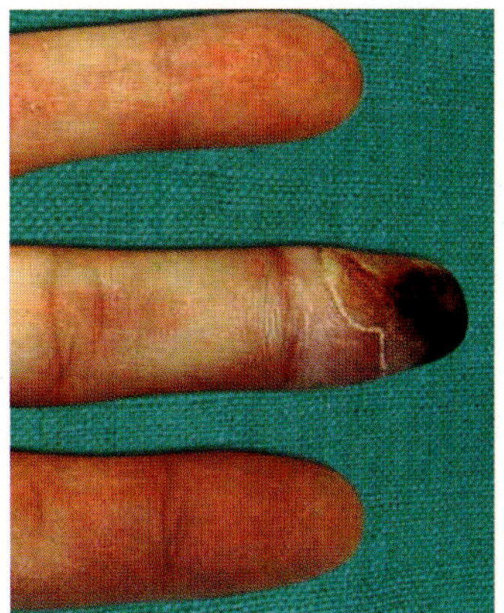

Fig. 38

Figs. 37 and 38: Cryoglobulinemia.

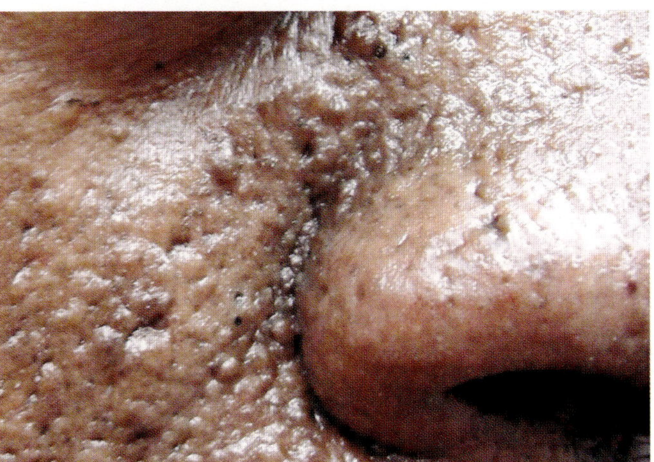

Fig. 39

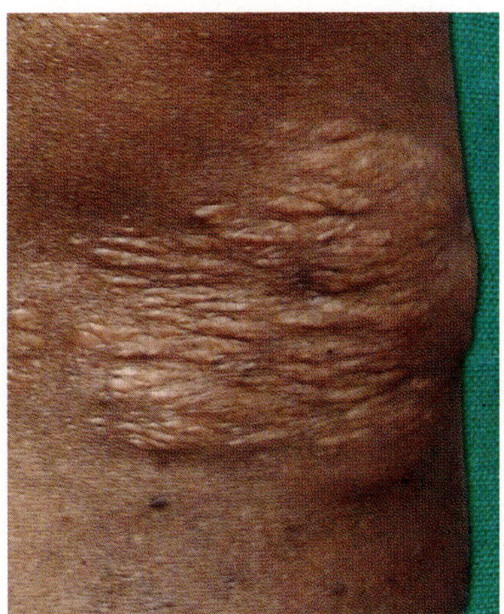

Fig. 40

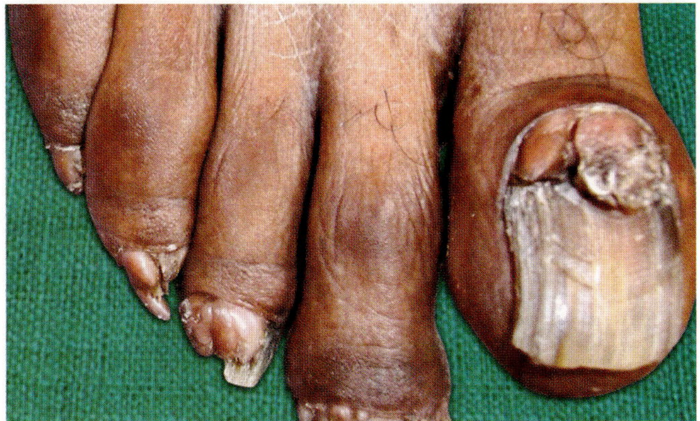

Fig. 41

Figs. 39 to 41: Tuberous sclerosis.

Cryoglobulinemia (Figs. 37 and 38): Cryoglobulinemia can cause disease through either an immune-complex-mediated phenomenon or cryoprecipitation resulting in vasculitis or thrombosis, respectively. Type I cryoglobulinemia is usually monoclonal and associated with a lymphoproliferative disorder such as myeloma. Types II and III, referred to as "mixed cryoglobulinemia (MC)," are associated with chronic inflammatory processes such as viral infections (predominately HCV) and autoimmune diseases. Various skin lesions can be seen in association with cryoglobulinemia: Type I, with its hyperviscosity, may cause livedo reticularis, acrocyanosis, digital ulceration or infarct, and/or purpura. Similar lesions can be found in MC, as well as cutaneous vasculitis. Figure 37 shows an ulcer that was a consequence of MC-induced thrombosis. The digital infarct demonstrated in Figure 38 was a result of vasculitis. Both of these cases had HCV as the underlying disease.

Genetic Disorders

A variety of genetic disorders affect the integument and the kidneys.

Tuberous sclerosis (TS) (Figs. 39 to 41): TS is an uncommon genetic disorder that affects multiple organ systems including the kidney and integument. The ash leaf hypopigmented macule is usually present at birth, but may not be recognized. The facial angiofibromas and shagreen patch (Figs. 39 and 40, respectively) appear in childhood or early adolescence. Periungual fibromas (Fig. 41) may affect the nails of the fingers or toes; they are cosmetically disfiguring and may cause some functional impairment. Patients with TS may have normal intelligence or impaired cognition. Various central nervous system abnormalities have been described including cortical tubers; seizures are common. Pulmonary effects may be delayed and include spontaneous pneumothorax and chylothorax.

Dermatologic Conditions Associated with the Uremic Condition

Some conditions seen in dialysis patients are unique to the uremic condition or more common in those who are uremic or on dialysis.

Pruritus (Figs. 42 to 47): Chronic pruritus is a significant problem for many dialysis patients and may be due to uremia or another underlying metabolic cause including HIV, HCV, chronic liver disease, and atopy. The cutaneous findings are a result of acute and chronic scratching and present as acute excoriations, atrophic and hypertrophic scars, hyperpigmentation or depigmentation, prurigo nodules, and lichen simplex chronicus. Figure 42 demonstrates excoriations that healed with mildly hyperpigmented atrophic scarring. Figure 43 represents classic prurigo nodules that are hyperkeratotic, distinct hyperpigmented papules. Figures 44 and 45 show dry, hyperkeratotic, hyperpigmented plaques that represent small but well-developed lesions of lichen simplex chronicus. Figures 46 and 47 illustrate various stages of lesions due to chronic scratching, ranging from depigmented atrophic healed

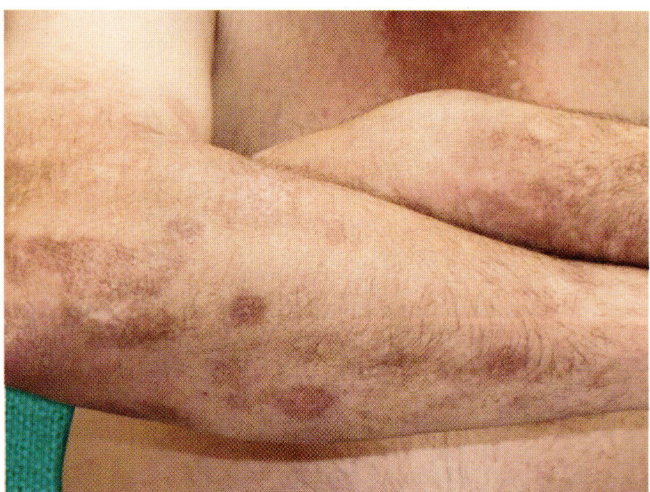

Fig. 42

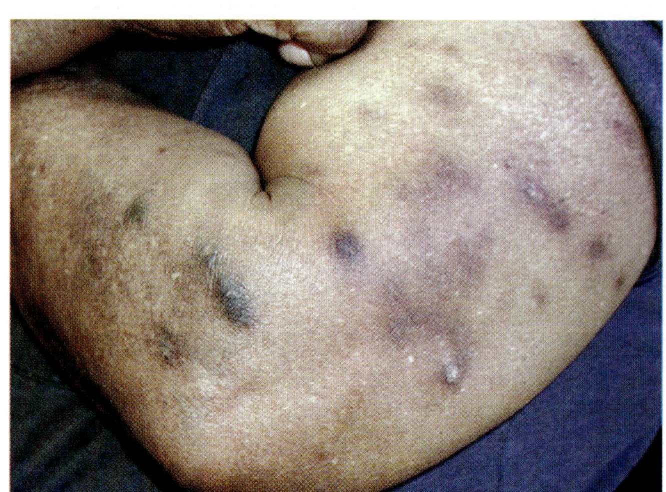

Fig. 43

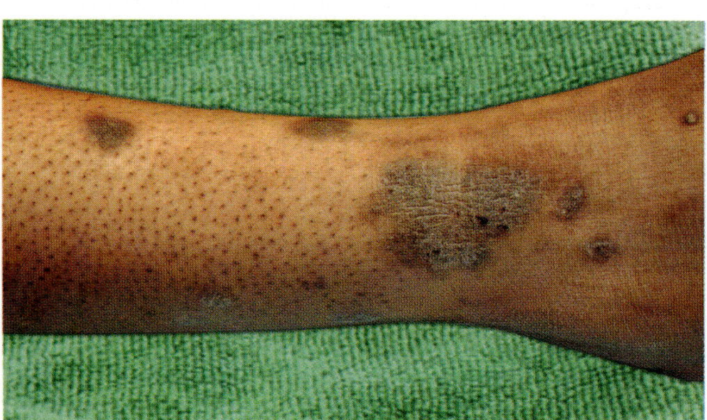

Fig. 44

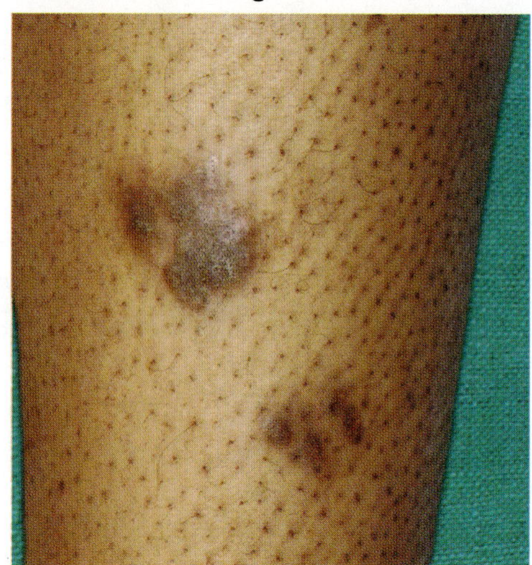

Fig. 45

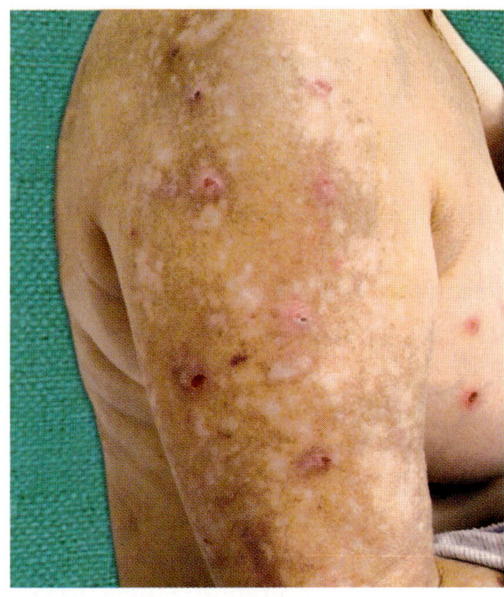

Fig. 46

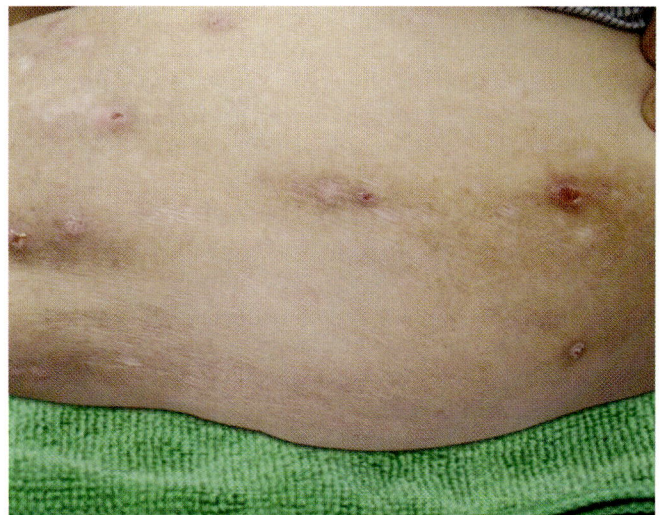

Fig. 47

Figs. 42 to 47: Pruritus.

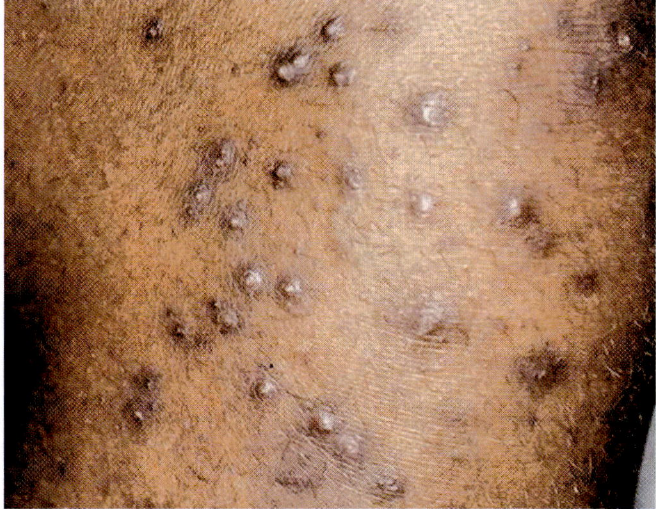

Fig. 48

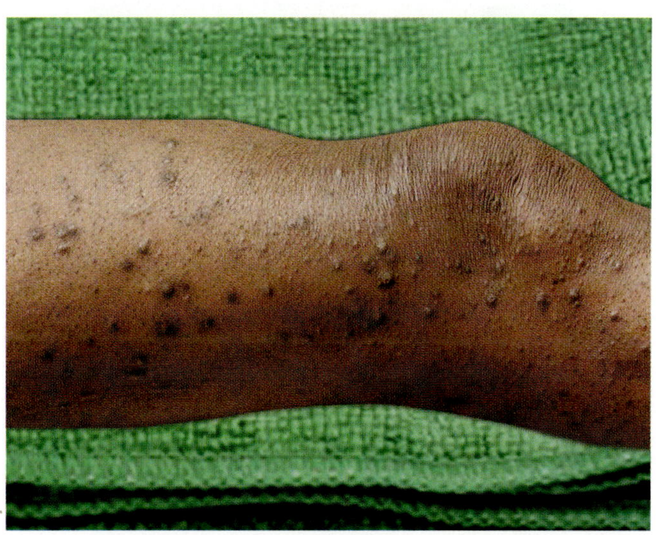

Fig. 49

Figs. 48 and 49: Kyrle disease.

scars to acutely excoriated prurigo nodules and erosions. Therapeutic options for uremic pruritus are inconsistently effective and include sedating antihistamines, emollients to alleviate xerosis, metabolic alterations to normalize calcium/phosphate levels, use of opiate-receptor antagonists, and UVB phototherapy. Over-the-counter topical antipruritics containing menthol, phenol, and pramoxine may be somewhat helpful as well.

Kyrle disease (Figs. 48 and 49): Kyrle disease is an acquired cutaneous perforating disorder that is most commonly found in diabetics on dialysis. The pathogenesis is poorly understood. Clinically one finds hyperkeratotic papules ranging in size from 2 to 10 mm. Intact papules contain a central keratin plug; however, chronic scratching may obliterate this clinical finding causing the lesion to resemble a prurigo nodule. Lesions are most common on the legs, though the arms, head, and neck may also be affected. Figure 48 demonstrates predominately undisturbed lesions with their conical shape; Figure 49 shows the variability that can be present due to scratching.

Nephrogenic systemic fibrosis (Fig. 50): The story of nephrogenic systemic fibrosis began with skin findings and was initially called nephrogenic fibrosing dermopathy; however, over time it was discovered to have extensive and devastating systemic effects as well. The skin findings were highly suggestive of a limited form of scleroderma with predominately acral cutaneous sclerosis as seen on the legs in the Figure here; but Raynaud's and other findings of CREST or systemic sclerosis were not present. Fortunately, it was rapidly recognized to be associated with the use of gadolinium in patients with functional renal impairment. Hopefully, with the avoidance of gadolinium in patients with renal compromise, there will be no new cases of this condition.

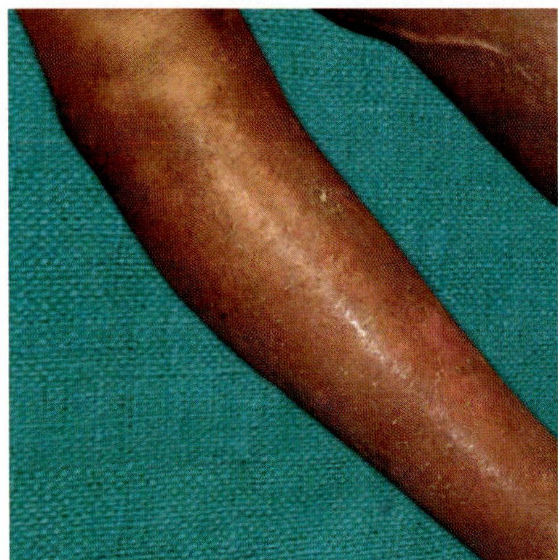

Fig. 50: Nephrogenic systemic fibrosis.

Calciphylaxis (Figs. 51 to 58): Calciphylaxis is a poorly understood, highly morbid condition seen in 1–4% of dialysis patients, although it may rarely be seen in patients with normal renal function as well. Though the pathogenesis is poorly understood, it is associated with vascular calcification, skin necrosis, and a high mortality rate. Because the end result of calciphylaxis is vascular ischemia, lesions are exquisitely painful. The most common first findings are deep, rock-hard, tender plaques, most commonly in the fatty areas of the thighs or abdomen; subtle epidermal changes may be present (Fig. 51). Hemorrhage may occur, presenting as stellate purpura, which is pathognomonic for vascular occlusion (Fig. 52). Since calciphylaxis is a vascular occlusive disorder, the skin findings may develop along the course of the affected vessels (Figs. 53 and 54). Ulceration (Fig. 55) is common and heralds a worse prognosis. Necrotic debris may be extensive (Figs. 56 and 57) and should be conservatively debrided to remove infected foci since the most common cause of death is overwhelming sepsis. In addition to debridement, the treatment options for calciphylaxis include normalization of the calcium/phosphate product, chemical or surgical parathyroidectomy, the use of oral bisphosphonates, and utilization of intravenous sodium thiosulfate. Patients should be evaluated for hypercoagulable states. The patient represented in Figure 58 had progressive disease despite using all of the listed modalities. Evaluation revealed an unsuspected antiphospholipid antibody syndrome. Initiation of heparin resulted in disease stabilization and the beginning of healing.

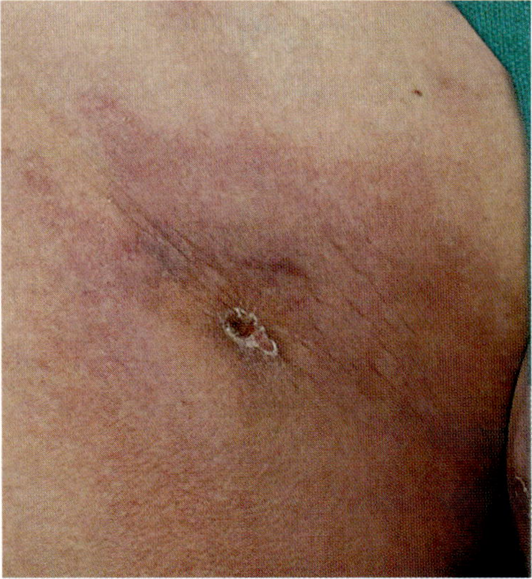

Fig. 51

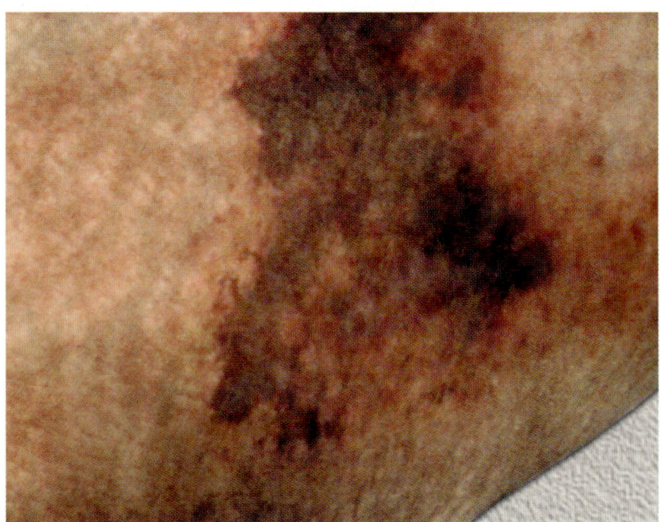

Fig. 52

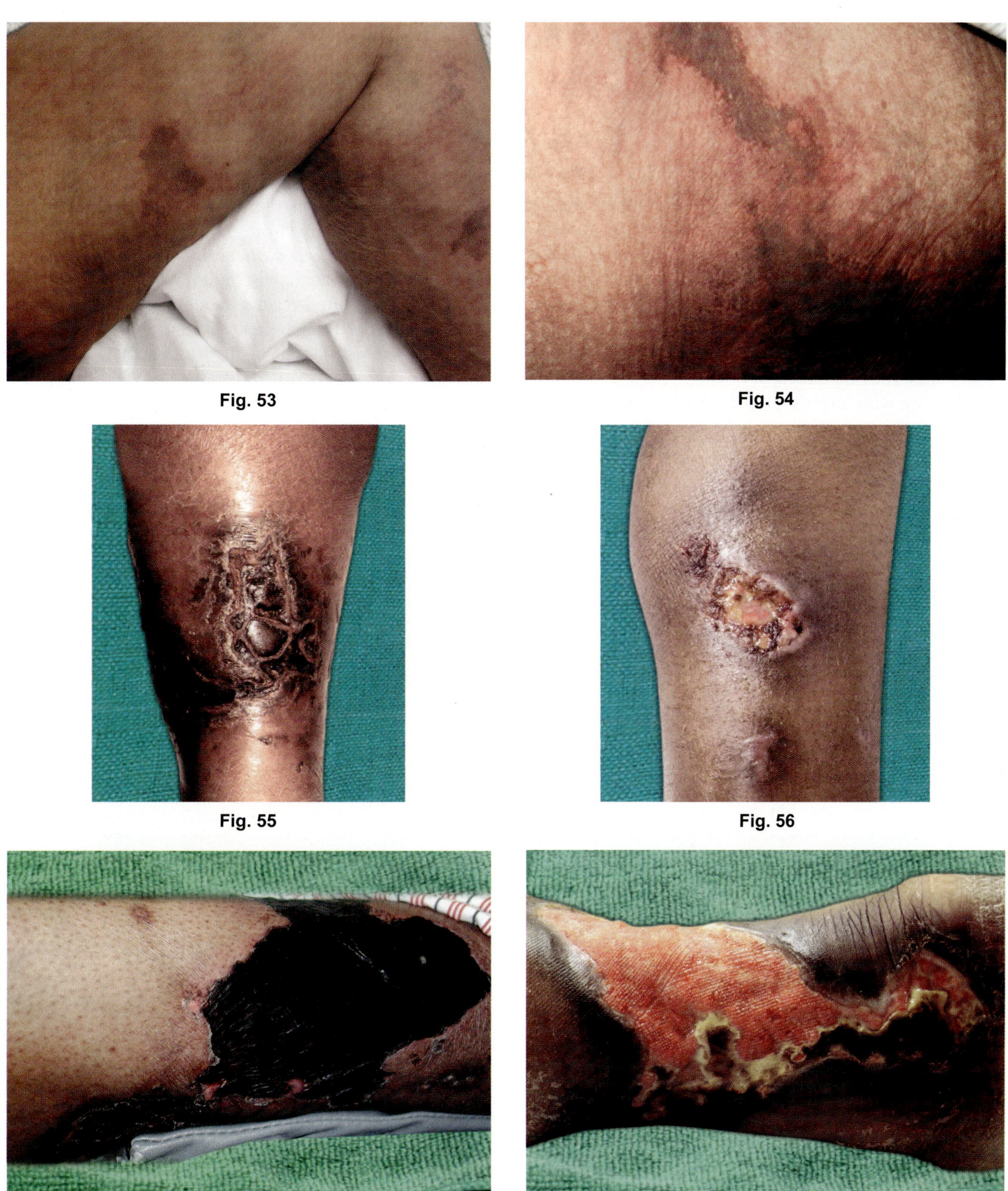

Fig. 53

Fig. 54

Fig. 55

Fig. 56

Fig. 57

Fig. 58

Figs. 51 to 58: Calciphylaxis.

Dermatologic Conditions Associated with Renal Transplantation

Medication Related

A variety of unique medication-related physiologic findings can be seen in solid organ recipients.

Cushingoid changes (Figs. 59 to 61): Cushing syndrome may result from excessive glucocorticoid administration. Commonly seen is thinning of the skin and the development of easy bruising and senile purpura (Figs. 59 and 60). Excessive lifetime sun exposure greatly increases the development of senile purpura, which is most prominent on the forearms, though any body surface area may be affected. Obesity and altered body morphology with the development of a dorsocervical hump (buffalo hump), supraclavicular fat pads, facial fullness, and plethora (Fig. 61) are frequent findings. Other skin changes include acanthosis nigricans, skin tags, hirsutism, and striae.

Steroid acne (Fig. 62): An acneiform eruption commonly follows high-dose glucocorticoid administration. Typically one sees monomorphous papulopustules on the torso (*see* Figure) and extremities, rarely affecting the face. This condition is distinct from acne vulgaris since it is more of a *Pityrosporum folliculitis* and lacks comedones, the primary lesions of acne. Discontinuation or lowering the dose of steroids often results in spontaneous regression. Acutely patients may benefit from the use of topical antifungal agents. Of note, at times true acne vulgaris may be triggered by glucocorticoid-induced hyperandrogenemia requiring more typical acne treatment.

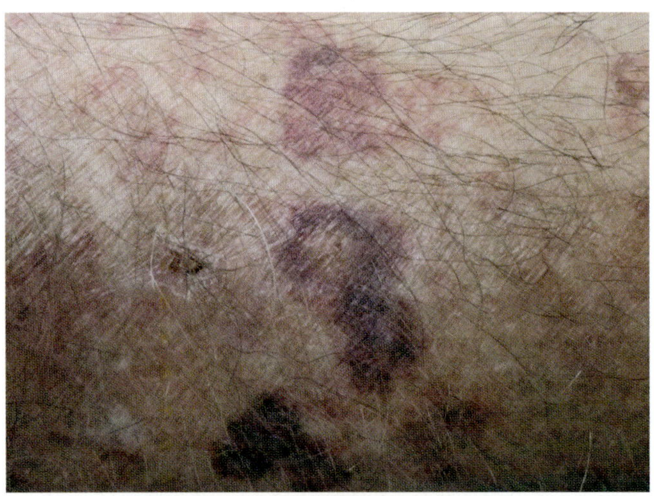

Fig. 59

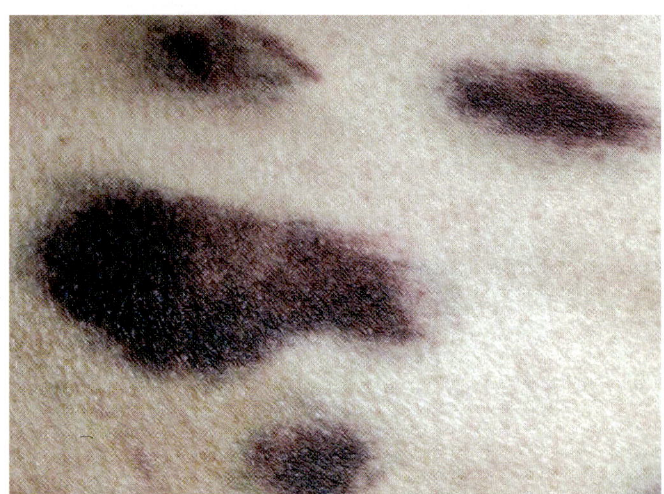

Fig. 60

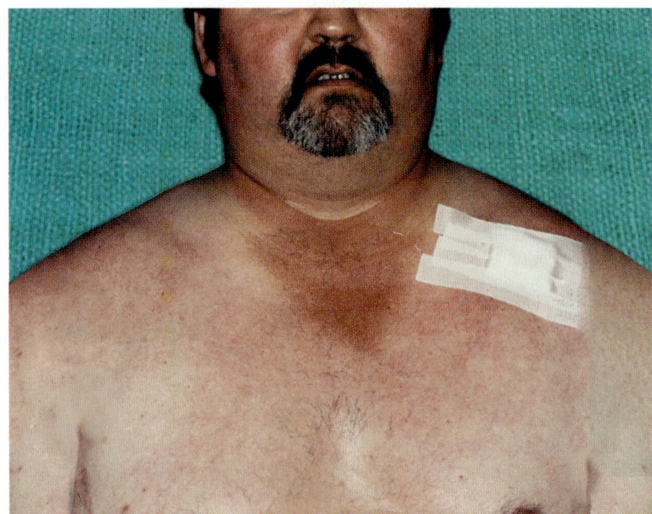

Fig. 61

Figs. 59 to 61: Cushingoid changes.

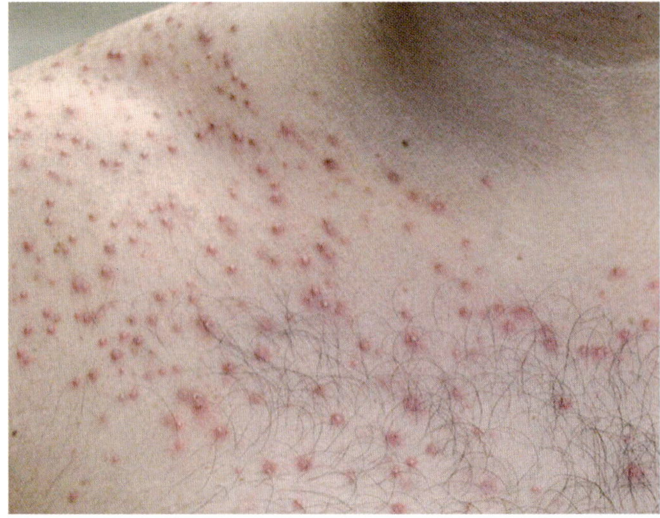

Fig. 62: Steroid acne.

Gingival hyperplasia (Fig. 63): Gingival hyperplasia is common in renal transplant recipients, especially in those receiving cyclosporine; its development may be augmented by concomitant use of other agents such as channel blockers or phenytoin. Though generally asymptomatic, it may be painful and unsightly. Some data suggest that gingival hyperplasia may be associated with earlier graft loss, probably related to toxic effects of cyclosporine.

Disorders of the pilosebaceous units (Fig. 64): Various disorders of the pilosebaceous unit are attributed to medications used to suppress organ rejection; acneiform disorders were discussed above. Similar to gingival hyperplasia, sebaceous gland hyperplasia is more commonly seen in cyclosporine-based regimens. Seen in this Figure are two roundish, yellowish papules with central depressions, typical for sebaceous gland hyperplasia. The yellowish rim is a result of the hyperplastic changes of the sebaceous globules and the central depression is the glandular opening. Lesions of sebaceous gland hyperplasia are frequently mistaken as basal cell carcinomas by the untrained eye.

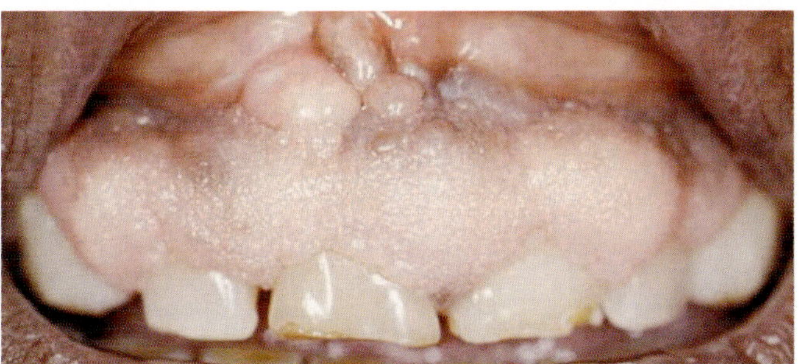

Fig. 63: Gingival hyperplasia.

Immunosuppression-Related Infections

Medications used to suppress organ rejection decrease cell-mediated immunity, predisposing patients to infection by a wide variety of organisms. Pictured here are some of these conditions.

Staphylococcal abscess (Fig. 65): Immune suppression and recurrent hospitalizations increase the risk of both methicillin-sensitive *Staphylococcus aureus* (MSSA) and methicillin-resistant *Staphylococcal aureus* (MRSA) skin infections. Seen here are multiple small abscesses in a patient chronically immunosuppressed and colonized with MRSA. Patients should be cultured and treated with appropriate antibiotics. Nares cultures should be performed and patients treated if found to be colonized with either MSSA or MRSA. Patients may benefit from decolonization regimens.

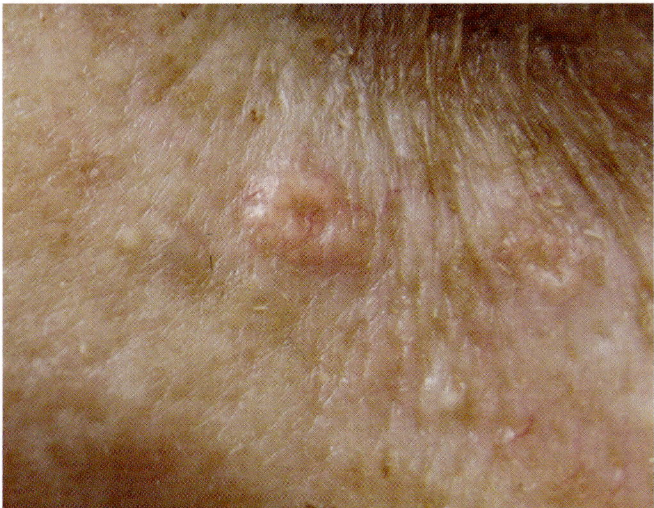

Fig. 64: Disorders of the pilosebaceous units.

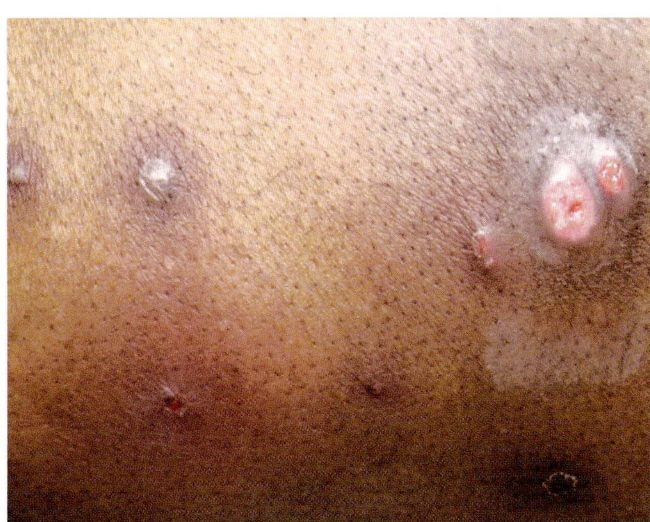

Fig. 65: Staphylococcal abscess.

Nocardiosis (Fig. 66): Nocardia are aerobic actinomycetes found in water, soil, and decaying organic matter. Over 30 species of Nocardia exist and at least 13 cause human disease. Localized disease can be seen in immune-competent individuals, whereas disseminated disease can occur in the immune suppressed. The morphology of this lesion is characterized by pseudoepithelial hyperplasia overlying dermal nodules draining purulent material. Histologic examination and cultures are necessary for proper diagnosis.

Oral candidiasis (Fig. 67): Candidiasis is common and probably more problematic in diabetics and otherwise immune-suppressed individuals. Commonly affected places are warm and wet—skin folds, groin, and mouth. Seen here is the classic white coating of thrush.

Human papilloma viruses (HPV) (Figs. 68 and 69): An adequate cell-mediated immunity is necessary for the host to adequately combat HPV; regrettably transplant patient have poor cell-mediated immunity due to antirejection medications. Seen here are two forms of HPV. Figure 68 shows classic plantar warts; visible is a collection of discrete verrucous papules. The dark dots represent thrombosed vessels within the wart. Figure 69 demonstrates the cosmetic devastation of flat warts in a renal transplant patient. Seen here is a confluence of the small hyperkeratotic, hyperpigmented, and verrucous papules. Unfortunately, little can be done to eradicate HPV when this extensive. Data suggest that after 5 years of immune suppression between 70% and 95% of kidney transplant patients are affected by HPV.

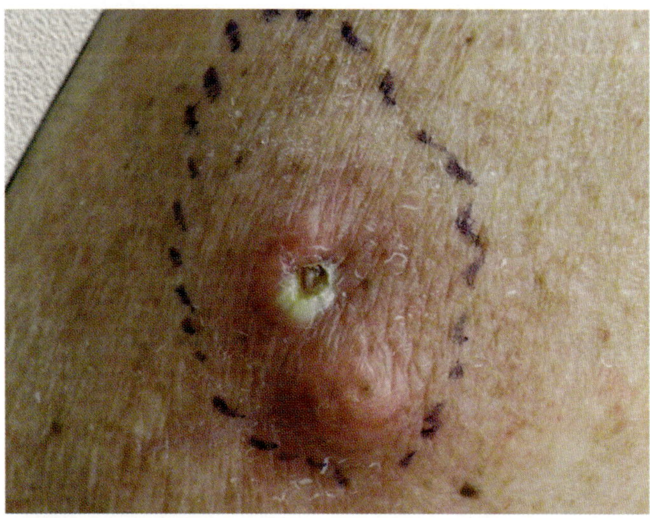

Fig. 66: Nocardiosis.

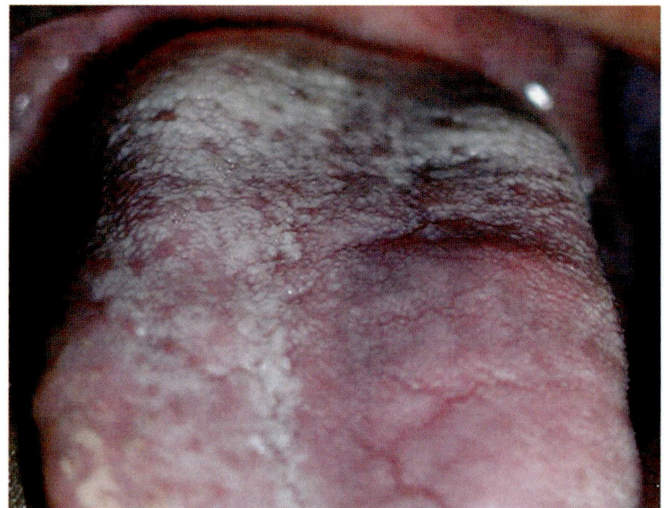

Fig. 67: Oral candidiasis.

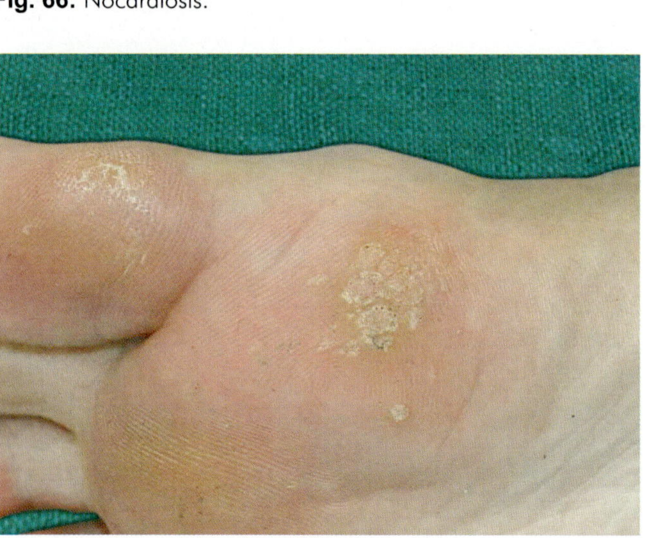

Fig. 68

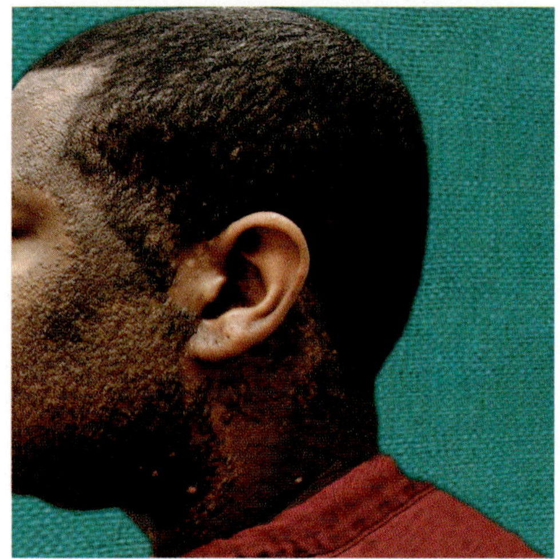

Fig. 69

Figs. 68 and 69: Human papilloma viruses.

Herpes simplex virus (HSV) (Figs. 70 and 71): HSV is common in immune-competent and immune-suppressed individuals. Figure 70 shows a typical outbreak for HSV1 in a male. Figure 71 shows a more widespread eruption not uncommon in immune-suppressed individuals. Confirming cultures and appropriate antiviral therapy are necessary.

Varicella zoster (Fig. 72): The primary infection of varicella zoster (herpes zoster) is typically chickenpox. After primary inoculation, the virus resides in a dorsal root ganglion awaiting reactivation. As a reaction to a trigger, which may be immune suppression, the virus reactivates, moves down the nerve, and causes a painful, blistering, dermatomal outbreak. Seen here are the unilateral, classic, grouped blisters affecting an isolated dermatome classic for "shingles." Immune-suppressed individuals are more likely to develop shingles in one or more dermatomes as well as disseminated zoster.

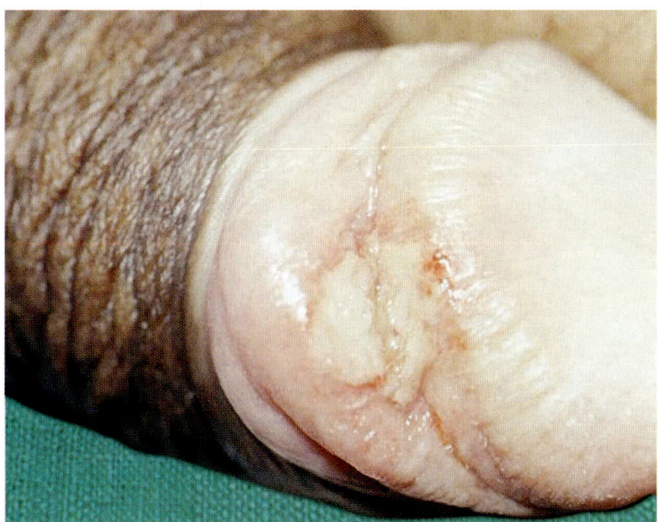

Fig. 70

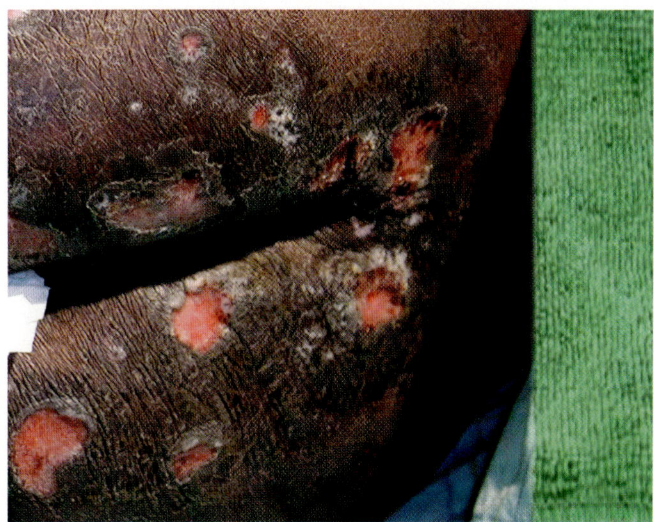

Fig. 71

Figs. 70 and 71: Herpes simplex virus.

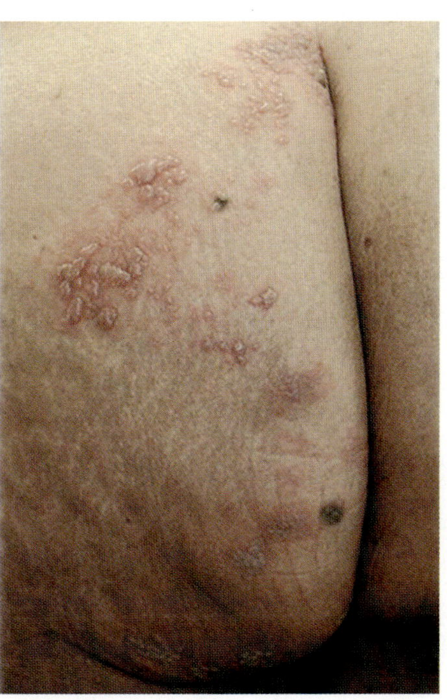

Fig. 72: Varicella zoster.

Tinea versicolor (Figs. 73 and 74): The most common fungal infection affecting renal transplant recipients is tinea versicolor; though immune-competent individuals may also be affected. The causative organism is a yeast, *Pityrosporum*. This yeast is part of normal cutaneous flora, but extensively overgrows in susceptible individuals; the chest and back are most commonly affected. Seen here are the typical scaly "confetti-like" macules of tinea versicolor coalescing into patches. Figure 73 shows a pinkish outbreak, whereas Figure 74 demonstrates hyperpigmentation. Hypopigmentation may also be seen. Diagnosis can be confirmed with microscopic analysis of a scraping treated with potassium hydroxide. Topical use of antifungals and dandruff shampoos can minimize the condition.

Dermatophyte infection—tinea corporis and tinea pedis (Figs. 75 to 77): Fungal infections with dermatophytes are also common in transplant patients. Figure 75 shows an intricate arrangement of concentric and confluent patches with trailing scale at the advancing edge of each lesion. This is a complex lesion of tinea corporis in a transplant patient due to *Trichophyton*. The source for the body infection is often an extensive *Trichophyton* infection (tinea pedis) on the foot (Fig. 76). Figure 77 shows the markedly scaly feet of a *Trichophyton* infection as well. Toe web maceration may be due to *Trichophyton*

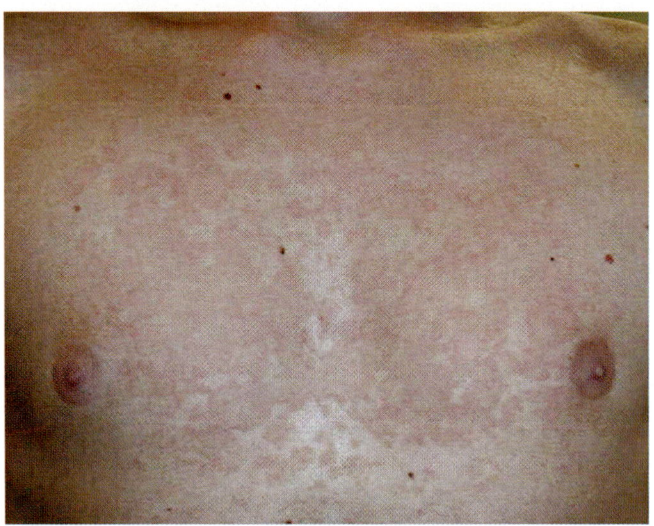

Fig. 73

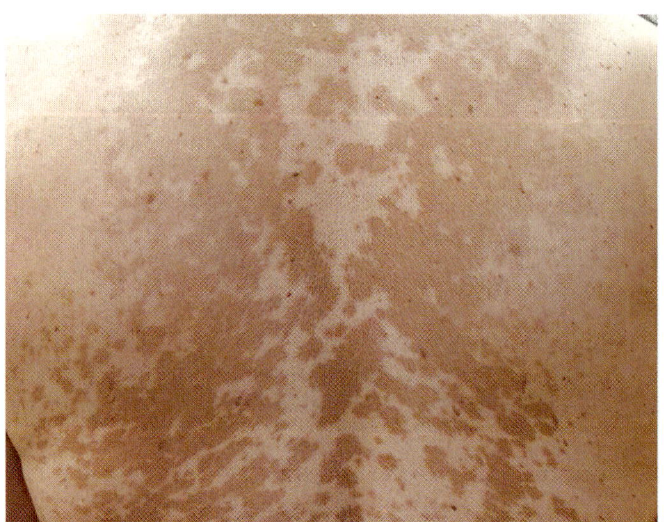

Fig. 74

Figs. 73 and 74: Tinea versicolor.

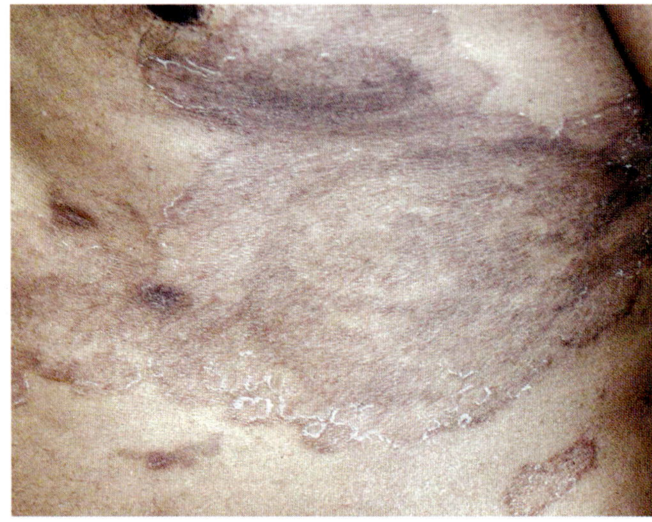

Fig. 75

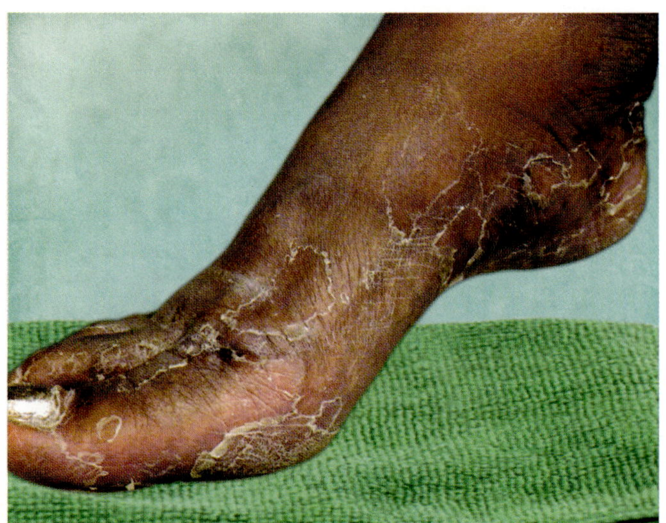

Fig. 76

or represent a more complex infection including yeasts and bacterial and should be cultured. Toe web infections causing epidermal barrier disruption may be associated with an increased risk of lower extremity cellulitis.

Deep fungal infections (Fig. 78): There are a myriad of fungi that can cause subcutaneous and systemic diseases. Some are isolated to various geographic sites and others are more ubiquitous; some infect immune competent as well as immune incompetent. The cutaneous findings are often alike, as is the histology. Special stains and culture determine the diagnoses. The cutaneous findings are that of pseudoepitheliomatous hyperplasia, intraepithelial abscesses, and suppurative and granulomatous inflammation. This lesion was due to *Exophiala jeanselmei*, a dematiaceous mold that is commonly found on walls of saunas and steam baths.

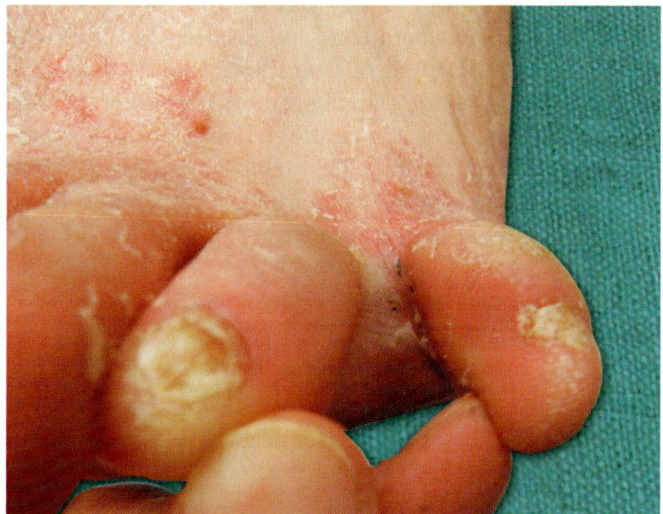

Fig. 77

Figs. 75 to 77: Dermatophyte infection.

Mycobacterial infections (Fig. 79): Transplant recipients are at an increased risk of infection with a variety of acid-fast bacilli (AFB), specifically typical or atypical mycobacteria. These infections are relatively unusual, but may be associated with significant morbidity. The more common of these are from the mycobacterium fortuitum/chelonae complex. The causative organism may be suspected from history, but it must be confirmed by biopsy and culture. Cutaneous findings for all of these are similar—chronic lesions have heaped up, pseudoepitheliomatous hyperplasia or hyperkeratotic papules and plaques and may be similar to that of *Nocardia* and deep fungal infections. Seen in this Figure is an extensive case of *Mycobacterium marinum.* The diagnosis must be made by biopsy and culture.

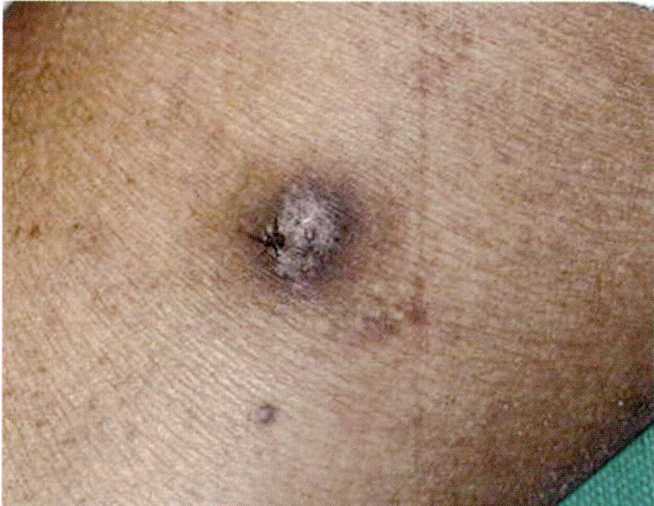

Fig. 78: Deep fungal infections.

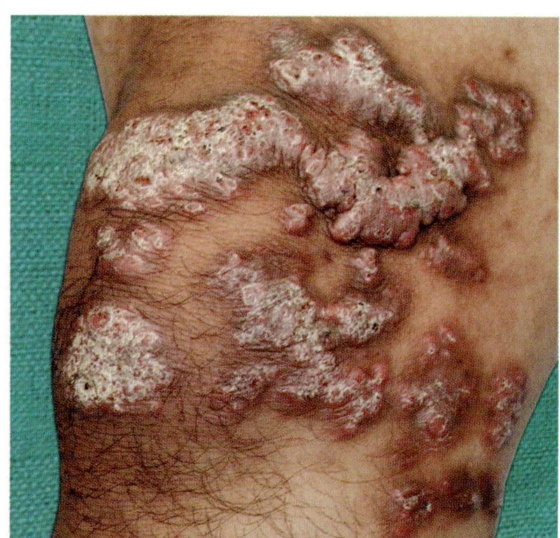

Fig. 79: Mycobacterial infections.

Immunosuppression-Related Malignancy

Solid organ transplant recipients develop cancers at a rate greater than the general population and most cancers are primary skin cancers. The incidence of nonmelanoma skin cancer in the renal transplant recipient is 20–40 times than that of the general population. The first skin cancer usually develops after 5 years of immune suppression and increases after that. Skin type, geographic location, extent of sun exposure, and other factors such as human papilloma viruses also play important roles in the development of skin cancers. It is strongly suggested that in addition to routine skin exams, all patients should be taught sun protection.

Nonmelanoma skin cancers: Basal cell carcinoma (BCC), the most common type of skin cancer, is four times more common than squamous cell carcinoma (SCC) in the general population. This ratio is reversed in the transplant population with SCC out numbering BCC at approximately 4:1. Metastatic disease is extremely rare from BCC but left untreated local destruction may be devastating; it has been estimated that the growth rate for BCC is such that each tumor may double in size over 2 years. SCCs are much more likely to cause metastatic disease and mortality. Excision with margin control is standard of care for most NMSC in the transplant patient. However, some patients with extensive disease may be challenging and require alternative options.

Melanoma: Melanoma occurs two to nine times more frequently in the transplant population than in the general population; rare cases have been transmitted by the donor. There is no consensus regarding the prognosis or risk of recurrence of melanoma in the transplant recipient.

Other skin cancers: Other skin cancers are more common in solid organ transplant recipients as well Two that must be recognized are Merkel cell carcinoma (MCC) and Kaposi sarcoma. Both of these malignancies are associated with infectious organisms: polyomavirus for MCC and human herpes virus type 8 for Kaposi sarcoma. The mortality rate of MCC exceeds that of melanoma.

Basal cell carcinoma (BCC) (Figs. 80 to 82): BCCs are typically translucent papules of various sizes. Starting in the lowest level of the epidermis, early and small lesions may be difficult to detect. Enlarging tumors may outgrow their blood supply allowing for central necrosis of the lesion—nicknamed a rodent ulcer. Figure 80 shows a classic BCC with a pearly translucent border and central crater. These same changes are present in Figure 81, but more difficult to discern. Figure 82 represents an early nodular BCC that is just beginning to form the central crater.

Basal cell carcinoma (BCC) (Figs. 83 and 84) (both Figures are courtesy of Dr. Erin Reese): Figure 83 demonstrates the translucent nature of a nodular BCC; the telangiectasia of the lesion can be well visualized. The vascularity of these lesions often account for the hemorrhage as seen in Figure 84.

Basal cell carcinoma (BCC) (Figs. 85 and 86) (both Figures are courtesy of Dr. Erin Reese): Active melanocytes may be present within BCC and produce melanin. The Figures here show large lesions with central ulceration and variable pigment. The pigment may cause the lesion to be mistaken for a melanoma.

Basal cell carcinoma (BCC) (Fig. 87): Untreated BCC may become very large and destructive. Removal of this extensive BCC will require wide excision with a complex repair.

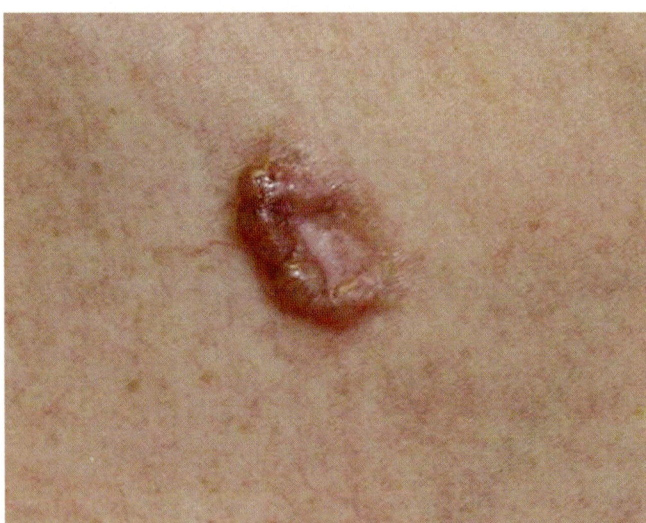

Fig. 80

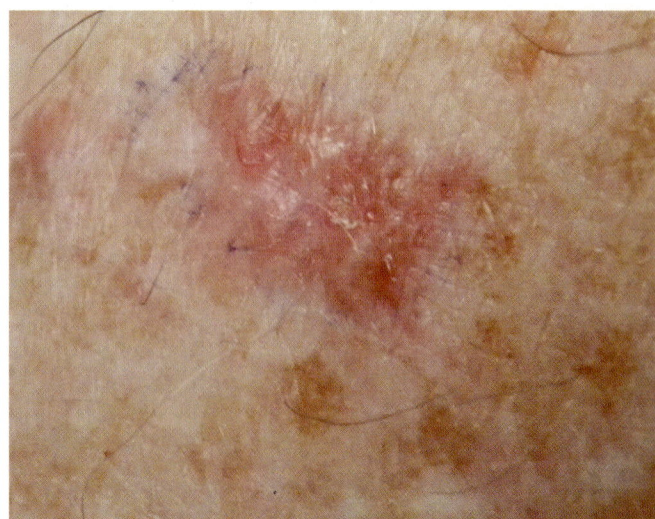

Fig. 81

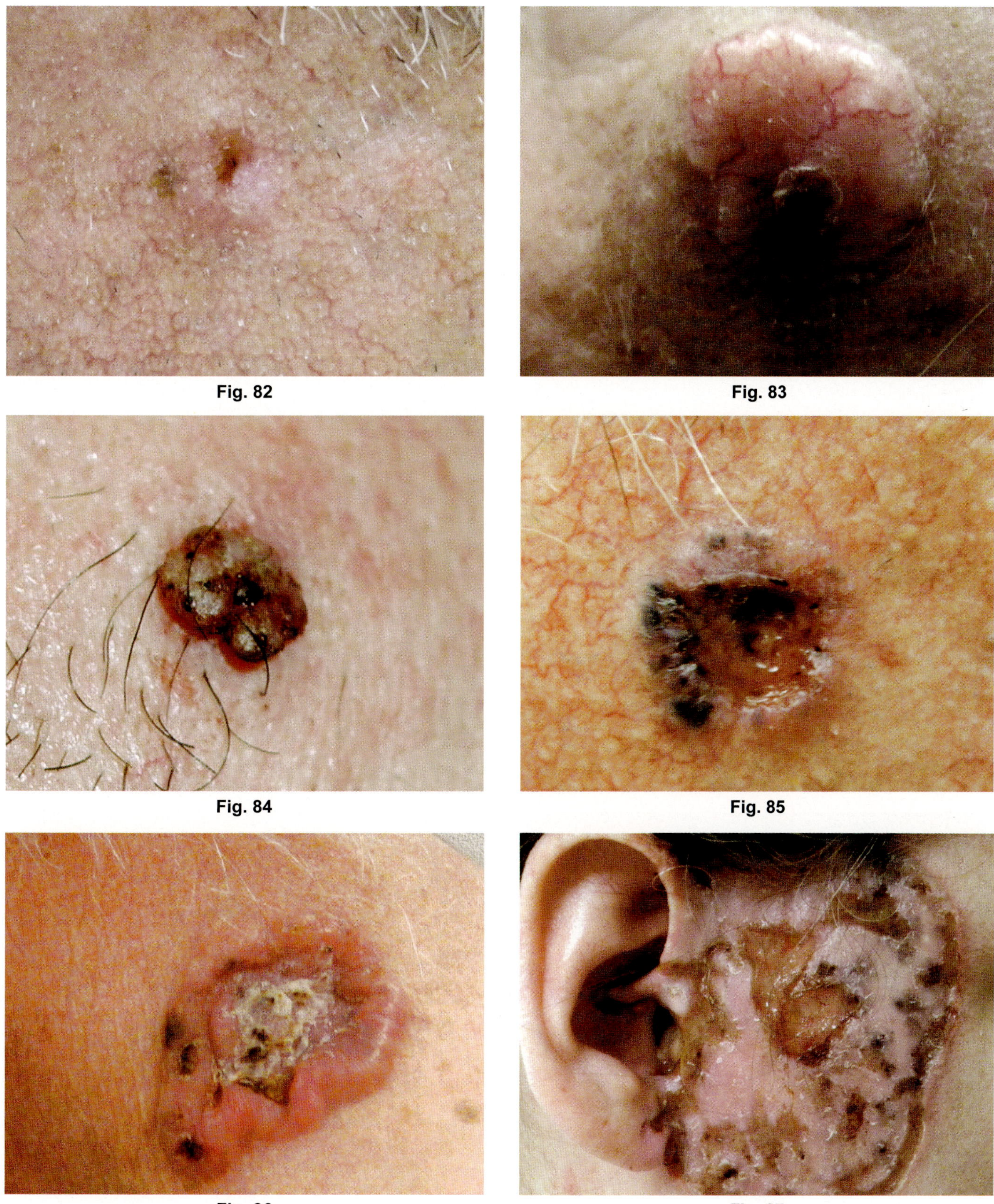

Fig. 82

Fig. 83

Fig. 84

Fig. 85

Fig. 86

Fig. 87

Figs. 80 to 87: Basal cell carcinoma.

Actinic keratosis (AK) (Figs. 88 and 89): The precursor to a squamous cell carcinoma (SCC) is a precancerous lesion called an AK. If left untreated, each AK has a small potential to develop into a SCC. Both AKs and SCCs may have hyperkeratosis as seen in these Figures. Clinically one may be able to differentiate between an AK and infiltrative SCC by palpation. The AK will be superficial—essentially sitting on top of the epidermis; a SCC will have more substance deep to the lesion. If unsure, a biopsy is needed.

Squamous cell carcinoma (SCC) (Fig. 90) (Courtesy of Dr. Algin Garrett): The Figure here shows a lot of chronic actinic damage with extensive hyperkeratotic papules and patches. Hidden in the center of this actinic milieu is a SCC.

Squamous cell carcinoma (SCC) (Fig. 91): Seen here is a classic example of a cutaneous horn. Although a cutaneous horn may overly benign lesions, one must always suspect the presence of a SCC in a transplant recipient.

Squamous cell carcinoma (SCC) (Fig. 92) (courtesy of Dr. Algin Garrett): The lesion in this Figure looks like a BCC; however, biopsy demonstrated it to be a SCC. This is an example of the importance of histologic evaluation for all suspicious lesions.

Squamous cell carcinoma (SCC) (Figs. 93 to 95) (Figs. 94 and 95 are courtesy of Dr. Algin Garrett): SCCs are commonly found on the hands in transplant recipients. Histologic findings in Figure 93 suggested that malignant

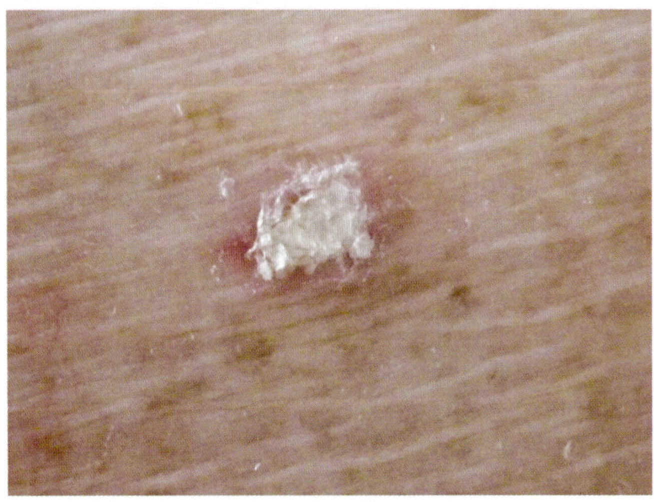

Fig. 88

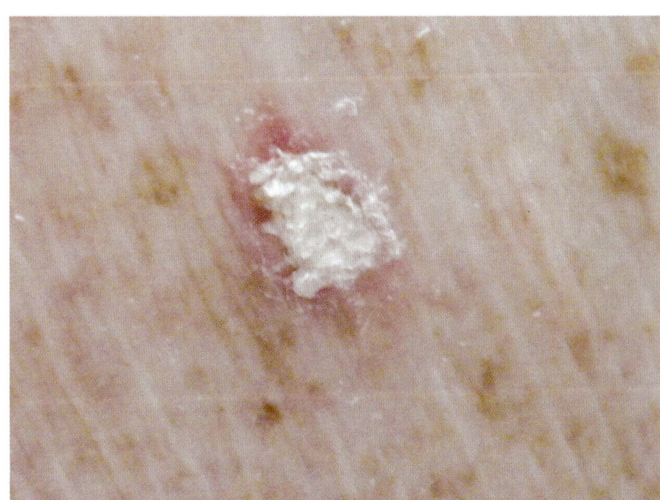

Fig. 89

Figs. 88 and 89: Actinic keratosis.

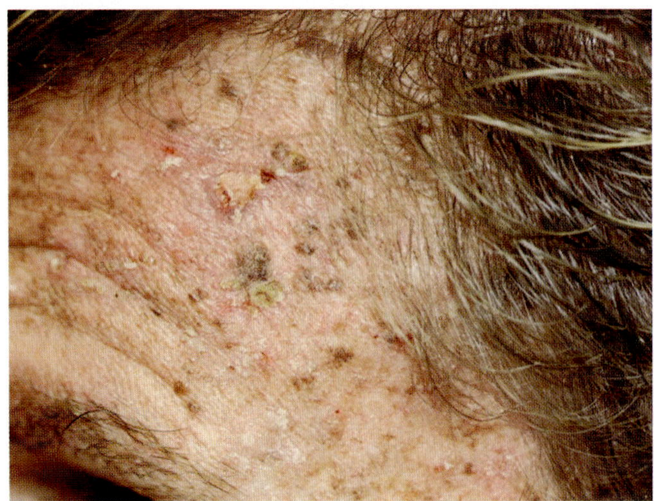

Fig. 90

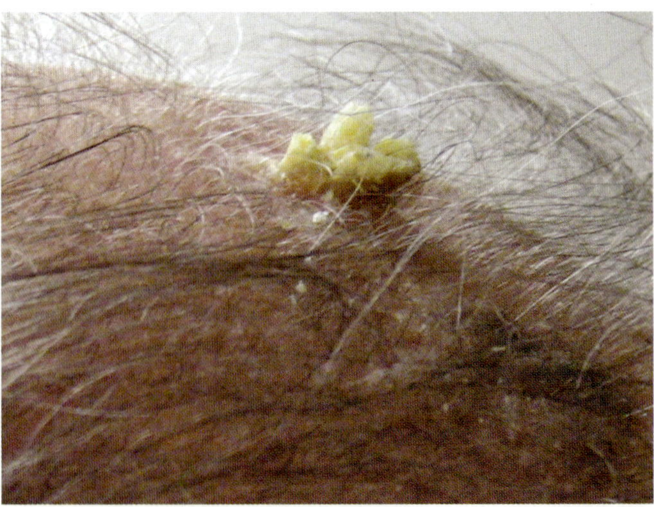

Fig. 91

transformation was associated with HPV infection. Figure 94 shows a typical small infiltrative SCC arising in an actinic keratosis. Figure 95 shows an extensive SCC that required digital amputation.

Squamous cell carcinoma (SCC) (Figs. 96 to 99) (Figs. 96 and 97 are courtesy of Dr. Algin Garrett): All of these lesions are due to an invasive SCC. Lesions of this magnitude have been present for many months to years. Surprisingly, patients don't report these lesions until they are quite problematic. Every patient should have a total body skin exam at least once per year.

Squamous cell carcinoma (SCC) (Figs. 100 to 102) (Figs. 100 and 101 are courtesy of Dr. Algin Garrett): Seen in these Figures are three additional cases of SCC—involving the lip, nose, and ear. Surgical removal is complicated by the anatomic locations of these tumors.

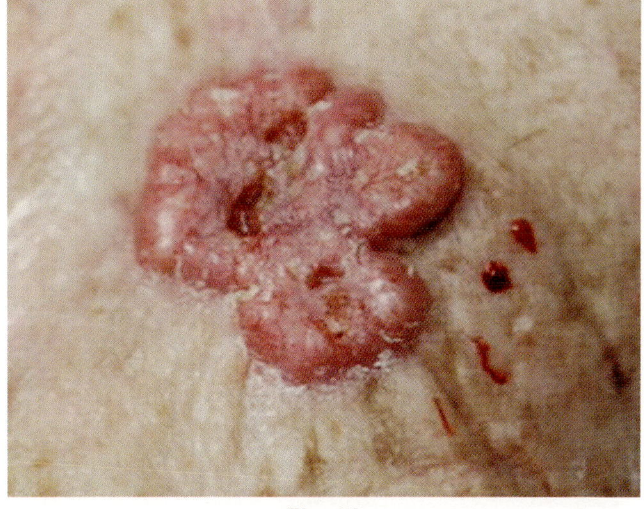

Fig. 92

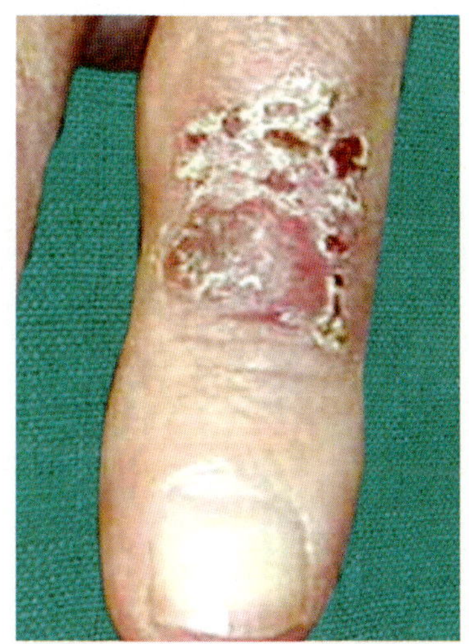

Fig. 93

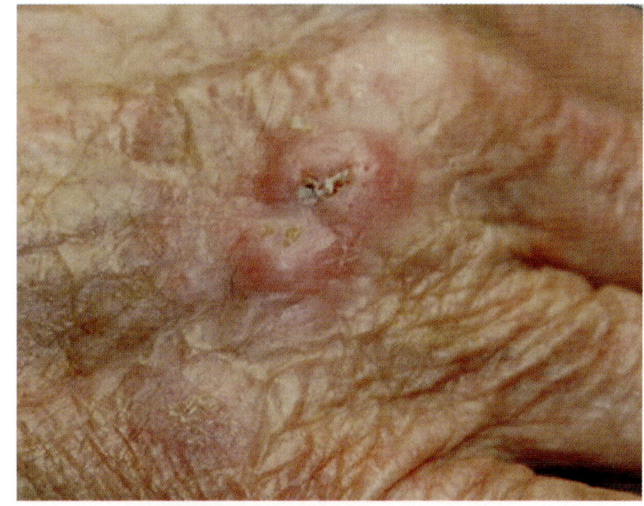

Fig. 94

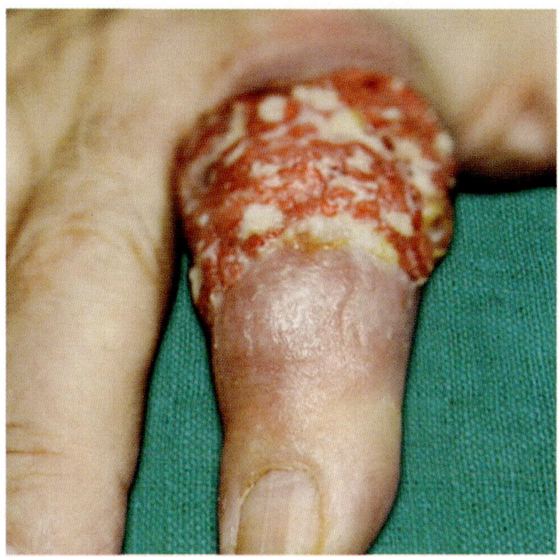

Fig. 95

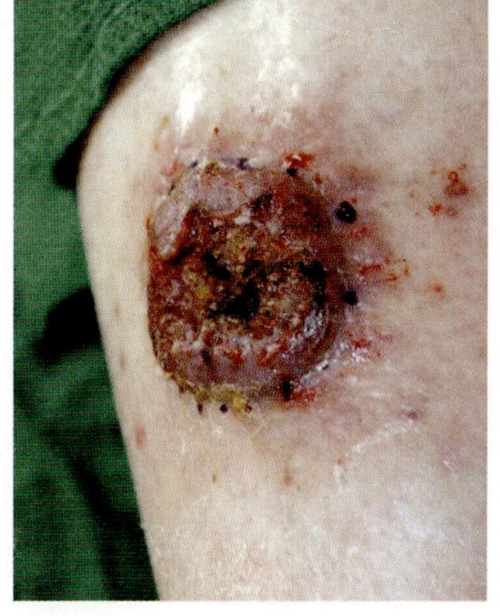

Fig. 96

Figs. 90 to 96: Squamous cell carcinoma.

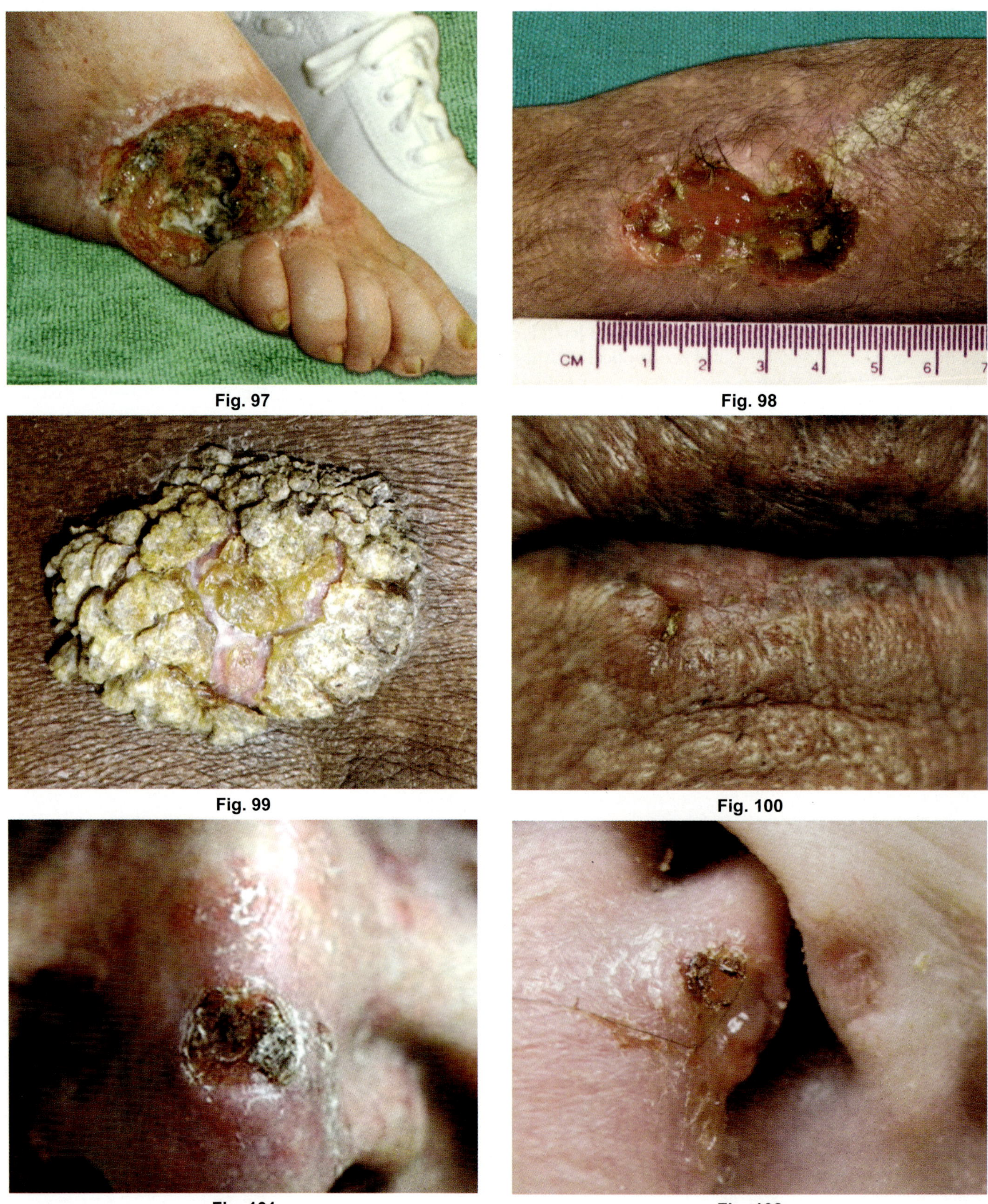

Fig. 97

Fig. 98

Fig. 99

Fig. 100

Fig. 101

Fig. 102

Figs. 97 to 102: Squamous cell carcinoma.

Kaposi sarcoma (Fig. 103): Seen here is a classic purple plaque of Kaposi sarcoma on the nose. Any mucocutaneous surface may be affected. Lesions range from violaceous to brown.

Malignant melanoma (Figs. 104 to 106): Every clinician should be aware of the ABCDEs of melanoma. A = asymmetry; visibly dissect the lesion and look at each half to determine if each half is identical, or if there are there marked differences between the two halves. B = border; determine if the borders are distinct and even or whether they are indistinct and/or notched. C = color; look for one or more colors. Multiple colors are suspicious for malignancy; so is color that seems to spread outside the margin of the lesion. Normal color appearing within a lesion is also of concern; it may represent regression of the melanoma, a poor prognostic sign. D = diameter; most melanomas are larger than 6 mm, although this is

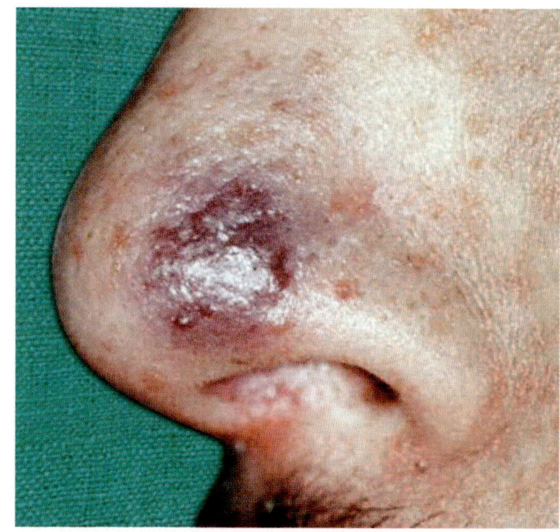

Fig. 103: Kaposi sarcoma.

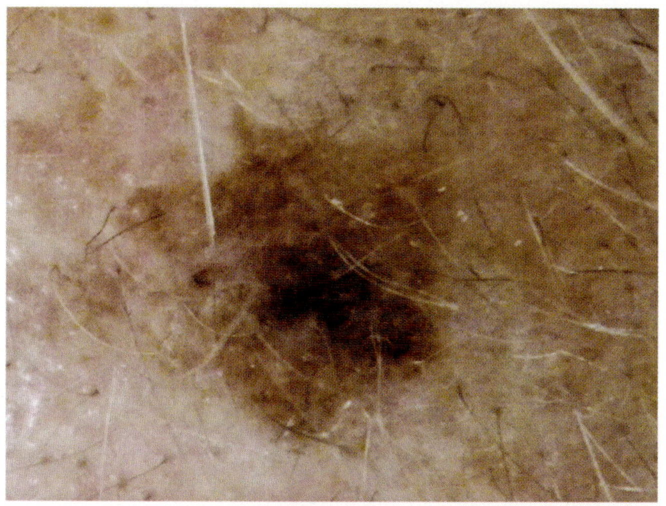

Fig. 104

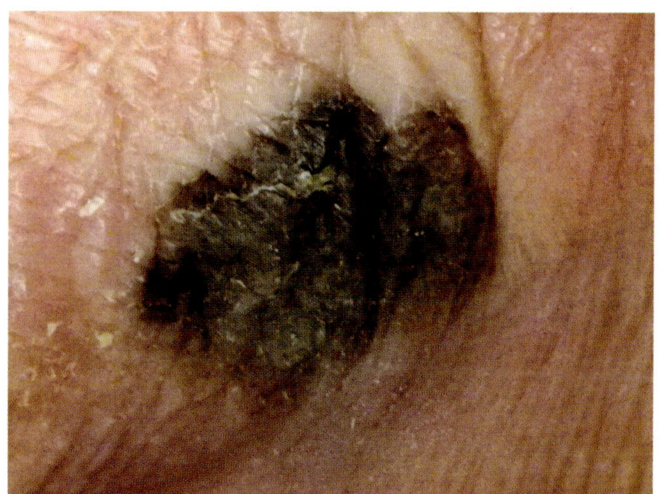

Fig. 105

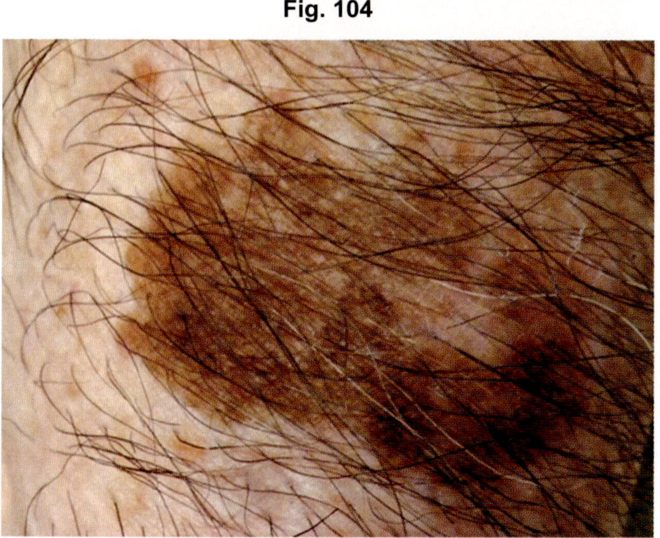

Fig. 106

Figs. 104 to 106: Malignant melanoma.

a very soft sign and melanomas may be much smaller. E = evolving. This is the newest of the parameters and is critically important. Tumors grow and changes. Not every tumor is cancerous, but every evolving lesion needs adequate attention.

Nail Changes Seen in Kidney Diseases

Nail fold capillary abnormalities (Fig. 107): An exam of the proximal nail fold may be quite helpful when suspecting the presence of a connective tissue disease. Tortuous capillary loops are commonly present in dermatomyositis, lupus, and systemic sclerosis, though it may be difficult to differentiate between these conditions by these changes alone. Seen here is an example of the abnormal capillary loops and irregular cuticle that belies an underlying connective tissue disease.

Half and half nails (Lindsey nails) (Fig. 108): Changes in nail beds may also be suggestive of an underlying systemic condition. Seen here is a classic example of half and half (Lindsey) nails. The proximal portion of the nail is white compared with the distal portion that can be pink, brown, or red. It is not pathognomonic of kidney disease but affects close to 70% of the dialysis population.

Beau lines (Fig. 109): Beau lines are grooves that run horizontally across the nail plate. They are thought to be caused by a temporary disruption of nail production associated with a significant systemic illness or stress, but not always related to kidney issues. When the systemic incident resolves or improves, nail production resumes. The nail plate before and after the incident is normal, but very thin during the time of illness. These nails will eventually grow out.

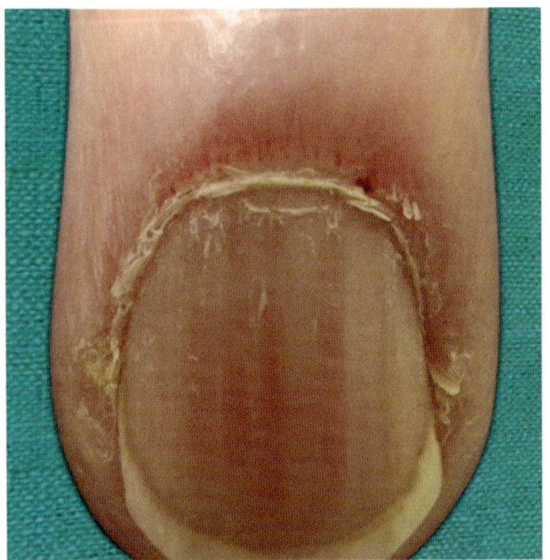

Fig. 107: Nail fold capillary abnormalities.

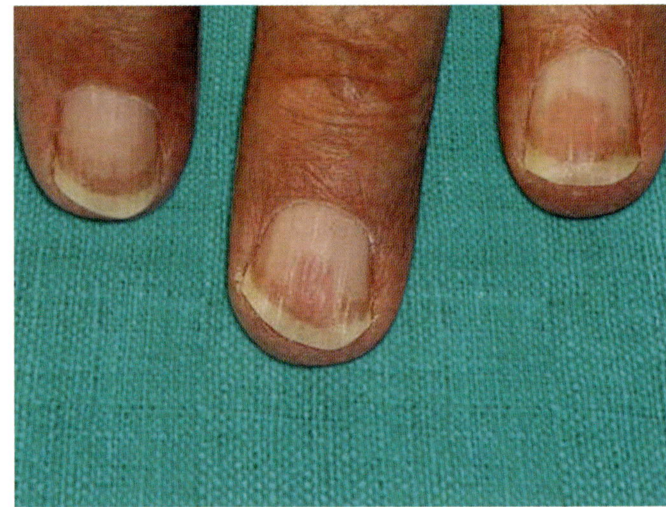

Fig. 108: Half and half nails (Lindsey nails).

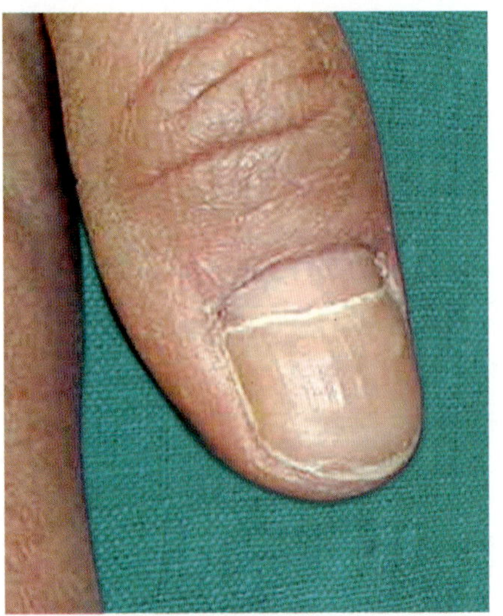

Fig. 109: Beau lines.

Cutaneous Drug Reactions

Drug reactions are not necessarily more common or more severe in patients with kidney disease or transplantation. However, in general, drug reactions are common and will be seen by practitioners caring for dialysis and transplant patients.

Exanthem (Figs. 110 and 111): The morbilliform drug eruption is by far the most common. It accounts for approximately 96% of all cutaneous adverse drug reactions. It begins most commonly on the back, progresses to the chest and abdomen, and then evolves peripherally to affect the upper and lower extremities. The head and neck and face are rarely affected. It consists of a blanchable maculopapular erythema. Patients are uniformly itchy. Figure 110 shows discrete blanchable lesions before they coalesce. Figure 111 shows the same process in a patient with color. The erythema can be difficult to see by those inexperienced with examining skin. Although antibiotics are the most common culprits, most any drug can cause an exanthem. A similar eruption may be seen with viral exanthems.

Fixed drug reaction (Fig. 112): A fixed drug eruption is a curious process. The term "fixed" refers to the location of the eruption in a given patient, meaning that each time the patient is exposed to the offending agent the same area will flair—the rash is "fixed" in location for that individual. However, if repetitive courses of the same agent are given, new areas, in addition to the old areas, will flair. When active, typical lesions are round to oval and reddish in color. Pigmentary alteration with marked residual hyperpigmentation is common. Although many drugs can cause this eruption, it is more common with nonsteroidal agents, laxatives, and sulfa antibiotics.

Lichenoid drug reaction (Fig. 113): Lichenoid drug eruptions clinically and histologically resemble lichen planus, although the drug-induced condition tends to be more severe with confluent lesions. The eruption

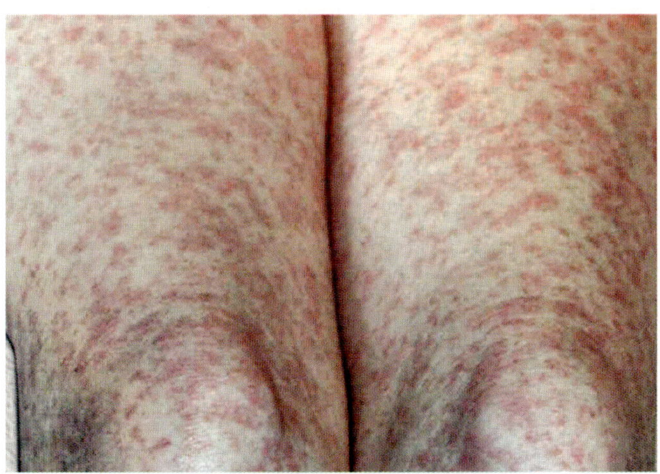

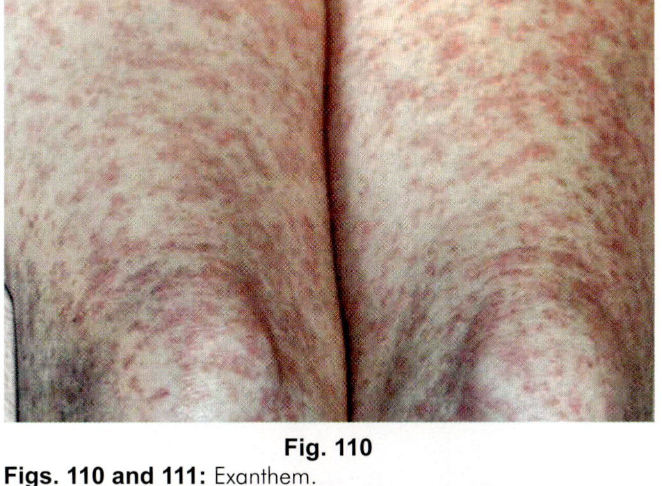

Fig. 110

Fig. 111

Figs. 110 and 111: Exanthem.

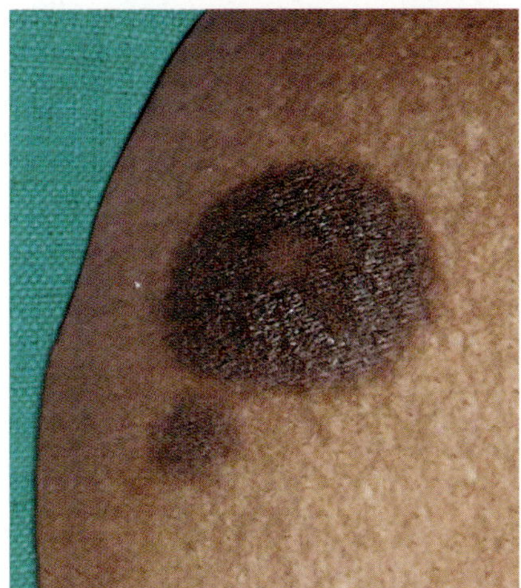

Fig. 112: Fixed drug reaction.

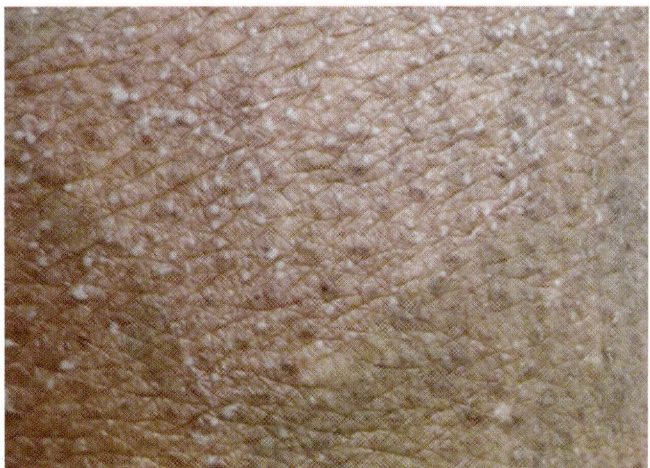

Fig. 113: Lichenoid drug reaction.

may start up to 1 year after the culprit drug was initiated. Seen here are confluent erythematous hyperpigmented papules and plaques in a statin-induced case of lichenoid drug eruption.

Leukocytoclastic vasculitis (LCV) (Fig. 114): LCV can occur in many settings. Seen here is a case of hemorrhagic LCV due to a β-lactam antibiotic in a hemodialysis patient.

Acute generalized exanthematous pustulosis (AGEP) (Fig. 115): AGEP develops as a rapid onset eruption consisting of generalized erythema studded with superficial small pustules. Patients are usually febrile and may or may not have a more significant systemic hypersensitivity reaction as well. The differential includes Stevens–Johnson syndrome (SJS), but unlike SJS, there is no mucosal involvement. The most common offending agents are antibiotics.

Erythema multiforme (EM) (Figs. 116 and 117): The two Figures here demonstrate some of the variability seen in EM. The classic example is a targetoid lesion with a dusky center. Lesions on the palms are significant; EM is one of only a few diseases that typically affect the palms and soles. The most common cause of EM is a recurring episode of herpes simplex. The second most common cause is a drug.

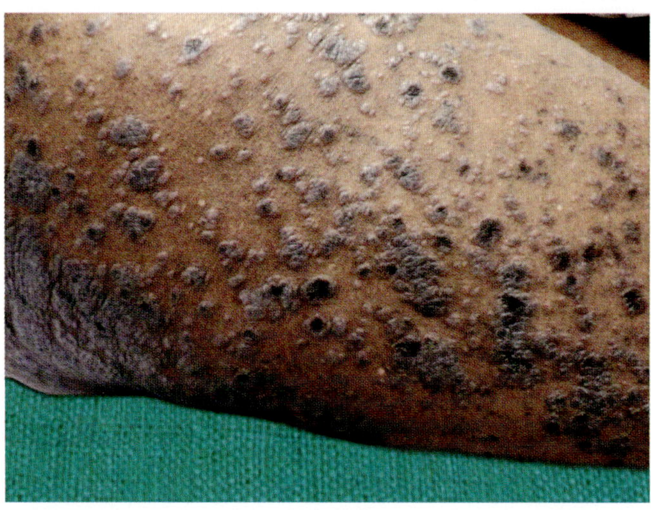

Fig. 114: Leukocytoclastic vasculitis.

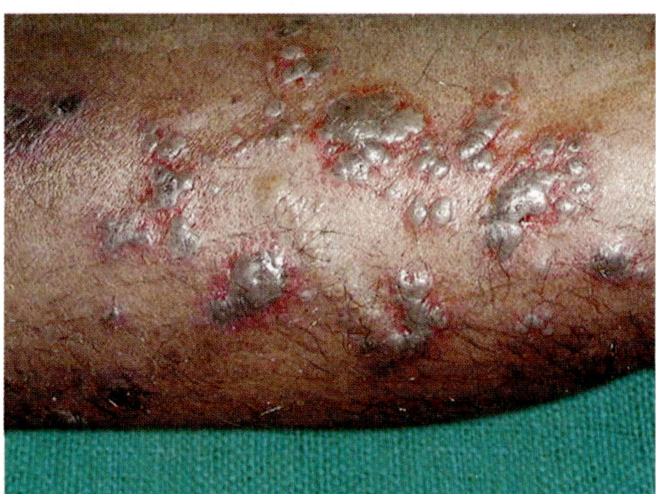

Fig. 115: Acute generalized exanthematous pustulosis.

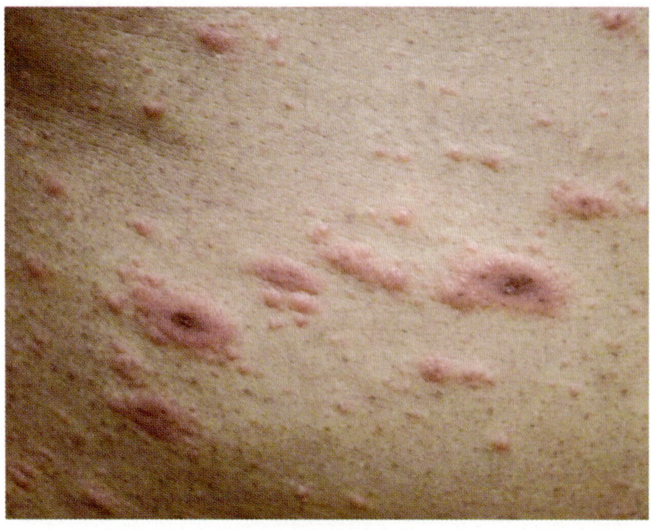

Fig. 116

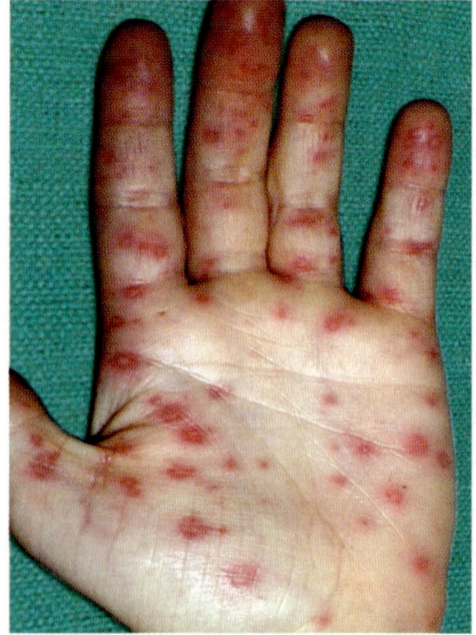

Fig. 117

Figs. 116 and 117: Erythema multiforme.

Stevens-Johnson syndrome (SJS) (Figs. 118 and 119): SJS is an immunologically mediated hypersensitivity reaction. Over the years, there has been much debate regarding SJS, toxic epidermal necrolysis (TEN), and EM. It is now mostly thought that erythema multiforme (EM) is one disease and SJS and TEN represent a disease spectrum. The diagnosis of SJS requires involvement of more than one mucosal surface. Figure 118 demonstrates atypical targetoid lesions suggestive of SJS; Figure 119 demonstrates the characteristic hemorrhagic-crusted oral mucosa of SJS and TEN.

Toxic epidermal necrolysis (TEN) (Figs. 120 and 121): TEN is the most severe of the cutaneous adverse drug reactions. By definition skin detachment is greater than 30% of the body surface area. Mortality rates range between 10% and 90%. Figure 120 demonstrates sloughing of skin over the lower leg. Figure 121 shows cutaneous hemorrhage preceding frank sloughing also on the lower extremity.

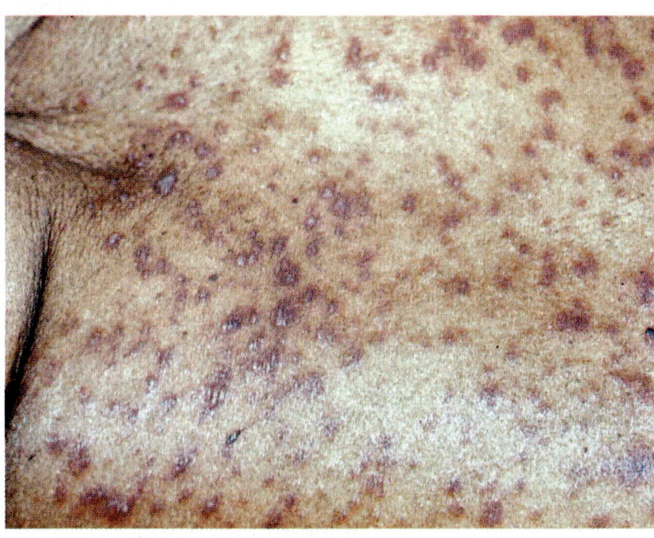

Fig. 118

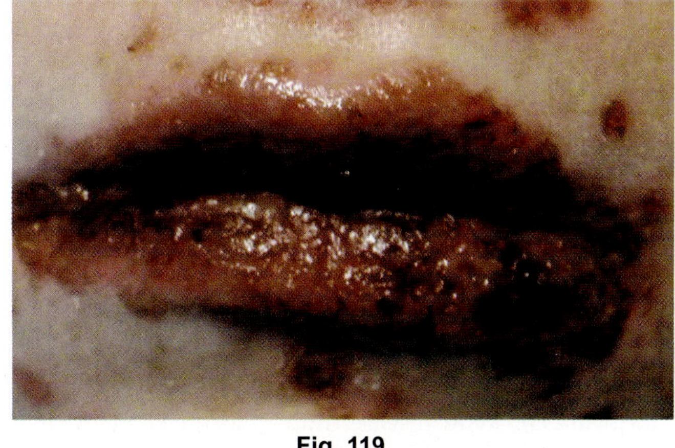

Fig. 119

Figs. 118 and 119: Stevens–Johnson syndrome.

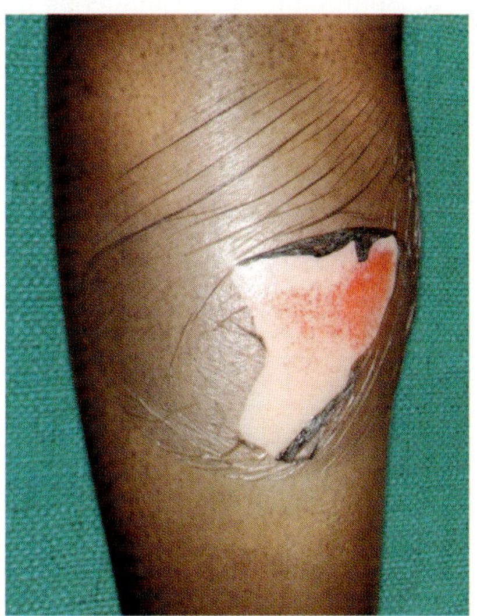

Fig. 120

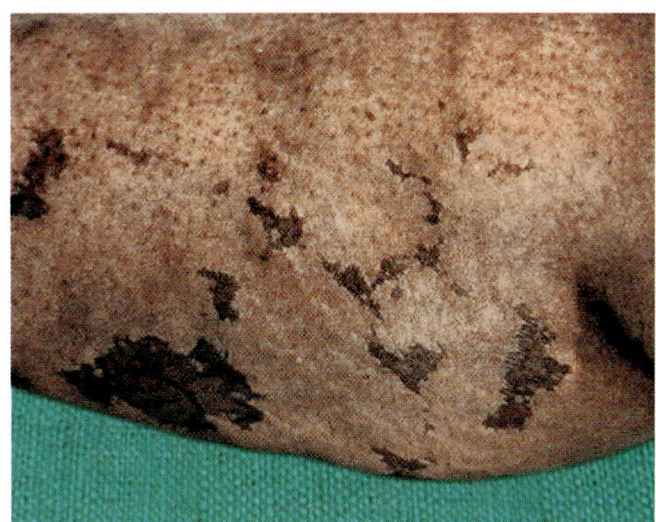

Fig. 121

Figs. 120 and 121: Toxic epidermal necrolysis.

FURTHER READING

1. Badiee P, Alborzi A. Invasive fungal infections in renal transplant recipients. Exp Clin Transplant. 2011; 9:355-62.
2. Bangash HK, Colegio OR. Management of non-melanoma skin cancer in immunocompromised solid organ transplant recipients. Curr Treat Options Oncol 2012; 13:354-76.
3. Bernstein EJ, Schmidt-Lauber C, Kay J, et al. Nephrogenic systemic fibrosis: a systemic fibrosing disease resulting from gadolinium exposure. Best Pract Res Clin Rheumatol 2012; 26:489-503.
4. Callen JP. Discoid lupus erythematosus. http://emedicine.medscape.com/article/1065529-overview
5. Dalianis T, Hirsch HH. Human polyomaviruses in disease and cancer. Virology 2013; 437:63-72.
6. Euvrard S, Morelon E, Rostaing L, et al. Sirolimus and secondary skin-cancer prevention in kidney transplantation N Engl J Med 2012; 367:329-39.
7. Feller L, Motswaledi MH, Chandran R, et al. Lupus erythematosus: a short account. SADJ 2011; 66:234-6.
8. Gera DN, Yadav DK, Patil SB, et al. Post-renal transplant Kaposi's sarcoma of the skin. Indian journal of nephrology. 2013; 23:78-80.
9. Hagen JW, Magro CM, Crowson AN, et al. Emerging adverse cutaneous drug reactions. Dermatol Clin. 2012; 30:695-730.
10. Hempel C, Martin C. Getting under the skin of adverse drug reactions. Orthopedics 2012; 35:872-6.
11. Hogan DJ. Kyrle disease. http://emedicine.medscape.com/article/1074469-overview
12. Jadali Z. Dermatologic manifestations of hepatitis C infection and the effect of interferon therapy: a literature review. Arch Iran Med 2012; 15:43-8.
13. Khan DA. Cutaneous drug reactions. J Allergy Clin Immunol 2012; 130:1225.e1-1225.e6
14. Ko HM, Hernandez-Prera JC, Zhu H, et al. Morphologic features of extrahepatic manifestations of hepatitis C virus infection. Clin Dev Immunol 2012; 2012:740138. doi: 10.1155/2012/740138. Epub 2012 Aug 5. Review. PMID: 22919404
15. Kuschal C, Thoms KM, Schubert S, et al. Skin cancer in organ transplant recipients: effects of immunosuppressive medications on DNA repair. Exp Dermatol 2012; 21:2-6.
16. Lodi G, Pellicano R, Carrozzo M, et al. Hepatitis C virus infection and lichen planus: a systematic review with meta-analysis. Oral Dis 2010; 16:601-12.
17. Motswaledi MH, Khammissa RA, Wood NH, et al. Discoid lupus erythematosus as it relates to cutaneous squamous cell carcinoma and to photosensitivity. SADJ 2011; 66:340-3.
18. Nunley JR. Dermatologic Manifestations of Renal Disease. http://emedicine.medscape.com/article/1094846-overview
19. Nunley, JR. Calciphylaxis. http://emedicine.medscape.com/article/1095481-overview
20. Ryan Caballes F, et al. Hepatitis C, porphyria cutanea tarda and liver iron: an update. Liver Int 2012; 32:880-93.
21. Shanmugam VK, Steen VD. Renal disease in scleroderma: an update on evaluation, risk stratification, pathogenesis and management. Curr Opin Rheumatol 2012; 24:669-76.
22. Tajbakhsh R, et al. Mucocutaneous manifestations and nail changes in patients with end-stage renal disease on hemodialysis. Saudi J Kidney Dis Transpl 2013; 24:36-40.
23. Tuttolomondo A, et al. Anderson-Fabry disease: a multiorgan disease. Curr Pharm Des 2013. [5Epub ahead of print] PMID: 23448451
24. Walling HW, Sontheimer RD. Cutaneous lupus erythematosus: issues in diagnosis and treatment. Am J Clin Dermatol 2009; 10:365-81.
25. Yu X, Han F, et al. Nocardia infection in kidney transplant recipients: case report and analysis of 66 published cases. Transplant Infect Dis 2011; 13:385-9.

PART 2 PANCREAS TRANSPLANTATION

CHAPTER 65

Overview

Christine Sardo Molmenti, Angelika Gruessner, Jeffrey Nicastro, Gene Coppa, Christine E Gruessner, Stefan A Gruessner, Horacio Rilo, Ernesto P Molmenti, Rainer Gruessner

The main goals of pancreas transplantation are:

- Insulin independence and normoglycemia with normal hemoglobin A1c levels
- Prolonged survival
- Improved quality of life

Over 50% of pancreas recipients have systemic dysfunctions at the time of transplantation.

Dysfunctions can be of varied nature, and include but are not limited to:

- Gastrointestinal
- Neurologic
- Ocular
- Renal
- Cardiac vascular

Pancreas transplantation:

- Is the only system able to achieve a continuous euglycemic environment (with normal glycosylated hemoglobin levels) in the absence of exogenous insulin
- Insulin independence is frequently achieved immediately after transplantation
- On a long-term basis, may prevent the progression (or development) of diabetic complications such as:
  - Retinopathy
  - Nephropathy
  - Lipid derangements
  - Cardiac dysfunction
  - Motor, sensory, and autonomic neuropathy

INDICATIONS AND PATIENT SELECTION

Candidates for pancreatic transplantation include:

- Type 1 diabetics (main indication)
- Selected type 2 diabetics
- Failed previous pancreas transplant recipients
- Diabetics due to total pancreatectomy, (for example, due to chronic pancreatitis)
- Diabetics due to cystic fibrosis (very rare)

A thorough preoperative workup is essential in order to optimize patient and graft outcome.

Cardiovascular complications (e.g., myocardial infarction or stroke) constitute the major source of morbidity and mortality.

PANCREATIC TRANSPLANT CATEGORIES

Simultaneous Pancreas Kidney (SPK) Transplantation (80% of Cases)

- Most frequent type of pancreas transplant
- Indicated for type 1 diabetics with renal failure
- Simultaneous implantation of both organs
- Immunosuppression similar for both organs

Pancreas After Kidney (PAK) Transplantation (15% of Cases)

- Most frequently indicated for type 1 diabetics who
  - Received a previous kidney transplant (such as from a live donor)
  - Received a previous SPK or PAK in which only the pancreas graft has failed

Pancreas Transplantation Alone (PTA) (5% of Cases)

- Indicated primarily in labile ("brittle") type 1 diabetics with hypoglycemic unawareness

- Also a consideration in type 1 diabetics who wish to eliminate (or diminish) the risk or progression of diabetic complications *in exchange for* immunosuppression

DONOR SELECTION AND PROCUREMENT

- When considering potential deceased donors, the accepting surgeon should determine the likelihood of function after implantation based on donor quality
- A history of diabetes in the donor should always be excluded
- Hyperglycemia in a brain dead donor does not constitute by itself a contraindication to pancreatic procurement
- At the time of procurement (and during the back table preparation), the organ should be inspected for the presence of detrimental factors such as inflammation, tumors, edema, fatty infiltration, fibrosis, necrosis, lacerations, and injuries
- During procurement, the dissection and mobilization of the pancreas, irrespective of the surgical approach, usually follows anatomical and embryological planes of adhesion
- The donor common, internal, and external iliac arteries and veins should be procured for the subsequent back table reconstruction

FURTHER READING

1. Gruessner AC, Sutherland DE, Gruessner RW. Long-term outcome after pancreas transplantation. Curr Opin Organ Transplant 2012;17:100–5.
2. Molmenti EP. Transplantation of the pancreas. In: Cameron JL, ed.: Current Surgical Therapy, 8th ed. Philadelphia: Elsevier Mosby, 2004;525-32.
3. Sutherland DE, Gruessner RW, Dunn DL, et al. Lessons learned from more than 1,000 pancreas transplants at a single institution. Ann Surg 2001;233:463–501.

CHAPTER 66

Operative Technique

Christine Sardo Molmenti, Angelika Gruessner, Jeffrey Nicastro, Gene Coppa, Christine E Gruessner, Stefan A Gruessner, Horacio Rilo, Ernesto P Molmenti, Rainer Gruessner

BACK TABLE PREPARATION

- Correct identification of donor organs and intended recipients following established protocols is essential to prevent potentially fatal errors
- Sterility is maintained at all times
- All specimens should preferably be sent for pathologic identification and evaluation
- During the back table preparation, the organ is prepared for implantation
- The reconstruction of the superior mesenteric and splenic arteries is undertaken with the donor iliac artery ("Y") graft obtained at the time of procurement
- The purpose of the back table preparation is to enable or facilitate the subsequent implantation of the organ
- The main task during the back table preparation is the arterial reconstruction. This is usually achieved with the Y-shaped iliac artery obtained from the donor (external iliac artery to superior mesenteric artery (SMA); internal iliac artery to splenic artery)
- In our experience, pancreas grafts rarely require elongation of the portal vein with donor iliac vein. However, some disagree with this view and routinely perform it
- Figure 1 shows a pancreas allograft ready for implantation

IMPLANTATION

- Immunosuppression therapy is started prior to implantation
- Some of us (RG) administer heparin on a routine basis toward the end of the case
- Some of us (EM) do not routinely administer intravenous heparin during the procedure. In these instances, intravenous (IV) dextran is started in the immediate postoperative period and continued for 48 hours
- Some of us (RG) administer insulin intraoperatively and postoperatively to maintain blood glucose levels less than or equal to 120 mg/dL
- Some of us (EM) do not provide any exogenous insulin and rather follow glucose levels as a way to monitor allograft function
- As the allograft produces insulin, glucose levels decrease
- Sudden increases in glucose levels should be viewed as a sign of allograft dysfunction, and an immediate evaluation of the allograft (primarily of its blood supply) should be undertaken
- Venous drainage of the pancreas graft can be systemic (usually iliac vein) or portal [superior mesenteric vein (SMV)]

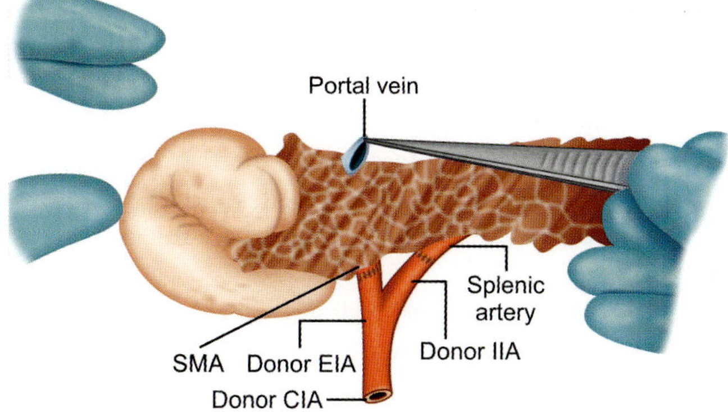

Fig. 1: Pancreas allograft ready for implantation. *Source:* Molmenti EP. Transplantation of the pancreas. In: Cameron JL (Ed). Current Surgical Therapy, 8th edition. Elsevier Mosby; 2004.

- Systemic venous drainage is associated with higher blood insulin levels than portal drainage (first pass effect on the liver)
- Exocrine pancreatic secretions can be diverted into the bladder or small bowel
- Bladder drainage:
  - Allows for pancreatic urinary amylase measurements
    - Low urinary amylase levels proceed to hyperglycemia by 5–7 days and allow for successful rejection treatment in about 90% cases
  - Allows for cystoscopic pancreas graft biopsies
  - Is usually associated with multiple metabolic and urologic complications
- In instances of enteric drainage, we perform an anastomosis of the donor duodenum to the recipient jejunum

IMPLANTATION OF THE PANCREATIC ALLOGRAFT

Preoperative Considerations

- We meet with the patient immediately prior to the procedure to address any pending questions
- In instances of a combined kidney pancreas, we usually perform the pancreatic implantation prior to the renal one, to minimize the pancreas cold ischemic time
  - In cases of systemic venous drainage (anastomosis to the external iliac vessels), the pancreas is preferably placed in the right lower quadrant:
    - Allows drainage of exocrine contents into the small bowel or bladder
    - Placing the pancreas in the right lower quadrant provides alignment of the iliac vessels and prevents topographic impediments (to the small bowel and bladder) associated with the left/sigmoid colon
    - Allows easier access to the bladder in instances where bladder drainage is desired
  - The kidney is routinely placed in the left lower quadrant
  - This sidedness may be altered depending on:
    - Surgeon preference
    - Vascular disease involvement of iliac vessels
    - Previous surgeries (transplants, ostomies, scars)
    - Other factors
- Verify that the correct allograft is available or will be available at the time of implantation
- The recipient should have adequates venous access—at least two large-bore peripheral IV
- Central venous lines *not* routinely placed
- Arterial lines *only* if needed based on recipient characteristics
- Urinary catheter *always* placed
- Oral aspirin is routinely administered prior to and after the procedure
- It is also our practice *not* to discontinue medications that recipients may have been taking on a routine basis such as clopidogrel and oral anticoagulants given the high risk of cardiovascular complications faced by most of our patients
- IV fluids:
  - Combined kidney pancreas transplant
    - We routinely administer 2–4 L of isotonic crystalloids during the entire procedure
    - We prefer normal saline
    - Lactated Ringer's solution is preferred by others
    - Adding potassium to IV fluids is discouraged
  - Isolated pancreas transplant
    - The volume of IV fluids administered is based on the physiologic needs of each individual patient
- We routinely administer subcutaneous heparin (unless therapeutically anticoagulated) immediately prior to the case, and maintain sequential compression devices on both lower extremities during the entire case to diminish the incidence of deep venous thromboses

Timeout

- Performed immediately prior to incision after the abdomen has been painted and draped
- Review all medications given preoperatively
- Intravenous antibiotics administered (assuring that they are received within minutes of incision)
- Other medications administered
  - Induction agents:
    - If combined kidney pancreas
      - 500 mg solumedrol (or other desired dosage)
      - 25 g mannitol
      - 100 mg of furosemide (alternatively, diuretics can be infused prior to reperfusion)

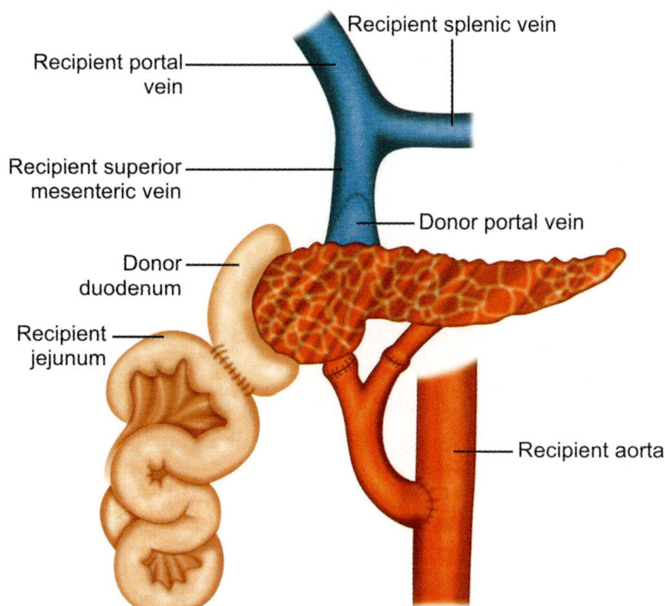

Fig. 2: Portal venous output with enteric drainage of exocrine secretions.
Source: Molmenti EP. Transplantation of the pancreas. In: Cameron JL (Ed). Current Surgical Therapy, 8th edition. Elsevier Mosby; 2004.

Portal Venous Output with Enteric Drainage of Exocrine Secretions

This is our preferred technique (EM). Figure 2 illustrates the portal venous output with enteric drainage of exocrine secretions technique.

Exposure

- Midline abdominal incision
- Superior mesenteric vein is dissected at the root of small bowel mesentery and exposed for the future anastomosis
- The abdominal aorta is dissected distal to the renal arteries making sure not to injure the inferior mesenteric artery
- The pancreatic allograft is brought into the operative field
- Our preference is to wrap it in a gauze with ice slush
  - The portal vein and reconstructed arterial vessels are exteriorized through an opening to allow for their anastomosis
  - The pancreas is clearly identified to prevent implantation mistakes
- Although we do not routinely do so, some surgeons prefer to systemically heparinize the recipient at the time of implantation

Vascular Implantation

- The venous anastomosis is performed first
  - A delicate semicircular clamp is placed on the dissected SMV
  - The vein is incised
  - The transplant portal vein is anastomosed end-to-side onto the recipient SMV
- The orientation of the donor portal vein should be carefully preserved in order to avoid torsions, kinks, and twists
- We routinely perform the venous anastomosis with a continuous nonresorbable monofilament suture (our preference is 6-0)
  - After completion of the anastomosis, a bulldog clamp is placed on the donor portal vein and the semicircular clamp on the recipient SMV is partially released
    - This allows for verification of hemostasis
  - The clamp on the SMV is subsequently released completely, allowing for continued enteric venous flow
- The arterial anastomosis is subsequently addressed
- The common iliac limb of the arterial graft used for the reconstruction is brought through an opening in the ascending colon mesentery
  - A semicircular clamp is placed on the infrarenal aorta at a site with as little atherosclerotic disease as possible
  - The aorta is incised. The opening can be enlarged and made round with an aortic hole puncher
- The transplant arterial graft is anastomosed end-to-side onto the recipient infrarenal aorta
  - Special attention has to be placed on preventing twist and/or kinks in the transplant arterial graft
  - We routinely perform the anastomosis with a continuous nonresorbable monofilament suture (our preference is 5-0)
    - Alternatively, the transplant arterial graft can be anastomosed
      - End-to-side onto the recipient common or external iliac artery
- After completion of the anastomosis, hemostasis is verified by placing a bulldog clamp on the transplant arterial graft and gently partially releasing the semicircular clamp on the aorta
- Prior to reperfusion, we verify that the recipient has:
  - Received adequate amounts of IV fluids
  - A systolic blood pressure of 120 mm Hg or higher
    - If this pressure is not achieved, options include
      - Additional IV fluids
      - Use of pressors
    - Hypotension can be an indicator of acute cardiac events

- The allograft is subsequently reperfused by releasing the clamps on the transplant portal vein and arterial graft
- Adequate reperfusion is characterized by:
  - The allograft becoming rapidly pink
  - Palpable pulses in the:
    - Transplant arterial graft
    - Transplant SMA
    - Transplant splenic vein
  - Adequate venous flow in the transplant portal vein
  - Distension of the transplant duodenum with newly produced exocrine secretions of the allograft
- If reperfusion is slow or poor:
  - Evaluate for vascular problems:
    - Kinks/twists
    - Defective anastomosis
    - Poor inflow/outflow involving native vessels
- If there are isolated areas of poor or no perfusion
  - Evaluate for:
    - Embolic events
    - Back table arterial reconstruction defects associated with impaired flow at the transplant SMA or splenic artery
  - Poor perfusion and ischemia of the transplant duodenum can be associated with subsequent anastomotic leaks/breakdown
- Place the pancreas in a position allowing for the vessels to lie in a comfortable way with no kinks or twists
- Perform an intraoperative Doppler evaluation of the:
  - Transplant arterial graft
  - Transplant SMA
  - Transplant splenic vein
  - Recipient aorta
  - Transplant portal vein
  - Recipient SMV

Enteric Drainage

- A proximal loop of jejunum that will reach the transplant duodenum is identified
- A side-to-side two layer tension-free anastomosis is constructed between the proximal jejunum and the transplant duodenum
  - Our preference is to have an outer interrupted 4-0 silk layer and an inner running 4-0 resorbable layer
  - This technique may be modified based on the technique of the operating surgeon, such as with the use of stapling devices
  - Alternatively, a defunctionalized Roux-en-Y loop can be constructed

Abdominal Closure

- Hemostasis is verified
- Muscles and fascia are closed as a single layer with interrupted nonabsorbable figure-of-8 stitches
  - Alternatively, long-term absorbable sutures can be used
    - Sutures with rapid resorption can lead to wound dehiscence
- We do not close the subcutaneous tissues
- The skin is closed with widely spaced interrupted simple 2-0 nylon stitches
  - In our experience this closure:
    - Is associated with a lower incidence of infections
    - Avoids the use of drains
    - Provides satisfactory cosmetic results

Portal Venous Output with Bladder Drainage of Exocrine Secretions

Given the location of the pancreas allograft, an anastomosis to the bladder would be very difficult or not possible.

Systemic Venous Output with Bladder Drainage of Exocrine Secretions

- A right lower quadrant incision is undertaken
- The pancreas allograft is implanted (usually) in the right lower quadrant into the external (or alternatively common) iliac vessels
- The pancreatic head and duodenum are oriented distally to provide a tension free anastomosis between duodenum and urinary bladder
- Figure 3 illustrates this technique

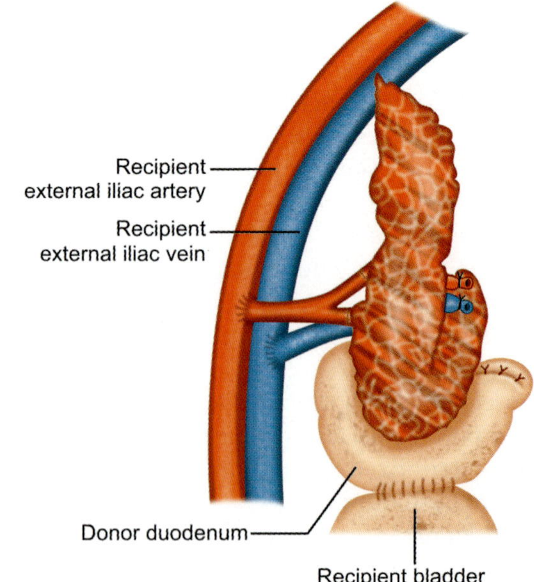

Fig. 3: Systemic venous output with bladder drainage of exocrine secretions.
Source: Molmenti EP. Transplantation of the pancreas. In: Cameron JL (Ed). Current Surgical Therapy, 8th edition. Elsevier Mosby; 2004.

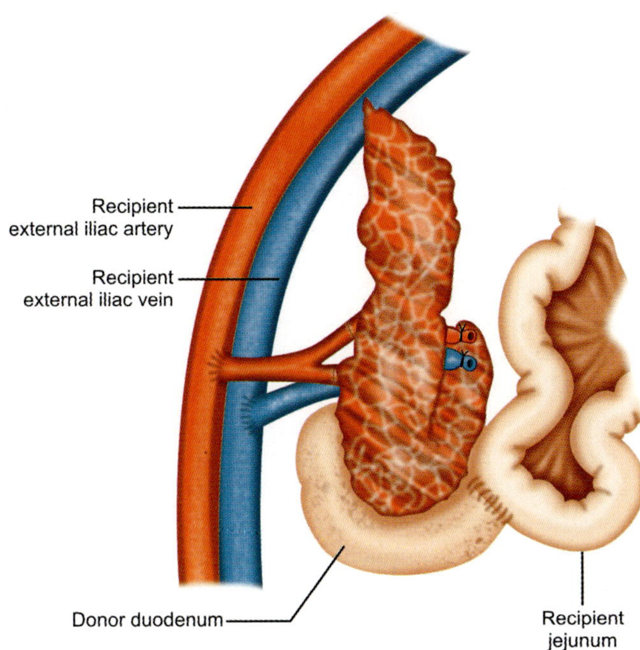

Fig. 4: Systemic venous output with enteric drainage of exocrine secretions.
Source: Molmenti EP. Transplantation of the pancreas. In: Cameron JL (Ed). Current Surgical Therapy, 8th edition. Elsevier Mosby; 2004.

Systemic Venous Output with Enteric Drainage of Exocrine Secretions

- A right lower quadrant incision is undertaken
- The pancreas allograft is implanted (usually) in the right lower quadrant into the external (or alternatively common) iliac vessels
- The pancreatic head and duodenum can be oriented either proximally or distally
- A jejunal loop or alternatively a Roux-en-Y reconstruction is anastomosed to the transplant duodenum
- Figure 4 illustrates this technique

SIMULTANEOUS KIDNEY PANCREAS TRANSPLANTATION

- The kidney is preferably implanted in a retroperitoneal fashion
- To gain access to the iliac vessels from a midline incision, we undertake a separation of the peritoneum from the abdominal wall musculature starting at the midline
- We continue this separation until the iliac vessels are exposed
- The implantation of the kidney allograft follows the steps previously described
- Alternatively, the kidney can be implanted intraperitoneally
  - In these instances special attention should be devoted to ensure that the vessels do not suffer any torsion

IMMEDIATE POSTOPERATIVE CONSIDERATIONS

- A duplex Doppler ultrasound imaging study of the transplanted pancreas (and kidney if combined kidney pancreas) is obtained in the postanesthesia care unit to document:
  - Adequate arterial and venous flow
  - Presence or absence of fluid collections
  - Baseline findings for future studies
    - In cases where the recipient had a previous kidney transplant, we obtain a Duplex Doppler ultrasound to verify that the kidney has not sustained any vascular injury associated with the pancreas transplant
- Although infrequent, positional changes at the time of closure can lead to poor allograft perfusion. If detected early, they can be addressed with limited or no organ damage
- Cardiology evaluation is obtained routinely in the immediate postoperative period
- We prefer to meet with family members/friends/others at the recipient's bedside to inform them of their outcome
  - In most instances, we have been updating them from the operating room as the case evolved
  - They should be reminded that no guarantees can be provided
- All recipients are followed by the multidisciplinary transplant team
- Referring physicians are welcome to participate in the immediate postoperative period as well
- In instances with no systemic anticoagulation, we continue with deep venous thrombosis prophylaxis (subcutaneous heparin and sequential compression devices) immediately after the procedure and throughout the entire hospital stay
- It is out preference to have computerized (or preprinted) order sets and protocols in order to decrease the incidence of mistakes and errors

POSTOPERATIVE MANAGEMENT

- Some of us (RG) usually start an intraoperative and postoperative heparin drip at about 200 units/hour, and continue it for the first 72 post-transplant hours to achieve partial thromboplastin time (PTT) levels between 35 and 45
- Some of us (EM) do not routinely administer intra- or postoperative heparin but rather start IV dextran in the immediate postoperative period and continue it for 48 hours
- Acetylsalicylic acid tablets are given orally starting in the immediate postoperative period and continued on a long-term basis
- Some of us (RG) administer exogenous insulin to keep levels less than 120 mg/dL (first 72 hours)
  - Alternatively, some of us (EM) do not administer any exogenous insulin and monitor glucose levels as a sign of pancreatic function. In these instances, glucose levels will decrease spontaneously in the immediate postoperative period simultaneous with insulin production. Sudden increases in glucose levels are indicative of pancreatic dysfunction (usually a catastrophic event such as pancreatic thrombosis). In such instances, flow to the allograft should be assessed (usually by means of a Duplex Doppler ultrasound study) immediately
- Normoglycemia is a marker of allografts with adequate function
- Sudden increases of glucose levels to 300 mg/dL or higher is a sign of allograft thrombosis
- Continuous hyperglycemia starting at the time of implantation is also encountered in instances of preservation injury and/or poor organ quality
- We routinely obtain a baseline duplex Doppler ultrasound examination of the pancreas transplant immediately after surgery, as well as daily until stable function is achieved
- In instances of sudden blood glucose elevations, an immediate duplex Doppler ultrasound examination of the allograft allows for evaluation of adequate blood flow
- Since the pancreas is a low blood flow organ, we aggressively prevent and treat hypotension in order to ensure adequate blood flow
- Postoperative complications represent an important cause of early morbidity and mortality

FURTHER READING

1. Gruessner AC, Sutherland DE, Gruessner RW. Long-term outcome after pancreas transplantation. Curr Opin Organ Transplant. 2012;17(1):100-5.
2. Molmenti EP. Transplantation of the Pancreas. In: Cameron JL (Ed). Current Surgical Therapy, 8th Edition. Elsevier Mosby; 2004.
3. Sutherland DE, Gruessner RW, Dunn DL, et al. Lessons learned from more than 1,000 pancreas transplants at a single institution. Ann Surg. 2001;233(4):463-501.

CHAPTER 67

Back Table Preparation

Ernesto P Molmenti, Christine Sardo Molmenti, and Collaborators

PREPARATION OF ILIAC ARTERY GRAFT AND PANCREATICODUODENAL COMPLEX (FIGS. 1 AND 2)

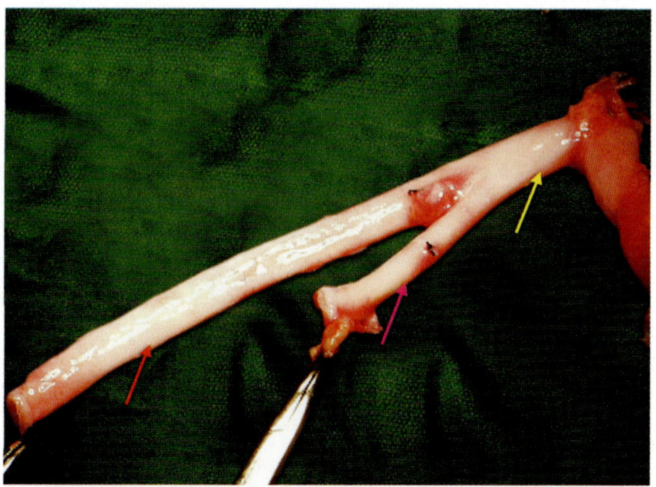

Fig. 1: The common (yellow arrow), external (red arrow), and internal (pink arrow) iliac arteries of the donor are obtained at the time of the procurement. They will be used in the arterial reconstruction of the pancreas allograft. The iliac veins should also be procured, for instances in which a venous graft is also required.

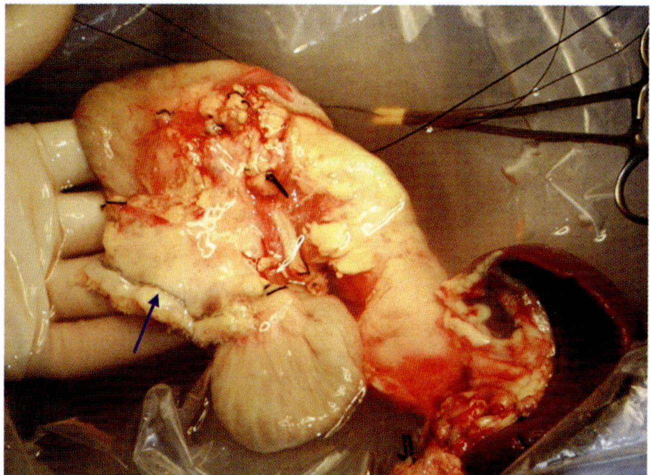

Fig. 2: Appearance of a pancreas allograft after procurement. Note that the duodenum and spleen have also been procured. We routinely remove the spleen during the back table preparation. The root of the small bowel mesentery has been stapled (arrow), and can be oversewn prior to implantation. Alternatively, the mesenteric vessels can be individually ligated (as shown in Figure 9).

PANCREAS BACK TABLE—RECONSTRUCTION OF SPLENIC AND SUPERIOR MESENTERIC ARTERIES (FIGS. 3 TO 6)

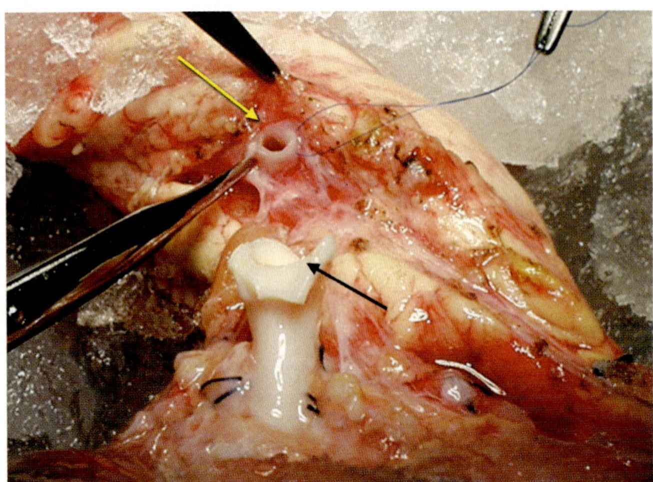

Fig. 3: The splenic artery (yellow arrow) and superior mesenteric artery (black arrow) are being prepared for reconstruction.

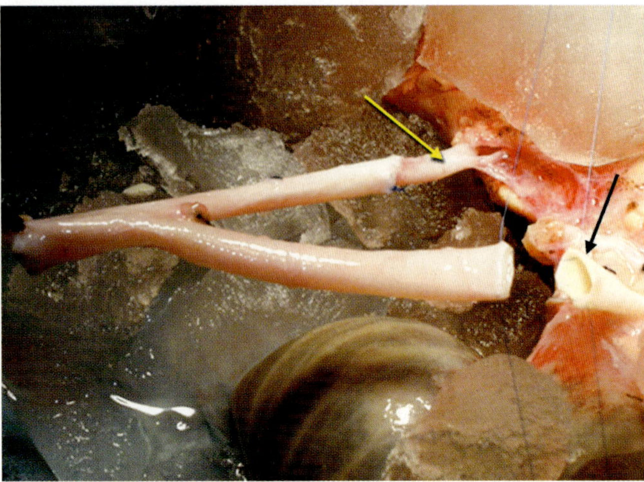

Fig. 4: The splenic artery (yellow arrow) has been dissected along its course up to its first major branch, and is already anastomosed to the internal iliac artery graft. The superior mesenteric artery (black arrow) is being anastomosed to the external iliac artery graft.

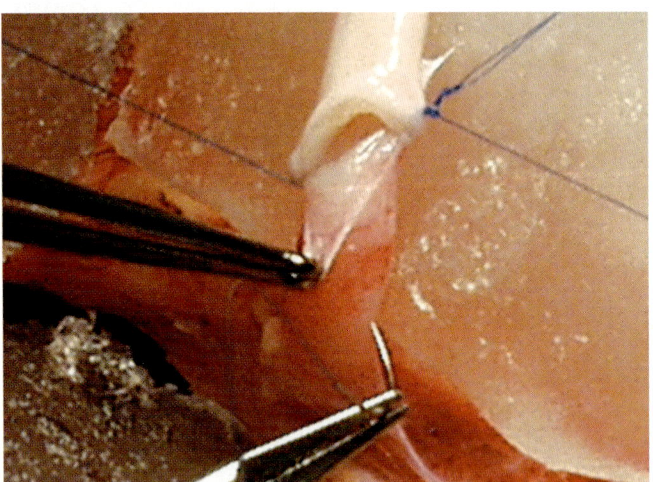

Fig. 5: The anastomosis is constructed.

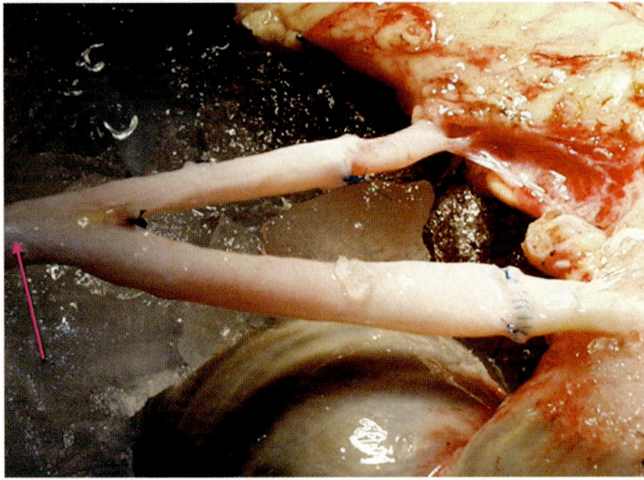

Fig. 6: The arterial reconstruction is finalized. The common iliac artery (pink arrow) of the arterial graft will subsequently be anastomosed onto the aorta at the time of implantation.

PANCREAS BACK TABLE—PORTAL VEIN (FIGS. 7 AND 8)

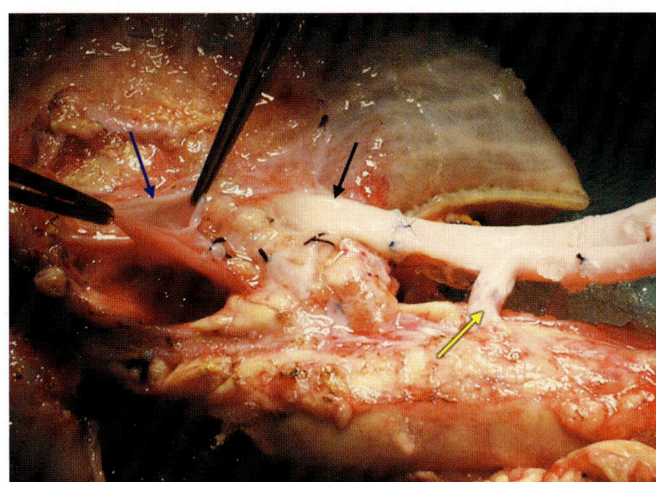

Fig. 7: The portal vein (blue arrow) is identified, and any small branches tied and transected in order to allow for its mobilization during implantation. Note the reconstructed splenic (yellow arrow) and superior mesenteric (black arrow) arteries.

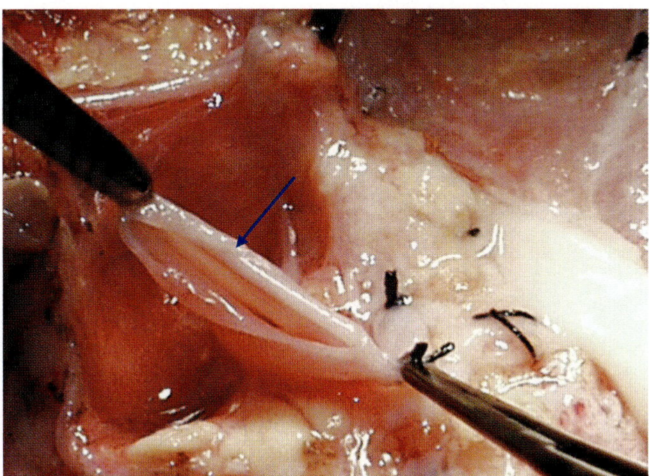

Fig. 8: The portal vein of the donor (blue arrow) is ready for implantation.

PANCREAS BACK TABLE—ALLOGRAFT READY FOR IMPLANTATION (FIGS. 9 AND 10)

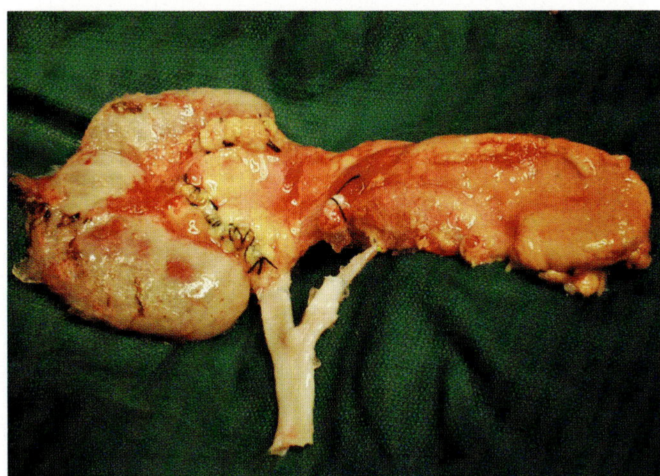

Fig. 9: Pancreas allograft prior to implantation. Note the reconstruction of the superior mesenteric and splenic arteries with the iliac artery graft, the removal of the spleen, and the vessels within the root of the mesentery that have been independently suture ligated.

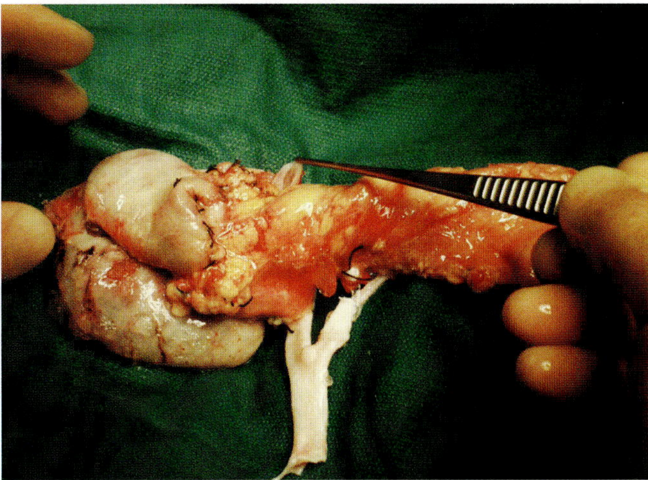

Fig. 10: The portal vein is being held with a surgical forceps. The duodenum has been reduced in length in order to prevent ischemic injuries and to reduce the volume of allograft tissue. Although not always done, in this specific case the stapled edges of the duodenum have been oversewn with silk sutures.

CHAPTER 68

Implantation

Ernesto P Molmenti, Christine Sardo Molmenti, and Collaborators

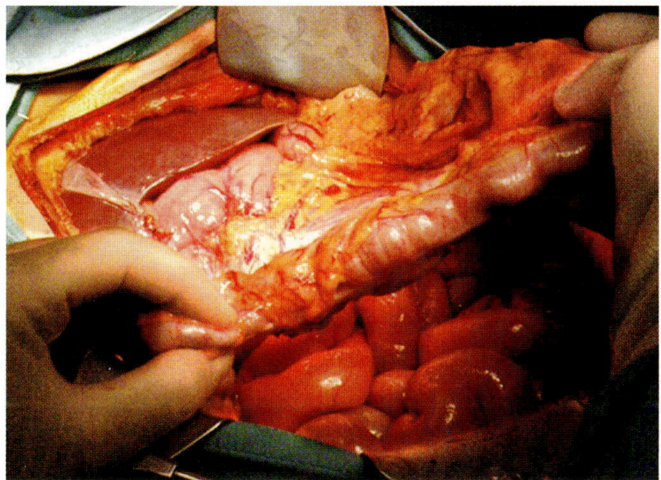

Fig. 1: A midline incision is made and the abdominal contents explored to exclude any unexpected pathologies.

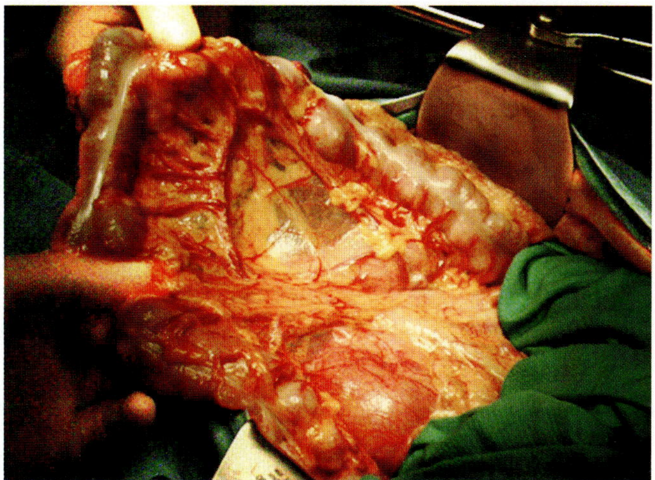

Fig. 2: The transverse colon is retracted proximally, and the root of the small bowel mesentery is exposed.

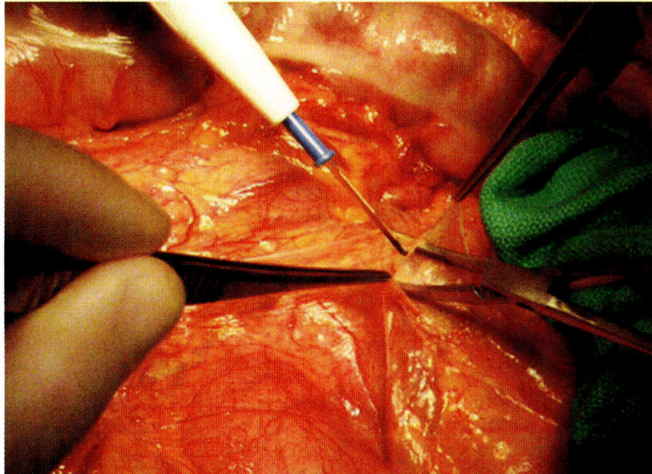

Fig. 3: The superior mesenteric vein, located ventral and to the right of the superior mesenteric artery, is dissected free of surrounding tissues.

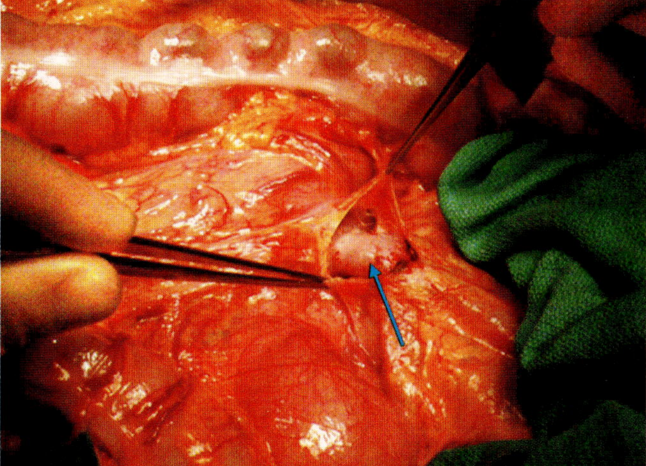

Fig. 4: The superior mesenteric vein (arrow) is exposed and readied for the anastomosis to the portal vein of the pancreas allograft.

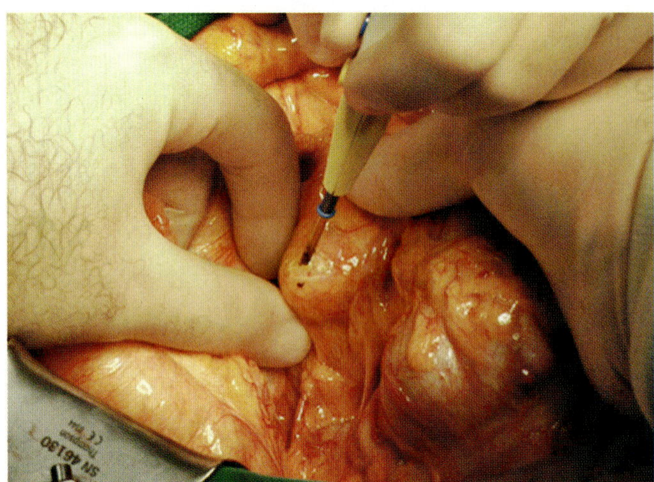

Fig. 5: The ascending colon and its mesentery are mobilized. An opening is made in an avascular site in the ascending colon mesentery to allow for the passage of the arterial graft.

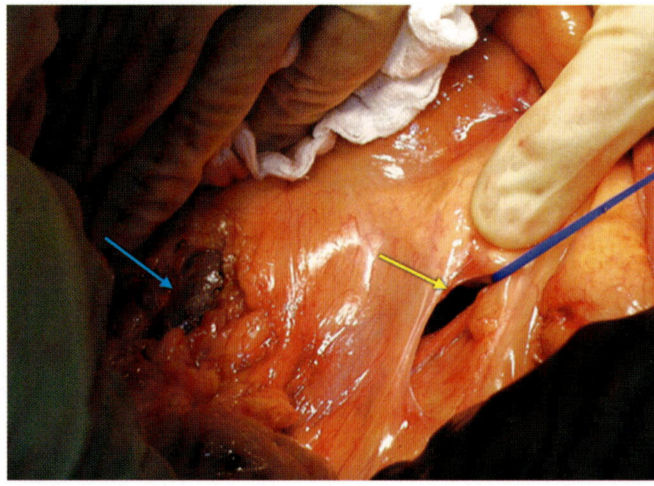

Fig. 6: Once the opening is made (yellow arrow), the surgeon may opt (as in this case) to thread a plastic loop through it for future identification. Note the superior mesenteric vein (blue arrow).

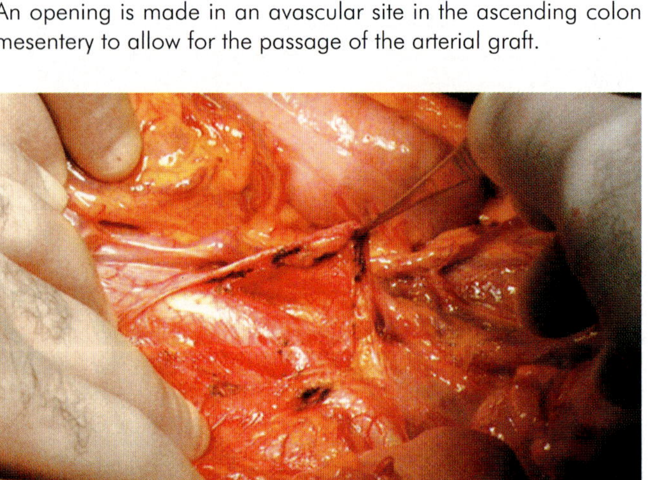

Fig. 7: The aorta is dissected in its infrarenal portion for its future anastomosis to the arterial graft.

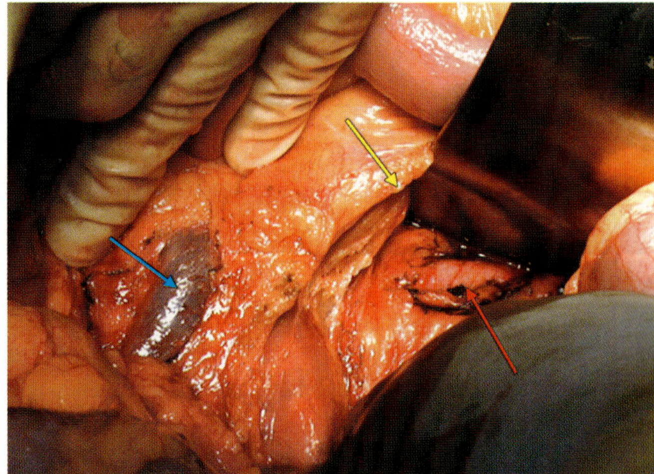

Fig. 8: View of the abdomen demonstrating the superior mesenteric vein (blue arrow), the aorta (red arrow), and the opening in the ascending mesocolon (yellow arrow). At this point, the abdomen is ready for the implantation of the pancreas graft.

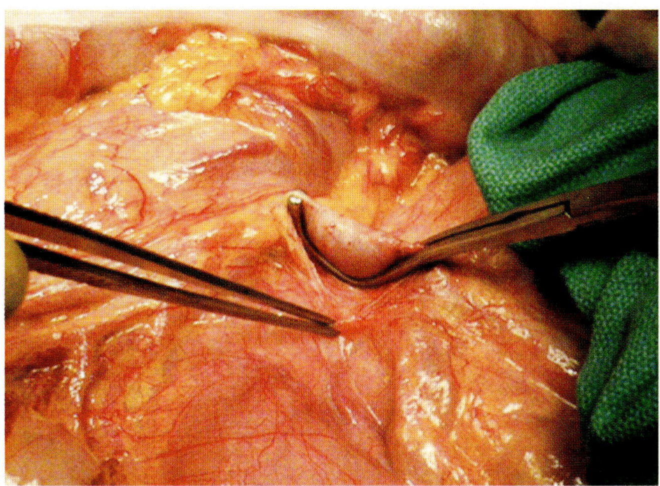

Fig. 9: The superior mesenteric vein is clamped close to its confluence into the portal vein.

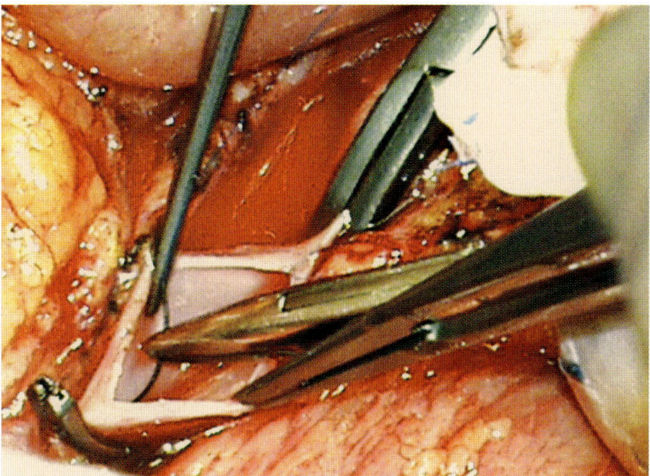

Fig. 10: Once the clamp is applied, the vein is opened longitudinally and corner stitches placed.

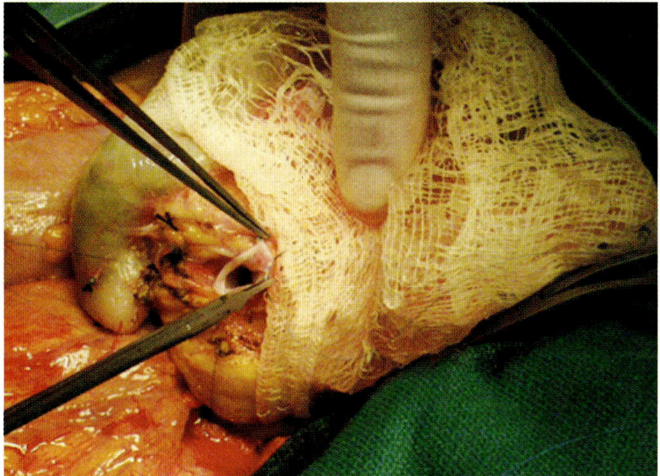

Fig. 11: The allograft is brought into the field, wrapped in a sponge with slush or fine ice. Corner stitches are placed in the donor portal vein, making sure that the orientation of the donor portal vein is consistent with that of the superior mesenteric vein of the recipient.

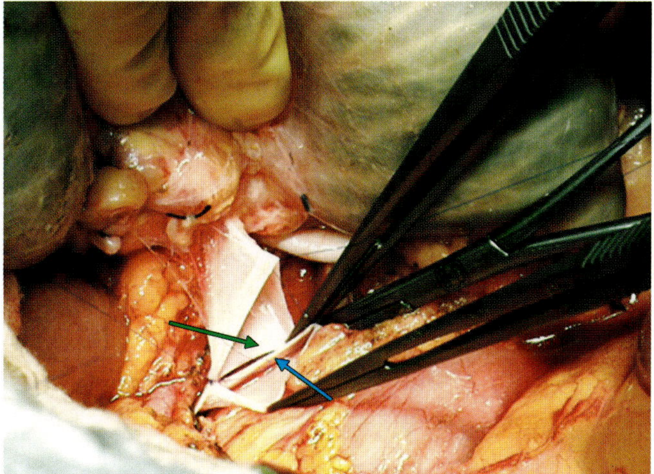

Fig. 12: The venous anastomosis is started, using the corner stitches as guides, between donor portal vein (green arrow) and recipient superior mesenteric vein (blue arrow).

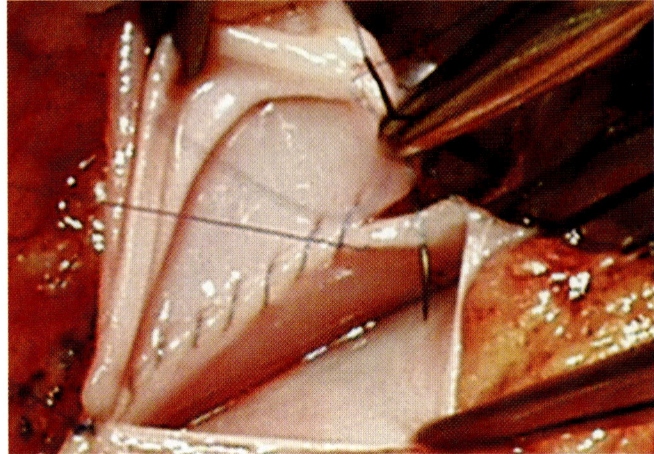

Fig. 13: We prefer to construct the left-side wall anastomosis from the inside, placing everting stitches that ensure an intima-to-intima apposition.

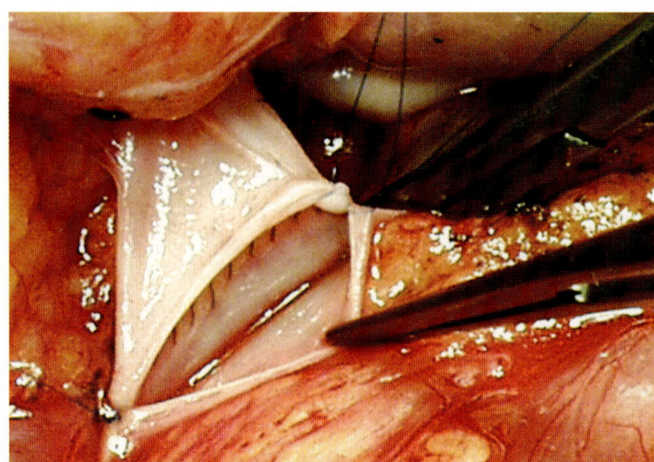

Fig. 14: Once the back wall is completed, we proceed to finalize the anastomosis.

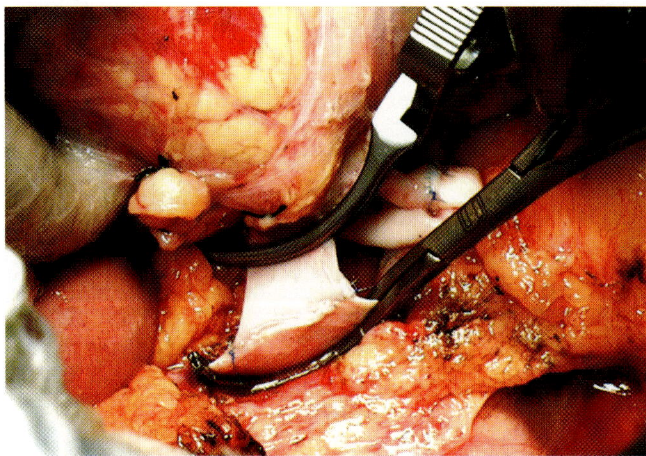

Fig. 15: Once the anastomosis is complete, a bulldog clamp is placed on the donor portal vein, and the clamp on the recipient superior mesenteric vein is released.

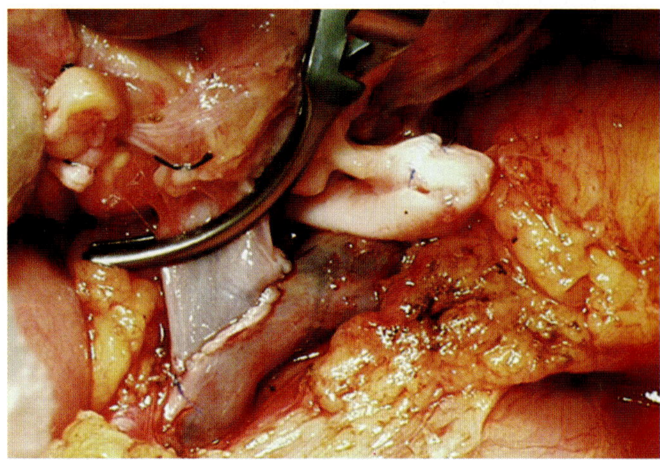

Fig. 16: Hemostasis and adequate patency of the anastomosis are verified.

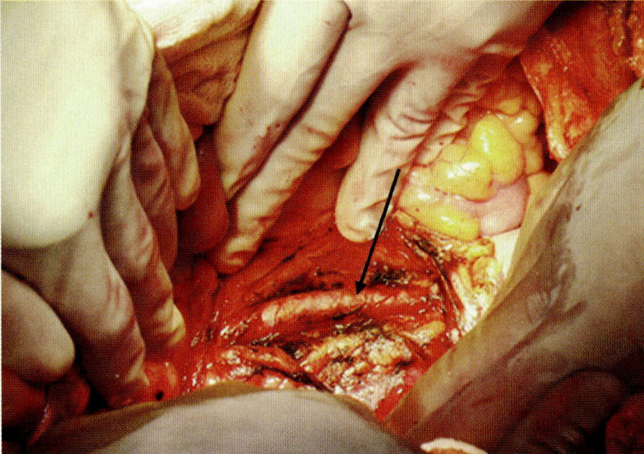

Fig. 17: The aorta (black arrow) had been previously dissected below the renal arteries.

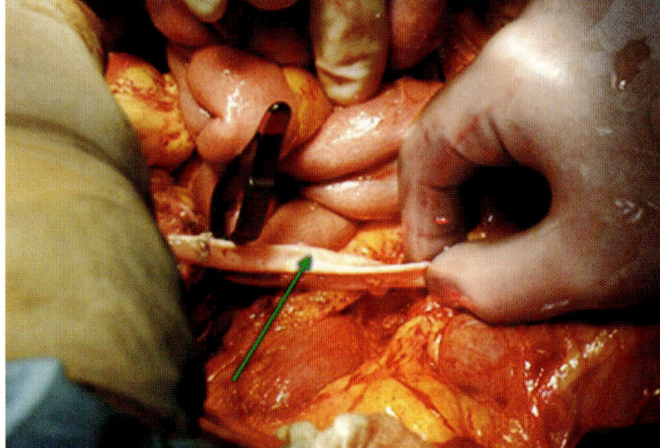

Fig. 18: The arterial graft (green arrow) is being prepared for its anastomosis to the aorta. Note the bulldog clamp on the portal vein of the pancreas graft.

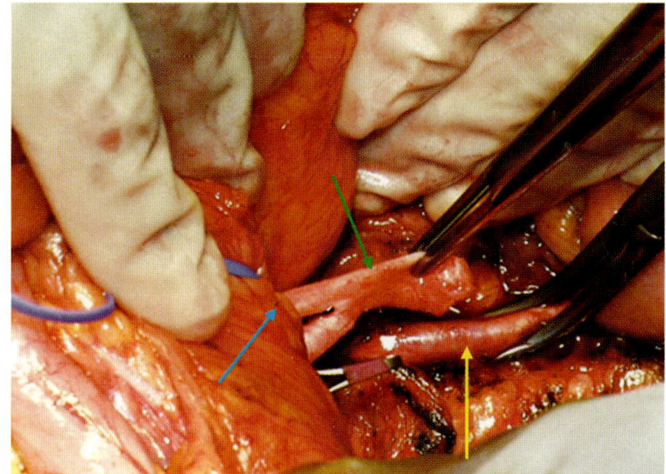

Fig. 19: The arterial graft (green arrow) traverses through the opening (blue arrow) in the mesentery of the right colon (note blue loop previously placed during the dissection) on its way to the aorta. A clamp partially occludes the aorta (yellow arrow) that will soon be incised.

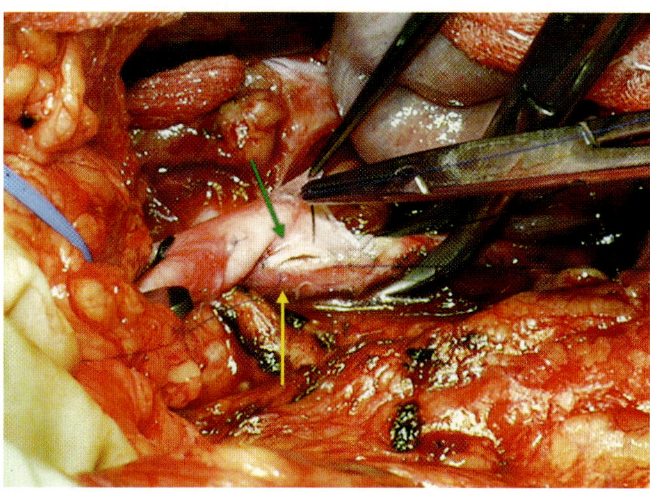

Fig. 20: The arterial graft (green arrow) to aorta (yellow arrow) anastomosis is constructed.

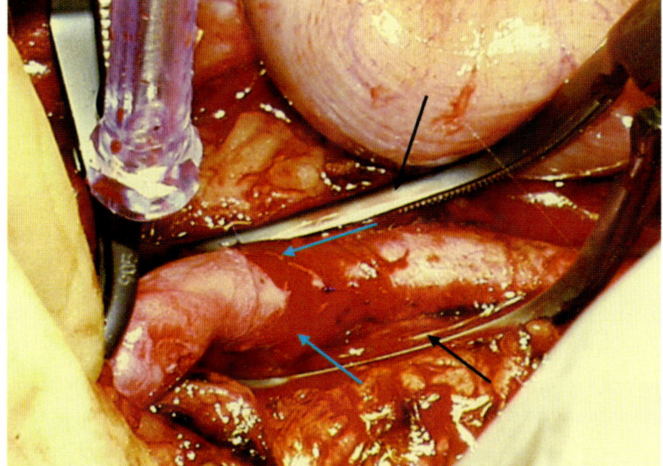

Fig. 21: The aortic clamp (black arrows) is released. The anastomosis (blue arrows) is inspected, and overall hemostasis verified.

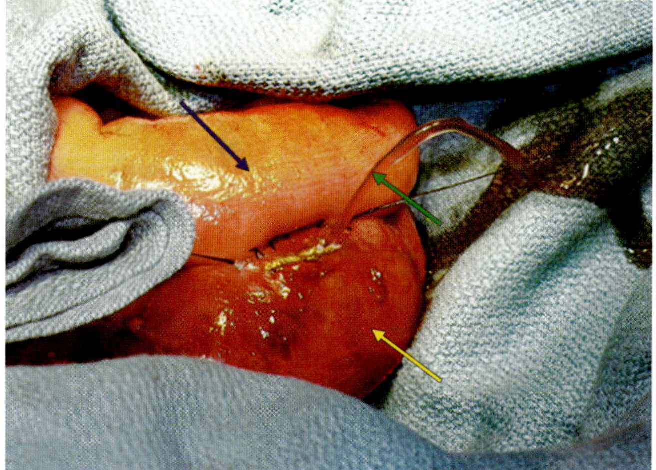

Fig. 22: The graft duodenum (yellow arrow) is anastomosed to the recipient proximal jejunum (blue arrow). Alternatively, a Roux-en-Y limb can be used for drainage of the pancreatic graft exocrine products. The flow of pancreatic juices (green arrow) from the allograft duodenum after it has been incised indicates that the implanted pancreas has started to work in a satisfactory fashion.

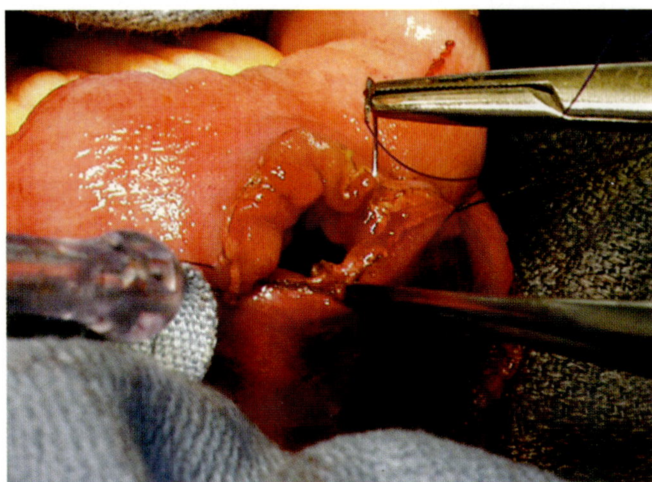

Fig. 23: We routinely construct a two-layered anastomosis, with an outer layer of interrupted silk stitches (previous picture) and a running layer of running absorbable sutures.

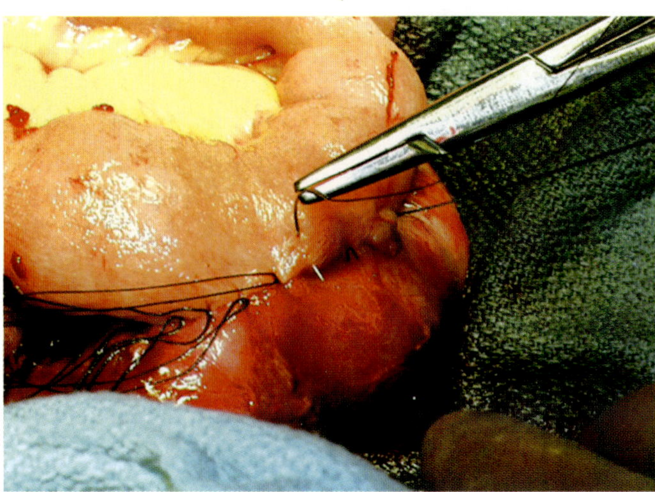

Fig. 24: An outer layer of interrupted stitches is used to finish the anastomosis.

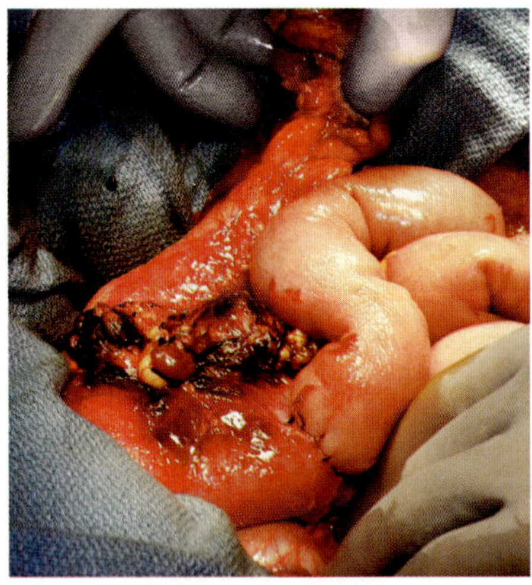

Fig. 25: View of the implanted graft. Dark areas within the head of the pancreas represent areas of hemostasis.

CHAPTER 69

Complications

Christine Sardo Molmenti, Angelika Gruessner, Jeffrey Nicastro, Gene Coppa, Christine E Gruessner, Stefan A Gruessner, Horacio Rilo, Ernesto P Molmenti, Rainer Gruessner

- In order to prevent unnecessary graft injury, we make every possible effort to minimize cold (preservation) and warm (implantation) ischemic times
- The pancreas low blood flow makes it prone to thrombosis
- Hemorrhage is not an infrequent complication, especially when heparin is administered
- Complications include but are not limited to rejection, thrombosis, necrosis, graft pancreatitis, leaks, bleeding, pseudocysts, abscesses, and small bowel obstruction
- Recipients can also develop complications that represent exacerbations of preexisting comorbidities rather than complications associated with the transplant itself

REJECTION

- Acute rejection is characterized by the presence of activated inflammatory cells in the parenchyma, in association with vascular and glandular injury
- Chronic rejection is characterized by atrophy and fibrosis of acini, vessels, and ducts
- There is currently no rejection serum/plasma marker with satisfactory sensitivity and specificity—urinary amylase levels are of the best practical value
- Biopsy represents the gold standard for diagnosis of pancreas graft rejection
- All surrogate markers (e.g., serum amylase levels, serum lipase levels, blood glucose levels, and C-peptide levels) have low sensitivity and/or specificity
- Decreases in urinary amylase (in bladder-drained grafts) are usually consistent with rejection, but could also be due to other etiologies such as drug toxicity and pancreatitis

PANCREATIC GRAFT IMAGING

- CT scanning and MRI imaging provide complete evaluation of the graft parenchyma, ducts, vessels, anastomoses, and intestinal status. The use of intravenous contrast should be carefully considered particularly in patients who received a simultaneous or previous kidney transplant
- Duplex Doppler ultrasound evaluation can be impaired by the presence of air-filled intestinal loops
- The role of angiography is diminished due to CTA/MRA/MRV—CT angiogram/MR arteriogram/MR venogram availability
- Percutaneous drainage and other interventions are of great use in addressing specific complications

VASCULAR COMPLICATIONS

- Thrombosis of the pancreas allograft is a feared vascular complication. Thrombosis results in pancreatic graft necrosis and usually requires graft pancreatectomy (Fig. 1)
- Pseudoaneurysms, hemorrhage, vascular/anastomotic stenosis, and torsion of the vascular grafts represent other potential complications
- In rare circumstances, and especially in instances of failed pancreatic allografts, an arterioenteric fistula may develop. Successful treatment of this complication that presents as massive gastrointestinal bleeding is dependent on a high degree of suspicion and rapid action

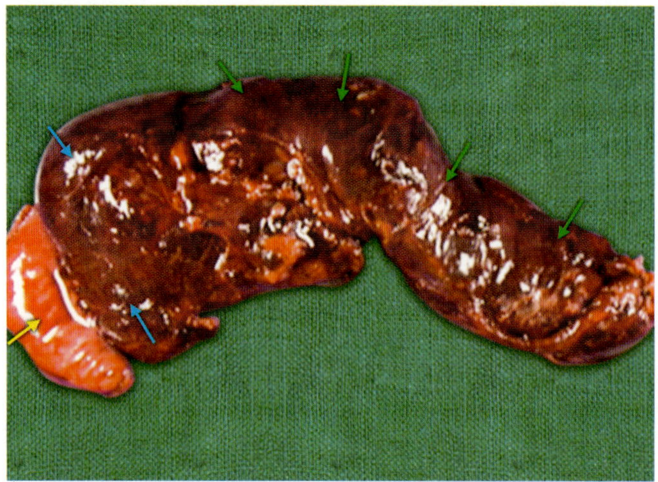

Fig. 1: Thrombosed pancreas allograft with attached segment of recipient jejunum. Note that the thrombosis involved only the pancreas (green arrows) and duodenal (light blue arrows) allografts. The recipient jejunum (yellow arrow), having a different blood supply, was resected in continuity with the graft duodenum to which it was anastomosed at the time of transplantation, but did not show any gross thrombotic changes.

COMPLICATIONS ASSOCIATED WITH ENTERIC-DRAINED PANCREATIC TRANSPLANTS

- Leaks and intra-abdominal abscesses
  - Usually manifested by infectious/septic findings
  - Diagnosis is based on clinical findings in conjunction with imaging studies
  - Treatment involves eradication of the septic focus and correction of the underlying pathology, including:
    - Drainage of abscesses
    - An initial period of non-surgical treatment in an attempt to allow for the leak to heal on its own can be considered in instances where the infection is controlled
    - Revision of the anastomosis
    - Removal of the pancreas transplant (very infrequent)
  - Monitor for the presence of infectious pseudoaneurysms (life-threatening complication that usually requires removal of the pancreatic graft)
- Anastomotic bleeds
  - Usually self-limited
  - Correct any predisposing factors such as anticoagulation
  - Rarely require surgical intervention

UROLOGICAL COMPLICATIONS ASSOCIATED WITH BLADDER-DRAINED PANCREATIC TRANSPLANTS

- Pancreas transplants with bladder drainage feature a variety of urological complications (most common: urinary tract infection, cystitis)
- Twenty to thirty percent of these cases eventually require surgical conversion to enteric drainage within 3 years
- Effective treatment is required in order to minimize allograft injury

PANCREATIC LEAKS

- Incidence: 5–15%
- Origin:
  - 35% duodenum-bladder anastomosis
  - 30% transplant duodenum
  - 35% no clearly identifiable site
- Timing:
  - Early (≤ 4 weeks post-transplant)
  - Late (> 4 weeks post-transplant)
- Clinical findings:
  - Pain
  - Fever
  - Distended abdomen
  - Diminished urinary output
  - Peritonitis
  - Vomiting
  - Improvement associated with urinary catheter placement
- Laboratory findings:
  - High serum amylase
  - Low urinary amylase
  - +/– increase in creatinine levels

EARLY PANCREATIC LEAKS (≤ 4 WEEKS POST-TRANSPLANT)

- Usually associated with technical complications
- Location:
  - Duodenum-bladder anastomosis
  - Duodenal graft
  - Ureter-bladder anastomosis (in instances of SPK—simultaneous pancreas kidney transplant)

- Diagnosis:
  - CT with retrograde injection of bladder contrast
  - Low-pressure cystogram
  - Voiding cystogram
  - Nuclear medicine
  - Sampling of collection fluid
- Treatment:
  - Small contained collections (30%)
    - Percutaneous drainage of collection in association with urinary catheter
  - Collections with associated peritonitis
    - Surgical exploration
      - Repair (80%, of which there is a 10% failure rate)
      - Conversion to enteric drainage (10%)
      - Allograft removal (10%)

LATE PANCREATIC LEAKS (> 4 WEEKS POST-TRANSPLANT)

- Usually associated with duodenal allograft pathologies
  - Ulcers
  - Perforations
  - Ischemia
  - Viral infections (such as CMV–cytomegalovirus)
- Rarely may result from injury sustained during instrumentation of the bladder
- Diagnosis:
  - CT with retrograde injection of bladder contrast
  - Low pressure cystogram
  - Voiding cystogram
  - Nuclear medicine
  - Sampling of collection fluid
- Treatment:
  - Usually require conversion to enteric drainage
  - Treatment of underlying conditions (such as viral infections and ischemia)

PANCREATIC FISTULAS

- Incidence: < 5%
- Usually associated with previous pancreatitis and/or pseudocysts (exocrine secretion volume: native normal pancreas 1.5 L/day, denervated pancreas 700–800 mL/day)
- Initial conservative approach, with treatment of associated infections (if present)
- Parenteral nutrition (if needed)
- Percutaneous drainage
- Urinary catheter (to prevent reflux in instances of bladder drained pancreas grafts)
- Octreotide

HEMATURIA

- Incidence: 10–50% in bladder-drained pancreas transplants
- Early
- Late

EARLY HEMATURIA (≤ 4 WEEKS POST-TRANSPLANT)

- Frequent finding
- Origin:
  - Allograft duodenum-bladder anastomosis (most frequent origin)
  - Allograft duodenitis (rejection, ischemia reperfusion injury)
  - Bladder catheter trauma
  - Post-biopsy
  - Reflux pancreatitis
  - Urinary infections
  - Cystitis (infectious, sterile)
  - Urethritis
  - Other
- Usually limited clinical findings
- Treatment:
  - Most cases respond to clinical management
    - Bladder irrigation
    - Discontinuation of anticoagulation
    - Correction of coagulopathies
  - Cystoscopy (in instances that don't respond to less invasive approaches)
    - Fulguration
    - Evacuation of clots
  - Surgical intervention (very rarely)

LATE HEMATURIA (> 4 WEEKS POST-TRANSPLANT)

- Etiology:
  - Usually associated with duodenal allograft pathologies
    - Ulcers (e.g., CMV)
    - Ischemia
    - Duodenitis (infectious)
    - Rejection
  - Urinary infections
  - Cystitis (infectious, sterile)
  - Urethritis
  - Reflux pancreatitis
  - Pseudoaneurysms
  - Bladder ulcers

- Stones
- Tumors
- Prostatitis
- Urethritis
- Diagnosis:
  - Imaging studies
  - Biopsy
- Treatment:
  - Based on the underlying pathology
    - Antivirals
    - Antibiotics
    - Immunosuppression
    - Conversion to enteric drainage
    - Percutaneous embolization
    - Allograft resection
    - Other

DYSURIA AND URETHRAL COMPLICATIONS

- Incidence: 2–20%
- Manifested as painful voiding
- Etiology:
  - Urethral (and/or glands/labia) injury as a result of exposure to pancreatic enzymes
  - In severe cases, urethral ulcers and disruption
  - Usually associated with mild urethral trauma (bladder catheters)
- Treatment:
  - Bladder catheterization (short term)
  - Urinary alkalinization
  - Suprapubic catheter (rarely required)
  - Conversion to enteric drainage (in severe cases)

RECURRENT URINARY TRACT INFECTIONS

- Incidence: 10–95%
- Treatment:
  - Antibiotics
  - Evaluation of underlying predisposing factors
    - Residual volume
    - Prostatic hypertrophy
    - Urethral strictures
    - Foreign bodies
    - Retained sutures
    - Bladder diverticulitis
    - Other

BLADDER DYSFUNCTION

- Forty-five percent of recipients have urodynamic abnormalities prior to transplantation
- Not a contraindication to transplantation
- Not necessarily associated with postoperative urological complications
- Treatment:
  - Conservative
    - Alpha blockers
    - Bladder training
    - Catheterization
  - Cystoscopy and further interventions based on individual findings:
    - Stone removal
    - Bladder neck procedures
    - Conversion to enteric drainage (infrequent)

Other potential complications include but are not limited to:

- Balanitis
- Cystitis
- Dehydration
- Metabolic acidosis (as a result of urinary losses of bicarbonate)
- Pancreatitis (secondary to urinary reflux or other causes)
- Stones
- Urethral disruption
- Urethral strictures
- Urethritis

FURTHER READING

1. Freund MC, Steurer W, Gassner EM, et al. AJR Am J Roentgenol 2004;182:919–25.
2. Gruessner AC, Sutherland DE, Gruessner RW. Long-term outcome after pancreas transplantation. Curr Opin Organ Transplant 2012;17:100–5.
3. Molmenti EP. Transplantation of the pancreas. In: Cameron JL, ed.: Current surgical therapy. 8th edn. Philadelphia: Elsevier Mosby, 2004;525-32.
4. Sutherland DE, Gruessner RW, Dunn DL, et al. Lessons learned from more than 1,000 pancreas transplants at a single institution. Ann Surg 2001;233:463–501.

CHAPTER 70

Pancreas Allograft Pathology

Cinthia B Drachenberg, Megan Troxell, John C Papadimitriou

GENERALITIES

Banff category 1: NORMAL PANCREAS ALLOGRAFT defined as absent or insignificant inflammation not involving ducts, veins, arteries, or acini. There is no graft sclerosis. The fibrous component is limited to normal septa and its amount is proportional to the size of the enclosed structures (ducts and vessels). The acinar parenchyma shows no signs of atrophy or injury (Figs. 1 to 5).

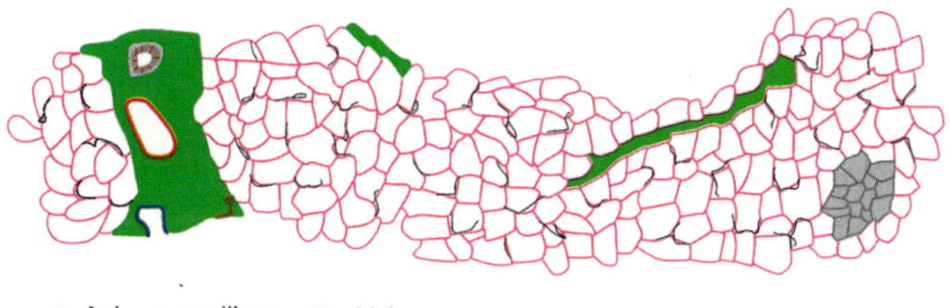

Fig. 1: Diagram representing normal pancreas parenchyma in a needle core biopsy. The bulk of the pancreas parenchyma is composed of exocrine acinar tissue arranged in lobules, separated by connective tissue fibrous septa (green areas). The delicate network of interacinar capillaries (black lines) is not evident on routine stains in normal tissue. The fibrous septa contain ducts, vessels, and nerves. Islets (light grey structure on the right) are distributed unevenly in the parenchyma and are occasionally absent in a needle core biopsy.

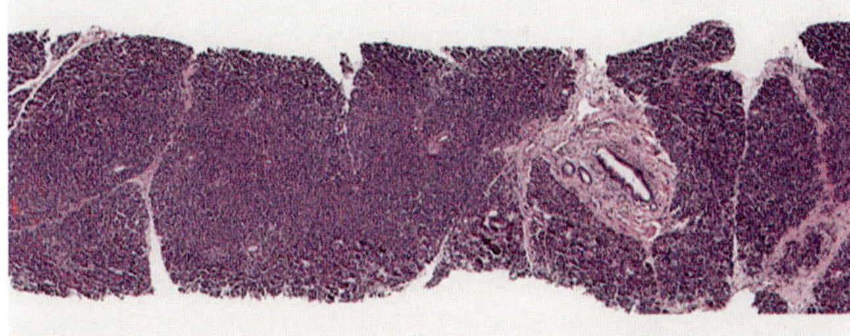

Fig. 2: Routine hematoxylin and eosin (H&E)-stained pancreas allograft biopsy. Several thin fibrous septa are present, one of which is more prominent and contains a duct and small ductal branches. In the normal acinar lobules, the individual acini are tightly packed together with minimal intervening connective tissue. The normal septal connective tissue is paucicellular (with few nuclear profiles evident on routine stain) and appears mostly pink.

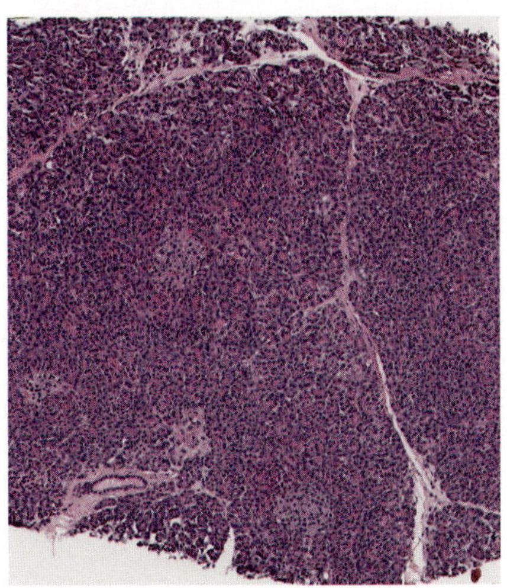

Fig. 3: This image also demonstrates the normal pancreatic architecture. Very thin fibrous septa intersect the lobular tissue. Note scattered islets of Langerhans as slightly paler round structures (lower center and left).

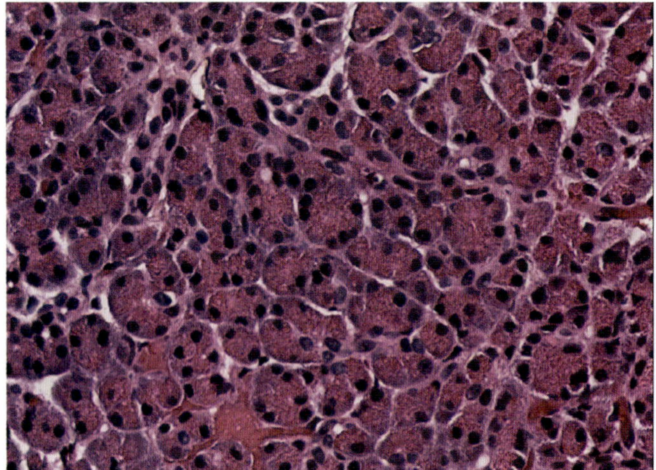

Fig. 4: The lobular tissue is composed of multiple acini that appear solid, although each acinus has a lumen (the lumina are inconspicuous in normal acini). The cytoplasm of acinar cells is brightly pink and granular due to their abundant secretory vesicles (pancreatic exocrine products). The normal acinar tissue lacks inflammation and fibrosis.

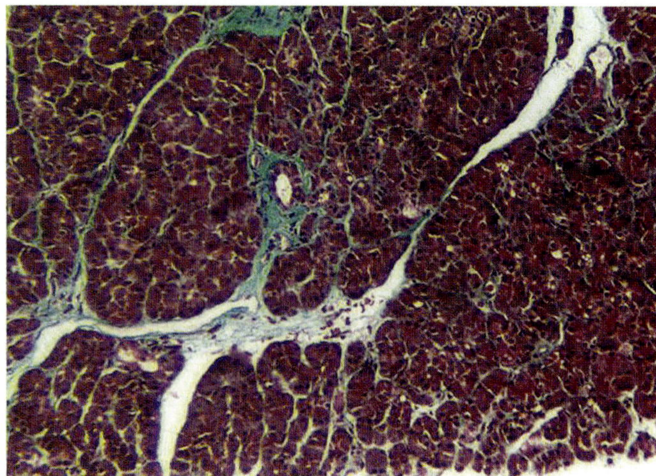

Fig. 5: In addition to H&E staining, pancreas allograft biopsies are routinely evaluated with a stain for collagen (Masson's trichrome stain). In this sample, the connective tissue is highlighted in green. Note that the periphery of the exocrine lobules is smooth and the edges are often rounded. There is minimal amount of connective tissue between lobules, but within the lobules the acini are tightly packed together with no appreciable connective between them. A duct is identified in a septal area (center).

Banff category 2: INDETERMINATE defined as septal inflammation that appears somehow active, but the overall features do not fulfill the criteria for mild T-cell mediated acute rejection (Fig. 6).

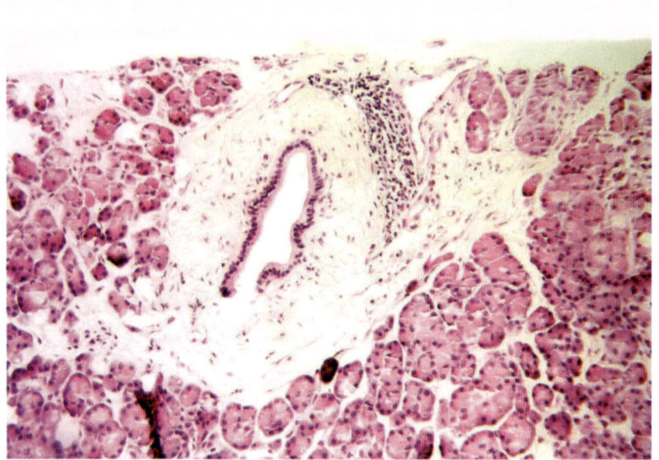

Fig. 6: Septal inflammation that does not fulfill the criteria for acute T-cell-mediated allograft rejection (ACMR) falls in the Banff category of "indeterminate." Note the normal duct with columnar epithelium. The inflammation is located by a vein with a triangular lumen to the upper right of the duct, but the venous endothelium lacks any evidence of injury.

ACUTE T-CELL MEDIATED ALLOGRAFT REJECTION

The main targets of ACMR in the pancreas are the acini, ducts, veins, and arteries. Perineural inflammation is also common.

Milder forms of ACMR are characterized by active septal infiltrates composed predominantly of T-cells, involving veins (venulitis) and ducts (ductitis). The acinar parenchyma is also affected either focally (in milder rejection) or extensively (in the more severe forms of rejection) (Figs. 11 to 19).

Arterial inflammation (intimal arteritis, transmural necrotizing arteritis) defines moderate and severe ACMR. Routine evaluation of C4d staining is necessary for an accurate diagnosis of ACMR versus AMR (Figs. 19 to 21, 38, and 39).

ACMR also manifests on the duodenal cuff segment as increased mucosal inflammation with various degrees of glandular inflammation (Fig. 22).

The Banff category 3: ACUTE T-CELL-MEDIATED REJECTION encompasses ACMR that is graded as follows:

Grade I/Mild ACMR (Figs. 7A, 8 to 10, and 12)—Active septal inflammation (activated, blastic lymphocytes, ± eosinophils) involving septal structures: venulitis (subendothelial accumulation of inflammatory cells and endothelial damage in septal veins, ductitis (epithelial inflammation and damage of ducts), and/or focal acinar inflammation. No more than two inflammatory foci per lobule with absent or minimal acinar cell injury.

Grade II/Moderate ACMR (Figs. 7B, 11, 13, 14, and 19)—Multifocal (but not confluent or diffuse) acinar inflammation (≥ 3 foci per lobule) with spotty (individual) acinar cell injury and dropout and/or mild intimal arteritis (with minimal, < 25% luminal compromise).

Grade III/Severe ACMR (Figs. 7C and 21)—Diffuse, (widespread, extensive) acinar inflammation with focal or diffuse multicellular/confluent acinar cell necrosis and/or moderate or severe intimal arteritis, > 25% luminal compromise and/or transmural inflammation, necrotizing arteritis.

C4d staining is negative in typical ACMR.

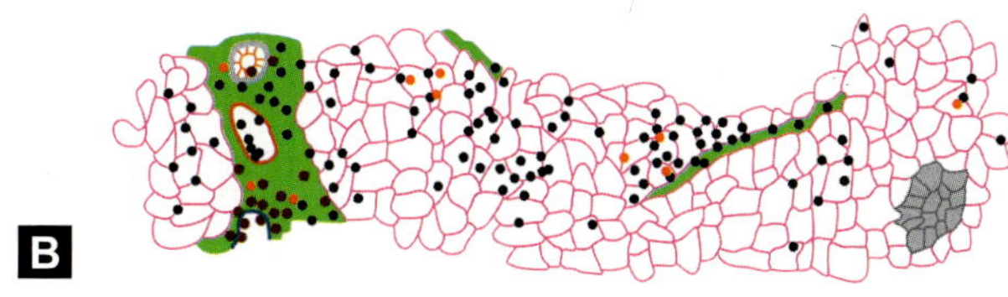

Figs. 7A to C: Schematic representation of ACMR. (A): Mild, Grade I; (B): Moderate, Grade II and (C): Severe, Grade III.

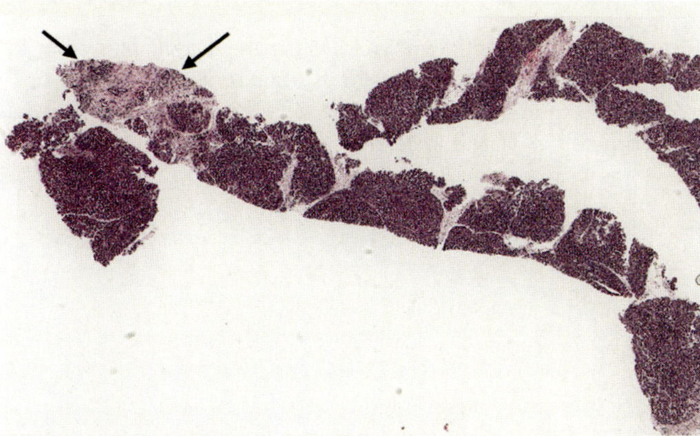

Fig. 8: Low-power view of a needle core biopsy. Although the tissue is slightly fragmented, multiple lobules can be identified, separated by fibrous septa. Even at low magnification it is possible to identify septal inflammation, particularly in the larger septal areas (arrows).

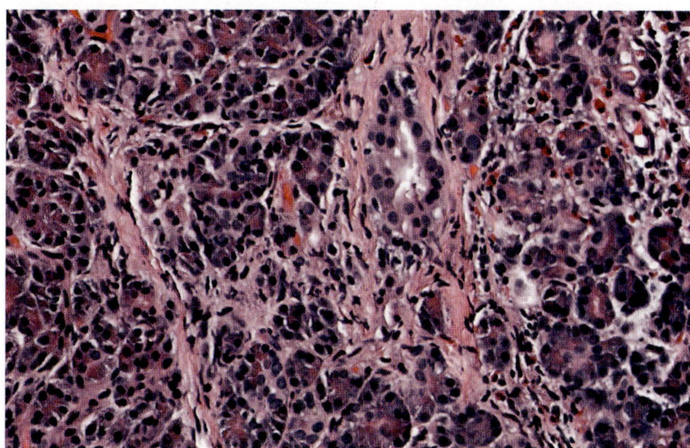

Fig. 9: This is an example of mild ACMR. This is one of focal areas of septal inflammation (see increased inflammatory cell nuclear profiles in the septal area), spilling into the adjacent acinar tissue (more seen on the right). Several eosinophils are present (top-right).

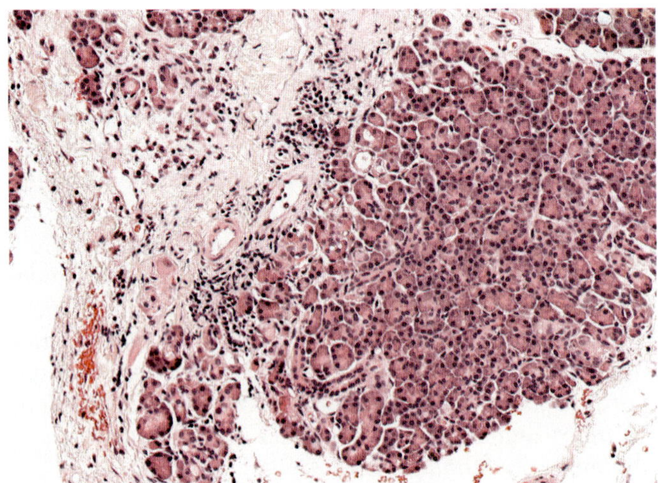

Fig. 10: Mild ACMR (Banff grade I). The septal area (left of image) shows lighter pink color and clear spaces indicating interstitial edema. In addition, clusters of lymphocytes characterized by their dark nuclei are evident mostly in the interface between the connective tissue and the adjacent lobule.

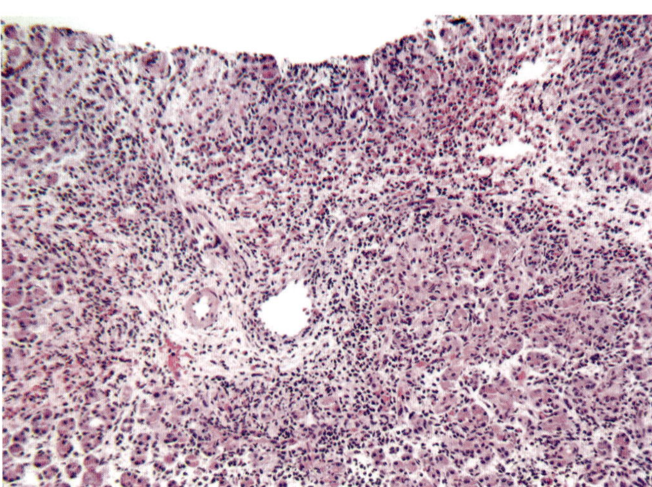

Fig. 11: Moderate ACMR (Banff grade II): Note extensive inflammatory infiltrates that involve the septal areas but also extend to all the acinar areas.

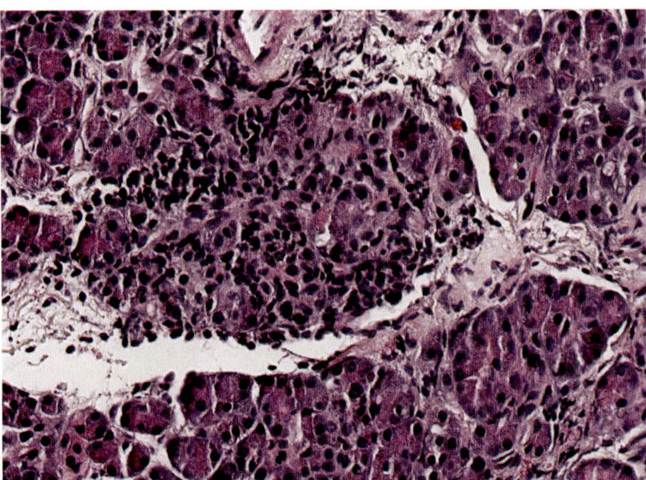

Fig. 12: Example of mild ACMR (Banff grade I). In this biopsy, only occasional lobular areas had patches of acinar inflammation as illustrated here. Note that in the inflamed area the lymphocytes tightly associate with the acinar tissue, blurring the boundaries of the individual acini (acinitis). A crack in the section (white spaces) separates the most inflamed from the less inflamed areas.

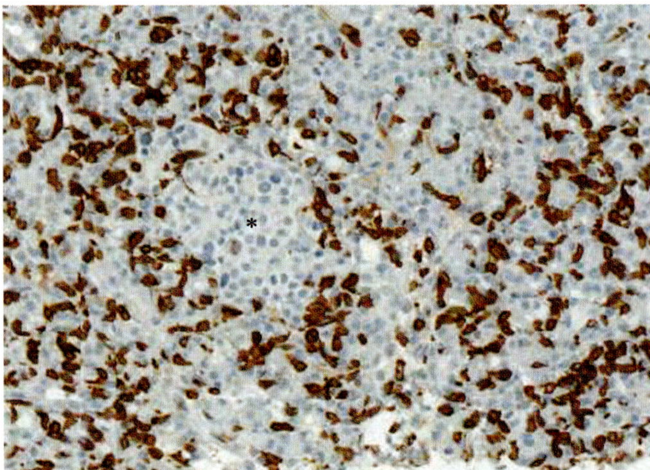

Fig. 13: The main effector in ACMR is the T cell. This stain for CD3 (pan-T-cell stain) demonstrates abundant T cells in the acini in a case of moderate-to-severe ACMR. The islets are not specifically targeted in ACMR (asterisk).

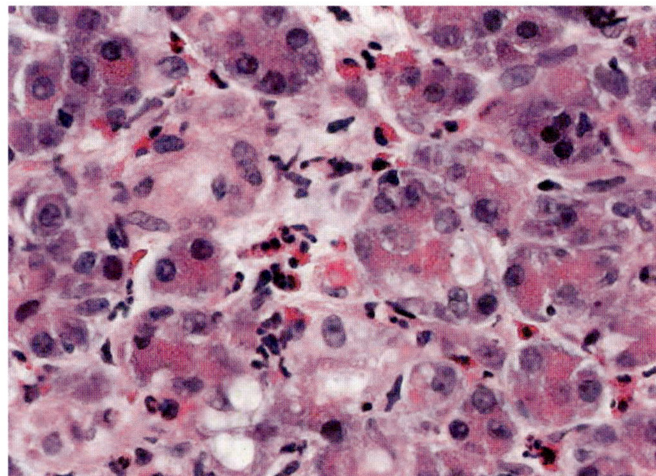

Fig. 14: In this example of ACMR, there are inflammatory cells in the interstitium and within the acini, including several eosinophils (characterized by their bright red cytoplasmic granules). The acinar cells show significant injury appearing mainly as cytoplasmic vacuolization. Rounded clear spaces represent acinar cell dropout (due to necrosis or apoptosis). Mild acinar inflammation can heal without sequela; however, severe acinar injury and cellular loss results in residual areas of fibrosis.

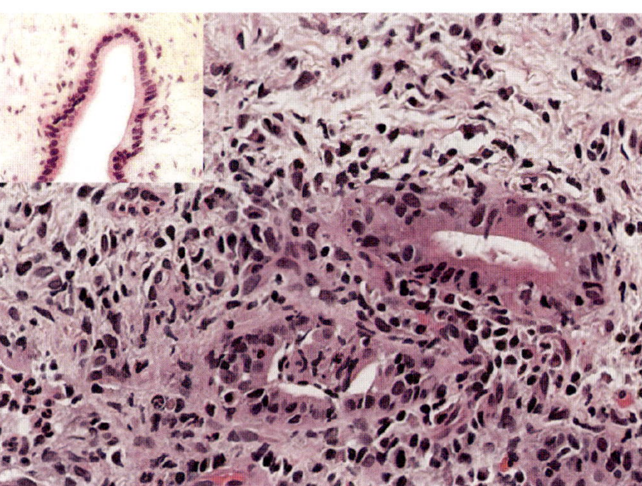

Fig. 15: Ductal inflammation (ductitis) in ACMR. The ductal epithelium shows features of cellular injury characterized by disarray of the cellular orientation (loss of cellular polarity) and nuclear atypia. Insert shows for comparison a normal duct with preserved columnar arrangement of the epithelium.

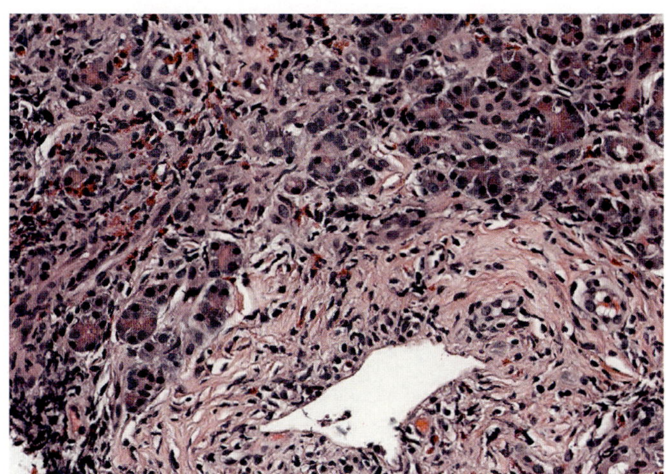

Fig. 16: In this example of moderate ACMR (Banff grade II), lymphocytic and eosinophilic infiltrates are seen in this image, involving most of the biopsy surface. The polygonal space (low-center) represents the wall of a duct in which the epithelium has been lost due to the marked inflammatory injury (severe ductitis).

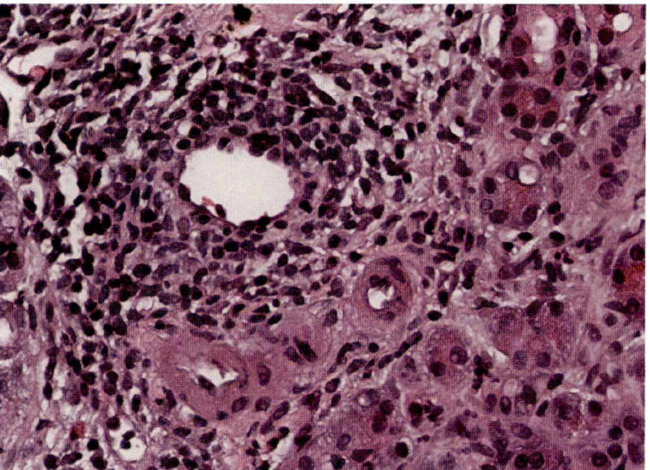

Fig. 17: High-power view of inflamed septal area and adjacent lobular tissue on the lower right. The oval space corresponds to a vein with venulitis. The latter is defined by cuffing by lymphocytes and infiltration of the venous endothelium with associated damage of the endothelial lining (typically detachment or lifting).

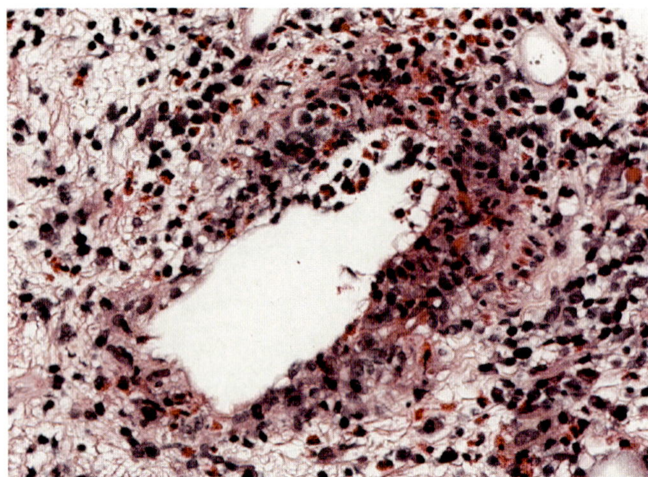

Fig. 18: Another example of venulitis; in this case the inflammation is mixed with lymphocytes and eosinophils. Note the endothelial cell sloughing on the upper part of the vein. There is severe interstitial edema in the surrounding connective tissue (clear spaces separating the collagen fibers).

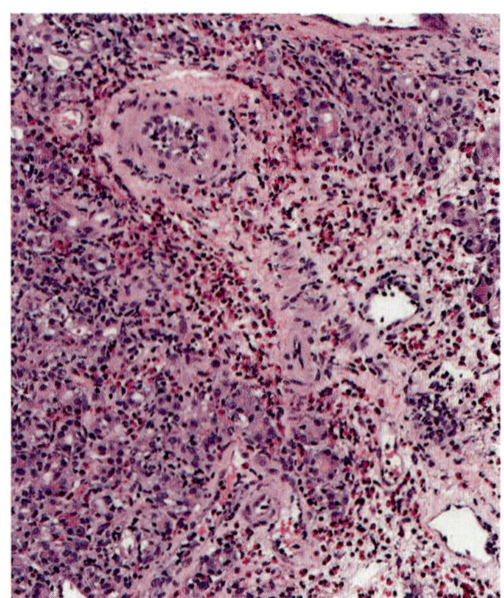

Fig. 19: Moderate ACMR (Banff grade II). The arterial lumen is occluded by intimal arteritis and the septa and acinar areas show prominent inflammation with numerous eosinophils.

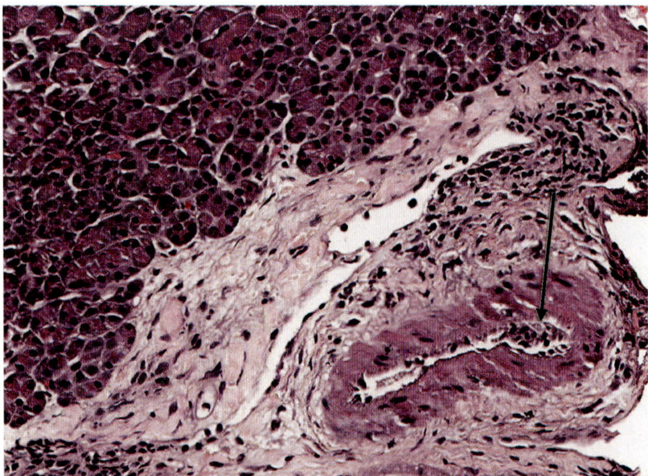

Fig. 20: Another example of intimal arteritis. Note the mononuclear inflammatory cells accumulating beneath the intima (arrow). If arterial inflammation is present, the rejection should be graded as moderate or severe, according to the severity of the arterial involvement (see Banff grading schema).

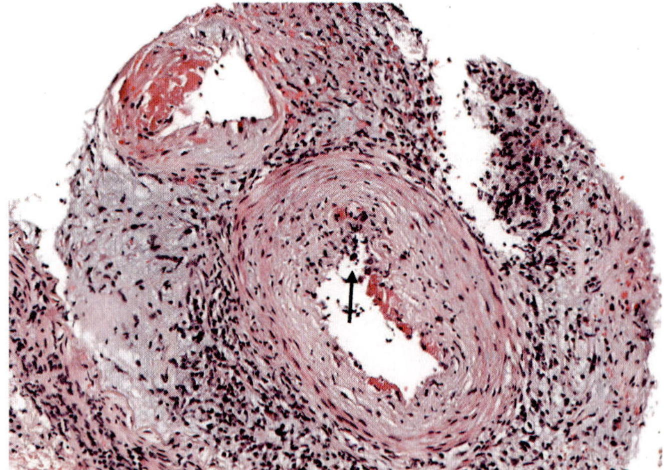

Fig. 21: Acute and chronic arterial rejection. The wall of the depicted arteries is very thick due to prominent intimal fibrosis. The areas of fibrosis are infiltrated by mononuclear cells indicating chronic ACMR (active transplant arteriopathy). In addition, there are features of acute rejection: inflammation of the intima (intimal arteritis) particularly in the upper area of the lower vessel where there is endothelial cell sloughing (arrow). Areas of fibrinoid necrosis/necrotizing arteritis (bright red pink discoloration) are noted particularly in the upper vessel.

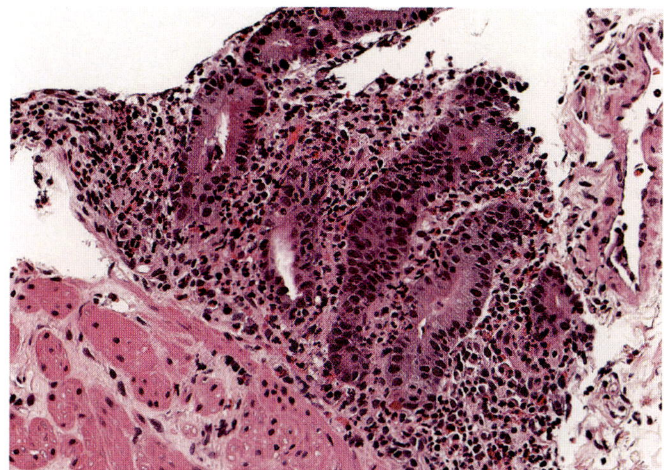

Fig. 22: Acute rejection in the graft duodenal cuff. ACMR manifests also in the segment of transplant duodenal cuff. This micrograph represents a fragment of duodenal mucosa and underlying smooth muscle (lower left). There is generalized increase in inflammatory cells in the mucosa with prominent inflammation permeating into the glandular structures (intestinal crypts). A large number of eosinophils and neutrophils are noted.

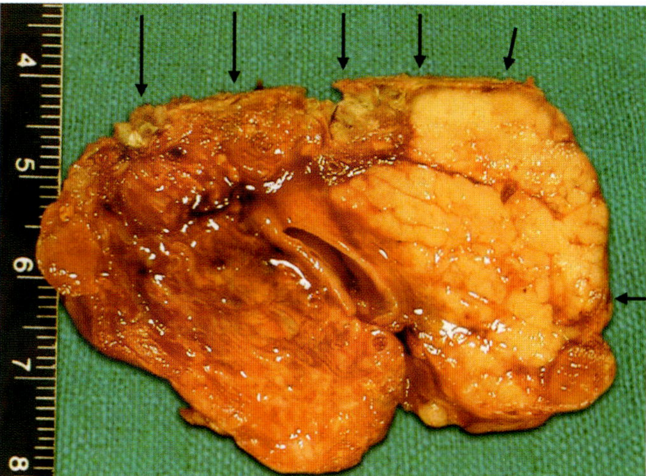

Fig. 23: Peripancreatic fluid collection/peripancreatitis. In the early post-transplant period, sterile or infected peripancreatic fluid collections are associated with inflammatory and fibroblastic reaction of the most peripheral parenchymal areas. The macroscopic picture represents a segment of a graft pancreatectomy; the upper edge of the specimen, in particular, has areas of yellow discoloration corresponding to areas graft peripancreatitis (arrows). A large vessel separates the parenchyma into left and right areas. Although the left parenchyma appears very congested, the right parenchyma appears normal. In most cases, the fibrosis and inflammation associated with peripancreatitis only involve the surface of the organ.

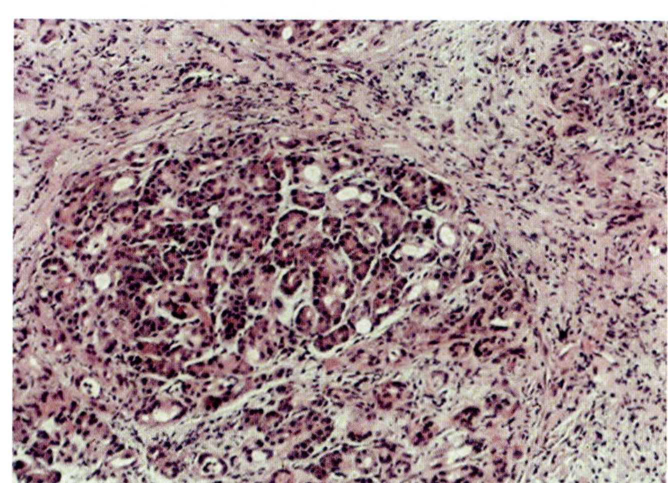

Fig. 24: Pancreas graft biopsy taken from an area of peripancreatitis. Acinar lobules are recognized, but the tissue architecture is markedly altered. Specifically, there are bands of connective tissue encircling and separating the lobular areas. The connective tissue is very cellular representing very active fibroblastic proliferation. In addition, because this is an inflammatory reaction, the connective tissue is typically inflamed (mixed inflammation including lymphocytes, macrophages, neutrophils, and occasional eosinophils). In the correct clinical setting (i.e., the context of a peripancreatic fluid collection or peripancreatitis), this pattern of active fibroblastic proliferation is very characteristic and can usually be distinguished from allograft rejection.

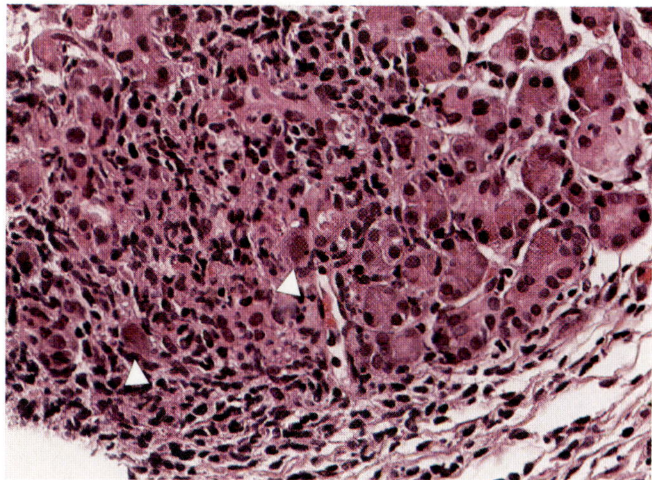

Fig. 25: Cytomegalovirus (CMV) pancreatitis is characterized by connective tissue and acinar inflammation that may resemble ACMR. In particular, the foci of acinar inflammation may be indistinguishable from rejection-related acinitis, except that CMV viral cytopathic changes will be identified if carefully searched for. White arrowheads mark cells with enlarged nuclei with the typical smudgy nuclear inclusions.

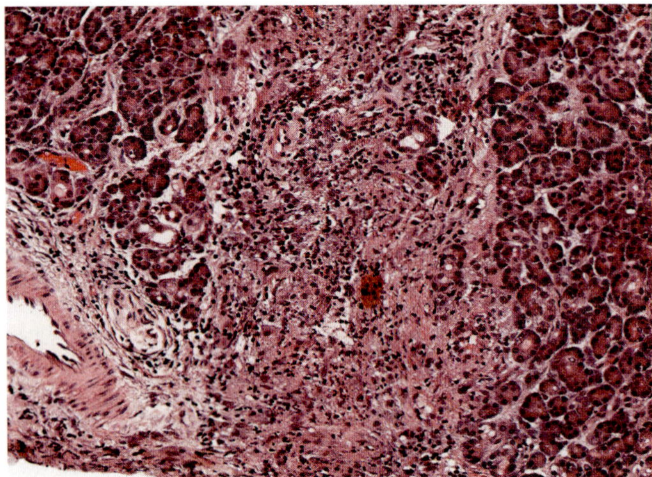

Fig. 26: Post-transplant lymphoproliferative disorder (PTLD) involving the graft also requires differentiation from ACMR. In PTLD, the lymphocytic or lymphoplasmacytic infiltrates do not particularly target the parenchymal structures (i.e., acini or vessels), but rather infiltrate the parenchyma randomly with areas of confluent growth.

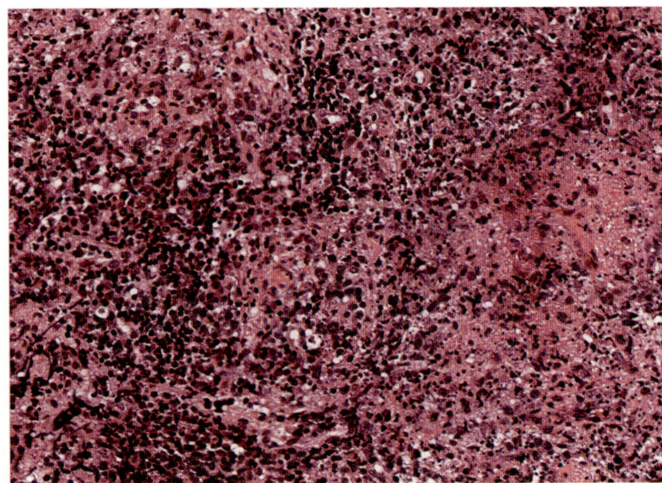

Fig. 27: In aggressive PTLD, the infiltrates appear monomorphic and cytologically atypical (composed of larger proportion of immunoblastic type cells versus a larger proportion of small lymphocytes seen in ACMR). Neoplastic growth in PTLD is associated with areas of necrosis as seen in the right areas of this image. Necrosis is characterized by loss of nuclear detail with accumulation of amorphous or granular cellular debris.

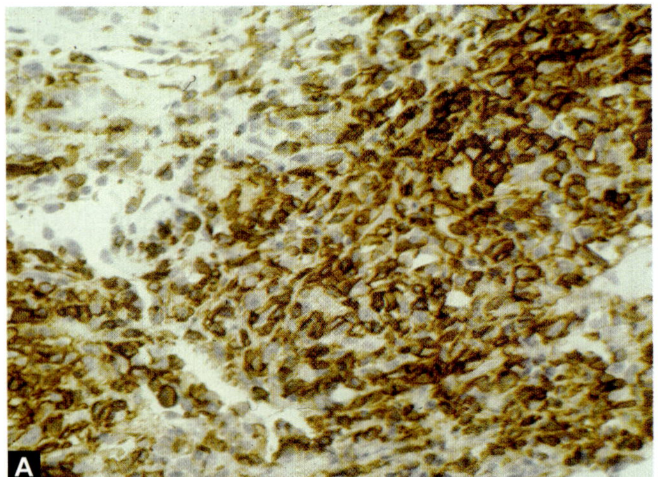

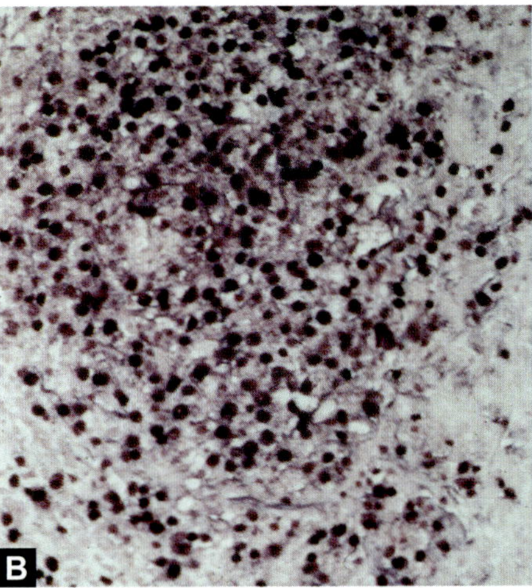

Figs. 28A and B: The vast majority of PTLD proliferations are composed predominantly of B cells. This is in contrast to the predominant T-cell proliferations of ACMR. A stain for B cells (CD79a) is positive in most cells in this case of PTLD (A). Evaluation of ancillary tests for EBV. In situ hybridization for EBV encoded RNA (EBER) is positive in the nuclei of most cells (B).

ANTIBODY-MEDIATED ALLOGRAFT REJECTION

Antibody-mediated allograft rejection (AMR) is characterized by injury to the vasculature due to deposition of antibodies in association with activation of the complement cascade. The most important morphological features of AMR are vascular injury and necrosis, often with thrombosis and secondary ischemic parenchymal necrosis. Hyperacute rejection, the most severe form of AMR, occurs in recipients with abundant preformed antibodies and leads to immediate graft loss. Less severe and/or more protracted forms of AMR can be diagnosed by evaluation of a needle allograft biopsy.

The Banff Category 4 refers to the Diagnosis of AMR. The diagnostic components used for the diagnosis of acute AMR are as follows:

- Confirmed circulating donor specific antibody (DSA)
- Morphological evidence of tissue injury such as interacinar inflammation (capillaritis), acinar cell damage (swelling/necrosis/apoptosis/dropout), vasculitis, thrombosis
- C4d positivity in interacinar capillaries (IAC, ≥5% of acinar lobular surface)

All 3 elements are required for a diagnosis of acute AMR.

A diagnosis of "consistent with acute AMR" is rendered when 2 of 3 diagnostic components are present. If only 1 of 3 diagnostic components is identified, the patient should be closely evaluated and followed-up for exclusion of evolving AMR.

Chronic, ongoing AMR presents as CHRONIC ACTIVE ANTIBODY-MEDIATED REJECTION which is diagnosed by the identification of features of acute AMR together with chronic changes (graft sclerosis, acinar atrophy, organizing vascular thrombosis), in the absence of features of ACMR or a previous diagnosis of ACMR.

Banff Grading of Acute AMR

Grade I/Mild Acute AMR

The diagram on the top represents mild AMR. There is preservation of the architecture and the changes are very subtle consisting only of mild monocytic-macrophagic or mixed (monocytic-macrophagic/neutrophilic) infiltrates in the interacinar capillaries. Acinar cell damage can be appreciated only at high magnification if searched with high degree of suspicion (Figs. 29A and 30 to 32).

Grade II/Moderate Acute AMR

Overall preservation of the architecture with interacinar monocytic-macrophagic or mixed (monocytic-macrophagic/neutrophilic) infiltrates (capillaritis). Other features include capillary dilatation, overall tissue congestion, foci of multicellular acinar cell dropout, and small foci of hemorrhage (Figs. 29B, 33, 34, and 40).

Grade III/Severe Acute AMR

Architectural disarray due to confluent foci hemorrhagic necrosis characterizes severe AMR. Scattered inflammatory infiltrates are present in the congested hemorrhagic background, as well as multifocal and confluent parenchymal necrosis. Arterial and venous wall necrosis and thrombosis can be present (as seen in cases of hyperacute rejection) (Figs. 29C, 35, and 38 to 40). Acute AMR should be differentiated from "technical failure" (Figs. 36 and 37).

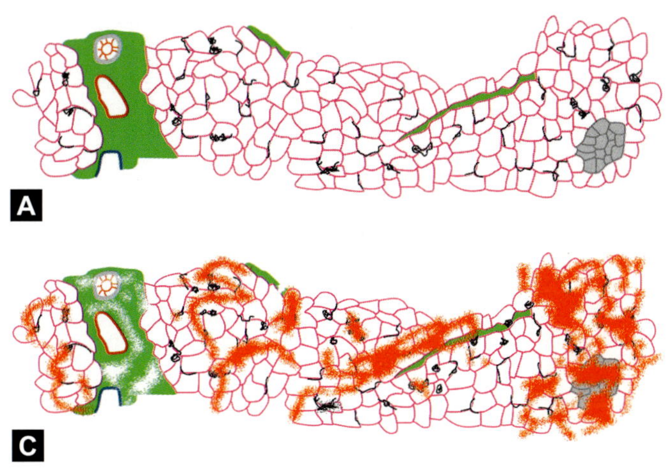

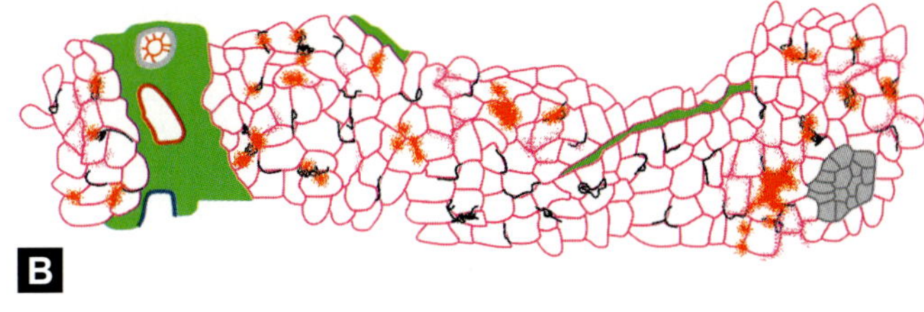

Figs. 29A to C: Schematic representation of AMR. (A): Mild, Grade I; (B): Moderate, Grade II; and (C): Severe, Grade III.

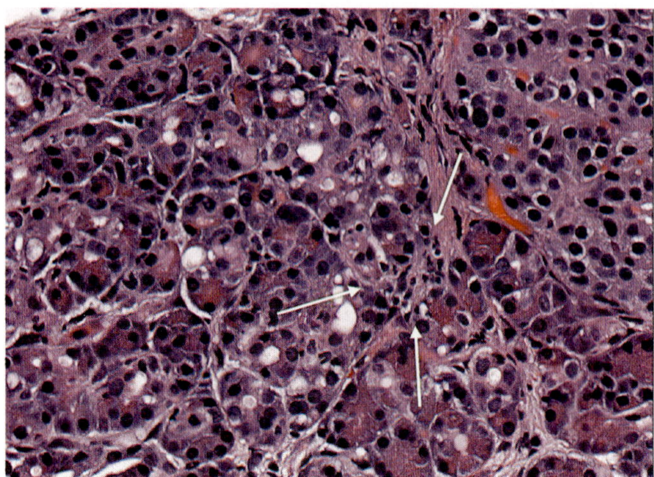

Fig. 30: This is an example of very mild acute AMR. On routine H&E stain, the inflammatory infiltrates are so subtle that can be easily missed (arrows).

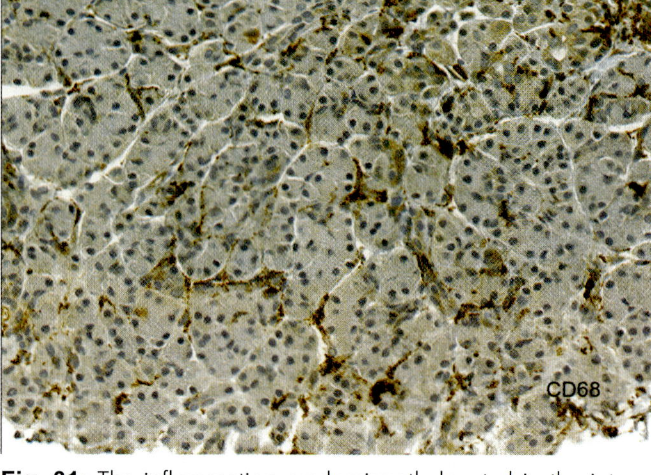

Fig. 31: The inflammation predominantly located in the interacinar capillaries can be easily identified with the aid of a special stain for macrophages (CD68).

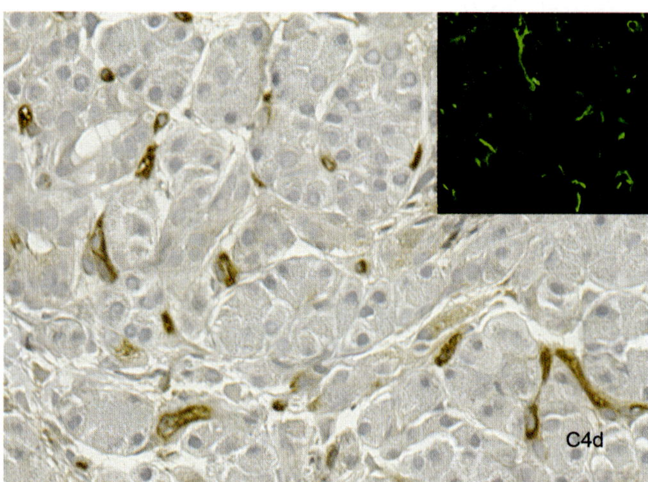

Fig. 32: As expected, the C4d stain highlights several interacinar capillaries. This C4d stain was performed on formalin fixed, paraffin embedded tissue. The insert demonstrates the same pattern of staining on immunofluorescence staining (performed in a frozen section from fresh rather than fixed tissue) (courtesy of Dr P Revelo).

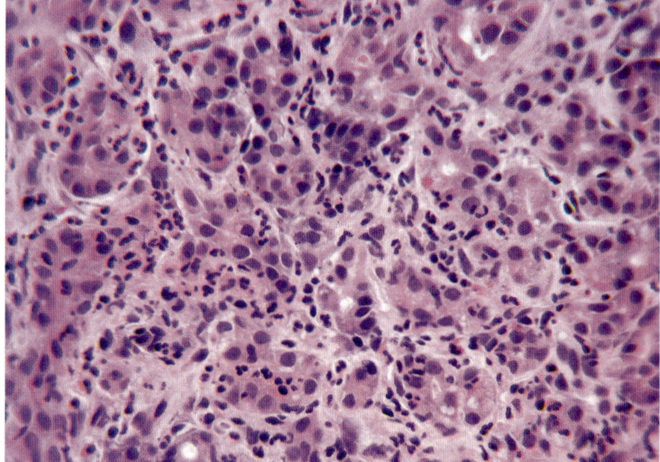

Fig. 33: In this example of moderate acute AMR, the inflammatory infiltrates that are composed of a mixture of macrophages and neutrophils are easily identified in between the acini. The inflammation in AMR predominates in between the acini (mostly within the microvasculature), in contrast to ACMR in which the infiltrates tend to infiltrate the individual acini (acinitis).

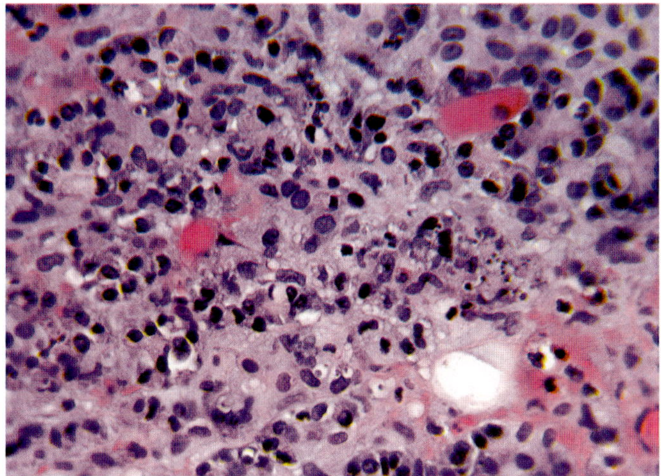

Fig. 34: High-power view of a case of moderate acute AMR with prominent acinar cell damage consisting of cytoplasmic vacuolization and multifocal cell necrosis appearing as a cluster of nuclear fragments on the center right.

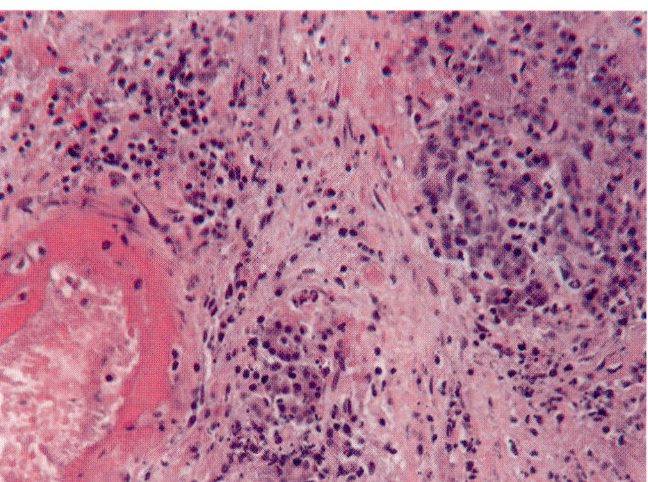

Fig. 35: Vascular necrosis (lower left corner) in a case of severe acute AMR. The background parenchyma appears congested with extravasation of red blood cells. Note the scattered inflammatory infiltrates as well as the loss of normal lobules. Rapid development of fibrosis is typical in cases of ongoing AMR; in this particular case the process progressed over the course of 6 weeks, and acute and chronic overlapping lesions were observed in the graft pancreatectomy.

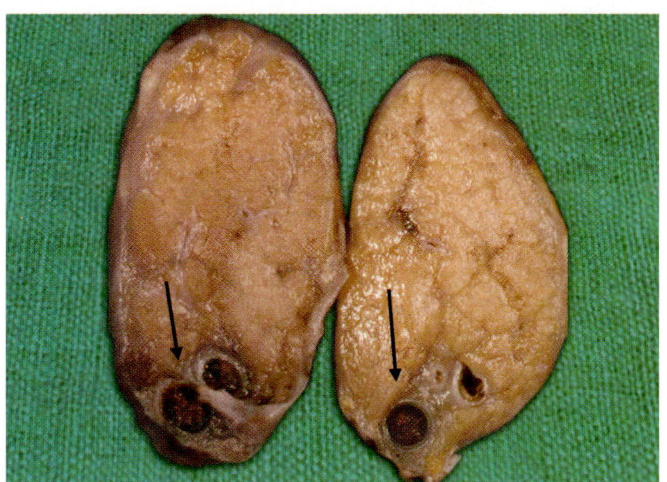

Fig. 36: Differential diagnosis of AMR. Acute AMR in the early post-transplantation period may present clinically with rapid graft thrombosis. Careful pathological evaluation with clinical and serological correlations can help differentiate graft thrombosis due to severe AMR from graft loss due to nonrejection causes such as "technical failure." Graft pancreatectomies performed due to thrombosis for "technical failure" lack features of acute rejection. Specifically intimal arteritis and arterial necrosis (transmural arteritis). In this example of graft thrombosis due to technical failure, the parenchyma is normal, but the vessels are occluded by thrombi (arrows).

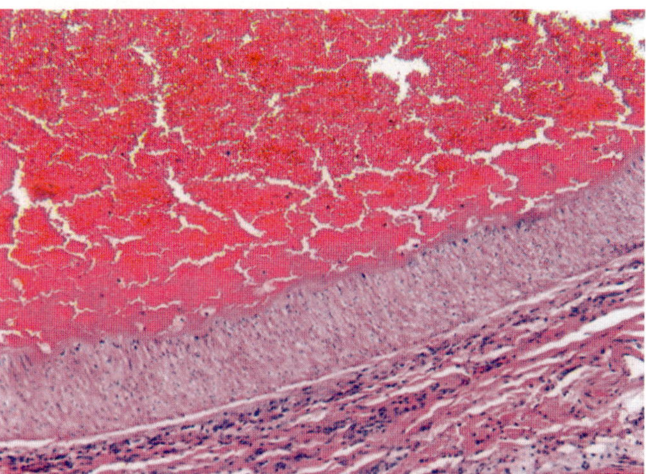

Fig. 37: Histological evaluation of grafts lost to technical failure shows normal arteries occluded by recently formed thrombi.

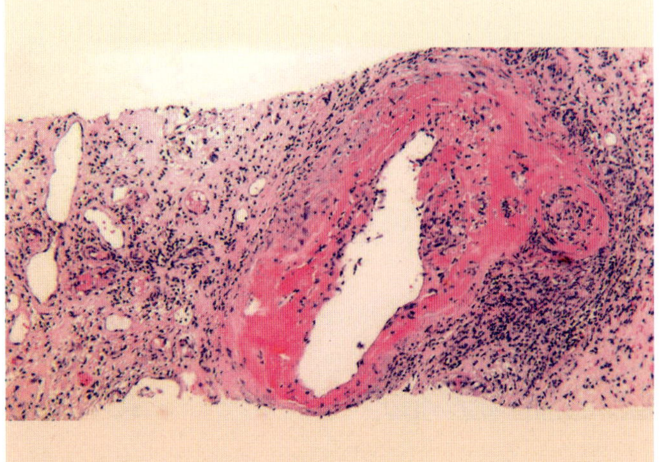

Fig. 38: Mixed acute and chronic T-cell rejection and AMR. Note the extensive parenchymal fibrosis with loss of recognizable acinar tissue. The arteries in the center show inflammation (intimal arteritis and active transplant arteriopathy) as well as extensive fibrinoid necrosis (bright red material in the arterial walls).

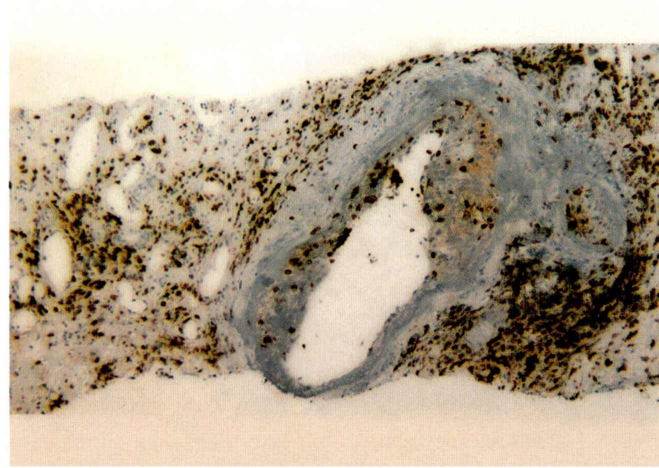

Fig. 39: A CD3 stain in the same field as the previous image demonstrates abundant T-cell infiltrates in the parenchyma, in the arterial intima (intimal arteritis), and in the areas of subintimal fibrosis (chronic allograft arteriopathy).

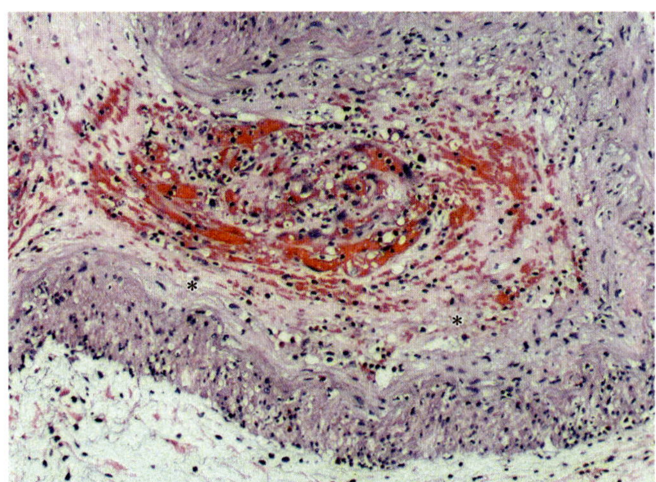

Fig. 40: Segment of artery with luminal obliteration due to ongoing ACMR. The lumen is essentially occluded by edematous and hemorrhagic fibrous tissue admixed with inflammatory cells.

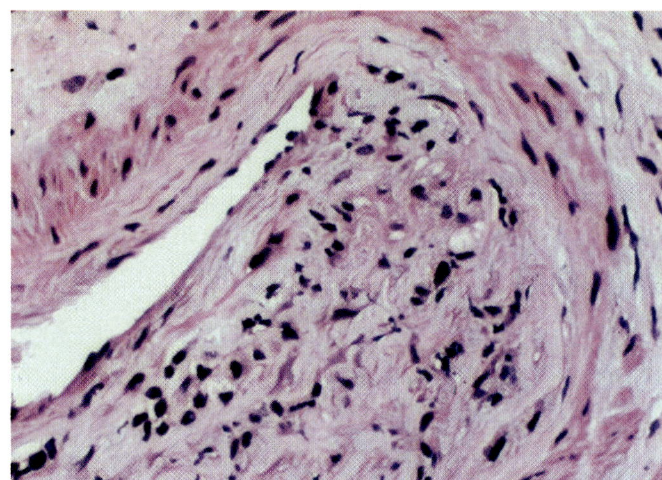

Fig. 41: *Banff category 5: Chronic allograft arteriopathy.* This artery shows asymmetrical luminal narrowing due to marked intimal fibrosis. Note that the fibrosis is cellular and there are numerous inflammatory cell nuclei within the fibrotic area fulfilling the criteria for allograft arteriopathy.

CHRONIC REJECTION GRAFT SCLEROSIS

Progression of graft sclerosis over time has been observed in patients with repeated or persistent rejection episodes.

The extent of fibrosis on pancreatic needle biopsies correlates with graft survival,that is, mild fibrosis is associated with prolonged graft survival, and severe fibrosis correlates with shortened remaining graft function.

The Banff category 5 refers to CHRONIC ALLOGRAFT ARTERIOPATHY. This is defined as arterial intimal fibrosis with mononuclear cell infiltration in the fibrotic areas (Fig. 41).

The Banff category 6 refers to CHRONIC ALLOGRAFT REJECTION/GRAFT FIBROSIS.

- Graft fibrosis is staged as follows:
  - Normal: The fibrous component (f) is limited to normal septa and its amount is proportional to the size of the enclosed structures (ducts and vessels; d, a, V). The acinar exocrine lobules (E/L) show no signs of atrophy or injury. The islets are preserved (i) (Fig. 42A)
  - Stage I (mild graft fibrosis): Expansion of fibrous septa; the fibrosis occupies less than 30% of the core surface but the acinar lobules have eroded, irregular contours. The central lobular areas are normal (Figs. 42B and 43)
  - Stage II (moderate graft fibrosis): The fibrosis occupies 30–60% of the core surface. The exocrine atrophy affects the majority of the lobules in their periphery (irregular contours) and in their central areas (thin fibrous strands criss-cross between individual acini) (Figs. 42C and 44)
  - Stage III (severe graft fibrosis): The fibrotic areas predominate and occupy more than 60% of the core surface with only isolated areas of residual acinar tissue and/or islets present (Figs. 42D and 45 to 49)

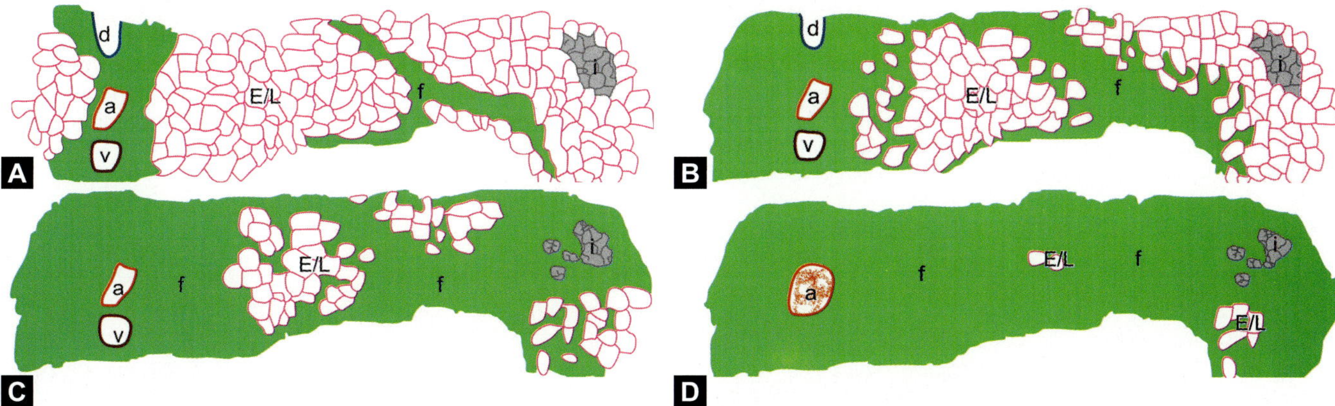

Figs. 42A to D: Normal, Stage I, Stage II, and Stage III graft fibrosis.

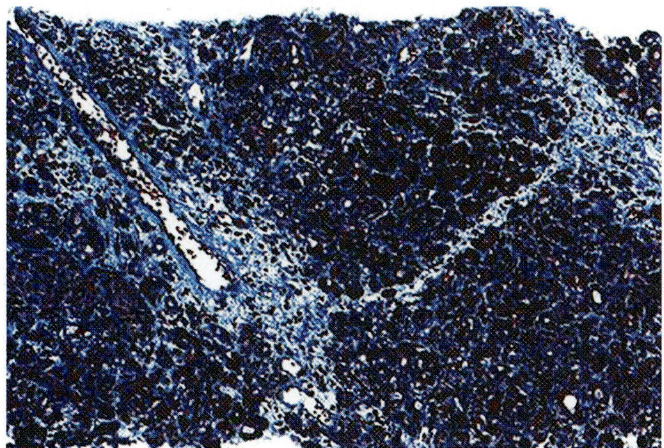

Fig. 43: Trichrome stain in a biopsy with acute allograft rejection. The septal areas show expansion, mostly due to interstitial edema (clear spaces separating the collagen fibers). The extent of the parenchymal inflammation diffusely involving the acini cannot be appreciated in this stain. After treatment with antilymphocytic globulin there was only partial clinical response.

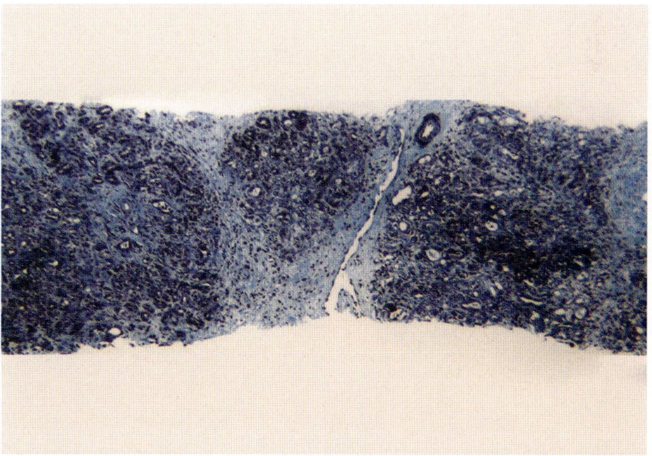

Fig. 44: Follow-up biopsy 1 month after treatment of moderate ACMR (Banff grade II) demonstrates marked decrease of the inflammatory infiltrates; however, the parenchyma shows prominent fibrosis that was not present at the time of the 1st biopsy. Note the expansion of the fibrous septa, as well as separation of the acini by interacinar connective tissue. Development of variable degrees of fibrosis as a sequela of moderate and/or severe acute rejection is the rule in pancreas allografts.

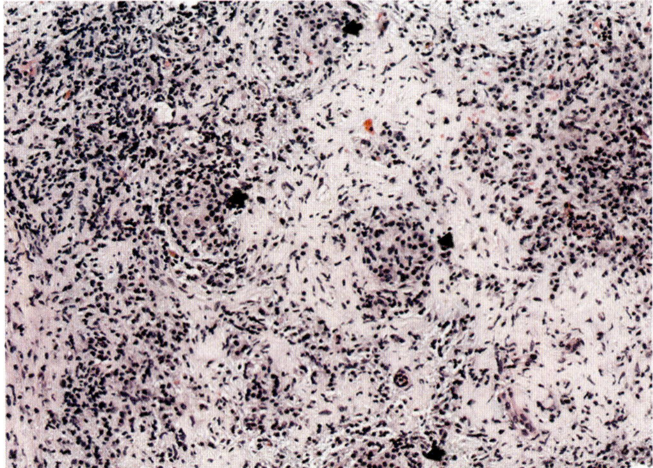

Fig. 45: This is an example of acute ACMR superimposed on chronic rejection/graft sclerosis. There are prominent inflammatory infiltrates in residual clusters of acinar parenchyma (top right area), as well as significant parenchymal fibrosis, also showing inflammation. Three residual islets of Langerhans are clearly identified (arrowheads).

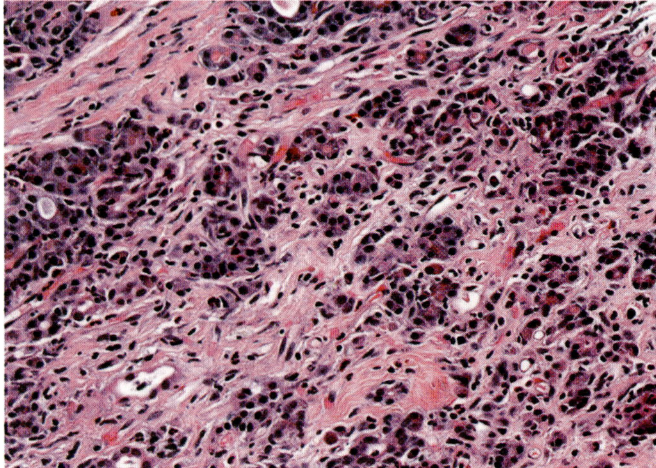

Fig. 46: Example of lobular fibrosis due to ongoing AMR. Compare the lobular architecture in this image to the normal lobular tissue seen in Figure 4. Parenchymal fibrosis results from both ACMR and AMR (ongoing, chronic).

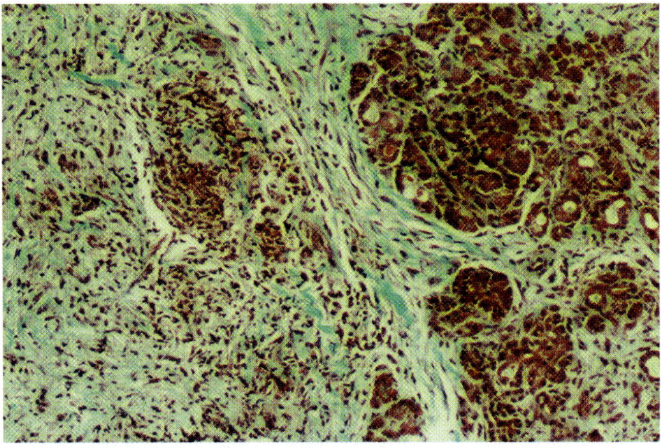

Fig. 47: Moderate fibrosis of pancreas allograft (Banff stage II). Extensive septal and partial acinar fibrosis are highlighted with the Masson's trichrome stain.

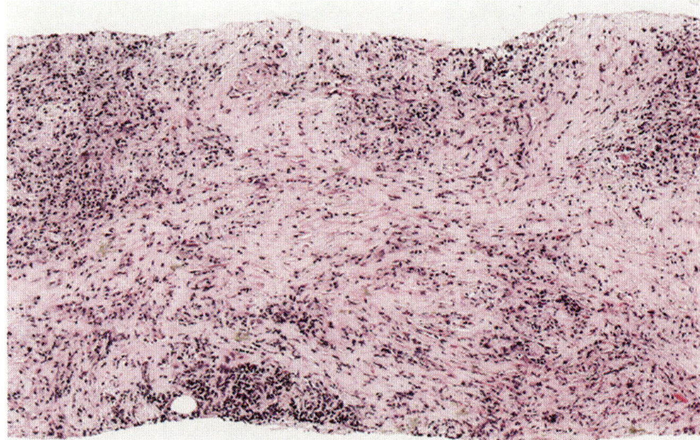

Fig. 48: H&E stain of severe graft sclerosis (Banff stage III). Abundant clusters of inflammatory cells are present but residual exocrine or endocrine parenchyma cannot be identified.

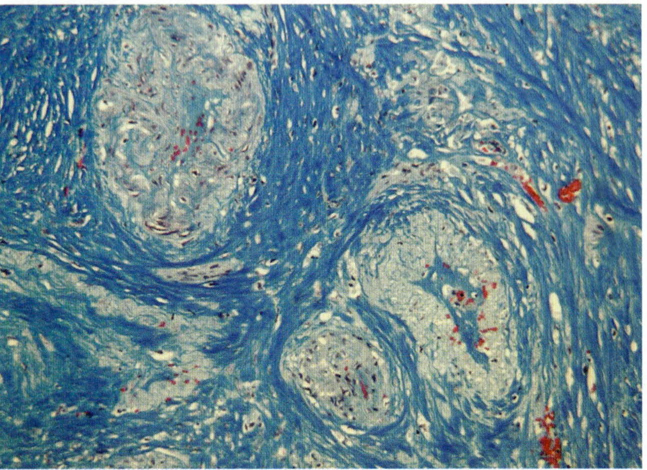

Fig. 49: Vascular obliteration is a common feature of advanced pancreas allograft sclerosis. This Masson's trichrome stain demonstrates arteries and a vein with total or subtotal occlusion of the vascular lumina by fibrous tissue.

ISLET ALLOGRAFT PATHOLOGY

The Banff category 7 refers to islet disorders including

- Recurrence of autoimmune DM (insulitis, selective B cell loss)
- Islet amyloid (amylin) deposition
- Islet cell drug toxicity

In patients biopsied for hyperglycemia, the possibility of an islet process should be ruled out with additional evaluation of insulin and glucagon stains that identify beta and alpha cells, respectively (Figs. 50 to 53).

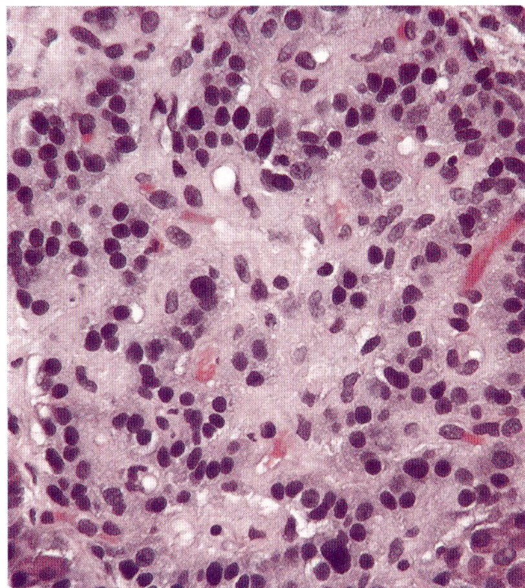

Fig. 50: Islet of Langerhans from a patient with recurrent autoimmune diabetes mellitus. The islet cells appear normal, although there is some degree of hyalinization (accumulation of pink amorphous tissue within the islet itself). It is not possible to distinguish alpha from beta cells without the aid of special stains.

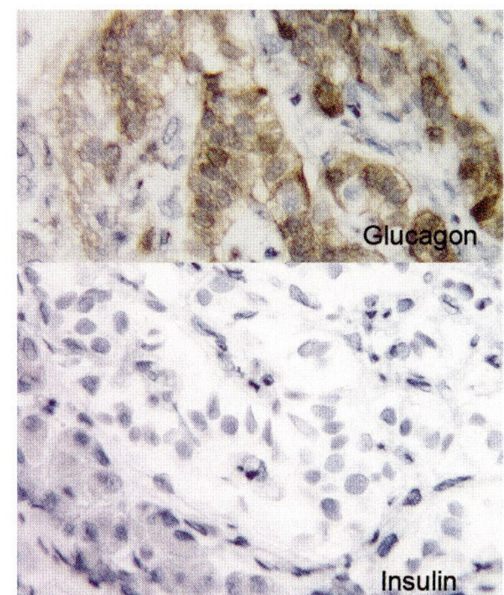

Fig. 51: Loss of the insulin producing beta cells is found in patients with recurrence of autoimmune diabetes mellitus. Beta cells are lost due to the inflammatory process specifically targeting them. The active inflammatory process presenting as insulitis (islet centered inflammation with destruction of beta cells) is typically transient and the islets may appear normal once the beta cells have been destroyed. An example of recurrent autoimmune DM is presented here in which the insulin stain is completely negative consistent with complete absence of beta cells, in contrast to the stain for glucagon stain that demonstrates abundant glucagon producing alpha cells.

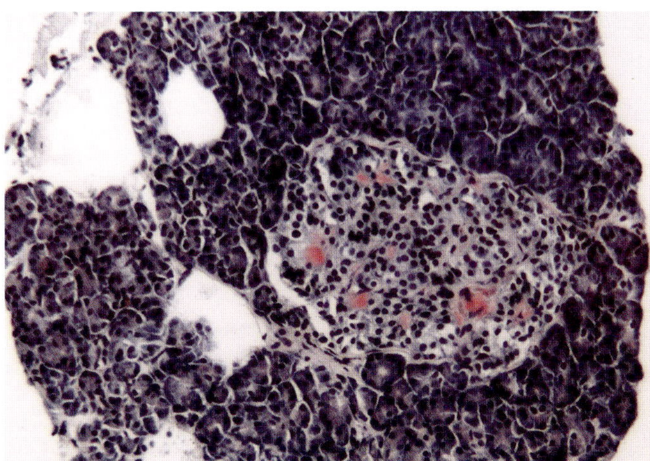

Fig. 52: A rare finding in patients biopsied due to hyperglycemia is the presence of islet amyloid (amylin). This material appears to deposit in patients with excessive insulin production (hyperinsulinemic state) leading to accumulation of amylin, a factor normally secreted together with insulin. Islet amyloid is identified with the Congo red stain that in this image identifies globular amyloid deposits within the islet. Note that the process only involves the islets and the adjacent parenchyma is not inflamed and lacks fibrosis. Mild fatty infiltration is noted (white spaces on left).

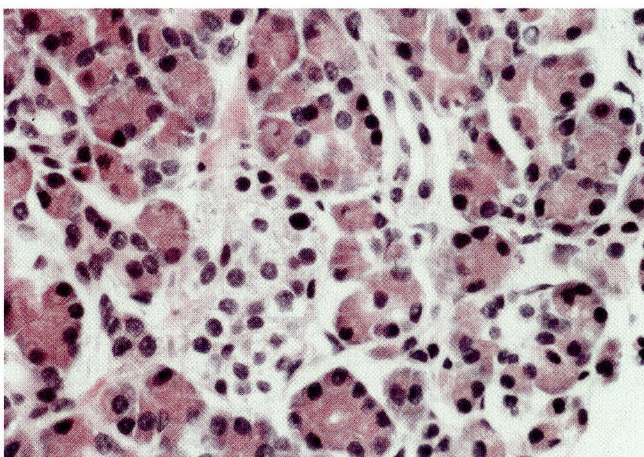

Fig. 53: Another cause of hyperglycemia due to islet cell injury is drug toxicity (in particular calcineurin inhibitor toxicity). The damaged islets cells appear clear due to cytoplasmic vacuolization. This process is typically reversible with adjustment of CNI dose.

FURTHER READING

1. Andersson A, Bohman S, Borg LA, et al. Amyloid deposition in transplanted human pancreatic islets: a conceivable cause of their long-term failure. Exp Diabetes Res. vol. 2008, doi:10.1155/2008/562985
2. Assalino M, Genevay M, Morel P, et al. Recurrence of type 1 diabetes after simultaneous pancreas-kidney transplantation in the absence of GAD and IA-2 autoantibodies. Am J Transplant. 2012;2:492-5.
3. Burke GW, 3rd, Vendrame F, Pileggi A, et al. Recurrence of autoimmunity following pancreas transplantation. Curr Diab Rep. 2011;11:413–9.
4. Cantarovich D, De Amicis S, Akl A, et al. Post-transplant donor-specific anti-HLA antibodies negatively impact pancreas transplantation outcome. Am J Transplant. 2011;11:2737–46.
5. Carbajal R, Karam G, Renaudin K, et al. Specific humoral rejection of a pancreas allograft in a recipient of pancreas after kidney transplantation. Nephrol Dial Transplant. 2007;22:942–4.
6. Carpenter HA, Engen DE, Munn SR, et al. Histologic features of rejection in cystoscopically directed needle biopsies of pancreatoduodenal allografts in dogs and humans. Transplant Proc. 1990;22:707–8.
7. de Kort H, Munivenkatappa RB, Berger SP, , et al. Pancreas allograft biopsies with positive C4d staining and anti-donor antibodies related to worse outcome for patients. Am J Transplant 201023;10:1660–7.
8. Drachenberg C, Klassen D, Bartlett S, et al. Histologic grading of pancreas acute allograft rejection in percutaneous needle biopsies. Transplant Proc. 1996;28:512–3.
9. Drachenberg CB, Abruzzo LV, Klassen DK, et al. Epstein-Barr virus-related post-transplantation lymphoproliferative disorder involving pancreas allografts: histological differential diagnosis from acute allograft rejection. Hum Pathol. 1998;29:569–77.
10. Drachenberg CB, Klassen DK, Weir MR, et al. Islet cell damage associated with tacrolimus and cyclosporine: morphological features in pancreas allograft biopsies and clinical correlation. Transplantation. 1999;68:396–402.
11. Drachenberg CB, Odorico J, Demetris AJ, et al. Banff schema for grading pancreas allograft rejection: working proposal by a multi-disciplinary international consensus panel. Am J Transplant: Official Journal of the American Society of Transplantation and the American Society of Transplant Surgeons. 2008;8:1237–49.
12. Drachenberg CB, Torrealba JR, Nankivell BJ, et al. Guidelines for the diagnosis of antibody-mediated rejection in pancreas allografts-updated Banff grading schema. Am J Transplant. 2011;11:1792–802.
13. Gaber LW. Pancreas allograft biopsies in the management of pancreas transplant recipients: histopathologic review and clinical correlations. Arch Pathol Lab Med [Review]. 2007;131:1192–9.
14. Klassen DK, Drachenberg CB, Papadimitriou JC, et al. CMV allograft pancreatitis: diagnosis, treatment, and histological features. Transplantation. 2000;69:1968–71.
15. Margreiter C, Aigner F, Resch T, et al. Enteroscopic biopsies in the management of pancreas transplants: a proof of concept study for a novel monitoring tool. Transplantation. 2012;93:207–13.
16. Papadimitriou JC, Drachenberg CB, Klassen DK, et al. Histological grading of chronic pancreas allograft rejection/graft sclerosis. Am J Transplant. 2003;3:599–605.
17. Papadimitriou JC, Wiland A, Drachenberg CB, et al. Effectiveness of immunosuppressive treatment for recurrent or refractory pancreas allograft rejection: correlation with histologic grade. Transplant Proc. 1998;30:3945.
18. Sibley RK, Sutherland DE. Pancreas transplantation. An immunohistologic and histopathologic examination of 100 grafts. Am J Pathol. 1987;128:151–70.
19. Torrealba JR, Samaniego M, Pascual J, et al. C4d-positive interacinar capillaries correlates with donor-specific antibody-mediated rejection in pancreas allografts. Transplantation. 2008;86:1849–56.
20. Troxell ML, Koslin DB, Norman D, et al. Pancreas allograft rejection: analysis of concurrent renal allograft biopsies and posttherapy follow-up biopsies. Transplantation. 2010; 90:75–84.
21. Vendrame F, Pileggi A, Laughlin E, et al. Recurrence of type 1 diabetes after simultaneous pancreas-kidney transplantation, despite immunosuppression, is associated with autoantibodies and pathogenic autoreactive CD4 T-cells. Diabetes. 2010;59:947–57.
22. Westermark P Amyloid in the islets of Langerhans: thoughts and some historical aspects. Ups J Med Sci. 2011;116:81–9.

CHAPTER 71

Radiology

Mariano Volpacchio, Catherine D'Agostino, Christopher Palestro, et al.

ORTHOTOPIC PANCREAS TRANSPLANT—PORTAL (SUPERIOR MESENTERIC) VENOUS DRAINAGE (FIGS. 1 TO 14)

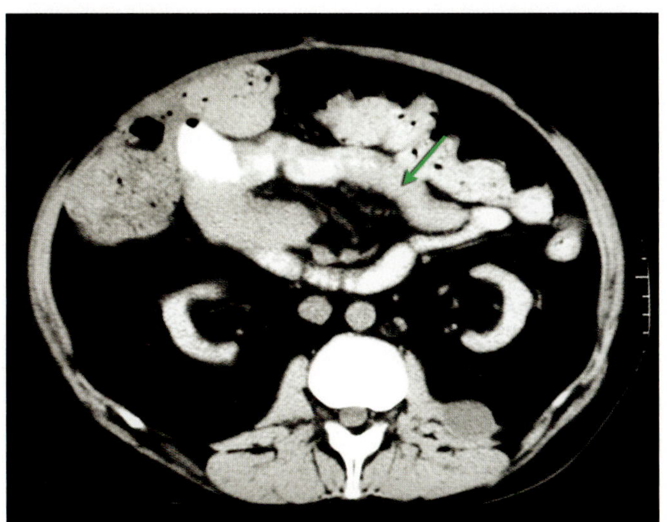

Fig. 1

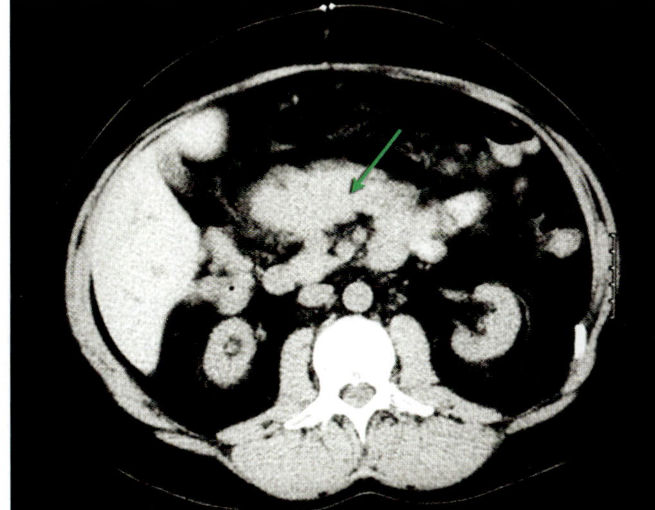

Fig. 2

Figs. 1 and 2: CT scans of pancreas (green arrows) transplants with venous drainage into the superior mesenteric and portal vein. Note that the pancreas is implanted onto the superior mesenteric vein close to its junction with the portal vein. The transverse colon and its mesentery lie ventral to the pancreas allograft, while the root of the small bowel mesentery lies dorsal to it. The native pancreas is also dorsal with respect to the allograft.

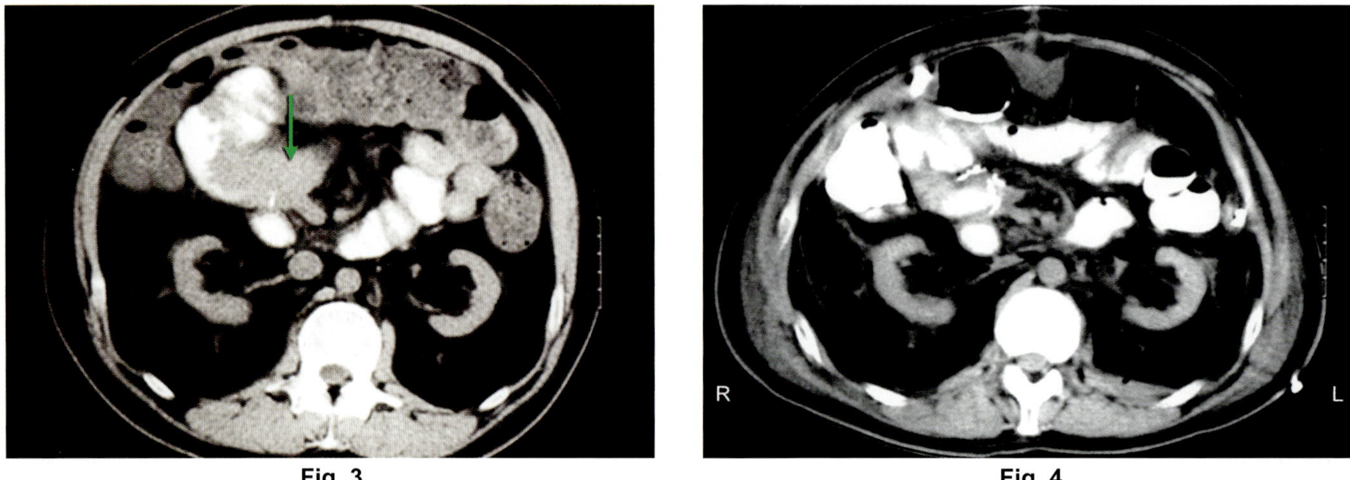

Fig. 3

Fig. 4

Figs. 3 and 4: In these images, it is possible to visualize the metallic clips in the duodenum, whose lumen is opacified with oral contrast in a pancreas transplant with portal venous drainage. The head of the transplanted pancreas is shown by an arrow (Fig. 3). Notice the atrophic native kidneys.

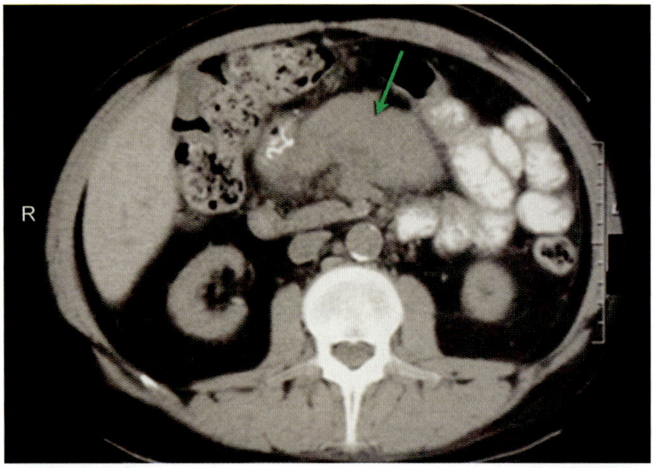

Fig. 5

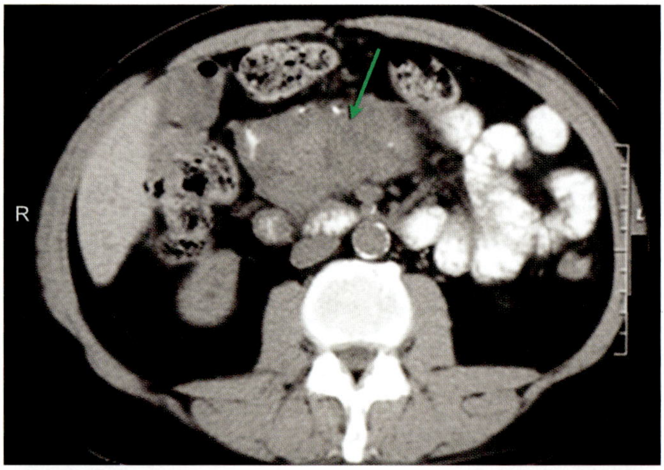

Fig. 6

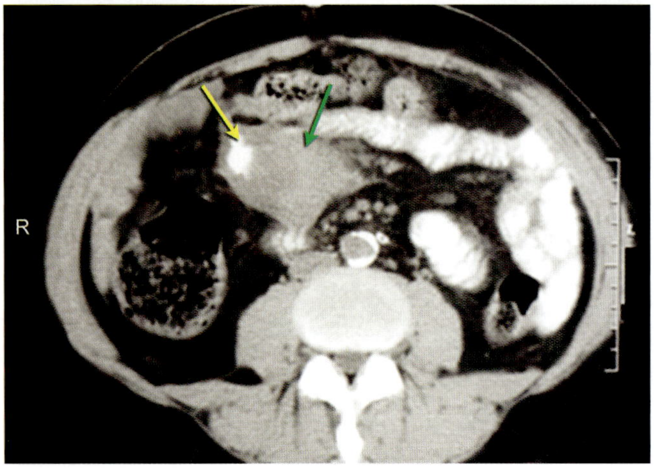

Fig. 7

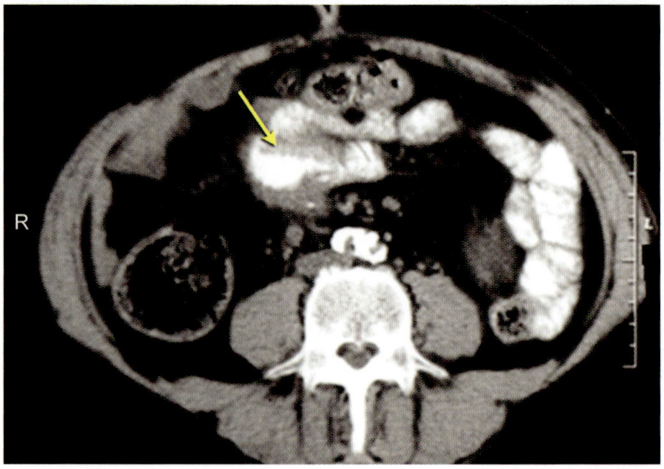

Fig. 8

Figs. 5 to 8: Sequential axial CT images showing a mildly enlarged pancreas allograft (green arrows) and its duodenal stump (yellow arrows). Notice the extensive aortoiliac atheromatous calcifications in this diabetic patient.

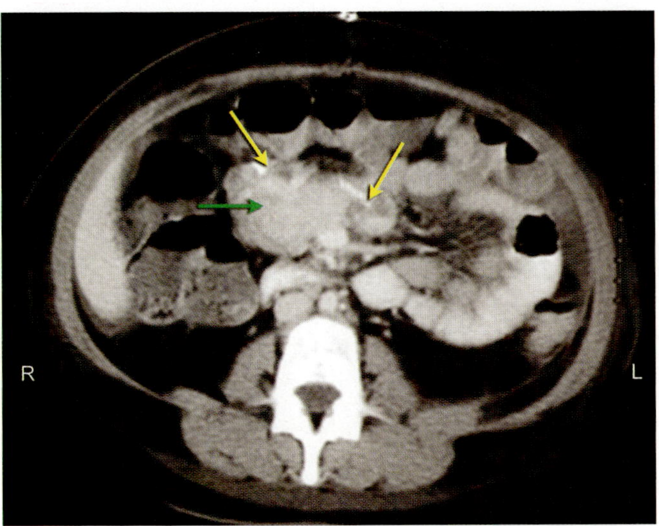

Fig. 9

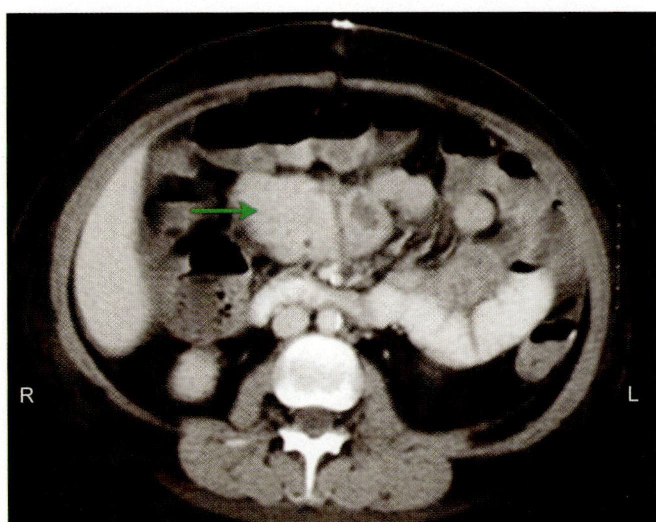

Fig. 10

Figs. 9 and 10: Axial contrast-enhanced CT images showing a normal-appearing well-perfused head of an orthotopic pancreatic graft (green arrows). The metallic staples (yellow arrows) indicate the edges of the duodenal stump.

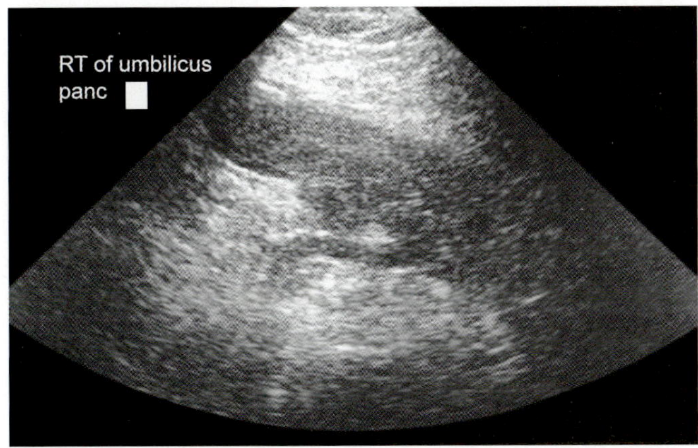

Fig. 11: Transverse ultrasound of a well-functioning pancreatic graft. Notice the normal-appearing uniform echotexture.

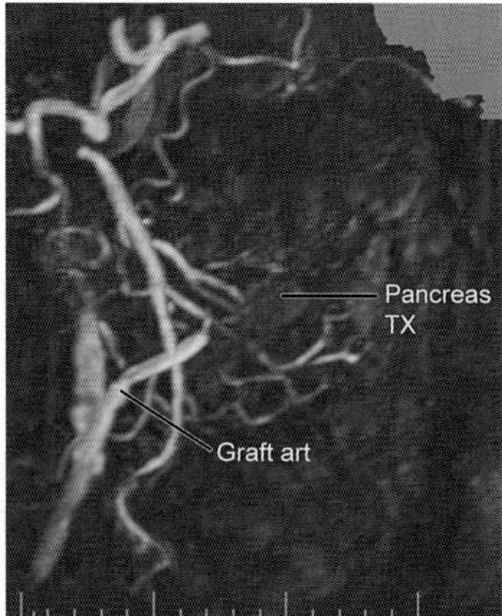

Fig. 12

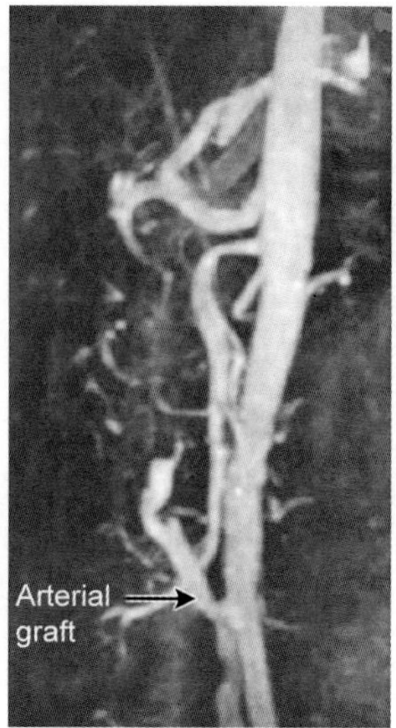

Fig. 13

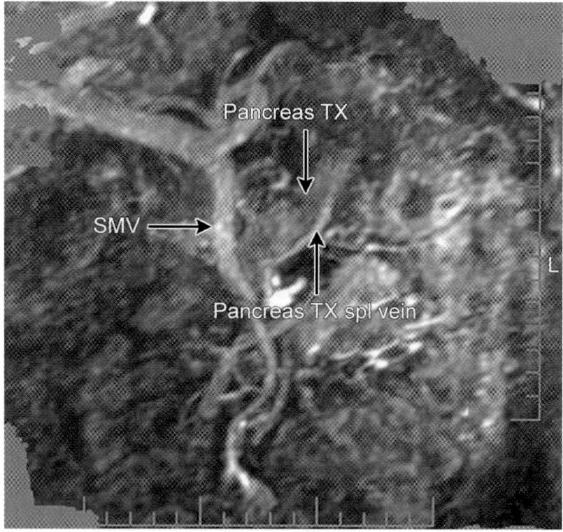

Fig. 14

Figs. 12 to 14: MRA images showing a normal-caliber patent arterial vessel graft emerging from the distal aorta/common iliac artery and supplying the pancreas graft. Notice also the patent portal vein draining the transplanted gland. MRI with its angiographic capabilities (MRA and MRV) provides a superb technique that allows for the evaluation of the graft vasculature in a noninvasive fashion.

HETEROTOPIC PANCREAS TRANSPLANT—SYSTEMIC VENOUS DRAINAGE (FIGS. 15 TO 17)

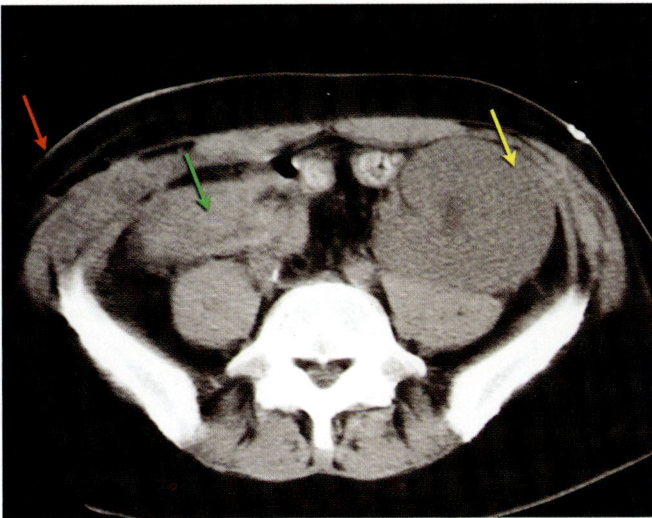

Fig. 15: CT scan of a pancreas (green arrow) transplant with systemic venous drainage. In this specific instance, a kidney (yellow arrow) was transplanted simultaneously. Note that the pancreas is implanted onto the iliac vein in the right lower quadrant. Placing the pancreas on the right side allows for better access to the small bowel or urinary bladder for exocrine drainage. Placing the pancreas on the left side is also possible, but the left and sigmoid colon could potentially make the bowel or bladder anastomoses more difficult. Note the abdominal wall defect (red arrow) on the right lower quadrant.

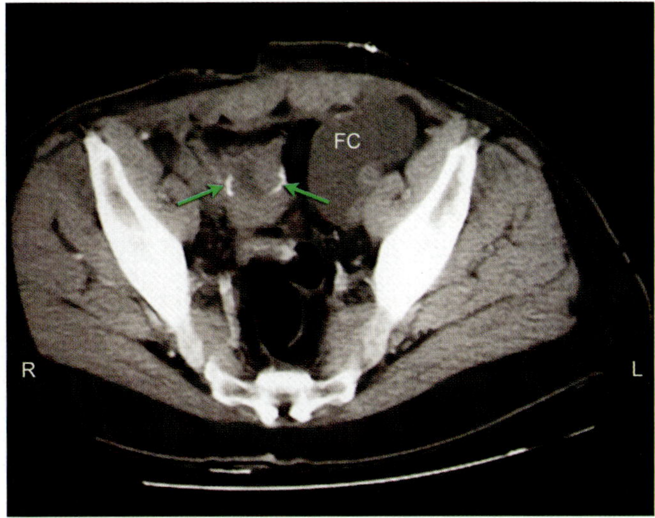

Fig. 16: Note the staple lines in the transplant duodenum (green arrows) and the fluid collection (FC) in the left lower quadrant.

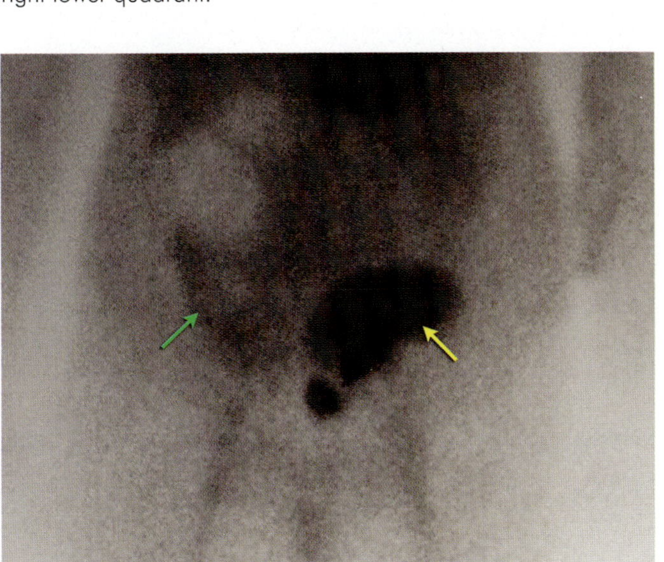

Fig. 17: Nuclear medicine study of a simultaneous pancreas (green arrow) and kidney (yellow arrow) transplant. In this instance, the pancreas transplant has systemic venous and enteric exocrine drainage. Radionuclide studies can provide useful information on blood flow and function.

DUPLEX DOPPLER ULTRASOUND IMAGING—ARTERIAL SUPPLY AND VENOUS DRAINAGE (FIGS. 18 TO 20)

- The first 24–48 hours after implantation are crucial for thrombosis of the pancreatic allograft
- We routinely obtain a baseline duplex Doppler ultrasound examination in the immediate post-operative period as well as in the first post-transplant day
- Further repeat studies are obtained based on clinical events

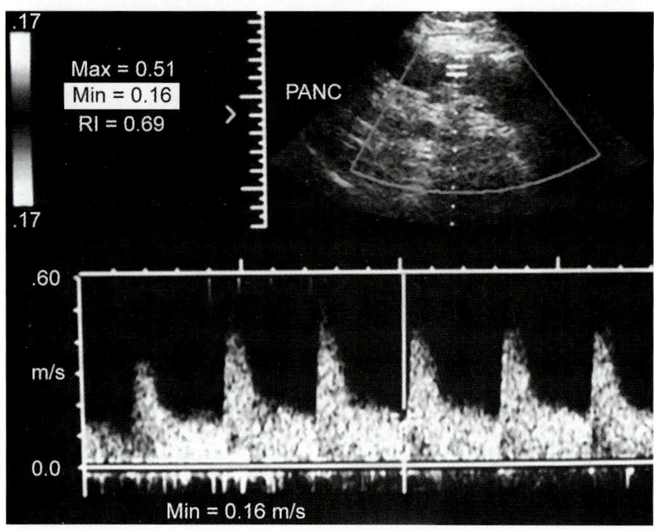

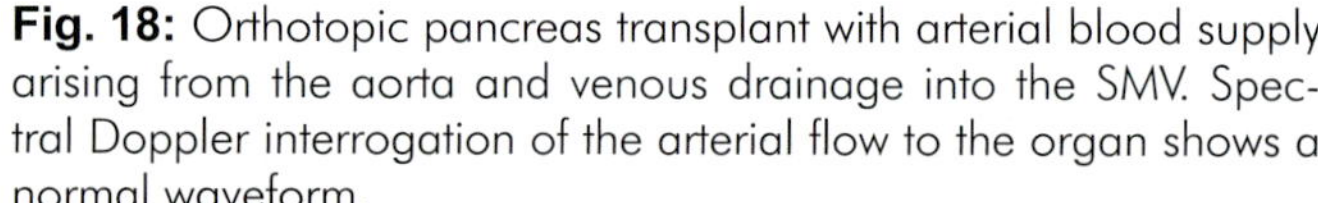
Fig. 18: Orthotopic pancreas transplant with arterial blood supply arising from the aorta and venous drainage into the SMV. Spectral Doppler interrogation of the arterial flow to the organ shows a normal waveform.

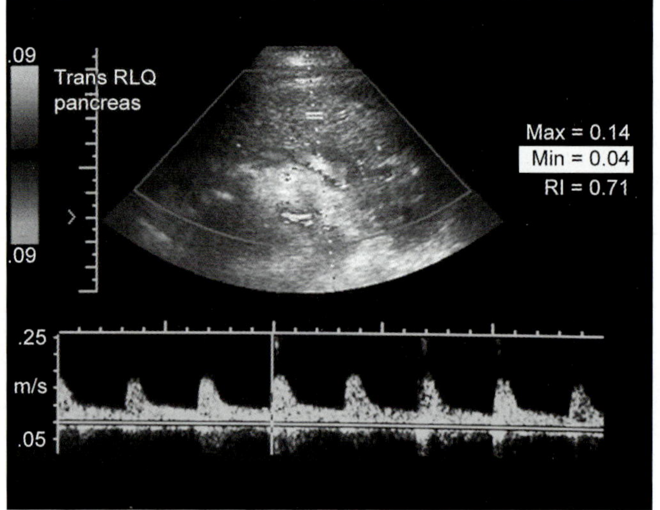

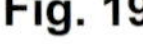
Fig. 19

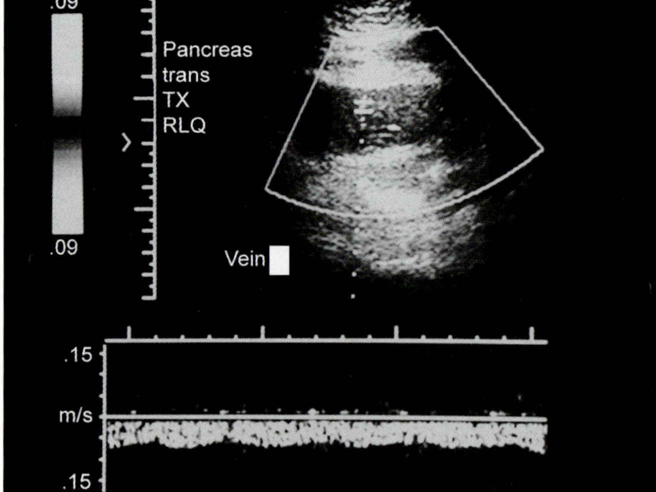

Fig. 20

Figs. 19 and 20: Heterotopic pancreas transplant with arterial supply from the iliac artery and venous drainage into iliac vein. Note the normal pancreatic arterial (Fig. 19) and venous (Fig. 20) waveforms.

PANCREATIC FISTULA (FIG. 21)

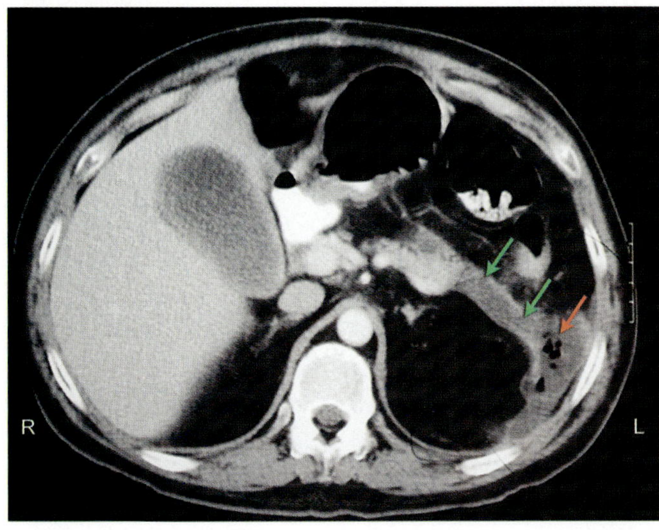

Fig. 21: Axial contrast-enhanced CT image showing a well-circumscribed fluid collection (green arrows) by the tail of the transplanted pancreas. Notice the presence of gas bubbles (red arrow) within the collection.

PERFORATION OF TRANSPLANTED DUODENUM (FIGS. 22 AND 23)

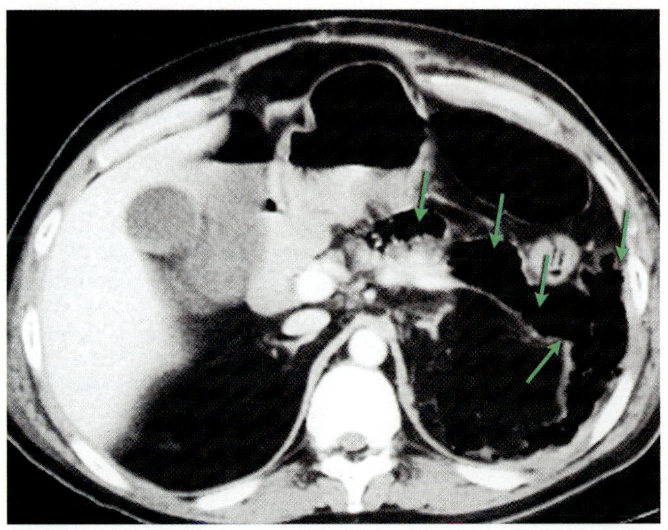

Fig. 22

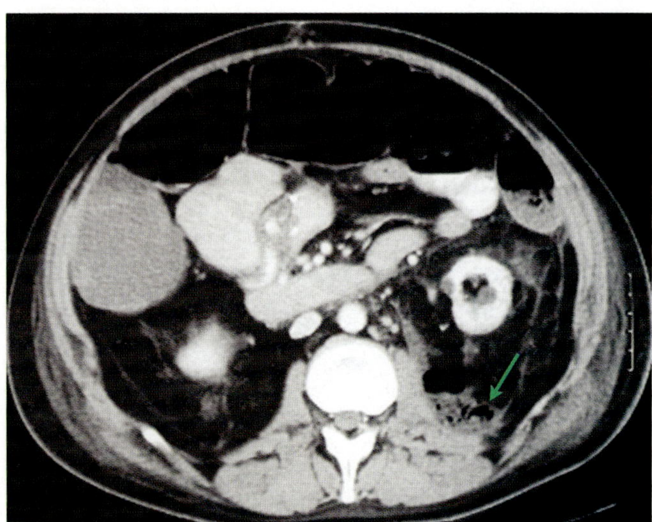

Fig. 23

Figs. 22 and 23: Isolated pancreas transplant with perforation of the transplant duodenum. Sequential axial contrast-enhanced CT images show a gas collection (arrows) arising from the duodenum (that proved to be perforated) and dissecting through the left retroperitoneal fat planes.

NORMAL BODY OF PANCREAS ALLOGRAFT (FIGS. 24 AND 25)

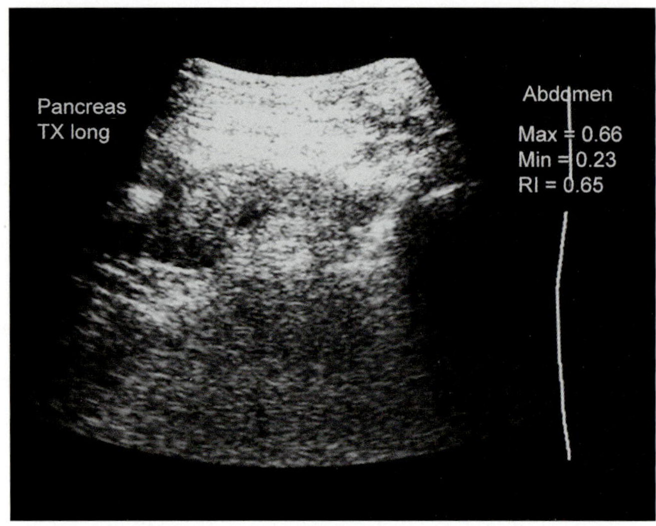

Fig. 24

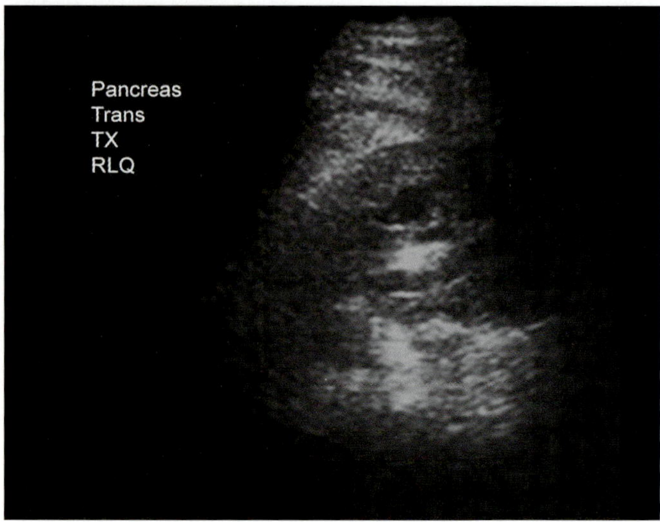

Fig. 25

Figs. 24 and 25: Two examples of normal pancreas grafts (portal venous drainage on Figure 24 and systemic venous drainage on Figure 25) on ultrasound imaging. Notice the homogeneous echotexture and the smooth margins surrounded by hyperechoic fat.

PANCREAS ALLOGRAFT EDEMA (FIGS. 26 AND 27)

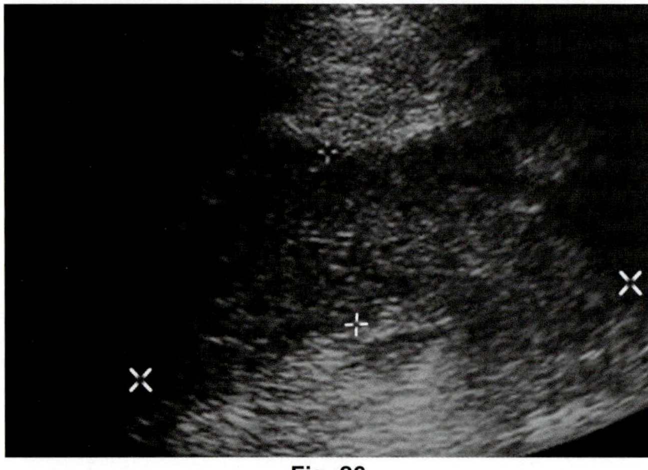

Fig. 26

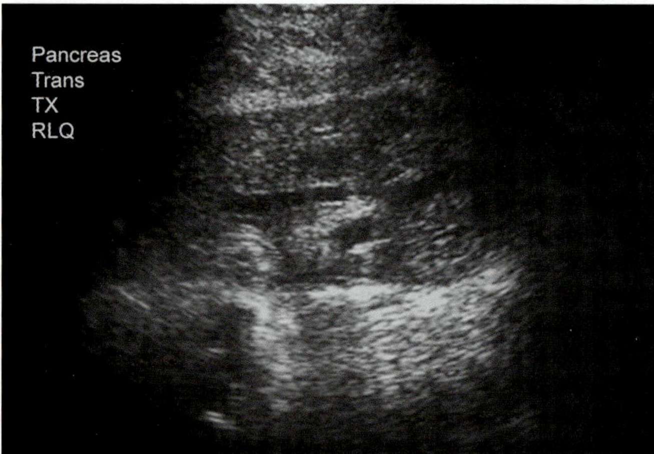

Fig. 27

Figs. 26 and 27: Transverse ultrasound images of enlarged edematous pancreatic grafts as evidenced by their decreased echogenicity.

ALLOGRAFT PANCREATITIS (FIGS. 28 TO 35)

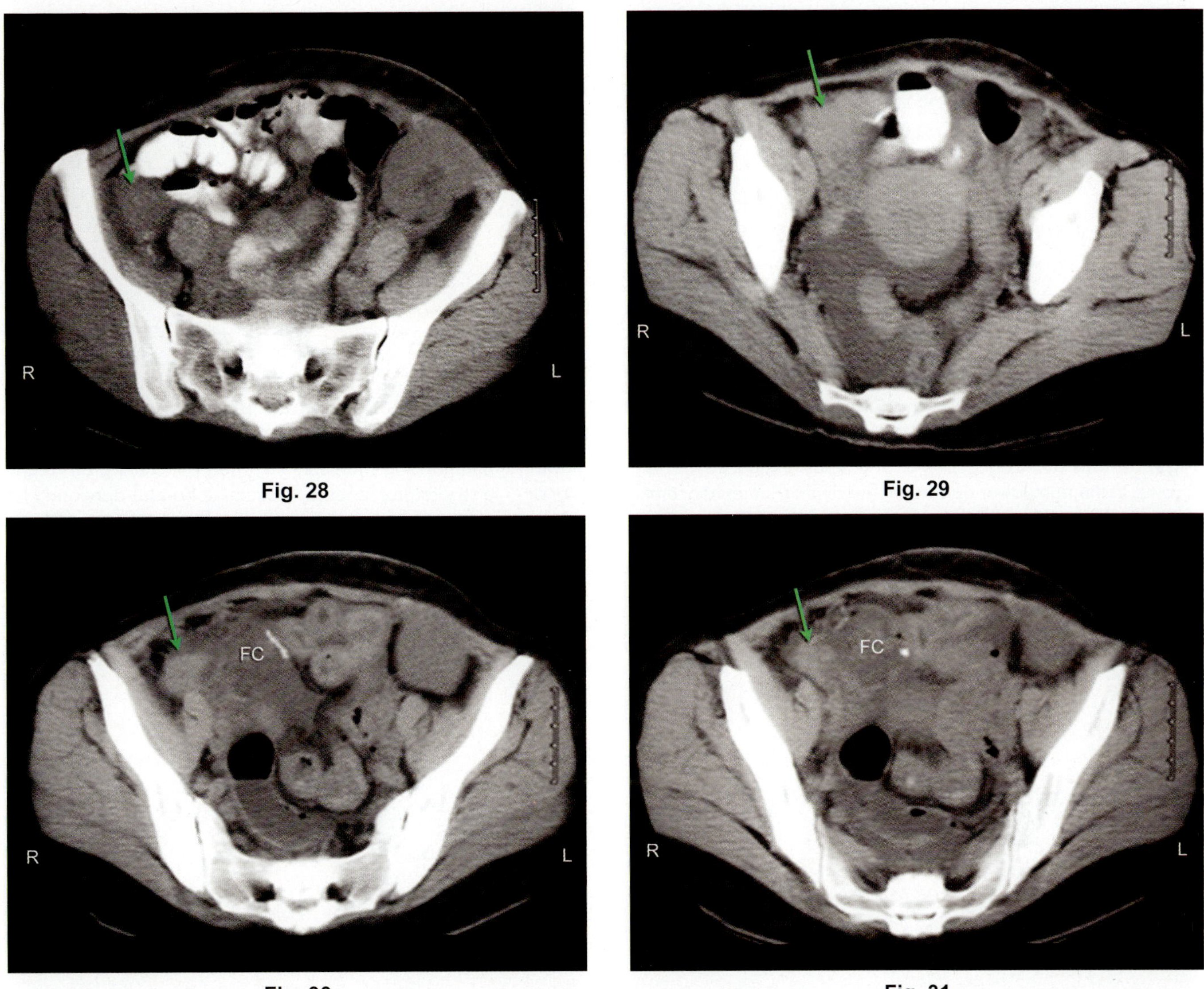

Fig. 28

Fig. 29

Fig. 30

Fig. 31

Figs. 28 to 31: Sequential axial CT images showing an enlarged heterogeneous right lower quadrant pancreatic graft (arrows) surrounded by a fluid collection (FC). Stranding of surrounding fat is also noted. The concept of gallstone pancreatitis is nonexistent in cases of allograft pancreatitis.

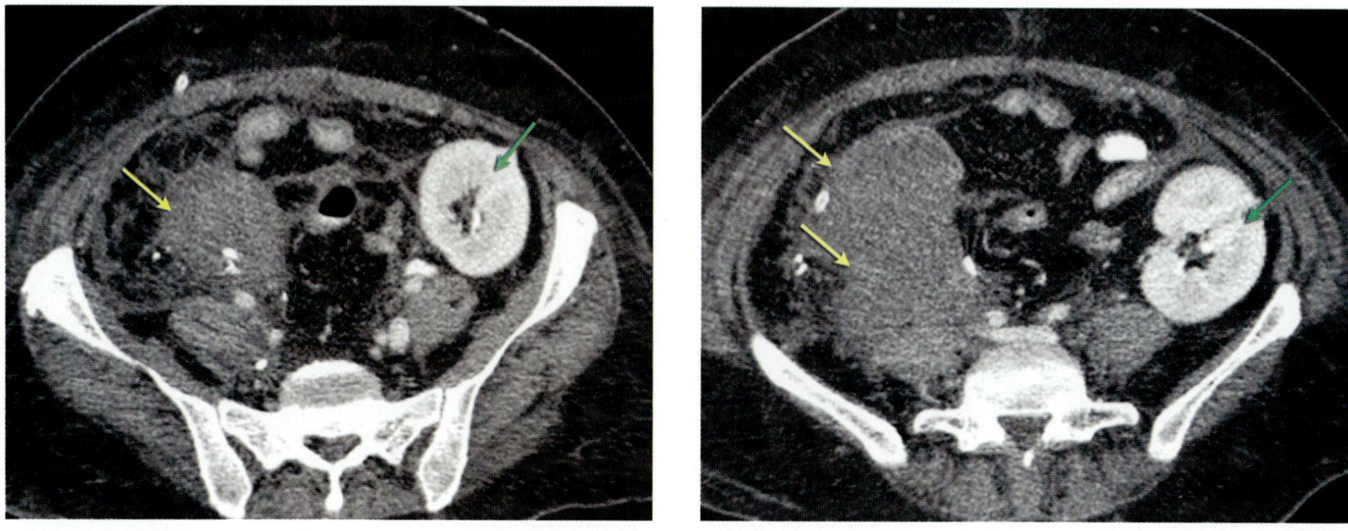

Fig. 32

Fig. 33

Figs. 32 and 33: Contiguous axial contrast-enhanced CT images showing nonenhancing markedly enlarged pancreas graft (yellow arrows) in the right lower quadrant. The diminished enhancement is secondary to severe graft edema. Notice the normal-appearing left lower quadrant kidney graft (green arrows).

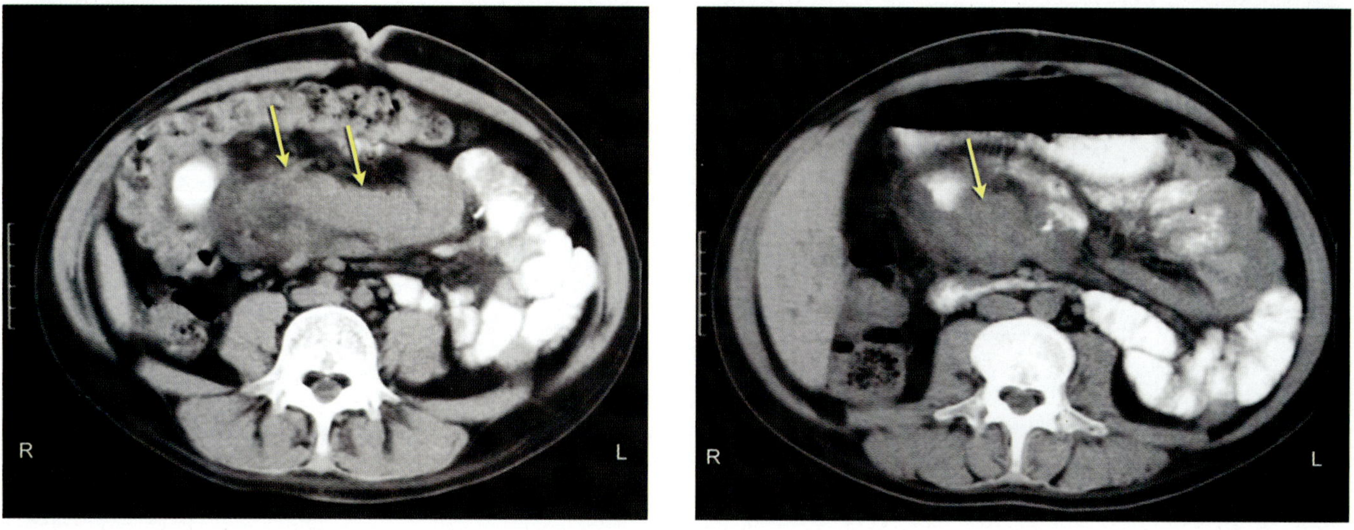

Fig. 34

Fig. 35

Figs. 34 and 35: Sequential axial CT images showing an edematous orthotopic pancreatic graft (arrows) with adjacent fat stranding. These findings are typical in both native and transplant pancreatitis.

ALLOGRAFT PANCREATITIS WITH NECROSIS (FIGS. 36 TO 38)

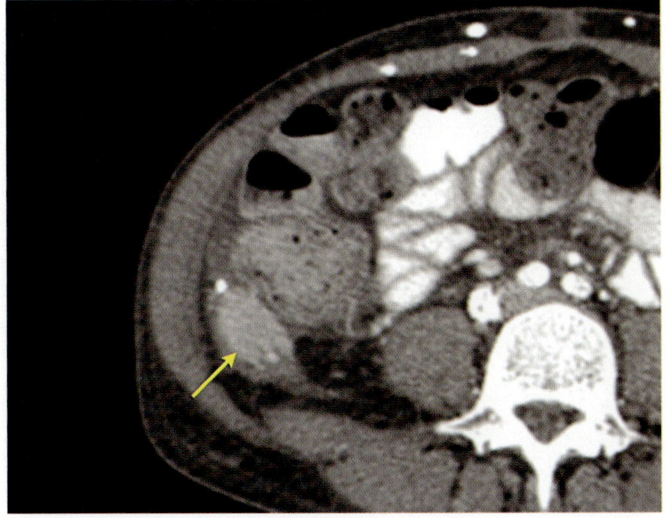

Fig. 36

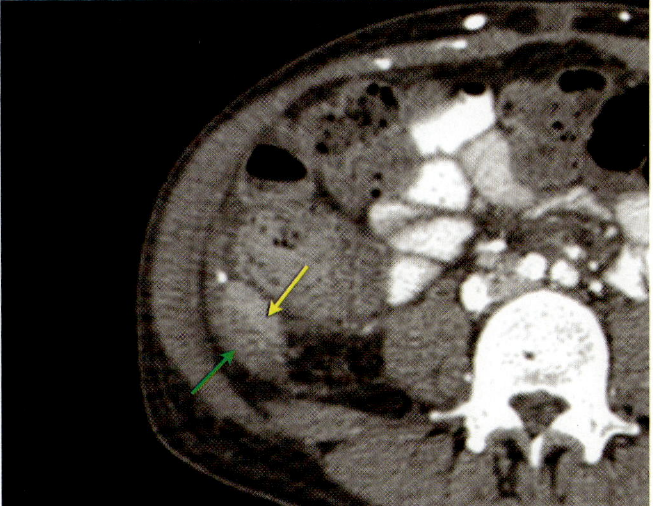

Fig. 37

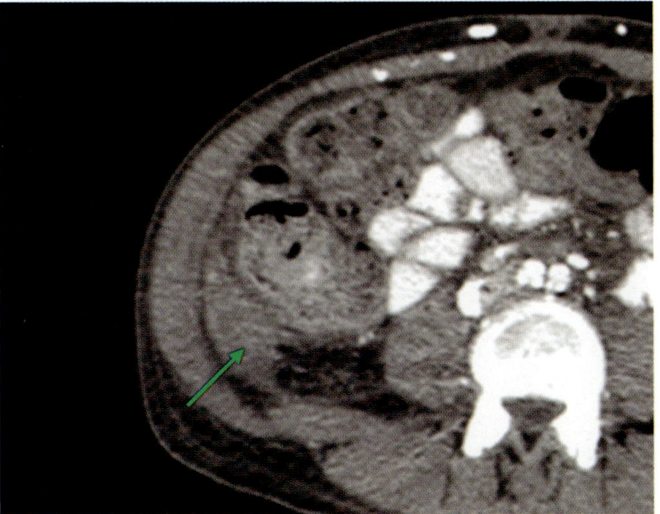

Fig. 38

Figs. 36 to 38: Contiguous contrast-enhanced axial CT images showing the transition between inflammed but well-perfused pancreas graft (yellow arrows) to a nonenhancing necrosed tail (green arrows) in this patient with graft pancreatitis. Notice the perigraft fat stranding.

PERIPANCREATIC COLLECTIONS (FIGS. 39 TO 46)

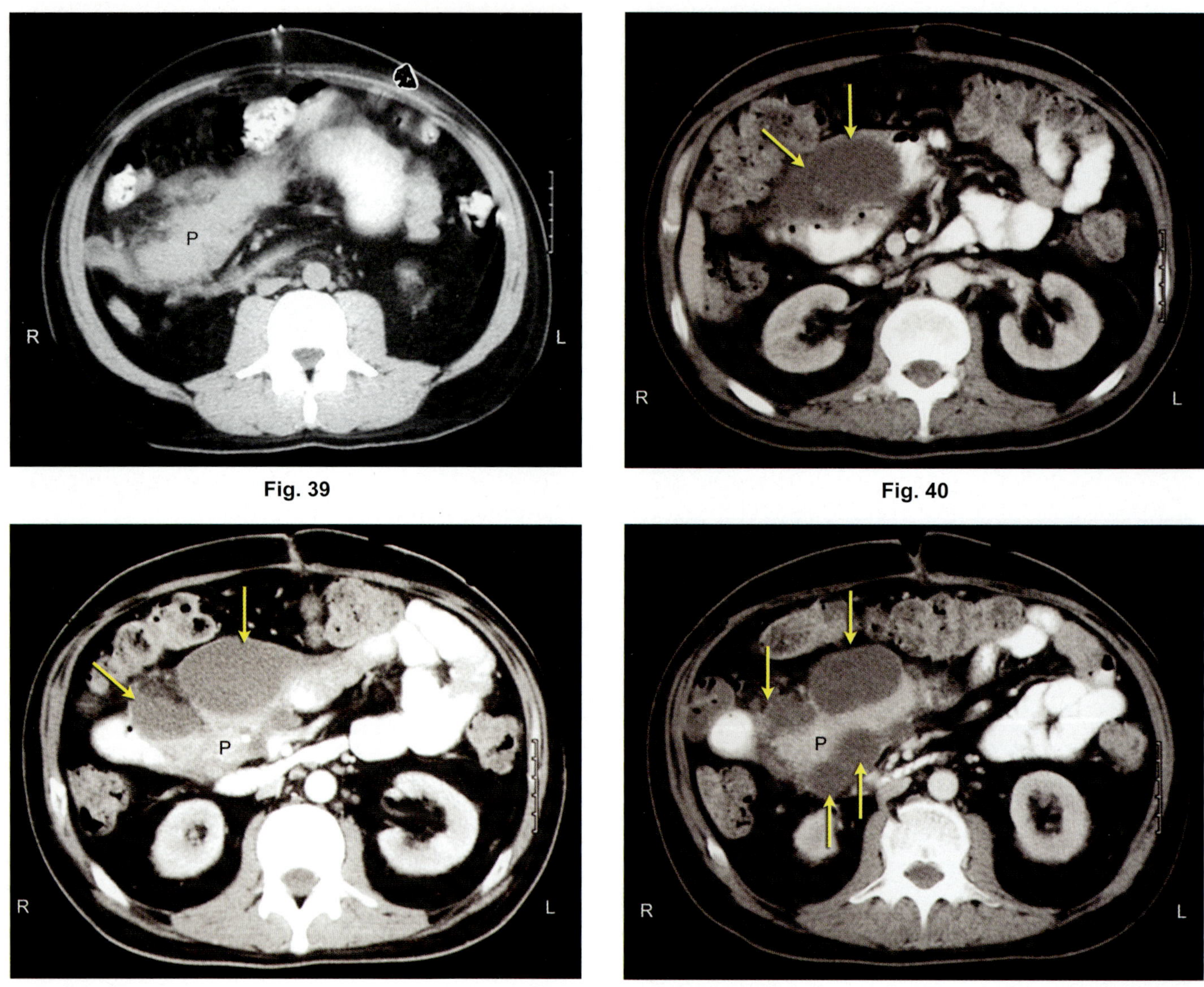

Fig. 39

Fig. 40

Fig. 41

Fig. 42

Figs. 39 to 42: Sequential axial contrast-enhanced CT images showing multiple, well-demarcated fluid collections (arrows) surrounding and indenting on the pancreas allograft. Notice the compressed pancreas (P) with normal density and enhancement.

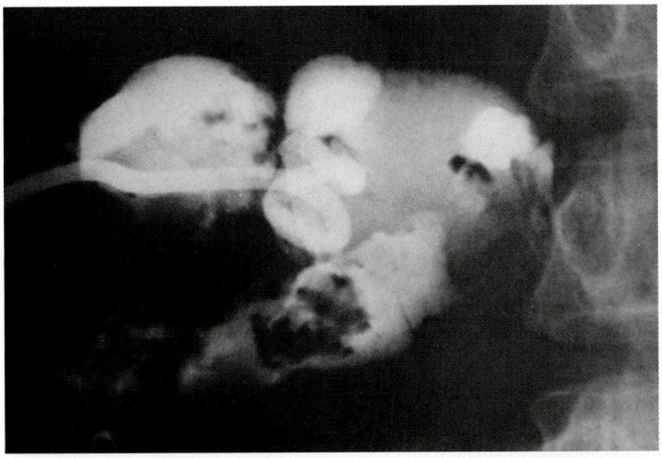

Fig. 43

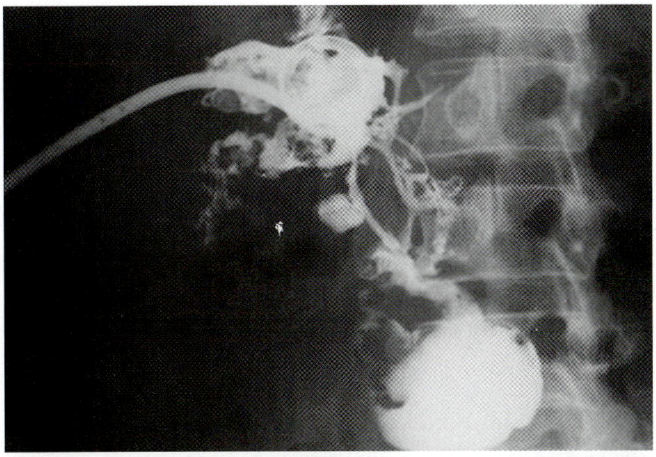

Fig. 44

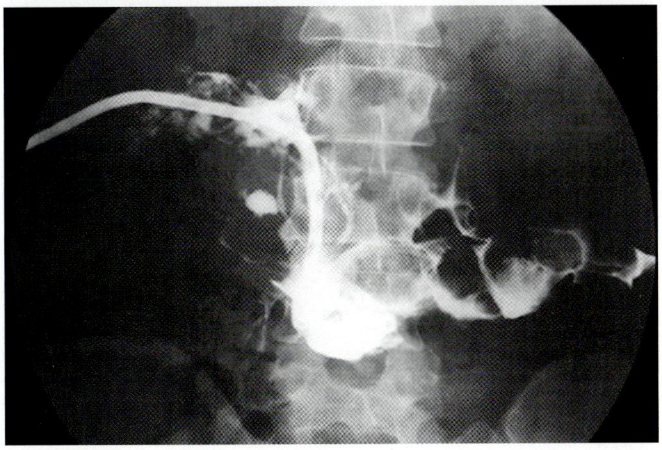

Fig. 45

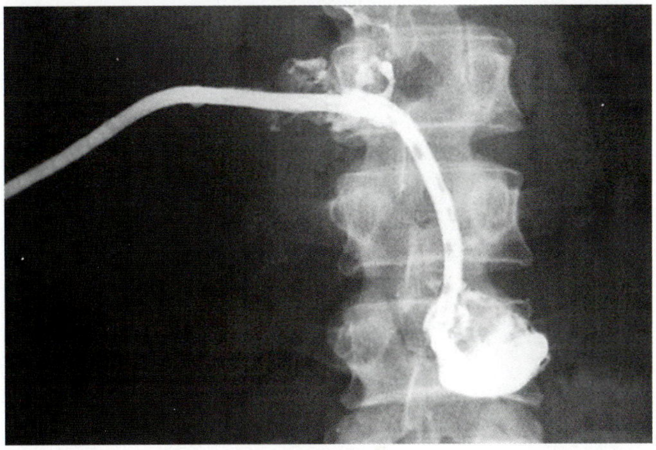

Fig. 46

Figs. 43 to 46: Percutaneous aspiration and drainage of the collections was performed under fluoroscopy. Notice how some of the collections communicated, and thus it was possible to attain drainage with the use of one catheter.

ALLOGRAFT PANCREATITIS WITH PERIPANCREATIC FLUID COLLECTION (FIGS. 47 TO 52)

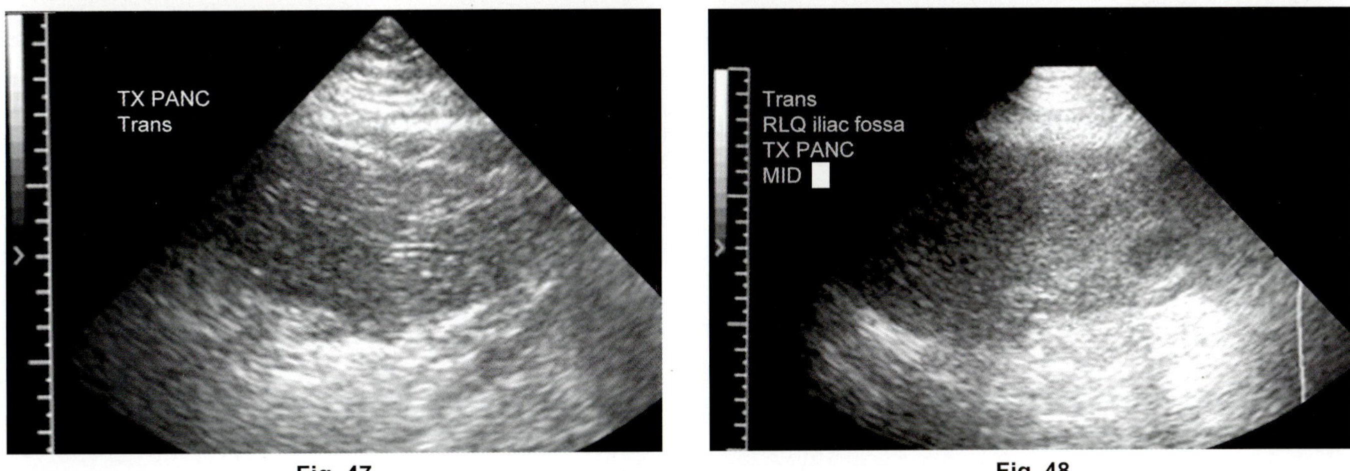

Fig. 47

Fig. 48

Figs. 47 and 48: Transverse ultrasound images show an enlarged pancreatic graft with decreased echogenicity consistent with pancreatitis.

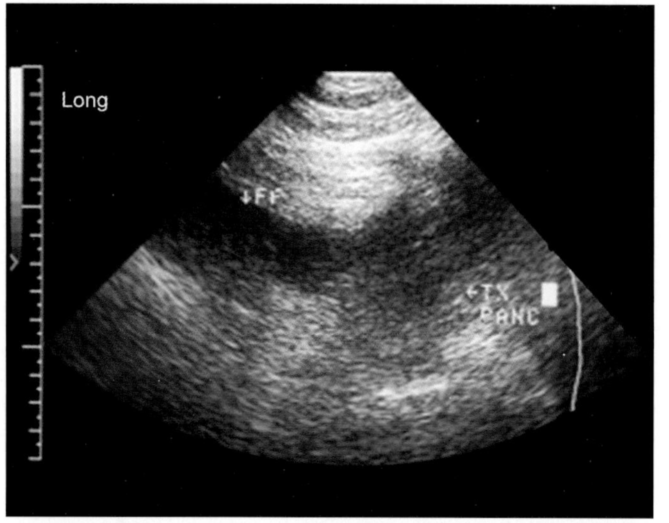

Fig. 49

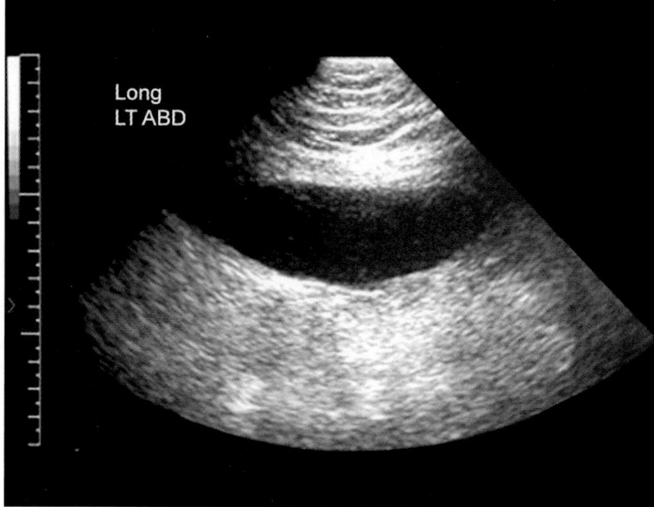

Fig. 50

Figs. 49 and 50: Additional images show an elongated fluid collection contiguous with the inflamed pancreatic graft.

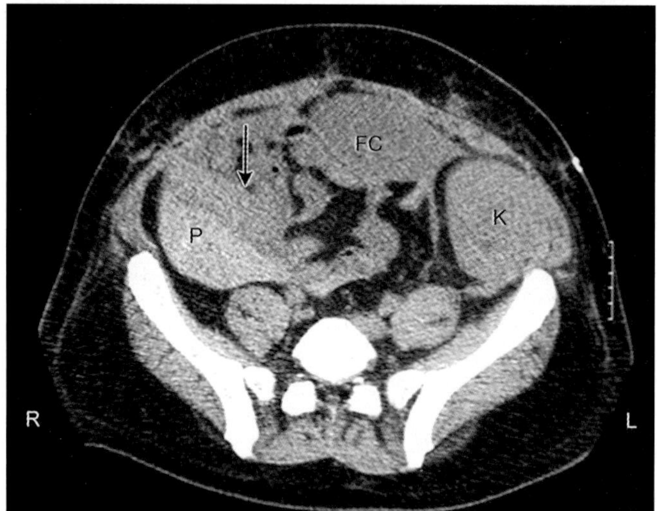

Fig. 51

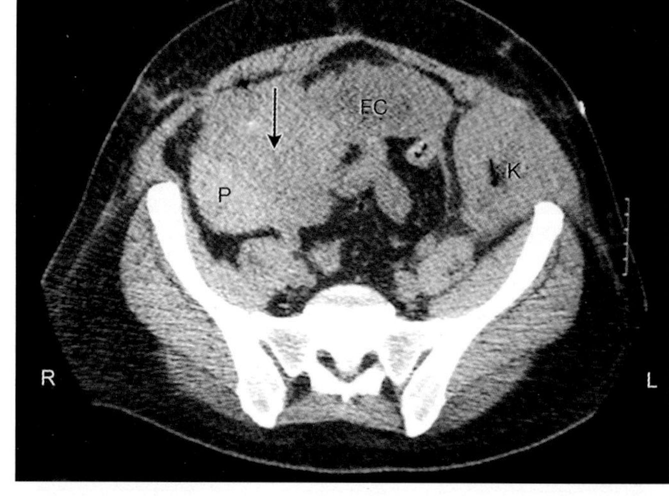

Fig. 52

Figs. 51 and 52: Axial CT images of the same patient with SPK transplantation show an enlarged, edematous pancreatic graft (P) in the right lower quadrant (RLQ) surrounded by a fluid collection (FC). Notice how the perigraft collection exhibits high attenuation (arrows) likely reflecting hemorrhagic fluid. A transplant kidney (K) is noted in the left lower quadrant (LLQ).

PANCREATIC GRAFT FISTULAS (FIGS. 53 AND 54)

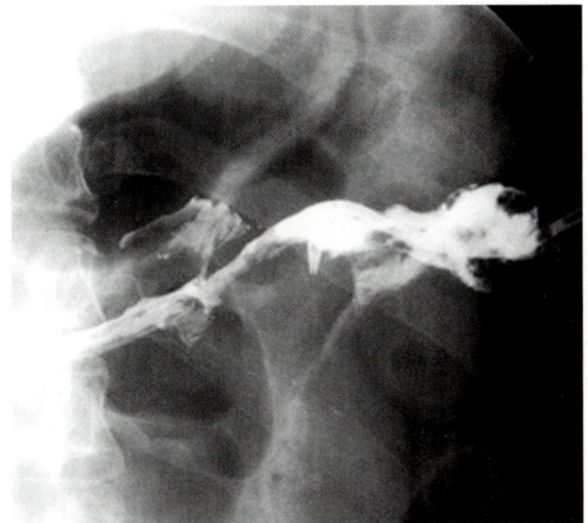

Fig. 53: Enteric drained pancreas: Abscessogram with fistulous tract to pancreatic bed.

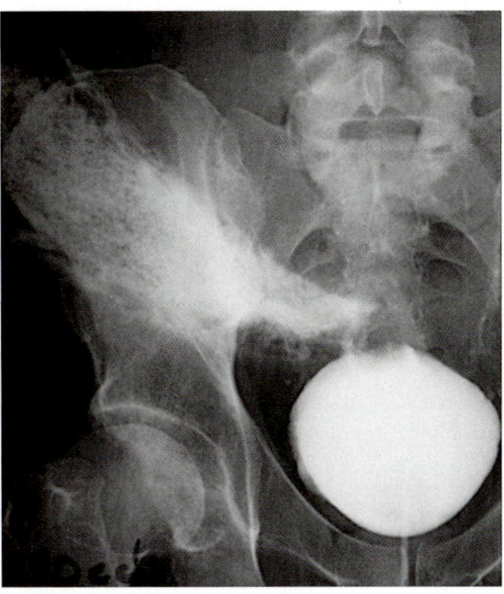

Fig. 54: Bladder drained pancreas. Contrast instilled into the bladder is seen in the peripancreatic area draining into the incision.

SIMULTANEOUS PANCREAS KIDNEY TRANSPLANT—BLADDER DRAINED—URETERAL OBSTRUCTION ASSOCIATED WITH BLADDER THICKENING SECONDARY TO IRRITATION FROM PANCREATIC EXOCRINE SECRETIONS (FIGS. 55 AND 56)

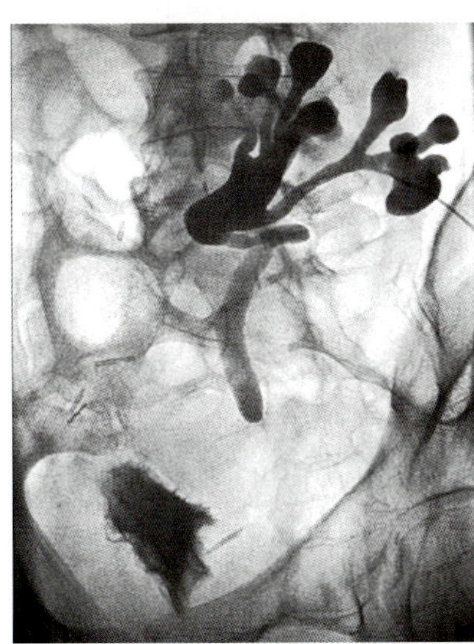

Fig. 55: Percutaneous nephrostogram shows hydronephrosis of the left lower quadrant (LLQ) kidney graft.

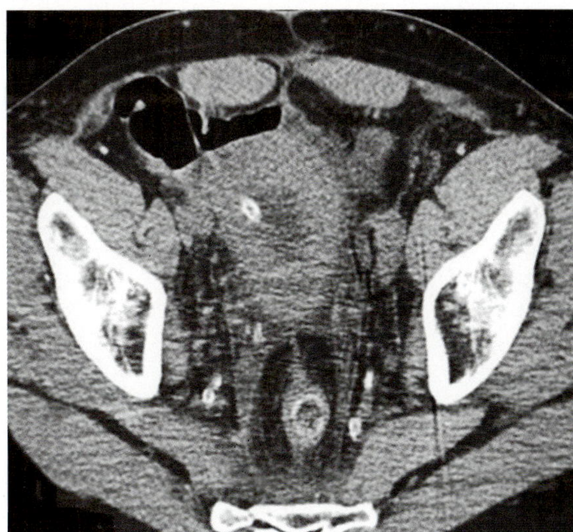

Fig. 56: Axial CT image of the same patient shows marked thickening of bladder wall secondary to inflammation as a result of irritation produced by pancreatic exocrine secretions. A urinary catheter is seen in the bladder lumen.

PART 3 ISLET CELL TRANSPLANTATION

CHAPTER 72

Islet Cell Transplantation

Horacio Rilo, George Georgiev, Christine Sardo Molmenti, Renee Cercone, Ernesto P Molmenti

- Chronic pancreatitis is a continuous inflammatory disease, characterized by irreversible morphologic changes that typically cause pain and permanent loss of function
- Incidence of chronic pancreatitis is 1.6–23 per 100,000 of the population—National Institute of Diabetes and Digestive and Kidney Diseases (NIDDK)
- Continuum of disease
  Acute pancreatitis → recurrent pancreatitis → chronic pancreatitis
- Risk Factors of Chronic Pancreatitis (TIGARO—based on the first letters of each risk factor)
  - Toxic-metabolic (alcohol, tobacco, medications)
  - Idiopathic
  - Genetic (mutations of the CFTR, SPINK1, PRSS genes)
  - Autoimmune
  - Recurrent
  - Obstructive (pancreas divisum, sphincter of Oddi dysfunction)
- Symptoms Chronic Pancreatitis
  - Fatigue
  - Steatorrhea
  - Vitamin deficiencies
  - Diabetes mellitus
  - Increased risk of pancreatic cancer
- Pain is the only sensation that can be elicited from the pancreas
  - Abdominal pain of severe intensity
  - Often radiates to the back and left shoulder
  - Produces strong autonomic responses
  - Alcohol or food consumption aggravates the symptoms
  - Ductal hypertension—Interstitial hypertension
  - Scarring of pancreatic nerves
  - Neuronal damage by bioactive substances released from inflammatory cells and activated pancreatic enzymes
- Pancreatitis-induced pain is intractable and difficult to manage clinically. Initial intervention is conservative:
  - Nonopioid analgesics (acetaminophen, non-steroidal anti-inflammatory drugs)
  - Opioid analgesics (morphine, meperidine)
  - Non-narcotic pain modulators (gabapentin, etc.)
  - Enzyme replacement therapy
  - Celiac nerve block
  - Pancreatic denervation
  - Endoscopic retrograde sphincterotomy
- 30–50% of patients require surgery due to:
  - Intractable pain not controlled by conservative intervention
  - Biliary obstruction
  - Gastrointestinal obstruction
  - Pseudocysts
  - Pancreatic fistula or ascites
  - Hemorrhage
  - Differentiation from carcinoma
- Up to fifty percent of patients require surgery: Denervation or resection
  - Puestow
  - Kausch (1909)-Whipple (1935)
  - Beger
  - Frey
  - Berne
  - Izbicki
- In patients in whom surgical intervention has failed, pancreatectomy can relieve pain; however, it is a drastic measure that leads to the development of "brittle diabetes"

- Auto islet transplantation following total pancreatectomy relieves severe abdominal pain associated with chronic pancreatitis and preserves endocrine function
- Auto islet transplant (AIT) (Fig. 1)
- Procedure (islet isolation)
- After removal of the organ, it is immediately submerged in UW organ preservation solution during initial resection of fat and fibrotic tissue and transport to clean room isolation facility
- The volume and weight of the pancreas are recorded
- The organ ducts are cannulated for perfusion of the enzyme (Figs. 2 to 5)
  - While introduction of the enzyme through the ducts is preferred, depending on the degree of fibrosis, intraparenchymal injection of the enzyme may be necessary for complete perfusion of the organ
- To maximize the surface area of the tissue exposed to enzymatic action during digestion, the pancreas is cut into smaller pieces

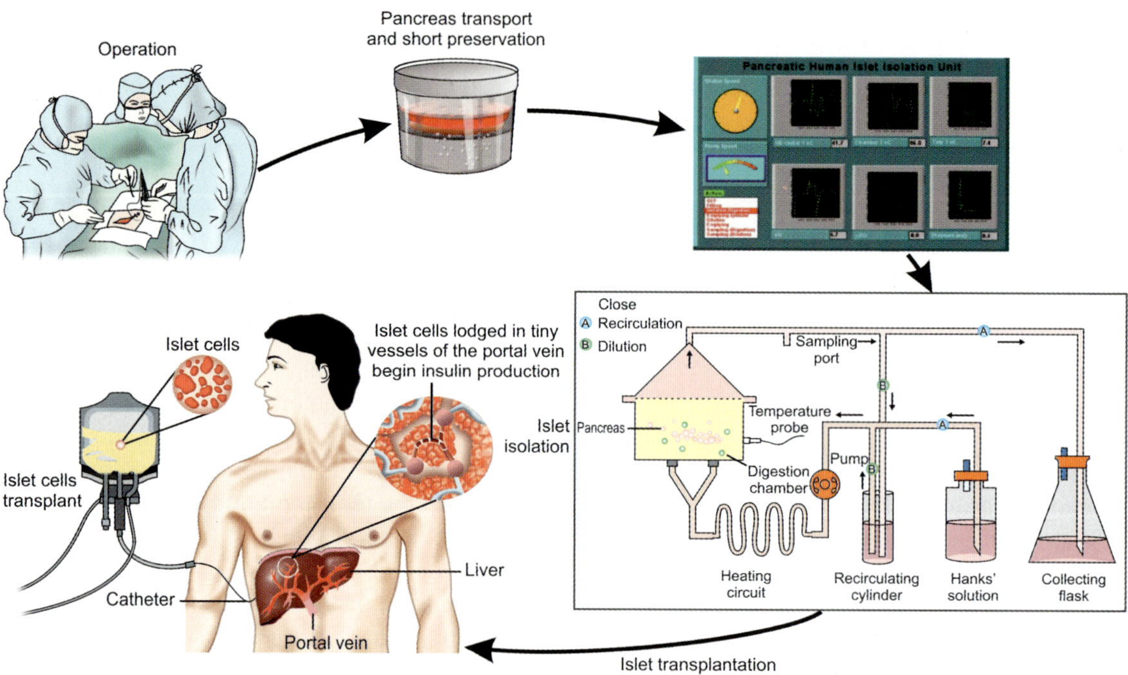

Fig. 1: Schematic representation of auto islet transplantation.

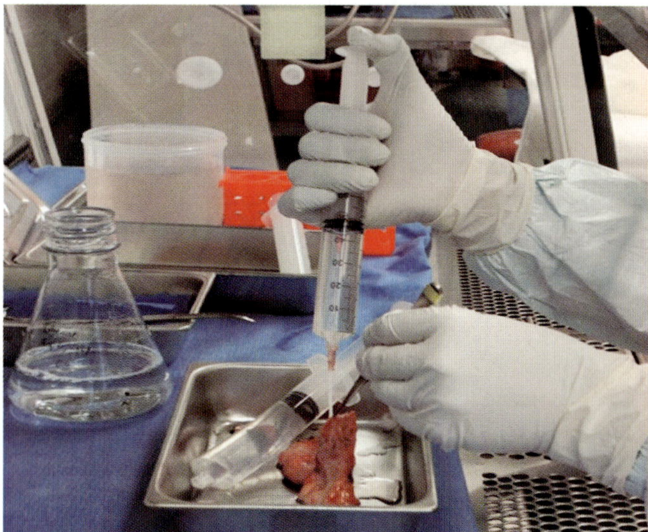

Fig. 2: Syringe perfusion of the organ.

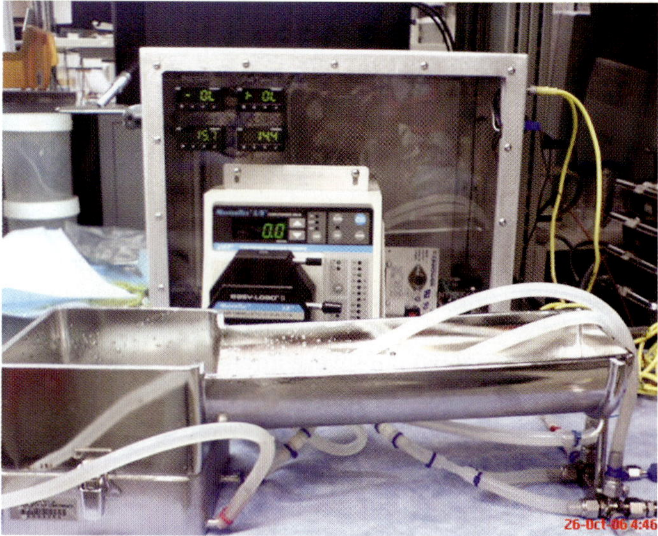

Fig. 3: Perfusion system.

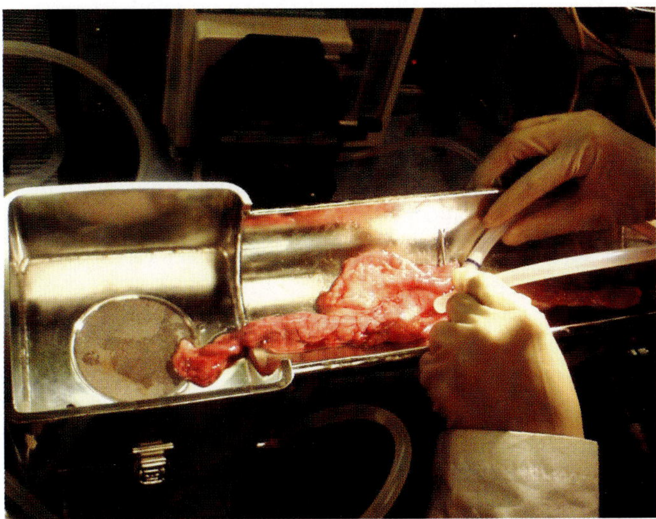

Fig. 4

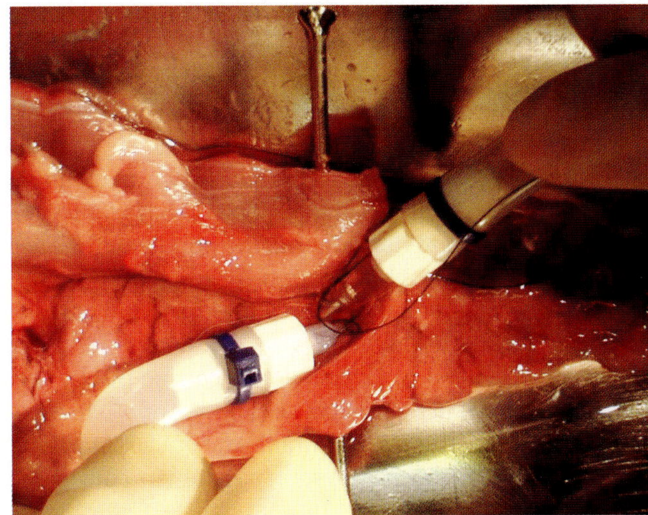

Fig. 5

Figs. 4 and 5: Pancreas perfusion with RILO device.

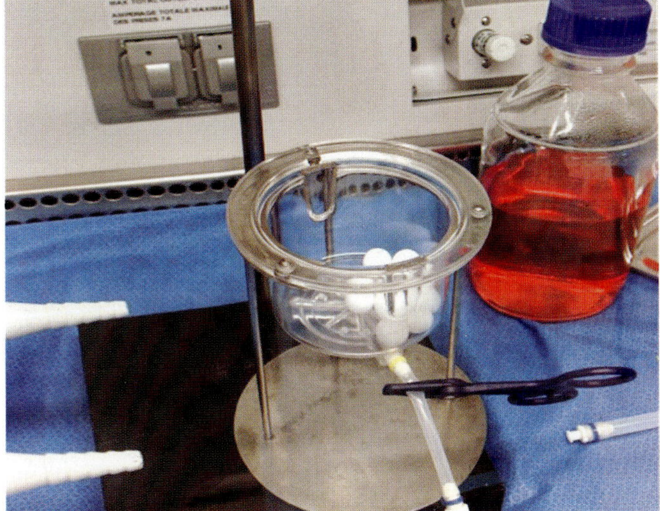

Fig. 6: Digestion chamber.

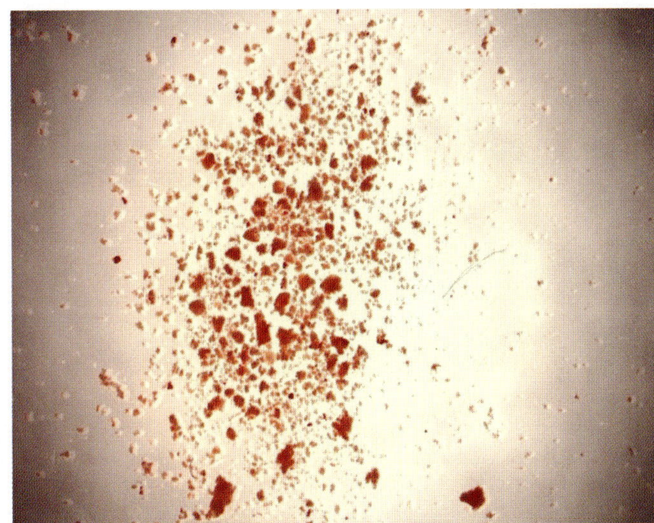

Fig. 7: Image of islets at ×10 magnification.

- The pancreas and enzyme mixture is loaded into the digestion chamber, containing several Teflon balls (Fig. 6)
  - Teflon balls provide mechanical forces during the digestion to facilitate the release of the islets and exocrine from the connective tissue
- Once the chamber is attached to the shaker arm and connected to automatic isolation system, the digestion can proceed
- Through precise control of the temperature of the system, the degree of digestion can be mediated
  - This aspect is critical and highly dependent on the degree of skill of the operator as overdigestion may fragment and damage the islets, while underdigestion may not harvest all of the islets present in the pancreas
    - In a normal organ, approximately 2% is composed of the Islets of Langerhans, while the rest is exocrine tissue
- To determine the extent of digestion, the system is periodically sampled and the amount of islets is quantified by Dithizone (DTZ) staining (Fig. 7)
  - DTZ is a Zn^{+2} receptor binding dye that selectively distinguishes islets from the non-islet tissue, such as exocrine, ducts, etc.
- Depending on the characteristics of the organ and the severity of the CP and extent of fibrosis, fat, the organ digestion time can vary accordingly
- Once the level of digestion is deemed sufficient to release the cells of interest without damaging them, the temperature of the system lowered to inactivate enzyme

- The system is flushed with cold media, and fractions of tissue are collected and centrifuged
- Fractions are recombined, and depending on the characteristics of the isolation may be treated with DNAse to prevent clumping of the tissue
- The final prep is resuspended in human serum albumin containing heparin and placed in blood bags for transport to the OR and infusion into the portal vein
- Prior to transport the final prep is sampled for determination of islet count (DTZ), endotoxin and assessments to test cell viability

The process of islet cell isolation is carried out by the automated islet isolation machine (Figs. 8 and 9) developed by Dr. Horacio Rilo, MD. An integrated user interface allows the precise control of system parameters (flow rate, pressure, and temperature) as well as sampling and collection of tissue. The design allows for precise control of digestion where the collagenase enzyme can be quickly inactivated by dilution and lowering the temperature to prevent over digestion and islet fragmentation.

ALLO = AUTO: Main differences between Allogeneic and Autologous Islet Tx

A schematic representation of the islet cell environment is depicted in Figure 10.

ISLET PURIFICATION AND CULTURE

For allogeneic islet Tx, purification of the islets is required to limit the volume infused (Figs. 11 to 15).

Purification is optional for auto islet transplantation.

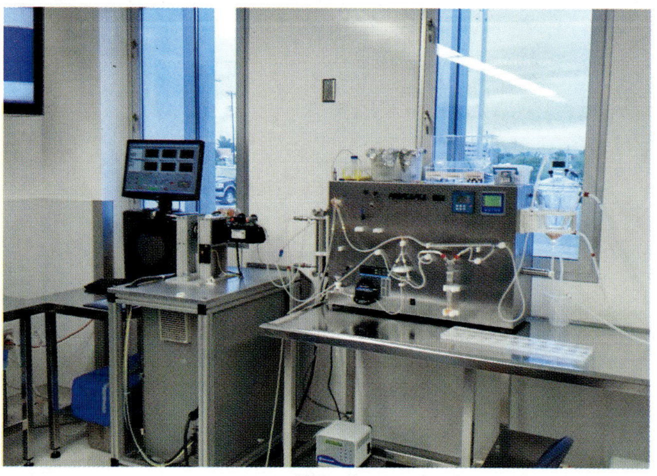

Fig. 8

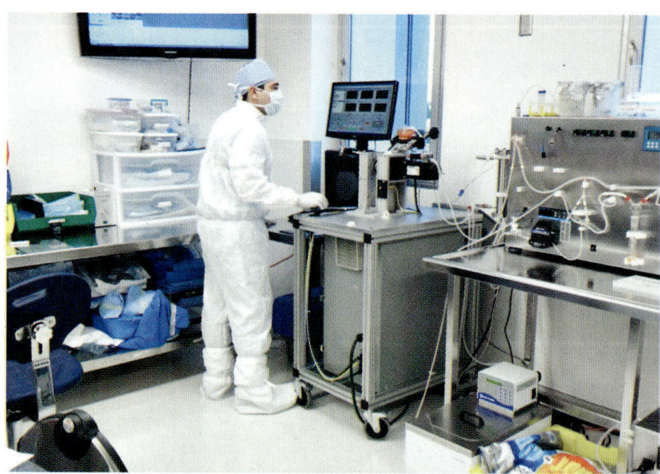

Fig. 9

Figs. 8 and 9: Automated islet isolation machine developed by Dr. Horacio Rilo, MD. An integrated user interface allows for precise control of system parameters (flow rate, pressure, and temperature) as well as sampling and collection of tissue. The design allows for precise control of digestion where the collagenase enzyme can be quickly inactivated to prevent over digestion and islet fragmentation.

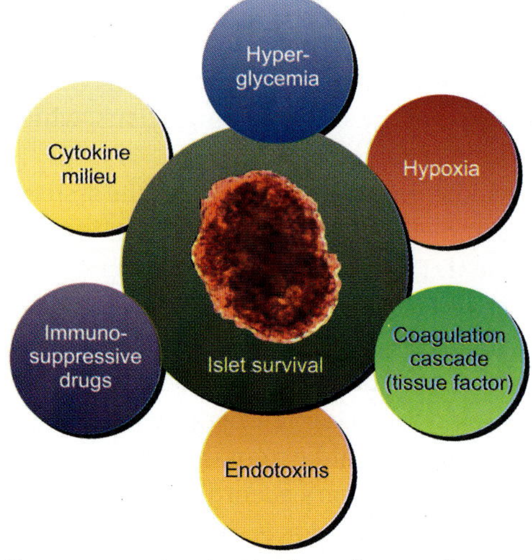

Fig. 10: Factors associated with islet cell survival.

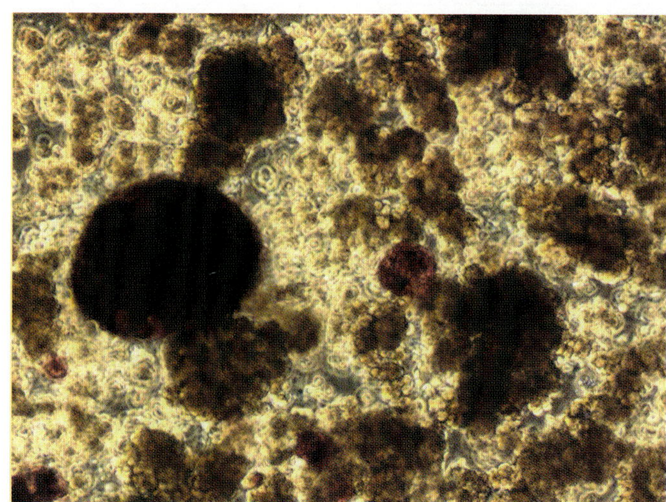

Fig. 11: Prepurification DTZ.

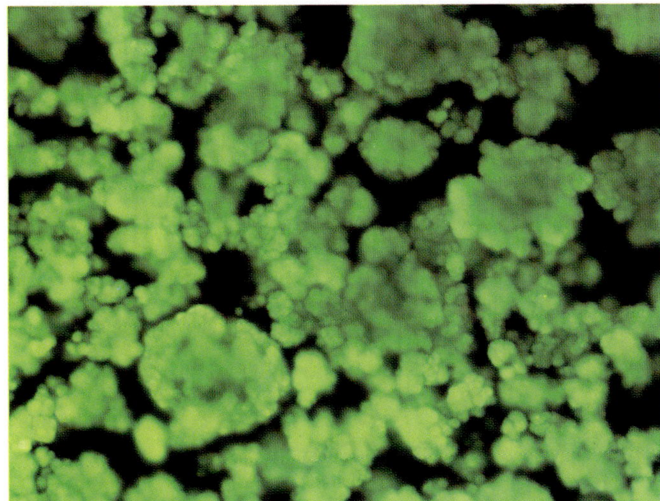

Fig. 12: Prepurification Acridine Orange (AO).

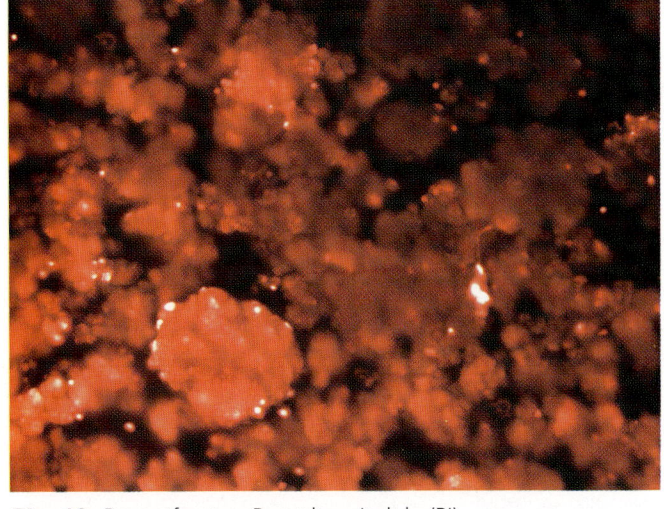

Fig. 13: Prepurification Propidium Iodide (PI).

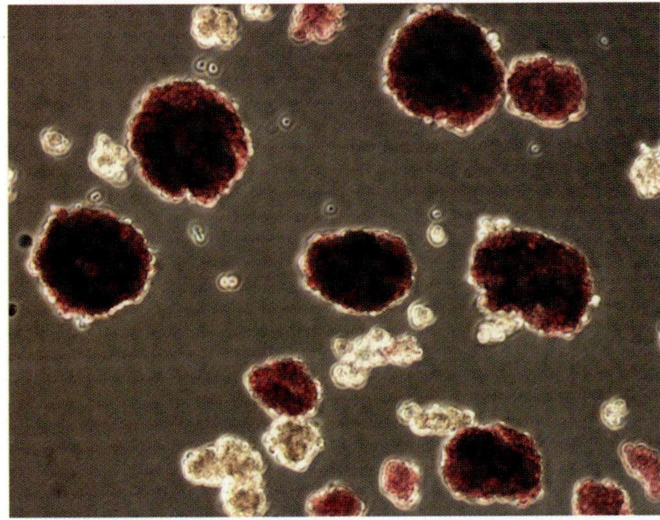

Fig. 14: Postpurification DTZ.

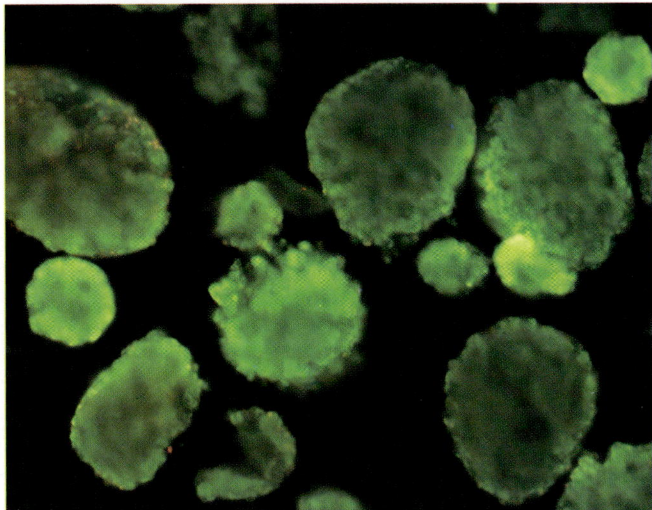

Fig. 15: Postpurification Acridine Orange (AO).

The purification is accomplished through the use of the Cobe 2991 cell sorter and continuous or discontinuous purification. Once purified the islets are cultured in complete, buffered medium at 37 °C 5% CO_2 for a period of several hours to days prior to infusion into the patient.

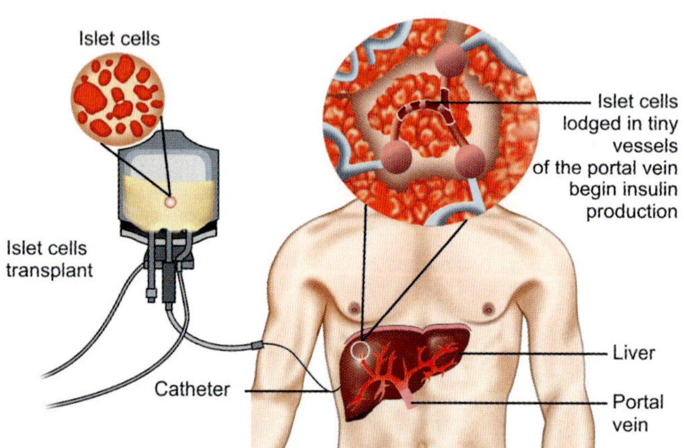

Fig. 16: Schematic representation of islet cell infusion.

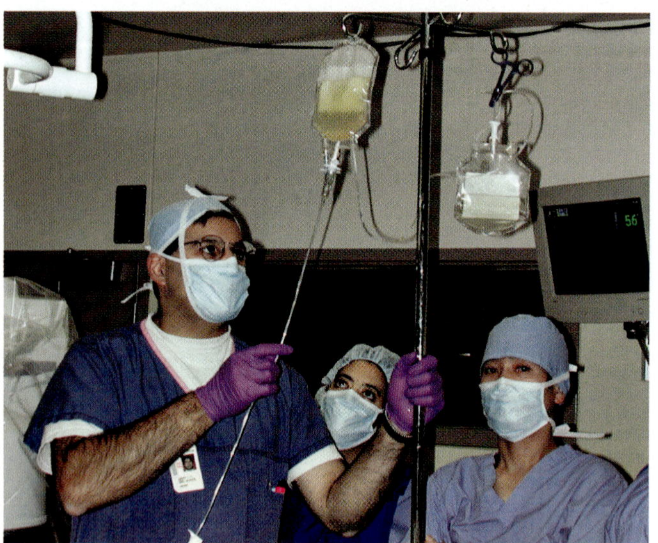

Fig. 18: Islet transplant surgeon.

ISLET CELL INFUSION

Figures 16 to 21 describe the process of islet cell infusion.

Figures 22 and 23 show glucose control in patient with pancreatectomy alone vs patient with auto islet transplant.

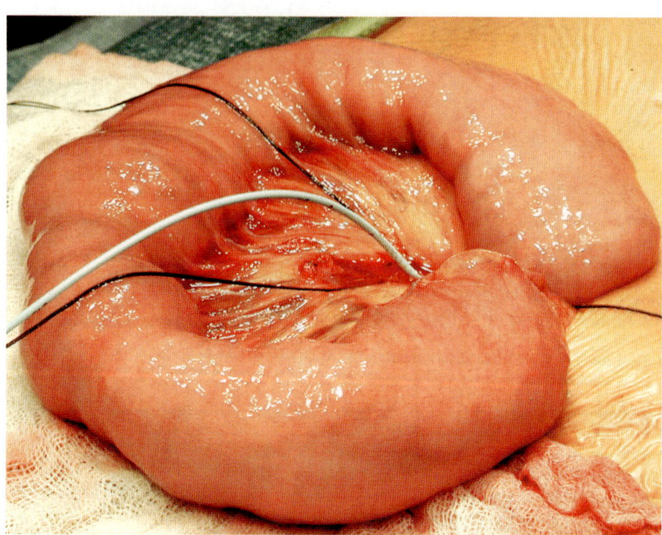

Fig. 17: Infusion catheter placement. Intraportal islet infusion: Changes in pressure.

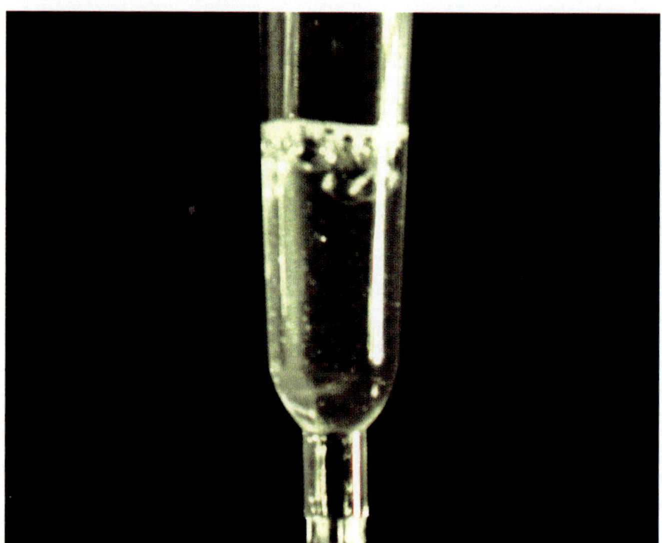

Fig. 19: Islet infusion and drip chamber.

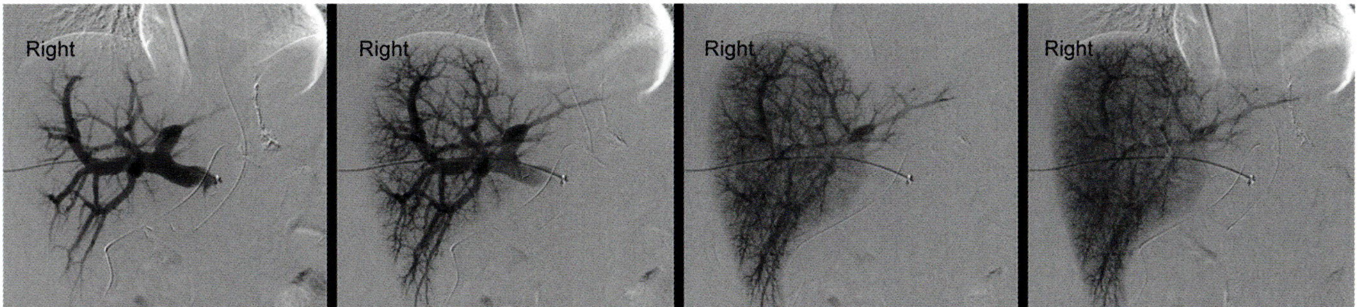

Fig. 20: Pre islet cell transplant portal pressure = 5 mm Hg.

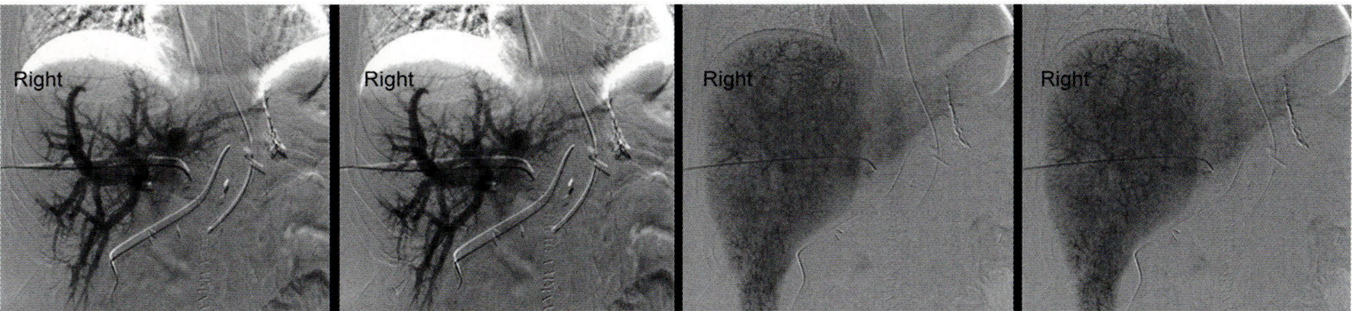

Fig. 21: Post islet cell transplant portal pressure = 24 mm Hg half bag infusion.

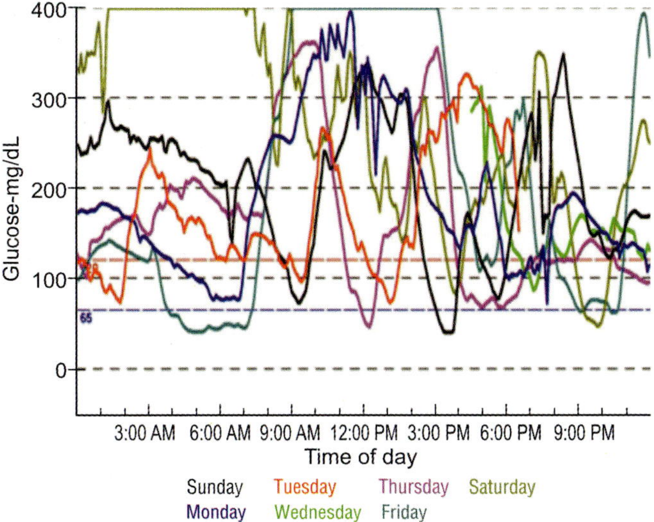

Fig. 22: Five day 24 hour glucose profile of patient with pancreatectomy alone, no islets, 6 months post surgery.

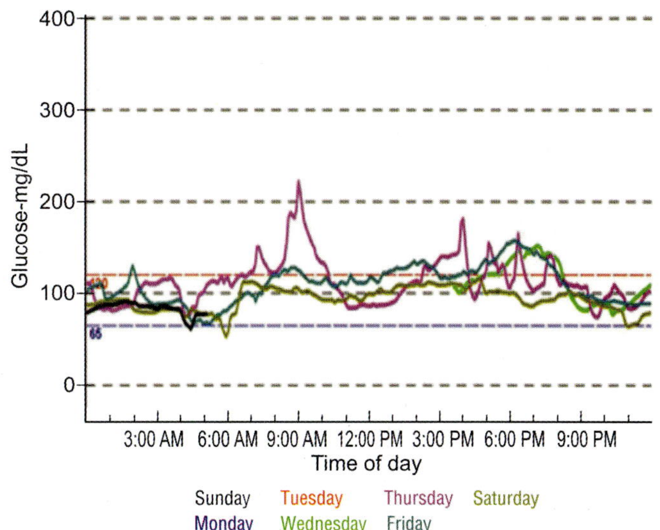

Fig. 23: Five day 24 hour glucose profile of auto islet patient 6 months post surgery.

RESULTS FROM AUTO TRANSPLANTATION

- Results from centers with the largest experiences show that in patients who undergo AIT:
  - Close to 85% experience dramatic pain relief
  - Up to one third of patients achieve insulin independence
  - Patients who do not experience normoglycemia require maintenance insulin but do not experience the abrupt and extreme glycemic excursions seen in patients undergoing pancreatectomy alone
  - Enjoy a significant improvement in quality of life

ISSUES WITH AUTO TRANSPLANTATION

- Most patients have had temporizing procedures prior to AIT and suffer from both exocrine and endocrine damage before surgery, which negatively impacts outcomes
- Few centers have the capability and resources to process islets for clinical transplantation
- The liver is the site of choice but may not be an ideal site for islets due to:
  - Intrahepatic islets are exposed to gastrointestinal toxins and medications in the portal circulation that are not seen in the native pancreas
  - Intrahepatic islets do not release glucagon in a physiologic response to hypoglycemia despite the fact that they appear to contain healthy alpha cells

FUTURE DIRECTIONS

- Performing AIT earlier in the course of treatment for the disease
- Evaluating alternate sites of islet implantation
- Strategies to improve islet survival, increase beta cell number and mass and to stimulate islet cell growth with the use of GLP-1 analogues and DDP4 inhibitors, and others

ADVANTAGES AND DISADVANTAGES TO PORTAL VEIN INFUSION (FIG. 24)

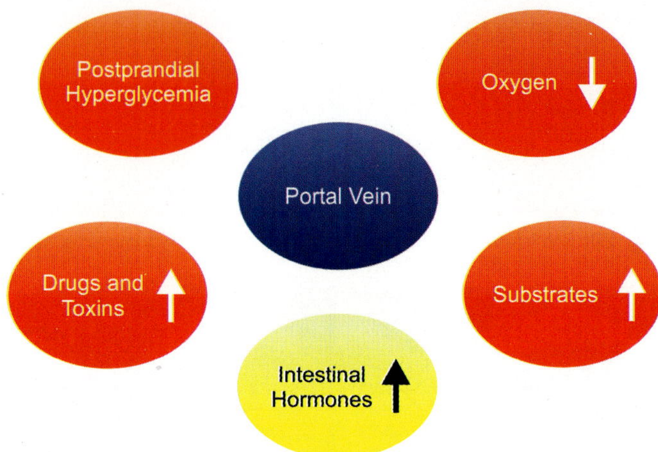

Fig. 24: Advantages and disadvantages of portal vein infusion.

CONCLUSIONS: AUTO TRANSPLANTATION

Chronic pancreatitis is a major medical problem with few effective medical therapies and limited surgical options. In patients with advanced chronic pancreatitis, auto islet transplant is very effective for relieving pain, improving quality of life and in maintaining endocrine function.

Index

Note: Page numbers followed by *f* and *t* indicate figures and tables respectively.

A

E

F

G

H

I

K

L

M

N

O

P

Q

R

S

T

U

V

W

X